All-in-One

Care Planning Resource

MEDICAL-SURGICAL,
PEDIATRIC,
MATERNITY,
& PSYCHIATRIC
NURSING CARE PLANS,
2nd EDITION

See What Nursing Students Have To Say About
All-in-One Care Planning Resource . . .

"The care plans are extremely thorough and well-organized. The rationale feature is a great asset to nursing students developing critical thinking skills and good, sound clinical judgment."
Jeffrey Waddell, Pittsburgh State University, Pittsburgh, Kansas

"Wonderful! Love the introductions that give you a complete picture of the signs and symptoms, assessments, and diagnostic tests you need to care for patients in clinicals."
Yvonne Gubersky, University of Arizona, Tucson, Arizona

"Rationales are clear and easy to read. It has lab values, and the teaching is specific to each diagnosis. It has everything! A great way to see the whole picture."
Brianna Chavez, Belmont University, Nashville, Tennessee

"I don't have to carry around four books anymore! This is one book with everything in it."
Leshia Gann, Belmont University, Nashville, Tennessee

"WOW!! Very thorough and complete in all aspects of patient care. I especially like the description of the condition with expected signs and symptoms and lab values."
James Green, Columbus State University, Columbus, Georgia

"The rationales that follow the interventions are great for planning your care and knowing why you are doing your interventions. Interventions and rationales are awesome! Patient and family teaching and discharge planning are very beneficial for clinical teaching."
Hattie McDowell, Truman State University, Kirksville, Missouri

"Well organized and easy to read. The student's best guide through nursing school!"
Jennifer Marler, Jacksonville University, Jacksonville, Florida

"An excellent source for not only completing accurate care plans, but providing holistic care for patients in prioritizing their health needs. I wish I had been able to utilize such a fantastic resource like this during my long care-plan-making nights!"
Nicole Colline, Quinnipiac University, Hamden, Connecticut

"More detail in the rationales makes the interventions more understandable! I definitely got my money's worth—covered all areas of nursing in one care plan book."
Ashley Zerwekh, Gateway Community College, Phoenix, Arizona

"I love how this book includes labs for specific disorders. It includes everything . . . a lot of good information! I wish I had this when I was a sophomore."
Vanessa Lincoln, Truman State University, Kirksville, Missouri

"Very thorough. Covered all aspects of the physiologic and psychosocial problems as well as listing of resources to refer patients to."
Cindy Green, Columbus State University, Columbus, Georgia

"I like the 'related-to' feature. And it's nice to have the lists of resources to send home with the families at discharge."
Suzanne Brown, Oklahoma State University, Oklahoma City, Oklahoma

"It's very handy to have a book that's all-in-one!"
Tanya Hentges, Truman State University, Kirksville, Missouri

"I wish I had this book for my first semester of clinicals. The material . . . pulls together related information that would usually be found in several separate textbooks. Nursing students can lighten their backpack for clinicals with this one book that includes it all."
Julie Wilner, University of Michigan, Ann Arbor, Michigan

All-in-One
Care Planning Resource

**MEDICAL-SURGICAL,
PEDIATRIC,
MATERNITY,
& PSYCHIATRIC**
Nursing Care Plans

2nd Edition

Pamela L. Swearingen, RN
Special Project Editor

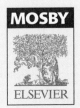
MOSBY
ELSEVIER

MOSBY
ELSEVIER

11830 Westline Industrial Drive
St. Louis, Missouri 63146

ALL-IN-ONE CARE PLANNING RESOURCE: MEDICAL-SURGICAL, PEDIATRIC, MATERNITY, AND PSYCHIATRIC NURSING CARE PLANS, SECOND EDITION

ISBN: 978-0-323-04416-5

Notice

Knowledge and best practice in this field are constantly changing. As new research and experience broaden our knowledge, changes in practice, treatment and drug therapy may become necessary or appropriate. Readers are advised to check the most current information provided (i) on procedures featured or (ii) by the manufacturer of each product to be administered, to verify the recommended dose or formula, the method and duration of administration, and contraindications. It is the responsibility of the practitioner, relying on their own experience and knowledge of the patient, to make diagnoses, to determine dosages and the best treatment for each individual patient, and to take all appropriate safety precautions. To the fullest extent of the law, neither the Publisher nor the Author assumes any liability for any injury and/or damage to persons or property arising out of or related to any use of the material contained in this book.

The Publisher

Previous edition copyrighted 2004

Library of Congress Control Number 2007924815

Acquisitions Editor: Kristin Geen
Developmental Editor: Jamie Horn
Publishing Services Manager: Deborah L. Vogel
Associate Project Manager: Brandilyn Tidwell
Designer: Julia Dummitt

Printed in United States of America

Last digit is the print number: 9 8 7 6 5 4 3 2 1

Working together to grow libraries in developing countries

www.elsevier.com | www.bookaid.org | www.sabre.org

ELSEVIER   BOOK AID International   Sabre Foundation

Dedication

To the memory of Mima M. Horne, RN, MS, CDE,
whose integrity, talent, and dedication
to the nursing profession live on.

MEDICAL-SURGICAL NURSING CARE PLANS

Lolita M. Adrien-Dunlap, RN, MS, CNS, CWOCN
Nursing Learning Specialist
Contra Costa College
San Pablo, California
Contributed care plans for Crohn's Disease, Fecal Diversions, and Ulcerative Colitis.

Linda S. Baas, RN, PhD, ACNP, CCRN
Professor and Director of Acute Care Graduate Program
University of Cincinnati College of Nursing
Cincinnati, Ohio
Contributed care plan for Prolonged Bedrest.

Marianne Baird, RN, MN
Clinical Nurse Specialist
Saint Joseph's Hospital of Atlanta
Atlanta, Georgia
Contributed Endocrine Care Plans.

Marie Bakitas, ARNP, DNSc, FAAN
Adult Nurse Practitioner, Palliative Care
Dartmouth-Hitchcock Medical Center
Lebanon, New Hampshire
Contributed care plan for Palliative and End-of-Life Care.

Lynda K. Ball, RN, BS, BSN, CNN
Quality Improvement Coordinator
Northwest Renal Network
Seattle, Washington
Contributed care plan for Care of the Renal Transplant Recipient.

Kathleen Barnett, RN, MA, APRN, BC-PCM
Palliative Care Nurse Educator – Project ENABLE II
Dartmouth College/Dartmouth-Hitchcock Medical Center
Lebanon, New Hampshire
Contributed care plan for Palliative and End-of-Life Care.

Michelle T. Bott, RN, BScN, MN
Director, Professional Practice
Guelph General Hospital
Guelph, Ontario
Contributed care plans for Acute Renal Failure, Chronic Kidney Disease, Hemodialysis, Peritoneal Dialysis, and Normal Laboratory Values appendix.

Jennifer Dunscomb, RN, MSN, CCRN
Clinical Nurse Specialist—Pulmonary, Cardiovascular, and Critical Care
Columbus Regional Hospital
Columbus, Indiana
Contributed care plans for Acute Respiratory Failure, Chronic Obstructive Pulmonary Disease, Pneumonia, Pneumothorax/ Hemothorax, and Pulmonary Embolus.

Karen Goff, RN, BSN
Senior Applications
Saint Joseph's Hospital of Atlanta
Atlanta, Georgia
Contributed care plans for Appendicitis, Cholelithiasis, Cholecystitis, Cholangitis, Cirrhosis, Hepatitis, Pancreatitis, Peptic Ulcers, and Peritonitis.

R. Mark Hovis, CRNA
Nurse Anesthetist
Washington University School of Medicine
St. Louis, Missouri
Contributed care plan for Perioperative Care.

Marguerite Jackson, RN, PhD, FAAN
Director, Administrative Unit, National Tuberculosis Curriculum Consortium
Associate Clinical Professor of Family and Preventive Medicine
University of California San Diego
San Diego, California
Contributed care plan for Pulmonary Tuberculosis and Infection Prevention and Control appendix.

Patricia Jansen, APRN, MSN, CS
Medical Surgical Clinical Nurse Specialist
Regional Medical Center of San Jose
San Jose, California
Contributed care plans for Benign Prostatic Hypertrophy, Older Adult Care, Ureteral Calculi, Urinary Diversions, and Urinary Tract Obstruction.

Suzanne Jed, APRN-BC, MSN, FNP
Clinical Education Coordinator
Mountain Plains AIDS Education and Training Center
Instructor, Division of Infectious Diseases, School of Medicine
University of Colorado at Denver and Health Sciences Center
Denver, Colorado
Contributed care plan for HIV.

Ingrid B. Mroz, RN, MS, CCRN
Clinical Nurse Specialist Adult Critical Care
Dartmouth-Hitchcock Medical Center
Lebanon, New Hampshire
Contributed care plan for Pain.

Barbara D. Powe, RN, PhD
Director, Underserved Populations Research
American Cancer Society
Atlanta, Georgia
Contributed care plan for Cancer Care, Psychosocial Support, and Psychosocial Support of the Patient's Family and Significant Others.

Dottie Roberts, RN, MSN, MACI, CMSRN, OCNS-C
Clinical Nurse Specialist
Palmetto Health Baptist
Columbia, South Carolina
Contributed Musculoskeletal Care Plans.

Sandra Rome, RN, MN, AOCN
Hematology/Oncology Clinical Nurse Specialist
Cedars-Sinai Medical Center
Assistant Clinical Professor, UCLA School of Nursing
Los Angeles, California
Contributed Hematologic Care Plans.

Nancy A. Stotts, RN, EdD, FAAN
Professor of Nursing
University of California San Francisco
San Francisco, California
Contributed care plan for Managing Wound Care.

Carol Monlux Swift, RN, BSN, CNRN
Staff Nurse Critical Care Unit
El Camino Hospital
Mountain View, California
Contributed Neurologic Care Plans.

Beth Taylor, RD, MS, CNSD, FCCM
Nutrition Support Specialist
Barnes-Jewish Hospital
St. Louis, Missouri
Contributed care plan for Providing Nutritional Support.

Mary Young, RN, ARNP, BC, MSN
Nurse Practitioner, Cardiology
Dartmouth-Hitchcock Medical Center
Lebanon, New Hampshire
Contributed care plans for Abdominal Trauma and Cardiac Care Plans.

Pediatric Nursing Care Plans

Sherry D. Ferki, RN, MSN
Adjunct Faculty, Pediatric Clinical Instructor
College of the Albemarle, ADN Program
Elizabeth City, North Carolina
Adjunct Faculty, Pediatric Clinical Instructor
Old Dominion University, School of Nursing
Norfolk, Virginia

Maternity Care Plans

Deborah E. Swenson, MSN, ARNP
OBSTETRIX Medical Group of Washington, Inc.
Seattle, Washington

Psychiatric Nursing Care Plans

Verna Benner Carson, APRN/PMH, PhD
National Director of RESTORE Family Behavioral Health
Tender Loving Care Home Health Care Services
Fallston, Maryland

Reviewers

JoAnn Acierno, RN, BSN
Instructor
Clarkson College
Omaha, Nebraska

Mike Aldridge, MSN, RN, CCRN, CNS
Instructor in Clinical Nursing
The University of Texas at Austin School of Nursing
Austin, Texas

Judith Ascenzi, RN, MSN
Unit Educator for the Johns Hopkins Hospital
Pediatric Intensive Care Unit
Baltimore, Maryland

Patricia W. Campbell, RN, MSN
Nursing Faculty
Carolinas College of Health Sciences
School of Nursing
Charlotte, North Carolina

Corine K. Carlson, MS, RN
Assistant Professor
Luther College
Decorah, Iowa

Jo Anne Carrick, RN, MSN, CEN
Instructor
Pennsylvania State University
School of Nursing
Sharon, Pennsylvania

Pattie G. Clark, RN, MSN, ABD
Associate Professor of Nursing and Nursing Outreach
  Coordinator
Abraham Baldwin College
Tifton, Georgia

Barbara Derwinski-Robinson, MSN, RNC
Associate Professor
Montana State University—Bozeman
College of Nursing
Billings, Montana

Nancy Eksterowicz, RN, MSN
Pain Services Coordinator
University of Virginia Health Systems
Afton, Virginia

Janice J. Hoffman, RN, PhD
Faculty
Johns Hopkins University School of Nursing
Baltimore, Maryland

Suzanne Jed, MSN, APRN-BC, FNP
Clinical Education Coordinator
Mountain Plains AIDS Education and Training Center
Instructor, Division of Infectious Diseases,
  School of Medicine
University of Colorado at Denver and Health
  Sciences Center
Denver, Colorado

Susie Kampfert, MSN, CCRN
Manager, Nursing Education
Metropolitan Hospital
Grand Rapids, Michigan

Merita Konstantacos, RN, MSN
Consultant
Clinton, Ohio

Lynn Woods Lowery, BSN, MSN
Instructor, Senior Nursing Program
Nurse Educator
Charity Delgado School of Nursing
New Orleans, Louisiana

Sarah Reidunn Pool, RN, MS
Nursing Education Specialist
Cardiac Surgery
Mayo Clinic
Rochester, Minnesota

Bruce Austin Scott, MSN, APRN, BC
Nursing Instructor
San Joaquin Delta College
Clinical Nurse IV
St. Joseph's Medical Center
Stockton, California

Phyllis Stout, MSN, APRN, BC
Associate Professor
St. John's College of Nursing of Southwest Baptist University
Springfield, Missouri

Allison J. Terry, RN, MSN, PhD
Nurse Consultant
Alabama Board of Nursing
Montgomery, Alabama

Susan Cook Vaughn, RN, MSN
Home Care Specialist
Gentiva Health Services
Charlotte, North Carolina

Lynette M. Wachholz, MN, ARNP, IBCLC
Pediatric Nurse Practitioner; Lactation Consultant
The Everett Clinic – Harbour Pointe
Mukilteo, Washington

Derek Wood, RN, BC, MS
Instructor
Aims Community College
Thornton, Colorado

Preface

All-in-One Care Planning Resource is a one-of-a-kind book featuring nursing care plans for all four core clinical areas. The inclusion of pediatric, maternity, and psychiatric nursing in addition to medical-surgical nursing care plans allows students to use one book throughout the nursing curriculum. This unique presentation—combined with solid content, an open and accessible format, and clinically relevant features—makes this a must-have care plans book for nursing students.

ORGANIZATION

This book is organized into four separate sections for medical-surgical, pediatric, maternal, and psychiatric care plans. Within each section, care plans are listed alphabetically by disorder or condition (the medical-surgical nursing care plans are organized alphabetically within each body system). General information that applies to more than one disorder can be found in the *General Care Plans* section, where nursing diagnoses and interventions for perioperative care, pain, prolonged bedrest, cancer care, psychosocial support for patients, psychosocial support for the patient's family and significant others, older adult care, and end-of-life care are discussed.

Each disorder uses the following consistent format:

- **Overview/Pathophysiology,** includes a synopsis of the disorder and its pathophysiology, where appropriate
- **Health Care Setting,** such as hospital, primary, community, or long-term care
- **Assessment,** covering signs and symptoms and physical assessment
- **Diagnostic Tests**
- **Nursing Diagnoses with Desired Outcomes**
- **Nursing Interventions and Rationales** in a clear two-column format
- **Related NIC Interventions and NOC Outcomes**
- **Patient-Family Teaching and Discharge Planning**

This book is organized to provide the most important information related to various disorders. By providing a consistent format for each disorder, key information that a nurse needs to know is fully covered. For example, the rationales given for the interventions are supported by supplemental information provided in the "Overview/Pathophysiology" and "Assessment" sections. This really is the most complete care planning book available!

FEATURES

The care plans in this book were written by clinical experts in each subject area to ensure the most current and accurate information. In addition to reliable content, the book offers the following special features:

- A **consistent, easy-to-use format** facilitates quick and easy retrieval of information.
- The **Health Care Setting** is specified for each care plan, since these conditions are treated in various settings such as hospital, primary care, long-term care facility, community, and home care.
- **Outcome criteria with specific timelines** assist in setting realistic goals for nursing outcomes and providing quality, cost-effective care.
- **Detailed, specific rationales** for each nursing intervention apply concepts to clinical practice.
- The **Patient-Family Teaching and Discharge Planning** section highlights key patient education topics, as well as resources for further information.
- The new **NANDA Taxonomy II** nursing diagnoses are included in each care plan.
- Related **NIC (Nursing Interventions Classification) interventions** and **NOC (Nursing Outcomes Classification) outcomes** are listed for each nursing diagnosis.
- Separate care plans on **Pain** and **End-of-Life Care** focus on palliative care for patients with terminal illnesses, as well as relief of acute and chronic pain.
- The **newest infection prevention and control guidelines** from the Centers for Disease Control and Prevention (CDC) are included in the appendix.
- **Normal laboratory values for adults** are listed in the appendix, including separate tables for Complete Blood Count; Serum, Plasma, and Whole Blood Chemistry; and Urine Chemistry. **Normal laboratory values** for pediatric patients are included at the end of the Pediatric Nursing Care Plans section.

This book was carefully prepared to meet the needs of today's busy nursing student. We welcome comments on how we can enhance its usefulness in subsequent editions.

Pamela L. Swearingen

Contents

Part I
MEDICAL-SURGICAL NURSING CARE PLANS

GENERAL CARE PLANS
1 Cancer Care, 1
2 Pain, 39
3 Perioperative Care, 45
4 Prolonged Bedrest, 61
5 Psychosocial Support, 73
6 Psychosocial Support for the Patient's Family and Significant Other, 87
7 Older Adult Care, 93
8 Palliative and End-of-Life Care, 105

RESPIRATORY CARE PLANS
9 Chronic Obstructive Pulmonary Disease, 117
10 Pneumonia, 123
11 Pneumothorax/Hemothorax, 131
12 Pulmonary Embolus, 137
13 Pulmonary Tuberculosis, 143
14 Respiratory Failure, Acute, 147

CARDIOVASCULAR CARE PLANS
15 Aneurysms, 149
16 Atherosclerotic Arterial Occlusive Disease, 151
17 Cardiac and Noncardiac Shock (Circulatory Failure), 157
18 Cardiac Surgery, 161
19 Coronary Artery Disease, 165
20 Dysrhythmias and Conduction Disturbances, 177
21 Heart Failure, 181
22 Hypertension, 193
23 Pulmonary Hypertension, 195
24 Venous Thrombosis/Thrombophlebitis, 201

RENAL-URINARY CARE PLANS
25 Benign Prostatic Hypertrophy, 207
26 Chronic Kidney Disease, 217
27 Care of the Patient Undergoing Hemodialysis, 223
28 Care of the Patient Undergoing Peritoneal Dialysis, 227
29 Renal Failure, Acute, 231
30 Care of the Renal Transplant Recipient, 239
31 Ureteral Calculi, 243
32 Urinary Diversions, 249
33 Urinary Tract Obstruction, 257

NEUROLOGIC CARE PLANS
34 General Care of Patients with Neurologic Disorders, 261
35 Bacterial Meningitis, 281
36 Guillain-Barré Syndrome, 287
37 Intervertebral Disk Disease, 295
38 Multiple Sclerosis, 305
39 Parkinsonism, 313
40 Seizures and Epilepsy, 323
41 Spinal Cord Injury, 333
42 Stroke, 349
43 Traumatic Brain Injury, 361

ENDOCRINE CARE PLANS
44 Diabetes Insipidus, 373
45 Diabetes Mellitus, 377
46 Diabetic Ketoacidosis, 387
47 Hyperosmolar Hyperglycemic Nonketotic Syndrome, 395
48 Hyperthyroidism, 399
49 Hypothyroidism, 407
50 Syndrome of Inappropriate Antidiuretic Hormone, 415

GASTROINTESTINAL CARE PLANS
51 Abdominal Trauma, 419
52 Appendicitis, 429
53 Cholelithiasis, Cholecystitis, and Cholangitis, 433
54 Cirrhosis, 437
55 Crohn's Disease, 445
56 Fecal Diversions: Colostomy, Ileostomy, and Ileal Pouch Anal Anastomoses, 455
57 Hepatitis, 463
58 Pancreatitis, 469
59 Peptic Ulcers, 477
60 Peritonitis, 481
61 Ulcerative Colitis, 487

HEMATOLOGIC CARE PLANS
62 Anemias of Chronic Disease, 495
63 Disseminated Intravascular Coagulation, 497
64 Polycythemia, 501
65 Thrombocytopenia, 505

MUSCULOSKELETAL CARE PLANS
66 Amputation, 509
67 Fractures, 515
68 Joint Replacement Surgery, 523
69 Osteoarthritis, 529
70 Osteoporosis, 535
71 Rheumatoid Arthritis, 541

SPECIAL NEEDS CARE PLANS
72 Caring for Individuals with Human Immunodeficiency Virus, 547
73 Managing Wound Care, 559
74 Providing Nutritional Support, 565

Part II
PEDIATRIC NURSING CARE PLANS
75 Asthma, 577
76 Attention Deficit Hyperactivity Disorder, 585
77 Bronchiolitis, 593
78 Burns, 599
79 Cerebral Palsy, 609
80 Child Abuse and Neglect, 615
81 Cystic Fibrosis, 621
82 Diabetes Mellitus in Children, 629
83 Fractures in Children, 637
84 Gastroenteritis, 641
85 Otitis Media, 647
86 Poisoning, 653
87 Sickle Cell Pain Crisis, 659

Part III
MATERNITY NURSING CARE PLANS
88 Bleeding in Pregnancy, 673
89 Cervical Insufficiency, 681
90 Diabetes in Pregnancy, 687
91 Hyperemesis Gravidarum, 695
92 Postpartum Wound Infection, 703
93 Preeclampsia, 711
94 Preterm Labor, 719
95 Preterm Premature Rupture of Membranes, 729

Part IV
PSYCHIATRIC NURSING CARE PLANS
96 Anxiety Disorders, 737
97 Bipolar Disorder (Manic Component), 745
98 Dementia—Alzheimer's Type, 751
99 Major Depression, 761
100 Schizophrenia, 769
101 Substance Abuse Disorders, 775

APPENDIX
A Infection Prevention and Control, 783
B Laboratory Tests Discussed in This Manual: Normal Values, 793

SELECTED BIBLIOGRAPHY, 799

INDEX, 813

All-in-One

Care Planning Resource

MEDICAL-SURGICAL,
PEDIATRIC,
MATERNITY,
& PSYCHIATRIC
NURSING CARE PLANS

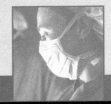

Cancer Care 1

OVERVIEW/PATHOPHYSIOLOGY

The term *cancer* refers to several disease entities, all of which have in common the proliferation of abnormal cells. To varying degrees, these cells have lost their ability to reproduce in an organized fashion, function normally, and die a natural death (apoptosis). As a result they may develop new functions not characteristic of their site of origin, spread and invade uncontrollably (metastasize), and cause dysfunction and death of other cells.

Cancer continues to be the second leading cause of death in the United States after cardiac disease (American Cancer Society, 2006). It can cause damage and dysfunction at the site of origin, regionally, or metastasize and cause problems at more distant body sites. Eventually a malignancy may cause irreversible systemic damage and failure.

HEALTH CARE SETTING

Medical or surgical floor in acute care; primary care, hospice, home care, long-term care

CARE OF PATIENTS WITH CANCER

Lung cancer

Lung cancer remains the most common cause of cancer death among men and women in the United States. American Cancer Society (ACS) statistics for 2004 indicate that 87% of lung cancer deaths may be attributed to smoking. Despite treatment advances in surgery, chemotherapy, and radiation therapy, the cure rate remains low. Although exposure to certain known carcinogens such as radon and asbestos may cause lung cancer, the greatest number of lung cancer cases is linked to tobacco smoking or exposure to secondhand smoke.

Most cases of lung cancer are classified as small cell or non–small cell, but a small portion of lung cancer cases are mesotheliomas, bronchial gland tumors, or carcinoids. The cell type, diagnosed via biopsy and pathologic staging, determines the appropriate treatment. Depending on the stage of lung cancer at presentation, surgery, chemotherapy, and/or radiation therapy may be part of the medical treatment plan. For patients with advanced disease for whom cure is not foreseen, palliative care should be initiated concurrently with other treatment modalities, but actually may be the only truly appropriate treatment course.

Screening: Currently there are no routine recommendations for screening for lung cancer, although clinical trials are in progress to evaluate efficacy of routine computerized axial tomography scanning for individuals at high risk for developing lung cancer. Lung cancer may be diagnosed through routine chest x-ray study, but diagnosis in early stages is usually incidental when the x-ray study is performed for other reasons. The ACS recommends current smokers be educated that the most important preventive strategy to avoid lung cancer is smoking cessation.

See also: "Perioperative Care" for appropriate nursing diagnoses, outcomes, and interventions, p. 45; and **Activity Intolerance,** p. 17, in this section.

Nervous system tumors

These tumors may be primary or secondary tumors of the central nervous system (CNS), which includes the brain and spinal cord. They are classified according to their cell of origin and graded according to their malignant behavior. Although histologically the tumor may be benign, the enclosed nature of the CNS may result in tumor effects causing significant damage or even death.

The primary CNS tumor, whether benign or malignant, can manifest with interrupted neuronal function, compression of the cord or brain and surrounding vasculature, cerebrospinal fluid (CSF) obstruction with resulting increased intracranial pressure, or degeneration of surrounding tissue. Treatment is initially surgical if the tumor site is accessible. For some tumors, complete resection is tantamount to cure. For very aggressive tumors or when a residual tumor is present postoperatively, radiation therapy and chemotherapy may be implemented.

Surgical excision of metastatic CNS tumors may be an option, but these tumors are more often treated with radiation therapy, including stereotactic surgery. Chemotherapy also may be an option for control.

Screening: Currently there are no recommendations for screening for CNS tumors.

See also: "Perioperative Care" for appropriate nursing diagnoses, outcomes, and interventions, p. 45, and "Traumatic Brain Injury" for **Deficient Knowledge:** Craniotomy Procedure, p. 367.

Gastrointestinal malignancies

Malignancies of the gastrointestinal (GI) system include carcinomas of the stomach, esophagus, bowel, anus, rectum, pancreas, liver, and gallbladder. Each disease site has its own staging criteria and prognostic factors. Most early stage tumors of all sites are surgically treated. Many treatment plans now begin with preoperative chemotherapy and/or concurrent radiation therapy in the weeks preceding surgery. This approach may eliminate the need for extensive surgeries, increase the chances for cure, or in the case of anorectal sparing approach, eliminate the necessity for a colostomy. Radiation therapy treatments are less common in gastric, colon, and liver tumors due to the toxicities associated with radiating these areas. Radiofrequency ablation is an interventional radiologic approach that is sometimes successful in managing metastatic liver tumors.

Screening: Currently the colon is the only GI site with recommended screening parameters. The ACS recommends screening individuals older than 50 years of age by one of five options: (1) annual fecal occult blood test (FOBT), (2) flexible sigmoidoscopy every 5 years, (3) annual FOBT plus flexible sigmoidoscopy every 5 years, (4) colonoscopy every 10 years, or (5) double-contrast barium enema every 5 years. When family history includes first-degree relatives with colorectal cancer, the ACS recommends screening begin sooner than age 50.

See also: "Perioperative Care," p. 45; "Fecal Diversions," p. 455; and "Managing Wound Care," p. 559, for appropriate nursing diagnoses, outcomes, and interventions.

Neoplastic diseases of the hematopoietic system

Hematopoietic system cancers include lymphomas, leukemias, plasma cell disorders, and myeloproliferative disorders.

Depending on cellular type, *lymphomas* are classified as Hodgkin and non-Hodgkin and are characterized by abnormal proliferation of lymphocytes. In addition to characteristic lymph node enlargement, involvement of other lymphoid organs such as the liver, spleen, and bone marrow does occur. Treatment planning, based on disease stage, usually involves chemotherapy and sometimes radiation therapy for eradication of local disease. Patients with Hodgkin lymphoma may have a chance for cure, whereas patients with certain grades of non-Hodgkin lymphoma may face treatment decisions for the remainder of their lives.

Screening: Currently there is no routine screening recommended for the lymphomas.

Leukemia is the abnormal proliferation and accumulation of white blood cells·(WBCs). Divided into two categories, leukemia presents as either acute or chronic, depending on cellular characteristics. Acute leukemia, characterized by abnormal proliferation of immature WBCs, also known as precursor or progenitor cells, is classified by the type of WBC involved. Treatment consists predominantly of chemotherapy and biologic therapy, with radiation therapy for CNS prophylaxis when indicated.

Chronic leukemia, characterized by abnormal proliferation of mature differentiated WBCs, is typically treated with chemotherapy; some forms of chronic leukemia may remain indolent for years, delaying treatment indefinitely. In both types of leukemia, abnormal cells may interfere with normal production of other WBCs, red blood cells (RBCs), and platelets.

Patients with chronic lymphocytic leukemia may have compromised immunity, resulting in frequent and possibly fatal infections.

Screening: No screening recommendations currently exist for leukemia. Diagnosis usually occurs when the presenting symptoms include fever, malaise, bruising or bleeding, infections, adenopathy, hepatosplenomegaly, weight loss, or night sweats but may also be initially noted on routine complete blood count (CBC). Diagnosis is confirmed with a CBC and peripheral smear and by bone marrow biopsy.

See also: "Hematologic Care Plans," p. 495, for appropriate nursing diagnoses, outcomes, and interventions related to care of patients with abnormal blood cells.

Head and neck cancers

Head and neck cancers include tumors of the tonsils, larynx, pharynx, tongue, and oral cavity. Incidence is greatest in men older than age 50, and incidence rates are double in men compared to women. By far the greatest risk factors are tobacco consumption through smoking or smokeless tobacco and alcohol consumption.

Screening: Although no formal recommendations regarding screening exist, routine dental examinations are one mechanism by which early detection occurs.

See also: "Pneumonia," p. 125, for outcomes and interventions in **Ineffective Airway Clearance.**

Breast cancer

According to the ACS, incidence of breast cancer continues to rise, occurring in one of seven women (lifetime risk) in the United States. Several factors must be taken into consideration to determine disease stage and prognosis and to establish a treatment plan upon diagnosis. Tumor differentiation is a prognostic factor, with poorly differentiated tumors foreboding a worse prognosis. Other factors considered in treatment and prognosis are rate of tumor growth (S-phase), DNA characteristics (ploidy), estrogen and progesterone receptors, other biochemical changes (e.g., HER-2/*neu*), lymph node metastases, and distant metastases. Treatment may include any, all, or a combination of the following: surgery, chemotherapy, radiation therapy, hormonal treatment, and biologic therapy. Metastatic breast cancer, considered a chronic disease in some women, may result in therapy spanning several years.

Screening: The ACS recommends all women older than age 40 have an annual mammogram and clinical breast examination (CBE) by a clinician. Women between the ages of 20 and 39 should have a CBE performed by a clinician every 3 years. Women deemed at higher risk for developing breast cancer may have mammography initiated earlier than age 40.

The ACS as a matter of routine no longer recommends monthly breast self-examination (BSE). Instead, it recommends educating women regarding potential benefits and limitations of BSE and allows women the choice of whether to perform BSE or not.

See also: "Perioperative Care," p. 45, for appropriate nursing diagnoses, outcomes, and interventions and **Risk for Disuse Syndrome,** p. 12, in this section.

Genitourinary cancers

Malignancies of the bladder, prostate gland, testicle, and kidneys comprise genitourinary cancers for men.

Bladder cancer is classified as superficial or invasive. Treatment is chosen based on extent of disease and may include surgery, local or systemic chemotherapy, laser surgery, or radiation. Metastases occur commonly in bone, liver, and lungs. Bladder cancer incidence is higher in men than in women.

Screening: No standards currently exist for screening for bladder cancer; however, survival may depend on prompt evaluation of early symptoms.

Prostate cancer occurs most commonly in men older than age 50. Treatment may consist of a combination of interstitial or external radiation therapy, chemotherapy, surgery, or hormonal therapy. Choice of treatment is determined in part by the disease stage and cellular histology at diagnosis and by clinician preference. In general, prostate cancers tend to grow slowly and metastasize late, enabling patients to live several years with the disease.

Screening: The ACS (American Cancer Society, 2006) believes that health care providers should offer the PSA (prostate-specific antigen) blood test and the DRE (digital rectal examination) yearly, beginning at age 50, to men who do not have any major medical problems and can be expected to live at least 10 more years. Men at high risk should begin testing at age 45. Men at high risk include African Americans and those who have a close relative (father, brother, or son) who had prostate cancer before age 65.

Testicular cancer occurs most often in men between ages 20 and 40. Tumors are classified as seminomas and nonseminomas, depending on their cellular line of differentiation, with many consisting of a mixed cellular type. Nonseminomas tend to grow and metastasize more aggressively. Treatment nearly always begins with surgery, and depending on histology, blood tumor markers, and bulk of disease, may be followed by chemotherapy and/or radiation therapy.

Screening: Surgical correction for cryptorchidism is recommended before age 6 to significantly reduce the risk of later development of testicular cancer. Screening programs are not routinely conducted, but a routine physical examination should include examination of the testes, which would detect an undescended testicle or mass. Any scrotal mass should be evaluated promptly.

Renal cell carcinomas, most predominantly classified as adenocarcinomas with histologic variants, occur in about 2% of all malignant diagnoses. Surgery is nearly always the treatment of choice for early stage renal cell cancers, and radiation therapy for control of symptoms is usually indicated for more advanced disease. Chemotherapy has a limited role with management of renal cell cancer. Biologic response modifiers are an option for more advanced disease. Incidence of renal cancer is higher in men than in women.

Screening: No screening programs exist to detect renal cell cancer, and incidence likely would be lowered if predominance of cigarette smoking could be reduced. Reports of hematuria should be investigated thoroughly. Presentation of any other symptoms compatible with renal cell carcinoma may forebode disease that is more advanced.

See also: "Perioperative Care," p. 45; "Urinary Diversions," p. 249; and "Benign Prostatic Hypertrophy," p. 207, for appropriate nursing diagnoses, outcomes, and interventions. Also see **Stress Urinary Incontinence,** p. 10, and **Sexual Dysfunction,** p. 10, in this section.

Sites of neoplasms of the female pelvis include the vulva, vagina, cervix, uterus, and ovaries. Discussion of bladder and kidney cancers occurs earlier in this section.

With increased use of the Papanicolaou (Pap) smear as a screening tool for *cervical cancer*, incidence of invasive cervical cancer has decreased, while incidence of preinvasive carcinoma in situ (CIS) has increased. Treated early, usually with surgery and sometimes with radiation therapy, cervical cancer is a curable disease. Surgery, chemotherapy, and/or radiation may manage stages that are more advanced.

Ovarian tumors occasionally detected during an annual pelvic examination are more commonly occult until symptoms of advanced disease are present. Treatment is initially surgical, which is a vital step for proper tumor staging. Survival, directly related to proper treatment, can only be determined by proper staging. Chemotherapy is commonly given after surgery.

Endometrial cancer, usually treated with surgery, is followed by radiation therapy in all but the earliest stages. Chemotherapy and hormonal therapy are usually reserved for advanced stages in which a surgical cure is not feasible and invasion of local or more distant tissues has occurred.

Screening: The ACS recommends an annual Pap smear and pelvic examination for women 3 years after beginning vaginal intercourse or by age 21. If using a liquid-based Pap test, women should be screened every 2 years. If using conventional Pap tests, screening should be done annually. At or after age 30, women who have had three normal consecutive annual examinations may elect to have screening every 2 or 3 years as recommended by their health care provider. Women age 70 or older who have had three consecutive normal Pap tests and no abnormal tests in the past 10 years may elect to discontinue annual Pap tests. Likewise, women with a total hysterectomy, including removal of the cervix, may elect no further Pap tests.

Endometrial biopsy remains the definitive standard to assess for endometrial cancer. Women at high risk for endometrial cancer should consider routine surveillance beginning at age 35, but currently the ACS has no definitive recommendations regarding screening for endometrial cancer.

See also: "Perioperative Care," p. 45, for appropriate nursing diagnoses, outcomes, and interventions.

NURSING DIAGNOSES AND INTERVENTIONS FOR GENERAL CANCER CARE

Note: *The following nursing diagnoses, desired outcomes, and interventions relate to generalized cancer care. Those for care specific to chemotherapy, immunotherapy, and radiation therapy follow this section.*

Nursing Diagnosis:
Ineffective Breathing Pattern

related to decreased lung expansion secondary to pulmonary fibrosis, cellular damage, and decreased lung capacity (pneumonectomy or lobectomy)

Note: For desired outcome and interventions, see this nursing diagnosis in "Perioperative Care," p. 50. Some chemotherapeutic agents (bleomycin, carmustine, busulfan, cytarabine, mitomycin, cyclophosphamide, methotrexate, melphalan, interferon alfa-2b, interleukin-2, fludarabine) can cause pulmonary toxicity, an inflammatory reaction that results in fibrotic lung changes, cellular damage, and decreased lung capacity. Radiation therapy can also cause pulmonary damage and changes resulting in decreased lung capacity.

Nursing Diagnosis:
Impaired Gas Exchange

related to altered oxygen supply secondary to anemia, pulmonary tumors, pneumonia, pulmonary emboli, pulmonary atelectasis, ascites, radiation, pericardial effusion, superior vena cava syndrome, or hepatomegaly

Note: For desired outcome and interventions, see this nursing diagnosis in "Pneumonia," p. 124, and on p. 139 in "Pulmonary Embolus."

Nursing Diagnosis:
Acute Pain

related to disease process, surgical intervention, or treatment effects

Note: For desired outcome and interventions, see "Pain," p. 39.

Nursing Diagnosis:
Chronic Pain

related to direct tumor involvement such as infiltration of tumor into nerves, bones, or hollow viscus; post chemotherapy pain syndromes (peripheral neuropathy, avascular necrosis of femoral or humeral heads, or plexopathy); or post radiation syndrome (plexopathy, radiation myelopathy, radiation-induced enteritis or proctitis, burning perineum syndrome, or osteoradionecrosis)

Desired Outcome: Patient participates in a prescribed pain regimen and reports that pain and side effects associated with the prescribed therapy are reduced to level of three or less within 1-2 hr of intervention, based on pain assessment tool (e.g., descriptive, numeric [on a scale of 0-10], or visual scale).

INTERVENTIONS	RATIONALES
After patient has undergone a complete medical evaluation for the causes of pain and the most effective strategies for pain relief, review evaluation and pain-relief strategies with patient and caregivers.	This review helps determine patient's level of understanding and reinforce findings, thereby promoting patient's knowledge and adherence to pain relief strategies. It also empowers patient as much as possible to participate in controlling his or her pain.
Assess patient's cultural beliefs and attitudes about pain. *Never* ignore a patient's report of pain, taking into consideration that a patient's definition of pain may be different from that of the assessing nurse. Promptly report *any* change in pain pattern or new complaints of pain to health care provider.	Cultural beliefs may influence how individuals describe their pain and its severity and their willingness to ask for pain medications. Pain is dynamic, and competent management requires frequent assessment at scheduled intervals.
Question patients regarding their level of "discomfort" or abnormal sensations in addition to your usual pain queries.	Patients with *neuropathic pain* may not describe their discomfort as pain; therefore, be sure to use additional terms.
	Nociceptive pain refers to the body's perception of pain and its corresponding response. It begins when tissue is threatened or damaged by mechanical or thermal stimuli that activate the peripheral endings of sensory neurons known as *nociceptors*. In contrast, neuropathic pain is caused by damage to central or peripheral nervous system tissue or from altered processing of pain in the CNS. The resulting pain is chronic, may be difficult to manage, and is often described differently (burning, electric, tingling, numbness, pricking, shooting) from nociceptive pain.
Include the following in your pain assessments:	
- Characteristics (e.g., "burning" or "shooting" often describes nerve pain).	Not all types of pain are managed solely by opioid therapy. Characterizing pain and documenting its location accurately will result in better pharmacologic intervention and assist nurses in developing a customized plan that incorporates nonpharmacologic measures as well.
- Location and sites of radiation.	
- Onset and duration.	Determining precipitating factors (as with onset) may assist in preventing or alleviating pain.
- Severity: Use a pain scale that is comfortable for patient (e.g., descriptive, numeric, or visual scale).	Severe pain can signal complications such as internal bleeding or leaking of visceral contents. Using a pain scale provides an objective measurement that enables the health care team to assess effectiveness of pain management strategies. Optimally, patient's rated pain on a 0-10 scale is 4 or less.
- Aggravating and relieving factors.	This information may assist in preventing or alleviating pain.
- Previous use of strategies that have worked to relieve pain.	Strategies that have worked in the past may work for current pain.
Assess patient's and caregiver's attitudes and knowledge about the pain medication regimen.	Many patients and their families have fears related to patient's ultimate addiction to opioids. It is important to dispel any misperceptions about opioid-induced addiction when chronic pain therapy is necessary. Fears of addiction may result in ineffective pain management.
Incorporate the following principles.	
- Administer nonopioid and opioid analgesics in correct dose, at correct frequency, and via correct route.	Pharmacologic management of pain is often the mainstay of treatment of chronic cancer pain.
	Chronic cancer analgesia is often administered orally. If pain is present most of the day, analgesia should be given around the clock (at scheduled intervals) rather than as needed because prolonged stimulation of the pain receptors increases the amount of drug required to relieve pain.
- Recognize and report/treat side effects of opioid analgesia early.	Side effects include respiratory depression, nausea and vomiting, constipation, sedation, and itching. The presence of these side effects does not necessarily preclude continued use of the drug.
- Use prescribed adjuvant medications.	Adjuvant medications (see p. 43) help increase efficacy of opioids and may minimize their objectionable side effects as well.

Continued

INTERVENTIONS	RATIONALES
- Monitor for signs and symptoms of tolerance, and when it occurs discuss treatment with health care provider.	Patients with chronic pain often require increasing doses of opioids to relieve their pain (tolerance). Respiratory depression occurs rarely in these individuals.
- Never stop opioids abruptly in patients who have been taking them for a prolonged period.	There is potential for physical dependence in patients taking opioids for a prolonged period, therefore they should be tapered gradually to prevent withdrawal discomfort.
- Use nonpharmacologic approaches, such as acupressure, biofeedback, relaxation therapy, and massage when appropriate. See "Pain," p. 43, for details.	Nonpharmacologic approaches are often effective in enhancing effects of opioid therapy.

••• **Related NIC and NOC labels:** *NIC:* Medication Management; Pain Management; Acupressure; Biofeedback; Simple Massage *NOC:* Comfort Level; Pain Control; Pain: Disruptive Effects

Nursing Diagnosis:

Ineffective Tissue Perfusion: Peripheral

related to interrupted blood flow secondary to lymphedema

Desired Outcome: Following intervention/treatment, patient exhibits adequate peripheral perfusion as evidenced by peripheral pulses greater than 2+ on a 0-4+ scale, normal skin color, decreasing or stable circumference of edematous site, equal sensation bilaterally, and ability to perform range of motion (ROM) in the involved extremity.

INTERVENTIONS	RATIONALES
Assess involved extremity for degree of edema, quality of peripheral pulses, color, circumference, sensation, and ROM.	This assessment helps determine presence/degree of lymphedema and potential threat to limb from hypoxia. Patient populations at risk include those who have had a radical mastectomy, lymph node dissection (upper and lower extremities), blockage of the lymphatic system from tumor burden, radiation therapy to the lymphatic system, or any combination of these.
Assess for tenderness, erythema, and warmth at edematous site.	These signs of infection need to be communicated to the provider for prompt intervention. A continuous supply of oxygen to the tissues through microcirculation is vital to the healing process and for resistance to infection.
Elevate and position involved extremity on a pillow in slight abduction. If surgery has been performed, instruct patient not to perform heavy activity with the affected limb during recovery period.	As blood collects, waiting to get into the heart, pressure in the veins increases. The veins are permeable, and the increased pressure causes fluid to leak out of the veins and into the tissue. Elevating the extremity helps reduce venous pressure.
Encourage patient to wear loose-fitting clothing.	Tight-fitting clothing may cause areas of constriction, reducing lymph and blood flow, as well as creating potential areas for impaired skin integrity.
Avoid BP readings, venipuncture, intravenous lines, and vaccinations in affected arm. As indicated, advise patient to get a medical alert bracelet that cautions against these actions.	Blood pressure cuffs can constrict lymphatic pathways, and injections or blood draws will cause an opening in the skin, providing an entrance for bacteria.
Consult physical therapist (PT) and health care provider about development of an exercise plan.	Exercise increases mobility, which promotes lymphatic flow. This in turn helps decrease edema.
As indicated, suggest use of elastic bandages.	Elastic bandages decrease edema in mild, chronic cases of lymphedema.
As indicated, suggest use of compression garments or sequential compression devices.	These garments/devices decrease edema in more severe cases of lymphedema.

••• **Related NIC and NOC labels:** *NIC:* Circulatory Precautions; Positioning; Skin Surveillance *NOC:* Tissue Perfusion: Peripheral

Nursing Diagnosis:

Ineffective Tissue Perfusion: Cardiopulmonary

related to interrupted venous flow secondary to deep venous thrombosis

Desired Outcome: Before hospital discharge, patient and/or caregivers competently administer anticoagulant therapy as prescribed and describe reportable signs and symptoms suggestive of progressive coagulopathy.

INTERVENTIONS	RATIONALES
Instruct patient in technique of self-administration of injectable low-molecular-weight heparin, if it is prescribed.	Individuals with certain malignancies (especially brain, breast, colon, renal, and lung) are at higher than average risk for deep venous thrombosis (DVT). Other possible contributing factors include recent surgery, presence of a venous access device, sepsis, obesity, concurrent cardiac disease, and underlying increased coagulability disorders.
If patient is taking oral anticoagulants, teach dietary modifications with warfarin therapy.	Foods high in vitamin K (antidote to warfarin) may interfere with achievement of therapeutic anticoagulation. These include green leafy vegetables, avocados, and liver. However, some prescribers do not restrict dietary intake of vitamin K–containing foods. Instead, patients are instructed to maintain dietary consistency in moderation without large variations, and the warfarin dose is adjusted accordingly. If patients are consistent in their dietary intake, the prothrombin time (PT)/international normalized ratio (INR) should remain stable and therapeutic.
Instruct patient regarding reportable signs and symptoms, such as unilateral edema of a limb with possible associated warmth, erythema, and tenderness.	DVT may reoccur.
Caution that a sudden increase in shortness of breath with or without chest pain also should be reported immediately.	DVT may progress to pulmonary embolism.
For additional desired outcomes and interventions, see **Ineffective Tissue Perfusion: Peripheral and Cardiopulmonary** on p. 202 in "Venous Thrombosis/Thrombophlebitis."	

••• **Related NIC/NOC labels:** *NIC:* Circulatory Precautions; Embolus Precautions; Medication Administration *NOC:* Circulation Status

Nursing Diagnosis:

Impaired Physical Mobility

related to musculoskeletal or neuromuscular impairment secondary to bone metastasis or spinal cord compression; pain and discomfort; intolerance to activity; or perceptual or cognitive impairment

Note: For desired outcome and interventions, see this nursing diagnosis in "Osteoarthritis," p. 529. Also see "Managing Wound Care" for discussions on care of patients at risk for pressure ulcers, p. 559.

Nursing Diagnosis:

Impaired Skin Integrity

related to malignant skin lesions

Desired Outcomes: Following instruction, patient verbalizes measures that promote comfort, preserve skin integrity, and promote competent management of and infection prevention of open wounds. Patient's skin remains intact.

INTERVENTIONS	RATIONALES
Identify if your patient is at risk for malignant lesions.	Individuals with breast, lung, colon, and renal cancers; T-cell lymphoma; melanoma; and extensions of head and neck cancers may be susceptible to developing skin metastases. These skin metastases often erode, providing challenges to wound care, patient dignity, body image, and odor control. Treatment may include radiation, systemic or local chemotherapy, cryotherapy, or excision.
Assess common sites of cutaneous metastases.	These sites include anterior chest, abdomen, head (scalp), and neck and should be assessed in patients at risk.
Inspect skin lesions.	The presence of skin lesions necessitates being alert to and documenting general characteristics, location and distribution, configuration, size, morphologic structure (e.g., nodule, erosion, fissure), drainage (color, amount, character), and odor so that changes can be detected and reported promptly.
Monitor for local warmth, swelling, erythema, tenderness, and purulent drainage.	These are indicators of infection, which can occur as a result of nonintact skin.
Perform the following skin care for nonulcerating lesions and teach these interventions to patient and significant other, as indicated:	Maintaining skin integrity reduces risk of infection.
- Wash affected area with tepid water and pat dry.	Excessively warm temperatures damage healing tissue.
- Avoid pressure on the area.	Pressure would further damage friable tissue.
- Apply dry dressing.	This dressing will protect the skin from exposure to irritants and mechanical trauma (e.g., scratching, abrasion).
- Apply occlusive dressings, such as Telfa, using paper tape.	An occlusive dressing promotes penetration of topical medications.
Teach patient to avoid wearing such fabrics as wool and corduroy.	These fabrics are irritating to the skin.
Perform the following skin care for ulcerating lesions and teach these interventions to patient and significant other, as indicated:	
For Cleansing and Débriding:	
Use ½-strength hydrogen peroxide and normal saline solution, followed by a normal saline rinse.	This solution will irrigate and débride the lesion. Rinsing removes peroxide and residual wound debris.
Use cotton swabs or sponges to apply gentle pressure. As necessary, gently irrigate using a syringe.	Using gentle pressure with these swabs or sponges débrides the ulcerated area and protects granulation tissue.
	If the ulcerated area is susceptible to bleeding, gentle pressure protects delicate granulation tissue.
Use soaks (wet dressings) of saline, water, Burrow's solution (aluminum acetate), or hydrogen peroxide on the involved skin.	These are methods of débridement, which will dislodge and remove bacteria and loosen necrotic tissue, foreign bodies, and exudate.
Be sure to rinse hydrogen peroxide or aluminum acetate off the skin.	Failure to do so may cause further skin breakdown.
As necessary, use wet-to-dry dressings.	These dressings will provide gentle débridement.
For Prevention and Management of Local Infection:	
Irrigate and scrub with antibacterial agents, such as acetic acid solution or povidone-iodine.	These antibacterial agents prevent/manage local infection.
Collect wound cultures, as prescribed.	A culture will determine presence of infection and optimal antibiotic therapy.
Apply topical antibacterial agents (e.g., sulfadiazine cream, bacitracin ointment) to open areas, as prescribed.	These agents prevent infection in open areas that are susceptible.
Administer systemic antibiotics, as prescribed.	Systemic antibiotics are used for wounds that are more extensively infected.
To Maintain Hemostasis:	
Use silver nitrate sticks for cautery.	These sticks help maintain hemostasis in the presence of capillary oozing.
Use oxidized cellulose or pack the wound with Gelfoam or similar product.	These products are used for bleeding in larger surface areas.

Continued

INTERVENTIONS	RATIONALES
To Control Odor:	
Cleanse wound and change dressings as often as necessary.	These actions control odor and promote patient comfort.
Collect specimens for culture and sensitivity of the wound drainage, as prescribed.	Culture and sensitivity of the wound will determine presence of infection and optimal antibiotic therapy.
Use antiodor agents (e.g., open a bottle of oil of peppermint or place a tray of activated charcoal).	This action will help control pervasive odor in patient's room.
Consult wound, ostomy, continence (WOC) enterostomal therapy (ET) nurse as needed on wound-healing techniques.	When wounds fail to respond to more traditional interventions, a WOC/ET nurse may provide alternative suggestions.
See also: "Providing Nutritional Support," p. 565, "Managing Wound Care," p. 559, and "Infection Prevention and Control," p. 783.	Wound healing depends on adequate intake of nutrients/protein for tissue synthesis.

••• **Related NIC** and **NOC labels:** *NIC:* Skin Surveillance; Infection Protection; Medication Administration: Skin; Skin Care: Topical Treatments; Wound Care: Closed Drainage; Wound Irrigation *NOC:* Tissue Integrity: Skin and Mucous Membranes; Wound Healing: Secondary Intention

Nursing Diagnosis:

Diarrhea

related to chemotherapeutic agents; biologic agents; antacids containing magnesium; radiation therapy to the abdomen or pelvis; tube feedings; food intolerance; and bowel dysfunction such as tumors, Crohn's disease, ulcerative colitis, and fecal impaction

Note: For desired outcomes and interventions, see "Ulcerative Colitis" for **Diarrhea,** p. 491 and **Risk for Impaired Skin Integrity: Perineal/Perianal** related to persistent diarrhea, p. 492; "Caring for Individuals with Human Immunodeficiency Virus" for **Diarrhea,** p. 551, and "Providing Nutritional Support" for **Diarrhea,** p. 571.

For patients receiving chemotherapy with potential to cause diarrhea (e.g., 5-fluorouracil, irinotecan), instruct patient regarding need to have appropriate antidiarrheal medications available and other methods used to combat effects of diarrhea (fluid replacement, addition of psyllium to the diet to provide bulk to stool, perineal hygiene). Instruct patient to notify health care provider if experiencing more than six loose stools per day.

Nursing Diagnosis:

Constipation

related to treatment with certain chemotherapy agents, opioids, tranquilizers, and antidepressants; less than adequate intake of food and fluids because of anorexia, nausea, or dysphagia; hypercalcemia; spinal cord compression; mental status changes; decreased mobility; or colonic disorders

Note: For desired outcomes and interventions, see "Perioperative Care" for **Constipation,** p. 56; "Prolonged Bedrest" for **Constipation,** p. 67; and "General Care of Patients with Neurologic Disorders" for **Constipation,** p. 277. Patients with cancer should not go more than 2 days without having a bowel movement. Patients receiving Vinca alkaloids are at

risk for ileus in addition to constipation. Preventive measures, such as use of senna products or docusate calcium with casanthranol, especially for patients taking opioids, are highly recommended. In addition, all individuals taking opioids should receive a prophylactic bowel regimen.

Nursing Diagnosis:

Stress Urinary Incontinence

related to loss of muscle tone in the urethral sphincter after radical prostatectomy

Desired Outcome: Within the 24-hr period before hospital discharge, patient relates understanding of incontinence cause and suggested regimen to promote bladder control.

INTERVENTIONS	RATIONALES
Before surgery, explain to patient that there is potential for permanent urinary incontinence after prostatectomy but that it may resolve within 6 months. Describe the reason for the incontinence.	A knowledgeable patient is not only less anxious but more likely to adhere to the treatment regimen. Aids such as anatomic illustrations will promote understanding.
Encourage patient to maintain adequate fluid intake of at least 2-3 L/day (unless contraindicated).	Dilute urine is less irritating to the prostatic fossa, as well as less likely to result in incontinence. Paradoxically, patients with urinary incontinence often reduce their fluid intake to avoid incontinence.
Teach patient to avoid caffeine and alcoholic beverages.	Caffeine and alcoholic beverages are examples of irritants that may increase stress incontinence.
Establish a bladder routine with patient before hospital discharge.	Documenting time, amount voided, amount of fluid intake, timing of fluid intake followed by voiding, and related information such as degree of wetness experienced (e.g., number of incontinence pads used in a day, degree of underwear dampness) and exertion factor causing the wetness (e.g., laughing, sneezing, bending, lifting) may help patient manage incontinence. This helps estimate amount of time patient can hold urine and avoid incontinence episodes.
	If successful, patient can then attempt to lengthen time intervals between voidings. **Note:** Patients need to empty their bladders at least q4h to reduce risk of urinary tract infection (UTI) caused by urinary stasis.
Teach patient Kegel exercises (see "Benign Prostatic Hypertrophy," p. 214) to promote sphincter control. Begin teaching before surgery if possible.	Kegel exercises strengthen pelvic area muscles, which will help regain bladder control. The patient must first identify the correct muscle groups in order to perform Kegel exercises correctly.
	These exercises require diligent effort to reverse incontinence and in fact may need to be done for several months before any benefit is obtained.
Remind patient to discuss any incontinence problems with health care provider during follow-up examinations.	Such a discussion will enable follow-up treatment for this problem.

••• **Related NIC** and **NOC labels:** *NIC:* Pelvic Muscle Control; Urinary Elimination Management; Urinary Habit Training *NOC:* Urinary Continence

Nursing Diagnosis:

Sexual Dysfunction

(erectile dysfunction, body changes, decreased libido, impaired sexual self-concept, infertility secondary to treatment) *related to* the disease process; psychosocial issues; radiation therapy to the lower abdomen, pelvis, and gonads; chemotherapeutic agents; or surgery

Desired Outcome: Following instruction, patient identifies potential treatment side effects on sexual and reproductive function and acceptable methods of contraception during treatment.

INTERVENTIONS	RATIONALES
Determine patient's readiness to discuss sexual concerns.	Gentle, sensitive, open-ended questions allow patients to signal their readiness to discuss concerns.
Initiate discussion about effects of treatment on sexuality and reproduction, using, for example, the PLISSIT model.	The PLISSIT model provides an excellent framework for discussion. This four-step model includes the following: (1) **P**ermission—give the patient permission to discuss issues of concern; (2) **L**imited **I**nformation—provide patient with information about expected treatment effects on sexual and reproductive function, without going into complete detail; (3) **S**pecific **S**uggestions—provide suggestions for managing common problems that occur during treatment; and (4) **I**ntensive **T**herapy—although most individuals can be managed by nurses using the first three steps in this model, some patients may require referral to an expert counselor.
Assess impact of diagnosis and treatment on patient's sexual functioning and self-concept.	Sexual dysfunction affects every individual differently. It is important not to assume its meaning but rather explore it with the individual and allow him or her to give meaning to the changes.
If female patient is of childbearing age, inquire if pregnancy is a possibility before treatment is initiated.	Pregnancy will cause a delay in treatment. If treatment cannot be delayed, a therapeutic abortion may be recommended.
Discuss possibility of decreased sexual response or desire.	This may result from side effects of chemotherapy. Informing patient may allay unnecessary anxiety.
Encourage patient to maintain open communication with partner about needs and concerns. Explore alternative methods of sexual fulfillment, such as hugging, kissing, talking quietly together, or massage.	Encouraging open dialogue promotes intimacy and helps prevent ill feelings or emotional withdrawal by either partner. In the presence of symptoms related to therapy, such interventions as taking a nap before sexual activity or use of pain or antiemetic medication may help decrease symptoms. Other suggestions include using a water-based lubricant for dyspareunia. If fatigue is a problem, partners might consider changing usual time of day for intimacy or using supine or side-lying positions, which require less energy expenditure.
Discuss possibility of temporary or permanent sterility resulting from treatment.	This discussion could open the door to explaining possibility of sperm banking for men before chemotherapy treatment or oophoropexy (surgical displacement of ovaries outside the radiation field) for women undergoing abdominal radiation therapy.
Teach patients importance of contraception during treatment if relevant. Discuss issues related to timing of pregnancy after treatment. Suggest that patients receive genetic counseling before attempting pregnancy, as indicated.	Healthy offspring have been born from parents who have received radiation therapy or chemotherapy, but long-term effects have not been clearly identified.
For patient undergoing lymphadenectomy for testicular cancer, explain that ejaculatory failure may occur if the sympathetic nerve is damaged, but erection and orgasm will be possible.	If ejaculatory failure does occur, patient should know that artificial insemination is possible because the semen flows back into the urine, from which it can be extracted, enabling the ovum to become impregnated artificially.
If appropriate, explain that a silicone prosthesis may be placed after orchiectomy. Consult health care provider about the potential for this procedure.	This will help the scrotum achieve a normal appearance.

••• **Related NIC and NOC labels:** *NIC:* Sexual Counseling; Self-Esteem Enhancement; Reproductive Technology Management *NOC:* Sexual Functioning

Nursing Diagnosis:

Risk for Disuse Syndrome

related to upper extremity immobilization secondary to discomfort, lymphedema, treatment or disease-related injury, or infection after breast surgery

Desired Outcomes: Before surgery, patient verbalizes knowledge about importance of and rationale for upper extremity movements and exercises. Upon recovery, patient has full or baseline level ROM of the upper extremity.

INTERVENTIONS	RATIONALES
Consult surgeon before breast surgery regarding such issues as wound healing, suture lines, and extent of the surgical procedure.	This consultation will determine type of surgery anticipated and enable development of an individualized exercise plan in collaboration with physical and occupational therapists specific to patient's needs.
Encourage finger, wrist, and elbow movement.	Such movements aid circulation, minimize edema, and maintain mobility in the involved extremity.
Elevate extremity as tolerated.	Elevation decreases edema.
Encourage progressive exercise by having patient use affected arm for personal hygiene and activities of daily living (ADLs). Initiate other exercises (e.g., clasping hands behind the head and "walking" fingers up the wall) as soon as patient is ready.	After drains and sutures have been removed (usually 7-10 days postoperatively), patient should begin exercises that will enhance external rotation and abduction of the shoulder. Ultimately patient should be able to achieve maximum shoulder flexion by touching fingertips together behind the back if patient was capable of this exercise before the surgery.
In patients who have had lymph node removal, avoid giving injections, measuring BP, or taking blood samples from affected arm. Remind patient about lowered resistance to infection and importance of promptly treating any breaks in the skin. Advise patient to treat minor injuries with soap and water after hospital discharge and to notify health care provider if signs of infection occur.	Loss of lymph nodes alters lymph drainage, which may result in edema of the arm and hand and increases risk of infection as well.
Advise patient to wear a medical alert bracelet that cautions against injections and tests in the involved arm.	Information on this bracelet optimally will help prevent infection caused by invasive procedures or ensure that patient receives prompt treatment if an infection occurs.
Advise patient to wear a thimble when sewing and a protective glove when gardening or doing chores that require exposure to harsh chemicals such as cleaning fluids.	This information promotes patient safety/infection prevention.
Explain that cutting cuticles should be avoided and lotion should be used to keep skin soft. An electric razor should be used for shaving the axilla.	This information promotes skin integrity and protects hand and arm from injury and subsequent infection.

••• **Related NIC and NOC labels:** *NIC:* Exercise Therapy: Joint Mobility; Exercise Therapy: Muscle Control; Exercise Promotion; Teaching: Prescribed Activity/Exercise *NOC:* Mobility Level

Nursing Diagnosis:

Deficient Knowledge:

Purpose, type, and management of venous access device (VAD)

Desired Outcome: Within the 24-hr period before hospital discharge, patient and significant other/caregiver verbalize understanding regarding the VAD, including its purpose, appropriate management measures, and reportable complications.

INTERVENTIONS	RATIONALES
Determine patient's and caregiver's level of understanding of the VAD that will be/has been inserted and intervene accordingly.	A VAD can be used for venipunctures and administration of drugs, fluids, and blood products. Determining patient's and caregiver's current knowledge base helps the nurse devise an individualized teaching plan. Three types of VADs are generally used: tunneled catheters, nontunneled catheters, and implanted ports.
Nontunneled catheters (peripheral or central):	These catheters are inserted by venipuncture into the vessel of choice, usually basilic, cephalic, or medial cubital vein, near or at the antecubital area, or jugular or subclavian vein in the upper thorax. A peripherally inserted central catheter (PICC) is an example of a nontunneled catheter. Maintenance involves daily flushing after each use with normal saline and/or heparinized solution. Sterile dressing and cap changes are necessary. Refer to institutional policies for specific instructions.
Tunneled central venous catheters:	These catheters are inserted into a central vein with a portion of the catheter tunneled through subcutaneous tissue and exiting the body at a convenient area, usually the chest. A Dacron cuff encircles the catheter about 2 inches from the exiting end of the catheter. Tissue grows into this cuff, helping prevent catheter dislodgement and decreasing risk of microorganisms migrating along the catheter surface and entering the bloodstream. Single-lumen or multi-lumen catheters are available. Examples of tunneled central venous catheters include Broviac, Hickman, and Groshong. Maintenance involves flushing per institutional protocol and after each use with saline and/or heparinized saline solution. A sterile dressing change is performed 24 hr after insertion and then every 5-7 days until healed. Cap changes are performed using sterile technique. Refer to institutional policies for specific instructions.
Implanted venous access ports:	Implanted ports are commonly inserted when long-term therapy is anticipated or lack of venous access is expected to be a chronic issue. They consist of a catheter attached to a plastic or metal port inserted into a central or peripheral vein and then sutured in place in a surgically created subcutaneous pocket, most commonly on the chest. Venous access ports are completely embedded under the skin and may have single or dual access ports. Access to the port may be from the top or side, depending on port style.
	Note: Noncoring needles must be used to access the port, which allows the system to reseal when the needle is removed.
	This catheter must not be flushed with any syringe smaller than 10 ml due to excess pressures generated by smaller syringes. When removing needle, pressure must be applied to sides of the port to promote ease of removal and patient comfort. Maintenance involves preparation of the site for access with an antibacterial preparation solution (e.g., povidone-iodine solution), optional local anesthetic, and flushing at least monthly or after each use with normal saline and/or heparinized solution. Refer to institutional policies for specific instructions. Dressings are not required after healing of the insertion site.
Teach patients to carry in their wallets the card provided by the manufacturer identifying type of catheter and recommended flushing solution.	There is a wide variety of catheter types, and the type of catheter determines the proper flushing solution.
Provide a model of the device during patient teaching.	Visual aids augment understanding.
Explain where the device will be inserted.	Nontunneled catheters may be inserted at the bedside or in the clinic under local anesthesia. Tunneled central venous catheters and implanted ports are inserted in the operating room under local anesthesia.
Teach patient that there may be mild discomfort, similar to a toothache, for 48 hr after the procedure but medication will ameliorate pain.	Explaining expected sensations and likely amelioration with analgesics reduces anxiety and provides patient with guidelines for reportable symptoms.

Continued

INTERVENTIONS	RATIONALES
If possible, introduce patient and caregiver to another individual who has the device.	Conversing with someone who has already undergone a procedure may increase knowledge, decrease anxiety, and provide another avenue of support.
Teach VAD maintenance care. Provide both verbal and written instructions, including educational materials provided by VAD manufacturer.	Maintenance care likely will be done while patient is at home, where written materials will serve as a reference.
Have patient or caregiver demonstrate dressing care, flushing technique, and cap-changing routine before hospital discharge. Provide 24-hr emergency number to call in case of problems.	This demonstration will reinforce previous teaching and when done correctly provides emotional support that this care can be done when at home.
Discuss potential complications associated with VADs, along with appropriate self-management measures.	
Infection:	Patient should be taught how to assess exit site for erythema, swelling, local increased temperature, discomfort, purulent drainage, and fever (temperature higher than 38° C [100.4° F]).
Bleeding:	Patient should be taught how to apply pressure to site and to notify health care team member if bleeding does not stop in 5 min.
Clot in the catheter:	Patient should be taught how to flush catheter without using excessive pressure, which could damage or dislodge catheter (particularly an implanted port). If flushing does not dislodge clot, patient or caregiver should notify health care team member.
Disconnected cap:	Patient should be taught how to tape all connections and importance of always carrying hemostats or alligator clamps with padded blades to prevent catheter from tearing.
Extravasation:	Although this is a relatively rare complication, it can cause severe damage if a chemotherapy agent with vesicant properties is involved. Patient should be taught to report pain, burning, and stinging in the chest, clavicle, and port pocket or along the subcutaneous tunnel during drug administration.

••• **Related NIC and NOC labels:** *NIC:* Teaching: Procedure/Treatment *NOC:* Knowledge: Treatment Regimen

Nursing Diagnosis:

Deficient Knowledge:

Side effects of antiandrogen therapy or bilateral orchiectomy

Desired Outcome: Within the 24-hr period before hospital discharge, patient verbalizes knowledge about the extent and duration of body changes.

INTERVENTIONS	RATIONALES
Assess patient's health care literacy (language, reading, comprehension). Assess culture and culturally specific information needs.	This assessment helps ensure that information is presented in a manner that is culturally and educationally appropriate. A knowledgeable patient likely will have less stress about his treatment, adhere to the treatment regimen accordingly, and report side effects promptly for timely treatment.
Inform patient of side effects of estrogen therapy and orchiectomy.	Breast enlargement, breast tenderness, loss of sexual desire, and hot flashes can occur.
For patients taking estrogen therapy, provide instruction about symptoms related to complications of thromboembolic disorders and myocardial infarction, which should be reported promptly to health care provider.	Shortness of breath; orthopnea; dyspnea; pedal edema; unilateral leg swelling or pain; and left arm, left jaw, or left-sided chest pain can occur with this therapy and should be reported promptly for timely intervention.
Explain that when therapy is discontinued, most side effects will resolve.	This knowledge may bring some reassurance to the patient.

Continued

INTERVENTIONS	RATIONALES
If appropriate, explain to patient that before initiating estrogen therapy, health care provider may prescribe radiation therapy to areolae of the breasts.	Radiation therapy will minimize painful gynecomastia. However, this procedure will not decrease other side effects.

••• **Related NIC and NOC labels:** *NIC:* Teaching: Procedure/Treatment *NOC:* Knowledge: Treatment Regimen

---

NURSING DIAGNOSES AND INTERVENTIONS SPECIFIC TO PATIENTS UNDERGOING CHEMOTHERAPY, IMMUNOTHERAPY, AND RADIATION THERAPY

Nursing Diagnosis:

Risk for Infection

related to inadequate defenses due to myelosuppression secondary to malignancy, chemotherapy, radiation therapy, and/or immunotherapy

Desired Outcomes: Patient is free of infection as evidenced by oral temperature 38° C (100.4° F) or less, BP 90/60 mm Hg or higher, and HR 100 bpm or less. Patient identifies risk factors for infection, verbalizes early signs and symptoms of infection and reports them promptly to health care professional if they occur, and demonstrates appropriate self-care measures to minimize risk of infection.

INTERVENTIONS	RATIONALES
Before administering chemotherapy, ensure that blood counts and other related laboratory studies are within accepted parameters per institutional policy. See Appendix B, p. 793, for normal values.	Chemotherapy causes predictable drops in WBC, RBC, and platelet counts because it can damage normal, healthy blood cells forming in the bone marrow. Administering chemotherapy to individuals with counts below specified parameters may put them at risk for infection, bleeding, or worsening anemia.
Identify patients at risk for infection by obtaining the absolute neutrophil count (ANC).	ANC may be used to determine if patient is at unacceptable risk for infection when administering chemotherapy.
Calculate ANC by using the following formula. ANC = (% of segmented neutrophils + % of bands) × Total WBC count	Neutropenia is a condition in which the number of neutrophils in the blood is too low. Because neutrophils are important in defending the body against bacterial and some viral infections, neutropenia places patients at increased risk for these infections. Severe neutropenia can lead to serious problems that require prompt care and attention inasmuch as the patient could develop bacterial, viral, fungal, or mixed infection at any time.
ANC of 1500-2000/mm³ = No significant risk.	
ANC of 1000-1500/mm³ = Minimal risk.	
ANC of 500-1000/mm³ = Moderate risk.	Neutropenic precautions need to be initiated.
ANC of less than 500/mm³ = Severe risk.	Neutropenic precautions need to be initiated.
Assess each body system.	This assessment will help determine potential for and actual sources of infection. Patients with severe neutropenia have a significantly increased risk of infection because of invasion of surface bacteria in the mouth, intestinal tract, and skin. These patients frequently exhibit mucosal inflammation, particularly of the gingival and perirectal areas.
Avoid invasive procedures when possible.	Invasive procedures increase risk of infection.
Monitor vital signs (VS), temperature, and invasive sites q4h.	Temperature 38° C (100.4° F) or higher, increased HR, decreased BP, and the following clinical signs: tenderness, erythema, warmth, swelling, and drainage at invasive sites; chills; and malaise are signs of infection.

Continued

INTERVENTIONS

Note: Temperature of 38° C (100.4° F) or higher may be the only sign of infection in the neutropenic patient.

Be alert to subtle changes in mental status: restlessness or irritability; warm and flushed skin; chills, fever, or hypothermia; increased urine output; bounding pulse; tachypnea; and glycosuria.

Place sign on patient's door indicating that neutropenic precautions are in effect for patients with ANC 1000/mm³ or less.

Instruct all persons entering patient's room to wash hands thoroughly and to follow other appropriate Centers for Disease Control and Prevention (CDC) guidelines.

Restrict individuals from entering who have transmissible illnesses.

Encourage patient to practice good personal hygiene, including good perineal care after elimination.

Notify health care provider immediately if patient's temperature is higher than 38° C (100.4° F).

Administer antibiotic therapy in a timely fashion (within 1 hr).

Implement routine oral care. Teach patient to use a soft-bristle toothbrush after meals and before bed (bristles may be softened further by running them under hot water).

Inspect oral cavity daily, noting presence of lesions, erythema, or exudate on the tongue or mucous membranes.

Encourage coughing, deep breathing, and turning.

Avoid use of rectal suppositories, rectal thermometer, or enemas. Caution patient to avoid straining at stool.

Suggest use of stool softener.

Teach patient to use electric shaver rather than razor blade; avoid vaginal douche and tampons; use emery board rather than clipper for nail care; check with health care provider before dental care; avoid invasive procedures.

Use antimicrobial skin preparations before injections, and change IV sites q48-72h or per protocol.

Instruct patient to use water-soluble lubricant before sexual intercourse and avoid oral and anal manipulation during sexual activities. Caution that patient should abstain from sexual intercourse during periods of severe neutropenia.

If indicated, advise patient to avoid foods with high bacterial count (raw eggs, raw fruits and vegetables, foods prepared in a blender that cannot adequately be cleaned); bird, cat, and dog excreta; plants, flowers, and sources of stagnant water. Follow institutional policy accordingly.

As prescribed, administer colony-stimulating factors.

See also: "Infection Prevention and Control," p. 783.

RATIONALES

Other signs of infection may be absent in the presence of neutropenia.

These are signs of impending sepsis, which often precede the classic signs of septic shock: cold, clammy skin; thready pulse; decreased BP; and oliguria. These signs should be reported promptly for timely intervention.

These patients are vulnerable to infection.

Washing hands is the most important form of infection prevention. Current CDC guidelines also state that individuals caring for patients at high risk for infection should not wear artificial nails and should consider keeping natural nails less than ¼ inch long.

Individuals with colds, influenza, chickenpox, or herpes zoster can transmit these illnesses to the patient.

Proper hygiene eliminates flora or bacteria that can easily lead to infection in an immunocompromised patient.

This is a possible sign of infection and necessitates an emergent CBC.

Inasmuch as the only sure sign of infection in a neutropenic patient is fever, initiation of antibiotic therapy in a timely fashion is imperative.

Gentle oral care helps prevent injury to oral mucosa that could result in infection.

Individuals with prolonged neutropenia are at risk for fungal, bacterial, and viral infections.

These actions decrease risk of pneumonia and of skin breakdown, which could lead to infection.

These actions could traumatize the rectal mucosa, thereby increasing risk of infection because of infectious flora in the rectum.

Patients with prolonged neutropenia are at increased risk for perirectal infection and should be monitored accordingly. Because the immune system is compromised, normal bacterial flora in the colon can be introduced to other parts of the body if perirectal abscesses are ruptured, leading to systemic infection.

These measures help maintain skin integrity, thereby minimizing risk for infection.

These actions help prevent infection.

These measures decrease risk of introducing infection because of nonintact skin.

Although scientifically unproved, tradition holds that patient be taught these measures to avoid these potential sources of infection during periods of neutropenia.

These agents minimize risk of myelosuppression associated with chemotherapy, especially for patients with a history of neutropenic fever.

••• **Related NIC and NOC labels:** *NIC:* Infection Protection; Medication Administration; Risk Identification; Teaching: Disease Process; Environmental Management; Skin Surveillance; Chest Physiotherapy; Nutrition Management; Oral Health Maintenance *NOC:* Immune Status; Infection Status

Nursing Diagnosis:

Activity Intolerance

related to decreased oxygen-carrying capacity of the blood secondary to anemia (caused by some chemotherapeutic drugs, radiation therapy, chronic disease such as renal failure, or surgery), or related to decreased oxygenation secondary to acute or chronic lung changes (e.g., occurring with lobectomy, pneumonectomy, pulmonary fibrosis)

Desired Outcome: After treatment, patient rates perceived exertion at 3 or less on a 0-10 scale and exhibits tolerance to activity as evidenced by RR 12-20 breaths/min with normal depth and pattern (eupnea), HR 100 bpm or less, and absence of dizziness and headaches.

INTERVENTIONS	RATIONALES
Advise patient that fatigue and activity intolerance are manifestations of decreased oxygen-carrying capacity of the blood and can be tempered by various interventions mentioned below.	Fatigue and activity intolerance are temporary side effects of chemotherapy or radiation therapy and will abate gradually when therapy has been completed. Understanding this relationship likely will help the patient cope better with the treatment.
Stress importance of good nutrition.	Vitamin and iron supplements and intake of foods high in iron such as liver and other organ meats, seafood, green vegetables, cereals, nuts, and legumes likely will help reverse the effects of anemia.
As prescribed, administer erythropoietin.	Epoetin alfa (Epogen, Procrit) is a synthetic form of erythropoietin that stimulates production of RBCs to treat anemia associated with cancer chemotherapy. (Erythropoietin will not be effective in patients who are iron deficient.)
As patient performs ADLs, be alert for dyspnea on exertion, dizziness, palpitations, headaches, and verbalization of increased exertion level.	These are signs of activity intolerance and decreased tissue oxygenation. If these signs are present, patient may be at risk for falls, which necessitates implementation of safety measures.
Ask patient to rate perceived exertion per Borg scale (see "Prolonged Bedrest" for **Risk for Activity Intolerance**, p. 61).	A rate of perceived exertion (RPE) greater than 3 is a sign of activity intolerance and usually necessitates stopping the activity.
Facilitate coordination of care providers to provide rest periods as needed between care activities.	Undisturbed rest periods of at least 90 min duration will help patient regain energy stores. Frequent activity periods without associated rest periods may result in depleted energy stores and emotional exhaustion.
Monitor oximetry and report significant findings.	O_2 saturation at 92% or less indicates need for oxygen supplementation and may be necessary only during periods of activity.
Administer oxygen as prescribed, and encourage deep breathing.	Augmenting oxygen delivery to the tissues will help decrease fatigue.
Administer blood components as prescribed.	Infusing RBCs increases hemoglobin level and treats anemia.
Doublecheck type and crossmatch with a colleague per institutional protocol; monitor for and report signs of transfusion reaction.	These actions help prevent/assess for life-threatening transfusion reactions.
Encourage gradually increasing activities to tolerance as patient's condition improves. Set mutually agreed upon goals with patient.	Mutually agreed-on goals promote adherence to increased activity levels, which will increase patient's tolerance.

••• Related NIC and NOC labels: *NIC:* Activity Therapy; Energy Management; Mutual Goal Setting; Nutrition Management; Oxygen Therapy *NOC:* Activity Tolerance; Endurance; Energy Conservation

Nursing Diagnosis:

Ineffective Protection

related to risk of bleeding/hemorrhage secondary to thrombocytopenia (for all patients receiving chemotherapy and radiation therapy, as well as those with cancers involving the bone marrow)

Desired Outcome: Patient is free of signs and symptoms of bleeding as evidenced by negative occult blood tests, HR 100 bpm or less, and SBP 90 mm Hg or greater.

INTERVENTIONS	RATIONALES
Identify platelet counts that place individuals at increased risk for bleeding.	- Platelets 150,000-300,000/mm³ = Normal risk for bleeding. - Platelets less than 50,000/mm³ = Moderate risk for bleeding. Initiate thrombocytopenic precautions. - Platelets less than 10,000/mm³ = Severe risk for bleeding. Patient may develop spontaneous hemorrhage.
Perform a baseline physical assessment, monitoring for evidence of bleeding.	Petechiae, ecchymosis, hematuria, hematemesis, tarry or bloody stools, hemoptysis, heavy menses, headaches, somnolence, mental status changes, confusion, and blurred vision signal bleeding and should be reported promptly for timely intervention.
Monitor VS at least every shift or with each appointment if patient is not hospitalized.	Hypotension and tachycardia are signs that signal bleeding and should be reported promptly for timely intervention.
Report SBP higher than 140 mm Hg.	In the presence of thrombocytopenia, patient is at risk for intracranial bleeding when SBP is elevated.
Avoid use of rectal thermometer (use a tympanic thermometer when available).	A rectal thermometer can damage rectal mucosa and cause rectal bleeding.
Test all secretions and excretions.	These may contain occult blood.
Perform a psychosocial assessment, including patient's past experience with thrombocytopenia; the effect of thrombocytopenia on patient's lifestyle; and changes in patient's work pattern, family relationships, and social activities.	This assessment identifies learning needs and necessity of skilled care after hospital discharge.
For patients with platelet count less than 50,000/mm³, place a sign on patient's door indicating that thrombocytopenia precautions are in effect.	Notifying all who enter patient's room that patient is at risk for bleeding optimally promotes patient's safety.
In the presence of bleeding, begin pad count for heavy menses (discourage use of tampons); measure quantity of vomiting and stool.	These actions quantify the amount of bleeding. Tampons may cause vaginal trauma during placement, resulting in bleeding.
Apply direct pressure and ice to site of bleeding (VAD, venipuncture).	Applying pressure and ice promote bleeding cessation.
Deliver platelet transfusion as prescribed.	Patients may lose blood from surgery, or the cancer may cause internal bleeding. In addition, both radiation and chemotherapy affect cells in the bone marrow, leading to low blood cell counts.
Initiate oral care at frequent intervals. Advise patient to brush with soft-bristle toothbrush after meals and before bed (hot water run over bristles may soften them further).	Gentle oral care promotes integrity of gingiva and mucosa and helps prevent bleeding and infection.
Avoid oral irrigation tools. In the presence of gum bleeding, teach patient to use sponge-tipped applicator rather than toothbrush, avoid dental floss, and avoid mouthwash with alcohol content.	**Caution:** Dental care should not be performed until platelet count approaches normal.
Suggest use of normal saline solution mouthwashes 4 times a day and water-based ointment for lubricating lips.	Alcohol-based products irritate impaired oral tissue and could promote bleeding.
Implement bowel program and check with patient daily for bowel movement.	Daily monitoring of bowel pattern promotes early intervention for constipation. If patient's platelet count is critically low, straining at stool must be avoided to prevent intraabdominal bleeding.
Assess need for stool softeners or psyllium.	These agents help prevent constipation and straining, which could result in bleeding.
Encourage adequate hydration (at least 2500 ml/day) and high-fiber foods.	Hydration and fiber promote stools that are soft with adequate bulk, both of which facilitate bowel movements without straining.
Avoid use of rectal suppositories, enemas, or harsh laxatives.	These products increase risk of bleeding/infection from inadvertent trauma to rectal mucosa.
Implement and teach patient measures that reduce risk of bleeding.	Patient should use electric shaver; apply direct pressure and elevation for 3-5 min after injections and venipuncture; and avoid vaginal douche and tampons and constrictive clothing. Alcohol is to be avoided as are medications that could induce bleeding, such as aspirin or aspirin-containing products, anticoagulants, and nonsteroidal antiinflammatory drugs (NSAIDs). Patient should perform gentle nose blowing and use emery board rather than clippers for nail care. Bladder catheterization should be avoided if possible.

Continued

INTERVENTIONS	RATIONALES
Instruct patient to abstain from sexual intercourse when the platelet count is less than 50,000/mm^3. Otherwise, instruct patient to use water-soluble lubrication during sexual intercourse. Caution patient to avoid anal intercourse.	Sexual intercourse could traumatize vaginal, anal, and penile tissue, causing bleeding or introduction of bacteria.
Caution patient to avoid activities that predispose to trauma or injury, and remove hazardous objects or furniture from patient's environment. Assist with ambulating if patient's physical mobility is impaired.	This information reduces possibility of trauma that could result in bleeding.
When patient's platelet count is less than 20,000/mm^3, teach importance of avoiding activities such as moving up in bed, straining at stool, bending at the waist, and lifting heavy objects (more than 10 lb). Suggest bedrest if patient's platelet count is less than 10,000/mm^3.	Valsalva's and other maneuvers that increase intracranial pressure put patient at risk for intracerebral bleeding.
Avoid invasive procedures when possible, including IM injections.	IM injections and invasive procedures increase risk of bleeding. If punctures are necessary, use of smaller-gauge needles and gentle pressure at puncture site until bleeding stops will help prevent hemorrhage.
See also: "Thrombocytopenia," p. 505.	

••• **Related NIC and NOC labels:** *NIC:* Bleeding Precautions; Bleeding Reduction; Blood Products Administration; Hemorrhage Control *NOC:* Coagulation Status

Nursing Diagnosis:

Impaired Skin Integrity and Impaired Tissue Integrity

(or risk for same) *related to* treatment with chemotherapy or biotherapy

Desired Outcome: Before chemotherapy, patient identifies potential skin and tissue side effects of chemotherapy and measures that will maintain skin integrity and promote comfort.

INTERVENTIONS	RATIONALES
Transient Erythema/Urticaria:	
Perform and document a pretreatment assessment of patient's skin.	Pretreatment assessment enables a more accurate assessment of the post-treatment reaction. Alterations of skin or nails that occur in conjunction with chemotherapy are a result of destruction of the basal cells of the epidermis (general) or of cellular alterations at the site of chemotherapy administration (local). Transient erythema/urticaria may be generalized or localized at the site of chemotherapy administration. It may be caused by several agents, including doxorubicin hydrochloride, bleomycin, L-asparaginase, mithramycin, and mechlorethamine.
If it is infusing, halt chemotherapy temporarily.	This action may prevent further skin/tissue damage until the nature of the reaction can be ascertained.
Assess and document onset, pattern, severity, and duration of the reaction after treatment.	Reactions are specific to the agent used and vary in onset, severity, and duration. Usually they occur soon after chemotherapy is administered and disappear in several hours.
Hyperpigmentation:	
Inform patient before treatment that this reaction is to be expected and may or may not disappear over the first few months when treatment is finished.	Hyperpigmentation is believed to be caused by increased levels of epidermal melanin-stimulating hormone. It can occur on the nail beds, on the oral mucosa, or along the veins used for chemotherapy administration, or it can be generalized. Hyperpigmentation is associated with many chemotherapeutic agents, but incidence is highest with alkylating agents and antitumor antibiotics. In addition, it can occur with tumors of the pituitary gland.
Caution patient to wear sunscreen with a high sun protection factor (SPF) and cover exposed areas.	Sunlight may exacerbate hyperpigmentation.

Continued

INTERVENTIONS	RATIONALES
Telangiectasis (Spider Veins):	
Inform patient that this reaction is permanent but that the vein configuration will become less severe over time.	Telangiectasis is believed to be caused by destruction of the capillary bed and occurs as a result of applications of topical carmustine and mechlorethamine.
Photosensitivity:	
Assess onset, pattern, severity, and duration of the reaction.	Photosensitivity is enhanced when skin is exposed to ultraviolet light. Acute sunburn and residual tanning may occur with very short exposure to the sun when receiving certain chemotherapy drugs. Photosensitivity can occur during the time the agent is administered, or it can reactivate a skin reaction caused by recent sun exposure before chemotherapy.
Teach patient to avoid exposing skin to the sun. Advise patient to wear protective clothing and use an effective sun-screening agent (SPF of 15 or higher).	Photosensitivity is enhanced when skin is exposed to ultraviolet light. Acute sunburn and residual tanning can occur with short exposure to the sun.
Teach patient to treat sunburns with comfort measures and to consult health care provider accordingly.	Such measures as taking a tepid bath and using moisturizing cream and aloe are usually effective.
Hyperkeratosis:	
For patients taking bleomycin, assess for presence of skin thickening and loss of fine motor function of the hands.	Hyperkeratosis presents as a thickening of the skin, especially over hands, feet, face, and areas of trauma. It is disfiguring and causes loss of fine motor function of the hands.
In the presence of skin thickening, assess for fibrotic lung changes: dyspnea, cough, tachypnea, and crackles.	Hyperkeratosis may be an indicator of more severe fibrotic changes in the lungs that usually are not reversible.
Reassure patient that skin thickening is usually reversible when bleomycin has been discontinued.	Patient will be less anxious knowing the condition is usually reversible.
Acne-Like Reaction:	
Suggest use of commercial acne preparations, such as benzoyl peroxide lotion, gel, or cream, to treat blemishes.	An acne-like reaction presents as erythema, especially of the face, and progresses to papules and pustules, which are characteristic of acne and will disappear when the drug is discontinued.
Teach proper skin care:	
- Avoid hard scrubbing.	Scrubbing can cause skin breaks that enable bacterial entry.
- Avoid use of antibacterial soap. Use a mild plain soap.	Removal of nonpathogenic bacteria on the skin results in replacement by pathogens, which are implicated in the genesis of acne.
- Avoid use of oil-based cosmetics.	Oil can clog pores and trap bacteria.
Ulceration:	
Assess for ulceration.	Ulceration presents as a generalized, shallow lesion of the epidermal layer and may be caused by several chemotherapeutic agents.
Treat ulcers with a solution of ¼ strength hydrogen peroxide and ¾-strength normal saline q4-6h.	This solution effectively cleanses the lesions.
Rinse with normal saline solution.	Normal saline rinses remove the cleansing solution from the skin.
Expose the ulcer to air, if possible.	A dark, moist, warm environment may promote bacterial growth and delay healing.
Be alert to signs of infection at the ulcerated site.	Local warmth, swelling, tenderness, erythema, and purulent drainage may be present at the site of ulceration and should be reported to health care provider for treatment.
Radiation Recall Reaction:	
Explain why radiation recall can occur and its signs and symptoms	Radiation recall can occur when chemotherapy is given after treatment with radiation therapy. Radiation enhancement occurs when radiation and chemotherapy are given concurrently. Both present as erythema, followed by dry desquamation at the radiation site. More severe reactions can progress to vesicle formation and wet desquamation. After the skin heals, it may be permanently hyperpigmented.

Continued

INTERVENTIONS	RATIONALES
Teach patient strategies to protect skin at the site of recall reaction.	Preventive strategies that may lessen severity of radiation recall reaction include the following: - Avoid sun exposure, which may precipitate a reaction similar to radiation recall. - Avoid wearing tight-fitting clothes and harsh fabrics. - Avoid excess heat or cold exposure to the area, salt water or chlorinated pools, deodorants, perfumed lotions, cosmetics, and shaving of the area. - Use mild detergents, such as Ivory Snow.
Dry, Pruritic Skin: Explain why dry, pruritic skin can occur and its signs and symptoms.	Dry, pruritic skin commonly occurs with biotherapy (e.g., Interferon, IL-2) or radiation recall reaction and should be treated aggressively. It may be accompanied by a rash and eventual desquamation.
Teach patient strategies for treating this condition.	Strategies that may lessen severity of dry, pruritic skin include the following: - Apply creams and water-based lotions several times a day, avoiding perfumed products. - Avoid hot bathing water and use only mild soaps. - Manage pruritus with antipruritic medications such as diphenhydramine or hydroxyzine hydrochloride. - Patients receiving IL-2 should check with their health care provider before using steroids because these may interfere with therapy.
See **Impaired Skin Integrity,** which follows, for more details about wound care.	

••• Related NIC and NOC labels: *NIC:* Skin Surveillance; Bathing; Medication Administration: Skin; Chemotherapy Management; Skin Care: Topical Treatments; Wound Care; Infection Protection; Infection Control; Teaching: Procedure/Treatment *NOC:* Tissue Integrity: Skin and Mucous Membranes; Wound Healing: Secondary Intention

Nursing Diagnosis:

Impaired Skin Integrity

related to radiation therapy

Desired Outcome: Within 24 hr of instruction, patient identifies potential skin reactions and management interventions that will promote comfort and skin integrity.

INTERVENTIONS	RATIONALES
Assess degree and extent of the skin reaction.	Severe skin reactions may necessitate a delay in radiation treatments. Skin reactions are graded as follows: *Grade 1:* Faint erythema or dry desquamation *Grade 2:* Moderate to brisk erythema or patchy moist desquamation, moderate edema *Grade 3:* Confluent moist desquamation, blisters, pitting edema *Grade 4:* Skin ulceration or necrosis of full thickness dermis (National Cancer Institute [NCI] Common Toxicity Criteria)

Continued

INTERVENTIONS	RATIONALES
Teach patient the following skin care for the treatment field:	This information enables the patient to self-treat or obtain specialized help for skin reaction stage.
- Cleanse skin gently and in a patting motion, using mild soap, tepid water, and soft cloth. Rinse the area and pat it dry.	Grade 1 reactions often do not require special interventions other than gentle, normal skin care.
- Apply cornstarch, A&D ointment, ointment containing aloe or lanolin, or mild topical steroids as prescribed.	This is the skin care protocol for a grade 2 reaction.
- Cleanse area with ½-strength hydrogen peroxide and normal saline, using irrigation syringe. Rinse with saline or water and pat dry gently.	This is the skin care protocol for grade 3 skin reaction.
- Use nonadhesive absorbent dressings for draining areas. Be alert to signs and symptoms of infection.	
- To promote healing, use moisture- and vapor-permeable dressings, such as hydrocolloids and hydrogels, on noninfected areas.	
- Topical antibiotics (e.g., sulfadiazine cream) may be applied to open areas susceptible to infection.	This is the skin care protocol for grade 4 reaction.
Débride wound of eschar.	This measure is necessary before healing can occur.
After removing eschar (results in yellow-colored wound), keep wound clean. (Wet-to-moist dressings often are used to keep the wound clean.)	This measure prevents infection.
Collaborate with WOT/ET nurse as needed.	This nurse is skilled in techniques necessary for wound healing.
Teach patient about the potential for altered pigmentation, atrophy, fragility, or ulceration.	These long-term skin changes are associated with radiation.

••• **Related NIC and NOC labels:** *NIC:* Skin Surveillance; Bathing; Medication Administration: Skin; Radiation Therapy Management; Skin Care: Topical Treatments; Wound Care; Infection Protection; Teaching: Procedure/Treatment *NOC:* Tissue Integrity: Skin and Mucous Membranes; Wound Healing: Secondary Intention

Nursing Diagnosis:

Impaired Tissue Integrity

(or risk for same) *related to* extravasation of vesicant or irritating chemotherapy agents

Desired Outcome: Patient's tissue remains intact without evidence of inflammation or tissue damage near the injection site.

Note: Only nurses experienced in venous access and knowledgeable about chemotherapy should administer vesicant drugs. It is vital for the nurse to be knowledgeable regarding any vesicant or irritant properties specific to a drug before the drug is administered.

INTERVENTIONS	RATIONALES
Ensure that vesicant chemotherapy is administered by a nurse who is experienced in venipuncture and knowledgeable about chemotherapy.	Vesicant agents have the potential to produce tissue damage and therefore should be administered by a nurse skilled in venipuncture. Vesicant agents include dactinomycin, daunomycin, doxorubicin, mitomycin C, epirubicin, estramustine, idarubicin, mechlorethamine, mitoxantrone, paclitaxel, vinblastine, vincristine, vindesine, and vinorelbine.
	The following irritants have the potential to produce pain along the injection site with or without inflammation: amsacrine, bleomycin, carmustine, dacarbazine, doxorubicin liposome, etoposide, ifosfamide, plicamycin, streptozocin, docetaxel, and teniposide.

Continued

INTERVENTIONS	RATIONALES
Select IV site carefully, using a new site if possible.	Ideally the IV site will be newly accessed for vesicant administration. A site older than 24 hr should be avoided because it will be difficult to ensure vessel integrity.
Avoid sites such as the antecubital fossa, wrist, or dorsal surface of the hand.	In these sites there is increased risk of damage to underlying tendons or nerves if extravasation occurs.
Assess patency of venous site before and during administration of the drug. Instruct patient to report burning, itching, or pain immediately.	Extravasation of vesicants often causes immediate symptoms. Prompt reporting of these symptoms by the patient will enable early intervention to minimize tissue damage.
Assess venous access site at frequent intervals.	Pain, burning, and stinging are common with extravasation, as are erythema and swelling around needle site. Blood return should not be used as the sole indicator to ascertain that extravasation has not occurred inasmuch as blood return is possible even in the presence of extravasation.
Keep extravasation kit readily available, along with institutional guidelines for extravasation management.	Not all vesicants have antidotes. When administering vesicants with known antidotes, the antidote should be readily available in combination with the extravasation kit. Because time is of the essence to minimize tissue destruction when extravasation occurs, institutional guidelines or extravasation kit must be readily accessible before initiating drug delivery.
In the event of extravasation, follow these general guidelines:	Early intervention at the site of extravasation minimizes tissue damage.
- Stop infusion immediately and aspirate any remaining drug from needle. To do this, first don latex gloves, then attach syringe to the tubing and aspirate the drug.	This action removes as much drug as possible from the extravasated site, thereby limiting tissue exposure.
- Consult chemotherapy infusion guidelines.	These guidelines provide specifics regarding management of extravasation of individual drugs.
- Leave needle in place if using an antidote.	The needle enables access if an antidote is to be used with the extravasated drug.
- Do not apply pressure to the site. Apply a sterile occlusive dressing, elevate site, and apply heat or cold as recommended by guidelines.	Pressure may cause added tissue damage.
- Document incident, noting date, time, needle insertion site, venous access device type and size, drug, drug concentration, approximate amount of drug extravasated, patient symptoms, extravasation management, and appearance of the site. Review institutional guidelines regarding necessity of photo documentation. Monitor site at frequent intervals.	Documentation of actions taken ensures accuracy in case questions arise later about how the extravasation was managed. Photos provide a reference point for evaluation.
- Provide patient with information about site care and follow-up appointments for evaluation of the extravasation. If appropriate, collaborate with health care provider regarding a plastic surgery consultation.	Tissue damaged by extravasation may take a long time to heal or may deteriorate so much that plastic surgery may be necessary. Patient needs to understand these possibilities to ensure optimum extravasation management.

••• **Related NIC and NOC labels:** *NIC:* Chemotherapy Management; Medication Management *NOC:* Tissue Integrity: Skin and Mucous Membranes

Nursing Diagnosis:

Risk for Injury

(to staff, patients, and environment) *related to* preparation, handling, administration, and disposal of chemotherapeutic agents

Desired Outcome: There is minimal chemotherapy exposure of staff and environment by proper preparation, handling, administration, and disposal of waste by individuals familiar with these agents.

Note: Pharmacists or specially trained and supervised personnel should prepare chemotherapy, and nurses familiar with these agents should administer them. Institutional guidelines should be readily available for safe preparation, handling, and potential complications such as spills or individual contact with these drugs. A chemotherapy administration certification course, which includes clinical mentoring, is highly recommended for nurses planning to administer chemotherapeutics.

Although no information is available regarding reproductive risks of handling chemotherapy drugs in workers who use a biologic safety cabinet and wear protective clothing, employees who are pregnant, planning a pregnancy (male or female), breastfeeding, or have other medical reasons prohibiting exposure to chemotherapy drugs may elect to refrain from preparing or administering these agents or caring for patients during their treatment and up to 48 hr after completion of therapy (OSHA, 1995).

INTERVENTIONS	RATIONALES
Implement the following measures when working with chemotherapy: use a biologic safety cabinet (laminar flow hood); an absorbent, plastic-backed pad placed on the work area; latex gloves (powder free and a minimum of 0.007 inch thick); full-length impervious (non-absorbent) gown with cuffed sleeves and back closure; and goggles. Wear gloves and gowns during all handling and disposal of these agents.	These measures minimize potential for aerosolization with resultant inhalation and direct skin contact with chemotherapeutic drugs during preparation.
Prime IV tubing with diluent rather than with fluid containing the chemotherapy agent.	This enables the nurse to challenge the vein before infusing potentially tissue-irritating or damaging agents.
Use syringes and IV administration sets with Luer-Lok fittings.	These fittings prevent accidental dislodgement of needles or tubing and thus an accidental chemotherapy spill.
When removing the IV administration set, wear latex gloves and wrap sterile gauze around the insertion port.	These actions prevent direct or aerosol contact with the drug.
Place all needles (that have not been crushed, clipped, or recapped), syringes, drugs, drug containers, and related material in a puncture-proof container that is clearly marked *Biohazardous Waste*. **Note:** Follow this procedure for disposal of immunotherapy waste as well.	Proper disposal of waste prevents accidental exposure to other workers and the environment.
Wear latex gloves (and impermeable gown and goggles if splashing is possible) when handling all body excretions for 48 hr after chemotherapy.	The drug is excreted through urine and feces and is present in blood and body fluids for approximately 48 hr after chemotherapy.
Ensure that only specially trained personnel clean a chemotherapy spill using a spill kit.	Chemotherapy spills could result in inadvertent exposure to other health care workers, the public, other patients, and the environment. Therefore only staff properly trained in handling these agents should be allowed to manage a spill. Double-gloves, eye protection, and an appropriate, full-length gown is worn. Absorbent pads are used to absorb liquid; solid waste is picked up with moist absorbent gauze; glass fragments are collected with a small scoop—never with hands. These areas are cleansed three times with a detergent solution. All waste is put in a biohazardous waste container.
Avoid any activity in which the hand goes to the mouth (e.g., eating, drinking, smoking) in any area in which the drug is prepared or administered.	Inadvertent ingestion of chemotherapeutic drugs may occur.
In the event of skin contact with the drug, wash the affected area with soap and water. Notify health care provider for follow-up care. If eye contact occurs, irrigate the eye with water for 15 min and notify health care provider for follow-up care.	Chemotherapeutic drugs may be absorbed through skin and mucous membranes.

••• **Related NIC and NOC labels:** *NIC:* Environmental Management: Worker Safety; Risk Identification; Area Restriction *NOC:* Safety Status: Physical Injury

Nursing Diagnosis:

Risk for Injury

(to staff, other patients, and visitors) *related to* risk of exposure to sealed sources of radiation, such as cesium-137 (^{137}Cs), iridium-192 (^{192}Ir), iodine-125 (^{125}I), palladium-103, strontium-90, or samarium-153 (^{153}Sm); or unsealed sources of radiation, such as iodine-131 (^{131}I) or phosphorus-32 (^{32}P)

Desired Outcome: Staff and visitors verbalize understanding about potential adverse effects of exposure to radiation and measures that must be taken to ensure personal safety.

INTERVENTIONS	RATIONALES
Assign patient a private room (with private bathroom), and place an appropriate radiation precaution sign on patient's chart, door, and ID bracelet. Be aware of appropriate radiation precautions (listed on safety precaution sheet) before beginning care of the patient.	These measures minimize radiation exposure risk to employees, other patients, and visitors. Most institutions have a radiation safety committee that assists in providing and enforcing guidelines to minimize radiation risks to employees and the environment (committee guidelines should be kept readily available). The committee approves certain rooms that may be used for patients undergoing radioactive treatment to minimize exposure to employees and other patients.
Follow radiologist or agency protocol for visitor restrictions.	Visitors usually are restricted to 1 hr/day and should stand 6 ft from the bed for their own protection.
Ensure that pregnant women and children younger than age 18 do not enter the room.	Rapidly dividing cells (e.g., those of a fetus) are more susceptible to effects of radiation.
Implement the two major principles involved in care of patients with radiation sources: *time* and *distance*.	These principles help ensure optimal care planning and staff and visitor safety by minimizing amount of time spent in room of patients with radiation sources, thus reducing exposure time and maximizing distance from implant (e.g., if the implant is in patient's prostate, stand at head of bed [HOB]).
	Time: Staff members should not spend more than 30 min/shift with patient and should not care for more than two patients with implants at the same time. Staff should perform nondirect care activities in the hall (e.g., opening food containers, preparing food tray, opening medications). Linen should be changed only when it is soiled, rather than routinely, and complete bed baths should be avoided.
	Distance: Radiation exposure is greater the closer one is to the source.
Wear gloves when in contact with secretions and excretions of all patients treated with unsealed radiation sources. Flush toilet at least three times after depositing urine or feces from commode.	Fluids from patients with unsealed radiation sources are a source of radiation exposure.
	Note: Urine from individuals with sealed radiation is not a source of radiation exposure and can be discarded in the usual manner. However, patients with implanted ^{125}I seeds should save all urine so that it may be assessed for presence of seeds.
Save all linen, dressings, and trash from patients with sealed sources of radiation.	The safety committee representative will analyze them before discard to ensure seeds have not been misplaced, which could result in accidental exposure to people or the environment.
Caution all staff members to use forceps, never the hands, to pick up seeds.	For protection against radiation exposure, long, disposable forceps and a sealed box should be kept in the room at all times in case displaced seeds are found.
Use disposable products for all patients with unsealed radiation. Cover all articles in the room with paper to prevent contamination.	These actions prevent inadvertent radiation exposure via body fluids, which will be radioactive for several days.
Attach a radiation badge (dosimeter) before entering room.	This badge monitors the amount of personal radiation exposure. According to federal regulations, radiation should not exceed 400 mrem/mo. Nurses who care for patients with radiation implants rarely receive this much exposure.

••• **Related NIC and NOC labels:** *NIC:* Environmental Management: Safety; Area Restriction *NOC:* Safety Status: Physical Injury

Nursing Diagnosis:

Imbalanced Nutrition: Less Than Body Requirements

related to nausea and vomiting or anorexia occurring with chemotherapy, radiation therapy, or disease; fatigue; or taste changes

Desired Outcome: At least 24 hr before hospital discharge, patient and caregiver verbalize understanding of basic nutritional principles to prevent further weight loss.

INTERVENTIONS	RATIONALES
For Anorexia:	
See "Providing Nutritional Support" for **Imbalanced Nutrition,** p. 568.	
Weigh patient daily.	Nausea, vomiting, anorexia, and taste changes all may contribute to weight loss.
Assess patient's food likes and dislikes, as well as cultural and religious preferences related to food choices.	Providing foods on patient's "like" list as often as feasible and avoiding foods on "dislike" list optimally will promote sufficient intake. However, foods previously enjoyed may become undesirable, whereas previously disliked foods may appeal.
Explain that anorexia may be caused by the pathophysiology of cancer and surgery or side effects of chemotherapy and radiation therapy.	Taste and olfactory receptors have a high rate of cell growth and may be sensitive to chemotherapy and radiation therapy.
Consult with nutritionist and teach importance of increasing caloric intake.	Increasing calories augments energy, minimizes weight loss, and promotes tissue repair.
Consult with nutritionist and teach importance of increasing protein intake.	Increasing protein facilitates repair and regeneration of cells.
Suggest that patient eat several small meals at frequent intervals throughout the day.	Smaller, more frequent meals are usually better tolerated than larger meals.
Encourage use of nutritional supplements.	Adequate protein and calories are important for healing, fighting infection, and providing energy.
If indicated, consult patient's health care provider regarding use of megestrol acetate and prednisone.	These agents have proved to have a positive influence on appetite stimulation and weight gain in individuals with cancer. Megestrol acetate is a progestogen similar to the hormone progesterone. It is used to treat breast cancer primarily, but because it is an appetite stimulant, it may be used for patients who have loss of appetite and weight loss in advanced cancer. Prednisone is a synthetic hormone called a "steroid" that is used in the treatment of many diseases and conditions, and it also has the effect of increasing appetite. These drugs must be monitored closely for adverse effects.
For Nausea and Vomiting:	Nausea and vomiting may occur with advanced cancer, bowel obstruction, some medications, and metabolic abnormalities.
Assess patient's pattern of nausea and vomiting: onset, frequency, duration, intensity, and amount and character of emesis.	Knowledge about the pattern of nausea and vomiting enables use of proper medication, route, and timing.
Explain to patient that nausea and vomiting may be side effects of chemotherapy and radiation therapy.	The pathophysiology of nausea and vomiting is complex and involves transmission of impulses to receptors in the brain. Various antiemetics work at different points in the nausea/vomiting cycle. This action helps ensure coverage of the expected emetogenic period of the chemotherapy agent given.
Teach patient to take antiemetic, if prescribed, 1 hr before chemotherapy and to continue to take the drug as prescribed. Consider duration of previous nausea and vomiting episodes following chemotherapy when recommending antiemetic administration schedule.	Nausea is better controlled when the goal is prevention.
Explain that antiemetics are most effective if taken prophylactically or at nausea onset.	
Teach patient to eat cold foods or foods served at room temperature.	The odor of hot food may aggravate nausea.

Continued

INTERVENTIONS	RATIONALES
Suggest intake of clear liquids and bland foods.	Strong odors and tastes can stimulate nausea or suppress appetite.
Teach patient to avoid sweet, fatty, highly salted, and spicy foods, as well as foods with strong odors, any of which may increase nausea.	Same as above.
Minimize stimuli such as smells, sounds, or sights, all of which may promote nausea.	Previous stimuli associated with nausea may provoke anticipatory nausea.
Encourage patient to eat sour or mint candy during chemotherapy.	These candies decrease unpleasant, metallic taste.
If not contraindicated, teach patient to take oral chemotherapy with antiemetics at bedtime.	This drug combination and its timing helps minimize incidence of nausea.
Encourage patient to explore various dietary patterns. Suggest that patient avoid eating or drinking for 1-2 hr before and after chemotherapy. Follow a clear liquid diet for 1-2 hr before and 1-24 hr after chemotherapy.	Some patients become nauseated in anticipation of chemotherapy. Reducing intake at this time may lessen this symptom.
Suggest that patient avoid contact with food while it is being cooked and avoid being around people who are eating.	Prolonged exposure to smells can extinguish appetite or promote nausea.
Advise eating small, light meals at frequent intervals (5-6 times/day).	Presenting large volumes of food can be overwhelming, thereby extinguishing the appetite or causing nausea.
Suggest that patient sit near an open window.	Breathing fresh air when feeling nauseated may relieve nausea.
Help patient find an appropriate distraction technique (e.g., music, television, reading).	Helping patient focus on things other than nausea may be helpful in nausea management.
Teach patient to use relaxation techniques, which may help prevent anticipatory nausea and vomiting. An example is found in **Health-Seeking Behaviors:** Relaxation technique effective for stress reduction, p. 172.	These techniques may help prevent anticipatory nausea and vomiting.
Instruct patient to slowly sip clear liquids such as broth, ginger ale, cola, tea, or gelatin; suck on ice chips; and avoid large volumes of water.	These actions help to increase oral moisture to relieve dry mouth.
For Fatigue:	
If patient is easily fatigued, encourage him or her to eat frequent, small meals and document intake.	The energy required to consume and digest a large meal may exacerbate fatigue and discourage further nutritional intake.
Provide foods that are easy to eat.	"Finger foods" (e.g., crackers with cheese or peanut butter, nuts, chunks of fruit, smoothies) require less energy expenditure to eat and enable patient to eat in a position of comfort rather than sitting at a table, which requires more energy.
If patient wears oxygen during exertion, encourage wearing it while eating.	Food consumption requires energy. A fatigued, hypoxic person likely will consume less food.
Avoid offering meals immediately after exertion.	A fatigued person will be less likely to want to eat and will tire quickly while eating, which also requires energy expenditure.
For Taste Changes:	
Suggest that patient try foods not previously enjoyed.	Previously enjoyed foods may no longer seem attractive, whereas foods that were once undesirable may now seem pleasant.
Encourage good mouth care; assess mucous membrane for thrush, lesions, or mucositis.	Thrush infections can cause taste alterations yet are easily treated. A coated tongue may interfere with ability to taste.
Suggest that patient try strongly flavored foods.	Patients often report that usual foods taste like sawdust.

••• **Related NIC and NOC labels:** *NIC:* Fluid Monitoring; Nutrition Monitoring; Teaching: Prescribed Diet; Weight Gain Assistance; Sustenance Support *NOC:* Nutritional Status: Nutrient Intake; Nutritional Status: Food and Fluid Intake

Nursing Diagnosis:

Impaired Oral Mucous Membrane

related to side effects of chemotherapy or biotherapy; radiation therapy to head and neck; ineffective oral hygiene; gingival diseases; poor nutritional status; tumors of the oral cavity and neck; and infection

Desired Outcomes: Patient complies with therapeutic regimen within 1 hr of instruction. Patient's oral mucosal condition improves as evidenced by intact mucous membrane; moist, intact tongue and lips; and absence of pain and lesions.

INTERVENTIONS	RATIONALES
For patients with myelosuppression, caution not to floss teeth or use oral irrigators or a stiff toothbrush.	The oral cavity is a prime site for infection in a myelosuppressed patient. Actions such as brushing with a stiff toothbrush and flossing could affect integrity of the oral mucous membrane and place patient at risk for infection. Patient should consult with a dentist as indicated.
Be aware that patient may require parenteral analgesics, such as morphine.	Parenteral analgesics may be necessary to relieve pain and promote adequate nutritional intake in patients with moderate to severe mucositis.
Suggest to patients with xerostomia (dryness of the mouth from a lack of normal salivary secretion) caused by radiation therapy that they may benefit from chewing sugarless gum; sucking on sugarless candy, frozen fruit juice pops, or sugar-free Popsicles or taking frequent sips of water. Saliva substitutes are another option, although they are expensive and do not last long.	These products replenish oral hydration and promote mucous membrane integrity. A dry mouth also interferes with nutritional intake.
Advise frequent dental follow-ups.	Lack of or decrease in salivary fluid predisposes patient to dental caries. Fluoride treatment is recommended for these patients for this reason.

••• **Related NIC and NOC labels:** *NIC:* Oral Health Restoration; Chemotherapy Management; Fluid Management; Pain Management; Oral Health Maintenance *NOC:* Oral Health; Tissue Integrity: Skin and Mucous Membranes

Nursing Diagnosis:

Impaired Swallowing

related to mucositis of the oral cavity or esophagus (esophagitis) secondary to radiation therapy to the neck, chest, and upper back; use of chemotherapy agents; obstruction (tumors); or thrush

Desired Outcomes: Before food or fluids are given, patient exhibits gag reflex and is free of symptoms of aspiration as evidenced by RR 12-20 breaths/min with normal depth and pattern (eupnea), normal skin color, and the ability to speak. Following instruction, patient verbalizes early signs and symptoms of esophagitis, alerts health care team as soon as they occur, and identifies measures for maintaining nutrition and comfort.

INTERVENTIONS	RATIONALES
Monitor patient for evidence of impaired swallowing with concomitant respiratory difficulties.	Esophagitis can occur with radiation therapy to the neck, chest, and upper back or be caused by chemotherapy agents, tumors, or thrush. Impaired swallowing places patient at risk for aspiration and necessitates aspiration precautions.
Teach patient early signs and symptoms of esophagitis and of stomatitis and importance of reporting symptoms promptly if they occur.	Sensation of a lump in the throat with swallowing, difficulty with swallowing solid foods, and discomfort or pain with swallowing occur early in esophagitis. Signs of stomatitis include generalized burning sensation of oral cavity, white patches on oral mucosa, ulcerations, and pain. Patient should report these indicators promptly to staff if they occur so that timely interventions can be made.

Continued

INTERVENTIONS	RATIONALES
Monitor patient's dietary intake and weight, teaching the following guidelines:	Impaired swallowing predisposes patient to nutritional deficits. Dietary intake should be monitored closely to evaluate early weight loss trends.
- Maintain a high-protein diet.	Protein promotes healing.
- Eat foods that are soft and bland.	These foods minimize pain while swallowing.
- Add milk or milk products to the diet (for individuals without excessive mucus production).	These products coat the esophageal lining to facilitate swallowing.
- Add sauces and creams to foods.	These foods may facilitate swallowing.
- Ensure adequate fluid intake of at least 2 L/day.	Patients with impaired swallowing are at risk for dehydration because they may avoid drinking and eating to prevent pain.
Implement the following measures that promote comfort, and discuss them with patient accordingly.	Reducing pain associated with swallowing will assist in maintaining adequate nutritional intake.
- Use a local anesthetic, as prescribed, to minimize pain with meals.	Lidocaine 2% and diphenhydramine may be taken by patient via swish and spit or swallow before eating. **Caution:** These anesthetics may decrease patient's gag reflex.
- Suggest patient sit in an upright position during meals and for 15-30 min after eating.	Esophageal reflux may occur with obstructions and can be distressing.
- Obtain prescription for analgesics and administer as prescribed. Teach patient importance of taking analgesics before eating or drinking to promote proper nutrition and hydration.	Discomfort may prevent patient from maintaining adequate nutritional intake. If pain is unrelieved with mild analgesics, an opioid such as oxycodone or morphine may be necessary.
Encourage frequent oral care with normal saline and sodium bicarbonate solution (1 teaspoon of each to 1 quart of water).	Impaired mucous membranes are at risk for infection with bacteria, yeast, and viruses.
Teach patient to avoid irritants, such as alcohol, tobacco, and alcohol-based commercial mouthwashes.	Irritants exacerbate discomfort and may prevent intake of adequate nutrients.
Have suction equipment readily available in case patient experiences aspiration. Educate patient about ways to manage oral secretions.	Esophageal reflux may occur with obstructions and can be distressing.
Suction mouth as needed, using low, continuous suction equipment.	Suction helps manage secretions and prevent aspiration.
Teach patient to expectorate saliva into tissues, and dispose of it per institutional policy.	This intervention helps patient manage oral secretions using proper infection control measures.
See also: "Providing Nutritional Support" for **Risk for Impaired Swallowing,** p. 574, for desired outcomes and interventions.	

••• **Related NIC and NOC labels:** *NIC:* Aspiration Precautions; Airway Suctioning; Positioning; Risk Identification; Nutrition Management *NOC:* Aspiration Control; Swallowing Status

Nursing Diagnosis:

Impaired Urinary Elimination

related to hemorrhagic cystitis secondary to cyclophosphamide/ifosfamide treatment, oliguria or renal toxicity secondary to cisplatin or high-dose methotrexate administration, renal calculi secondary to hyperuricemia, or dysuria secondary to cystitis

Desired Outcomes: Patients receiving cyclophosphamide/ifosfamide test negative for blood in their urine, and patients receiving cisplatin exhibit urinary output of 100 ml/hr or more 1 hr before treatment and 4-12 hr after treatment. Patients with leukemia and lymphomas and those taking methotrexate exhibit urine pH 7.5 or higher.

INTERVENTIONS	RATIONALES
Ensure adequate hydration during treatment and for at least 24 hr after treatment for patient taking cyclophosphamide, ifosfamide, methotrexate, or cisplatin. Teach patient importance of drinking at least 2-3 L/day. IV hydration also may be required, especially with high-dose chemotherapy.	Adequate hydration ensures sufficient dilution of the drug by urine in the urinary system and prevents exposure of renal cells to high drug concentrations and possible toxicity. Renal failure also may ensue when cellular breakdown products deposit in the renal tubules when patient has been inadequately hydrated before chemotherapy given for leukemia or lymphoma.
Administer cyclophosphamide early in the day. Encourage patient to urinate q2h during the day and before going to bed.	These actions help minimize retention of metabolites in the bladder, especially during the night.
Test urine for presence of blood, and report positive results to health care provider.	Hemorrhagic cystitis can occur in patients taking cyclophosphamide/ifosfamide and should be reported promptly to ensure timely intervention.
Monitor input and output (I&O) at least q8h during high-dose treatment for 48 hr after treatment. Be alert to decreasing urinary output.	Most chemotherapy drugs are eliminated from the body within a 48-hr period. Maintaining adequate urine output for 48 hr prevents high drug metabolite concentrations in the kidneys and bladder.
Ensure that mesna is administered before ifosfamide or cyclophosphamide and then 4 hr and 8 hr after the infusion (or via a continuous infusion).	Mesna inhibits the hemorrhagic cystitis caused by ifosfamide/cyclophosphamide. The half-life of mesna is shorter than the half-life of ifosfamide/cyclophosphamide. Therefore multiple doses or continuous infusion of mesna beyond the end of the ifosfamide/cyclophosphamide infusion is required to prevent urotoxicity.
Test all urine for presence of blood.	Ifosfamide and cyclophosphamide can cause hemorrhagic cystitis.
Promote fluid intake to maintain urine output at approximately 100 ml/hr. Monitor I&O during infusion and for 24 hr after therapy to ensure that this level of urinary output is attained.	Adequate fluid intake and resultant urinary output ensure that drug metabolites in high concentrations do not stay within the urinary system for prolonged periods.
For patient receiving cisplatin, prehydrate with IV fluid (150-200 ml/hr). Monitor I&O hourly for 4-12 hr after therapy.	This amount of hydration helps ensure that urine output is maintained at 100-150 ml/hr or more, which decreases potential for nephrotoxicity, a potential side effect of cisplatin. Patients may require diuretics to maintain this output. Cisplatin can be administered as soon as urine output is 100-150 ml/hr.
Promote fluid intake for at least 24 hr after treatment, especially for patient taking diuretics. Notify health care provider promptly if urine output drops to less than 100 ml/hr.	Continual flushing of the urinary system prevents concentration of cisplatin metabolites in the kidneys and potential associated nephrotoxicity. Urine output should be kept at a relatively high level.
In patients with leukemia and lymphoma, monitor I&O q8h, being alert to decreasing output. Test urine pH with each voiding to ensure that it is 7.5 or higher.	If cellular breakdown products that occur from the chemotherapy effect on tumor cells are allowed to concentrate in the renal tubules, renal failure can occur. Proper hydration prevents this potential cause of renal failure. Alkaline urine promotes excretion of uric acid that results from tumor lysis associated with treatment of leukemia and lymphoma.
Administer sodium bicarbonate or acetazolamide (Diamox) as prescribed.	These agents alkalinize the urine.
Administer allopurinol as prescribed.	Allopurinol prevents uric acid formation and is often administered before chemotherapy for patients with leukemia or lymphoma.
Monitor leukemia and lymphoma patients for the presence of urinary calculi. For more information, see "Ureteral Calculi," p. 243.	Hyperuricemia may be caused by chemotherapy treatment for leukemia and lymphoma. The rapid cell lysis and increased excretion of uric acid may result in renal calculi.
Teach patient signs of cystitis: fever, pain with urination, malodorous or cloudy urine, blood in the urine, and urinary frequency and urgency. Instruct patient to notify health care professional if these signs and symptoms occur.	Cystitis can occur secondary to cyclophosphamide and ifosfamide treatment and should be reported to health care provider for timely intervention.

••• **Related NIC and NOC labels:** *NIC:* Urinary Elimination Management; Fluid Management; Medication Management *NOC:* Urinary Elimination

Nursing Diagnosis:

Deficient Knowledge:

Type of, procedure for, and purpose of radiation implant (internal radiation) and measures for preventing and managing complications

Desired Outcome: Before radiation implant is inserted, patient and significant other/caregiver verbalize understanding of implant type and procedure and identify measures for preventing and managing complications.

INTERVENTIONS	RATIONALES
Assess patient's health care literacy (language, reading, comprehension). Assess culture and culturally specific information needs.	This assessment helps ensure that materials are presented in a manner that is culturally and educationally appropriate.
Determine patient's and caregiver's level of understanding of the radiation implant. Explain the following, as indicated.	Knowledge level will determine content of the individualized teaching plan.
- Afterloading	Implant carrier is inserted in the operating room, and radioactive source is inserted later.
- Preloading	Radioactive source is implanted with carrier.
Explain that the implant is used to provide high doses of radiation therapy to one area.	This method spares normal tissue from radiation.
Explain that radiation precautions (see **Risk for Injury,** p. 25) are required.	These precautions protect patient, health care team, other patients, and visitors.
Explain the following assessment guidelines and management interventions for specific types of implants:	
Gynecologic Implants:	
Explain that the following may occur: vaginal drainage, bleeding, or tenderness; impaired bowel or urinary elimination; and phlebitis. Instruct patient to report any of these or any associated signs and symptoms.	An informed patient likely will report untoward signs and symptoms promptly to ensure timely treatment.
Explain that complete bedrest is required.	Bedrest helps prevent displacement of implants. HOB may be elevated to 30-45 degrees, and patient may logroll from side to side. A urinary catheter is placed to facilitate urinary elimination.
Advise that a low-residue diet and medications to prevent bowel elimination may be prescribed.	These interventions help prevent bowel movements during implant period. Generally a bowel clean-out (oral cathartics and/or enemas until clear) is prescribed.
Teach patient to perform isometric exercises while on bedrest.	Isometric exercises minimize risk of contractures and muscle atrophy and promote venous return during bedrest.
Encourage patient to take analgesics routinely for pain or to request analgesic before pain becomes severe.	These actions help keep pain at a minimal level. Prolonged stimulation of pain receptors results in increased sensitivity to painful stimuli and increase amount of drug required to relieve pain.
Explain importance of and rationale for wearing antiembolism hose and performing calf-pumping and ankle-circling exercises while on bedrest. If prescribed, describe rationale for and use of sequential compression devices or pneumatic foot pumps.	These actions help prevent the lower extremity venostasis, thrombophlebitis, and emboli that can occur during enforced bedrest.
Explain that ambulation will be increased gradually when bedrest no longer is required (see "Prolonged Bedrest," p. 61, for guidelines after prolonged immobility).	Gradual increments in ambulation will promote return to normal body function without undue stress on the body.
Explain that after radiation source has been removed, patient should dilate her vagina either through sexual intercourse or a vaginal dilator.	These actions help prevent vaginal fibrosis or stenosis.

Continued

INTERVENTIONS	RATIONALES
Head and Neck Implants:	
After a complete nutritional assessment, discuss measures for nutritional support during the implantation, such as a soft or liquid diet, a high-protein diet, and optimal hydration (more than 2500 ml/day).	Irradiated tissues may be swollen, irritated, and painful, which may interfere with nutritional intake. A high-protein diet promotes healing.
Teach signs and symptoms of infection at site of implantation.	Fever, pain, swelling, local increased warmth, erythema, and purulent drainage at the implantation site may occur. Patient should report these indicators promptly to ensure timely treatment.
When appropriate, advise need for careful and thorough oral hygiene while implant is in place.	Irradiated tissues are vulnerable to infection by bacteria, yeast, and viruses.
	Note: When implants are placed within tongue, palate, or other structures of the buccal cavity, patient should not perform oral hygiene. Oral hygiene will be specifically prescribed by health care provider and generally accomplished by the nurse. Improper mouth care could result in dislodgement of the device, pain, or improper cleansing.
Encourage patient to take analgesics routinely for pain or to request analgesic before pain becomes severe.	These actions help ensure optimal pain management. Prolonged stimulation of pain receptors results in increased sensitivity to painful stimuli and increases amount of drug required to relieve pain.
Advise patient to use a humidifier.	A humidifier will aid in maintaining moist mucous membranes and secretions. The patient should be instructed in procedures for cleaning the humidifier to avoid introduction of bacteria.
Identify alternative means for communication if patient's speech deteriorates. Consult speech therapist as appropriate.	Patient should be aware that cards, Magic Slate, pencil and paper, and picture boards are potential communication measures. Preparing patient before impairment likely would reduce anxiety.
Breast Implants:	
Teach signs of infection that may appear in the breast.	Pain, fever, swelling, erythema, warmth, and drainage at insertion site are indicators of infection and should be reported immediately for timely treatment.
Teach importance of avoiding trauma at implant site and keeping skin clean and dry.	These actions will help maintain skin integrity, prevent infection, and promote healing.
Encourage patient to take analgesics routinely for pain or to request analgesic before pain becomes severe.	Pain is more efficiently managed when pain medications are administered promptly and before it becomes severe. Prolonged stimulation of pain receptors results in increased sensitivity to painful stimuli and will increase amount of drug required to relieve pain.
Prostate Implants:	
Explain need for patient to use a urinal for voiding.	Use of a urinal will help ensure that urinary output is measured every shift and enable inspection of urine for presence of radiation seeds.
Instruct patient or caregiver to report dysuria, decreasing caliber of stream, difficulty urinating, voiding small amounts, feelings of bladder fullness, or hematuria.	Localized inflammation from radiation may cause urinary obstruction.
Inform patient that linen, dressings, and trash need to be saved.	This information helps ensure that all radiation seeds will be accounted for.
Encourage patient to take analgesics routinely for pain or to request analgesic before pain becomes severe.	Pain is more efficiently managed when pain medications are administered promptly and before it becomes severe. Prolonged stimulation of pain receptors results in increased sensitivity to painful stimuli and will increase amount of drug required to relieve pain.
Caution that caregiver should limit amount of time spent close to implant site.	This precaution helps ensure caregiver's protection from the radiation source.

••• **Related NIC and NOC labels:** *NIC:* Preparatory Sensory Information; Teaching: Procedure/ Treatment; Radiation Therapy Management; Learning Readiness Enhancement *NOC:* Knowledge: Treatment Procedures; Knowledge: Treatment Regimen

Nursing Diagnosis:

Deficient Knowledge:

Purpose and procedure for external beam radiation therapy, appropriate self-care measures after treatment, and available educational and community resources

Desired Outcome: Before external radiation beam therapy is initiated, patient and significant other/caregiver identify its purpose and describe the procedure, appropriate self-care measures, and available educational and community resources.

INTERVENTIONS	RATIONALES
See first eight interventions under **Deficient Knowledge:** Chemotherapy, p. 34.	
Provide information about treatment schedule, duration of each treatment, and number of treatments planned.	Outlining the plan of care reduces anxiety and assists patient and family with planning their lives and activities accordingly.
	Radiation therapy usually is given 5 days/wk, Monday through Friday. The treatment itself lasts only a few minutes; the majority of the time is spent preparing patient for treatment. Immobilization devices and shields are positioned before treatment to ensure proper delivery of radiation and to minimize radiation to surrounding normal tissue.
Explain that the skin will be marked with pinpoint dots called *tattoos*. However, if gentian violet is used, explain importance of not washing the marks (see **Impaired Skin Integrity,** p. 21, for more information).	Tattoos, which are permanent, assist technician in positioning radiation beam accurately and ensuring precise delivery of the radiation.
Caution patient that it is important not to use skin lotions, deodorants, or soaps unless approved by the radiation therapy provider.	Some products may interfere with radiation.
Discuss side effects that may occur with radiation treatment and appropriate self-care measures. See other nursing diagnoses and interventions in this section for more detail about local side effects.	Systemic side effects include fatigue and anorexia; however, the most commonly occurring side effects appear locally (e.g., side effects associated with head and neck radiation include mucositis, xerostomia, altered taste sensation, dental caries, sore throat, hoarseness, dysphagia, headache, and nausea and vomiting).
Teach strategies that help prevent skin breakdown.	These strategies include preventing local irritation by clothing, belts, or collars; avoiding chemical irritants such as alcohol, deodorants, or lotions; avoiding sun exposure of irradiated areas; and avoiding tape application to radiation field.
Provide patient with written materials that list radiation side effects and their management.	Supplemental written materials enhance knowledge and understanding.
Provide information about community resources for transportation to and from the radiation center and for skilled nursing care, as needed.	Stress associated with travel to a radiation center may interfere significantly with the lives of family members and may even give patient cause to terminate treatment. Home care nurses can assist patient and family at home as treatment progresses and side effects become more pronounced.

••• **Related NIC and NOC labels:** *NIC:* Preparatory Sensory Information; Teaching: Procedure/Treatment; Radiation Therapy Management; Learning Readiness Enhancement *NOC:* Knowledge: Treatment Procedures; Knowledge: Treatment Regimen

Nursing Diagnosis:

Deficient Knowledge:

Chemotherapy and purpose, expected side effects, and potential toxicities related to chemotherapy drugs; appropriate self-care measures for minimizing side effects; and available community and educational resources

Desired Outcome: Before the nurse administers specific chemotherapeutic drugs, patient and caregiver(s) verbalize knowledge about potential side effects and toxicities, appropriate self-care measures for minimizing side effects, and available community and educational resources.

INTERVENTIONS	RATIONALES
Assess patient's health care literacy (language, reading, comprehension). Assess culture and culturally specific information needs.	This assessment helps ensure that information is presented in a manner that is culturally and educationally appropriate.
Establish patient's and caregiver's current level of knowledge about patient's health status, goals of therapy, and expected outcomes.	Understanding knowledge level of patient and caregiver will facilitate development of an individualized teaching plan.
Assess patient's and caregiver's cognitive and emotional readiness to learn.	To facilitate learning, teaching must be tailored to patient's comprehensive abilities. The denial process may prevent comprehension of teaching content.
Recognize barriers to learning. Define all terminology as needed. Correct any misconceptions about therapy and expected outcomes.	Barriers, including ineffective communication, inability to read, neurologic deficit, sensory alterations, fear, anxiety, or lack of motivation will affect patient's learning and the teaching plan.
Provide written materials to reinforce information taught.	The ACS, NCI, pharmaceutical companies, and other organizations publish quality patient education materials the nurse may use to complement any verbal teaching.
Assess patient's and caregiver's learning needs and establish short-term and long-term goals. Identify preferred methods of learning and amount of information they would like to receive.	Identifying preferred methods of learning and amount of information they would like to receive enables the nurse to develop a teaching plan based on this information.
Use individualized verbal and audiovisual strategies. Give simple, direct instructions; reinforce this information often.	These strategies promote learning and comprehension. Because anxiety may interfere with comprehension, repetition will help reinforce teaching.
Provide an environment free of distractions and conducive to teaching and learning.	A quiet setting free of distraction facilitates learning and retention.
Discuss drugs patient will receive. Provide both written and verbal information.	To help ensure that retention has occurred, patient should be able to verbalize accurate knowledge about route of administration, duration of treatment, schedule, frequency of laboratory tests, most common side effects and toxicities, follow-up care, and appropriate self-care.
Provide emergency phone numbers.	These numbers should be used in case patient develops fever or side effects of chemotherapy that require emergent intervention.
Identify appropriate community resources to assist with transportation, costs of care, emotional support, and skilled care as appropriate.	Community resources may provide comfort for families under stress and prevent psychosocial issues from interfering with the plan of care.

••• **Related NIC and NOC labels:** *NIC:* Teaching: Procedure/Treatment; Learning Facilitation; Learning Readiness Enhancement; Chemotherapy Management *NOC:* Knowledge: Treatment Regimen; Knowledge: Treatment Procedures

Nursing Diagnosis:

Deficient Knowledge:

Immunotherapy and its purpose, potential side effects and toxicities, appropriate self-care measures to minimize side effects, and available community and education resources

Desired Outcome: Before immunotherapy is administered, the patient and significant other/caregiver verbalize understanding of its purpose, potential side effects and toxicities, appropriate self-care measures to minimize side effects, injection technique and site rotation (if appropriate), and available community and education resources.

INTERVENTIONS	RATIONALES
See first eight interventions under **Deficient Knowledge:** Chemotherapy, earlier.	
Teach proper injection technique and site rotation schedule. Teach importance of recording site of injection, time of administration, side effects, self-management of side effects, and any medications taken, as well as proper disposal of needles.	These patients often give their own injections of interferon. A diary or log will facilitate self-care.
Teach proper handling and storage of medication (e.g., refrigeration). As appropriate, arrange for community nursing follow-up for additional supervision and instruction.	Home care nursing support may reinforce teaching, assist with patient monitoring, and provide emotional support to patient and family.
Teach importance of being alert to the side effects of interferon.	Fever, chills, and flulike symptoms are expected side effects of interferon.
Suggest that patient take acetaminophen, with health care provider's approval, to manage these symptoms, but avoid aspirin and NSAIDs.	Aspirin and NSAIDs may interrupt action of interferon.
Monitor I&O and weight closely for hospitalized patients and teach these assessments to patients.	Fluid shifts may occur with IL-2 treatment.
Teach patient to monitor and record temperature twice daily and to drink 2000-3000 ml fluid/day.	These actions enable detection of fever, an expected interferon side effect, and replace fluid losses that can occur as a result.
Provide information regarding nutritional supplementation.	Dose-related anorexia and weight loss are other common side effects of interferon.
See also: "Providing Nutritional Support," p. 565.	

••• **Related NIC and NOC labels:** *NIC:* Teaching: Procedure/Treatment; Learning Facilitation; Learning Readiness Enhancement; Medication Management; Teaching: Prescribed Medication *NOC:* Knowledge: Treatment Regimen; Knowledge: Treatment Procedures

Nursing Diagnosis:

Disturbed Body Image

related to alopecia secondary to radiation therapy to head and neck or administration of certain chemotherapeutic agents

Desired Outcome: Patient discusses the effects alopecia may have on self-concept, body image, and social interaction and identifies measures to cope satisfactorily with alopecia.

INTERVENTIONS	RATIONALES
Discuss potential for hair loss with patient before treatment.	Patient needs to be informed about expected hair loss, depending on type of therapy, to develop strategies for coping and adaptation.
- Radiation therapy of 1500-3500 cGy to the head and neck will produce either partial or complete hair loss.	Hair loss is usually temporary and loss onset usually occurs 14-21 days from initiation of treatment. Regrowth begins as early as 2-3 months after final treatment but in some cases may take longer. This knowledge is likely to be reassuring to the patient.
- Radiation therapy of more than 4000 cGy usually results in permanent hair loss.	Patient may need to develop strategies for permanent hair loss.
- Hair loss associated with chemotherapy is temporary and related to specific agent, dose, and duration of administration.	Regrowth usually begins 1-2 mo after last treatment and often temporarily grows back a different texture. Common chemotherapeutic agents that cause alopecia include actinomycin D, amsacrine, bleomycin, cyclophosphamide, daunomycin, docetaxel, doxorubicin, epirubicin, etoposide (VP-16), topotecan (Hycamtin), idarubicin, ifosfamide, irinotecan (CPT-11), paclitaxel, teniposide, vinblastine, and vincristine.
Explore impact hair loss has on patient's self-concept, body image, and social interaction.	Alopecia is an extremely stressful side effect for most people. For some men, beard loss is disturbing as well.
Caution patient about inadvisability of scalp hypothermia and tourniquet applications during IV chemotherapy.	These measures have not proved to be effective in minimizing hair loss and are contraindicated with some malignancies.
Suggest measures that may help minimize the psychological impact of hair loss on women, such as cutting the hair short before treatment. Selecting a wig before hair loss occurs enables patient to match color and style of own hair. Wearing a hair net or turban during hair loss assists with collecting hair as it falls out. Wearing scarves, hats, caps, turbans, makeup, and accessories may enhance self-concept.	These measures may help minimize the psychological impact of hair loss. Being prepared by having head coverings available when hair loss actually occurs may reduce anxiety surrounding the event.

Note: Wigs are tax deductible and often are reimbursed by insurance with appropriate prescriptions. Some centers and communities have wig banks that provide used and reconditioned wigs at no cost. |
Inform patient that hair loss may occur on body parts other than the head.	Areas such as the axillae, groin, legs, eyes (eyelashes and eyebrows), and face also may lose hair. Loss of facial hair makes it difficult for makeup to stay on.
Instruct patient to keep head covered during summer and winter.	Covering the head minimizes sunburn during summer and prevents heat loss during winter. Certain chemotherapy agents and radiation therapy may sensitize skin to sun exposure.
Suggest resources that promote adaptation to alopecia.	For example, ACS hosts the "Look Good Feel Better" program, which provides women with encouragement and tips for managing body image changes during treatment.

••• **Related NIC and NOC labels:** *NIC:* Body Image Enhancement; Coping Enhancement; Counseling; Emotional Support; Self-Esteem Enhancement; Support Group *NOC:* Body Image; Self-Esteem

Nursing Diagnosis:

Disturbed Sensory Perception: Auditory, Kinesthetic, Tactile

related to neuropathies associated with certain chemotherapeutic drugs

Desired Outcome: Patient reports early signs and symptoms of ototoxicity and peripheral neuropathy (functional disturbance of the peripheral nervous system) and measures are implemented promptly to minimize these side effects.

INTERVENTIONS	RATIONALES
Teach patient to report early symptoms of hearing loss. Instruct caregivers to observe for early symptoms inasmuch as they may notice signs before patient does.	Cumulative doses of cisplatin can result in irreversible loss of high-frequency range hearing or tinnitus.
Suggest that patient face speaker and watch speaker's lips during conversation while being aware that background noise may interfere with hearing ability.	This information promotes skills with which to cope with hearing loss.
Suggest a trial before purchasing a hearing aid.	A hearing aid may be helpful, or it may amplify background noise and worsen speech comprehension.
In instances of cisplatin-induced hearing loss, refer patient to community resources for hearing-impaired persons.	Hearing loss from cisplatin is usually irreversible. A baseline audiogram may be done before cisplatin administration.
Monitor patient for development of peripheral neuropathy. Suggest consultation with PT or occupational therapist (OT) to assist with maintaining function. Teach patient that severity of symptoms may abate when treatment is halted; however, recovery may be slow and is usually incomplete.	Peripheral neuropathy can occur with several antineoplastic agents. Neurotoxicity is cumulative with some chemotherapy drugs, and therefore assessment of symptoms is done before delivery of each dose. Numbness and tingling (paresthesias) of fingers and toes occur initially and can progress to difficulty with fine motor skills, such as buttoning shirts or picking up objects. The most severely affected individuals may lose sensation at hip level and have difficulty with balance and ambulation. Instruct patient to report early signs and symptoms.
Assess patient for neuropathic pain. See "Chronic Pain," p. 4, for desired outcomes and interventions.	Patients with neuropathies may experience neuropathic pain, which is often described and treated differently than nociceptive pain.
Monitor bowel elimination daily in individuals at risk for paralytic ileus associated with neuropathy.	Patients receiving vinca alkaloids are at risk for paralytic ileus and require monitoring for this problem.
Administer stool softeners, psyllium, or laxatives daily if patient does not have bowel movements at least every other day. Instruct patient to increase dietary fiber and fluid intake.	If constipation is a problem, patient should be placed on a bowel regimen. Prevention of constipation is easier than treating constipation.

••• **Related NIC and NOC labels:** *NIC:* Communication Enhancement: Hearing Deficit; Environmental Management; Active Listening; Exercise Therapy: Balance; Peripheral Sensation Management; Exercise Therapy: Ambulation *NOC:* Communication: Receptive Ability; Balance; Muscle Function; Neurologic Status: Motor Function

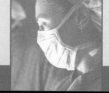

Pain 2

Nursing Diagnosis:

Acute Pain/Chronic Pain

related to disease process, injury, or surgical procedure

Desired Outcome: Patient's subjective report of pain using a pain scale, family's report, and behavioral and/or physiologic indicators reflect that pain is either reduced or at an acceptable level within 1-2 hr.

INTERVENTIONS	RATIONALES
Obtain history about ongoing/previous pain experiences and previously used methods of pain control. Elicit what was/was not effective. Consider whether pain is acute, chronic, or acute with an underlying chronic component.	A pain history enables development of a systematic approach to pain management for each patient, using information gathered from pain history and the hierarchy of pain measurement (self-report, pathologic conditions or procedures that usually cause pain, behavioral indicators, report of family, and physiologic indicators). Agency for Health Care Policy and Research (AHCPR) and American Pain Society (APS) state self-report of pain is the single most reliable indicator of pain.
Teach patients that pain assessment and management are not only a part of their treatment but also their right.	Patients have the right to appropriate assessment and management of their pain (TJC, 2001).
Use a formal patient-specific method of assessing self-reported pain when possible, including description, location, intensity, and aggravating/alleviating factors.	The first step of effective pain management is accurate assessment of pain. A numerical rating scale (NRS) of 0 (no pain) to 10 (worst possible pain), descriptive scales, and visual analog scale (VAS) are commonly used to assess intensity in adults who are cognitively intact. Pain intensity scales are available in many different languages when language barriers are present. The Wong-Baker FACES scale may be useful to measure pain in children (Wong & Baker, 1988). Consider using the Faces Pain Scale (Bieri, et al. 1990) in older adults (Taylor and Herr, 2001). **Use the selected scale consistently.** **Note:** Although pain is multidimensional in nature, it is the subjective intensity of pain that is most often measured in clinical practice.
Evaluate patient's health history for alcohol and drug (prescribed and nonprescribed) use, which could affect effective doses of analgesics (i.e., patient may require more or less). Ensure that surgeon, anesthesiologist, and other health care providers are aware of any significant findings. Consult a pain management team if available.	Other drug use could alter effective doses of analgesics or lead to undertreatment. All care providers must be consistent in setting limits while providing effective pain control through pharmacologic and nonpharmacologic methods. Psychiatric or clinical pharmacology consultation may be necessary.

Continued

INTERVENTIONS	RATIONALES
Assess for behavioral and physiologic indicators of pain at frequent intervals (e.g., during scheduled vital signs [VS] assessments). Document responses.	Behavioral and physiologic responses are potential indicators of pain in patients who are unable to self-report. This assessment optimizes reassessment and treatment intervals.
	Note: Not all patients demonstrate the same response to pain, nor does the lack of response negate the presence of pain.
	Behavioral responses: Examples include facial expression (grimacing, facial tension), vocalization (moaning, groaning, sighing, crying), verbalization (praying, counting), body action (rocking, rubbing, restlessness), and behaviors (massaging, guarding, short-attention span, irritability, sleep disturbance). Behavioral examples may be seen in patients with impaired communication, including those who are cognitively impaired, unconscious, or conscious but unable to communicate.
	Physiologic responses: Examples include diaphoresis, vasoconstriction, increased or decreased blood pressure (15% or more from baseline), increased pulse rate (15% or more from baseline), pupillary dilation, change in respiratory rate (RR) (usually increased to greater than 20 breaths/min), muscle tension or spasm, and decreased intestinal motility (evidenced by nausea, vomiting). Physiologic indicators may reflect pain as a result of autonomic stimulation of the sympathetic and parasympathetic responses.
Develop a systematic and collaborative approach to pain management for each patient, using information gathered from pain history and the hierarchy of pain measurement.	American Nurses Association Standards of Pain Management Nursing Practice (2005) identifies importance of involvement of patient, family, and other health care providers in data collection, formulation of outcomes, and development of the pain management plan.
	The AHCPR and APS state self-report of pain is the single most reliable indicator of pain.
Use at least two identifiers (e.g., patient's name, medical record number) before administering medications.	Using two or more identifiers improves accuracy of patient identification in keeping with TJC National Patient Safety Goals promoting the right patient receiving the right medication.
Use a preventive approach: administer prn pain medications before pain becomes severe as well as before painful procedures, ambulation, and bedtime.	Prolonged stimulation of pain receptors results in increased sensitivity to painful stimuli and the need to increase the amount of drug required to relieve pain.
Administer analgesics according to the World Health Organization (WHO, 1996) three-step analgesic ladder.	The WHO analgesic ladder focuses on selecting analgesics and adjuvants based on pain intensity. The WHO analgesic ladder has been endorsed by the AHCPR Guidelines (1994) and the American Pain Society (1999). **Note:** Not all patients start with the first step; the process is determined by the etiology and severity of the pain.
	The three steps include:
	- Level one: nonopioid, $\pm$ adjuvant
	- Level two: opioid for mild to moderate pain, $\pm$ nonopioid, $\pm$ adjuvant
	- Level three: opioid for moderate to severe pain, $\pm$ nonopioid, $\pm$ adjuvant
Recognize that choice of analgesic agent is based on three general considerations: therapeutic goal, patient's medical condition, and drug cost.	Individualized therapeutic goal and the stage of illness/disease process are important factors in agent selection to maximize pain relief and minimize potential of adverse side effects. The difference in cost of different drugs used to accomplish the same goal may be large. Where there is no proven or expected benefit of using one drug in preference to another to accomplish a desired goal, the less costly drug should be considered. **The right drug is the one that works with the fewest side effects.**
Also consider convenience, anticipated analgesic requirements, side effects, and patient's previous experience with a specific agent or patient's recall of side effects experienced with a specific agent, including route.	The preferred route is the one that is least invasive while achieving adequate relief. Aversion to painful routes of delivery (e.g., subcutaneous, IM) may lead to underreporting of pain by patients and to undermedication by nurses.

Continued

INTERVENTIONS	**RATIONALES**
	- IM analgesia is inconsistent; less titratable; and can cause complications such as hematoma, granuloma, infection, aseptic tissue necrosis, and nerve injury. APS suggests that this route be used rarely, and the AHCPR Acute Pain Practice Guidelines suggest that it be avoided when possible.
	- Oral route is least invasive; is convenient and flexible; and produces relatively steady analgesia.
	- IV route is used for agents with quick time to onset of analgesia and for severe pain.
For relief of mild-moderate pain that may be associated with surgery, trauma, soft tissue and muscle injury, and inflammatory conditions, administer nonopioid agents, such as:	**Note:** These agents also may be administered in conjunction with opioids.
- Salicylates (acetylsalicylic acid [aspirin])	
- Para-aminophenolderivatives (acetaminophen)	
- Nonsteroidal antiinflammatory drugs (NSAIDs) (ibuprofen, ketorolac)	Ketorolac may be given IM or IV for patients unable to tolerate oral agents. Undesirable side effects such as gastrointestinal (GI) disturbances (epigastric pain, nausea, dyspepsia), platelet dysfunction, bleeding, and renal compromise may occur.
- Indoleacetic acids (indomethacin)	
- **Caution:** Be certain that GI function has returned (e.g., presence of bowel sounds, absence of vomiting) before administering oral agents.	NSAIDs have peripheral effects and a different mechanism of action and thus are very effective when combined or used with centrally acting opioid analgesics. They also have a dose-sparing effect and may contribute to the reduction of opioid side effects. Unless contraindicated, APS recommends use of nonopioid agents even if pain is severe enough to require addition of an opioid. Another advantage of NSAIDs is their dual antipyretic and antiinflammatory actions.
- Use COX-2 selective NSAIDs with caution.	Recent Food and Drug Administration alerts and manufacturers' withdrawals of rofecoxib (Vioxx) and valdecoxib (Bextra) mandate all health care providers remain current and assess risks/benefits based on current information, safety data, and availability.
As prescribed, administer opioid analgesics (e.g., morphine) for pain of greater severity.	Morphine is the standard of comparison for opioid analgesics, and morphine or related "mu" (μ) receptor agonists are preferred when possible.
Use meperidine and normeperidine, a metabolite of meperidine, with caution.	Normeperidine is a central nervous system (CNS) excitotoxin, which with repetitive dosing may produce anxiety, muscle twitching, and seizures. Patients with impaired renal function and those taking monoamine oxidase (MAO) inhibitors are particularly at risk. Recommended use is for less than 48 hr for acute pain in patients without renal or CNS dysfunction or dose less than 600 mg/24 hr (APS, 1999).
Note: Do not use naloxone (Narcan) to attempt to reverse normeperidine toxicity.	Naloxone does not reverse normeperidine and may potentiate hyperexcitability.
If use of naloxone is necessary, titrate with caution.	Too much too fast can precipitate severe pain, hypertension, tachycardia, and even cardiac arrest (Brimacombe et al., 1991).
Do not administer mixed agonist-antagonist analgesics concurrently with morphine or other pure agonists because reversal of analgesic effects may occur.	Mixed agonist-antagonist agents such as butorphanol (Stadol) and pentazocine (Talwin) produce analgesia by binding to opioid receptors, while blocking or remaining neutral to the μ receptors. To date, there is no convincing evidence that agonist-antagonists offer any advantage over morphine-like agonists in the treatment of acute pain. Mixed agonist-antagonist agents may be useful in patients who are unable to tolerate other opioids.

Continued

INTERVENTIONS	RATIONALES
Assess patients receiving opioid analgesics for level of pain relief and potential side effects, including evidence of excessive sedation or respiratory depression (i.e., RR less than 10 breaths/min or Spo$_2$ less than 90%-92%). In the presence of respiratory depression, reduce amount or frequency of the dose as prescribed. Have naloxone readily available to reverse severe respiratory depression.	Sedative effects precede respiratory depression. Close monitoring of sedation level may prevent respiratory depression.
Monitor older adults and individuals with chronic obstructive pulmonary disease, asthma, and other respiratory disorders closely for respiratory depression and excessive sedation when they are receiving opioid analgesics. Consider using reduced doses and titrate carefully.	Older adults who are opioid naive and patients with coexisting conditions are at higher risk of respiratory depression (Pasero & McCaffrey, 1994). Increased tolerance to respiratory depression occurs over days to weeks. Therefore patients who are opioid naive (or have coexisting conditions) are at greater risk of respiratory depression than the patient who has been receiving an opioid for a week or more.
Wean patient from opioid analgesics by decreasing dose or frequency.	In general, doses should be reduced by no more that 10%-20% per day with vigilant assessment for withdrawal signs and symptoms.
Convert to oral therapy as soon as possible. When changing route of administration or medication, be certain to use equianalgesic doses of the new drug.	**Note:** Changing route of medication administration often results in inadequate pain relief because of ineffective equianalgesic conversion.
Reassess pain level and assess for side effects: - Routinely at scheduled intervals (e.g., q2-4h with VS) - With each report of pain - Following administration of pain medication based on time to onset, time to peak effect, and duration of action	More opioid is required to produce respiratory depression than to produce sedation. Sedative effects precede respiratory depression. Close monitoring of the level of sedation and respiratory status may prevent respiratory depression.
Consult with health care provider to discuss converting to scheduled dosing with supplemental prn analgesics when pain exists for 12 hr out of 24 hr.	Experts recommend around-the-clock (ATC) dosing for patients with continuous pain because it provides superior pain relief with fewer side effects (APS, 1999). Prolonged stimulation of pain receptors results in increased sensitivity to painful stimuli and the need to increase the amount of drug required to relieve pain. Addiction to opioids occurs infrequently in hospitalized patients.
Titrate the dose to achieve the desired effect.	The initial effect and duration of action of analgesics may differ vastly in acutely ill older adults who may require lower doses, whereas higher doses may be required for those with chronic substance abuse. It is important to consider factors such as these that can influence the initial effect and duration of action due to variations in the metabolism of analgesics. The goal is to develop a safe and effective pain management plan.
Provide patient-controlled analgesia (PCA) as prescribed.	PCA is a patient-activated system for pain control that uses an infusion pump to deliver specified doses of analgesics with options of continuous infusions, bolus dosing, or both. Patient selection is important because patients must be capable of understanding and activating the device and be willing to participate in their own treatment. Morphine, fentanyl, and hydromorphone are examples of opioids available for PCA use.
Increase patient monitoring following initiation, during initial 24 hr, and at night when patient may hypoventilate. Do not assume pain is controlled; assess patient to determine if relief has been obtained.	Monitoring involves pain, sedation, and respiratory assessments and may include Spo$_2$ and capnography. Safety issues with PCA have been described with suggested strategies to reduce risk in ISMP Medication Safety Alerts (Acute Care 2003, Nurse Advise-ERR, 2005).
Monitor patients in whom neuraxial analgesia is used based on drug(s) being administered, catheter placement, and drug concentration and volume.	Neuraxial analgesia (spinal, epidural, and caudal) is a widely used option for regional analgesia. It decreases many side effects associated with intravenous opioids, and there is evidence it can lead to increased mobility and postoperative recovery. Local anesthetics, opioids, steroids, and clonidine are examples of agents that may be used.

Continued

INTERVENTIONS	RATIONALES
For *local anesthetics,* monitor motor examination/sensory level and pain intensity. For *opioids,* monitor respiratory rate, sedation level, and pain intensity.	Assessments may include sensory level and motor examination evaluations, level of pain intensity, sedation level, VS, and side effects. Potential side effects/complications include catheter migration, occlusion, hematoma, respiratory depression, hypotension, nausea/vomiting, urinary retention, and pruritus. For local anesthetics sensory assessments are performed bilaterally along dermatomes.
As prescribed, use analgesic adjuvants/co-analgesics.	These agents are used to prolong and enhance analgesia, not specifically to treat isolated incidents of anxiety or depression.
Note: Avoid substituting sedatives and tranquilizers for analgesics.	Sedatives and tranquilizers are not analgesics. Tricyclic antidepressant agents primarily used for neuropathic pain produce analgesia while improving mood and sleep. **Caution:** Concomitant use with opioids may lead to sedation and orthostatic hypotension. Amitriptyline has the best-documented analgesia but is the least tolerated because of anticholinergic effects, including dry mouth, blurred vision, and constipation. Benzodiazepines are anxiolytic/sedatives with little to no analgesic effect. They are useful for decreasing recall, treating acute anxiety, and decreasing muscle spasm associated with acute pain. They may decrease opioid requirement by decreasing pain perception. If administered without an analgesic, the patient's perception of pain may increase. Antiepileptics may be prescribed for pain associated with nerve injury from tumors or other destructive processes. Although the specific mechanism of action for pain reduction is unknown, it is believed to be the result of suppression of the paroxysmal discharges and reduction of neuronal hyperexcitability. Antihistamines potentiate the effect of opioid analgesics. **Note:** Phenergan may increase perceived pain intensity and increase restlessness.
Assess for and report analgesia side effects. For management of constipation, see **Constipation** in "Prolonged Bedrest," p. 67.	Other analgesia side effects can include sedation, respiratory depression, nausea/vomiting, pruritus, and hypotension.
Augment action of the medication by using nonpharmacologic methods of pain control, including weight reduction, physical therapy, cognitive behavioral therapies, acupuncture, massage, and biofeedback. Other methods include reflexology, acupressure, Reiki, thermotherapy, back and foot massage, range-of-motion exercises, transcutaneous electrical nerve stimulation, distraction, relaxation exercises, and guided imagery.	Patients in whom nonpharmacologic interventions may be most successful include those who express interest in the approach, express anxiety or fear, or those with inadequate relief with pharmacologic management (AHCPR, 1992). Many of these techniques may be taught to and implemented by the patient and significant other.
Maintain a quiet environment and plan nursing activities to enable long periods of uninterrupted rest at night.	Promoting rest and sleep may decrease level of pain.
Evaluate for and correct nonoperative sources of discomfort.	Such sources including uncomfortable positioning, full bladder, and infiltrated IV site can be corrected readily without resorting to drug use.
Carefully evaluate patient if sudden or unexpected changes in pain intensity occurs, and notify health care provider immediately should this occur.	This may signal complications such as internal bleeding or leakage of visceral contents.
Document efficacy of analgesics and other pain control interventions using a pain scale or other formalized method.	This documentation communicates level of pain relief obtained, interventions, effectiveness of the interventions, and ongoing follow-up to meet the analgesic goal.

••• Related NIC and NOC labels: *NIC:* Medication Management; Pain Management; Analgesic Administration; Medication Administration; Positioning; Acupressure; Biofeedback; Simple Massage; Simple Relaxation Therapy; Transcutaneous Electrical Nerve Stimulation (TENS); Distraction; Heat/Cold Application; Hypnosis *NOC:* Comfort Level; Pain Control; Pain: Disruptive Effects; Pain Level

Perioperative Care   3

Nursing Diagnosis:

Deficient Knowledge:

Surgical procedure, preoperative routine, and postoperative care

Desired Outcome: Patient verbalizes knowledge about the surgical procedure, including preoperative preparations and sensations and postoperative care and sensations, and demonstrates postoperative exercises and use of devices before surgical procedure or during immediate postoperative period for emergency surgery.

INTERVENTIONS	RATIONALES
Preoperatively:	
Evaluate patient's desire for knowledge about diagnosis and procedure.	Some individuals find detailed information helpful; others prefer very brief and simple explanations.
Assess patient's understanding about the diagnosis, surgical procedure, preoperative routine, and postoperative regimen.	Assessment should include patient's primary language and whether an interpreter is needed, patient's readiness to learn, limitations on patient's ability to learn such as blindness or decreased hearing, and patient's self-assessment as to which modes of learning he or she finds most helpful, such as reading, listening, visual aids, or demonstration.
Determine past surgical experiences and their positive or negative effect on patient. Assess the nature of any concerns or fears related to surgery. Document and communicate these assessment data to others involved in patient's care.	Assessing patient's knowledge, past experiences, and concerns about the surgical procedure will enable the nurse to focus on individual areas in need of greatest intervention.
Based on your assessment, clarify and explain diagnosis and surgical procedure accordingly. When possible, emphasize associated sensations (e.g., dry mouth, thirst, muscle weakness). Provide ample time for instruction and clarification and reinforce health care provider's explanation of the procedure.	This information provides a knowledge base from which patient can make informed therapy choices and consent for procedures and presents an opportunity to clarify misconceptions.
Use anatomic models, diagrams, and other audiovisual aids when possible. Provide simply written information to reinforce learning. Provide written and verbal information in patient's native language for non–English-speaking patients. **Note:** Evaluate patient's reading comprehension before providing written materials.	Because individuals learn differently, using more than one teaching modality will provide teaching reinforcement of verbal information given.
Document if patient provides an advance directive (see p. 105).	Laws about advance directives differ for each state.
Explain perioperative course of events. Review the following with patient and significant other:	These measures increase patient's knowledge of the surgical procedure, which optimally will promote adherence and minimize stress.
- Procedures for required preoperative assessment and testing and when and where they will be performed. Issue written directions, phone numbers, and maps as indicated. Discuss location and proper arrival time for the surgery.	Patient will need information regarding location of the preoperative testing center, parking arrangements, and expected length of time such testing will require.

Continued

45

INTERVENTIONS	RATIONALES
- Where patient will be before, during, and immediately after surgery.	Patient may be in postanesthesia care unit (PACU), intensive care unit (ICU), or specialty unit.
- Clarify sounds and other sensations (e.g., sore throat, cool temperature, hard stretcher) patient may experience during immediate postoperative period. If possible, take patient to the new unit and introduce him or her to nursing staff.	Including sensory information in patient teaching is consistent with current nursing research that has determined patient outcomes are improved when expected sensations are explained.
- Preoperative medications and timing of surgery (scheduled time, expected duration).	
- If indicated, preoperative bowel preparation.	
- Pain management, including sensations to expect and methods of relief. If patient-controlled analgesia (PCA) or patient-controlled epidural anesthesia (PCEA) will be prescribed, have patient give a return demonstration of use of the delivery device.	This information increases likelihood of successful pain management. Some patients mistakenly expect to be pain free; others fear becoming addicted to narcotics (opioids).
- Use of pain assessment tools such as the numeric pain rating scale or the Wong-Baker FACES pain rating scale.	Pain assessment tools aid in the evaluation of pain and effectiveness of interventions.
- Placement of tubes, catheters, drains, cooling systems (Cryocuff), continuous passive motion (CPM) units, oxygen delivery devices, and similar devices routinely used for patient's surgery. Show these devices to patient when possible.	Patient may be unfamiliar with use and purpose of these devices. Learning about them and seeing them in advance of surgery may help decrease fears and anxieties perioperatively.
- Use of antiembolism stockings, sequential compression devices (SCDs), pneumatic foot pumps, or similar devices.	These garments/devices prevent venous stasis and decrease risk of thrombus formation.
- Dietary alterations and progression, including NPO (nothing by mouth) status followed by clear liquids until return of full gastrointestinal (GI) function.	Traditionally, health care providers have progressed patients from clear liquids to a regular diet after surgery for a variety of reasons, including ease of swallowing and digestion and liquid diet being more readily tolerated in the presence of an ileus. However, practitioners are questioning the scientific basis of this diet advancement. Recent studies are indicating that a clear liquid diet may not always be indicated.
- Restrictions of activity and positions, as indicated by specific surgical procedure.	For example, patients undergoing hip arthroplasty have specific positional limitations.
- Need to refrain from smoking during perioperative period.	Inhalation of toxic fumes/chemical irritants can damage lung tissue by decreasing cilia, which line the respiratory tract and carry particles to the lower pharynx. Damaged lung tissue increases likelihood of hypoxemia and lung infections, including pneumonia.
- Visiting hours and location of waiting room.	Families may feel less anxious when they are aware of a designated area where they can wait and receive updates on progress of the surgery. Knowledge of visiting hours likely will reassure them they will have access to patient after surgery.

Postoperatively:

Explain postoperative activities, exercises, and precautions. Have patient give a return demonstration of the following devices and exercises, as appropriate:	Adherence is enhanced when patients are knowledgeable about activities, exercises, and precautions. Patients gain confidence when they practice new skills before surgery and gain feedback on their technique.
- Deep-breathing and coughing exercises (see **Ineffective Airway Clearance,** p. 48).	These actions help prevent atelectasis, pneumonia, and other respiratory disorders that can occur during the postoperative period.
Caution: Individuals for whom increased intracranial, intrathoracic, or intraabdominal pressure is contraindicated should not cough.	Coughing increases intracranial, intrathoracic, and intraabdominal pressure. Patients undergoing intracranial surgery, spinal fusion, eye and ear surgery, and similar procedures should avoid vigorous coughing because it raises intracranial pressure, which could cause harm. Coughing after a herniorrhaphy and some thoracic surgeries should be done in a controlled manner, with the incision supported carefully, to avoid raising intraabdominal and intrathoracic pressure dramatically.
- Use of incentive spirometry and other respiratory devices.	This device, when used with coughing and deep breathing, expands alveoli and mobilizes secretions, which helps prevent atelectasis, pneumonia, and other respiratory disorders.

Continued

INTERVENTIONS

INTERVENTIONS	RATIONALES
- Calf-pumping, ankle-circling, and footboard-pressing exercises (see "Venous Thrombosis/Thrombophlebitis," p. 203, for more information).	These exercises promote circulation and help prevent thrombophlebitis in the legs.
- Use of PCA/PCEA device.	Adequate pain management increases mobility, which decreases risk of nosocomial pneumonia and thrombosis formation and aids in the return of gastrointestinal peristalsis.
- Movement in and out of bed.	Logrolling, raising self by using a trapeze device, and gradual movement are techniques that may be required.
Before patient is discharged, teach prescribed activity precautions.	This teaching helps prevent excessive strain on the operative site. A patient who has a total hip replacement, for example, will need to follow activity precautions to prevent dislocation of the new joint.
	Increasing exercises gradually to tolerance, avoiding heavy lifting (more than 10 lb), and avoiding driving a car (often for as long as 4-6 wk) are precautions given to most surgical patients for safety because of potential for decreased attention span and impaired reflexes resulting from opioid use. Lifting precautions may reduce stress on surgical incisions. Restrictions on sexual activity are indicated by the surgical procedure. Returning progressively to preoperative activity level promotes physical and psychosocial well-being.
Provide time for patient to ask questions and express feelings of anxiety; be reassuring and supportive. Be certain to address patient's main concerns.	Expressing feelings of anxiety and having questions answered are essential ways of reducing anxiety while learning new information.

••• **Related NIC and NOC labels:** *NIC:* Teaching: Preoperative; Preparatory Sensory Information; Teaching: Procedure; Anxiety Reduction; Teaching: Prescribed Activity/Exercise *NOC:* Knowledge: Treatment Procedures; Knowledge: Prescribed Activity; Knowledge: Treatment Regimen

Nursing Diagnosis:

Risk for Injury

related to exposure to pharmaceutical agents and other external factors during the perioperative period

Desired Outcome: Patient does not experience injury or untoward effects of pharmacotherapy or other external factors.

INTERVENTIONS	RATIONALES
Assess need for holding, administering, or adjusting patient's maintenance medications before or immediately after surgery. Consult health care provider as necessary.	Some medications, such as anticonvulsants and cardiac medications, should be continued throughout the perioperative period. Sometimes patients need to be weaned from medications such as baclofen for the perioperative period because stopping them suddenly could result in seizures or hallucinations. Other medications may require increased dosages during surgery (i.e., hydrocortisone in place of prednisone and with increased dosage for steroid-dependent patients) or alternative routes.
Reinforce importance of NPO status.	Maintaining NPO status reduces risk of aspiration postoperatively. Clear liquids may be allowed up to 2 hr before surgery in patients with low risk of pulmonary aspiration.
Verify completion of preoperative activities and procedures, and document on preoperative checklist or nursing documentation.	Documentation on patient's preoperative checklist or inpatient's medical record helps ensure communication among health care team members, continuity, and optimum patient outcomes.

Continued

INTERVENTIONS	RATIONALES
The preoperative verification process must confirm the correct patient, procedure, and site of operation.	This verification process should take place upon admission to the facility, before patient leaves the preoperative area, upon entry to the surgical room, and anytime responsibility for patient care is transferred to another caregiver. The verification process should involve the patient while still awake and aware if possible.
Verify that an appropriate member of the surgical team has used a sufficiently permanent-type marker that will remain visible after completion of skin prep and has marked the operative site.	The mark should be at or near the incision site and be unambiguous (i.e., use of initials or "YES" and/or a line representing proposed incision).
Document allergies, any evidence of skin breakdown, bruises, rashes, or wounds, and presence of dressings, drains, or ostomy.	Documentation decreases risk of untoward outcomes. Noting patient's preexisting wounds, dressings, and drains also helps ensure appropriate intraoperative positioning.
Assess for and document patient's exposure to actual or potential abuse or neglect.	All states require health care providers to report suspected abuse and neglect of children and vulnerable adults who are in their care.
Document patient's access to care and transportation upon discharge.	Surgery, pain, and analgesic medications may impede the patient's ability to care for self adequately after discharge.
Be sure that consent has been signed and witnessed and patient appears to understand what the procedure involves. Answer questions, or call health care provider to answer patient's questions. Ensure that patient's identification bracelet, blood transfusion bracelet, and allergy alert bracelet are in place.	These interventions help ensure that all appropriate documentation is present and that all steps have been taken to provide for patient's safety and well-being.
Review medical record to ensure that all appropriate documentation is present; report untoward findings to health care provider.	Health care provider may not be aware of recent abnormal electrocardiogram (ECG), suspicious chest radiograph, or abnormal laboratory findings.
Prepare surgical site and perform additional presurgical procedures as prescribed.	This may involve clipping of hair or use of depilatory agent (shaving is not usually recommended) and patient showering with antimicrobial agent. Additional presurgical procedures may involve, for example, douche, enema, or eye drops.
Administer preoperative analgesia, sedation, or other medications as prescribed and on time.	This intervention helps ensure adequate serum levels of the prescribed drug. Giving antibiotics preoperatively may decrease risk of infection postoperatively.
Make provisions for patient safety following administration (e.g., bed in lowest position, side rails up, and reminding patient not to get out of bed without assistance).	Sedatives administered preoperatively may alter mental status and coordination, increasing patient's risk for injury.
Be aware that once patient is in the location in which the procedure will be conducted and just before the procedure is started, a "time out" must be performed.	"Time out" must involve the entire operative team and confirm correct patient identity, procedure, site, and position and availability of any special equipment, implants, and other requirements that help ensure patient's safety and well-being.

••• **Related NIC and NOC labels:** *NIC:* Risk Identification; Environmental Management: Safety; Surgical Precautions; Fall Prevention
NOC: Risk Control; Safety Status: Physical Injury

<u>Nursing Diagnosis:</u>

Ineffective Airway Clearance

related to alterations in pulmonary physiology and function secondary to anesthetics, narcotics, mechanical ventilation, hypothermia, and surgery; increased tracheobronchial secretions secondary to effects of anesthesia combined with ineffective coughing; and decreased function of the mucociliary clearance mechanism

Desired Outcome: Patient's airway is clear as evidenced by normal breath sounds to auscultation, RR 12-20 breaths/min with normal depth and pattern (eupnea), normothermia, normal skin color, and O_2 saturation greater than 92% on room air.

INTERVENTIONS	RATIONALES
Assess respiratory status, including breath sounds, q1-2h during immediate postoperative period and q8h during recovery.	This assessment will determine presence of rhonchi that do not clear with coughing, labored breathing, tachypnea (RR more than 20 breaths/min), mental status changes, restlessness, cyanosis, and presence of fever (38.3° C [101° F] or higher, which are all signs of respiratory system compromise).
Use oximetry to assess oxygen saturation as indicated, and report saturation 92% or less to health care provider.	Pulse oximetry is a noninvasive measure of arterial oxygen saturation. Values 92% or less are consistent with hypoxia and probably signal need for oxygen supplementation or workup to determine cause of desaturation. Oximetry is especially indicated in patients with chronic obstructive pulmonary disease (COPD), respiratory or cardiovascular disease, morbid obesity, cardiothoracic surgery, major surgery, prolonged general anesthesia, and surgery for a fractured pelvis or long bone, as well as in debilitated patients and older adults, all of whom are at increased risk for desaturation.
Administer humidified oxygen as prescribed.	This intervention supplements oxygen and prevents further drying of respiratory passageways and secretions via added humidity.
Keep emergency airway equipment (e.g., Ambu bag and mask, intubation tray, endotracheal tubes, suctioning equipment, tracheostomy tray) readily available.	This ensures their availability in the event of sudden airway obstruction or ventilatory failure.
Encourage deep breathing and coughing q2h or more often for the first 72 hr postoperatively. In the presence of fine crackles (rales) and if not contraindicated, have patient cough to expectorate secretions. Facilitate deep breathing and coughing by demonstrating how to splint abdominal and thoracic incisions with hands or a pillow. If indicated, medicate ½ hr before deep breathing, coughing, or ambulation to promote adherence.	These actions expand alveoli and mobilize secretions. The effects of anesthesia and immobility may collapse alveoli and place patient at risk for nosocomial pneumonia and atelectasis. Proper positioning promotes chest expansion and ventilation of basilar lung fields.
If patient has a weak cough or poor reserve, try the "step-cough" technique. Coach patient to cough in rapid succession.	A few weak coughs in a row may stimulate a larger, productive cough at the end of the cycle to clear the bronchial tree of secretions. **Caution:** Vigorous coughing may be contraindicated for some individuals (e.g., those undergoing intracranial surgery, spinal fusion, eye and ear surgery, and similar procedures). Coughing after a herniorrhaphy and some thoracic surgeries should be done in a controlled manner, with incision supported carefully.
Consider whether patient may be more motivated to perform pulmonary toilet with incentive spirometer or positive expiratory pressure (PEP) device.	Devices may be a motivating factor because patient has a visual indicator of effectiveness of the breathing effort.

●●● **Related NIC and NOC labels:** *NIC:* Respiratory Monitoring; Vital Signs Monitoring; Chest Physiotherapy; Airway Suctioning; Oxygen Therapy; Aspiration Precautions *NOC:* Respiratory Status: Gas Exchange; Respiratory Status: Airway Patency

Nursing Diagnosis:

Risk for Aspiration

related to entry of gastric secretions, food, or fluids into tracheobronchial passages secondary to central nervous system (CNS) depression, depressed cough and gag reflexes, decreased GI motility, abdominal distention, recumbent position, presence of gastric tube, diabetes, gastroesophageal reflux disease (GERD), obesity, and possible impaired swallowing in individuals with oral, facial, or neck surgery

Desired Outcome: Patient's upper airway remains unobstructed as evidenced by clear breath sounds, RR 12-20 breaths/min with normal depth and pattern (eupnea), normal skin color, and a return to preoperative O_2 saturation.

INTERVENTIONS	RATIONALES
If sedated patient experiences nausea or vomiting, turn immediately into a side-lying position.	This position minimizes potential for aspiration.
Encourage fully alert patients to remain in an upright position.	Maintaining a sitting position after meals decreases risk of aspiration by facilitating gravity drainage from the stomach to the small bowel. An upright position also helps prevent reflux.
As necessary, suction oropharynx with Yankauer or similar suction device to remove vomitus.	Suctioning enables immediate removal of vomitus, which could be aspirated. Patients at high risk for aspiration should have suctioning apparatus immediately available for this life-saving intervention.
Administer antiemetics, histamine H_2-receptor blocking agents, omeprazole, metoclopramide, and similar agents as prescribed.	These agents decrease nausea, vomiting, and acidity of gastric contents and stimulate GI motility. H_2-receptor antagonists increase gastric pH, and nonparticulate antacids (e.g., Bicitra, Citra pH, and Alka Seltzer Gold) act as aspiration pneumonitis prophylaxis. Neutralizing gastric acidity may reduce severity of pneumonia if aspiration occurs.
Check placement and patency of gastric tubes q8h and before instillation of feedings and medications. Consult health care provider before irrigating tubes for these individuals.	These actions prevent instillation of anything into patient's airway.
Note: Use caution when irrigating and otherwise manipulating GI tubes of patients with recent esophageal, gastric, or duodenal surgery.	The tube may be displaced or the surgical incision disrupted by such activity.
Assess abdomen q4-8h by inspection, auscultation, palpation, and percussion for evidence of distention (increasing size, firmness, increased tympany, decreased bowel sounds).	A distended and rigid abdomen along with increased or absent bowel sounds may indicate an ileus, which places patient at increased risk for vomiting and aspiration. Increased tympany or high-pitched bowel sounds may signal mechanical obstruction, which also places patient at increased risk for vomiting and aspiration.
Notify health care provider if distention is of rapid onset or if it is associated with pain.	Rapid abdominal distention postoperatively may indicate intraabdominal hemorrhage and can lead to a sometimes fatal condition called *abdominal compartment syndrome*.
Encourage early and frequent ambulation.	Ambulation improves GI motility and reduces abdominal distention caused by accumulated gases.
Introduce oral fluids cautiously, especially in patients with oral, facial, and neck surgery.	Swelling and irritation in the oropharynx may cause dysphagia and pain postoperatively. Nasal packing or intranasal splint aspiration also may cause airway obstruction.
For additional information, see "Providing Nutritional Support" for **Risk for Aspiration,** p. 570.	

••• **Related NIC and NOC labels:** *NIC:* Aspiration Precautions; Vomiting Management; Positioning; Postanesthesia Care; Respiratory Monitoring; Vital Signs Monitoring; Gastrointestinal Intubation *NOC:* Aspiration Control

Nursing Diagnosis:

Ineffective Breathing Pattern (or risk of same)

related to decreased lung expansion secondary to CNS depression, pain, muscle splinting, recumbent position, obesity, narcotics, and effects of anesthesia

Desired Outcome: Patient exhibits effective ventilation as evidenced by relaxed breathing, RR 12-20 breaths/min with normal depth and pattern (eupnea), clear breath sounds, normal color, return to preoperative O_2 saturation on room air, Pao_2 80 mm Hg or greater, pH 7.35-7.45, $Paco_2$ 35-45 mm Hg, and HCO_3^- 22-26 mEq/L.

INTERVENTIONS

RATIONALES

See interventions under **Ineffective Airway Clearance**, p. 48.

INTERVENTIONS	RATIONALES
Perform preoperative baseline assessment of patient's respiratory system, noting rate, rhythm, degree of chest expansion, quality of breath sounds, cough, and sputum production, as well as smoking history and current respiratory medications. Note preoperative O_2 saturation and arterial blood gas (ABG) values if available.	Baseline assessment enables rapid detection of subsequent postoperative problems and timely intervention for same.
If appropriate, encourage patient to refrain from smoking for at least 1 wk after surgery. Explain effects of smoking on the body.	Inhalation of toxic fumes/chemical irritants can damage lung tissue, increasing likelihood of hypoxemia and respiratory infection.
Monitor O_2 saturation continuously via oximetry in high-risk individuals (e.g., patients who are heavily sedated, patients with preexisting lung disease, morbidly obese patients, patients having undergone upper airway surgery, or older patients) and at periodic intervals in other patients as indicated.	Pulse oximetry is a noninvasive method of measuring saturated hemoglobin in tissue capillaries.
Notify health care provider of O_2 saturation 92% or less.	O_2 saturation of 92% or less may signal need for supplemental oxygen.
Evaluate ABG values, and notify health care provider of low or decreasing Pao_2 and high or increasing $Paco_2$. Also assess for signs of hypoxia.	Declining Pao_2 may signal hypoxemia and need for supplemental oxygen. Early signs of hypoxia include restlessness, dyspnea, tachycardia, tachypnea, and confusion. Cyanosis, especially of the tongue and oral mucous membranes, and extreme lethargy or somnolence are late signs of hypoxia. Hypercapnia combined with acidemia and hypoxemia may result in pulmonary vasoconstriction that may be severe and life threatening.
Assist patient with turning and deep-breathing/coughing exercises q2h for the first 72 hr postoperatively.	These activities promote expansion of lung alveoli and prevent pooling of secretions, which could lead to nosocomial pneumonia.
If patient has an incentive spirometer *or* PEP device, provide instructions and ensure adherence to its use q2h or as prescribed.	These devices promote expansion of the alveoli and aid in mobilizing secretions to the airways; subsequent coughing further mobilizes and clears secretions.
Unless contraindicated, assist patient with ambulation by second postoperative day.	Ambulation promotes circulation and ventilation, which helps prevent formation of deep vein thrombosis and pulmonary embolus.

••• **Related NIC and NOC labels:** *NIC:* Respiratory Monitoring; Vital Signs Monitoring; Postanesthesia Care; Teaching: Prescribed Activity/Exercise *NOC:* Vital Signs Status

Nursing Diagnosis:

Risk for Deficient Fluid Volume

related to postoperative bleeding/hemorrhage

Desired Outcomes: Patient is normovolemic as evidenced by BP 90/60 mm Hg or higher (or within patient's preoperative baseline), HR 60-100 bpm, RR 12-20 breaths/min with normal depth and pattern (eupnea), brisk capillary refill (less than 2 sec), warm extremities, distal pulses greater than 2+ on a 0-4+ scale, urinary output 30 ml/hr or more, and urine specific gravity less than 1.030. Patient does not demonstrate significant mental status changes and verbalizes orientation to person, place, and time.

INTERVENTIONS	RATIONALES
Monitor vital signs (VS) and physical indicators at frequent intervals during the first 24 hr of the postoperative period for signs of internal hemorrhage and impending shock. See "Cardiac and Noncardiac Shock," p. 157, for management.	There is greater potential for postoperative bleeding/hemorrhage during this period. Decreasing pulse pressure (difference between SBP and DBP), decreasing BP, increasing HR, and increasing RR are indicators of internal hemorrhage and impending shock.
	Physical indicators include pallor, diaphoresis, cool extremities, delayed capillary refill, diminished intensity of distal pulses, restlessness, agitation, mental status changes, and disorientation, as well as subjective complaints of thirst, anxiety, or a sense of impending doom.
Inspect surgical dressing; record saturated dressings and report significant findings to health care provider.	Rapid saturation of the dressing with bright red blood is evidence of frank bleeding, which necessitates prompt intervention.
If initial postoperative dressing becomes saturated, reinforce and notify health care provider.	Health care provider may want to perform the initial dressing change.
Monitor wound drains and drainage systems, and report significant findings to health care provider.	Excessive drainage (more than 50 ml/hr for 2-3 hr) should be reported promptly for timely intervention.
Note amount and character of drainage from gastric and other tubes at least q8h. **Note:** After gastric and some other GI surgeries, patient will have small amounts of bloody or blood-tinged drainage for the first 12-24 hr. Be alert to large or increasing amounts of bloody drainage.	If drainage appears to contain blood (e.g., bright red, burgundy, or dark coffee ground appearance), it will be necessary to perform an occult blood test (may be performed in the laboratory). If the test is newly or unexpectedly positive, results should be reported to health care provider for timely intervention.
Monitor and measure urinary output q4-8h during initial postoperative period. Report significant findings to health care provider.	Average hourly output less than 30 ml/hr and specific gravity 1.030 or more are indicators of deficient fluid volume, which can signal bleeding/hemorrhage.
Review complete blood count (CBC) values for evidence of bleeding.	Evidence of bleeding may be indicated by decreases in hemoglobin (Hgb) from normal (male 14-18 g/dl; female 12-16 g/dl); and decreases in hematocrit (Hct) from normal (male 40%-54%; female 37%-47%). Significant decreases occur with active bleeding, an emergency situation.
Maintain patent 18-gauge or larger IV catheter.	The gauge of this catheter will enable repeat infusions of blood products if hemorrhagic shock develops.

••• Related NIC and NOC labels: *NIC:* Bleeding Precautions; Blood Products Administration; Hemorrhage Control; Shock Prevention; Venous Access Devices Maintenance; Vital Signs Monitoring; Laboratory Data Interpretation *NOC:* Fluid Balance

Nursing Diagnosis:

Risk for Deficient Fluid Volume

related to active loss secondary to presence of indwelling drainage tubes, wound drainage, or vomiting; inadequate intake of fluids secondary to nausea, NPO status, CNS depression, or lack of access to fluids; or failure of regulatory mechanisms with third spacing of body fluids secondary to the effects of anesthesia, endogenous catecholamines, blood loss during surgery, and prolonged recumbency

Desired Outcomes: Patient is normovolemic as evidenced by BP 90/60 mm Hg or higher (or within patient's preoperative baseline), HR 60-100 bpm, distal pulses greater than 2+ on a 0-4+ scale, urinary output 30 ml/hr or more, urine specific gravity 1.030 or less, stable or increasing weight, good skin turgor, warm skin, moist mucous membranes, and normothermia. Patient does not demonstrate significant mental status changes and verbalizes orientation to person, place, and time.

INTERVENTIONS	RATIONALES
Monitor VS q4-8h during recovery phase.	Decreasing BP, increasing HR, and slightly increased body temperature are indicators of dehydration.
Monitor urinary output q4-8h. Be alert for concentrated urine.	Concentrated urine (specific gravity more than 1.030) and low or decreasing output (average normal output is 60 ml/hr or 1400-1500 ml/day) are indicators of deficient fluid volume.
Administer and regulate IV fluids and electrolytes as prescribed until patient is able to resume oral intake. When IV fluids are discontinued, encourage intake of oral fluids, at least 2-3 L/day in nonrestricted patient. As possible, respect patient's preference in oral fluids, and keep them readily available in patient's room.	Oral fluids usually are restricted until peristalsis returns and nasogastric (NG) tube is removed. However, ice chips or small sips of clear liquids may be allowed.
Measure and record output from drains, ostomies, wounds, and other sources. Ensure patency of gastric and other drainage tubes. Record quality and quantity of output.	Both sensible and insensible losses need to be determined to ensure complete estimation of patient's fluid volume status.
Measure, describe, and document any emesis.	Same as above.
Be alert to and document excessive perspiration along with documentation of urinary, fecal, and other drainage.	
Report excessive losses.	Replacement fluids likely will be indicated.
Monitor patient's weight daily. Always weigh patient at same time every day, using same scale and same type and amount of bed clothing.	Daily weight measurement is an effective means of evaluating patient's hydration and nutritional status. Weighing patient at the same time and under the same conditions avoids discrepancies that could reflect inaccurate losses or gains.
Be aware that weighing patient daily is not useful in detecting intravascular fluid loss due to third spacing.	Movement of fluid from one area of the body to another will not change the total body weight.
If nausea and vomiting are present, assess for potential causes.	Potential causes include administration of opioid analgesics, loss of gastric tube patency, and environmental factors (e.g., unpleasant odors or sights).
Administer antiemetics (e.g., hydroxyzine, ondansetron, prochlorperazine, promethazine), metoclopramide, or similar agents as prescribed.	These agents combat nausea and vomiting, which could impair intake and add to fluid losses.
Instruct patient to request medication *before* nausea becomes severe.	Postoperative vomiting is significantly less when patients receive nausea/vomiting prophylaxis (Curr Med Res Opin 2006:22[6]:1093-1099).
Monitor serum electrolytes.	Fluid loss may cause electrolyte imbalances.
Be alert to K^+ less than 3.5 mEq/L and to the following: lethargy, irritability, anorexia, vomiting, muscle weakness and cramping, paresthesias, weak and irregular pulse, and respiratory dysfunction.	These are signs of hypokalemia, which must be detected and reported promptly to prevent potentially life-threatening cardiac dysrhythmias.
Also assess for Ca^{++} less than 8.5 mg/dl and the following: tetany, muscle cramps, fatigue, irritability, personality changes, and Trousseau's or Chvostek's sign.	These are signs of hypocalcemia. If detected and treated promptly, cardiac emergency may be prevented. Trousseau's sign is elicited by applying BP cuff to the arm, inflating it to slightly higher than SBP, and leaving it inflated for 1-4 min. Carpopedal spasms are indicative of hypocalcemia. Chvostek's sign is assessed by tapping the face just below the temple (where the facial nerve emerges). The sign is positive if twitching occurs along side of nose, lip, or face.

••• **Related NIC and NOC labels:** *NIC:* Fluid/Electrolyte Management; Hypovolemia Management; Vital Signs Monitoring; Electrolyte Management: Hypocalcemia; Electrolyte Management: Hypokalemia *NOC:* Electrolyte & Acid/Base Balance; Hydration

Nursing Diagnosis:

Excess Fluid Volume

related to compromised regulatory mechanisms after major surgery

Desired Outcome: Following intervention/treatment, patient becomes normovolemic as evidenced by BP within normal range of patient's preoperative baseline, distal pulses less than 4+ on a 0-4+ scale, presence of eupnea, clear breath sounds, absence of or barely detectable edema (1+ or less on a 0-4+ scale), urine specific gravity at least 1.010, and body weight near or at preoperative baseline.

INTERVENTIONS	RATIONALES
Assess for and report any indicators of fluid overload, including elevated BP, bounding pulses, dyspnea, crackles (rales), and pretibial or sacral edema.	An increase in BP and an S_3 galloping rhythm may indicate impending heart failure. Crackles and dyspnea may signal a shift of fluid from the vascular space to the pulmonary interstitial space and alveoli causing pulmonary edema.
Maintain record of 8-hr and 24-hr input and output (I&O). Note and report significant imbalance. Monitor urinary specific gravity and report consistently low (less than 1.010) findings.	Normal 24-hr output is 1400-1500 ml, and normal 1-hr output is 60 ml/hr or 480 ml per 8 hr. Decreased urinary output could be a sign of fluid volume excess.
Weigh patient daily, using same scale and same type and amount of bed clothing. Note significant weight gain.	Weight changes reflect changes in body fluid volume. One L of fluid equals approximately 2.2 lb. Weighing patient at the same time and under the same conditions avoids discrepancies that could reflect inaccurate losses or gains.
Administer furosemide as prescribed.	Furosemide mobilizes interstitial fluid and decreases excess fluid volume.
Caution: Monitor patients carefully who are on diuretic therapy. See **Risk for Deficient Fluid Volume, p. 53,** for signs and symptoms of hypokalemia.	Diuretic therapy may cause dangerous K^+ depletion that could result in cardiac dysrhythmias. As well, diuretic therapy can lead to hyponatremia because of sodium losses.
Monitor older adults and individuals with cardiovascular disease especially carefully.	These individuals are especially at risk for developing postoperative fluid volume excess. Older adults have age-related changes of decreased glomerular filtration rate (GFR). Decreased kidney function and increased probability of chronic illness such as cardiac disease may signal higher risk of postoperative excessive fluid volume.
Anticipate postoperative diuresis approximately 48-72 hr after surgery.	This may occur because of mobilization of third-space (interstitial) fluid.

••• **Related NIC and NOC labels:** *NIC:* Fluid/Electrolyte Management; Vital Signs Monitoring; Electrolyte Management: Hypokalemia *NOC:* Fluid Balance; Electrolyte and Acid/Base Balance

Nursing Diagnosis:

Risk for Infection

related to inadequate primary defenses (e.g., broken skin, traumatized tissue, decrease in ciliary action, stasis of body fluids), invasive procedures, or chronic disease

Desired Outcome: Patient is free of infection as evidenced by normothermia; HR 100 bpm or less; RR 20 breaths/min or less with normal depth and pattern (eupnea); negative cultures; clear and normal-smelling urine; clear and thin sputum; no significant mental status changes; orientation to person, place, and time; and absence of unusual tenderness, erythema, swelling, warmth, or drainage at the surgical incision.

INTERVENTIONS	RATIONALES
Monitor VS for evidence of infection, such as elevated HR and RR and increased body temperature.	With onset of infection, the immune system is activated, causing symptoms of infection to appear. Sustained temperature elevation after surgery may signal presence of pulmonary complications, urinary tract infection, wound infection, or thrombophlebitis.
Notify health care provider if these are new findings.	Presence of a fever affects treatment decisions.
Evaluate mental status, orientation, and level of consciousness q8h.	Consider infection the likely cause if altered mental status or LOC is unexplained by other factors, such as age, medication, or disease process.

Continued

INTERVENTIONS	RATIONALES
Encourage and assist patient with coughing, deep breathing, incentive spirometry, and turning q2-4h, and note quality of breath sounds, cough, and sputum.	These activities expand alveoli in the lung and mobilize secretions, which will decrease potential for respiratory infection/pneumonia. Optimally they will promote cough and improve quality of breath sounds.
Evaluate IV sites for erythema, warmth, swelling, tenderness, unusual drainage.	These are signs of infection. The body may be mounting a response to ward off offending pathogens.
Change IV line and site if evidence of infection is present and according to agency protocol (q48-72h).	These are standard infection control guidelines to prevent/ameliorate infection.
Evaluate patency of all surgically placed tubes or drains. Irrigate, gently "milk," or attach to low-pressure suction as prescribed. Promptly report unrelieved loss of patency.	These actions prevent stasis and reflux of body fluids, which can result in infection. "Milking" the tube, however, may not be allowed in some facilities.
Assess stability of tubes/drains.	Movement of improperly secured tubes and drains enables access of pathogens at insertion site.
Note color, character, and odor of all drainage. Report significant findings.	Foul-smelling, purulent, or abnormal drainage are indicators of infection.
Evaluate incisions and wound sites for unusual erythema, warmth, tenderness, induration, swelling, delayed healing, and purulent or excessive drainage.	These are indicators of localized infection.
Change dressings as prescribed, using "no touch" and sterile techniques. Prevent cross-contamination of wounds in same patient by changing one dressing at a time and washing hands between dressing changes.	These are standard infection control guidelines to prevent infection.
Be alert to patient complaints of a feeling of "letting go" or to a sudden profusion of serous drainage on or a bulge in the dressing.	It is likely that a wound dehiscence or evisceration has occurred. Wound infection and poor wound healing put patient at risk for wound dehiscence.
If patient develops evisceration, do not reinsert tissue or organs. Place a sterile, saline-soaked gauze over eviscerated tissues and cover with a sterile towel until the wound can be evaluated by health care provider.	Keeping viscera moist with a sterile towel increases viability of tissues and reduces risk of contamination and further infection.
Maintain patient on bedrest, usually in semi-Fowler's position with knees slightly bent. Keep patient NPO and anticipate need for IV therapy.	These actions provide comfort, prevent further evisceration, and prepare patient for surgery.
When appropriate, encourage use of intermittent catheterization q4-6h instead of indwelling catheter.	In most cases there is less risk of infection with intermittent than with indwelling catheterization, especially in patient's own home. Emptying the bladder routinely prevents stasis of urine and decreases presence of pathogens.
Keep drainage collection container below bladder level, avoiding kinks or obstructions in drainage tubing.	This intervention prevents both reflux of urine (and potential pathogens) into bladder and urinary stasis, either of which could lead to infection.
Do not open closed urinary drainage system unless absolutely necessary, and irrigate catheter only with health care provider's prescription and when obstruction is the known cause.	Keeping the system closed decreases risk of contamination and infection.
Assess patient for chills; fever (temperature higher than 37.7° C [100° F]); dysuria; urgency; frequency; flank, low back, suprapubic, buttock, inner thigh, scrotal, or labial pain; and cloudy or foul-smelling urine.	These are indicators of urinary tract infection (UTI), which signal that the body is mounting a response to ward off offending pathogens.
Encourage intake of 2-3 L/day in nonrestricted patients.	Increasing hydration minimizes potential for UTI by diluting the urine and maximizing urinary flow.
Ensure that perineum and meatus are cleansed during daily bath and perianal area is cleansed after bowel movements. Do not hesitate to remind patient of these hygiene measures.	Microorganisms can be introduced into the body via the catheter. Good hygiene decreases the number of microorganisms.
Be alert to meatal swelling, purulent drainage, and persistent meatal redness. Intervene if patient is unable to perform self-care.	These are indicators of meatal infection and potential UTI.
Change catheter according to established protocol or sooner if sandy particles can be felt in distal end of catheter or patient develops UTI. Change drainage collection container according to established protocol or sooner if it becomes foul smelling or leaks.	Because the catheter can be a source of infection, changing the system per protocol (usually every month) is customary.

Continued

INTERVENTIONS	RATIONALES
Obtain cultures of suspicious drainage or secretions (e.g., sputum, urine, wound) as prescribed. For urine specimens, be certain to use sampling port, which is at proximal end of drainage tube.	Cultures determine if an infection is present and direct therapy with an appropriate antibiotic if it is.
Cleanse area with an antimicrobial wipe and use a sterile syringe with 25-gauge needle to aspirate urine.	Larger-gauge needles form larger puncture holes that increase risk of compromising the sterile system.
Prevent transmission of infectious agents by washing hands well before and after caring for patient and by wearing gloves when contact with blood, drainage, or other body substance is likely.	Handwashing is an effective means of preventing microbial transmission. Wearing gloves protects the caregiver from the patient's body substances.
Use precautions (see "Infection Prevention and Control," Appendix A, p. 783, for patients colonized with methicillin-resistant *Staphylococcus aureus* (MRSA), vancomycin-resistant *Enterococcus* (VRE), or other epidemiologically important organisms.	Such precautions prevent cross contaminating from infectious sources to uninfected patients.

••• Related NIC and NOC labels: *NIC:* Infection Control; Infection Protection; Environmental Management; Incision Site Care; Infection Control: Intraoperative; Laboratory Data Interpretation; Respiratory Monitoring; Skin Surveillance; Specimen Management; Wound Care; Chest Physiotherapy; Perineal Care; Tube Care; Urinary Retention Care *NOC:* Infection Status; Wound Healing: Primary Intention

Nursing Diagnosis:

Constipation

related to immobility, opioid analgesics and other medications, dehydration, lack of privacy, disruption of abdominal musculature, or manipulation of abdominal viscera during surgery

Desired Outcome: Patient returns to his or her normal bowel elimination pattern as evidenced by return of active bowel sounds within 48-72 hr after most surgeries, absence of abdominal distention or sensation of fullness, and elimination of soft, formed stools.

INTERVENTIONS	RATIONALES
Monitor for and document elimination of flatus or stool.	This signals return of intestinal motility.
Assess for abdominal distention, tenderness, absent or hypoactive bowel sounds, and sensation of fullness. Report gross distention, extreme tenderness, and prolonged absence of bowel sounds.	Gross distention, extreme tenderness, and prolonged absence of bowel sounds are signs of decreased GI motility and possible ileus. High-pitched bowel sounds may indicate impending bowel obstruction.
Encourage in-bed position changes, exercises, and ambulation to patient's tolerance unless contraindicated.	These activities stimulate peristalsis, which promotes bowel elimination.
If an NG tube is in place, perform the following:	
- Check placement of tube after insertion, before any instillation, and q8h. For a larger-bore tube, aspirate gastric contents and assess for pH less than 5.0 for gastric tube placement. If the tube is in the trachea, patient may exhibit signs of respiratory distress or consistently low O_2 saturation levels, or there may be absence of drainage. Reposition tube immediately. Once assured of placement, mark tube to easily assess tube migration, and secure tubing in place. For smaller-bore tubes, check recent x-ray film to confirm position before instilling anything.	A malpositioned NG tube will be ineffective in relieving gastric distention.
- Keep tube securely taped to patient's nose and reinforce placement by attaching tube to patient's gown with safety pin or tape.	Securing the tube prevents its migration into the patient's airway.
- Measure and record quantity and quality of output, including color.	Typically the color will be green. For patients who have undergone gastric surgery, output may be brownish initially because of small amounts of bloody drainage but should change to green after about 12 hr.

Continued

INTERVENTIONS	RATIONALES
- Test reddish, brown, or black output for presence of blood. Reposition tube as necessary.	These colors may signal GI bleeding.
- **Note:** For patient with gastric, esophageal, or duodenal surgery, notify health care provider before manipulating tube.	Manipulation of NG tubes in these patients could result in disruption of the surgical anastomosis.
- Gently instill normal saline as prescribed.	This action helps maintain patency of GI tube.
- Ensure low, intermittent suction of gastric sump tubes by maintaining patency of sump port (usually blue). If sump port becomes occluded by gastric contents, flush sump port with air until a *whoosh* sound is heard over epigastric area.	When the port is open and air is entering the stomach, continuous suction is safe. If the port becomes occluded, the tube essentially becomes a single lumen tube and the continuous suction could damage the lining of the stomach.
- **Caution:** Never clamp or otherwise occlude sump port. For patient with gastric, esophageal, or duodenal surgery, notify health care provider before irrigating tube.	Excessive pressure may accumulate and damage gastric mucosa or disrupt the surgical anastomosis.
- When tube is removed, monitor patient for abdominal distention, nausea, and vomiting.	These are signs that GI motility is still decreased and requires further intervention.
Monitor and document patient's response to diet advancement from clear liquids to a regular or other prescribed diet.	Poor response to diet advancement as evidenced by abdominal distention, nausea, and vomiting may signal continued decreased GI motility and should be reported for timely intervention. Postoperatively, decreased GI motility can result from stress (autonomic), surgical manipulation of the intestine, immobility, and effects of medications.
Encourage oral fluid intake (more than 2500 ml/day), especially intake of prune juice.	Increased hydration, including prune juice, helps promote soft stools that will minimize need to strain.
Administer stool softeners, mild laxatives, senna-based herbal teas, and enemas as prescribed. As appropriate, encourage high-fiber diet (fresh vegetables and fruits). Monitor and record results.	These interventions promote bulk and softness in stools for easier evacuation.
Arrange periods of privacy during patient's attempts at bowel elimination.	Privacy promotes relaxation and success with defecation.

••• **Related NIC and NOC labels:** *NIC:* Bowel Management; Diet Staging; Exercise Promotion; Fluid Management; Medication Management; Enteral Tube Feeding *NOC:* Bowel Elimination; Hydration; Symptom Control

Nursing Diagnosis:

Disturbed Sleep Pattern

related to preoperative anxiety, stress, postoperative pain, noise, and altered environment

Desired Outcome: Following intervention/treatment, patient relates minimal or no difficulty with falling asleep and describes a feeling of being well rested.

INTERVENTIONS	RATIONALES
Administer sedative/hypnotic as prescribed. Monitor for CNS and respiratory depressant effects of opioid analgesics.	Sedative/hypnotics may cause CNS depression and contribute to the respiratory depressant effects of opioid analgesics. Active metabolites of many of the benzodiazepines may accumulate and result in greater physiologic effects or toxicity. As well, there is a greater incidence of sleep disruption in older adults with chronic illnesses who take this combination of drugs.
Caution: Use special caution when administering sedative/hypnotic to patients with COPD. Monitor respiratory function, including oximetry, at frequent intervals in these patients.	Sedative hypnotics could cause respiratory depression in patients who already have inadequate ventilation.

Continued

INTERVENTIONS	RATIONALES
After administering sedative/hypnotic, be certain to raise side rails, lower bed to its lowest position, and caution patient not to smoke in bed.	Patient will become drowsy, which necessitates these safety measures.
Administer analgesics at bedtime.	This action reduces nighttime pain and augments effects of hypnotic to promote sleep.
Be certain that consent for surgery is signed before administering sedative/hypnotic.	Patient should sign legal document only when alert and cognizant of its contents.
Use nonpharmacologic measures to promote sleep.	Behavioral interventions are the preferred method for insomnia because of their established efficacy and absence of drug side effects.

••• **Related NIC and NOC labels:** *NIC:* Sleep Enhancement; Environmental Management; Medication Administration; Pain Management
NOC: Sleep

Nursing Diagnosis:

Impaired Physical Mobility

related to postoperative pain, decreased strength and endurance secondary to CNS effects of anesthesia or blood loss, musculoskeletal or neuromuscular impairment secondary to disease process or surgical procedure, perceptual impairment secondary to disease process or surgical procedure (e.g., ocular surgery, neurosurgery), or cognitive deficit secondary to disease process or effects of opioid analgesics and anesthetics

Desired Outcome: Optimally, by hospital discharge (depending on type of surgery), patient returns to preoperative baseline physical mobility as evidenced by ability to move in bed, transfer, and ambulate independently or with minimal assistance.

INTERVENTIONS	RATIONALES
Assess patient's preoperative physical mobility by evaluating coordination and muscle strength, control, and mass.	Preoperative/baseline assessments enable accurate measurements of postoperative mobility problems.
Be aware of medically imposed restrictions against movement, especially with conditions or surgeries that are orthopedic, neurosurgical, or ocular.	Restricting movement and certain positions can prevent disruption of the surgical repair.
Evaluate and correct factors limiting physical mobility.	Factors such as oversedation with opioid analgesics, failure to achieve adequate pain control, and poorly arranged physical environment can be corrected.
Initiate movement from bed to chair and ambulation as soon as possible after surgery, depending on postoperative prescriptions, type of surgery, and patient's recovery from anesthetics.	Patient usually can tolerate a graduated progression in activity and ambulation.
Assist patient with moving slowly to a sitting position in bed and then standing at bedside before attempting ambulation. For more information, see **Ineffective Tissue Perfusion: Cerebral,** p. 66.	Many anesthetic agents depress normal vasoconstrictor mechanisms and can result in sudden hypotension with quick changes in position.
Encourage frequent movement and ambulation by postoperative patients. Provide assistance as indicated.	These actions reduce potential for postoperative complications, including atelectasis, pneumonia, thrombophlebitis, skin breakdown, muscle weakness, and depressed GI motility.
Teach exercises that can be performed in bed and explain their purpose.	Exercises such as gluteal and quadriceps muscle sets (isometrics) and ankle circling and calf pumping promote muscle strength, increase venous return, and prevent stasis.
For additional information, see "Prolonged Bedrest" for **Risk for Activity Intolerance,** p. 61, and **Risk for Disuse Syndrome,** p. 63.	

••• **Related NIC and NOC labels:** *NIC:* Exercise Promotion: Ambulation; Energy Management; Fall Prevention; Pain Management
NOC: Mobility Level

Nursing Diagnosis

Risk for Trauma

related to weakness, balancing difficulties, and reduced muscle coordination secondary to anesthetics and postoperative opioid analgesics

Desired outcome: Patient does not fall and remains free of trauma as evidenced by absence of bruises, wounds, and fractures.

INTERVENTIONS	RATIONALES
Orient and reorient patient to person, place, and time during initial postoperative period. Inform patient that surgery is over. Repeat information until patient is fully awake and oriented (usually several hours but may be days in heavily sedated or otherwise obtunded individuals).	Orientation and repeated explanations increase mental awareness and alertness, which decrease risk of trauma caused by disorientation. These measures also help patient cope with unfamiliar surroundings.
Maintain side rails on stretchers and beds in upright and locked positions.	Side rails help prevent trauma to head and extremities. Some individuals experience agitation and thrash about as they emerge from anesthesia.
Secure all IV lines, drains, and tubing.	This action prevents their dislodgement.
Maintain bed in its lowest position when leaving patient's room.	This action protects patient from major trauma in case he or she falls out of bed.
Place call mechanism within patient's reach; instruct patient in its use.	Patient can call for help when it is needed, for example, when needing to use the toilet. This will reduce risk of falls and injury.
Identify patients at risk for falling. Correct or compensate for risk factors.	Risk factors include the following:
	- *Time of day:* Night shift, peak activity periods such as meals, bedtime.
	- *Medications:* Opioid analgesics, sedatives, hypnotics, and anesthetics.
	- *Impaired mobility:* Individuals requiring assistance with transfer and ambulation.
	- *Sensory deficits:* Diminished visual acuity caused by disease process or environmental factors; changes in kinesthetic sense because of disease or trauma.
Use restraints and protective devices if necessary and prescribed.	These devices provide protection during an emergent state. However, because they can cause agitation, their use should be infrequent and as a last resort. Behavioral intervention or a patient sitter is preferred.

••• **Related NIC and NOC labels:** *NIC:* Environmental Management: Safety; Fall Prevention; Risk Identification *NOC:* Safety Status: Physical Injury

Nursing Diagnosis:

Risk for Impaired Skin Integrity

related to presence of secretions/excretions around percutaneous drains and tubes

Desired Outcome: Patient's skin around percutaneous drains and tubes remains intact and nonerythematous.

INTERVENTIONS	RATIONALES
Change dressings as soon as they become wet. (The health care provider may prefer to perform the first dressing change at the surgical incision.) Use sterile technique for all dressing changes.	These interventions protect the wound from contamination and accumulation of fluids that may cause excoriation.
Keep area around drains as clean as possible.	Intestinal secretions, bile, and similar drainage can lead quickly to skin excoriation (pepsin, conjugated bile acids, gastric acid, and lysolecithin all have a low [acidic] pH of 1-3). Sterile normal saline or a solution of saline and hydrogen peroxide or other prescribed solution may be used to clean around drain site.
If some external drainage is present, position a pectin-wafer skin barrier around drain or tube. Ointments, such as zinc oxide, petrolatum, and aluminum paste, also may be used.	Skin barriers and ointments are used to protect the skin from drainage that could cause breakdown because of caustic enzymes, especially from the small bowel.
Consult wound, ostomy, continence (WOC) enterostomal therapy (ET) nurse as indicated.	These nurses provide specialized interventions if drainage is excessive, skin excoriation develops, or a collection bag needs to be placed over drains and incisions.
For additional information, see "Managing Wound Care," p. 559.	

••• **Related NIC and NOC labels:** *NIC:* Skin Surveillance; Incision Site Care; Infection Control; Infection Protection; Skin Care: Topical Treatments; Wound Care *NOC:* Tissue Integrity: Skin & Mucous Membranes

Nursing Diagnosis:

Impaired Oral Mucous Membrane

related to NPO status and/or presence of NG or endotracheal tube

Desired Outcome: At time of hospital discharge, patient's oral mucosa is intact, without pain or evidence of bleeding.

INTERVENTIONS	RATIONALES
Provide oral care and oral hygiene q4h and prn. Arrange for patient to gargle, brush teeth, and cleanse mouth with sponge-tipped applicators as necessary.	Oral care provides comfort and prevents excoriation and excessive dryness of oral mucous membrane.
Use a moistened cotton-tipped applicator to remove encrustations. Carefully lubricate lips and nares with antimicrobial ointment or emollient cream.	These interventions provide comfort and decrease risk of tissue breakdown caused by dry tissues.
If indicated, obtain a prescription for lidocaine gargling solution.	This solution provides comfort if patient's throat tissue is irritated from presence of an NG tube.

••• **Related NIC and NOC labels:** *NIC:* Oral Health Maintenance *NOC:* Tissue Integrity: Skin & Mucous Membranes

ADDITIONAL NURSING DIAGNOSES/ PROBLEMS:

"Pain"	p. 39
"Pneumonia"	p. 123
"Venous Thrombosis/Thrombophlebitis"	p. 201
"Managing Wound Care"	p. 559
"Providing Nutritional Support"	p. 565

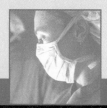

Prolonged Bedrest   4

OVERVIEW/PATHOPHYSIOLOGY

Patients on prolonged bedrest face many potential physiologic problems. Some are short term and easily corrected. Others, such as joint contractures, may result in permanent disability. This section reviews the most common physiologic and psychosocial problems that may occur. With patients being discharged from the hospital sooner than they used to be, many of these problems now are seen when the patient is transferred to a long-term care facility or when discharged to home.

HEALTH CARE SETTING

Extended care, acute care, home care

Nursing Diagnosis:

Risk for Activity Intolerance

related to deconditioned status

Desired Outcomes: Within 48 hr of discontinuing bedrest, patient exhibits cardiac tolerance to activity or exercise as evidenced by HR 20 bpm or less over resting HR; SBP 20 mm Hg or less over or under resting SBP; RR 20 breaths/min or less with normal depth and pattern (eupnea); normal sinus rhythm; warm and dry skin; and absence of crackles (rales), new murmurs, new dysrhythmias, gallop, or chest pain. Patient rates perceived exertion (RPE) at 3 or less on a scale of 0 (none) to 10 (maximal).

INTERVENTIONS	RATIONALES
Perform range-of-motion (ROM) exercises 2-4 times/day on each extremity. Individualize the exercise plan based on the following guidelines.	These exercises build stamina by increasing muscle strength and endurance and prevent physiologic problems such as contractures and pressure damage to skin caused by inactivity.
Caution: Avoid isometric exercises in cardiac patients.	These exercises can increase systemic arterial blood pressure.
Mode or type of exercise: Begin with passive exercises, moving the joints through the motions of abduction, adduction, flexion, and extension. Progress to active-assisted exercises in which you support the joints while patient initiates muscle contraction. When patient is able, supervise him or her in active isotonic exercises, during which patient contracts a selected muscle group, moves the extremity at a slow pace, and then relaxes the muscle group. Have patient repeat each exercise 3-10 times.	Beginning with passive movement, progressing to active-assisted, and continuing with active isotonic takes patient from the least exerting to the most exerting exercises over a period of time, thus enabling gradual tolerance.
Caution: Stop any exercise that results in muscular or skeletal pain. Consult a physical therapist (PT) about necessary modifications.	This action prevents injury in a joint too inflamed or diseased to tolerate this type of exercise intensity.
Intensity: Begin with 3-5 repetitions as tolerated by patient.	Starting with minimal intensity and progressing step-by-step to more intensity enables gradual tolerance.
- Measure HR and BP at rest, peak exercise, and 5 min after exercise.	These assessments help determine tolerance to the exercise. If HR or SBP increases more than 20 bpm or more than 20 mm Hg over resting level, the number of repetitions should be decreased. If HR or SBP decreases more than 10 bpm or more than 10 mm Hg at peak exercise, this could be a sign of left ventricular failure, denoting that the heart cannot meet this workload. For other adverse signs and symptoms, see *Assessment of exercise tolerance.*

Continued

INTERVENTION	RATIONALES
Duration: Begin with 5 min or less of exercise. Gradually increase the exercise to 15 min as tolerated.	Starting with minimal duration and progressing to greater duration enables gradual tolerance.
Frequency: Begin with exercises 2-4 times/day.	As duration increases, the frequency can be reduced.
Assessment of exercise tolerance: Be alert to signs and symptoms that the cardiovascular and respiratory systems are unable to meet the demands of the low-level ROM exercises.	Excessive shortness of breath may occur if (1) transient pulmonary congestion occurs secondary to ischemia or left ventricular dysfunction, (2) lung volumes are decreased, (3) oxygen-carrying capacity of the blood is reduced, or (4) there is shunting of blood from the right to the left side of the heart without adequate oxygenation. If cardiac output does not increase to meet the body's needs during modest levels of exercise, SBP may fall; the skin may become cool, cyanotic, and diaphoretic; dysrhythmias may be noted; crackles (rales) may be auscultated; or a systolic murmur of mitral regurgitation may occur.
If patient tolerates the exercise, increase intensity or number of repetitions each day.	Tolerance is a sign that cardiovascular and respiratory systems are able to meet the demands of these low-level ROM exercises.
Ask patient to rate perceived exertion experienced during exercise, basing it on the following scale developed by Borg (1982). 0 = Nothing at all 1 = Very weak effort 2 = Weak (light) effort 3 = Moderate effort 4 = Somewhat stronger effort 5 = Strong effort 7 = Very strong effort 9 = Very, very strong effort 10 = Maximal effort	Exercises to prevent deconditioning should be performed at low levels of effort. Patient should not experience an RPE greater than 3 while performing ROM exercises. Intensity of the exercise should be reduced and the frequency increased until an RPE of 3 or less is attained.
As patient's condition improves, increase activity as soon as possible to include sitting in a chair.	To promote optimal conditioning, activity should be increased to correspond to patient's increased tolerance.
Assess for orthostatic hypotension. Prepare patient for this change by increasing the amount of time spent in high Fowler's position and moving patient slowly and in stages.	Orthostatic hypotension can occur as a result of decreased plasma volume and difficulty in adjusting immediately to postural change. For more information about orthostatic hypotension, see **Ineffective Tissue Perfusion: Cerebral.**
Progress activity in hospitalized patients as follows. **Level I: Bedrest** • Flexion and extension of extremities 4 times/day, 15 times each extremity • Deep breathing 4 times/day, 15 breaths • Position change from side to side q2h **Level II: Out of bed to chair** • As tolerated, 3 times/day for 20-30 min • May perform ROM exercises 2 times/day while sitting in chair **Level III: Ambulate in room** • As tolerated, 3 times/day for 3-5 min in room **Level IV: Ambulate in hall** • Initially, 50-200 ft 2 times/day, progressing to 600 ft 4 times/day • May incorporate slow stair climbing in preparation for hospital discharge • Monitor for signs of activity intolerance	Signs of activity intolerance include decrease in BP more than 20 mm Hg, increase in HR to more than 120 bpm (or more than 20 bpm above resting HR in patients receiving beta-blocker therapy), and shortness of breath (discussed earlier).

Continued

INTERVENTION	RATIONALES
Have patient perform self-care activities as tolerated.	Self-care activities such as eating, mouth care, and bathing may increase patient's activity level.
Teach patient's significant other the purpose of and interventions for preventing deconditioning. Involve him or her in patient's plan of care.	Significant others can promote and participate in patient's activity/exercises once they understand the rationale and are familiar with the interventions.
Provide emotional support to patient and significant other as patient's activity level is increased.	Emotional support helps allay fears of failure, pain, or medical setbacks.

••• **Related NIC and NOC labels:** *NIC:* Energy Management; Exercise Promotion: Strength Training; Exercise Therapy: Ambulation; Exercise Therapy: Joint Mobility; Exercise Therapy: Muscle Control; Vital Signs Monitoring; Emotional Support; Teaching: Prescribed Activity/Exercise *NOC:* Activity Tolerance; Endurance

Nursing Diagnosis:

Risk for Disuse Syndrome

related to paralysis, mechanical immobilization, prescribed immobilization, severe pain, or altered level of consciousness

Desired Outcomes: When bedrest is discontinued, patient exhibits complete ROM of all joints without pain, and limb girth measurements are congruent with or increased over baseline measurements.

Note: ROM exercises should be performed at least 2 times/day for all immobilized patients with normal joints. Modification may be required for patient with flaccidity (e.g., immediately after stroke or spinal cord injury [SCI]) to prevent subluxation, or for patient with spasticity (e.g., during the recovery period for patient with stroke or SCI) to prevent an increase in spasticity. Consult PT or occupational therapist (OT) for assistance in modifying the exercise plan for these patients. Also, be aware that ROM exercises are restricted or contraindicated for patients with rheumatologic disease during the inflammatory phase and for joints that are dislocated or fractured.

INTERVENTIONS	RATIONALES
During assessment of patient's joints, pay special attention to the following areas: shoulder, wrist, fingers, hips, knees, and feet.	These areas are especially susceptible to joint contracture. Shoulders can become "frozen" to limit abduction and extension; wrists can "drop," prohibiting extension; fingers can develop flexion contractures that limit extension; hips can develop flexion contractures that affect the gait by shortening the limb or develop external rotation or adduction deformities that affect the gait; knees may have flexion contractures that can develop to limit extension and alter the gait; and feet can "drop" as a result of prolonged plantar flexion, which limits dorsiflexion and alters the gait.
Ensure that patient changes position at least q2h. Post a turning schedule at patient's bedside.	Position changes not only maintain correct body alignment, thereby reducing strain on the joints, but also prevent contractures, minimize pressure on bony prominences, decrease venostasis, and promote maximal chest expansion.
Try to place patient in a position that achieves proper standing. Maintain this position with pillows, towels, or other positioning aids.	A position in which the head is neutral or slightly flexed on the neck, hips are extended, knees are extended or minimally flexed, and feet are at right angles to the legs achieves proper standing alignment, which helps promote ambulation when patient is ready to do so.
Ensure that patient is prone or side lying, with hips extended, for the same amount of time that patient spends in the supine position or, at a minimum, 3 times/day for 1 hr.	These positions prevent hip flexion contractures.
When the head of bed (HOB) must be elevated 30 degrees, extend patient's shoulders and arms, using pillows to support the position.	This position maintains proper spinal posture.
Allow patient's fingertips to extend over pillow's edge.	This position maintains normal arching of the hands.

Continued

INTERVENTIONS	RATIONALES
Caution: Ensure that patient spends time with hips in extension (see preceding intervention).	This position helps prevent hip flexion contracture.
When patient is in the side-lying position, extend the lower leg from the hip.	This position helps prevent hip flexion contracture.
When patient can be placed in the prone position, move him or her to the end of the bed and allow the feet to rest between the mattress and footboard.	This prevents not only plantar flexion and hip rotation, but also injury to heels and toes.
Place thin pads under the angles of the axillae and lateral aspects of the clavicles.	These pads help prevent internal rotation of the shoulders and maintain anatomic position of the shoulder girdle.
Use positioning devices liberally.	Using pillows, rolled towels, blankets, sandbags, antirotation boots, splints, and orthotics helps maintain joints in neutral position, which helps ensure that they remain functional when activity is increased.
When using adjunctive devices, monitor involved skin at frequent intervals.	Assessing for alterations in skin integrity enables prompt interventions that prevent skin breakdown.
Assess for footdrop by inspecting the feet for plantar flexion and evaluating patient's ability to pull toes upward toward the head. Document this assessment daily.	Footdrop may occur with prolonged plantar flexion. However, because feet lie naturally in plantar flexion, assess for patient's inability to dorsiflex (pull the toes up toward the head). This is a sign of footdrop, and it requires prompt intervention to prevent or ameliorate permanent damage.
Teach patient and significant other the rationale and procedure for ROM exercises, and have patient give return demonstrations. Review **Risk for Activity Intolerance,** p. 61, to ensure that patient does not exceed his or her tolerance. Provide passive exercises for patients unable to perform active or active-assisted exercises. In addition, incorporate movement patterns into care activities, such as position changes, bed baths, getting patient on and off the bedpan, or changing patient's gown. Ensure that joints especially susceptible to contracture are exercised more stringently.	These actions facilitate adherence to the exercise regimen and help prevent contracture formation.
Provide patient with a handout that reviews exercises and lists repetitions for each. Instruct the significant other to encourage patient to perform exercises as required.	These actions facilitate learning and adherence to the exercise program.
Perform and document limb girth measurements, dynamography, and ROM, and establish exercise baseline limits.	This assessment of existing muscle mass, strength, and joint motion enables subsequent evaluation and promotes exercise and ROM appropriate for patient.
Explain to patient how muscle atrophy occurs. Emphasize the importance of maintaining or increasing muscle strength and periarticular tissue elasticity through exercise. If there are complicating pathologic conditions, consult the health care provider about the appropriate form of exercise for patient.	Muscle atrophy occurs because of disuse or failure to use the joint, often caused by immediate or anticipated pain. This explanation encourages patient to perform exercises inasmuch as disuse eventually may result in decreased muscle mass and blood supply and a loss of periarticular tissue elasticity, which in turn can lead to increased muscle fatigue and joint pain with use.
Explain the need to participate maximally in self-care as tolerated.	Self-care helps maintain muscle strength and promote a sense of participation and control.
For noncardiac patients needing greater help with muscle strength, assist with resistive exercises (e.g., moderate weight lifting to increase size, endurance, and strength of the muscles). For patients in beds with Balkan frames, provide a means for resistive exercise by implementing a system of weights and pulleys.	Resistance increases the force needed to perform the exercise and promotes the maintenance or rebuilding of muscle strength.
First, determine patient's baseline level of performance on a given set of exercises, then set realistic goals with patient for repetitions (e.g., if patient can do 5 repetitions of lifting a 5-lb weight with the biceps muscle, the goal may be to increase repetitions to 10 within 1 wk, to an ultimate goal of 20 within 3 wk, and then advance to 7.5-lb weights).	Well-planned goals provide markers for assessing effectiveness of the exercise plan and progress made.

Continued

INTERVENTIONS	RATIONALES
If the joints require rest, teach isometric exercises.	In these exercises, patient contracts a muscle group and holds the contraction for a count of 5 or 10. The sequence is repeated for increasing counts or repetitions until an adequate level of endurance has been achieved. Thereafter, maintenance levels are performed.
Provide a chart to show patient progress, and combine this with large amounts of positive reinforcement.	Attaining progress and having positive reinforcement promote continued adherence to the exercise plan.
Post the exercise regimen at the bedside. Instruct the significant other in the exercise regimen, and elicit his or her support and encouragement of patient's performance of the exercises.	These actions ensure consistency by all health care personnel and involvement and support of significant others.
As appropriate, teach transfer or crutch-walking techniques and use of a walker, wheelchair, or cane. Include the significant other in demonstrations, and stress the importance of good body mechanics.	These interventions help ensure that patient can maintain highest possible level of mobility.
Provide periods of uninterrupted rest between exercises/activities.	Rest enables patient to replenish energy stores.
Seek referral to PT or OT as appropriate.	Such a referral will help patient who has special needs or who is not in a care facility to attain the best ROM possible.

••• **Related NIC and NOC labels:** *NIC:* Activity Therapy; Energy Management; Exercise Promotion; Risk Identification; Sleep Enhancement; Teaching: Prescribed Activity/Exercise; Exercise Therapy: Joint Mobility; Exercise Therapy: Muscle Control; Exercise Therapy: Ambulation; Positioning *NOC:* Endurance; Immobility Consequences: Physiological; Mobility Level

Nursing Diagnosis:

Ineffective Tissue Perfusion: Peripheral

related to interrupted venous flow secondary to prolonged immobility

Desired Outcomes: At least 24 hr before hospital discharge, patient has adequate peripheral perfusion as evidenced by normal skin color and temperature and adequate distal pulses (greater than 2+ on a 0-4+ scale) in peripheral extremities. Patient performs exercises independently, adheres to the prophylactic regimen, and maintains intake of 2-3 L/day of fluid unless contraindicated.

INTERVENTIONS	RATIONALES
Teach patient that pain, redness, swelling, and warmth in the involved area and coolness, edema, unnatural color or pallor, and superficial venous dilation distal to the involved area should be reported to a staff member promptly if they occur.	These are indicators of deep vein thrombosis (DVT). A knowledgeable patient is likely to report these indicators promptly for timely intervention.
Monitor for indicators just listed, along with routine vital sign (VS) checks. If patient is asymptomatic for DVT, assess for positive Homans' sign: flex knee 30 degrees and dorsiflex the foot.	Pain elicited with dorsiflexion may be a sign of DVT, and patient should be referred to his or her health care provider for further evaluation.
	Additional signs of DVT may include fever, tachycardia, and elevated erythrocyte sedimentation rate (ESR). Normal ESR (Westergren method) in males younger than 50 yr is 0-15 mm/hr, and older than 50 yr is 0-20 mm/hr; in females younger than 50 yr it is 0-20 mm/hr, and older than 50 yr it is 0-30 mm/hr.
Perform passive ROM or encourage active ROM exercises.	These exercises increase circulation, which promotes peripheral tissue perfusion.
Teach patient calf-pumping (ankle dorsiflexion-plantar flexion) and ankle-circling exercises.	Same as above. Patient should repeat each movement 10 times, performing each exercise hourly during extended periods of immobility, as long as the patient is free of symptoms of DVT.
Encourage deep breathing.	Deep breathing increases negative pressure in the lungs and thorax to promote emptying of large veins and thus increase peripheral tissue perfusion.

Continued

INTERVENTIONS	RATIONALES
When not contraindicated by peripheral vascular disease (PVD), ensure that the patient wears antiembolism hose, pneumatic foot pump devices, or pneumatic sequential compression stockings.	These garments/devices prevent venous stasis, the precursor to DVT. The pneumatic devices, which provide more compression than antiembolism hose, are especially useful in preventing DVT in patients who are mostly immobile.
Remove hose for 10-20 min q8h. Reapply hose after elevating patient's legs at least 10 degrees for 10 min.	Removing hose enables inspection of underlying skin for evidence of irritation or breakdown. Elevating the legs before reapplying the hose promotes venous return and decreases edema, which otherwise would remain and cause discomfort when the hose are reapplied.
Instruct patient not to cross the feet at the ankles or knees while in bed.	These actions may cause venous stasis.
If patient is at risk for DVT, elevate the foot of the bed 10 degrees.	Elevating the foot of the bed increases venous return.
In nonrestricted patient, increase fluid intake to at least 2-3 L/day. Educate patient about the need to drink large amounts of fluid (9-14 8-oz glasses) daily. Monitor input and output (I&O) to ensure adherence.	Increased hydration reduces hemoconcentration, which can contribute to development of DVT.
Administer anticlotting medication as prescribed.	Patients at risk for DVT, including those with chronic infection and history of PVD and smoking, as well as patients who are older, obese, and anemic, may require anticoagulants to minimize risk of clotting. Drugs such as aspirin, sodium warfarin, phenindione derivatives, heparin, or low-molecular-weight heparin (LMWH; e.g., enoxaparin sodium) may be given. Many patients are taught how to self-administer LMWH injections after hospital discharge.
Monitor appropriate laboratory values (e.g., prothrombin time [PT], partial thromboplastin time [PTT]).	Optimal laboratory values are 10-13.5 sec for PT and 60-70 sec or 1.5-2.5 × control value if on anticoagulant therapy for PTT. Values higher than these signify that patient is at increased risk for bleeding.
Educate patient to self-monitor for and report bleeding.	Anticoagulant drugs increase risk of bleeding. It is important for patient to know signs of bleeding so that he or she can report them as soon as they are noted to ensure timely intervention. Possible types of bleeding include epistaxis, bleeding gums, hematemesis, hemoptysis, melena, hematuria, hematochezia, menometrorrhagia, and ecchymoses.
Teach medication and food interactions that can affect warfarin.	This information will reduce the possibility of drug and/or food interactions in patients taking warfarin. Examples include foods high in vitamin K (interfere with anticoagulation) and drugs such as aspirin (enhance response to warfarin) and diuretics (decrease response to warfarin). Many over-the-counter herbals can prolong bleeding.
In patients susceptible to DVT, acquire bilateral baseline measurements of mid-calf, knee, and mid-thigh, and record them on patient's Kardex. Monitor these measurements daily and compare them with baseline measurements.	These assessments monitor for extremity enlargement caused by DVT.

●●● **Related NIC and NOC labels:** *NIC:* Circulatory Care: Venous Insufficiency; Skin Surveillance; Bed Rest Care; Circulatory Precautions; Positioning; Pressure Management; Fluid Management; Pneumatic Tourniquet Precautions; Embolus Care: Peripheral *NOC:* Tissue Integrity: Skin and Mucous Membranes; Tissue Perfusion: Peripheral

Nursing Diagnosis:

Ineffective Tissue Perfusion: Cerebral

(orthostatic hypotension) *related to* interrupted arterial flow to the brain secondary to prolonged bedrest

Desired Outcome: When getting out of bed, patient has adequate cerebral perfusion as evidenced by HR less than 120 bpm and BP 90/60 mm Hg or greater (or within 20 mm Hg of patient's normal range) immediately after position change, dry skin, normal skin color, and absence of vertigo and syncope, with return of HR and BP to resting levels within 3 min of position change.

INTERVENTIONS	**RATIONALES**
Assess patient for recent diuresis, diaphoresis, or change in vasodilator therapy.	These are factors that increase risk of orthostatic hypotension because of fluid volume changes. For example, bedrest incurs a diuresis of about 600-800 ml during the first 3 days. Although this fluid decrease is not noticed when patient is supine, the lost volume will be evident (i.e., with orthostatic hypotension) when the body tries to adapt to sitting and standing.
Also be alert to diabetic cardiac neuropathy, denervation after heart transplantation, advanced age, or severe left ventricular dysfunction.	These are factors that increase risk of orthostatic hypotension because of altered autonomic control.
Explain cause of orthostatic hypotension and measures for preventing it.	Patients who are informed as to cause and ways of preventing orthostatic hypotension are more likely to avoid it. Measures to prevent orthostatic hypotension are discussed in subsequent interventions.
Apply antiembolism hose once patient is mobilized.	Used to prevent DVT, antiembolism hose also may be useful in preventing orthostatic hypotension by promoting venous return once patient is mobilized. It may be necessary to supplement the hose with elastic wraps to the groin when patient is out of bed. These wraps should encompass the entire surface of the legs.
When patient is in bed, provide instructions for leg exercises as described under **Risk for Activity Intolerance,** p. 61. Encourage patient to perform leg exercises immediately before mobilization.	Leg exercises promote venous return, which help prevent orthostatic hypotension.
Prepare patient for getting out of bed by encouraging position changes within necessary confines.	Position changes help reacclimate patient to upright position. It is sometimes possible and advisable to use a tilt table.
Follow these guidelines for mobilization:	
Check BP in any high-risk patient for whom this will be the first time out of bed. Instruct patient to report immediately symptoms of lightheadedness or dizziness.	Low BP, lightheadedness, and dizziness are signs of orthostatic hypotension and necessitate a return to the supine position.
Be alert to a drop in SBP of 20 mm Hg or greater and an increased pulse rate, combined with symptoms of vertigo and impending syncope.	These are signs of orthostatic hypotension that signal the need for return to the supine position.
Have patient dangle the legs at bedside. Be alert to indicators of orthostatic hypotension, including diaphoresis, pallor, tachycardia, hypotension, and syncope. Question patient about the presence of lightheadedness or dizziness. Again, encourage performance of leg exercises.	This action provides for a gradual adjustment to the possible effects of venous pooling and related hypotension in persons who have been supine or in Fowler's position for some time. Dangling of the legs may be necessary until intravascular fluid volume is restored. It also provides an opportunity for leg exercises that can reduce risk of venous stasis.
If leg dangling is tolerated, have patient stand at the bedside with two staff members in attendance. If no adverse signs or symptoms occur, have patient progress to ambulation as tolerated.	This intervention helps ensure patient's safety in the event of a fall.

••• **Related NIC and NOC labels:** *NIC:* Circulatory Care: Arterial Insufficiency; Cerebral Perfusion Promotion; Positioning; Vital Signs Monitoring; Circulatory Care: Venous Insufficiency *NOC:* Circulation Status; Tissue Perfusion: Cerebral

Nursing Diagnosis:

Constipation

related to less than adequate fluid or dietary intake and bulk, immobility, lack of privacy, positional restrictions, and use of opioid analgesics

Desired Outcomes: Within 24 hr of this diagnosis, patient verbalizes knowledge of measures that promote bowel elimination. Patient relates return of normal pattern and character of bowel elimination within 3-5 days of this diagnosis.

INTERVENTIONS	RATIONALES
Assess patient's bowel history.	This assessment determines patient's normal bowel habits and interventions that are used successfully at home.
Monitor and document patient's bowel movements, diet, and I&O.	This information tracks bowel movements and factors that promote or prevent constipation.
	Indications of constipation include the following: fewer than patient's usual number of bowel movements, abdominal discomfort or distention, straining at stool, and patient complaints of rectal pressure or fullness. Fecal impaction may be manifested by oozing of liquid stool and confirmed via digital examination.
Auscultate each abdominal quadrant for at least 1 min to determine presence of bowel sounds.	Bowel sounds are gurgles occurring normally at a rate of 5-32/min. Bowel sounds are decreased or absent with paralytic ileus. High-pitched rushing sounds or "tinkles" may be heard during abdominal cramping and may signal intestinal obstruction.
If rectal impaction is suspected, use a gloved, lubricated finger to remove stool from the rectum.	Digital stimulation may be adequate to promote bowel movement. Oil retention enemas may soften impacted stool.
Teach patient the importance of a high-fiber diet and a fluid intake of at least 2-3 L/day (unless this is contraindicated by a renal, hepatic, or cardiac disorder).	These measures increase peristalsis and likelihood of normal bowel movements. High-fiber foods include bran, whole grains, nuts, and raw and coarse vegetables and fruits with skins.
	Good hydration softens the stool, making it easier to evacuate. Patients with renal, hepatic, or cardiac disorders may be on fluid restrictions.
Maintain patient's normal bowel habits whenever possible by offering a bedpan; ensuring privacy; and timing medications, enemas, or suppositories so that they take effect at the time of day when patient normally has a bowel movement.	These actions may facilitate regularity of bowel movements.
Provide warm fluids before breakfast, and encourage toileting.	These measures take advantage of patient's gastrocolic and duodenocolic reflexes.
Maximize patient's activity level within limitations of endurance, therapy, and pain.	Increased activity promotes peristalsis, which helps prevent constipation.
Request pharmacologic interventions from the health care provider when necessary. To help prevent rebound constipation, make a priority list of interventions to ensure minimal disruption of patient's normal bowel habits.	Starting with the gentlest interventions helps prevent rebound constipation and ensures minimal disruption of patient's normal bowel habits.
	The following is a suggested hierarchy of interventions:
	- Bulk-building additives (psyllium), bran
	- Mild laxatives (apple or prune juice, milk of magnesia)
	- Stool softeners (docusate sodium, docusate calcium)
	- Potent laxatives and cathartics (bisacodyl, cascara sagrada)
	- Medicated suppositories
	- Enemas
Discuss the role that opioid agents and other medications play in causing constipation.	Opioids, antidepressants, anticholinergics, iron supplements, diuretics, and muscle relaxants are known to cause constipation.
Teach nonpharmacologic methods of pain control. See discussion in "Pain," p. 43.	Alternative, nontoxic methods of pain control may decrease the need for opioid analgesics and hence the likelihood of constipation caused by opioid analgesics.

●●● **Related NIC and NOC labels:** *NIC:* Bowel Management; Constipation/Impaction Management; Exercise Promotion; Fluid Management; Medication Management; Nutrition Management; Self-Care Assistance: Toileting *NOC:* Bowel Elimination; Hydration

Nursing Diagnosis:
Deficient Diversional Activity

related to prolonged illness and hospitalization

Desired Outcome: Within 24 hr of intervention, patient engages in diversional activities and relates absence of boredom.

INTERVENTIONS	RATIONALES
Be alert to patient wishing for something to read or do, daytime napping, and expressed inability to perform usual hobbies because of hospitalization.	These are indicators of boredom.
Assess patient's activity tolerance as described on p. 62.	Activity tolerance will determine the amount of activity a patient can engage in within limits of his or her diagnosis.
Collect a database by assessing patient's normal support systems and relationship patterns with significant others. Question patient and significant other about patient's interests.	This enables the nurse to explore diversional activities that may be suitable for the health care setting and patient's level of activity tolerance.
Personalize patient's environment with favorite objects and photographs of significant others.	This intervention provides visual stimulation.
Provide low-level activities commensurate with patient tolerance.	These activities promote mental stimulation and reduce boredom. Examples include providing books or magazines pertaining to patient's recreational or other interests, providing computer games, supplying television, and supplying writing implements for short intervals of activity.
Initiate activities that require little concentration, and proceed to more complicated tasks as patient's condition allows (e.g., if reading requires more energy or concentration than patient is capable of, suggest that the significant other read to patient or bring audiotapes of books).	Initially patient may find difficult tasks frustrating. Physiologic problems such as anemia and pain may make concentration difficult.
Encourage discussion of past activities or reminiscence.	This could serve as a substitute for performing favorite activities during convalescence.
As patient's endurance improves, obtain appropriate diversional activities such as puzzles, model kits, handicrafts, and computerized games and activities; encourage patient to use them.	Watching television, listening to the radio, and playing cards or backgammon often are good diversions.
Suggest that significant other bring in a radio or, if appropriate, rent a television or radio from the hospital if not part of the standard room charge.	
If appropriate for patient, arrange for hospital volunteers to visit, play cards, read books, or play board games.	
Encourage significant other to visit within limits of patient's endurance and to involve patient in activities that are of interest to him or her. Encourage significant other to stagger visits throughout the day.	Visiting and partaking in activities with loved ones likely would reduce boredom.
As appropriate for patient who desires social interaction, consider relocation to a room in an area of high traffic.	People watching can be a good diversion.
As patient's condition improves, assist him or her with sitting in a chair near a window so that outside activities can be viewed. When patient is able, provide opportunities to sit in a solarium so that he or she can visit with other patients. If physical condition and weather permit, take patient outside for brief periods.	New scenery, whether within the same room or in another area, can reduce boredom, as can meeting and speaking with other people.
Request consultation from OT, social services, pastoral services, and psychiatric nurse.	Such referrals may yield other diversional activities/interventions.
Increase patient's involvement in self-care to provide a sense of purpose, accomplishment, and control.	Performing in-bed exercises (e.g., deep breathing, ankle circling, calf pumping), keeping track of I&O, and similar activities can and should be accomplished routinely by patients to provide a sense of purpose, accomplishment, and control, which likely will diminish boredom.

••• Related NIC and NOC labels: *NIC:* Activity Therapy; Socialization Enhancement; Therapeutic Play; Bibliotherapy; Reminiscence Therapy; Role Enhancement; Support System Enhancement *NOC:* Social Involvement

Nursing Diagnosis:

Ineffective Sexuality Pattern

related to actual or perceived physiologic limitations on sexual performance secondary to disease, therapy, or prolonged hospitalization

Desired Outcome: Within 72 hr of this diagnosis, patient relates satisfaction with sexuality and/or understanding of ability to resume sexual activity.

INTERVENTIONS	RATIONALES
Assess patient's normal sexual function, including importance placed on sex in the relationship, frequency of interaction, normal positions used, and the couple's ability to adapt or change to meet requirements of patient's limitations.	This assessment helps determine patient's normal sexual function and adaptations that will be necessary under current conditions.
Identify patient's problem diplomatically, and clarify it with patient.	This assessment helps determine if patient suffers from sexual dysfunction resulting from lack of privacy, current illness, or perceived limitations. Indicators of sexual dysfunction can include regression, acting-out with inappropriate behavior such as grabbing or pinching, sexual overtures toward staff members, self-enforced isolation, and similar behaviors.
Encourage patient and significant other to verbalize feelings and anxieties about sexual abstinence, having sexual relations in the hospital, hurting patient, or having to use new or alternative methods for sexual gratification.	Open communication is the foundation for maintaining a strong, intimate relationship.
Develop strategies in collaboration with patient and significant other.	This information will promote understanding of ways to achieve sexual satisfaction.
Encourage acceptable expressions of sexuality by patient.	Examples of positive and acceptable behaviors may eliminate inappropriate behaviors. Examples for a woman could include wearing makeup and jewelry and for a man, shaving and wearing own shirts and shorts.
Inform patient and significant other that it is possible to have time alone together for intimacy. Provide that time accordingly by putting a *Do not disturb* sign on the door, enforcing privacy by restricting staff and visitors to the room, or arranging for temporary private quarters.	These actions will facilitate intimacy by ensuring privacy.
Encourage patient and significant other to seek alternative methods of sexual expression when necessary.	Accustomed methods of sexual expression may not work under current circumstances. Alternative methods may include mutual masturbation, altered positions, vibrators, and identification of other erotic areas for the partner.
Refer patient and significant other to professional sexual counseling as necessary.	Counseling may improve communication and acceptance of alternative therapies.

••• **Related NIC and NOC labels:** *NIC:* Sexual Counseling; Self-Esteem Enhancement *NOC:* Sexual Functioning

Nursing Diagnosis:

Ineffective Role Performance: Dependence vs. independence

Desired Outcome: Within 48 hr of this diagnosis, patient collaborates with caregivers in planning realistic goals for independence, participates in own care, and takes responsibility for self-care.

INTERVENTIONS	RATIONALES
Encourage patient to be as independent as possible within limitations of endurance, therapy, and pain.	Optimally, such encouragement will facilitate independence as much as feasible. However, temporary periods of dependence are appropriate because they enable the individual to restore energy reserves needed for recovery.
Ensure that all health care providers are consistent in conveying expectations of eventual independence.	Consistency in message facilitates trusting relationships with health care providers and realistic goal setting.
Alert patient to areas of excessive dependence, and involve him or her in collaborative goal setting to achieve independence.	Although there are times when dependence is needed and desired, it is healthy to begin to foster a degree of independence as recovery progresses.
Do not minimize patient's expressed feelings of depression. Allow patient to express emotions, but provide support, understanding, and realistic hope for a positive role change.	Minimizing patient's expressed feelings of depression can add to anger and depression. Offering realistic hope and encouragement can provide needed emotional support in movement toward independence.
If indicated, provide self-help devices.	These devices increase patient's independence with self-care.
Provide positive reinforcement when patient meets or advances toward goals.	Positive reinforcement builds on patient's strengths and promotes self-efficacy.

●●● **Related NIC and NOC labels:** *NIC:* Coping Enhancement; Counseling; Role Enhancement; Body Image Enhancement; Emotional Support; Normalization Promotion *NOC:* Coping; Role Performance

ADDITIONAL NURSING DIAGNOSES/ PROBLEMS:

"Psychosocial Support," for psychosocial nursing interventions	p. 73
"Pneumonia" for interventions related to prevention of pneumonia	p. 123
"Pressure Ulcers" for **Impaired Tissue Integrity** (or risk for same)	p. 563

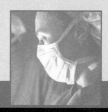

Psychosocial Support 5

Nursing Diagnosis:

Fatigue

related to disease process, treatment, medications, depression, or stress

Desired Outcome: Before hospital discharge, patient and caregivers describe interventions that conserve energy resources.

INTERVENTIONS	RATIONALES
Assess patient's patterns of fatigue and times of maximum energy.	This information helps identify areas for teaching energy conservation, relaxation, and diversional activities to reduce fatigue.
Assess how fatigue affects patient's emotional status and ability to perform activities of daily living (ADLs). Suggest activity schedules to maximize energy expenditures (e.g., "After you eat lunch, take a 15-minute rest before you go to x-ray").	Developing an activity plan (e.g., rescheduling activities, allowing rest periods, asking for assistance, exercise) will help conserve energy, reduce fatigue, and maintain ADLs.
Help patient maintain a regular sleep pattern by allowing for uninterrupted periods of sleep. Encourage patient to rest when fatigued rather than attempting to continue activity. Encourage naps during the day.	Lack of effective sleep can lead to psychosocial distress (e.g., inability to concentrate, anxiety, uncertainty, and depression).
Reduce environmental stimulation overload (e.g., noise level, visitors for long periods of time, lack of personal quiet time).	This action helps promote uninterrupted sleep patterns.
Discuss with patient how to delegate chores to family and friends who are offering to assist.	This action helps conserve energy and enables family and friends to feel a part of patient's care.
Encourage patient to maintain a regular schedule once discharged, recognizing that attempting to continue previous activity levels may not be realistic.	This information helps patient engage in a realistic activity schedule to minimize fatigue and avoid frustration if his or her physical functioning does not return to baseline levels.
Encourage mild exercise such as short walks and stretching, which may begin in the hospital if not contraindicated.	Such exercise will promote flexibility, muscle strength, and cardiac output and reduce stress.
Evaluate patient for signs and symptoms of anemia.	Anemia can result from cancer or its treatments. Fatigue can occur because of decreased oxygen-carrying capacity of blood. Pharmacologic agents or transfusions may be needed to increase red blood cells.

••• **Related NIC and NOC labels:** *NIC:* Energy Management; Environmental Management; Exercise Promotion: Stretching; Exercise Promotion: Ambulation; Sleep Enhancement *NOC:* Activity Tolerance; Endurance; Energy Conservation

Nursing Diagnosis:

Disturbed Sleep Pattern

related to environmental changes, illness, therapeutic regimen, pain, immobility, psychologic stress, altered mental status, or hypoxia

Desired Outcomes: After discussion, patient identifies factors that promote sleep. Within 8 hr of intervention, patient attains 90-min periods of uninterrupted sleep and verbalizes satisfaction with ability to rest.

INTERVENTIONS	RATIONALES
Assess patient's usual sleeping patterns (e.g., bedtime routine, hours of sleep per night, sleeping position, use of pillows and blankets, napping during the day, nocturia).	Some or all of patient's usual sleep pattern may be incorporated into the plan of care. A routine as similar to patient's normal routine as possible will help promote sleep.
Explore relaxation techniques that promote patient's rest/sleep.	Imagining relaxing scenes, listening to soothing music or taped stories, and using muscle relaxation exercises are relaxation techniques that are known to promote rest/sleep.
Administer sleep medicines at a time appropriate to induce sleep, taking into consideration time to onset and half-life.	Simulating patient's usual sleep/wake pattern aids in uninterrupted sleep.
As indicated, administer pain medications before sleep.	This intervention decreases the likelihood that pain will interfere with patient's sleep.
Identify causative factors and activities that contribute to patient's insomnia, awaken patient, or adversely affect sleep patterns.	Factors such as pain, anxiety, hypoxia, therapies, depression, hallucinations, medications, underlying illness, sleep apnea, respiratory disorder, caffeine, and fear may contribute to sleep pattern disturbance. Some may be ameliorated, and others may be modified.
Promote physical comfort via such measures as massage, back rubs, bathing, and fresh linens before sleep.	These measures help relieve stress and promote relaxation.
Organize procedures and activities to allow for 90-min periods of uninterrupted rest/sleep. Limit visiting during these periods.	Ninety minutes of sleep allows complete progression through the normal phases of sleep.
Whenever possible, maintain a quiet environment.	Excessive noise and light can cause sleep deprivation. Providing earplugs, reducing alarm volume, and using white noise (i.e., low-pitched, monotonous sounds: electric fan, soft music) may facilitate sleep. Dimming the lights for a period of time, drawing the drapes, and providing blindfolds are other ways of promoting sleep.
If appropriate, put limitations on patient's daytime sleeping. Attempt to establish regularly scheduled daytime activity (e.g., ambulation, sitting in chair, active range of motion), which may promote nighttime sleep.	Napping less during the day will promote a more normal nighttime pattern. Physical activity causes fatigue and may facilitate nighttime sleeping.
Investigate and provide nonpharmacologic comfort measures that are known to promote patient's sleep.	Nonpharmacologic comfort measures such as earplugs, anxiety reduction, and use of patient's own bed clothing and pillows may promote sleep.
Also see this nursing diagnosis in "Perioperative Care," p. 57.	

••• **Related NIC and NOC labels:** *NIC:* Energy Management; Sleep Enhancement; Exercise Promotion; Environmental Management: Comfort; Music Therapy; Progressive Muscle Relaxation; Simple Relaxation Therapy; Simple Guided Imagery *NOC:* Rest; Sleep

Nursing Diagnosis:

Anxiety

related to actual or perceived threat of death, change in health status, threat to self-concept or role, unfamiliar people and environment, medications, preexisting anxiety disorder, or the unknown

Desired Outcome: Within 1-2 hr of intervention, patient's anxiety has resolved or decreased as evidenced by patient's verbalization of same, HR 100 bpm or less, RR 20 breaths/min or less, and absence of or decrease in irritability and restlessness.

INTERVENTIONS	RATIONALES
Engage in honest communication with patient, providing empathetic understanding. Listen closely.	These actions help establish an atmosphere that allows free expression.
Assess patient's level of anxiety. Be alert to verbal and nonverbal cues.	Being cognizant of patient's level of anxiety enables nurse to provide appropriate interventions, as well as modify the plan of care accordingly. Levels of anxiety include: - *Mild:* Restlessness, irritability, increased questions, focusing on the environment. - *Moderate:* Inattentiveness, expressions of concern, narrowed perceptions, insomnia, increased HR. - *Severe:* Expressions of feelings of doom, rapid speech, tremors, poor eye contact. Patient may be preoccupied with the past; may be unable to understand the present; and may have tachycardia, nausea, and hyperventilation. - *Panic:* Inability to concentrate or communicate, distortion of reality, increased motor activity, vomiting, tachypnea.
For patients with severe anxiety or panic state, refer to psychiatric clinical nurse specialist, case manager, or other health care team members as appropriate.	Patients in severe anxiety or panic state may require more sophisticated interventions or pharmacologic management.
Approach patient with a calm, reassuring demeanor. Show concern and focused attention while listening to patient's concerns. Provide a safe environment and stay with patient during periods of intense anxiety.	These actions reassure patient that you are concerned and will assist in meeting his or her needs.
Restrict patient's intake of caffeine, nicotine, and alcohol.	Caffeine is a stimulant that may increase anxiety in persons who are sensitive to it. Cessation of caffeine, nicotine, and alcohol can lead to physiologic withdrawal symptoms including anxiety.
Avoid abrupt discontinuation of anxiolytics.	Abrupt withdrawal can cause headaches, tiredness, and irritability.
If patient is hyperventilating, have him or her concentrate on a focal point and mimic your deliberately slow and deep breathing pattern.	Modeling provides patient with a focal point for learning effective breathing technique.
Validate assessment of anxiety with patient.	Validating patient's anxiety level provides confirmation of nursing assessment, as well as openly acknowledges patient's emotional state. In so doing, patient is given permission to share feelings. For example, "You seem distressed. Are you feeling uncomfortable now?"
After an episode of anxiety, review and discuss with patient the thoughts and feelings that led to the episode.	This action validates with patient the cause of the anxiety and explores interventions that may avert another episode.
Identify patient's current coping behaviors. Review coping behaviors patient has used in the past. Assist patient with using adaptive coping to manage anxiety.	Identifying maladaptive coping behaviors (e.g., denial, anger, repression, withdrawal, daydreaming, or dependence on narcotics, sedatives, or tranquilizers) helps establish a proactive plan of care to promote healthy coping skills. For example, "I understand that your wife reads to you to help you relax. Would you like to spend a part of each day alone with her?"
Encourage patient to express fears, concerns, and questions.	Encouraging questions gives patient an avenue in which to share concerns. For example, "I know this room looks like a maze of wires and tubes; please let me know when you have any questions."
Provide an organized, quiet environment (see **Disturbed Sensory Perception,** p. 82).	Such an environment reduces sensory overload that may contribute to anxiety.
Introduce self and other health care team members; explain each individual's role as it relates to patient's care.	Familiarity with staff and their individual roles may increase patient's comfort level and decrease anxiety.
Teach patient relaxation and imagery techniques. See **Health-Seeking Behaviors:** Relaxation Technique Effective for Stress Reduction, p. 172.	Teaching relaxation and imagery skills empowers patient to manage anxiety-provoking episodes more skillfully and fosters a sense of control.
Enable support persons to be in attendance whenever possible.	Many people benefit from support of others and find that it reduces their stress level.

••• **Related NIC and NOC labels:** *NIC:* Anxiety Reduction; Active Listening; Behavior Management; Calming Technique; Coping Enhancement; Presence; Environmental Management; Progressive Muscle Relaxation; Simple Relaxation Therapy; Support Group
NOC: Anxiety Control; Coping

Nursing Diagnosis:

Fear

related to separation from support systems, unfamiliarity with environment or therapeutic regimen, loss of sense of control, recurrence of the disease, or uncertainty about the future

Desired Outcome: Following intervention, patient expresses fears and concerns and reports feeling greater psychologic and physical comfort.

INTERVENTIONS	RATIONALES
Validate patient's fears and concerns and provide opportunities for patient to express them.	These actions help determine factors contributing to patient's feelings of fear. For example, "You seem very concerned about receiving more blood today."
Listen closely to patient.	Reactions such as anger, denial, occasional withdrawal, and demanding behaviors may be coping responses.
Encourage patient to ask questions and gather information about the unknown. Provide information about equipment, therapies, and routines according to patient's ability to understand.	Increasing knowledge level about therapies and procedures reduces/eliminates fear of the unknown and affords a sense of control.
Acknowledge fears in an empathetic manner.	Acknowledging feelings encourages communication and hence reduces fear. For example, "I understand this equipment frightens you, but it is necessary to help you breathe."
	An empathic response promotes expression of fears and provides reassurance that concerns are acknowledged. For example, "You seem very concerned about receiving more blood today."
Encourage patient to participate in and plan care whenever possible.	Participation promotes an increased sense of control, which helps decrease fears.
Provide continuity of care by establishing a routine and arranging for consistent caregivers whenever possible. Appoint a case manager or primary nurse.	Consistency in care providers promotes familiarity and trust.
Discuss with health care team members the appropriateness of medication therapy for patients with disabling fear or anxiety.	Pharmacologic interventions are sometimes necessary in assisting patients to cope with fears/anxieties about treatment, diagnosis, and prognosis.
Explore patient's desire for spiritual or psychologic counseling.	Exploring spiritual/psychologic dimension of the current experience may assist patient to cope with fear and stress.
Consult health care provider regarding a visit by another individual with the same disorder or situation who has experienced the same treatment.	Many people benefit from outside sources of support in decreasing fears. Interaction with another person who has had a similar experience provides hope and encouragement.

••• **Related NIC and NOC labels:** *NIC:* Anxiety Reduction; Active Listening; Coping Enhancement; Presence; Support System Enhancement; Support Group *NOC:* Anxiety Control; Fear Control

Nursing Diagnosis:

Ineffective Coping

related to health crisis, sense of vulnerability, or inadequate support systems

Desired Outcome: Before hospital discharge, patient verbalizes feelings, identifies strengths and coping behaviors, and does not demonstrate ineffective coping behaviors.

INTERVENTIONS	RATIONALES
Assess patient's perceptions and ability to understand current health status. Discuss meaning of disease and current treatment with patient, actively listening with a nonjudgmental attitude.	Evaluation of patient's comprehension enables development of an individualized care plan.
Establish honest, empathetic communication with the patient.	This promotes effective therapeutic communication, for example, "Please tell me what I can do to help you."
Support positive coping behaviors and explore effective coping behaviors used in the past.	These actions identify, reinforce, and facilitate positive coping behaviors, for example, "I see that reading that book seems to help you relax."
Identify factors that inhibit patient's ability to cope.	This enables patient to identify areas such as unsatisfactory support system, deficient knowledge, grief, and fear that may contribute to anxiety and ineffective coping and to consider modification of these factors.
Help patient identify previous methods of coping with life problems.	How patient has handled problems in the past may be a reliable predictor of how he or she will cope with current problems.
Recognize maladaptive coping behaviors. If appropriate, discuss these behaviors with patient.	Examples of maladaptive behaviors include severe depression; dependence on narcotics, sedatives, or tranquilizers; hostility; violence; and suicidal ideation. Patient may have used substances and other maladaptive behaviors in controlling anxiety. This pattern can interfere with ability to cope with current situation. If appropriate, nurses should discuss these behaviors with patient. For example, "You seem to be requiring more pain medication. Are you having more physical pain, or does it help you cope with your situation?"
Refer patient to psychiatric liaison, clinical nurse specialist, case manager, or clergy as appropriate.	Professional intervention may assist with altering maladaptive behaviors.
Help patient identify or develop a support system.	Many people benefit from outside support systems in helping them cope.
As patient's condition allows, assist with reducing anxiety. See **Anxiety,** p. 74.	Anxiety makes effective coping more difficult to achieve.
Maintain an organized, quiet environment. See **Disturbed Sensory Perception,** p. 82.	Such an environment helps reduce patient's sensory overload to aid with coping.
Encourage frequent visits by family and caregiver if visits appear to be supportive to patient.	Visitors may help minimize patient's emotional and social isolation, thereby promoting coping behaviors.
As appropriate, explain to caregiver that increased dependency, anger, and denial may be adaptive coping behaviors used by patient in early stages of crisis until effective coping behaviors are learned.	Lack of understanding about patient's maladaptive coping can lead to unhealthy interaction patterns and contribute to anxiety within the family.
Arrange community referrals, as appropriate.	Support in the home environment promotes healthier adaptations and may avert crises.

••• **Related NIC and NOC labels:** *NIC:* Coping Enhancement; Anxiety Reduction; Emotional Support; Support System Enhancement; Family Involvement Promotion; Referral *NOC:* Coping; Social Support

Nursing Diagnosis:

Powerlessness

related to absence of a sense of control over events

Desired Outcome: Before hospital discharge, patient begins to make decisions about care and therapies and reports onset of an attitude of realistic hope and sense of self-control.

INTERVENTIONS	RATIONALES
Assess patient's personal preferences, needs, values, and attitudes. Before providing information, assess patient's knowledge and understanding of condition and care.	This assessment helps develop a care plan individualized for patient's needs, which optimally will decrease sense of powerlessness.
Assess for expressions of fear, lack of response to events, and lack of interest in information.	These are signals of patient's feelings of powerlessness.
Evaluate caregiver practices, and adjust them to support patient's sense of control.	For example, if patient always bathes in the evening to promote relaxation before bedtime, modify the care plan to include an evening bath rather than follow the hospital routine of giving a morning bath.
Ask patient to identify activities that may be performed independently.	Self-care activities likely will promote sense of control.
Whenever possible, offer alternatives related to routine hygiene, diet, diversional activities, visiting hours, and treatment times.	Offering alternatives promotes a sense of control and power over daily routine.
When distant relatives and casual acquaintances request information about patient's status, check with patient for consent before sharing information.	This action ensures privacy and preserves patient's territorial rights whenever possible.
Avoid overprotection and parenting behaviors toward patient. Instead, act as an advocate for patient and significant other.	Discouraging patient's dependency on staff will help promote independent behaviors.
Assess support systems; involve significant other in patient care whenever possible. Refer to clergy and other support persons or systems as appropriate.	Many people feel empowered by outside support systems. Promoting family involvement reduces their feelings of powerlessness as well.
Offer realistic hope for the future, realizing that within any situation there is always a reason to be hopeful, even if it is a "good" or peaceful death.	This likely will increase sense of control and power and promote hopefulness.
Determine patient's wishes about end-of-life decisions, and document advance directives as appropriate.	These actions help promote patient's sense of control and power over these decisions.

••• Related NIC and NOC labels: *NIC:* Decision-Making Support; Family Involvement Promotion; Patient Rights Protection; Active Listening; Coping Enhancement; Referral *NOC:* Family Participation in Professional Care; Participation: Health Care Decisions

Nursing Diagnosis:

Spiritual Distress

related to disturbances in belief and value systems that give meaning and a sense of hope

Desired Outcome: Before hospital discharge, patient begins to verbalize religious or spiritual beliefs, continues previous practices, and expresses less distress and feelings of anxiety and fear.

INTERVENTIONS	RATIONALES
Assess patient's spiritual or religious beliefs, values, and practices.	This assessment will assist in development of an individualized care plan. For example, "Do you have a religious preference?" "How important is it to you?" "Are there any religious or spiritual practices in which you wish to participate while in the hospital?"
Inform patient of availability of spiritual resources, such as a chapel or chaplain.	This information increases awareness of available spiritual resources and promotes a sense of acceptance of patient's spirituality.
Display a nonjudgmental attitude toward patient's religious or spiritual beliefs and values.	This action creates an environment that is conducive to free expression.
Identify available support persons or systems that may assist in meeting patient's religious or spiritual needs (e.g., clergy, fellow church members, support groups).	Many people derive an increased sense of hope from religious and spiritual counselors.

Continued

INTERVENTIONS	RATIONALES
Be alert to comments related to spiritual concerns or conflicts.	Comments such as "I don't know why God is doing this to me" and "I'm being punished for my sins" suggest that patient is feeling some degree of spiritual distress.
Listen closely and ask questions.	These actions help patient resolve conflicts related to spiritual issues and help the nurse plan how best to assist patient. For example, "I understand that you want to be baptized. We can arrange to do that here."
Provide privacy and opportunities for spiritual practices such as prayer and meditation.	Many people find prayer and meditation difficult in a nonprivate setting.
If spiritual beliefs and therapeutic regimens are in conflict, provide patient with honest, substantiated information.	Such information promotes informed decision making. For example, "I understand your religion discourages receiving blood transfusions. We respect your position; however, it does not allow us to give you the best care possible."
Refer patient for help with decision making if he or she is struggling with treatment-related decisions.	Such help assists in resolving care dilemmas, if appropriate. Many hospitals provide assistance in the form of educational materials and counseling in order to help resolve such dilemmas.

••• Related NIC and NOC labels: *NIC:* Spiritual Support; Emotional Support; Referral; Support System Enhancement *NOC:* Spiritual Well-Being

Nursing Diagnosis:

Anticipatory Grieving/Risk for Dysfunctional Grieving

related to actual or potential loss of physiologic well-being (e.g., expected loss of body function or body part, changes in self-concept or body image, illness, death)

Desired Outcome: Following intervention, patient and caregiver express grief, participate in decisions about the future, and discuss concerns with health care team members and one another.

INTERVENTIONS	RATIONALES
Assess and accept patient's behavioral response.	Reactions such as disbelief, denial, guilt, anger, and depression are normal reactions to grief.
Determine patient's stage of grieving.	Comprehension of patient's stage of grief enables more effective therapeutic interventions. It is normal for a person to move from one stage to another and then revert to a previous stage. The time required to do so varies from individual to individual. If a person is unable to move into the next stage, referral for professional intervention may be indicated.
	- *Protest stage:* denial, disbelief, anger, hostility, resentment, bargaining to postpone loss, appeal for help to recover loss, loud complaints, altered sleep and appetite.
	- *Disorganization stage:* depression, withdrawal, social isolation, psychomotor retardation, silence.
	- *Reorganization stage:* acceptance of loss, development of new interests and attachments, restructuring of lifestyle, return to preloss level of functioning.
Assess spiritual, religious, and sociocultural expectations related to loss.	Helping patients find meaning in their experience may facilitate the grieving process. For example, "Is religion an important part of your life?" "How do you and your family deal with serious health problems?"
Refer to clergy or community support groups as appropriate.	Such a referral reinforces that there are support systems and resources to help work through grief.

Continued

INTERVENTIONS	RATIONALES
Demonstrate empathy.	Empathetic communication (including respecting desire not to communicate) promotes a trusting relationship and open dialogue. For example, "This must be a very difficult time for you and your family" or "Is there anything you'd like to talk about today?"
In selected circumstances, explain the grieving process.	This approach may help patient and family better understand and acknowledge their feelings and help family members better understand behaviors and verbalizations expressed by patient.
When appropriate, provide referral for bereavement care.	Such a referral helps patient and family grieve their loss.
Assess grief reactions of patient and significant other, and identify those individuals with potential for dysfunctional grieving reactions (e.g., absence of emotion, hostility, avoidance).	This assessment helps identify and reduce dysfunctional grieving, if present.
If potential for dysfunctional grieving is present, refer the individual to psychiatric clinical nurse specialist, case manager, clergy, or other source of counseling as appropriate.	Promoting normal progression through the grieving stages may allay unnecessary emotional suffering.

••• **Related NIC and NOC labels:** *NIC:* Coping Enhancement; Grief Work Facilitation; Anticipatory Guidance; Emotional Support; Family Support; Hope Installation; Spiritual Support; Counseling; Grief Work Facilitation *NOC:* Coping; Family Coping; Psychosocial Adjustment: Life Change; Grief Resolution

Nursing Diagnosis:

Disturbed Body Image

related to loss or change in body parts or function or physical trauma

Desired Outcomes: Within 24-hr period before hospital discharge, patient begins to acknowledge bodily changes and demonstrates movement toward incorporating changes into self-concept. Patient does not demonstrate maladaptive response, such as severe depression.

INTERVENTIONS	RATIONALES
Establish open, honest communication with patient. Give patient permission to grieve loss.	These actions promote an environment conducive to free expression in which patient is comfortable talking about body image concerns. For example, "Please feel free to talk to me whenever you have any questions."
Assess patient for indicators suggesting body image disturbance.	Patient may exhibit nonverbal indicators (avoidance of looking at or touching body part, hiding or exposing body part) or verbal indicators (expression of negative feeling about body, expression of feelings of helplessness, personalization or depersonalization of missing or mutilated part, or refusal to acknowledge change in structure or function of body part).
When planning patient's care, be aware of therapies that may influence patient's body image, and educate patient accordingly before they are implemented.	Various drugs and surgical procedures can cause body changes. Monitoring equipment and invasive procedures can cause a diminished image of self and feelings of helplessness.
Assess patient's knowledge of the pathophysiologic process that has occurred and present health status.	This assessment promotes patient's understanding of health status and clarifies misconceptions that may be contributing to disturbed body image.
Discuss the loss or change with patient. Practice nonjudgmental acceptance of patient's reality.	Loss of any type has meaning of differing magnitudes for each individual. Talking about these issues may be a first step in accepting changes. What may seem to be a small change may be of great significance to the patient (e.g., arm immobilizer, catheter, hair loss, ecchymoses, facial abrasions).

Continued

INTERVENTIONS	RATIONALES
Explore with patient concerns, fears, and feelings of guilt.	Some body changes may reverse with time, and this information may lessen stress and concern. Assessing emotional reactions to the loss may help the nurse provide therapeutic support. For example, "I understand you are frightened. Your face looks different now, but you will see changes and it will improve. Gradually you will begin to look more like yourself."
Encourage patient and family members to interact with one another. Help family avoid reinforcement of their loved one's unhappiness over a changed body part or function.	Support and encouragement from loved ones help many people cope better with body changes. Guiding family members appropriately in their dealings with patients promotes healthy interactions that foster well-being. For example, "I know your son looks very different to you now, but it would help if you speak to him and touch him as you would normally."
Encourage patient to participate gradually in self-care activities as he or she becomes physically and emotionally able.	Self-care activities and a sense of getting back to normal can contribute to a sense of wholeness and control. Assisting patient with resuming a sense of normalcy promotes progression through the stages of grief.
Allow for some initial withdrawal and denial behaviors.	This is normal. For example, when changing dressings over traumatized part, explain what you are doing but do not expect patient to watch or participate initially.
Discuss opportunities for reconstruction or rehabilitation of the loss or change. Offer realistic hope for the future.	These actions promote a realistic sense of hope and help patient plan for the future. Examples include surgery, prosthesis, grafting, physical therapy, cosmetic therapies, modified clothing, and organ transplant.
Recognize manifestations of severe depression (e.g., sleep disturbances, change in affect, and change in communication pattern). As appropriate, refer to psychiatric clinical nurse specialist, case manager, clergy, or support group.	This knowledge enables referral of patient who is at risk for self-harm, including suicide. See **Risk for Suicide**, p. 763, in "Major Depression."
Offer choices and alternatives whenever possible. Emphasize patient's strengths, and encourage activities that interest patient.	These actions help patient attain a sense of autonomy and control.
If possible, refer patient to a support group or another patient who has had a similar experience (e.g., Reach to Recovery volunteer for a breast surgery patient).	Many people benefit from outside support systems and sharing experiences with another person who has had a similar experience.
Be aware that touch may enhance a patient's self-concept and reduce his or her sense of isolation.	Touch may mitigate a sense that patient is hideous or unattractive because of the body change.

See also: Disturbed Body Image, p. 459, in "Fecal Diversions."

••• Related NIC and NOC labels: *NIC:* Body Image Enhancement; Active Listening; Coping Enhancement; Self-Care Assistance; Support Group; Self-Esteem Enhancement *NOC:* Body Image; Psychosocial Adjustment: Life Change; Self-Esteem

Nursing Diagnosis:

Impaired Verbal Communication

related to neurologic or anatomic deficit, psychologic or physical barriers (e.g., tracheostomy, intubation), or cultural or developmental differences

Desired Outcome: At the time of intervention, patient communicates needs and feelings and reports decreased or absent feelings of frustration over communication barriers.

INTERVENTIONS	RATIONALES
Assess cause of impaired communication (e.g., tracheostomy, stroke, cerebral tumor, Guillain-Barré syndrome).	Determining cause of communication impairment will enable nur__ develop a customized plan of care that incorporates commun__ skills patient can use, given his or her disability.
Involve patient and/or caregiver in assessing patient's ability to read, write, and understand English. If patient speaks a language other than English, collaborate with English-speaking family member or an interpreter to establish effective communication.	This assessment helps establish effective communication and en__ teaching materials provided are at a level appropriate for patie__
When communicating, face patient; make direct eye contact; and speak in a clear, normal tone of voice.	A visual or hearing-impaired person often develops compensatory methods, for example, lip reading for a person who is hearing-impaired.
When communicating with a deaf person about the treatment plan, arrange to have an interpreter present if possible.	An interpreter facilitates effective communication, promotes informed consent, and enables patient to ask questions.
If patient cannot speak because of a physical barrier (e.g., tracheostomy, wired mandibles), provide reassurance and acknowledge his or her frustration.	These actions will help decrease frustration caused by inability to communicate verbally. For example, "I know this is frustrating for you, but please do not give up. I want to understand you."
Provide slate, word cards, pencil and paper, alphabet board, pictures, or other device to assist patient with communication. Adapt call system to meet patient's needs. Document meaning of signals used by patient to communicate.	These actions will enable effective communication, promote continuity of care, and lessen patient's anxiety.
Explain source of patient's communication impairment to caregiver; teach caregiver effective communication alternatives (see previous list).	Inability to communicate with ease may cause feelings of isolation that can be intensified if patient has difficulty communicating with caregiver.
Be alert to nonverbal messages. Validate their meaning with patient.	Nonverbal response, such as facial expressions, hand movements, and nodding of the head, is a valid means of communication, and its meaning must be validated to facilitate understanding.
Encourage patient to communicate needs; reinforce independent behaviors.	Inability to speak may foster maladaptive behaviors, and this reinforces need for patient to be understood.
Be honest with patient; do not pretend to understand if you are unable to interpret patient's communication.	Pretending to understand patient will only add to his or her frustration and diminish trust.
If surgery is expected to create a physical condition that will cause interference with communication, begin teaching preoperatively. Facilitate postoperative referrals for speech and swallowing.	These actions will help ensure that an effective method of communication will be in place postoperatively so that the patient's needs will be met.

••• **Related NIC and NOC labels:** *NIC:* Active Listening; Communication Enhancement: Hearing Deficit; Communication Enhancement: Speech Deficit; Communication Enhancement: Visual Deficit; Presence; Environmental Management; Cognitive Stimulation; Cultural Brokerage; Reality Orientation *NOC:* Communication Ability; Communication: Expressive Ability; Communication: Receptive Ability

Nursing Diagnosis:

Disturbed Sensory Perception

related to therapeutically or socially restricted environment; psychologic stress; altered sensory reception, transmission, or integration; or chemical alteration

Desired Outcome: Within 24 hours of diagnosis, patient verbalizes orientation to person, place, and time; reports the ability to concentrate; and expresses satisfaction with degree and type of sensory stimulation being received.

INTERVENTIONS	RATIONALES
Assess factors contributing to patient's sensory-perceptual alteration.	Some factors may be readily reversible. Others will require palliative measures. Modifying environmental stimulation and intervening for physiologic factors as much as feasible may reduce patient stress, promote normal sleep patterns, and assist in maintaining orientation. These factors may include the following: - *Environmental:* Excessive noise in the environment; constant, monotonous noise; restricted environment (immobility, traction, isolation); social isolation (restricted visitors, impaired communication); therapies. - *Physiologic:* Altered organ function, sleep or rest pattern disturbance, medication, history of altered sensory perception.
Avoid constant lighting (maintain day/night patterns); and reduce noise whenever possible (decrease alarm volumes, avoid loud talking, keep room door closed, provide earplugs).	These actions will manage or ameliorate factors contributing to environmental stimulus overload.
Determine sensory stimulation appropriate for patient and plan care accordingly.	This assessment enables a plan of care suitable for patient's needs.
If appropriate, provide meaningful sensory stimulation. - As needed, orient patient to surroundings and reason for hospitalization. Display clocks, large calendars, and meaningful photographs and objects from home. - Depending on patient preference, provide a radio, music, reading materials, and tape recordings of family and significant other. - Position patient to look toward window when possible. Stimulate patient's vision with mirrors, colored decorations, and pictures. - Discuss current events, time of day, holidays, and topics of interest during patient care activities. - Stimulate patient's sense of taste with sweet, salty, and sour substances as allowed. - When providing information, use simple terminology and maintain eye contact. Avoid talking "down" to the patient. - Always advise patient before initiating any procedures or personal contact. - Establish personal contact by touch, if appropriate, to help promote and maintain patient's contact with the real environment. - Encourage significant other to communicate with patient often, using a normal tone of voice. - Convey concern and respect for patient. Introduce yourself and call patient by name. - Encourage use of eyeglasses and hearing aids.	Sensory stimulation may help patient attain/maintain orientation.
Maintain proper lighting, position call bell within reach, and keep bed in the lowest position with side rails up.	These actions promote patient's safety during period of disorientation.
Assess patient's sleep/rest pattern to evaluate its contribution to the sensory/perceptual disorder. Make sure that patient attains at least 90 min of uninterrupted sleep as often as possible. For more information, see **Disturbed Sleep Pattern,** p. 73.	Sleep deprivation causes increased stress that can lead to irritability and disorientation.

●●● **Related NIC and NOC labels:** *NIC:* Cognitive Stimulation; Reality Orientation; Communication Enhancement: Hearing Deficit; Communication Enhancement: Visual Enhancement; Speech Deficit; Environmental Management; Sleep Enhancement *NOC:* Cognitive Orientation; Communication: Receptive Ability; Hearing Compensation Behavior; Sensory Function: Vision

Nursing Diagnosis:

Social Isolation

related to altered health status, inability to engage in satisfying personal relationships, altered mental status, body image change, or altered physical appearance

Desired Outcome: Before hospital discharge, patient demonstrates movement toward interaction and communication with others.

INTERVENTIONS	RATIONALES
Assess factors contributing to patient's social isolation.	This assessment will help determine causes of social isolation and modify those factors. These may include: - Restricted visiting hours - Absence of or inadequate support system - Inability to communicate (e.g., presence of intubation/tracheostomy) - Physical changes that affect self-concept - Denial or withdrawal - Hospital environment
Recognize patients at risk for social isolation.	Individuals most at risk for social isolation include older adults and disabled, chronically ill, and economically disadvantaged persons.
Help patient identify feelings associated with loneliness and isolation.	This information facilitates interventions based on individual need. For example, "You seem very sad when your family leaves the room. Can you tell me more about your feelings?"
Determine patient's need for socialization, and identify available and potential support person or systems. Explore methods for increasing social contact.	Assessing need for interaction and developing a care plan accordingly will reduce sense of isolation surrounding the illness. Methods for increasing social contact include TV, radio, tapes of loved ones, intercom system, more frequent visitations, and scheduled interaction with nurse or support staff.
Provide positive reinforcement for socialization that lessens patient's feelings of isolation and loneliness.	Encouraging interaction gives patient permission to ask for social interaction from the nurse while decreasing sense of isolation. For example, "Please continue to call me when you need to talk to someone. Talking will help both of us better understand your feelings."
Facilitate patient's ability to communicate with others (see **Impaired Verbal Communication,** p. 81).	Impaired communication may be the cause of social isolation.

●●● Related NIC and NOC labels: *NIC:* Socialization Enhancement; Support System Enhancement; Active Listening; Emotional Support; Presence; Visitation Facilitation; Communication Enhancement; Family Involvement Promotion *NOC:* Social Involvement; Social Support; Well-Being

Nursing Diagnosis:

Deficient Knowledge:

Current health status and prescribed therapies

Desired Outcome: Before procedures or hospital discharge (as appropriate), patient verbalizes understanding regarding current health status and therapies.

INTERVENTIONS

INTERVENTIONS	RATIONALES
Assess patient's health care literacy (language, reading, comprehension). Assess culture and culturally specific information needs as well as cognitive and emotional readiness to learn.	This assessment helps ensure that information is presented in a manner that is culturally and educationally appropriate.
Recognize other barriers to learning.	Barriers to learning include ineffective communication, educational deficit, neurologic deficit, sensory alterations, fear, anxiety, and lack of motivation.
Assess patient's current level of knowledge regarding health status.	This assessment enables development of an individualized teaching plan, as well as correction of misperceptions and misinformation.
Assess learning needs and establish short-term and long-term goals.	Well-planned goals provide markers for assessing effectiveness of the teaching plan and progress made.
Use individualized verbal or written information to promote learning and enhance understanding. Give simple, direct instructions. As indicated, use audiovisual tools as supplemental information.	Because individuals learn differently, using more than one teaching modality will provide more opportunities to assimilate information.
Include caregiver in all patient teaching, and encourage reinforcement of correct information regarding diagnosis and treatments.	Anxiety often filters the information given. Involving a spouse or other family member provides teaching reinforcement.
Encourage patient's involvement in care information by planning care collaboratively. Explain rationale for care and therapies.	Involving patient in his or her own care planning promotes adherence to the treatment plan and engenders a sense of control and ownership.
Communicate often with patient. Request feedback regarding what has been taught.	Anxiety may interfere with reception, comprehension, and retention. Individuals in crisis often need repeated explanations before information can be understood. Creating an environment of permission in which patient feels comfortable asking questions and revealing knowledge deficits facilitates learning.
Provide written information appropriate to patient's comprehension level.	Written material reinforces teaching and enables review at a later time.
As appropriate, assess understanding of informed consent.	Patient will use information received to make informed decisions regarding care.

••• **Related NIC and NOC labels:** *NIC:* Teaching: Disease Process; Health System Guidance; Learning Readiness Enhancement; Active Listening; Teaching: Procedure/Treatment; Preparatory Sensory Information; Decision-Making Support; Patient Rights Protection *NOC:* Knowledge: Disease Process; Knowledge: Illness Care; Knowledge: Treatment Regimen

ADDITIONAL NURSING DIAGNOSES/ PROBLEMS:

"Palliative and End-of-Life Care," as appropriate for issues facing patients who are dying — p. 105

"Anxiety Disorders" for **Ineffective Coping** related to anxiety — p. 740

"Bipolar Disorder" for **Risk for Other-Directed Violence** — p. 746

"Major Depression" for **Hopelessness** — p. 763

Risk for Suicide — p. 763

Dysfunctional Grieving — p. 765

Psychosocial Support 6 for the Patient's Family and Significant Other

Note: *The Health Insurance Portability and Accountability Act of 1996 (HIPAA) restricts who may request and receive health care–related information about a patient in order to protect confidentiality. Health care providers must be sensitive to and aware of expressed patient preferences before discussing patient with others, including family. This includes divulging information regarding patient's presence in the hospital.*

Nursing Diagnosis:

Fear

related to patient's life-threatening condition and knowledge deficit

Desired Outcome: Following intervention, significant others/family members report that fear has lessened.

INTERVENTIONS	RATIONALES
Assess family's fears and their understanding of patient's clinical situation.	Some fears may be realistic; others may not be and need clarification.
Evaluate verbal and nonverbal responses.	Some family members may not readily verbalize their fears but may give nonverbal cues such as withdrawing emotionally (evidenced by body position, facial expression, attitude of disinterest), refusing to be present during discussion, or disrupting discussion.
Acknowledge family's fear.	Simple acknowledgement and giving more information can go a long way toward decreasing fear. For example, "I understand these tubes must frighten you, but they are necessary to help nourish your son."
Assess family's history of coping behavior.	How a family has coped with fear in the past often is a reliable predictor of how they will cope in the current situation. For example, "How does your family react to difficult situations?" Awareness of maladaptive responses may assist nurse in fostering more productive methods of coping.
Provide opportunities for family members to express fears and concerns.	Verbalizing feelings in a nonthreatening environment can help them deal with unresolved/unrecognized issues that may be contributing to the current stressor. Anger, denial, withdrawal, and demanding behavior may be adaptive coping responses during the initial period of crisis.
	Identifying fears also enables the nurse to dispel inaccuracies, which will help the family cope with the situation as it exists.

Continued

INTERVENTIONS	RATIONALES
Provide information at frequent intervals about patient's status, treatments, and equipment used.	This information increases family's knowledge of patient's health status, helping alleviate fear of the unknown.
Encourage family to use positive coping behaviors by identifying fears, developing goals, identifying supportive resources, facilitating realistic perceptions, and promoting problem solving.	When under stress, family may not recall sources of support without being reminded. For example, "Who usually helps your family during stressful times?"
Recognize anxiety, and encourage family members to describe their feelings.	Before family members can learn coping strategies, they must first clarify their feelings. For example, "You seem very uncomfortable tonight. Can you describe your feelings?"
Be alert to maladaptive responses to fear. Provide referrals to psychiatric clinical nurse specialist or other staff member as appropriate.	Violence, withdrawal, severe depression, hostility, and unrealistic expectations for staff or of patient's recovery are maladaptive responses to fear, and they require expert guidance.
Offer *realistic* hope, even if it is hope for patient's peaceful death.	Even though family members may have feelings of hopelessness, it sometimes helps to hear realistic expressions of hope.
Explore family's desire for spiritual or other counseling.	People often derive hope and experience a decrease in fear and dread from spiritual counseling.
Assess your own feelings about patient's life-threatening illness.	Without personal awareness of one's beliefs, a health care provider's attitude and fears may be reflected inadvertently to the family.
For other interventions, see **Interrupted Family Processes** and **Disabled Family Coping** listed later in this care plan.	

●●● **Related NIC and NOC labels:** *NIC:* Anxiety Reduction; Active Listening; Coping Enhancement; Support System Enhancement; Counseling *NOC:* Anxiety Control; Fear Control

Nursing Diagnosis:

Interrupted Family Processes

related to situational crisis (patient's illness)

Desired Outcome: Following intervention, family members demonstrate effective adaptation to change/traumatic situation as evidenced by seeking external support when necessary and sharing concerns within the family unit.

INTERVENTIONS	RATIONALES
Assess family's character: social, environmental, ethnic, and cultural factors; relationships; and role patterns.	Having this detailed information will assist nurse in developing an individualized care plan.
Identify family's developmental stage.	The family may be dealing with other situational or maturational crises, such as managing an elderly parent or a teenager with a learning disability.
Assess previous adaptive behaviors.	How the family has dealt with problems in the past may be a reliable predictor of how they will adapt to current issues. For example, "How does your family react in stressful situations?"
Discuss observed conflicts and communications.	Awareness of this information will assist with development of an individualized plan of care, including referral for specialized care if appropriate. For example, "I noticed that your brother would not visit your mother today. Has there been a problem we should be aware of? Knowing about it may help us better care for your mother."
Acknowledge family's involvement in patient care and promote strengths. Encourage family to participate in patient care conferences. Promote frequent, regular patient visits by family members.	This reinforces positive ways of dealing with the crisis and promotes a sense of involvement and control for the family. For example, "You were able to encourage your wife to turn and cough. That is very important to her recovery."

Continued

INTERVENTIONS	RATIONALES
Provide family with information and guidance related to patient. Discuss the stresses of hospitalization, and encourage family to discuss feelings of anger, guilt, hostility, depression, fear, or sorrow. Refer to clergy, clinical nurse specialist, or social services as appropriate.	Encouraging expressions of emotion assists family members in beginning the process of grieving. For example, "You seem to be upset since being told that your husband is not leaving the hospital today." Acknowledging their feelings promotes acceptance and facilitates therapeutic communication.
Evaluate patient and family responses to one another. Encourage family to reorganize roles and establish priorities as appropriate.	These actions will help facilitate family's adaptation to the situation regarding patient and prevent unnecessary conflict. Assisting family members to redefine their roles may reduce confusion and provide direction. For example, "I know your husband is concerned about his insurance policy and seems to expect you to investigate it. I'll ask the financial counselor to talk with you."
Encourage family to schedule periods of rest and activity outside the hospital and to seek support when necessary.	Persons undergoing stress sometimes require guidance of others to promote their own self-care. For example, "Your neighbor volunteered to stay in the waiting room this afternoon. Would you like to rest at home? I'll call you if anything changes."

••• **Related NIC and NOC labels:** *NIC:* Coping Enhancement; Family Support; Emotional Support; Grief Work Facilitation; Respite Care
NOC: Family Coping

Nursing Diagnosis:

Compromised Family Coping

related to inadequate or incorrect information or misunderstanding, temporary family disorganization and role change, exhausted support persons or systems, unrealistic expectations, fear, or anxiety

Desired Outcome: Following intervention, family members begin to verbalize feelings, identify ineffective coping patterns, identify strengths and positive coping behaviors, and seek information and support from nurse or other support persons or systems outside the family.

INTERVENTIONS	RATIONALES
Establish open, honest communication within the family. Assist family members with identifying strengths, stressors, inappropriate behaviors, and personal needs.	These actions will help promote positive, effective communication among family members while enabling family to examine areas that contribute both to effective and ineffective coping in a nonthreatening environment. For example, "I understand your mother was very ill last year. How did you manage the situation?" "I know your loved one is very ill. How can I help you?"
Assess family members for ineffective coping and identify factors that inhibit effective coping.	Ineffective methods of coping (e.g., depression, chemical dependency, violence, withdrawal) can interfere with ability to deal with the current situation. Awareness of barriers to effective coping (e.g., inadequate support system, grief, fear of disapproval by others, and deficient knowledge) is the first step toward promoting changes and healthy adaptation. For example, "You seem to be unable to talk about your husband's illness. Is there anyone with whom you can talk about it?"
Assess family's knowledge about patient's current health status and treatment. Provide information often, and allow sufficient time for questions. Reassess family's understanding at frequent intervals.	By providing information frequently and answering questions, stress, fear, and anxiety can be attenuated.

Continued

INTERVENTIONS	RATIONALES
Provide opportunities in a private setting for family members to talk and share concerns with nurses. If appropriate, refer family to psychiatric clinical nurse specialist for therapy.	Family may need additional assistance in working through family issues.
Offer realistic hope. Help the family to develop realistic expectations for the future and to identify support persons or systems that will assist them.	These actions will foster realistic expectations about patient's future health status and promote adaptation to impending changes.
Assist family with reducing anxiety by encouraging diversional activities (e.g., time spent outside the hospital) and interaction with support persons or systems outside the family.	Promoting respites enhances coping and assists family members in remaining focused and supportive of patient. For example, "I know you want to be near your son, but if you would like to go home to rest, I will call you if any changes occur."

●●● **Related NIC and NOC labels:** *NIC:* Coping Enhancement; Caregiver Support; Family Support; Respite Care *NOC:* Family Coping

Nursing Diagnosis:

Disabled Family Coping

related to unexpressed feelings, ambivalent family relationships, or disharmonious coping styles among family members

Desired Outcome: Within the 24-hr period before hospital discharge, family members begin to verbalize feelings; identify sources of support, as well as ineffective coping behaviors that create ambivalence and disharmony; and do not demonstrate destructive behaviors.

INTERVENTIONS	RATIONALES
Establish open, honest communication and rapport with family members.	An atmosphere in which family can express honest feelings and needs will help move them toward healthy coping and adaptation. For example, "I am here to care for your mother and to help your family as well."
Identify ineffective coping behaviors. Refer to psychiatric clinical nurse specialist, case manager, clergy, or support group as appropriate.	Ineffective coping behaviors (e.g., violence, depression, substance misuse, withdrawal) can interfere with learning effective strategies. Awareness of ineffective or destructive coping behaviors is the first step toward promoting change. For example, "You seem to be angry. Would you like to talk to me about your feelings?"
Identify perceived or actual conflicts.	This information enables family to examine areas that require change in a nonthreatening environment and identify potential sources of support. For example, "Are you able to talk freely with your family members?" "Are your brothers and sisters able to help and support you during this time?"
Assist family in the quest for healthy functioning and adaptations within the family unit (e.g., facilitate open communication among family members and encourage behaviors that support family cohesiveness).	Facilitating open communication among family members and encouraging behaviors that support family cohesiveness promote skill acquisition in a nonthreatening environment and identify existing coping strengths. For example, "Your mother enjoyed your last visit. Would you like to see her now?"
Assist family members in developing realistic goals, plans, and actions. Refer them to clergy, psychiatric nurse, social services, financial counseling, and family therapy as appropriate.	These actions help provide direction in making necessary changes and adaptations.

Continued

INTERVENTIONS	RATIONALES
Encourage family members to spend time outside the hospital and to interact with support individuals. Respect family's need for occasional withdrawal.	A life out of balance adds to stress and promotes maladaptive coping.
Include family members in patient's plan of care. Offer them opportunities to become involved in patient care.	Becoming involved in patient's care (e.g., range-of-motion exercises, patient hygiene, and comfort measures such as back rubs) may decrease feelings of powerlessness, thereby increasing coping ability.

••• **Related NIC and NOC labels:** *NIC:* Coping Enhancement; Family Support; Family Integrity Promotion; Respite Care; Support System Enhancement; Referral; Spiritual Support *NOC:* Caregiver Emotional Health; Caregiver-Patient Relationship; Family Coping

Nursing Diagnosis:

Readiness for Enhanced Family Coping

related to use of support persons or systems, referrals, and choosing experiences that optimize wellness

Desired Outcomes: Family members express intent to use support persons, systems, and resources, and identify alternative behaviors that promote family communication and strengths. Family members express realistic expectations and do not demonstrate ineffective coping behaviors.

INTERVENTIONS	RATIONALES
Assess family relationships, interactions, support persons or systems, and individual coping behaviors.	This assessment facilitates development of an individualized care plan using existing family structure.
Permit movement through stages of adaptation. Encourage further positive coping.	Such an environment allows family members to process events surrounding patient's illness in a healthy manner.
Acknowledge expressions of hope, plans, and growth among family members.	A sense of hopefulness is essential to process painful events in a healthy manner.
Provide opportunities in a private setting for family interactions, discussions, and questions.	Discussions and sharing of emotions in a nonpublic forum encourages development of open, honest communication within the family. For example, "I know the waiting room is very crowded. Would your family like some private time together?"
Refer family to community or support groups (e.g., ostomy support group, head injury rehabilitation group).	Many people benefit from support of other people who have had similar experiences in learning new coping strategies.
Encourage family to explore outlets that foster positive feelings.	Examples of outlets that foster positive feelings and thus promote effective coping include periods of time outside the hospital area, meaningful communication with patient or support individuals, and relaxing activities such as showering, eating, exercising.

••• **Related NIC and NOC labels:** *NIC:* Family Support; Normalization Promotion; Coping Enhancement; Support Group; Support System Enhancement *NOC:* Family Coping; Caregiver Well-Being

Nursing Diagnosis:

Deficient Knowledge:

Patient's current health status or therapies

Desired Outcome: Following intervention, family members/significant others begin to verbalize knowledge and understanding about patient's current health status and treatment.

INTERVENTIONS	RATIONALES
Assess family's health care literacy (language, reading, comprehension). Assess culture and culturally specific education needs.	This assessment helps ensure that information is presented in a manner that is culturally and educationally appropriate.
At frequent intervals, inform family about patient's current health status, therapies, and prognosis. Use individualized verbal, written, and audiovisual strategies to promote family's understanding.	Being informed frequently promotes family's accurate understanding of patient's health status and allays unnecessary anxiety. In turn, this enables family members to process and plan.
At frequent intervals, evaluate family's comprehension of information provided. Assess factors for misunderstanding, and adjust teaching as appropriate.	Some individuals in crisis need repeated explanations before comprehension can be ensured. For example, "I have explained many things to you today. Would you mind summarizing what I've told you so that I can be sure you understand your husband's status and what we are doing to care for him?"
Encourage family to relay correct information to patient.	This will reinforce comprehension for both the family and patient and promote open communication.
Inquire of family members if their information needs are being met.	This action reinforces understanding by family members and assures them that the information/support they desire will be met. For example, "Do you have any questions about the care your mother is receiving or about her condition?"
Help family members use the information they receive to make health care decisions about patient.	Family members may require assistance in processing information and applying it appropriately (e.g., regarding surgery, resuscitation, organ donation).

••• **Related NIC and NOC labels:** *NIC:* Teaching: Disease Process; Learning Readiness Enhancement; Teaching: Procedure/Treatment *NOC:* Knowledge: Disease Process; Knowledge: Illness Care; Knowledge: Treatment Procedures

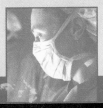

Older Adult Care 7

Nursing Diagnosis:

Acute Confusion

related to decreased cerebral perfusion secondary to age-related decreased physiologic reserve or cardiac dysfunction, electrolyte imbalance secondary to age-related decreased renal function, altered sensory/perceptual reception secondary to poor vision or hearing, or decreased brain oxygenation secondary to illness state and decreased functional lung tissue

Desired Outcomes: Patient's mental status returns to normal for patient within 3 days of treatment. Patient sustains no evidence of injury or harm as a result of mental status.

INTERVENTIONS	RATIONALES
Assess patient's baseline level of consciousness (LOC) and mental status on admission. Obtain preconfusion functional and mental status abilities from significant other. Ask patient to perform a three-step task. For example, "Raise your right hand, place it on your left shoulder, and then place the right hand by your right side."	A component of the Mini-Mental Status Examination, this assessment of a three-step task provides a baseline for subsequent assessments of patient's confusion. A three-step task is complex and is a gross indicator of brain function. Because it requires attention, it can also test for delirium.
Test short-term memory by showing patient how to use call light, having patient return the demonstration, and then waiting at least 5 min before having patient demonstrate use of call light again. Document patient's actions in behavioral terms. Describe the "confused" behavior.	Inability to remember beyond 5 min indicates poor short-term memory.
Identify cause of acute confusion.	Acute confusion is caused by physical and psychosocial conditions and not by age alone. For example, oximetry or arterial blood gas (ABG) values may reveal low oxygenation levels, serum glucose or fingerstick glucose may reveal high or low glucose level, and electrolytes and complete blood count (CBC) will ascertain imbalances and/or presence of elevated white blood cell (WBC) count as a determinant of infection. Hydration status may be determined by pinching skin over sternum or forehead for turgor (tenting occurs with fluid volume deficit) and checking for dry mucous membranes and furrowed tongue.
Assess for pain using a rating scale of 0-10. If patient is unable to use a scale, assess for behavioral cues such as grimacing, clenched fists, frowning, and hitting. Ask family or significant other to assist in identifying pain behaviors.	Acute confusion can be a sign of pain.
Treat patient for pain, as indicated, and monitor behaviors.	If pain is the cause of the confusion, patient's behavior should change accordingly.
Review cardiac status. Assess apical pulse and notify health care provider of an irregular pulse that is new to the patient. If patient is on a cardiac monitor or telemetry, watch for dysrhythmias; notify health care provider accordingly.	Dysrhythmias and other cardiac dysfunctions may result in decreased oxygenation, which can lead to confusion.
Review current medications, including over-the-counter (OTC) drugs, with pharmacist.	Toxic levels of certain medications, such as digoxin or theophylline, cause acute confusion. Drugs that are anticholinergic also can cause confusion, as can drug interactions.

Continued

INTERVENTIONS	RATIONALES
Monitor intake and output (I&O) at least q8h.	Optimally, output should match intake. Dehydration can result in acute confusion.
Review patient's creatinine clearance test to assess renal function.	Renal function plays an important role in fluid balance and is the main mechanism of drug clearance. Blood urea nitrogen (BUN) and serum creatinine are affected by hydration status and in older patients reveal only part of the picture. Therefore, to fully understand and assess renal function in older patients, creatinine clearance must be tested.
Have patient wear glasses and hearing aid, or keep them close to the bedside and within easy reach for patient use.	Glasses and hearing aids are likely to help decrease sensory confusion.
Keep patient's urinal and other routinely used items within easy reach for patient.	A confused patient may wait until it is too late to seek assistance with toileting.
If patient has short-term memory problems, toilet or offer urinal or bedpan q2h while awake and q4h during the night. Establish a toileting schedule and post it on patient care plan and, inconspicuously, at the bedside.	A patient with a short-term memory problem cannot be expected to use the call light.
Check on patient at least q30min and every time you pass the room. Place patient close to nurses' station if possible. Provide an environment that is nonstimulating and safe.	A confused patient requires extra safety precautions.
Provide music but not TV.	Patients who are confused regarding place and time often think the action on TV is happening in the room.
Attempt to reorient patient to surroundings as needed. Keep a clock with large numerals and a large print calendar at the bedside; verbally remind patient of date and day as needed.	Reorientation may decrease confusion.
Tell patient in simple terms what is occurring. For example, "It's time to eat breakfast," "This medicine is for your heart," "I'm going to help you get out of bed."	Sentences that are more complex may not be understood.
Encourage patient's significant other to bring items familiar to patient, including blanket, bedspread, pictures of family and pets.	Familiar items may promote orientation while also providing comfort.
If patient becomes belligerent, angry, or argumentative while you are attempting to reorient, *stop this approach.* Do not argue with patient or patient's interpretation of the environment. State, "I can understand why you may [hear, think, see] that."	This approach prevents escalation of anger in a confused person.
If patient displays hostile behavior or misperceives your role (e.g., nurse becomes thief, jailer), leave the room. Return in 15 min. Introduce yourself to patient as though you had never met. Begin dialogue anew.	Patients who are acutely confused have poor short-term memory and may not remember the previous encounter or that you were involved in that encounter.
If patient attempts to leave the hospital, walk with patient and attempt distraction. Ask patient to tell you about the destination For example, "That sounds like a wonderful place! Tell me about it." Keep tone pleasant and conversational. Continue walking with patient away from exits and doors around the unit. After a few minutes, attempt to guide patient back to the room. Offer refreshments and a rest. For example, "We've been walking for a while and I'm a little tired. Why don't we sit and have some juice while we talk?"	Distraction is an effective means of reversing a behavior in the patient who is confused.
If patient has a permanent or severe cognitive impairment, check on her or him at least q30min and reorient to baseline mental status as indicated; however, do not argue with patient about his or her perception of reality.	Arguing can cause a cognitively impaired person to become aggressive and combative. **Note:** Individuals with severe cognitive impairment (e.g., Alzheimer's disease or dementia) also can experience acute confusional states (i.e., delirium) and can be returned to their baseline mental state.
If patient tries to climb out of bed, offer urinal or bedpan or assist to the commode.	Patient may need to use the toilet.
Alternatively, if patient is not on bedrest, place him or her in chair or wheelchair at nurses' station.	This action provides added supervision to promote patient's safety while also promoting stimulation and preventing isolation.

Continued

INTERVENTIONS

INTERVENTIONS	RATIONALES
Bargain with patient. Try to establish an agreement to stay for a defined period, such as until health care provider, meal, or significant other arrives.	This is a delaying strategy to defuse anger. Because of poor memory and attention span, patient may forget he or she wanted to leave.
Have patient's significant other talk with patient by phone or come in and sit with patient if patient's behavior requires checking more often than q30min.	These actions by significant other may help promote patient's safety.
If patient is attempting to pull out tubes, hide them (e.g., under blankets). Put a stockinette mesh dressing over IV lines. Tape feeding tubes to side of patient's face using paper tape, and drape the tube behind patient's ear.	Remember: Out of sight, out of mind.
Evaluate continued need for certain therapies.	Such therapies may become irritating stimuli. For example, if patient is now drinking, discontinue IV line; if patient is eating, discontinue feeding tube; if patient has an indwelling urethral catheter, discontinue catheter and begin toileting routine.
Use restraints with caution and according to agency policy.	Patients can become more agitated when wrist and arm restraints are used.
Use medications cautiously for controlling behavior.	Follow the maxim "start low and go slow" with medications because older patients can respond to small amounts of drugs.
	Neuroleptics, such as haloperidol, can be used successfully in calming patients with dementia or psychiatric illness (contraindicated for individuals with parkinsonism). However, if patient is experiencing acute confusion or delirium, short-acting benzodiazepines (e.g., lorazepam) are more effective in reducing anxiety and fear. Anxiety or fear usually triggers destructive or dangerous behaviors in acutely confused older patients. **Note:** Neuroleptics can cause akathisia, an adverse drug reaction evidenced by increased restlessness.

Also see "Dementia—Alzheimer's Type," p. 751, as appropriate.

••• **Related NIC and NOC labels:** *NIC:* Dementia Management; Reality Orientation; Cerebral Perfusion Promotion; Environmental Management: Safety; Neurologic Monitoring *NOC:* Information Processing; Identity; Distorted Thought Control; Decision Making; Cognitive Orientation; Cognitive Ability

Nursing Diagnosis:

Impaired Gas Exchange (or risk for same)

related to decreased functional lung tissue secondary to age-related changes

Desired Outcomes: Patient's respiratory pattern and mental status remain normal for patient. Patient's ABG or pulse oximetry values are within patient's normal limits.

INTERVENTIONS	RATIONALES
Assess and document the following upon admission and routinely thereafter: respiratory rate (RR), pattern, and depth; breath sounds; cough; sputum; and sensorium.	This assessment establishes a baseline for subsequent assessments of patient's respiratory system.
Assess patient for subtle changes in mentation such as increased restlessness, anxiety, disorientation, and presence of hostility. If available, monitor oxygenation status via ABG findings (optimally Pao_2 80%-95% or greater) or pulse oximetry (optimally greater than 92%).	Mentation changes such as increased restlessness, anxiety, disorientation, and presence of hostility can signal decreased oxygenation.
Assess lungs for presence of adventitious sounds.	The aging lung has decreased elasticity. The lower part of the lung is no longer adequately aerated. As a result, crackles commonly are heard in individuals 75 years of age and older. This sign alone does not mean that a pathologic condition is present. Crackles (rales) that do not clear with coughing in an individual with no other clinical signs (e.g., fever, increasing anxiety, changes in mental status, increasing respiratory depth) are considered benign.

Continued

INTERVENTIONS	RATIONALES
Encourage patient to cough and breathe deeply. When appropriate, instruct patient in use of incentive spirometry.	These actions promote alveolar expansion and clear the secretions from the bronchial tree, thereby helping ensure better gas exchange.
Unless contraindicated by a cardiac or renal condition, encourage fluid intake to greater than 2.5 L/day.	Hydration helps ensure less viscous pulmonary secretions, which are more easily mobilized.
Treat fevers promptly, decrease pain, minimize pacing activity, and lessen anxiety.	These interventions reduce potential for increased oxygen consumption.
Instruct patient in use of support equipment such as oxygen masks or cannulas.	Knowledge helps promote adherence to therapy.

••• **Related NIC and NOC labels:** *NIC:* Vital Signs Monitoring; Laboratory Data Interpretation; Oxygen Therapy; Respiratory Monitoring; Chest Physiotherapy; Cough Enhancement *NOC:* Vital Signs Status; Tissue Perfusion: Pulmonary; Respiratory Status: Gas Exchange

Risk for Aspiration

related to loss of muscle mass or dysfunction in body parts necessary for optimal swallowing secondary to age-related changes

Desired Outcomes: Patient swallows independently without choking. Patient's airway is patent and lungs are clear to auscultation both before and after meals.

INTERVENTIONS	RATIONALES
Perform a baseline assessment of patient's ability to swallow by asking if he or she has any difficulty swallowing or if any foods or fluids are difficult to swallow or cause gagging. If patient is unable to answer, consult patient's caregiver or significant other. Document findings.	This assessment helps determine patient's ability to swallow without choking and should be compared with subsequent assessments to document improvements or deficits.
Assess patient's ability to swallow by placing thumb and index finger on both sides of the laryngeal prominence and asking patient to swallow. Check for the gag reflex by gently touching one side and then the other of the posterior pharyngeal wall using a tongue blade. Document both findings.	Ability to swallow and an intact gag reflex are necessary to prevent aspiration and choking before patient takes foods or fluids orally.
Place patient in an upright position with chin tilting down slightly while eating or drinking, and support upright position with pillows on patient's sides.	This position minimizes risk of choking and aspirating by closing off the airway and facilitating gravitational flow of foods and fluids into the stomach and through the pylorus.
Monitor patient when he or she is swallowing.	This assessment will help determine patient's ability to swallow without choking. Deficits may necessitate aspiration precautions.
Watch for drooling of saliva or food, or inability to close lips around a straw.	These are signs of limited lip, tongue, or jaw movement.
Check for retention of food in sides of mouth.	This is an indication of poor tongue movement.
Monitor intake of food. Document consistencies and amounts of food patient eats, where patient places food in the mouth, how patient manipulates or chews before swallowing, and length of time before patient swallows the food bolus.	Other caregivers will find this information useful during subsequent feedings.
Monitor patient for coughing or choking before, during, or after swallowing.	Coughing or choking may occur up to several minutes following placement of food or fluid in the mouth and signals aspiration of material into the airway.
Monitor patient for changes in lung auscultation (e.g., crackles [rales], wheezes, rhonchi), shortness of breath, dyspnea, decreasing LOC, increasing temperature, and cyanosis.	These are signs of silent aspiration. For example, some older patients, especially those in declining health, have increased risk for silent aspiration when the esophageal sphincter fails to close completely between swallows.
Monitor patient for a wet or gurgling sound when talking after a swallow.	This sound indicates aspiration into the airway and signals delayed or absent swallow and gag reflexes.

Continued

INTERVENTIONS	RATIONALES
For patients with poor swallowing reflex, tilt their head forward 45 degrees during swallowing. **Note:** For patients with hemiplegia, tilt head toward unaffected side.	This head position will help prevent inadvertent aspiration by closing off the airway.
As indicated, request evaluation by speech therapist.	This evaluation will enable specialized assessment of gag and swallow reflexes.
Anticipate swallowing video fluoroscopy in evaluation of patient's gag and swallow reflexes.	This procedure is used to determine whether patient is aspirating, consistency of materials most likely to be aspirated, and aspiration cause.
	Using four consistencies of barium, the radiologist and speech therapist watch for the presence of reduced or ineffective tongue function, reduced peristalsis in the pharynx, delayed or absent swallow reflex, and poor or limited ability to close the epiglottis that protects the airway.
Based on results of the swallowing video fluoroscopy, thickened fluids may be prescribed.	Agents are added to the fluid to make it more viscous and easier for patient to swallow. Similarly, mechanical soft, pureed, or liquid diets may be prescribed to enable patient to ingest food with less potential for aspiration.
Provide adequate rest periods before meals.	Fatigue increases risk for aspiration.
Remind patients with dementia to chew and swallow with each bite. Check for retained food in sides of mouth.	Patients with dementia might forget to chew and swallow.
Ensure that patient has dentures in place, if appropriate, and that they fit correctly.	Chewing well minimizes risk of choking.
Ensure that someone stays with patient during meals or fluid intake.	This ensures added safety in the event of choking or aspiration.
Provide adequate time for patient to eat and drink.	Generally, patients with swallowing deficits require twice as much time for eating and drinking as those whose swallowing is adequate.
Be aware of location of suction equipment to be used in the event of aspiration.	If patient is at increased risk for aspiration, suction equipment should be available at the bedside.
If patient aspirates, implement the following:	
- Follow American Heart Association (AHA) standards if patient displays characteristics of complete airway obstruction (i.e., choking).	This is an emergency situation.
- For partial airway obstruction, encourage patient to cough as needed.	This action will clear the airway.
- For partial airway obstruction in unconscious or nonresponsive individual who is not coughing, suction airway with a large-bore catheter such as Yankauer or tonsil suction tip.	Suctioning clears the airway.
- For either a complete or partial aspiration, inform health care provider and obtain prescription for chest x-ray examination.	X-ray will determine if food/fluid remains in the airway.
- Implement NPO (nothing by mouth) status until diagnosis is confirmed.	NPO prevents further risk to patient.
- Monitor breathing pattern and RR q1-2h after a suspected aspiration for alterations (i.e., increased RR).	This assessment helps determine that a change in patient's condition has occurred.
- Anticipate use of antibiotics.	There is risk for infection/pneumonia after aspiration.
Encourage patient to cough and deep breathe q2h while awake and q4h during the night.	These measures promote expansion of available lung tissue and help prevent infection.

••• **Related NIC and NOC labels:** *NIC:* Aspiration Precautions; Respiratory Monitoring; Vital Signs Monitoring; Airway Suctioning
NOC: Aspiration Control; Swallowing Status

Nursing Diagnosis:

Risk for Deficient Fluid Volume

related to inability to obtain fluids by self secondary to illness, placement of fluid, or presence of chronic illness; or related to use of osmotic agents during radiologic tests

Desired Outcomes: Patient's mental status; VS; and urine specific gravity, color, consistency, and concentration remain within normal limits for patient. Patient's mucous membranes remain moist, and there is no "tenting" of skin. Patient's intake equals output.

INTERVENTIONS	RATIONALES
Monitor fluid intake. In nonrestricted individuals, encourage fluid intake of 2-3 L/day. Specify intake goals for day, evening, and night shifts.	These actions help ensure that patient's hydration status is adequate.
Assess and document skin turgor. Check hydration status by pinching skin over sternum or forehead.	Skin that remains in the lifted position (tenting) and returns slowly to its original position indicates dehydration. A furrowed tongue signals severe dehydration.
Assess and document color, amount, and frequency of any fluid output, including emesis, urine, diarrhea, or other drainage.	This assessment enables comparison of intake to output amounts. Urine that is dark in color signals concentration and thus dehydration.
Monitor patient's orientation, ability to follow commands, and behavior.	Loss of ability to follow commands, decrease in orientation, and confused behavior can signal a dehydrated state.
Weigh patient daily at the same time of day (preferably before breakfast) using same scale and bed clothing.	Using comparable measurements ensures more accurate comparisons. Wide variations in weight (e.g., 2.5 kg [5 lb] or greater) can signal increased or decreased hydration status.
In patient who is dehydrated, anticipate elevation in serum Na^+, BUN, and serum creatinine levels.	These elevations often occur with dehydration.
If patient is receiving IV therapy, monitor cardiac and respiratory systems for signs of overload. Assess apical pulse and listen to lung fields during every VS assessment.	Overload could precipitate heart failure or pulmonary edema. Rising HR, crackles, and bronchial wheezes can be signals of heart failure or pulmonary edema.
Carefully monitor I&O when patient is receiving tube feedings or dyes for contrast. Watch for evidence of third spacing of fluids, including increasing peripheral edema, especially sacral; output significantly less than intake (1:2); and urine output less than 30 ml/hr.	These agents act osmotically to pull fluid into interstitial tissue.
Whenever in the room, offer patient fluid. Offer a variety of drinks that patient likes, but limit caffeine because it acts as a diuretic.	Older persons have a decreased sense of thirst and need encouragement to drink.
Assess patient's ability to obtain and drink fluids by himself or herself. Place fluids within easy reach. Use cups with tops to minimize concern over spilling.	These actions remove barriers to adequate fluid intake.
Ensure access to toilet, urinal, commode, or bedpan at least q2h when patient is awake and q4h at night. Answer call light quickly.	The time between recognition of the need to void and urination decreases with age.

••• Related NIC and NOC labels: *NIC:* Fluid/Electrolyte Management; Intravenous Therapy; Vital Signs Monitoring; Cardiac Care: Acute; Urinary Elimination Management; Self-Care Assistance: Feeding *NOC:* Nutritional Status: Food & Fluid Intake; Hydration; Fluid Balance Electrolyte & Acid/Base Balance

Nursing Diagnosis:

Risk for Infection

related to age-related changes in immune and integumentary systems, suppressed inflammatory response secondary to long-term medication use (e.g., antiinflammatory agents, steroids, analgesics), slowed ciliary response, or poor nutrition

Desired Outcome: Patient remains free of infection as evidenced by orientation to person, place, and time and behavior within patient's normal limits; RR and pattern within patient's normal limits; urine that is straw colored, clear, and of characteristic odor; core temperature and HR within patient's normal limits; sputum that is clear to whitish in color; and skin that is intact and of normal color and temperature for patient.

INTERVENTIONS	RATIONALES
Assess patient's baseline VS, including LOC and orientation. Also be alert to HR greater than 100 bpm and RR greater than 24 breaths/min. Auscultate lung fields for adventitious sounds. Be aware, however, that crackles (rales) may be a normal finding when heard in the lung bases.	A change in mentation is a leading sign of infection in older patients. Other signs of infection include tachycardia and tachypnea. Adventitious breath sounds may or may not be seen until late in the course of illness.
Monitor patient's temperature, using a low-range thermometer if possible.	Older adults may run lower temperatures because of decreasing metabolism in individuals who are inactive and sedentary. They also tend to lose heat readily to the environment and may not be kept at the right temperature. A temperature of 35.5° C (96° F) may be normal, whereas a temperature of 36.67°-37.22° C (98°-99° F) may be considered febrile.
Obtain temperature readings rectally if the oral reading does not match the clinical picture (i.e., patient's skin is very warm, patient is restless, mentation is depressed), or if the temperature reads 36.11° C (97° F) or higher.	If the oral reading seems unreliable, rectal readings may help ensure that patient's core temperature is accurately determined.
If possible, avoid use of a tympanic thermometer.	Reliability of the electronic tympanic thermometer may be inconsistent because of improper use.
Assess patient's skin for tears, breaks, redness, or ulcers. Document condition of patient's skin on admission and as an ongoing assessment (refer to **Risk for Impaired Skin Integrity,** p. 100).	Skin that is not intact is susceptible to infection.
Assess quality and color of patient's urine. Document changes when noted, and report findings to health care provider. Also be alert to urinary incontinence, which can signal urinary tract infection (UTI).	UTI, as manifested by cloudy, foul-smelling urine without painful urination and urinary incontinence is the most common infection in older adults.
Avoid insertion of urinary catheters when possible.	Urinary catheter use increases risk of infection.
Obtain drug history in reference to use of antiinflammatory or immunosuppressive drugs or long-term use of analgesics or steroids.	These drugs mask fever, a sign of infection.
If infection is suspected, anticipate initiation of IV fluid therapy.	Fluid therapy will help maintain optimal hydration as well as replace losses caused by fever and thin the secretions for easier expectoration.
Anticipate blood cultures, urinalysis, and urine culture.	Cultures will isolate the bacteria type.
Anticipate WBC count.	WBC count 11,000/mm³ or higher can be a late sign of infection in older patients because the immune system is slow to respond to insult.
Expect a chest x-ray examination if patient's chest sounds are not clear.	This will be performed to rule out pneumonia.
If infection is present, prepare for initiation of broad-spectrum antibiotic therapy, oxygen therapy, and use of acetaminophen.	These interventions will eliminate infection, promote oxygenation to the brain, and decrease fever. Fever increases cardiac workload (i.e., HR rises) as the body responds to infection. Because of decreased physiologic reserve, older patients may have increased risk of heart failure or pulmonary edema from prolonged tachycardia.

••• **Related NIC and NOC labels:** *NIC:* Respiratory Monitoring; Vital Signs Monitoring; Skin Surveillance; Specimen Management *NOC:* Infection Status

Nursing Diagnosis:

Hypothermia

related to age-related changes in thermoregulation and/or environmental exposure

Desired Outcome: Patient's temperature and mental status remain within patient's normal limits, or they return to patient's normal limits at a rate of 1° F/hr, after interventions.

INTERVENTIONS	RATIONALES
Monitor patient's temperature, using a low-range thermometer if possible.	This assessment will determine if patient has hypothermia. Older adults can have a normal temperature of 35.5° C (96° F).
Assess patient's temperature orally by placing thermometer far back in patient's mouth.	This method provides the most accurate assessment of patient's core temperature.
Note: Do not take axillary temperature in the older adult. If unable to measure patient's temperature orally, measure temperature via ear but note that reliability of electronic tympanic thermometers may be inconsistent because of improper use.	Older persons have decreased peripheral circulation and loss of subcutaneous fat in the axillary area, resulting in formation of a pocket of air that may make readings inaccurate.
Assess and document patient's mental status.	Increasing disorientation, mental status changes, or presence of atypical behavior can signal hypothermia.
Be alert to patients taking sedatives, hypnotics (including anesthetics), and muscle relaxants.	These drugs decrease shivering and therefore place patients at risk for environmental hypothermia. In addition, all older adults are at risk for environmental hypothermia at ambient temperatures of 22.22°-23.89° C (72°-75° F).
Ensure that patients going for testing or x-ray examination are sent with enough blankets to keep warm.	This intervention will help prevent hypothermia.
If patient is mildly hypothermic, initiate slow rewarming.	To reverse mild hypothermia, one method of slow rewarming is raising room temperature to at least 23.89° C (75° F). Other methods of external warming include use of warm blankets, head covers, and warm circulating air blankets.
If patient's temperature falls below 35° C (95° F), warm patient internally by administering warm oral or IV fluids.	To reverse moderate to severe hypothermia, patient is warmed internally by administering warm oral or IV fluids. Warmed saline gastric or rectal irrigations or introduction of warmed humidified air into the airway are other methods of internal warming.
Be alert to signs of too rapid rewarming.	Signs of too rapid rewarming include irregular HR, dysrhythmias, and very warm extremities caused by vasodilation in the periphery, which causes heat loss from the core.
If patient's temperature fails to rise 1° F/hr using these techniques, anticipate laboratory tests, including WBC count for possible sepsis, thyroid test for hypothyroidism, and glucose level for hypoglycemia.	Causes other than environmental ones may be responsible for the hypothermia.
As prescribed, administer antibiotics for sepsis, initiate thyroid therapy, or administer glucose for hypoglycemia.	The patient's temperature will not return to normal unless the underlying condition has been treated.

••• **Related NIC and NOC labels:** *NIC:* Hypothermia Treatment; Vital Signs Monitoring; Environmental Management; Heat Application; Fluid Management *NOC:* Thermoregulation

Nursing Diagnosis:

Risk for Impaired Skin Integrity

related to decreased subcutaneous fat and decreased peripheral capillary networks secondary to age-related changes in the integumentary system

Desired Outcome: Patient's skin remains nonerythremic and intact.

INTERVENTIONS	RATIONALES
Assess patient's skin on admission and routinely thereafter.	This assessment provides a baseline for subsequent assessments of patient's skin integrity.
Note any areas of redness or any breaks in the skin surface.	Redness or breaks in skin integrity necessitate aggressive skin care interventions to prevent further breakdown and infection.
Ensure that patient turns frequently (at least q2h).	Turning alternates sites of pressure and pressure relief.
Lift or roll patient across sheets when repositioning.	Pulling, dragging, or sliding across sheets can lead to shear (cutaneous or subcutaneous tissue) injury.
Monitor skin over bony prominences for erythema.	Skin that lies over the sacrum, scapulae, heels, spine, hips, pelvis, greater trochanter, knees, ankles, costal margins, occiput, and ischial tuberosities is at increased risk for breakdown because of excessive external pressure.
Use pillows or pads around bony prominences, even when patient is up in a wheelchair or sits for long periods.	This intervention maintains alternative positions and pads bony prominences, thereby protecting overlying skin. The ischial tuberosities are susceptible to breakdown when patient is in the seated position. Gel pads for chair or wheelchair seats aid in distributing pressure.
Use lotions liberally on dry skin.	Lotions promote moisture and suppleness. Lanolin-containing lotions are especially useful.
Use alternating-pressure mattress, air-fluidized mattress, waterbed, air bed, or other pressure-sensitive mattress for older patients who are on bedrest or unable to get out of bed.	These mattresses protect skin from injury caused by prolonged pressure.
Avoid placing tubes under patient's limbs or head. Place pillow or pad between patient and tube for cushioning.	Excess pressure from tubes can create a pressure ulcer.
Get patient out of bed as often as possible. Liberally use mechanical lifting devices to aid in safe patient transfers. If patient is unable to get out of bed, assist with position changes q2h.	These actions promote blood flow, which helps prevent skin breakdown.
Establish and post a turning schedule on the patient care plan and at the bedside.	Schedules increase awareness of staff and patient/family of turning schedule.
Ensure that patient's face, axillae, and genital areas are cleansed daily.	Complete baths dry out older adults' skin and should be given every other day instead.
Use tepid water (90°-105° F [32.2°-40.5° C]) and super-fatted, nonperfumed soaps.	Hot water can burn older adults, who have decreased pain sensitivity and decreased sensation to temperature. Super-fatted soaps help decrease dryness of skin.
Minimize use of plastic protective pads under patient. When used, place at least one layer of cloth (drawsheet) between patient and plastic pad to absorb moisture. For incontinent patient, check pad at least q2h.	These pads trap moisture and heat and can lead to skin breakdown.
Document percentage of food intake with meals. Encourage significant other to provide patient's favorite foods. Suggest nutritious snacks if patient's diet is not restricted. Obtain nutritional consultation with dietitian as needed.	Food/snacks high in protein and vitamin C help prevent skin breakdown.
For more information, see "Providing Nutritional Support," p. 565, and "Pressure Ulcers," p. 562.	

••• **Related NIC and NOC labels:** *NIC:* Skin Surveillance; Positioning; Circulatory Precautions; Pressure Management; Skin Care: Topical Treatments; Bathing *NOC:* Tissue Integrity: Skin & Mucous Membranes; Immobility Consequences: Physiologic

Nursing Diagnosis:

Disturbed Sleep Pattern

related to unfamiliar surroundings and hospital routines

Desired Outcomes: Within 24 hr of interventions, patient reports attainment of adequate rest. Mental status remains normal for the patient.

INTERVENTIONS	RATIONALES
Assess and document patient's sleeping pattern, obtaining information from patient or patient's caregiver or significant other.	Older adults typically sleep less than they did when they were younger and often awaken more frequently during the night.
Ask questions about naps and activity levels.	Individuals who take naps and have a low level of activity frequently sleep only 4-5 hr/night.
Determine patient's usual nighttime routine and attempt to emulate it.	Following patient's usual nighttime rituals may facilitate sleep.
Attempt to group together activities such as medications, VS, and toileting.	This reduces the number of interruptions and facilitates rest and sleep.
Provide pain medications, back rub, and pleasant conversation at sleep time.	These comfort measures may facilitate sleep.
Monitor patient's activity level.	If patient complains of being tired after activities or displays behaviors such as irritability, yelling, or shouting, encourage napping after lunch or early in the afternoon. Otherwise, discourage daytime napping, especially in the late afternoon, because it can interfere with nighttime sleep.
Discourage caffeinated coffee, cola, and tea after 6 PM.	Stimulants can make it difficult to fall asleep and stay asleep as well as increase nighttime awakenings to urinate.
Provide a quiet environment and minimize interruptions during sleep hours.	Excessive noises, bright overhead lights, noisy roommates, and loud talking can cause sleep deprivation. Use of sound generators (e.g., of ocean waves) or white noise (e.g., fan) may promote sleep.

••• **Related NIC and NOC labels:** *NIC:* Energy Management; Sleep Enhancement; Exercise Promotion; Environmental Management: Comfort; Simple Massage; Pain Management *NOC:* Rest; Sleep

Nursing Diagnosis:

Constipation

related to changes in diet, activity, and psychosocial factors secondary to hospitalization

Desired Outcomes: Patient states that bowel habit has returned to normal pattern within 3-4 days of this diagnosis. Stool appears soft, and patient does not strain in passing stools.

INTERVENTIONS	RATIONALES
On admission, assess and document patient's normal bowel elimination pattern. Include frequency, time of day, associated habits, and successful methods used to correct constipation in the past. Consult patient's caregiver or significant other if patient is unable to provide this information.	This assessment establishes baseline and determines patient's normal bowel elimination pattern.
Inform patient that changes occurring with hospitalization may increase potential for constipation. Urge patient to institute successful nonpharmacologic methods used at home as soon as this problem is noticed or prophylactically as needed.	Constipation is easier to treat preventively than it is when present and/or prolonged.
Teach patient the relationship between fluid intake and constipation. Unless otherwise contraindicated, encourage fluid intake that exceeds 2500 ml/day. Monitor and record bowel movements (date, time, consistency, amount).	A high fluid intake promotes soft stool and decreases risk/degree of constipation. A high fluid volume may be contraindicated in patients with renal, cardiac, or hepatic disorders who may have fluid restrictions.
Encourage patient to include roughage (e.g., raw fruits and vegetables, whole grains, nuts, fruits with skins) as a part of each meal when possible. For patients unable to tolerate raw foods, encourage intake of bran via cereals, muffins, and breads.	Eating roughage reduces potential for constipation by promoting bulk in the stool.
Titrate amount of roughage to the degree of constipation.	Too much roughage taken too quickly can cause diarrhea, gas, and distention.

Continued

INTERVENTIONS	RATIONALES
Teach patient the relationship between constipation and activity level. Encourage optimum activity for all patients. Establish and post an activity program to enhance participation; include devices necessary to enable independence.	Exercise can prevent or decrease constipation by promoting peristalsis.
If patient's bowel movement occurs in the early morning, use patient's gastrocolic or duodenocolic reflex to promote colonic emptying. If patient's bowel movement occurs in the evening, ambulate patient just before the appropriate time.	Scheduling interventions that coincide with patient's bowel habit are more likely to promote bowel movements. Drinking hot liquids in the morning, for example, also promotes peristalsis. Digital stimulation of the inner anal sphincter also may facilitate bowel movement.
Attempt to use methods patient has used successfully in the past. Follow the maxim "go low, go slow" (i.e., use lowest level of nonnatural intervention and advance to more powerful interventions slowly).	Aggressive interventions may result in rebound constipation and interfere with patient's subsequent bowel movements.
When requesting a pharmacologic intervention, use the more benign, oral methods first.	Older persons tend to focus on the loss of habit as an indicator of constipation rather than on the number of stools. Do not intervene pharmacologically until the older adult has not had a stool for 3 days. The following hierarchy is suggested. - Bulk-building additives such as psyllium or bran - Mild laxatives (apple or prune juice, Milk of Magnesia) - Stool softeners (docusate sodium, docusate calcium) - Potent laxatives or cathartics (bisacodyl, cascara sagrada) - Medicated suppositories (glycerin, bisacodyl) - Enema (tap water, saline, sodium biphosphate/phosphate)
After diagnostic imaging of the gastrointestinal tract with barium, ensure that patient receives a postexamination laxative.	The laxative facilitates removal of the barium. After any procedure involving a bowel clean-out, there may be rebound constipation from the severe disruption of bowel habit.
Monitor hydration status for signs of dehydration. Emphasize diet, fluid, activity, and resumption of routines. If no bowel movement occurs in 3 days, begin with mild laxatives to try to regain normal pattern.	Dehydration can occur as a result of osmotic agents used. Deficient fluid volume can result in hard stools, which are more difficult to evacuate.

See Also: "Prolonged Bedrest," for **Constipation,** p. 67.

••• **Related NIC and NOC labels:** *NIC:* Constipation Management; Fluid Management; Exercise Promotion; Nutrition Management *NOC:* Bowel Elimination; Hydration; Symptom Control

Nursing Diagnosis:

Hopelessness

related to slow recovery from illness or surgery secondary to decreased physiologic reserve

Desired Outcome: Within 2-4 days of interventions, patient verbalizes knowledge of his or her strengths, feelings about health, and the understanding of a potentially long recovery.

INTERVENTIONS	RATIONALES
Monitor patient for signs of depression.	Behavior such as refusal to participate in own care; refusal to eat or marked decline in appetite or intake; refusal to answer questions; and statements such as "I don't care," "Leave me alone," and "Let me die." are signs of hopelessness and depression.
Encourage patient to verbalize feelings of despair, frustration, fear, and anger and concerns regarding hospitalization and health. Reassure patient and significant other that such feelings and concerns are normal.	Verbalization of feelings and the knowledge that these feelings are normal often help minimize feelings of despair.

Continued

INTERVENTIONS	RATIONALES
Discuss normal age changes with patient.	Recovery periods are longer for older adults because of decreased physiologic reserve. More energy is spent in maintaining normal status, and thus the body has less capacity to rebuild strength and endurance.
Encourage short-term goals and praise small steps, such as participation in own care.	These actions may help decrease frustrations caused by slow recovery.
Arrange a care conference to discuss discharge requirements specific to patient. Involve patient and significant other in the conference.	Reassurance about continuity of care may help diminish feelings of frustration and hopelessness.
Set realistic goals with patient based on patient's condition and desires.	A decrease in physiologic reserve increases recovery time.

••• **Related NIC and NOC labels:** *NIC:* Active Listening; Emotional Support; Mutual Goal Setting; Family Support; Role Enhancement
NOC: Quality of Life; Hope; Decision Making; Depression Control

Nursing Diagnosis:

Powerlessness

related to hospital environment

Desired Outcome: Within 2-4 days after interventions, patient participates in care and verbalizes feelings of control over his or her environment.

INTERVENTIONS	RATIONALES
Encourage patient to verbalize feelings about hospitalization and illness.	This will help determine if patient is experiencing feelings of powerlessness.
Assist patient in identifying factors that contribute to feelings of powerlessness.	Identifying causative factors is the first step in eliminating them.
Encourage patient to participate in activities of daily living (ADL) as much as possible. Provide adequate time for patient to complete ADL.	Participating in self-care will help decrease feelings of powerlessness.
As often as possible, enable patient to participate in scheduling of activities.	Having a "say so" in scheduling may decrease feelings of powerlessness.
Discuss with patient and significant other realistic goals of care, and encourage patient's participation in care planning.	Participating in care planning helps promote some sense of control and power.
Explain procedures and routines to patient. Inform patient when changes in the plan of care are necessary.	Staying well informed decreases sense of powerlessness.
Provide flexibility in patient's plan of care when possible (e.g., if patient wants to wear his or her own clothes, enable patient to do so).	Having flexibility promotes a sense of having some control and power.

••• **Related NIC and NOC labels:** *NIC:* Active Listening; Decision-Making Support; Self-Responsibility Facilitation; Mutual Goal Setting
NOC: Participation: Health Care Decisions

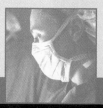

Palliative and End-of-Life Care 8

OVERVIEW/PATHOPHYSIOLOGY

According to the World Health Organization (2003) and the National Consensus Project for Quality Palliative Care (2004), palliative care is the active total care of patients whose disease is not responsive to curative treatment. Control of pain and other symptoms and of psychologic, social, and spiritual problems is paramount. The goal of palliative care is achievement of the best quality of life for patients and their families. The following nursing diagnoses relate specifically to issues, outcomes, and interventions that are common across medical diagnoses for patients in an advanced phase of illness.

HEALTH CARE SETTING

Primary care, hospitalization, hospice or palliative care, home health care

---

NURSING DIAGNOSES EARLIER IN THE DISEASE PROCESS

Nursing Diagnosis:

Deficient Knowledge:

Choices regarding disease management when cure is unrealistic, including data about advance directives and comfort-focused care

Desired Outcome: Patient and family express knowledge about advance directives, complete documents in accordance with state laws, and have discussion with health care team within weeks of diagnosis of life-limiting illness or before an acute crisis occurs.

INTERVENTIONS	RATIONALES
Assess patient's health care literacy (language, reading, comprehension). Assess culture and culturally specific information needs.	This assessment helps ensure that information is presented in a manner that is culturally and educationally appropriate.
Advise patient of need for prompt legal preparations (will, trusts, Durable Power of Attorney for Health Care [DPOA-HC]). Discuss role/ limitations of DPOA-HC. Secure copies of legal documents and place in patient's medical record.	This information ensures that patient, family, and staff are aware of legal preparations and promotes understanding of ability to make choices and maintain control when illness becomes advanced.
Ensure that patient's preferences for hydration and nutrition are addressed specifically in DPOA-HC or living will documents as required by state law.	These documents make patient's wishes regarding autopsy, organ donation/transplantation, hydration and feeding tubes, use of antibiotics, chemotherapy, radiation therapy, diagnostic procedures, blood transfusions, and IVs known to family members and health care providers and ensures that those wishes are clear.
Assist patient in completion of advance directives documents, which might also include "Five Wishes."	"Five Wishes," a program currently available in most states, is a style of advance directives that outlines the type of care a patient desires, not just what should be withheld.
Discuss meaning of "do not resuscitate" (DNR) Order and preferences for withholding or withdrawing other life-sustaining therapies.	This information helps ensure that patient and family/significant others understand what will occur during this phase of care.

Continued

INTERVENTIONS	RATIONALES
Explain what is meant by "comfort measures only."	This information will help patient make decisions regarding care and nutrition outlined in advance directives.
Encourage professional counseling if any of the previous cause discord within the family.	Patients should select a DPOA-HC that is capable of carrying out their wishes. The patient's wishes may not be the wishes of the person who is the closest relative.

••• **Related NIC and NOC labels:** *NIC:* Teaching: Disease Process; Teaching: Procedure/Treatment; Patients Rights Protection; Decision-Making Support *NOC:* Knowledge: Treatment Procedure(s)

Nursing Diagnosis:

Deficient Knowledge:

Progressive disease process and expectations as death approaches

Desired Outcome: Patient and family verbalize understanding of the palliative care approach to management of disease progression and express preferences for care, care goals, and preferred site of death.

INTERVENTIONS	RATIONALES
Assess patient's/family's health care literacy (language, reading, comprehension). Assess culture and culturally-specific information needs.	This assessment helps ensure that information is presented in a manner that is culturally and educationally appropriate.
Educate patient and family about signs and symptoms of disease progression, including appetite loss, changes in respiratory and mental status, and potential for pain to increase in intensity and severity.	Understanding physiologic changes may alleviate patient/family fear or anxiety as changes occur.
Describe principles of palliative care to patient and family.	This information promotes understanding that palliative care is not "giving up" but rather focuses on achieving the best possible quality of life for patient and family when the disease is no longer curable.
Discuss interventions for managing symptoms as death approaches.	Aggressive symptom management and ensuring best quality of life are very active treatments that can be provided. For example, "You should not feel 'there is nothing more to be done' because curative treatment is no longer effective."
Refer patients to palliative care or hospice care providers, while maintaining relationships with family/primary care physicians, community, and specialist care providers as appropriate.	These actions help ensure that patient and family do not feel abandoned as care shifts to a palliative focus.
Understand practical insurance and financial issues related to hospice care vs. home care.	There is a wide variation of reimbursement for hospice and palliative care provided by private insurers and HMOs. For example, Medicare hospice benefits provide a package of services via approved hospice programs; whereas the "plain" Medicare plan (Parts A & B) does not cover these services unless the patient is homebound.
Provide alternatives to calling for emergency care when death is imminent, such as calling hospice or palliative care team for home visit and/or symptom management suggestions. Obtain an out-of-hospital DNR bracelet for patient if this is consistent with his or her wishes.	These are alternatives to calling for emergency care (e.g., calling 911). However, calling 911 for an individual receiving home care can enable emergency personnel to provide comfort measures rather than resuscitation interventions.
Keep patient and family informed about any changes in treatment plan.	Patient and family should be at the center of the treatment plan.

••• **Related NIC and NOC labels:** *NIC:* Teaching: Disease Process; Health System Guidance *NOC:* Knowledge: Disease Process; Knowledge: Treatment Regimen

NURSING DIAGNOSES RELATED TO SYMPTOM MANAGEMENT

Nursing Diagnosis:

Acute Pain and/or Chronic Pain

related to progressive disease state, immobility, obstructions, organ failure, or neuropathy

Desired Outcomes: Within 4 hr of this nursing diagnosis, patient expresses or exhibits acceptable level of physical comfort with minimal side effects from analgesics. Family assists patient with maintaining, responding to, and titrating analgesia as patient's condition changes.

INTERVENTIONS	RATIONALES
Distinguish between physical pain and suffering.	The nurse may consider the cause of distress to be other than physical suffering if rapid, appropriate titration of analgesics does not relieve distress. In this case, sedation may be the only means to relieve suffering.
Assess regularly and use behavioral cues for patient unable to communicate.	Many patients are unable to communicate verbally as death nears. Joint Commission on Accreditation of Healthcare Organizations (TJC) standards (2004) calls for "optimizing comfort and dignity" for patients dying in a hospital.
Enable patient to define balance between discomfort and analgesics.	Many symptoms (e.g., dry mouth) cause discomfort and are managed in ways other than by using analgesics.
Address addiction concerns of patient and family.	Pain is an appropriate indication for use of opioids, and under these circumstances, patients are not "addicted" to medications.
Address fears of respiratory depression from increasing opioid use.	Most patients receive opioid analgesics at end of life. Decreasing levels of consciousness and respirations are expected as part of the dying process and are not a toxicity of opioids.
Implement nonpharmacologic treatments of pain, e.g., massage and soft music.	Nonpharmacologic measures may provide additive relief from symptoms not achieved with pharmacologic approaches alone.
Discuss with health care provider the advisability of stopping medications that are no longer necessary (e.g., vitamins, lipid-reducing agents, hypoglycemics) or that require a different route of administration.	Most patients are unable to take medications orally during the last days or hours of life.
See "Pain," p. 39, for more information.	

••• **Related NIC and NOC labels:** *NIC:* Pain Management; Dying Care *NOC:* Comfort Level

Nursing Diagnosis:

Ineffective Breathing Pattern (Dyspnea)

related to progression of disease process

Desired Outcome: Within 1 hr of this nursing diagnosis, patient states that he or she does not perceive difficulty with breathing.

INTERVENTIONS	RATIONALES
Assess patient's perception of dyspnea.	Patient's perception should guide treatment interventions. However, objective parameters may not coincide with patient's perception of dyspnea (e.g., patient may have low oxygen saturation as measured by pulse oximetry but not feel dyspneic, and vice versa).
Assess for treatable causes of dyspnea. Consider least invasive interventions first (e.g., antibiotics, steroids, diuretics) to relieve underlying pathology causing dyspnea.	Anemia, heart failure, pleural effusion, ascites, and pneumonia, for example, are causes of ineffective breathing pattern (other than simply end of life) that can be treated.

Continued

INTERVENTIONS	RATIONALES
Carefully evaluate risk/benefit of more invasive techniques such as thoracentesis, paracentesis, radiation therapy.	This evaluation helps ensure that invasive therapies will have time to offer relief, not simply cause undue discomfort during dying process.
Advise family that although breathing changes are common and distressing, they are manageable.	Breathing changes in the patient can be upsetting to the family.
Maintain room at cool temperature.	Cooler temperatures help minimize feelings of suffocation.
Place a cool cloth on patient's face or forehead as indicated.	This intervention is likely to promote comfort.
Administer oxygen by nasal cannula only if this offers subjective relief of dyspnea. Use lowest flow rate possible and offer humidification if technically possible.	A face mask is usually uncomfortable and can interfere with ability to communicate with significant others.
Administer morphine or other opioid regularly by least invasive available route to relieve dyspnea.	The oral route (pills or elixir) is preferred, but if this is not possible, rectal, sublingual, nebulized, subcutaneous, or IV route can be used. Opioids are the drug of choice to relieve dyspnea.
Place fan close to patient's face.	The face contains baroreceptors that respond to air movement and can effectively relieve perception of dyspnea.
Position patient with head/upper body elevated. Suggest sleeping in chair, if needed.	Elevation of the head may make breathing easier and provide comfort.
Administer nebulized bronchodilators, steroids, and/or opioids.	These agents help relieve dyspnea.
Teach relaxation breathing techniques to patient and family. Encourage physical touch/massage as a calming technique.	These activities help relieve anxiety, which may improve breathing pattern.
Consider need for pharmacologic management of anxiety (e.g., use of anxiolytics).	Such agents may help alleviate fear and concomitant breathlessness.
Discuss principle of "double effect" of medications. Elicit patient preferences and values about alertness vs. sedation or discomfort if both goals cannot be achieved. Honor patient's choices for symptom management.	Some medicines may relieve symptoms but at the expense of the unintended side effect of sedation or hastened death. See ANA Position Statement (2005): Pain Management and Control of Distressing Symptoms in Dying Patients.

••• **Related NIC and NOC labels:** *NIC:* Positioning; Respiratory Monitoring; Anxiety Reduction; Oxygen Therapy; Teaching: Prescribed Activity/Exercise *NOC:* Respiratory Status: Ventilation; Vital Signs Status

Nursing Diagnosis:

Ineffective Airway Clearance

related to increased pulmonary secretions and congestion secondary to diminishing level of consciousness as death approaches

Desired Outcomes: Patient does not show signs of struggle or discomfort when "death rattle" is present. The family expresses understanding that these noisy respirations are more distressing to them than to the (unconscious) patient.

INTERVENTIONS	RATIONALES
Explain etiology of the noisy breathing.	Noisy breathing is a result of secretions in the upper airway in patients who are too weak to cough effectively.
Reassure family and significant others that patient's breathing, though noisy, is peaceful and unlabored.	Noisy breathing can be distressing to family and friends of the patient.
Attempt to position patient laterally and recumbent, rather than supine.	This position will help maintain as patent an airway as possible.
Use oxygen only if it enables patient to have unlabored respirations.	If respirations are not improved with oxygen, its use may further discomfort the patient.
Avoid suctioning, other than in the oral cavity.	Aggressive, deep suctioning will increase, not decrease, secretions and can cause trauma.

Continued

INTERVENTIONS	RATIONALES
Maintain patient in a relatively dehydrated state.	Such a state will minimize accumulation of pulmonary secretions.
If death rattle persists despite dehydration, administer prescribed anticholinergics via least invasive route.	Anticholinergics decrease secretions and are much more effective when administered early in the onset of this symptom. Effective agents include scopolamine patch, glycopyrrolate (IV, subcutaneous, PO), atropine, and hyoscine butylbromide.
Reassure family that patients are often unaware of discomfort at this point.	This information will help relieve anxiety of family and significant others about possible discomfort resulting from dehydration to manage pulmonary secretions.

••• **Related NIC and NOC labels:** *NIC:* Airway Management; Positioning *NOC:* Aspiration Control; Respiratory Status: Airway Patency

Nursing Diagnosis:

Disturbed Thought Processes (Delirium)

related to disease progression, infection, altered metabolic state, or symptom management side effects

Desired Outcomes: Reversible etiologies of delirium are treated within hours of onset. When delirium is irreversible, agitation is reduced or minimized.

INTERVENTIONS	RATIONALES
Recognize etiologies of delirium in the terminally ill. Assess for and correct, if possible, common treatable causes. For example, discuss with health care provider decreasing or eliminating medications that are not directed at comfort.	Common causes of delirium in the terminally ill that may be reversed or treated with relatively noninvasive measures include brain metastasis, steroid use, opioid toxicity, anticholinergics, benzodiazepines, withdrawal from drug/ethanol, unrelieved pain, pruritus, constipation, urinary retention, infection, hepatic encephalopathy, hypoglycemia, hyperglycemia, hypoxia, hypercalcemia, and dehydration.
Maintain a quiet, well-lighted environment.	This will help relieve anxiety, which optimally will reduce agitation.
Role-model soft-spoken language for the family.	Patient likely maintains sense of hearing even when other senses are impaired. A quiet environment will help reduce agitation.
Pad side rails, and keep bed in low position. Use patient companion or other environmental safety measures (e.g., bed alarms).	These actions help ensure physical safety for patient who has delirium, while avoiding measures such as restraints that promote agitation.
Assess if gentle massage is appropriate as a calming measure.	Some benefits of massage include reducing pain, decreasing anxiety and depression, and relaxing muscles and nerve tissue.
Reorient patient frequently. Have large-faced clocks and calendars within sight. Encourage family to provide familiar and comforting items from patient's home, such as a favorite pillow or blanket.	Reminding patient of person, place, and time may help reorient and mitigate delirium.
If the current opioid regimen is believed to be the cause of delirium, suggest a different opioid in an equianalgesic dose.	This intervention likely will manage delirium and control agitation.
Consider palliative sedation if this is consistent with patient and family preferences and values. Administer benzodiazepine medications (e.g., continuous infusion of midazolam) as prescribed.	These interventions manage delirium and control agitation as death approaches.

Continued

INTERVENTIONS	RATIONALES
Avoid use of phrase "terminal sedation" and instead use "sedation in imminently dying."	The former phrase implies sedation to end patient's life rather than intent of sedation for symptom management and alleviation of distress in the patient who is dying.
Advise family that delirium may signal imminent death.	This information helps prepare family for patient's death.

••• **Related NIC and NOC labels:** *NIC:* Reality Orientation; Delirium Management; Medication Management; Calming Technique; Environmental Management; Decision-Making Support; Counseling; Patients Rights Protection; Family Support *NOC:* Cognitive Orientation; Decision Making

Nursing Diagnosis:

Risk for Imbalanced Fluid Volume (Dehydration or Edema)

related to inability to regulate fluid intake and output secondary to disease progression

Desired Outcomes: Patient's desires for fluid intake are determined by subjective feelings of thirst. Patient receives hydration according to stated preferences. Hydration goals are realistic with appropriate endpoints such as correction of a metabolic disorder that results in enhanced subjective well-being.

INTERVENTIONS	RATIONALES
Do not attempt to manage perception of dry mouth by achieving normal hydration.	This perception is often the result of mouth breathing or other cause that is unresponsive to oral hydration.
Be alert to peripheral edema, urinary incontinence, pleural effusion, ascites, pulmonary congestion, enhanced "death rattle."	These are signs of uncomfortable fluid overload.
Address issues of artificial hydration and nutrition/feeding tubes on advanced directives before patient's inability to communicate preferences.	This helps ensure that patient's wishes are followed.
Advise and encourage family not to insist that patient eat.	It is normal to eat and drink less at end of life. Dehydration results in a peaceful, painless death.
Administer rectal acetaminophen regularly.	This medication reduces discomfort of dehydration-related fever.
Perform meticulous oral care using mouth/lip moisturizers.	This intervention minimizes discomfort of dry mouth (xerostomia).
If family wishes to continue oral feedings, encourage frequent meals, small portions, use of small plates, and companionship during meals.	This intervention recognizes cultural/ethnic implications of oral intake of foods/beverages and eating/drinking while providing for smaller portions that are more realistic for patients at end of life.
Prepare soft, easily swallowed foods such as soup, milkshake, yogurt, custard, ice cream.	These types of foods help promote comfort during the feeding process.
Provide nonirritating fluids that contain electrolytes if patient/family so request, using least invasive route (e.g., via oral, subcutaneous, hypodermoclysis, or IV as last resort).	These fluids treat negative effects of dehydration (e.g., delirium).
Advise family to expect urine to become scant and dark in color.	This information will help relieve family's anxiety about urine color and output.

••• **Related NIC and NOC labels:** *NIC:* Fluid Management; Medication Administration; Nutrition Management; Feeding; Oral Health Restoration *NOC:* Fluid Balance; Nutritional Status: Food and Fluid Intake

Nursing Diagnosis:

Impaired Oral Mucous Membrane (Dry Mouth/Xerostomia)

related to reduced saliva, mouth breathing, oral infections, mucositis, and/or dehydration

Desired Outcomes: Patient's oral mucous membrane becomes moist. Patient does not report/exhibit discomfort from dry mouth.

INTERVENTIONS	RATIONALES
Use topical interventions such as a misting spray bottle with saline to moisten oral mucous membrane; apply emollients on lips.	Studies have shown that dry mouth is the most common and distressing symptom of a conscious person at end of life. IV fluids and interventions directed at a normal hydration status rarely relieve dry mouth.
Encourage family to assist with mouth care.	This involves family in patient care.
If patient is on oxygen, add humidifier.	Humidity helps relieve dry oral mucous membrane.
Rule out oral thrush, herpes; treat if necessary.	Thrush is a potential cause of dry or painful mouth.
Provide fluid intake via frequent sips of water, Popsicles, ice chips. Encourage intake of soups, sauces, gravies, ice cream, and frozen yogurt in patients able to eat.	These fluids and foods provide comfort and relieve oral dryness.
Avoid caffeine, alcohol, alcohol-based products (e.g., mouthwash, cough syrups), and acidic and spicy foods.	These substances can cause oral dryness.
Offer spray bottle filled with water and a few drops of vegetable oil. Suggest use of lemon drops or other sour candy if patient can tolerate without aspiration. Administer saliva substitutes.	These substances help keep mucous membrane moist.
Encourage good dental hygiene (soft-bristled toothbrush, regular brushing, and flossing).	Gentle oral care relieves unpleasant taste while helping maintain oral mucous membrane.

••• **Related NIC and NOC labels:** *NIC:* Oral Health Maintenance; Fluid Management; Dying Care *NOC:* Oral Health

Nursing Diagnosis:

Risk for Imbalanced Nutrition: Less Than Body Requirements

related to anorexia, nausea and vomiting, cachexia, intestinal obstruction, impaired swallowing, and aspiration risk secondary to disease progression

Desired Outcomes: Patient does not report presence of hunger. Family honors patient's wishes regarding artificial nutrition.

INTERVENTIONS	RATIONALES
Remind family that eating will not reverse the underlying disease state. Identify other ways family can express love.	Many families see food as an expression of love and will become distressed when patient is no longer able to have a "normal" nutritional intake.
Help patient and family understand that a normal nutritional status is unrealistic as the disease progresses and the body no longer processes ingested nutrients.	Loss of interest in food is normal near death.
Explain that artificial nutrition such as parenteral nutrition does not relieve feelings of hunger if present, nor does it prolong survival in a terminal state.	The body only takes in what it needs.

Continued

INTERVENTIONS	RATIONALES
If appropriate, obtain a nutritional consult to determine the most digestible feedings, given patient's underlying disease.	Oral nutrition is the method of choice for patients who can swallow and who have intact gastrointestinal (GI) systems. Enteral routes include nasogastric, gastrostomy, and jejunostomy tubes. However, these routes can result in harm (e.g., bloating, nausea/vomiting, edema, diarrhea) if the GI system cannot absorb and digest nutrients.
Avoid giving commercial nutritional supplements.	They likely will suppress patient's appetite and may be unpalatable. Giving supplements may result in inability to ingest foods patient likes and enjoys.

•••• Related NIC and NOC labels: *NIC:* Nutrition Management; Sustenance Support *NOC:* Nutritional Status

PSYCHOSOCIAL NURSING DIAGNOSES

Nursing Diagnoses:

Fear/Anxiety

related to life-threatening condition, pain, the unknown (death), and patient's concern that he or she will be forgotten

Desired Outcomes: Patient's (and family's) fears are acknowledged and addressed. Patient states that fear has lessened.

INTERVENTIONS	RATIONALES
Distinguish between anxiety and fear. Identify appropriate interventions (see **Death Anxiety,** which follows).	Anxiety is a state of apprehension and dread whose source the patient cannot identify. Fear often has a realistic, definable cause. Distinguishing between the two will enable appropriate interventions.
Reassure patient that pain and other discomforts will be managed.	This information will help relieve anxiety and fear.
Identify and address family's fears and concerns. Keep family informed of physical symptoms to expect as death approaches (e.g., changes in breathing, decreased level of consciousness [LOC], coolness and mottling of skin).	Physical symptoms of death can be distressing to the family. Knowing what to expect may help them cope with their anxieties and fears related to patient's approaching death.
If appropriate, encourage patient and family to seek support from pastoral counselors in addressing religious beliefs about the meaning of suffering, death, and afterlife.	Spiritual guidance can help the family cope with anxieties and fears about loss of their loved one and for the patient may help resolve anxieties and fears related to spiritual concerns and conflicts.
Assist patient and family with creating videos or audiotapes and scrapbooks for recalled memories.	Recalled memories can help facilitate the grieving process and mitigate fears for the patient that he or she will be forgotten.
Encourage patient to use this time to create a legacy.	For examples, see www.alegacytoremember.com/HowTo.html.

•••• Related NIC and NOC labels: *NIC:* Anxiety Reduction; Active Listening; Counseling; Support System Enhancement; Support Group; Emotional Support; Dying Care *NOC:* Anxiety Control; Fear Control

Nursing Diagnosis:

Death Anxiety

related to impending death, fear of unmanaged physical symptoms, and fear of unknown

Desired Outcomes: Patient states (or exhibits) that he or she is free of physical discomforts and emotional distress. Family members verbalize understanding of the dying process.

INTERVENTIONS	RATIONALES
Provide aggressive symptom management of physical discomforts before attempting to assess anxiety.	Physical symptoms can cause anxiety.
Help patient recognize early physical manifestations of anxiety (e.g., racing heart, sweating, feeling flushed, wheezing).	Recognizing these symptoms early and using a preemptive strategy will minimize escalation of anxiety.
Support patient and family in expressing fears and anxieties related to previous experiences with the dying. Listen carefully to stories to anticipate special needs during current death event. For instance, if family members tell you they feel guilty about not saying "I love you" before the death of another individual, encourage them to say or write down what they most want the dying patient to know, even if the patient is not conscious.	Such discussions may help reduce anxiety.
Review age-appropriate guidelines for child participation in care and presence with dying family member, and encourage family to allow children to be present consistent with these guidelines.	Participation/presence likely would help children cope with their fears and anxieties about the death of their family member.
Ask about content of bad dreams or nightmares.	These occurrences may be a sign of anxiety-related sleep disturbance or opioid toxicity.
Obtain referrals to or guidance of specific religious counselors.	Such counselors will help support patient through anxiety regarding death.
Encourage use of relaxation techniques such as imagery, progressive muscle relaxation, relaxation breathing. Administer anxiolytics as appropriate.	These measures are known to reduce anxiety.

••• **Related NIC and NOC labels:** *NIC:* Anxiety Reduction; Coping Enhancement; Emotional Support; Spiritual Support; Reminiscence Therapy; Dying Care; Family Involvement Promotion; Grief Work Facilitation; Simple Relaxation Therapy *NOC:* Anxiety Control; Dignified Dying

Nursing Diagnosis:

Powerlessness

related to actual debility and inability to carry out normal role functions

Desired Outcome: Patient makes choices for end-of-life care.

INTERVENTIONS	RATIONALES
Reinforce use of patient's advance directives and advance care planning activities in guiding care.	Ensuring that patient's wishes are followed minimizes sense of powerlessness.
Remind patient and family of their continuing ability to make choices around end-of-life care.	Having control over these decisions will reduce feelings of powerlessness. Some examples include patient's right to choose whether to eat or drink, have certain care procedures performed, have or decline treatments, and actualize preferences around site of dying (e.g., home vs. institution).
Encourage open communication with family. Suggest resources that facilitate conversations within the family.	Example: Byock, Ira. (2004). *The Four Things That Matter Most: A Book About Living.* New York: Free Press.

••• **Related NIC and NOC labels:** *NIC:* Decision-Making Support; Health System Guidance; Patients Rights Protection; Family Involvement Promotion *NOC:* Participation: Health Care Decisions

Nursing Diagnosis:

Spiritual Distress

related to religious, cultural, and existential beliefs about dying

Desired Outcome: Patient states that he or she has ability to connect with spiritual/pastoral counselors to discuss issues of spirituality, existential concerns, and their meanings.

INTERVENTIONS	RATIONALES
Support patient's religious customs around end-of-life issues in the following ways:	These measures help provide a supportive, open environment in which patient can discuss these issues if he or she chooses.
- Offer to pray with patient and family if appropriate.	
- Remember that being "spiritual" is not necessarily synonymous with being "religious."	
- Ask patient what has brought his or her life satisfaction, joy, and sorrow.	
- Assist family in creation of rituals (e.g., letting go, remembering, forgiving).	
- Suggest planning of funeral/memorial service, music, readings.	
- Include pastoral/spiritual counselor (e.g., priest/minister/rabbi) as integral member of care giving team as appropriate.	This intervention helps provide spiritual guidance and counseling during periods of distress.

••• **Related NIC and NOC labels:** *NIC:* Dying Care; Spiritual Support; Forgiveness Facilitation; Reminiscence Therapy; Referral *NOC:* Dignified Dying; Spiritual Well-Being

Nursing Diagnosis:

Risk for Caregiver Role Strain

related to multiple demands on family members and resources when caring for dying loved one

Desired Outcome: Caregivers are assisted with providing care, given respite, and reassured that they are doing a good job.

INTERVENTIONS	RATIONALES
Identify available resources (e.g., hospice, friends, community, church members) to assist with care giving in patient's and family members' preferred site of death.	Such resources may relieve some of the strain of caregiving.
Suggest counseling and other psychosocial support resources (e.g., social worker, case manager) that assist family with maintaining integrity, dealing with practical issues, and avoiding conflict during strain of illness.	There may be lack of insurance funding for many activities of care (e.g., childcare, transportation, housekeeping) and other worries that caregivers may have regarding loss of time from work, loss of savings, and loss of income of ill family member.
Remind caregivers of their own health care needs. Encourage family to take breaks for meals, relaxation, and attention to non-ill family members, especially young children.	These measures may reduce stress and anxiety in caregivers and family members.
Offer family members unrestricted access to patient as death approaches but also encourage them to take frequent rest periods.	These actions provide flexibility in visiting and opportunities for rest as well, which will help alleviate strain.
If family members are unable to be present for a period of time, provide phone numbers so that they can stay in contact with staff.	This action will help relieve stress and anxiety if family members have to be away and may reduce guilt about not being there.

••• **Related NIC and NOC labels:** *NIC:* Caregiver Support; Emotional Support; Respite Care; Anticipatory Guidance; Active Listening; Coping Enhancement; Grief Work Facilitation; Referral; Support System Enhancement; Family Integrity Promotion; Risk Identification *NOC:* Caregiver Emotional Health; Caregiver Physical Health; Caregiver Stressors

Nursing Diagnosis:

Anticipatory Grieving

related to impending loss of loved one

Desired Outcome: Family/significant others identify and express feelings appropriately and demonstrate balancing caregiving with their own physical and emotional respite needs.

INTERVENTIONS	RATIONALES
Encourage grieving and expressions of feelings by patient, family, and staff. Permit expressions of anger and silence—do not try to say something meaningful or profound.	Anticipatory grieving is valuable. Anger is often substituted for grief.
Assist family with recalling successful past coping strategies.	Strategies that have worked in the past also may work in the present.
Be available to actively listen, and respect need to use denial occasionally.	Denial can be an effective coping mechanism for grief.
Give family permission to express ambivalence about impending death.	These feelings are normal, and acknowledging them may help minimize feelings of guilt about having them. For instance, "Many people in your circumstance don't want to lose their loved one, yet they wish for the suffering to be over. I wonder if you've had feelings like this?"
Suggest locks of hair and other tangible mementos to survivors.	Mementos may facilitate the grieving process.
Permit family to stay with patient after death.	This enables them to say "good-bye" and express grief.

Continued

INTERVENTIONS	RATIONALES
Arrange bereavement follow-up for family members. For example, inform them about availability of bereavement groups, books on grieving, and available counseling resources.	This intervention provides support to the family in their grief after the death has occurred. Families whose loved ones have received hospice care will have formal bereavement follow-up, but such programs are rare in hospital and non-hospice settings.
Recommend judicious use of anxiolytics/sedatives for acutely grieving survivors.	These agents promote rest and help alleviate anxiety during their grief.
Provide phone numbers or concrete information regarding funeral arrangements.	This information assists family in beginning process of identifying funeral plans. Participating in such tasks may help assuage grief.
Notify other health care providers (e.g., primary care provider, surgeon, ambulatory care nurses) of patient's death so that they can express their sympathy to family. Consider making a bereavement phone call or sending a sympathy card.	Condolences from health care providers are meaningful to survivors and help with grief.

••• **Related NIC and NOC labels:** *NIC:* Coping Enhancement; Grief Work Facilitation; Dying Care; Counseling; Support System Enhancement; Visitation Facilitation *NOC:* Family Coping; Grief Resolution; Psychosocial Adjustment: Life Change

ADDITIONAL NURSING DIAGNOSES/ PROBLEMS:

"Pain"	p. 1
"Cancer Care"	p. 39
"Psychosocial Support"	p. 73
"Psychosocial Support for the Patient's Family and Significant Other"	p. 87
"Managing Wound Care"	p. 559
"Providing Nutritional Support"	p. 565

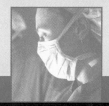

Chronic Obstructive Pulmonary Disease

9

OVERVIEW/PATHOPHYSIOLOGY

Chronic obstructive pulmonary disease (COPD) is the fourth leading cause of death in the United States. It is a disease state characterized by airflow limitation that is not fully reversible. Airflow limitation usually is progressive and associated with an abnormal inflammatory response of the lungs to noxious particles or gases and characterized by chronic inflammation throughout the airways, parenchyma, and pulmonary vasculature.

In the central airways, inflammatory cells infiltrate the surface epithelium. Enlarged mucus-secreting glands and an increased number of goblet cells lead to mucus hypersecretion. In smaller airways, chronic inflammation leads to repeated cycles of injury to the airway wall. Repair of the airway wall results in increased collagen content and scar tissue formation that narrow the lumen and produce fixed airway obstruction.

Destruction of lung parenchyma in COPD patients typically occurs as emphysema, which involves dilation and destruction of the bronchioles. An imbalance of proteinases and antiproteinases in the lungs is believed to be a major mechanism causing this disorder.

HEALTH CARE SETTING

Primary care or long-term care, with possible hospitalization resulting from complications

ASSESSMENT

Signs and symptoms: Chronic cough, which is usually the first symptom to develop. Dyspnea is the main reason patients seek medical attention. As lung function deteriorates, work of breathing increases, and wheezing and chest tightness may be accompanying symptoms.

Physical assessment: Use of accessory muscles of respiration, prolonged expiratory phase, digital clubbing, decreased thoracic expansion, barrel chest appearance, dullness over areas of consolidation, adventitious breath sounds (especially coarse rhonchi and wheezing), ankle edema, distended neck veins, bloated appearance.

Risk factors: Include both genetic and environmental factors. Genetic factors (e.g., hereditary deficiency of alpha-1 antitrypsin) increase risk for disease development and progression. Environmental factors include cigarette smoking and other outdoor/indoor air pollutants. Cigarette smokers have a high prevalence of lung function abnormalities and a greater decline of lung function than nonsmokers. Passive exposure to cigarettes also may contribute to COPD.

DIAGNOSTIC TESTS

Chest x-ray: Will reveal normal anteroposterior (AP) diameter, nearly normal diaphragm position, and increased peripheral lung markings.

ABG values: Important in advanced COPD and should be obtained when there are signs of right-sided (diastolic) heart failure (e.g., jugular vein distention, peripheral edema) or respiratory failure (Pao_2 less than 60 mm Hg with or without $Paco_2$ greater than 50 mm Hg).

Oximetry: Will reveal decreased O_2 saturation (90% or less).

Alpha-1 antitrypsin deficiency screen: Performed in patients who develop COPD at a young age (younger than 45 years) or who have a strong family history of the disease.

Spirometry: Confirms diagnosis of COPD. Clinical indicators and a forced expiratory volume in 1 second (FEV_1) diagnose and classify severity of COPD.

Sputum culture: May reveal presence of infective organisms. Sputum specimens are best collected when the patient first wakes in the morning.

Differential diagnosis: COPD may mimic many other diseases.

<u>**Nursing Diagnosis:**</u>

Ineffective Breathing Pattern

related to decreased lung expansion secondary to chronic airflow limitations

Desired Outcome: Following treatment/intervention, patient's breathing pattern improves as evidenced by reduction in or absence of dyspnea and movement toward a state of eupnea with O_2 saturation greater than 90% with or without oxygen therapy, pH higher than 7.35, and $Paco_2$ less than 50 mm Hg.

INTERVENTIONS	RATIONALES
Assess respiratory status q2-4h.	Restlessness, anxiety, mental status changes, shortness of breath, tachypnea, and use of accessory muscles of respiration are signs of respiratory distress, which should be reported promptly for immediate intervention.
Auscultate breath sounds q2-4h.	A decrease in breath sounds or an increase in adventitious breath sounds (crackles, wheezes, rhonchi) may precede respiratory distress and necessitate prompt intervention.
Administer bronchodilator therapy as prescribed.	Bronchodilators open airways by relaxing smooth muscles of the airways.
Monitor for tachycardia and dysrhythmias.	These are side effects of bronchodilator therapy.
Administer steroids as prescribed.	Steroid therapy may decrease airway obstructions, decrease inflammation, and improve dyspnea.
Monitor patient's response to prescribed O_2 therapy. Titrate oxygen to keep oxygen saturation greater than 90%.	High concentrations of O_2 can depress the respiratory drive in individuals with chronic CO_2 retention.
Monitor oximetry readings.	O_2 saturation 90% or less can indicate need for O_2 therapy.
Monitor serial arterial blood gas (ABG) values.	Pao_2 likely will continue to decrease as patient's disease progresses. Patients with chronic CO_2 retention may have chronically compensated respiratory acidosis with a low normal pH (7.35-7.38) and a $Paco_2$ greater than 50 mm Hg.

••• **Related NIC and NOC labels:** *NIC:* Respiratory Monitoring; Oxygen Therapy; Acid-Base Monitoring *NOC:* Respiratory Status: Ventilation

<u>**Nursing Diagnosis:**</u>

Impaired Gas Exchange

related to altered oxygen supply secondary to decreased alveolar ventilation as a result of collapsed terminal airways and hyperinflated alveoli

Desired Outcomes: Optimally within 1-2 hr following treatment/intervention, patient has adequate gas exchange as evidenced by RR 12-20 breaths/min (or values consistent with patient's baseline). Before discharge from care facility, patient's ABG values are as follows: Pao_2 60 mm Hg or higher, $Paco_2$ 35-45 mm Hg, and pH 7.35-7.45; or oximetry readings demonstrating O_2 saturation greater than 90% or values consistent with patient's baseline.

INTERVENTIONS	RATIONALES
Observe for signs and symptoms of hypoxia.	Hypoxia (evidenced by agitation, anxiety, restlessness, changes in mental status or level of consciousness [LOC]) indicates oxygen deficiency and necessitates prompt treatment.
Recognize that cyanosis of the lips and nail beds is a late indicator of hypoxia.	Treatment is less complicated when symptoms are treated early.
Auscultate breath sounds q2-4h or more frequently as indicated by patient's condition.	Decreased or adventitious sounds (e.g., crackles, rhonchi, wheezes) necessitate prompt treatment.
Monitor oximetry readings; report significant findings.	O_2 saturation 90% or less can indicate oxygenation problems and a possible need for O_2 therapy.
Monitor ABG results.	Decreasing Pao_2 and increasing $Paco_2$ can signal respiratory compromise.
Position patient in high Fowler's position, with patient leaning forward and elbows propped on the over-the-bed table. Pad the over-the-bed table with pillows or blankets. Record patient's response to positioning.	This position promotes comfort and optimal gas exchange by enabling maximal chest expansion. Leaning forward with diaphragm positioned against over-the-bed table may increase pressure of gastric contents and promote diaphragm contraction, thereby decreasing dyspnea.
Deliver and monitor O_2 and humidity as prescribed. Titrate oxygen to keep oxygen saturations greater than 90%.	Oxygen therapy for COPD will help decrease hypoxia and mortality. Delivering O_2 with humidity will help minimize convective losses of moisture.
Administer noninvasive positive pressure ventilation (NIPPV) as prescribed.	NIPPV has been shown to increase blood pH, reduce $Paco_2$, and reduce severity of dyspnea in the first 4 hr of treatment, eliminating need for mechanical ventilation in some patients.

••• **Related NIC and NOC labels:** *NIC:* Acid-Base Monitoring; Laboratory Data Interpretation; Respiratory Monitoring; Positioning; Oxygen Therapy *NOC:* Respiratory Status: Gas Exchange

Nursing Diagnosis:

Imbalanced Nutrition: Less Than Body Requirements

related to decreased intake secondary to fatigue and anorexia

Desired Outcome: For a minimum of 24 hr before hospital discharge, patient has adequate nutrition as evidenced by stable weight and positive nitrogen (N) state on N studies.

INTERVENTIONS	RATIONALES
Monitor food and fluid intake.	This assessment provides data that will determine need for dietary consultation.
Request consultation with dietitian as indicated.	Such a consultation will facilitate calorie counts and enable patient to verbalize likes and dislikes within the parameters of allowable foods.
Provide diet in small, frequent meals that are nutritious and easy to consume.	Small meals are easier to consume in individuals who are fatigued.
Unless otherwise indicated, provide calories more from unsaturated fat sources than from carbohydrate sources.	During the process of carbohydrate metabolism, the body uses O_2 and produces CO_2, which is then excreted by the lungs. Patients with COPD take in less O_2 and retain CO_2. A high-fat diet minimizes this problem because fat generates the least amount of CO_2 for a given amount of O_2 used, whereas carbohydrates generate the most. Foods high in unsaturated fats and proteins that should be encouraged include nuts, lean meat, poultry, and fish. High-carbohydrate sources that should be discouraged include cakes, cookies, jams, pastries, and sugar-concentrated snacks.

Continued

INTERVENTIONS	RATIONALES
When not otherwise indicated, encourage fluid intake (2.5 L/day or more).	Adequate hydration helps decrease sputum viscosity for patients with chronic sputum production.
Discuss with patient and significant others the importance of good nutrition in the treatment of COPD.	This information optimally will promote adequate nutrition and stable body weight. A knowledgeable patient is more likely to adhere to the treatment plan.

••• **Related NIC and NOC labels:** *NIC:* Nutritional Monitoring; Nutrition Therapy; Nutritional Counseling; Teaching: Prescribed Diet; Weight Management *NOC:* Nutritional Status; Nutrient Intake

Nursing Diagnosis:

Activity Intolerance

related to imbalance between oxygen supply and demand secondary to inefficient work of breathing

Desired Outcome: Patient reports decreasing dyspnea during activity or exercise and rates his or her perceived exertion at 3 or less on a 0-10 scale.

INTERVENTIONS	RATIONALES
Monitor patient's respiratory response to activity including assessment of oxygen saturations.	Activity intolerance is indicated by excessively increased respiratory rate (RR) (e.g., more than 10 breaths/min above baseline) and depth, dyspnea, and use of accessory muscles of respiration. Ask patient to rate perceived exertion (see **Risk for Activity Intolerance**, p. 61, in "Prolonged Bedrest" for a description). If activity intolerance is noted, instruct patient to stop the activity and rest. COPD patients may become hypoxic during increased activity and require oxygen therapy to prevent hypoxemia, which increases the risk for exacerbations of COPD.
Maintain prescribed activity levels, and explain rationale to patient.	Prescribed activity levels will increase patient's stamina while minimizing dyspnea. COPD is a progressive disease, and affected individuals can become totally disabled because they must use all available energy for breathing.
Allow 90 min for undisturbed rest. Facilitate coordination across health care providers.	Ninety minutes of undisturbed rest decreases oxygen demand and enables adequate physiologic recovery.
Assist patient with active range-of-motion (ROM) exercises. For more information, see **Risk for Activity Intolerance** in "Prolonged Bedrest," p. 61.	ROM exercises help build stamina and prevent complications of decreased mobility.
Request consultation from pulmonary rehabilitation.	A comprehensive program includes exercise training, nutrition counseling, and education. Patients who have completed a pulmonary rehabilitation program have been shown to have improved quality of life and slowed progression of the disease.

••• **Related NIC and NOC labels:** *NIC:* Activity Therapy; Energy Management; Exercise Therapy: Joint Mobility *NOC:* Endurance

ADDITIONAL NURSING DIAGNOSES/ PROBLEMS:

"Psychosocial Support" for **Anxiety**   p. 74

"Heart Failure" for **Excess Fluid Volume**   p. 184

 PATIENT-FAMILY TEACHING AND DISCHARGE PLANNING

When providing patient-family teaching, focus on sensory information, avoid giving excessive information, and initiate a visiting nurse referral for necessary follow-up teaching. Include verbal and written information about the following.

✓ Use of home O_2, including instructions for when to use it, importance of not increasing prescribed flow rate, precautions, and community resources for O_2 replacement when necessary. Request respiratory therapy consultation to assist with teaching related to O_2 therapy, if indicated.

✓ Medications, including drug name, route, purpose, dosage, schedule, precautions, and potential side effects. Also discuss drug-drug, herb-drug, and food-drug interactions. If patient will take corticosteroids while at home, provide instructions accordingly to ensure patient takes the correct amount.

✓ Smoking cessation: Single most effective way of reducing risk of development and progression of COPD. Nicotine replacement therapy also should be considered to assist with withdrawal from tobacco.

✓ Signs and symptoms of heart failure that necessitate medical attention: increased dyspnea, fatigue, and coughing; changes in amount, color, or consistency of sputum; swelling of ankles and legs; fever; and sudden weight gain. Patients with COPD often have right-sided (diastolic) heart failure secondary to cardiac effects of the disease. For more information, see "Heart Failure," p. 181.

✓ Importance of avoiding contact with infectious individuals, especially those with respiratory infections.

✓ Recommendation that patient receive a pneumococcal vaccination and annual influenza vaccination.

✓ Review of sodium-restricted diet and other dietary considerations as indicated.

✓ Importance of pacing activity level to conserve energy.

✓ Follow-up appointment with health care provider; confirm date and time of next appointment.

✓ Introduction to pulmonary rehabilitation programs. Physical training programs may improve ventilation and cardiac muscle function, which may compensate for nonreversible lung disease.

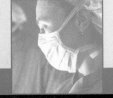

Pneumonia 10

OVERVIEW/PATHOPHYSIOLOGY

Pneumonia is an acute bacterial or viral infection that causes inflammation of the lung parenchyma (alveolar spaces and interstitial tissue). As a result of the inflammation involved, lung tissue becomes edematous and air spaces fill with exudate (consolidation), gas exchange cannot occur, and nonoxygenated blood is shunted into the vascular system, causing hypoxemia. Bacterial pneumonias involve all or part of a lobe, whereas viral pneumonias appear diffusely throughout the lungs.

Influenza, which can cause pneumonia, is the most serious viral airway infection for adults. Patients more than 65 years old, residents of extended care facilities, and individuals with chronic health conditions have the highest mortality rate from influenza.

Pneumonias generally are classified into two types: community acquired and hospital associated (nosocomial). A third type is pneumonia in the immunocompromised individual.

Community acquired: The most common. Individuals with community-acquired pneumonia generally do not require hospitalization unless an underlying medical condition, such as chronic obstructive pulmonary disease (COPD), cardiac disease, or diabetes mellitus, or an immunocompromised state complicates the illness.

Hospital associated (nosocomial): Nosocomial pneumonias usually occur following aspiration of oropharyngeal flora or stomach contents in an individual whose resistance is altered or whose coughing mechanisms are impaired (e.g., a patient who has decreased LOC, dysphagia, diminished gag reflex, or a nasogastric tube or who has undergone thoracoabdominal surgery or is on mechanical ventilation). Bacteria invade the lower respiratory tract via three routes: (1) gastric acid aspiration (the most common route) causing toxic injury to the lung, (2) obstructions (foreign body or fluids), and (3) infections (rare). Gram-negative pneumonias are associated with a high mortality rate, even with appropriate antibiotic therapy. *Aspiration pneumonia* is a nonbacterial (anaerobic) cause of hospital-associated pneumonia that occurs when gastric contents are aspirated. If the alveolar-capillary membrane is affected, adult respiratory distress syndrome (ARDS) may be seen.

Pneumonia in the immunocompromised individual: Immunosuppression and neutropenia are predisposing factors in the development of nosocomial pneumonias from both common and unusual pathogens. Severely immunocompromised patients are affected not only by bacteria but also by fungi (*Candida, Aspergillus*), viruses (cytomegalovirus), and protozoa (*Pneumocystis carinii*). Most commonly, *P. carinii* is seen in persons with human immunodeficiency virus infection or in persons who are immunosuppressed therapeutically following organ transplantation.

HEALTH CARE SETTING

Primary care, with acute care hospitalization resulting from complications

ASSESSMENT

Findings are influenced by patient's age, extent of the disease process, underlying medical condition, and pathogen involved. Generally, any factor that alters integrity of the lower airways, thereby inhibiting ciliary activity, increases the likelihood of developing pneumonia.

General signs and symptoms: Cough (productive and nonproductive), increased sputum (rust colored, discolored, purulent, bloody, or mucoid) production, fever, pleuritic chest pain (more common in community-acquired bacterial pneumonias), dyspnea, chills, headache, myalgia. Older adults may be confused or disoriented and run low-grade fevers but may present with few other signs and symptoms.

General physical assessment findings: Restlessness; anxiety; decreased skin turgor and dry mucous membranes secondary to dehydration; presence of nasal flaring and expiratory grunt; use of accessory muscles of respiration (scalene, sternocleidomastoid, external intercostals); decreased chest expansion caused by pleuritic pain; dullness on percussion over affected (consolidated) areas; tachypnea (respiratory rate [RR] more than 20 breaths/min); tachycardia (HR more than 90 bpm); increased vocal fremitus; egophony ("e" to "a" change) over area of consolidation; decreased breath sounds; high-pitched and inspiratory crackles (rales) (increased by or heard only after coughing); low-pitched inspiratory crackles (rales) caused by airway secretions; and circumoral cyanosis (a late finding). **Note:** Findings may be normal, even with abnormal chest x-ray results.

Diagnostic Tests

Chest x-ray examination: To confirm presence of pneumonia (i.e., infiltrate appearing on the film).

123

Sputum for Gram stain and culture and sensitivity tests: Sputum is obtained from the lower respiratory tract before initiation of antibiotic therapy to identify causative organism. It can be obtained via expectoration, suctioning, transtracheal aspiration, bronchoscopy, or open-lung biopsy.

WBC count: Will be increased (more than 12,000/mm^3) in the presence of bacterial pneumonias. Normal or low white blood cell (WBC) (less than 4000/mm^3) count may be seen with viral or mycoplasma pneumonias.

Chemistry panel: To detect presence of hypernatremia and/or hyperglycemia.

Blood culture and sensitivity: To determine presence of bacteremia and aid in identification of causative organism. To attain the best yield, two sets of blood cultures should be drawn before administration of antibiotics.

Oximetry: May reveal decreased O_2 saturation (92% or less).

ABG values: May vary, depending on presence of underlying pulmonary or other debilitating disease. Findings may demonstrate hypoxemia (Pao$_2$ less than 80 mm Hg) and hypocarbia (Paco$_2$ less than 32-35 mm Hg), with a resultant respiratory alkalosis (pH more than 7.45) in the absence of an underlying pulmonary disease.

Serologic studies: Acute and convalescent antibody titers drawn to diagnose viral pneumonia. A relative rise in antibody titers suggests viral infection.

Acid-fast stains and cultures: To rule out tuberculosis.

NURSING DIAGNOSES FOR PATIENTS *WITH* PNEUMONIA

Nursing Diagnosis:

Impaired Gas Exchange

related to altered oxygen supply and alveolar-capillary membrane changes secondary to inflammatory process in the lungs

Desired Outcome: Hospital discharge is anticipated when patient exhibits at least five of the following indicators: temperature 37.8° C or less, HR 100 bpm or less, RR 24 breaths/min or less, SBP 90 mm Hg or more, oxygen saturation more than 90%, and ability to maintain oral intake.

INTERVENTIONS	RATIONALES
Observe for and promptly report signs and symptoms of respiratory distress.	Signs and symptoms of respiratory distress include restlessness, anxiety, mental status changes, shortness of breath, tachypnea, and use of accessory muscles of respiration. Cyanosis of the lips and nail beds may be a late indicator of hypoxia. Respiratory distress necessitates prompt medical intervention.
Auscultate breath sounds at least q2-4h or as indicated by patient's condition. Report significant findings.	Decreased or adventitious sounds (e.g., crackles, wheezes) can signal potential airway obstruction that would further aggravate hypoxia and necessitate prompt intervention.
Monitor and document vital signs (VS) q2-4h.	A rising temperature and other changes in VS (e.g., increased HR and RR) may signal presence of worsening inflammatory response in the lungs. This could cause further hypoxia contributing to adult respiratory distress syndrome and need for mechanical ventilation.
Administer antibiotics within 4 hr of hospital admission and ongoing as prescribed.	Early administration of antibiotics decreases inflammatory response in the lung, promoting healing, and reducing risk of mortality. Typical antibiotic therapy for community-acquired pneumonia includes use of cephalosporins (ceftriaxone and cefotaxime) along with macrolides (azithromycin and erythromycin). Cephalosporins alone will not provide coverage against atypical bacteria without the addition of a macrolide. Fluoroquinolones (gatifloxacin, levofloxacin, moxifloxacin, and gemifloxacin) may be used solely because of their broad-spectrum coverage. However, they are not routinely the first drug of choice because of concerns about increasing resistance. Proper identification of the organism and determination of sensitivity to specific antibiotics are critical for appropriate therapy.

Continued

INTERVENTIONS	RATIONALES
Monitor oximetry readings; report O_2 saturation of 90% or less.	O_2 saturation of 90% or less is a sign of a significant oxygenation problem and can indicate need for O_2 therapy.
Administer oxygen as prescribed.	Oxygen is administered when oxygen saturation or arterial blood gas (ABG) results demonstrate hypoxemia. Special consideration must be given to patients with chronic CO_2 retention. (Normally, the respiratory drive is stimulated by increasing $Paco_2$ levels. In patients with CO_2 retention, the respiratory drive is paradoxically stimulated by decreasing Pao_2 levels. Therefore in the presence of high concentrations of oxygen, the respiratory drive actually may be depressed in these patients.) Initially, oxygen is delivered in low concentrations, and oxygen saturation or ABG levels are watched closely. If O_2 saturation or Pao_2 does not rise to acceptable levels (92% or 60 mm Hg or more, respectively), Flo_2 is increased in small increments, with concomitant checks of ABG values or oxygen saturations.
Monitor ABG results.	Acute hypoxemia (Pao_2 less than 80 mm Hg) often indicates need for oxygen therapy. Hypocarbia ($Paco_2$ less than 35 mm Hg), with a resultant respiratory alkalosis (pH greater than 7.45) in the absence of an underlying pulmonary disease, is consistent with pneumonia.
Position patient for comfort (usually semi-Fowler's position).	This position provides comfort, promotes diaphragmatic descent, maximizes inhalations, and decreases work of breathing. Gravity and hydrostatic pressure when patient is in this position promote perfusion and ventilation-perfusion matching. In patients with unilateral pneumonia, positioning on unaffected side (i.e., "good side down") promotes ventilation-perfusion matching.
Facilitate coordination across health care providers to provide rest periods between care activities. Allow 90 min for undisturbed rest.	Rest decreases oxygen demand in a patient whose reserves are likely limited.

••• **Related NIC and NOC labels:** *NIC:* Oxygen Therapy; Acid-Base Monitoring; Positioning; Energy Management; Respiratory Monitoring; Vital Signs Monitoring *NOC:* Respiratory Status: Gas Exchange; Vital Signs Status

Nursing Diagnosis:

Ineffective Airway Clearance

related to presence of tracheobronchial secretions secondary to infection or related to pain and fatigue secondary to lung consolidation

Desired Outcomes: Patient demonstrates effective cough. Following intervention, patient's airway is free of adventitious breath sounds.

INTERVENTIONS	RATIONALES
Auscultate breath sounds q2-4h (or as indicated by patient's condition), and report changes in patient's ability to clear pulmonary secretions.	This assessment determines presence of adventitious breath sounds (e.g., crackles, wheezes). If coarse crackles are present, this is a sign patient needs to cough. Fine crackles at lung bases likely will clear with deep breathing. Wheezing is a sign of airway obstruction, which necessities prompt intervention to ensure effective gas exchange.
Inspect sputum for quantity, odor, color, and consistency; document findings.	As patient's condition worsens, sputum can become more copious and change in color from clear → white → yellow → green, or it may show other discoloration characteristic of underlying bacterial infection (e.g., rust colored; "currant jelly").
Ensure that patient performs deep breathing with coughing exercises at least q2h.	These exercises help clear airways of secretions. Controlled coughing (tightening upper abdominal muscles while coughing 2 to 3 times) ensures a more effective cough because it uses the diaphragmatic muscles, which increases forcefulness of the effort.

Continued

INTERVENTIONS	RATIONALES
Assist patient into position of comfort, usually semi-Fowler's position.	This position provides comfort and facilitates ease and effectiveness of these exercises by promoting better lung expansion (there is less lung compression by abdominal organs) and gas exchange.
Assess need for hyperinflation therapy.	Patient's inability to take deep breaths is a sign of the need for this therapy. Deep inhalation with hyperinflation device expands alveoli and aids in mobilizing secretions to the airways, and coughing further mobilizes and clears the secretions. Emphasis of this therapy is on inhalation to expand the lungs maximally. Patient inhales slowly and deeply 2 × normal tidal volume and holds the breath at least 5 sec at the end of inspiration. To maintain adequate alveolar inflation, 10 such breaths/hr is recommended.
Report complications of hyperinflation therapy to health care provider.	Complications include hyperventilation, gastric distention, headache, hypotension, and signs and symptoms of pneumothorax (shortness of breath, sharp chest pain, unilateral diminished breath sounds, dyspnea, cough).
Teach patient to splint chest with pillow, folded blanket, or crossed arms.	This action reduces pain while coughing, thereby promoting a more effective cough.
Instruct patients who are unable to cough effectively in cascade cough.	A cascade cough removes secretions and improves ventilation via a succession of shorter and more forceful exhalations than are done with usual coughing exercise.
Deliver oxygen with humidity as prescribed.	This intervention provides oxygenation while decreasing convective losses of moisture and assisting with mobilization of secretions.
Assist patient with position changes q2h. If patient is ambulatory, encourage ambulation to patient's tolerance.	Movement and activity help mobilize secretions to facilitate airway clearance.
Suction as prescribed and indicated.	Suctioning maintains a patent airway by removing secretions.
When not contraindicated, encourage fluid intake (2.5 L/day or more).	Increasing hydration decreases viscosity of the sputum, which will make it easier to raise and expectorate.

••• **Related NIC and NOC labels:** *NIC:* Respiratory Monitoring; Chest Physiotherapy; Positioning; Airway Suctioning; Cough Enhancement; Medication Administration: Inhalation *NOC:* Respiratory Status: Gas Exchange; Respiratory Status: Ventilation

Nursing Diagnosis:

Deficient Fluid Volume

related to increased insensible loss secondary to tachypnea, fever, or diaphoresis

Desired Outcome: At least 24 hr before hospital discharge, patient is normovolemic as evidenced by urine output 30 ml/hr or more, stable weight, HR less than 100 bpm, SBP greater than 90 mm Hg, fluid intake approximating fluid output, moist mucous membranes, and normal skin turgor.

INTERVENTIONS	RATIONALES
Monitor intake and output (I&O). Be alert to and report urinary output less than 30 ml/hr or 0.5 ml/kg/hr.	This assessment monitors trend of fluid volume. An indicator of deficient fluid volume is urinary output less than 30 ml/hr for 2 consecutive hr. Consider insensible losses if patient is diaphoretic and tachypneic.
Weigh patient daily at the same time of day and on the same scale; record weight. Report weight decreases of 1-1.5 kg/day.	These actions ensure consistency and accuracy of weight measurements. Weight changes of 1-1.5 kg/day can occur with fluid volume excess or deficit.

Continued

INTERVENTIONS	RATIONALES
Encourage fluid intake (at least 2.5 L/day in unrestricted patients).	These actions help ensure adequate hydration.
Maintain IV fluid therapy as prescribed.	
Promote oral hygiene, including lip and tongue care.	Oral hygiene moistens dried tissues and mucous membranes in patients with fluid volume deficit.
Provide humidity for oxygen therapy.	Humidity helps minimize convective losses of moisture during oxygen therapy.

••• **Related NIC and NOC labels:** *NIC:* Fluid Management; Fluid Monitoring; Intravenous Therapy *NOC:* Fluid Balance; Hydration

NURSING DIAGNOSIS FOR PATIENTS *AT RISK* FOR DEVELOPING PNEUMONIA

Nursing Diagnosis:

Risk for Infection

(nosocomial pneumonia) *related to* inadequate primary defenses (e.g., decreased ciliary action), invasive procedures (e.g., intubation), and/or chronic disease

Desired Outcome: Patient is free of infection as evidenced by normothermia, WBC count 12,000/mm^3 or less, and sputum clear to whitish in color.

INTERVENTIONS	RATIONALES
Perform good handwashing technique before and after contact with patient (even though gloves were worn).	This intervention helps prevent spread of infection by removing pathogens from hands. Hand hygiene involves using alcohol-based waterless antiseptic agent if hands are not visibly soiled or using soap and water if hands are dirty or contaminated with proteinaceous material.
Identify presurgical candidate who is at increased risk for nosocomial pneumonia.	This assessment helps ensure that at-risk surgical patients remain free of infection because nosocomial pneumonia has a high morbidity and mortality rate. Factors that increase risk for nosocomial pneumonia in surgical patients include the following: older adult (older than 70 yr), obesity, COPD, other chronic pulmonary conditions (e.g., asthma), history of smoking, abnormal pulmonary function tests (especially decreased forced expiratory flow rate), intubation, and upper abdominal/thoracic surgery.
Provide preoperative teaching, explaining and demonstrating pulmonary activities that will be used postoperatively to prevent respiratory infection.	Pulmonary activities that help to prevent infection/pneumonia include deep breathing, coughing, turning in bed, splinting wounds before breathing exercises, ambulation, maintaining adequate oral fluid intake, and use of hyperinflation device.
Make sure patient verbalizes knowledge of these activities and their rationales and returns demonstrations appropriately.	These actions help ensure patient is knowledgeable and capable of performing these activities. Learning how to apply information via a return demonstration is more helpful than receiving verbal instruction alone. A knowledgeable patient is more likely to adhere to therapy.
Advise individuals who smoke to discontinue smoking, especially during preoperative and postoperative periods. Refer to a community-based smoking cessation program as needed.	Inhalation of toxic fumes/chemical irritants can damage cilia and lung tissue and is a factor that increases likelihood of developing pneumonia.
When appropriate, discuss possibility of health care provider's prescription of transdermal nicotine patches.	These patches help promote smoking cessation.
Administer analgesics ½ hr before deep breathing exercises. Support (splint) surgical wound with hands, pillows, or folded blanket placed firmly across site of incision.	These interventions help control pain, which otherwise would interfere with lung expansion.

Continued

INTERVENTIONS	RATIONALES
Identify patients who are at increased risk for aspiration.	Individuals with depressed level of consciousness (LOC), dysphagia, or a nasogastric (NG) or enteral tube in place are at risk for aspiration, which predisposes them to pneumonia.
Maintain head of bed (HOB) at 30- to 45-degree elevation, and turn patient onto side rather than back. When patient receives enteral alimentation, recommend continuous rather than bolus feedings. Hold feedings when patient is lying flat.	Aspiration is one of the two leading causes of nosocomial pneumonia. Aspiration precautions include maintaining HOB at 30-degree elevation, turning patient onto side rather than back, and using continuous rather than bolus feedings when patient receives enteral alimentation.
Recognize risk factors for infection in patients with tracheostomy and intervene as follows.	Risk factors include presence of underlying lung disease or other serious illness, increased colonization of oropharynx or trachea by aerobic gram-negative bacteria, greater access of bacteria to lower respiratory tract, and cross-contamination caused by manipulation of tracheostomy tube.
- Wear gloves on both hands when handling tube or when handling mechanical ventilation tubing.	Loss of skin integrity or space around the tube would enable ingress of pathogens via the wound or tube.
- Suction as needed rather than on a routine basis.	Frequent suctioning increases risk of trauma and cross-contamination.
- Always wear gloves on both hands to suction. Use sterile catheter for each suctioning procedure. Consider use of closed suction system; replace closed suction system if soiled, for mechanical failure, or per agency policy. Always replace suction system between patients. Use only sterile fluids and dispense them using sterile technique. Replace (rather than replenish) solutions and equipment at frequent intervals. Change breathing circuits every week unless circuits are soiled, a mechanical failure occurs, or agency policy states otherwise.	These practices further decrease risk of contamination.
- Fill fluid reservoirs immediately before use (not far in advance).	
- Avoid saline instillation during suctioning. If patient has tenacious secretions, increase heat and humidity.	Saline instillation can cause dislodgement of bacteria into lower lung fields, increasing the risk of inflammation and invasion of sterile tissue. It can also stimulate coughing.
- Avoid the following when working with nebulizer reservoirs: introduction of nonsterile fluids or air, manipulation of nebulizer cup, or backflow of condensate from delivery tubing into reservoir or into patient when tubing is manipulated.	These are ways in which nebulizer reservoirs can contaminate patient.
- Discard any fluid that has condensed in tubing; do not allow it to drain back into reservoir or into patient.	

••• **Related NIC and NOC labels:** *NIC:* Infection Control; Infection Prevention; Incision Site Care; Aspiration Precautions; Environmental Management; Infection Control: Intraoperative; Artificial Airway Management; Cough Enhancement; Tube Care *NOC:* Infection Status

ADDITIONAL NURSING DIAGNOSIS FOR PATIENTS ON MECHANICAL VENTILATION

See *"General Care of Patients with Neurologic Disorders"* for **Risk for Infection** related to *inadequate primary defenses secondary to intubation, p. 264.*

✓ PATIENT-FAMILY TEACHING AND DISCHARGE PLANNING

When providing patient-family teaching, focus on sensory information, avoid giving excessive information, and initiate a visiting nurse referral for necessary follow-up teaching. Include verbal and written information about the following:

✓ Techniques that promote gas exchange and minimize stasis of secretions (e.g., deep breathing, coughing, use of hyperinflation device, increasing activity level as appropriate for patient's medical condition, percussion, and postural drainage as necessary).

✓ Medications, including drug name, purpose, dosage, frequency or schedule, precautions, and potential side effects, particularly of antibiotics. Also discuss drug-drug, herb-drug, and food-drug interactions. Instruct patient to complete full dose of antibiotics to prevent reinfection and subsequent readmission.

✓ Signs and symptoms of pneumonia and importance of reporting them promptly to health care professional should they recur. Teach patient's significant others that changes in mental status may be the only indicator of pneumonia if patient is elderly.

✓ Importance of preventing fatigue by pacing activities and allowing frequent rest periods.

✓ Importance of avoiding exposure to individuals known to have flu and colds.

✓ Recommendation that the following individuals receive a pneumococcal vaccination: patients who are more than 65 years old, have chronic health conditions, and/or are residents of an extended care facility and have not received the vaccine within the last 5 years. Vaccine history should be assessed on admission and vaccine(s) given to patients who meet criteria without contraindications (allergy).

✓ Recommendation that the following individuals receive an influenza vaccination annually: those who are older than 50 years old, have chronic health conditions, and/or are residents of an extended care facility and have not received the vaccine within the year. Influenza vaccines are routinely administered from the months of October through March. Vaccine history should be assessed on admission and given to patients who meet criteria without contraindications (e.g., allergy, history of Guillain-Barré).

✓ Minimizing factors that can cause reinfection, including close living conditions, poor nutrition, and poorly ventilated living quarters or work environment.

✓ Importance of smoking cessation education and community resources to assist in cessation.

✓ Phone numbers to call in case questions or concerns arise about therapy or disease after discharge. Additional general information can be obtained by visiting www.lungusa.org.

✓ Information in the following free brochures that outline ways to help patients stop smoking:

- *How to Help Your Patients Stop Using Tobacco: A National Cancer Institute Manual for the Oral Health Team*, from the Smoking and Tobacco Control Program of the National Cancer Institute; call (800) 4-CANCER.

- *Clinical Practice Guideline: A Quick Reference Guide for Smoking Cessation Specialists*, from the Agency for Health Care Policy and Research (AHCPR); call (800) 358-9295.

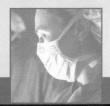

Pneumothorax/Hemothorax 11

PNEUMOTHORAX
OVERVIEW/PATHOPHYSIOLOGY

Pneumothorax is an accumulation of air in the pleural space that leads to increased intrapleural pressure. Risk factors include blunt or penetrating chest injury, chronic obstructive pulmonary disease (COPD), previous pneumothorax, and positive pressure ventilation. The three types of pneumothorax are as follows.

Spontaneous: Also referred to as *closed pneumothorax* because the chest wall remains intact with no leak to the atmosphere. It results from rupture of a bleb or bulla on the visceral pleural surface, usually near the apex. Generally, the cause of the rupture is unknown, although it may result from a weakness related to a respiratory infection or from an underlying pulmonary disease (e.g., COPD, tuberculosis, malignant neoplasm). The affected individual is usually young (20-40 yr), previously healthy, and male. Generally, onset of symptoms occurs at rest rather than with vigorous exercise or coughing. Potential for recurrence is great, with the second pneumothorax occurring an average of 2-3 yr after the first.

Traumatic: Can be open or closed. An open pneumothorax occurs when air enters the pleural space from the atmosphere through an opening in the chest wall, such as with a gunshot wound, stab wound, or invasive medical procedure (e.g., lung biopsy, thoracentesis, or placement of a central line into a subclavian vein). A sucking sound may be heard over the area of penetration during inspiration, accounting for the classic wound description as a "sucking chest wound." A closed pneumothorax occurs when the visceral pleura is penetrated but the chest wall remains intact with no atmospheric leak. This usually occurs following blunt trauma that results in rib fracture and dislocation. It also may occur from use of positive end expiratory pressure (PEEP) or after cardiopulmonary resuscitation.

Tension: Generally occurs with closed pneumothorax; also can occur with open pneumothorax when a flap of tissue acts as a one-way valve. Air enters the pleural space through the pleural tear when the individual inhales, and it continues to accumulate but cannot escape during expiration because the tissue flap closes. With tension pneumothorax, as pressure in the thorax and mediastinum increases, it produces a shift in the affected lung and mediastinum toward the unaffected side, which further impairs ventilatory efforts. The increase in pressure also compresses the vena cava, which impedes venous return, leading to a decrease in cardiac output and, ultimately, to circulatory collapse if the condition is not diagnosed and treated quickly. Tension pneumothorax is a life-threatening medical emergency.

HEMOTHORAX
OVERVIEW/PATHOPHYSIOLOGY

Hemothorax is an accumulation of blood in the pleural space. Hemothorax generally results from blunt trauma to the chest wall, but it can also occur following thoracic surgery, after penetrating gunshot or stab wounds, as a result of anticoagulant therapy, after insertion of a central venous catheter, or following various thoracoabdominal organ biopsies. Mediastinal shift, ventilatory compromise, and lung collapse can occur, depending on the amount of blood accumulated.

HEALTH CARE SETTING

Acute care, primary care

ASSESSMENT

Clinical presentation will vary, depending on type and size of the pneumothorax or hemothorax.

DIAGNOSTIC TESTS

Chest x-ray examination: Will reveal presence of air or blood in the pleural space on the affected side, pneumothorax/hemothorax size, and any shift in the mediastinum.

Oximetry: Will reveal decreased O_2 saturation (90% or less).

ABG values: Hypoxemia (Pao_2 less than 80 mm Hg) may be accompanied by hypercarbia ($Paco_2$ greater than 45 mm Hg) with resultant respiratory acidosis (pH less than 7.35). Arterial oxygen saturation may be decreased initially but usually returns to normal within 24 hr.

CBC: May reveal decreased hemoglobin proportionate to amount of blood lost in a hemothorax.

Assessment			
Spontaneous or Traumatic Pneumothorax		**Tension Pneumothorax**	**Hemothorax**
Closed	**Open**		
Signs and Symptoms			
Shortness of breath, cough, chest tightness, chest pain	Shortness of breath, sharp chest pain	Dyspnea, chest pain	Dyspnea, chest pain
Physical Assessment			
Tachypnea, decreased thoracic movement, cyanosis, subcutaneous emphysema, hyperresonance over affected area, diminished breath sounds, paradoxical movement of chest wall (may signal flail chest), change in mental status	Agitation, restlessness, tachypnea, cyanosis, presence of chest wound, hyperresonance over affected area, sucking sound on inspiration, diminished breath sounds, change in mental status	Anxiety, tachycardia, cyanosis, jugular vein distention, tracheal deviation toward the unaffected side, absent breath sounds on affected side, distant heart sounds, hypotension, change in mental status	Tachypnea, pallor, cyanosis, dullness over affected side, tachycardia, hypotension, diminished or absent breath sounds, change in mental status

Nursing Diagnosis:

Ineffective Breathing Pattern (or risk for same)

related to decreased lung expansion secondary to malfunction of chest drainage system

Desired Outcome: Following intervention, patient becomes eupneic; lung expansion is noted on chest x-ray after chest tube removal.

INTERVENTIONS	RATIONALES
Assess patient's mental, respiratory, and cardiac status at frequent intervals (q2-4h, as appropriate).	This assessment monitors patient's status while chest drainage system is in place. The purpose of a chest drainage system is to drain air or fluid and reexpand the lung. Diminished breath sounds, along with tachycardia, restlessness, anxiety, and changes in mental status, are signs of respiratory distress that may occur as a result of chest drainage system malfunction. If these signs are present, prompt intervention is necessary to prevent further hypoxia and distress.
Assess and maintain closed chest drainage system as follows:	These actions help ensure maintenance of closed chest drainage system and facilitate drainage.
- Tape all connections and secure chest tube to thorax with tape.	
- Avoid all tubing kinks, and ensure that the bed and equipment are not compressing any component of the system. Eliminate all dependent loops in tubing.	
- Maintain fluid in underwater-seal chamber and suction chamber at appropriate levels.	The suction apparatus does not regulate the amount of suction applied to closed chest drainage system. The amount of suction is determined by the water level in the suction control chamber.
- Monitor bubbling in the underwater-seal chamber.	Intermittent bubbling in this chamber is normal and signals that air is leaving the pleural space. Absence of bubbling indicates the system is malfunctioning and suction is not being maintained.
- Locate and seal any leak in the system if possible.	Continuous bubbling in the underwater-seal chamber may be a signal that air is leaking into the drainage system.
- Dial the level of dry suction per health care provider's recommendation.	This action maintains air and fluid removal from the pleural space.
	Note: Suction aids in lung reexpansion, but removing suction for short periods, such as for transporting, will not be detrimental or disrupt the closed chest drainage system.

Continued

INTERVENTIONS	RATIONALES
- Monitor fluctuations in the underwater-seal chamber.	These fluctuations are characteristic of a patent chest tube. Fluctuations stop when either the lung has reexpanded or there is a kink or obstruction in the chest tube.
- Avoid stripping of chest tubes with mechanical or handheld tube-stripping devices.	This mechanism for maintaining chest tube patency is controversial and has been associated with creating high negative pressures in the pleural space, which can damage fragile lung tissue.
- If approved by health care provider, squeeze alternately hand-over-hand along the drainage tube.	This gentler method of chest tube milking may generate sufficient pressure to move fluid along the tube.
Keep the following necessary emergency supplies at the bedside.	
- Petrolatum gauze pad.	This gauze pad is applied over the insertion site if the chest tube becomes dislodged. Use of this dressing provides an airtight seal to prevent recurrent pneumothorax.
- A bottle of sterile water.	Submerging chest tube in a bottle of sterile water if it becomes disconnected from the underwater-seal system provides for a temporary closed chest drainage system.
Never clamp a chest tube without a specific directive from health care provider.	Clamping may lead to tension pneumothorax because air in the pleural space no longer can escape.

••• **Related NIC and NOC labels:** *NIC:* Airway Management; Respiratory Monitoring; Ventilation Assistance *NOC:* Respiratory Status: Airway Patency; Respiratory Status: Ventilation

Nursing Diagnosis:

Impaired Gas Exchange

related to altered oxygen supply secondary to ventilation-perfusion mismatch

Desired Outcomes: Following treatment/intervention, patient exhibits adequate gas exchange and ventilatory function as evidenced by RR 20 breaths/min or less with normal depth and pattern (eupnea); no significant mental status changes; and orientation to person, place, and time. At a minimum of 24 hr before hospital discharge, patient's ABG values are as follows: Pao_2 80 mm Hg or more and $Paco_2$ 35-45 mm Hg (or values within patient's acceptable baseline parameters), or oximetry readings demonstrate O_2 saturation greater than 90%.

INTERVENTIONS	RATIONALES
Monitor serial arterial blood gas (ABG) results or oximetry readings. Report significant findings to health care provider.	These assessments detect decreasing Pao_2 or O_2 saturation and increasing $Paco_2$, which can signal impending respiratory compromise and necessitate prompt intervention.
Observe for indicators of hypoxia. Report significant findings.	Increased restlessness, anxiety, tachycardia, and changes in mental status are early indicators of hypoxia and can signal impending respiratory compromise, which would necessitate prompt intervention.
Assess vital signs and breath sounds q2h or as indicated by patient's condition. Report significant findings.	These assessments monitor patient's trend. Significant changes such as increased heart rate (HR), increased respiratory rate (RR), and unilateral decreased breath sounds signal a worsening or unresolved condition.
Following tube or exploratory thoracotomy, check patient q15min until stable. Report significant findings.	These assessments enable prompt detection of respiratory distress for timely intervention, including increased RR, diminished or absent movement of chest wall on affected side, paradoxical movement of the chest wall, increased work of breathing, use of accessory muscles of respiration, complaints of increased dyspnea, unilateral diminished breath sounds, and cyanosis.

Continued

INTERVENTIONS	RATIONALES
	Chest tubes may be placed in any patients who are symptomatic to remove air or fluid from the pleural space and enable reexpansion of the lung. A thoracotomy may be indicated if patient has had 2 or more spontaneous pneumothoraces or if the current pneumothorax does not resolve within 7 days. In the presence of a hemothorax, a thoracotomy may be indicated to locate the source and control the bleeding if loss exceeds 200 ml/hr for 2 hr.
Evaluate HR and blood pressure for tachycardia and hypotension. Report significant findings.	Tachycardia, along with tachypnea, is a compensatory mechanism that occurs due to hypoxia/hypoxemia. Tachycardia and hypotension are indicators of shock.
Support patient in optimal position (e.g., semi-Fowler's).	This position provides comfort and enables full expansion of unaffected lung, adequate expansion of chest wall, and descent of diaphragm.
Change patient's position q2h.	This intervention promotes drainage and lung reexpansion and facilitates alveolar perfusion.
Encourage patient to take deep breaths, providing necessary analgesia to decrease discomfort during deep breathing exercises. Instruct patient in splinting thoracotomy site with arms, pillow, or folded blanket.	Deep breathing promotes full lung expansion and decreases risk of atelectasis. Analgesia and splinting decrease discomfort during deep-breathing exercises. Coughing facilitates mobilization of tracheobronchial secretions, if present.
Deliver and monitor oxygen and humidity as indicated for patients with oxygen saturations of 90% or less.	This intervention ensures adequate oxygen levels if patient has hypoxemia, which is likely to be present if the pneumothorax/hemothorax is large. Humidity minimizes convective losses of moisture.

••• **Related NIC and NOC labels:** *NIC:* Acid-Base Management; Oxygen Therapy; Ventilation Assistance; Positioning; Respiratory Monitoring; Cough Enhancement; Vital Signs Monitoring *NOC:* Respiratory Status: Gas Exchange; Respiratory Status: Ventilation; Vital Signs Status

Nursing Diagnosis:

Acute Pain

related to impaired pleural integrity, inflammation, or presence of a chest tube

Desired Outcomes: Within 1 hr of intervention, patient's subjective perception of pain decreases, as documented by pain scale. Objective indicators, such as grimacing, are absent or diminished.

INTERVENTIONS	RATIONALES
At frequent intervals, assess patient's degree of discomfort, using patient's verbal and nonverbal cues. Devise a pain scale with patient, rating pain from 0 (no pain) to 10 (worst pain).	These assessments monitor trend of pain and help determine success of subsequent pain interventions. Because of rich innervation of the pleura, chest tube placement is painful; significant analgesia is usually required.
Medicate with analgesics as prescribed, using pain scale to evaluate and document medication effectiveness.	These actions provide pain relief and determine effectiveness of the analgesia.
Encourage patient to request analgesic before pain becomes severe or, alternatively, administer at scheduled intervals.	Prolonged stimulation of pain receptors results in increased sensitivity to painful stimuli and increases amount of drug required to relieve pain.
Premedicate patient 30 min before initiating coughing, exercising, or repositioning and 30 min before, during, and after chemical pleurodesis.	This intervention provides comfort during painful exercises and repositioning and facilitates compliance. Chemical pleurodesis is extremely painful and requires diligent pain management.
Teach patient to splint affected side when coughing, moving, or repositioning.	This action reduces discomfort and promotes adherence to treatment plan.
Facilitate coordination among health care providers to provide rest periods between care activities. Allow 90 min for undisturbed rest.	Relaxation and rest decrease oxygen demand and may decrease level of pain.

Continued

INTERVENTIONS	RATIONALES
Stabilize chest tube. Tape chest tube securely to thorax.	These actions reduce pull or drag on latex connector tubing, prevent discomfort, and help facilitate drainage and appropriate functioning.
Position tube to ensure there are no dependent loops.	
For additional interventions, see "Pain," p. 39.	

••• **Related NIC and NOC labels:** *NIC:* Analgesic Administration; Pain Management; Environmental Management: Comfort; Splinting
NOC: Pain Level; Pain Control

ADDITIONAL NURSING DIAGNOSES/ PROBLEMS:

"Psychosocial Support"	p. 73
"Abdominal Trauma" for **Deficient Fluid Volume**	p. 421

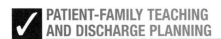

PATIENT-FAMILY TEACHING AND DISCHARGE PLANNING

When providing patient-family teaching, focus on sensory information, avoid giving excessive information, and initiate a visiting nurse referral for necessary follow-up teaching. Include verbal and written information about the following.

✓ Purpose for chest-tube placement and maintenance.

✓ Potential for recurrence of spontaneous pneumothorax. Average time between occurrences is 2-3 yr. Explain importance of seeking medical care immediately if symptoms recur (see Assessment).

✓ Medications, including drug name, purpose, dosage, schedule, precautions, and potential side effects. Also discuss drug/drug, herb/drug, and food/drug interactions.

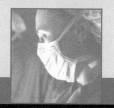

Pulmonary Embolus 12

OVERVIEW/PATHOPHYSIOLOGY

The most common pulmonary perfusion abnormality is a pulmonary embolus (PE). PE is caused by passage of a foreign substance (blood clot, fat, air, or amniotic fluid) into the pulmonary artery or its branches, with resulting obstruction of the blood supply to lung tissue and subsequent collapse. The most common source is a dislodged blood clot from the systemic circulation, typically the deep veins of the legs or pelvis. Thrombus formation is the result of the following factors: blood stasis, alterations in clotting factors, and injury to vessel walls. A fat embolus is the most common nonthrombotic cause of pulmonary perfusion disorders. It is the result of release of free fatty acids causing a toxic vasculitis, followed by thrombosis and obstruction of small pulmonary arteries by fat.

Total obstruction leading to pulmonary infarction is rare because the pulmonary circulation has multiple sources of blood supply. Early diagnosis and appropriate treatment reduce mortality to less than 10%. Although most pulmonary emboli resolve completely and leave no residual deficits, some patients may be left with chronic pulmonary hypertension.

HEALTH CARE SETTING

Acute care

ASSESSMENT

Signs and symptoms often are nonspecific and variable, depending on extent of obstruction and whether patient has infarction as a result of the obstruction.

Pulmonary embolus: Sudden onset of dyspnea and sharp chest pain, restlessness, anxiety, nonproductive cough or hemoptysis, palpitations, nausea, and syncope. With a large embolism, oppressive substernal chest discomfort and signs of diastolic (right-sided) heart failure will be present. See "Heart Failure," p. 181, for signs and symptoms.

Pulmonary infarction: Fever, pleuritic chest pain, and hemoptysis.

Physical assessment: Tachypnea, tachycardia, hypotension, crackles (rales), decreased chest wall excursion secondary to splinting, S_3 and S_4 gallop rhythms, transient pleural friction rub, jugular venous distention, diaphoresis, edema, and cyanosis. Temperature may be elevated if infarction has occurred.

HISTORY AND RISK FACTORS

Immobility: Especially significant when it coexists with surgical or nonsurgical trauma, carcinoma, or cardiopulmonary disease. Risk increases as duration of immobility increases.

Cardiac disorders: Atrial fibrillation, heart failure, myocardial infarction, rheumatic heart disease.

Surgical intervention: Risk increases in prolonged surgeries of more than 30 min duration or during the postoperative period, especially for patients with orthopedic, pelvic, thoracic, or abdominal surgery and for those with extensive burns or musculoskeletal injuries of the hip or knee.

Pregnancy: Especially during postpartum period.

Chronic pulmonary and infectious diseases

Trauma: Especially lower extremity fractures and burns. The degree of risk is related to severity, site, and extent of trauma.

Mechanical ventilation: Risk increases because of immobility and inflammatory processes.

Carcinoma: Particularly neoplasms involving the breast, lung, pancreas, and genitourinary and alimentary tracts.

Obesity: A 20% increase in ideal body weight is associated with an increased incidence of PE.

Varicose veins or prior thromboembolic disease

Age: Risk of thromboembolism is greatest for patients older than 55 yr of age.

Specific findings for fat embolus: Typically, patient is asymptomatic for 12-24 hr following embolization. This period ends with sudden cardiopulmonary and neurologic deterioration: apprehension, restlessness, mental status changes, confusion, delirium, coma, and dyspnea.

Physical assessment for fat embolus: Tachypnea, tachycardia, and hypertension; fever; petechiae, especially of conjunctivae, neck, upper torso, axillae, and proximal arms; inspiratory crowing; pulmonary edema; profuse tracheobronchial secretions; fat globules in sputum; and expiratory wheezes.

History and risk factors for fat embolus

Multiple long bone fractures, especially fractures of the femur and pelvis; trauma to adipose tissue or liver; burns; osteomyelitis; sickle cell crisis.

Diagnostic Tests

General findings for pulmonary emboli

ABG values: Hypoxemia (Pao_2 less than 80 mm Hg), hypocarbia ($Paco_2$ less than 35 mm Hg), and respiratory alkalosis (pH more than 7.45) usually are present. A normal Pao_2 does not rule out presence of pulmonary emboli.

D-dimer: A degradation product produced by plasmin-mediated proteolysis of cross-linked fibrin. D-dimer is measured by an enzyme-linked immunosorbent assay. The higher the result (with less than 250 ng/ml considered negative in most laboratories), the more likely it is patient has PE. This test is not sensitive or specific enough to diagnose PE, but it may be used in conjunction with other diagnostic tests.

Chest x-ray examination: Initially findings are normal, or an elevated hemidiaphragm may be present. After 24 hr, x-ray examination may reveal small infiltrates secondary to atelectasis that result from the decrease in surfactant. If pulmonary infarction is present, infiltrates and pleural effusions may be seen within 12-36 hr.

ECG results: If PEs are extensive, signs of acute pulmonary hypertension may be present: right-shift QRS axes, tall and peaked P waves, ST-segment changes, and T-wave inversion in leads V_1-V_4.

Spiral or helical CT: Enables image acquisition of pulmonary arteries during a single breath hold and with optimal contrast enhancement. Spiral computed tomography (CT) is rapidly becoming the test of choice in diagnosing PE because of its higher specificity and sensitivity.

Pulmonary ventilation-perfusion scan: Used to detect abnormalities of ventilation or perfusion in the pulmonary system. Radiopaque agents are inhaled and injected peripherally. Images of distribution of both agents throughout the lung are scanned. If the scan shows a mismatch of ventilation and perfusion (i.e., pattern of normal ventilation with decreased perfusion), vascular obstruction is suggested.

Pulmonary angiography: The definitive study for PE, this is an invasive procedure that involves right heart catheterization and injection of dye into the pulmonary artery (PA) to visualize pulmonary vessels. An abrupt vessel "cutoff" may be seen at the site of embolization. Usually, filling defects are seen. More specific findings are abnormal blood vessel diameters (i.e., obstruction of right PA would cause dilation of left PA) and shapes (i.e., affected blood vessel may taper to a sharp point and disappear).

Findings specific for fat emboli

ABG values: Should be drawn on patients at risk for fat embolus for the first 48 hr following injury because early hypoxemia indicative of fat embolus is apparent only with laboratory assessment. Hypoxemia (Pao_2 less than 80 mm Hg) and hypercarbia ($Paco_2$ more than 45 mm Hg) will be present with a respiratory acidosis (pH less than 7.35).

Chest x-ray examination: A pattern similar to adult respiratory distress syndrome is seen: diffuse, extensive bilateral interstitial and alveolar infiltrates.

CBC: May reveal decreased hemoglobin (Hgb) and hematocrit (Hct) secondary to hemorrhage into the lung. In addition, thrombocytopenia (platelets $150,000/mm^3$ or less) is indicative of fat embolism.

Serum lipase: Will rise with fat embolism.

Urinalysis: May reveal fat globules following fat embolus.

Nursing Diagnosis:

Risk for Injury

related to venous stasis, hypercoagulable state, and/or vessel injury contributing to venous thromboembolism (VTE)

Desired Outcome: Following intervention/treatment, patient exhibits no venous thromboembolic events (see descriptions under Assessment).

INTERVENTIONS	RATIONALES
Assess patient for risk factors relating to VTE.	Risk factors alone or in combination increase the risk for developing VTE. Examples include advanced age, orthopedic surgery, and immobility.
Collaborate with health care provider regarding appropriate treatment with prophylaxis.	Prophylaxis may include but is not limited to pneumatic compression devices and/or medical prophylaxis with low-dose heparin or low-molecular-weight heparin (LMWH).
	Unfractionated heparin (UFH) therapy: Started immediately in patients without bleeding.
	LMWH: Used as an alternative to low-dose heparin. LMWH is administered subcutaneously daily (prophylaxis). Most LMWH is excreted by the kidneys, and therefore dose must be adjusted for individuals with renal impairment. LMWH has been shown to be safe if given during pregnancy.

Continued

INTERVENTIONS	RATIONALES
Encourage ambulation and monitor activity.	Increased ambulation prevents venous stasis, a major risk factor for development of VTE.

••• **Related NIC and NOC labels:** *NIC:* Health education; Risk identification *NOC:* Risk control

Nursing Diagnosis:

Impaired Gas Exchange

related to altered oxygen supply secondary to ventilation-perfusion mismatch

Desired Outcomes: Following intervention/treatment, patient exhibits adequate gas exchange and ventilatory function as evidenced by RR 12-20 breaths/min with normal pattern and depth (eupnea); no significant changes in mental status; and orientation to person, place, and time. At a minimum of 24 hr before hospital discharge, patient has O_2 saturation greater than 90% or Pao_2 80 mm Hg or higher, $Paco_2$ 35-45 mm Hg, and pH 7.35-7.45 (or values consistent with patient's acceptable baseline parameters).

INTERVENTIONS	RATIONALES
Monitor patient for respiratory rate (RR) increased from baseline and increasing dyspnea, anxiety, restlessness, confusion, and cyanosis. Report significant findings.	These signs and symptoms of increasing respiratory distress and indicators of PE necessitate prompt intervention.
As indicated, monitor oximetry readings; report O_2 saturation of 90% or less.	A low O_2 saturation may indicate need for O_2 therapy. Hypoxia is common with PE, although its absence does not mean that patient does not have a PE.
Instruct patient not to cross legs when lying in bed or sitting in a chair.	These positions impede venous return from the legs and can increase risk of PE.
Pace patient's activities and procedures.	Pacing activities and procedures decreases metabolic demands for oxygen and prevents further complications related to immobility.
	Note: It is safe for patient to ambulate once anticoagulation has been started.
Ensure that patient performs deep breathing and coughing exercises 3-5 times q2h.	These exercises mobilize secretions and improve ventilation.
Ensure delivery of prescribed concentrations and humidity of oxygen.	Supplemental oxygen helps maintain a Pao_2 greater than 60 mm Hg and optimally 80 mm Hg or greater. Humidifying the oxygen minimizes convective losses of moisture.
Monitor oxygen saturations. Report lack of response to treatment or worsening oxygen saturations.	A poor response to treatment or worsening oxygen saturation necessitates prompt reporting for timely evaluation and further treatment.

••• **Related NIC and NOC labels:** *NIC:* Oxygen Therapy; Respiratory Monitoring; Acid-Base Monitoring; Positioning; Cough Enhancement; Embolus Care: Pulmonary; Energy Management *NOC:* Tissue Perfusion: Pulmonary; Respiratory Status: Ventilation; Respiratory Status: Gas Exchange

Nursing Diagnosis:

Ineffective Protection

related to risk of prolonged bleeding or hemorrhage secondary to anticoagulation therapy

Desired Outcome: Patient is free of frank or occult bleeding; body secretions/excretions test negative for blood.

INTERVENTIONS	RATIONALES
Monitor vital signs for indicators of profuse bleeding or hemorrhage. Report significant findings.	Hypotension, tachycardia, and tachypnea are signs of bleeding/hemorrhage, which can occur with anticoagulant therapy and necessitate prompt intervention.
At least once each shift inspect wounds, oral mucous membranes, any entry site of an invasive procedure, and nares.	This assessment helps determine if blood is present at any of these sites.
At least once each shift inspect torso and extremities.	The presence of petechiae or ecchymoses signals bleeding within the tissues.
If parenteral medications are mandatory, attempt to administer subcutaneously using a small-gauge needle.	Bleeding and hematoma formation are more likely to occur with larger puncture wounds, such as with IM injections.
Apply pressure to all venipuncture or arterial puncture sites until bleeding stops completely.	To ensure that all bleeding stops completely, it is necessary to apply pressure for a longer than usual amount of time.
Ensure easy access to the following antidotes for prescribed treatment:	
- Protamine sulfate	1 mg counteracts 100 U of heparin. Usual initial dose is 50 mg. Fatal hemorrhage occurs in 1%-2% of patients undergoing heparin therapy.
- Vitamin K (vitamin K_1 [phytonadione] or K_3 [menadione])	20 mg is given subcutaneously to counteract effects of oral anticoagulants.
- Fresh frozen plasma	This product may be required in cases of serious bleeding.
	Note: Reversal agents should not be the first line of therapy unless a patient is actively bleeding.
If patient is receiving heparin therapy, monitor serial partial thromboplastin time (PTT).	This will confirm that PTT is in the desired range (1.5-2.5 $\times$ control).
If patient is receiving warfarin therapy, monitor serial prothrombin time (PT).	This will confirm that PT is in the desired range (1.25-1.5 $\times$ control, or international normalization ratio value of 2.0-3.0).
Report values outside desired range. Establish compatibility of all drugs before administering them.	These actions help ensure patient's physiologic safety.
Consult pharmacist about compatibility before infusing other IV drugs through heparin IV line.	For patients on heparin therapy, the following agents decrease the effect of heparin therapy: digitalis, tetracycline, nicotine, and antihistamines.
For patients on warfarin therapy, consult pharmacist to obtain specific information about patient's medication profile.	Numerous drugs result in a decrease or increase in response to treatment with warfarin.
Note: Consult a pharmacist before infusing any medication through the same IV line.	For patients on thrombolytic therapy, although no specific drug interactions are currently known for thrombolytic therapy, new drugs are always coming on the market.
Discuss with patient and significant others the effects of anticoagulant therapy and importance of reporting promptly the presence of bleeding.	Hematuria, melena, frank bleeding from the mouth, epistaxis, hemoptysis, and excessive vaginal bleeding (menometrorrhagia) are potential effects of anticoagulant therapy and necessitate timely intervention to prevent further blood loss.
Teach necessity of using soft toothbrush and mouthwash for oral care. Instruct patient to shave with electric rather than straight or safety razor.	These measures minimize risk of bleeding.
If patient is restless and combative, provide a safe environment. Use extreme care when moving patient.	These actions help prevent falls and avoid bumping extremities into side rails, which could result in severe bleeding.

●●● **Related NIC and NOC labels:** *NIC:* Bleeding Precautions; Hemorrhage Control *NOC:* Coagulation Status

Nursing Diagnosis:

Deficient Knowledge:

Oral anticoagulant therapy, potential side effects, and foods and medications to consider during therapy

Desired Outcome: Before hospital discharge, patient verbalizes knowledge of prescribed anticoagulant drug, potential side effects, and foods and medications to consider while receiving oral anticoagulant therapy.

INTERVENTIONS	RATIONALES
Assess patient's health care literacy (language, reading, comprehension). Assess culture and culturally specific learning needs.	This assessment helps ensure that information is presented in a manner that is culturally and educationally appropriate.
Determine patient's knowledge of oral anticoagulant therapy. As appropriate, discuss drug name; purpose; dose; schedule; precautions; food-drug, herb-drug, and drug-drug interactions; and potential side effects.	Knowledgeable patients are more likely to adhere to the therapeutic regimen.
Teach potential side effects/complications of anticoagulant therapy: easy bruising, prolonged bleeding from cuts, spontaneous nosebleeds, bleeding gums, black and tarry or bloody stools, vaginal bleeding, and blood in urine and sputum.	This information increases patient's awareness of side effects and complications to report to health care provider for timely intervention.
Discuss importance of laboratory testing and follow-up visits with health care provider.	Laboratory testing helps ensure that patient's blood clotting time stays within therapeutic range. To promote safety, patient needs close management by health care provider while undergoing anticoagulant therapy.
Explain importance of informing all health care providers (including dentist) that patient is taking an anticoagulant. Suggest that patient wear a medical alert tag or otherwise carry identification informing health care providers about the anticoagulant therapy.	These actions help ensure that patient is not given drugs or therapies that will have adverse effects on anticoagulant therapy, causing greater risk for hemorrhaging or clotting.
Teach patient to notify health care provider when ingesting large amounts of foods high in vitamin K.	Foods high in vitamin K (e.g., asparagus, avocados, beef liver, broccoli, cabbage, soybeans, lettuce, olive oil, and canola oil) can interfere with anticoagulation.
Caution patient that soft-bristled rather than hard-bristled toothbrush and electric rather than straight or safety razor should be used during anticoagulant therapy.	These devices minimize risk of injury that could cause severe bleeding.
Instruct patient to consult health care provider before taking over-the-counter or prescribed drugs that were used before initiating anticoagulant therapy.	Aspirin, cimetidine, trimethaphan, and macrolides are among the many drugs that enhance response to warfarin. Drugs that decrease response include antacids, diuretics, oral contraceptives, and barbiturates, among others.

••• **Related NIC and NOC labels:** *NIC:* Teaching: Prescribed Medication; Medication Management *NOC:* Knowledge: Medication

ADDITIONAL NURSING DIAGNOSES/ PROBLEMS:

"Perioperative Care"	p. 45
"Prolonged Bedrest"	p. 61

✓ PATIENT-FAMILY TEACHING AND DISCHARGE PLANNING

When providing patient-family teaching, focus on sensory information, avoid giving excessive information, and initiate a visiting nurse referral for necessary follow-up teaching. Include verbal and written information about the following. **Note:** Rehabilitation and family teaching concepts for fat emboli are nonspecific.

✓ Risk factors related to development of thrombi and embolization and preventive measures to reduce the risk.

✓ Signs and symptoms of thrombophlebitis: calf swelling; tenderness or warmth in the involved area; slight fever; and distention of distal veins, coolness, edema, and pale color in the distal affected leg.

✓ Signs and symptoms of pulmonary embolism: sudden onset of dyspnea and anxiety, nonproductive cough or hemoptysis, palpitations, nausea, syncope.

✓ Importance of preventing impairment of venous return from the lower extremities by avoiding prolonged sitting, crossing legs, and constrictive clothing.

✓ Medications, including drug name, dosage, purpose, schedule, precautions, and potential side effects. Also discuss drug-drug, herb-drug, and food-drug interactions.

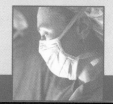

Pulmonary Tuberculosis 13

OVERVIEW/PATHOPHYSIOLOGY

Tuberculosis (TB) is an infectious disease caused primarily by *Mycobacterium tuberculosis*. In the United States an estimated 10 to 15 million persons are infected with this organism, the majority of whom have latent tuberculosis infection (LTBI) in which the bacteria are in the body (usually the lungs) in a dormant form that neither causes disease nor is communicable to other persons. A small proportion of persons (about 10%) with LTBI will develop active TB in their lifetimes.

For many years (from 1953 to 1984), reported cases of TB in the United States decreased almost 6% each year, and there was a general perception that TB was no longer a problem. This decline was due to many factors, including improved living conditions (less crowding and better ventilation), better nutrition, and antituberculosis drugs. As a result, the public health infrastructure to support TB control weakened as other diseases, for example, human immunodeficiency virus (HIV)/acquired immunodeficiency syndrome (AIDS), became more prominent. It was not until the late 1980s that the link between TB and HIV/AIDS became apparent as was manifested partially by multidrug-resistant (MDR) TB outbreaks occurring in seven hospitals between 1990 and 1992, resulting in many cases of LTBI, TB disease, and death. In addition, reported cases of TB increased 20% between 1985 and 1992. After the hospital outbreaks and other changes in administrative and legislative support to control TB, cases have steadily declined again in most areas of the country. In 2005, there were fewer than 15,000 reported cases of TB in the United States, more than half of which were among foreign-born persons. Worldwide, TB remains a leading cause of death in undeveloped countries, with the World Health Organization estimating that approximately one third of the world's population is infected with *Mycobacterium tuberculosis*.

M. *tuberculosis* is transmitted by the airborne route via minute, invisible particles called *droplet nuclei*. When individuals with TB disease of the lungs or throat cough, sneeze, speak, or sing, their respiratory secretions harbor TB organisms that are expelled into the air and transform quickly into tiny droplet nuclei that can remain suspended in air for several hours, depending on the environment (especially ventilation). In order to become infected, another person must breathe the air containing the droplet nuclei. A person's natural defenses of the nose and upper airway and immune system will often prevent sufficient numbers of organisms to reach the alveoli to cause infection. In fact, it generally takes 5 to 200 organisms implanted in the alveoli to cause LTBI. When organisms reach the alveoli, they are ingested by macrophages. Some of the bacilli spread through the bloodstream when the macrophages die; however, the immune system response usually prevents the individual from developing TB disease. Although the majority of TB cases are pulmonary (85%), TB can occur in almost any part of the body or as disseminated disease. About half of people with LTBI who develop active tuberculosis (5%) will do so within the first year or two after infection. The remainder (5%) will develop active TB within their lifetimes.

HEALTH CARE SETTING

Primary care or long-term care, with possible hospitalization (acute care) resulting from complications

ASSESSMENT

For an accurate diagnosis of TB, a complete medical and psychosocial history should be taken along with a physical examination that includes a tuberculin skin test or an interferon gamma release assay (IGRA) blood test (one such blood test is called the QuantiFERON-TB Gold test), chest x-ray examination, and sputum examination (including acid-fast bacilli [AFB] smears, cultures, and drug sensitivity studies).

Signs and symptoms: Tuberculosis is often diagnosed based on a group of symptoms that may include commonly described early symptoms, such as productive prolonged cough, fever, and night sweats as well as chest pain, hemoptysis, chills, loss of appetite, unintended weight loss over a short period of time, and tiredness.

Note: *Close contacts of the patient require identification so that they can undergo evaluation for the presence of LTBI. TB is reportable to the Public Health Department.*

History/risk factors for developing active TB: Immunocompromised state, especially HIV infection; injection drug use; radiographic evidence of prior, healed TB; weight loss of 10% or more of ideal body weight; and other medical conditions, including diabetes mellitus, silicosis, end-stage renal disease, some types of cancers, and certain immunosuppressive therapies. Persons who have emigrated from areas of the world with high rates of TB are also more likely to have LTBI than persons born in the United States.

DIAGNOSTIC TESTS

Tuberculin skin test or intradermal injection of antigen (purified protein derivative): This test uses a purified protein derivative (PPD) of mycobacterial organisms that is administered intradermally and interpreted as positive or negative using measured millimeters of induration. The test is considered positive when an area of induration 10 mm or greater is present within 48-72 hr after injection. High-risk categories such as persons with HIV infection and recent exposure are considered positive with 5 mm or greater induration. Those who are immunocompromised and some patients with active TB may have a negative PPD test, even in the presence of active TB disease. A positive PPD test indicates LTBI and is not diagnostic for active disease.

QuantiFERON-TB Gold (QFT) blood test: Until recently, the only way to diagnose LTBI was with the tuberculin skin test (TST). Since 2001, an alternative to the TST, the QFT, has been approved by the Food and Drug Administration (FDA). This whole-blood interferon gamma assay requires only one patient visit for a blood specimen to assess for LTBI (rather than for active disease) and will become more widely used as laboratories implement the requirements for specimen evaluation. Other whole-blood interferon gamma assays are also under development.

Acid-fast stain: Detection of AFB in stained smears examined under a microscope usually provides the first bacteriologic clue of TB. Smear results should be available within 24 hr of specimen collection. AFB in the smear may be mycobacteria other than M. *tuberculosis*; many patients can have TB and have a negative smear. Specimens are generally collected by asking the patient to expectorate sputum into a cup; however, tracheal washing, thoracentesis of pleural fluid, and lung biopsy are other options.

Chest x-ray examination: Involvement is most characteristically evident in the apex and posterior segments of the upper lobes. Although not diagnostically definitive, it will reveal calcification at original site, enlargement of hilar lymph nodes, parenchymal infiltrate, pleural effusion, and cavitation. Patients with HIV infection may have an atypical radiographic presentation of TB. Any abnormality on an AIDS patient's chest x-ray film should be considered possible TB until ruled out.

Gastric washings: May reveal presence of tubercle bacilli secondary to swallowed sputum. Gastric washings are usually used for children who cannot expectorate sputum.

Nursing Diagnosis:

Deficient Knowledge:

The spread of TB and procedure for Airborne Infection Isolation

Desired Outcome: Following instruction, patient and significant others verbalize how TB is spread and measures necessary to prevent the spread.

INTERVENTIONS	RATIONALES
Assess patient's health care literacy (language, reading, comprehension). Assess culture and culturally specific information needs. Then teach patient about TB and the mechanism by which it is spread (respiratory droplet nuclei).	This assessment helps ensure that information is presented in a manner that is culturally and educationally appropriate. A well-informed patient is more likely to adhere to precautions against spreading the disease.
Explain Airborne Infection Isolation (AII) to patient and significant others. Post a notice of isolation/airborne precautions on patient's room door.	Until antimicrobial therapy is successful as indicated by AFB smears, AII (or "airborne precautions" in the nomenclature of Standard Precautions) requires a private room with special ventilation that dilutes and removes airborne contaminants and controls the direction of airflow. The negative pressure is monitored continuously or checked and recorded daily while patient is isolated in this room. Patient should wear a regular surgical mask if it is necessary to leave the room.
Remind staff and visitors of need to keep patient's door closed.	A closed door enables effective function of the ventilation system.

Continued

INTERVENTIONS	RATIONALES
Explain to staff and visitors the importance of wearing N-95 or other high-efficiency respirators, including proper fit and use. Provide appropriate respirators at doorway or other convenient place.	N-95 respirators, designed to provide a tight face seal and filter particles in the 1- to 5- $\times$ m range, are worn by all individuals entering patient's room to reduce possibility of infection.
Teach patient importance of covering mouth and nose with tissue when sneezing or coughing and of disposing used tissue in appropriate waste container.	These actions reduce the possibility of spreading infection.

••• **Related NIC and NOC labels:** *NIC:* Infection Protection; Infection Control; Teaching: Disease Process *NOC:* Knowledge: Disease Process; Knowledge: Infection Control

PATIENT-FAMILY TEACHING AND DISCHARGE PLANNING

When providing patient-family teaching about tuberculosis, focus on sensory information, avoid giving excessive information, and initiate a referral to the public health department for investigation and follow-up of household members and other contacts exposed to the patient with TB. Include verbal and written information about the following:

✓ Antituberculosis medications, including drug name, purpose, dosage, schedule, precautions, and potential side effects. Also discuss drug-drug, herb-drug, and food-drug interactions. Remind patient that medications are to be taken without interruption for the prescribed period. Remind patient of the need for continued laboratory monitoring for complications of pharmacotherapy. Describe directly observed therapy (DOT) if that is the medication administration method selected.

✓ Importance of periodic reculturing of sputum.

✓ Importance of basic hygiene measures, including handwashing, covering cough with tissues, and proper disposal of contaminated items.

✓ Phone numbers to call in case questions or concerns arise about therapy or disease after discharge. Additional general information can be obtained by contacting the following:
- www.cdc.gov/tb
- www.lungusa.org
- www.thoracic.org
- www.umdnj.edu/ntbcweb (Northeastern National Tuberculosis Center at the University of Medicine and Dentistry of New Jersey)
- http://ntcc.ucsd.edu (National Tuberculosis Curriculum Consortium at the University of California San Diego)

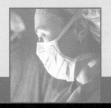

Respiratory Failure, Acute 14

OVERVIEW/PATHOPHYSIOLOGY

Acute respiratory failure (ARF) develops when the lungs are unable to exchange O_2 and CO_2 adequately. Clinically, respiratory failure exists when Pao_2 is less than 50 mm Hg with the patient at rest and breathing room air. $Paco_2$ of 50 mm Hg or more or pH less than 7.35 is significant for respiratory acidosis, which is the common precursor to ARF.

Although a variety of disease processes can lead to development of respiratory failure, four basic mechanisms are involved.

Alveolar hypoventilation: Occurs secondary to reduction in alveolar minute ventilation. Because differential indicators (cyanosis, somnolence) occur late in the process, the condition may go unnoticed until tissue hypoxia is severe.

Ventilation-perfusion mismatch: Considered the most common cause of hypoxemia. Normal alveolar ventilation occurs at a rate of 4 L/min, with normal pulmonary vascular blood flow occurring at a rate of 5 L/min. Normal ventilation/perfusion ratio is 0.8:1. Any disease process that interferes with either side of the equation upsets physiologic balance and can lead to respiratory failure as a result of reduction in arterial O_2 levels.

Diffusion disturbances: Processes that physically impair gas exchange across the alveolar-capillary membrane. Diffusion is impaired because of the increase in anatomic distance the gas must travel from alveoli to capillary and capillary to alveoli.

Right-to-left shunt: Occurs when the previously mentioned processes go untreated. Large amounts of blood pass from the right side of the heart to the left and out into the general circulation without adequate ventilation; therefore blood is poorly oxygenated. This mechanism occurs when alveoli are atelectatic or fluid filled, inasmuch as these conditions interfere with gas exchange. Unlike the first three responses, hypoxemia secondary to right-to-left shunting does not improve with O_2 administration because the additional Fio_2 is unable to cross the alveolar-capillary membrane.

HEALTH CARE SETTING

Primary care; acute care resulting from complications.

ASSESSMENT

Clinical indicators of ARF vary according to the underlying disease process and severity of the failure. ARF is one of the most common causes of impaired level of consciousness. Often it is misdiagnosed as heart failure, pneumonia, or stroke.

Early indicators: Restlessness, changes in mental status, anxiety, headache, fatigue, cool and dry skin, increased blood pressure, tachycardia, cardiac dysrhythmias.

Intermediate indicators: Confusion, increased agitation, and increased oxygen requirements with decreased oxygen saturations. Patients who have hypoventilation respiratory failure often exhibit lethargy and bradypnea. Patients with ventilation-perfusion mismatch often exhibit tachypnea.

Late indicators: Cyanosis, diaphoresis, coma, respiratory arrest.

DIAGNOSTIC TESTS

ABG analysis: Assesses adequacy of oxygenation and effectiveness of ventilation and is the most important diagnostic tool. Typical results are Pao_2 60 mm Hg or less, $Paco_2$ 45 mm Hg or more, and pH less than 7.35, which are consistent with severe respiratory acidosis.

Chest x-ray examination: Ascertains presence of underlying pathophysiology or disease process that may be contributing to the failure.

NURSING DIAGNOSES/PROBLEMS: (THE LISTED DISORDERS MAY BE PRECURSORS TO ARF)	
"Psychosocial Support"	p. 73
"Chronic Obstructive Pulmonary Disease"	p. 117
"Pneumonia" for **Impaired Gas Exchange**	p. 124
Deficient Fluid Volume	p. 126
"Pneumothorax/Hemothorax"	p. 131
"Pulmonary Embolus"	p. 137
"Guillain-Barré Syndrome"	p. 287
"Multiple Sclerosis"	p. 305

✓ **PATIENT-FAMILY TEACHING AND DISCHARGE PLANNING**

ARF is an acute condition that is symptomatically treated during patient's hospitalization. Discharge planning and teaching should be directed at educating patient and significant others about underlying pathophysiology and treatment specific for that process. See sections in this chapter that relate specifically to the underlying pathophysiology contributing to development of ARF.

Aneurysms 15

OVERVIEW/PATHOPHYSIOLOGY

An aneurysm is a pathologic enlargement of a section of an artery. The most common cause is atherosclerosis, which weakens the vessel wall, causing it to expand. Other causes include hereditary lack of elastin, vessel wall trauma, congenital connective tissue disorders (e.g., Marfan's syndrome), and infection. Undiagnosed and untreated aneurysms place affected individuals at risk for rupture and embolization. Although aneurysms can develop in any vessel, abdominal aortic aneurysms (AAA) are the most common. Rupture is common in aneurysms larger than 6 cm.

Aneurysms in the thoracic aorta are a degenerative process of the aorta, often caused by hypertension and cigarette smoking, and are more susceptible to dissection. *Dissecting aneurysms* have atherosclerotic lesions and develop intimal tears, allowing bleeding into the layers of the vessel, which causes false lumens to form that can obstruct or limit blood flow in the true lumen of the vessel and other vital organs. This pathology is distinctly different from that of AAAs.

Aneurysms are often referred to as "silent killers" because many times patients do not realize they have one, and acute rupture is life threatening. However, there has been an increase in the detection of AAAs due to increased screening of patients at risk with ultrasound and computerized axial tomography (CT) scans.

HEALTH CARE SETTING

Chronic aneurysms in which surgery is not imminent may be followed in primary care. When there is rupture or dissection, preoperative and immediate postoperative care may be done in intensive care, followed by a step-down or progressive care unit for postoperative care. Some patients may require home care assistance after they are discharged.

ASSESSMENT

Abdominal aortic aneurysm: A pulsatile, nontender mass may be palpated and felt on both sides of the midline. Acute abdominal pain, often radiating to the back, of sudden onset, and severe in nature is indicative of aneurysm rupture and must be treated emergently. However, some can rupture without symptoms. AAAs occur most often in men and represent approximately 80% of all aneurysms. They may be difficult to assess in patients who are obese.

Thoracic aneurysm: Patient may be asymptomatic for years. Pressure from the aneurysm on adjacent structures can result in dull pain in the upper back, dyspnea, cough, dysphagia, hemoptysis, tracheal deviation, and hoarseness. If there is pain associated with these aneurysms, it is more likely to be nonradiating central chest pain.

Femoral aneurysm: Signs of decreased distal arterial blood flow occur. These aneurysms can rupture or thrombose. See indicators discussed under "Atherosclerotic Arterial Occlusive Disease," p. 151.

Acute indicators (rupture or dissection): Sudden onset of severe pain often described as "tearing" or "ripping," pallor, diaphoresis, and sudden loss of consciousness.

Physical assessment with acute rupture: Decreased blood pressure (BP) and weakened peripheral pulses, tachycardia, cyanosis, and cool and clammy skin. Hypovolemic shock and death can ensue, depending on the severity of bleeding.

DIAGNOSTIC TESTS

CT scan: Preferred method of AAA diagnosis. Three-dimensional CT scans are also available in many areas. These scans take a two-dimensional picture and by looking at density give a clear view of an aneurysm all the way around, making measurements more accurate for endograft repairs.

Ultrasound: Sound waves may help determine aneurysm size, shape, and location. This is an inexpensive, noninvasive, quick, and simple screening examination.

Abdominal x-ray examination: May detect calcifications in the vessel wall.

Contrast arteriography: Rarely used now that diagnostic imaging with CT scans is widely available. Contrast arteriography will show the size of the aneurysm as well as the origin of blood vessels arising from the aorta.

Nursing Diagnosis

Ineffective Tissue Perfusion (or risk of same)

related to interrupted arterial flow secondary to rupture or embolization of artery

Desired Outcome: Patient has adequate perfusion as evidenced by peripheral pulse amplitude greater than 2+ on a 0-4+ scale and brisk capillary refill (less than 2 sec) and exhibits baseline extremity sensation, motor function, color, and temperature.

INTERVENTIONS	RATIONALES
Assess peripheral pulses at least hourly, and report decreases or absence of a pulse.	This provides ongoing assessment of peripheral perfusion trend in a patient who has had surgical resection of an aneurysm.
	Pulse amplitude 2+ or less (or other than "N") could signal embolization. Some health care centers use A (absent), D (requires Doppler), W (weak), N (normal), and B (bounding) to describe peripheral pulses.
Assess peripheral sensation with vital signs. Instruct patient to report impaired sensation promptly to staff members. Report significant findings to health care provider.	Impaired sensation could signal embolization or bleeding, and it must be reported promptly for timely intervention.
Ensure accurate intake and output measurements, and pay special attention to urine output.	Severe hypotension or renal artery occlusion can decrease renal perfusion. Optimally the patient has an output of 30 ml/hr or greater.
Report to health care provider any changes in extremity color, capillary refill, temperature, and motor function as well as presence of or increasing pain.	These are assessments of peripheral perfusion; changes from baseline (e.g., capillary refill 3 sec or greater, coolness, pallor, or mottling, decreased motor function, and pain) may signal embolization or bleeding. Arterial obstruction, if present, must be treated emergently to prevent loss of the extremity.
Maintain patient in neutral position and on bedrest until otherwise directed.	These interventions maintain BP and perfusion. If patient is postoperative for AAA repair, this position will maintain integrity of graft and minimize risk of postprocedure embolization.
Report any bloody diarrhea to health care provider.	This may be a sign of bowel ischemia.
As prescribed, administer beta-blockers (i.e., metoprolol, atenolol, propanolol) to decrease myocardial irritability and contractility.	These agents slow heart rate and decrease blood pressure, which will aid in preventing dissection.

••• **Related NIC and NOC labels:** *NIC:* Circulatory Care: Arterial Insufficiency; Embolus Care: Peripheral; Positioning; *NOC:* Tissue Perfusion: Peripheral; Circulation Status

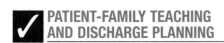

PATIENT-FAMILY TEACHING AND DISCHARGE PLANNING

When providing patient-family teaching, focus on sensory information, avoid giving excessive information, and initiate a visiting nurse referral for necessary follow-up teaching. Include verbal and written information about the following:

✓ Importance of regular medical follow-up to ensure graft patency and prompt identification of the development of a new aneurysm.

✓ Prevention of recurrence of aneurysm by avoiding factors that accelerate atherosclerosis, such as cigarette smoking, obesity, and hypertension.

✓ Necessity of a regularly scheduled exercise program that alternates exercise with rest.

✓ Indicators of wound infection and thrombus or embolus formation, and need to report them promptly to health care provider should they occur.

✓ Medications, including drug name, purpose, dosage, schedule, precautions, and potential side effects. Also discuss drug-drug, herb-drug, and food-drug interactions. Caution patient about importance of antibiotic use similar to that for heart patients for any minor procedures or dental work.

✓ Phone number of nurse available to discuss concerns and questions or clarify unclear instructions.

✓ Importance of follow-up visits with health care provider; confirm date and time of next appointment.

✓ Potential for aneurysm rupture if surgery is not immediately planned.

✓ Importance of seeking immediate medical attention if aneurysm is not fixed and any signs and symptoms of rupture occur. Provide numbers of emergency services in the area.

✓ Potential need for ultrasound for other family members to rule out aneurysm.

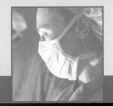

Atherosclerotic Arterial Occlusive Disease 16

OVERVIEW/PATHOPHYSIOLOGY

Inflammation is central to the pathogenesis of *atherosclerosis*, peripheral artery disease. Injury to cell walls may occur secondary to hypertension, diabetes, infection, hyperlipidemia, nicotine use, or hereditary factors. Atherosclerotic lesions can develop from accumulation of plaque, hemorrhage, calcium deposits, or lipids. *Arteriosclerosis* generally defines any process that causes wall thickening.

Occlusive disease is diagnosed when 75% or more of a cross section of artery becomes blocked. In the presence of other comorbidities, such as myocardial infarction, hypertension, chronic obstructive pulmonary disease, or diabetes, loss of limb and life may be threatened.

HEALTH CARE SETTING

Acute care or primary care

ASSESSMENT

Signs and symptoms: Severe, cramping pain (intermittent claudication) with exercise that is relieved by rest. This is indicative of ischemia secondary to decreased blood flow. Patient also may have delayed healing, decreased sensory or motor function, swelling, leg ulcers, gangrene, and pallor, followed by dependent rubor. The patient also may have paresthesia, pulselessness, and paralysis in the affected extremity.

Physical assessment: Decreased pulse amplitude, decreased hair distribution, and bluish discoloration of the extremities and areas of decreased circulation. Skin may appear shiny and atrophied while the nails may appear thickened. Audible bruits may be assessed with a stethoscope over partially occluded vessels. Capillary filling will be 2 or more sec (with normal circulation, capillary filling occurs in less than 2 sec), and amplitude of peripheral pulses will be decreased or only detected by Doppler examination.

Risk factors: Hypertension, cigarette smoking, diabetes mellitus, trauma, family history of atherosclerotic disease, and hyperlipidemia.

DIAGNOSTIC TESTS

Ankle-brachial index: Determines degree of arterial occlusion and subsequent ischemia. Blood pressure is determined at the ankle (using either posterior tibial or dorsalis pedis pulse) and at the brachial artery. The pressure obtained at the ankle is divided by that at the brachial artery. Normally ankle-brachial index (ABI) is greater than 1.0; resting pain occurs with an ABI 0.3 or less.

Doppler flow studies: Uses a transducer that emits sound waves through a probe to determine amount of blood flow through arteries in which palpable pulses are difficult to obtain. Waveforms also can be assessed similar to an electrocardiogram. The more normal or triphasic waveform looks like a regular heart rhythm. A flatter line with lengthening, called *monophasic*, indicates more severe disease. Pressures also can be obtained for ABIs.

Duplex imaging: Uses ultrasound and Doppler to assess arteries for measuring flow and velocities. Originally used in carotid disease, this method is now useful for other arteries and veins in the body.

Pulse-volume recording: Blood pressure cuffs are placed over the thighs, calves, or feet to obtain pulse-volume recordings and pulse waveforms.

Exercise testing: Determines amount of exercise that precipitates claudication.

Angiography of peripheral vasculature: Locates obstruction and reveals extent of vascular lesions by injecting dye into arteries and taking pictures of the arteries in a timed sequence. This imaging study is useful in patients in whom angioplasty or stenting may be possible.

Digital subtraction angiography: Arteriogram in which the computer subtracts early images from late images, deleting bone and soft tissue, so that only contrast-filled arteries appear.

Magnetic resonance imaging: Demonstrates vessels in multiple projections and can be used with or without contrast. It is used widely but is more expensive and not suitable for all patients. Implanted metal (e.g., pacemakers, automatic defibrillators) and prosthetic joint replacements can distort the image.

Nursing Diagnosis

Impaired Tissue Integrity (or risk of same): Lower Extremity

related to altered arterial circulation secondary to atherosclerotic process

Desired Outcome: Patient's lower extremity tissue remains intact.

INTERVENTIONS	RATIONALES
Assess legs, feet, and between toes for ulcerations.	Ulcerations can occur with decreased arterial circulation. A decrease in circulation significantly decreases oxygen delivery to the tissues and subsequently impairs healing of even the most minor break in the skin. A baseline assessment of a worsening condition enables timely interventions.
Teach patient the importance of walking and range-of-motion (ROM) exercises for hip, knee, and ankle.	Walking is the best activity and patients can be instructed to walk until they have pain, rest until recovery, and then resume walking.
	Walking and exercise improve collateral circulation. This is especially useful for patients who claudicate, along with other risk factor modifications. Activity may be contraindicated for some patients with severe disease.
Discuss an exercise program with health care provider, and describe routine to patient.	Exercise promotes circulation.
	Note: Bedrest without exercise may be prescribed in acute, severe cases to decrease oxygen demand to the tissues, which optimally will decrease pain.
Teach patient how to assess peripheral pulses, warmth, sensation, and color of lower extremities (LE). Encourage daily foot inspections by patient or by family members if patient's vision is compromised.	Monitoring status of the LE keeps patient and health care provider informed of changes in circulatory status as well as infection.
Encourage cessation of smoking and other tobacco use. Provide smoking and tobacco cessation literature. Discuss with health care provider use of medication for smoking cessation.	Stopping tobacco use helps prevent increased vasoconstriction and severity of the circulation deficit, as well as the effects of nicotine on the lungs and other body organs.
Discuss importance of keeping feet warm and protected by wearing socks when walking or in bed.	Decreased circulation because of vasoconstriction results in cooler blood to the LE and hence hypothermia. Keeping warm promotes vasodilatation and more optimal blood supply.
Caution patient about using heating pads.	Heating pads increase metabolism and may promote ischemia if circulation is limited. Also, patient's sensitivity to temperature is often decreased and burns can result.
Discuss importance of nightlights being placed in bedrooms and bathrooms.	Nightlights promote vision and thereby help avoid tissue trauma at night when getting up.
Caution patient to avoid pressure over areas of bony prominence.	Pressure increases the risk of skin breakdown; areas over bony prominence are particularly susceptible.
Caution patient to cover all exposed areas when going outside in cooler weather.	This action helps prevent hypothermia, to which patient with decreased circulation may be susceptible. Cold temperatures cause vasoconstriction, which results in decreased tissue perfusion.

••• **Related NIC and NOC labels:** *NIC:* Circulatory Care: Arterial Insufficiency; Circulatory Precautions; Medication Administration; *NOC:* Tissue Integrity: Skin & Mucous Membranes; Wound Healing: Secondary Intention

Nursing Diagnosis:

Chronic Pain

related to atherosclerotic obstructions and ischemia

Desired Outcomes: By hospital discharge, patient's subjective perception of chronic pain decreases as documented by pain scale. Objective indicators, such as grimacing, are absent.

INTERVENTIONS	RATIONALES
Assess for presence of pain, using a pain scale from 0 (no pain) to 10 (worst pain).	This assessment helps determine degree and trend of pain.
Administer pain medications as prescribed.	Usually mild analgesics are given to reduce pain. Opioids may be given for postoperative pain control or rest pain before surgery. They may not be effective in some patients for rest pain, and they are used cautiously in older adults.
Document pain relief obtained using the pain scale.	This documentation helps determine effectiveness of the medication.
Teach patient to rest when claudication (severe, cramping pain) occurs. If claudication occurs at rest, encourage patient to position legs so that they are dependent, and ensure warmth with socks and blankets, as appropriate.	Intermittent claudication from activity is relieved by rest. Claudication at rest implies severe circulatory compromise; measures such as leg dependency and warmth may reduce pain.
Explore alternative methods of pain relief, such as visualization, guided imagery, biofeedback, meditation, and relaxation exercises or tapes. See "Coronary Artery Disease," **Health-Seeking Behaviors**, p. 172, for an example of a relaxation exercise.	Because the pain may be chronic and continuous, pain relief should be augmented with nonpharmacologic methods, which do not have side effects.
Institute measures such as walking and use of medications (see **Impaired Tissue Integrity**, earlier) as directed by health care provider.	These measures increase circulation to ischemic extremities, which optimally will increase patient's comfort level.

••• **Related NIC and NOC labels:** *NIC:* Pain Management; Analgesic Administration; Simple Relaxation Therapy; Biofeedback; Exercise Therapy: Ambulation; Exercise Promotion: Stretching; Simple Guided Imagery *NOC:* Pain Control; Pain: Disruptive Effects

Nursing Diagnosis:

Deficient Knowledge:

Potential for infection and impaired tissue integrity caused by decreased arterial circulation

Desired Outcome: By hospital discharge, patient verbalizes knowledge about the potential for infection and impaired tissue integrity, as well as measures to prevent these problems.

INTERVENTIONS	RATIONALES
Assess patient's health care literacy (language, reading, comprehension). Assess culture and culturally specific information needs.	This assessment helps ensure that information is presented in a manner that is culturally and educationally appropriate.
Teach how to assess for signs of infection or problems with skin integrity and to report significant findings to health care provider.	This information facilitates understanding of symptoms that occur with infection or impaired skin integrity and describes symptoms that should be reported for timely intervention.
Caution about increased potential for easily traumatizing skin (e.g., from bumping lower extremities).	Decreased circulation in the legs diminishes the healing process after tissue trauma.
Instruct patient to inspect both feet each day for any open wounds or bruises. If necessary, suggest that patient use a long-handled mirror to see bottoms of feet. Advise patient to report any open areas to health care provider.	Open wounds can lead to infection, which should be reported promptly for timely intervention.
Stress importance of wearing shoes or slippers that fit properly without areas of stress or friction.	Improper fit can lead to traumatized tissues. Bare feet in an individual with decreased sensation can lead to trauma.
Instruct patient to cut toenails straight across or have them cut by a podiatrist.	Ingrown toenails can lead to infection.
Advise patient to cover corns or calluses with pads.	This action helps prevent further injury.
Encourage patient to keep feet clean and dry, using mild soap and warm water for cleansing, and apply a mild lotion.	These actions promote hygiene and prevent dryness, which could result in skin breakdown that could lead to infection.

Continued

INTERVENTIONS	RATIONALES
Advise patient not to scratch feet.	These actions can result in abrasions that can easily become infected.
Suggest that patient keep feet warm with warm soaks and loose-fitting socks.	Decreased circulation leaves patient vulnerable to hypothermia. Keeping warm promotes vasodilatation and increased blood supply to the area.
Caution patient to check temperature of warm soaks and bath water carefully.	Too hot a temperature can cause burns in an individual whose temperature sensitivity is decreased.

●●● **Related NIC and NOC labels:** *NIC:* Infection Protection; Teaching: Disease Process *NOC:* Knowledge: Infection Control

Nursing Diagnosis:

Ineffective Tissue Perfusion: Peripheral (or risk of same)

related to decreased arterial flow to secondary progressive thickening of intimal walls and narrowing of arterial lumen, or acute occlusion secondary to postsurgical graft embolus

Desired Outcome: Patient has adequate peripheral perfusion as evidenced by BP within 15-20 mm Hg of baseline BP and absence of the six Ps in the involved extremities: pain, pallor, pulselessness, paresthesia, poikilothermia (coolness), and paralysis.

INTERVENTIONS	RATIONALES
Administer the following drugs as prescribed:	
- Antiplatelet agents (e.g., aspirin, clopidogrel, or ticlopidine)	These drugs help prevent platelet adherence and thromboembolism.
- Anticoagulants (e.g., heparin or warfarin)	These drugs may be used in situations in which thinning the blood to prevent thrombus formation is as important as decreasing platelet aggregation.
- Thrombolytics (e.g., urokinase or tissue plasminogen activator)	These drugs may be used to lyse clot formation.
- Blood viscosity-reducing/antiplatelet agent (e.g., pentoxifylline or cilostazol)	These drugs may increase flexibility of erythrocytes, thereby enhancing their movement through the microcirculation and preventing aggregation of red blood cells and platelets. This therapy has the potential to increase circulation at the capillary level and reduce or alleviate symptoms caused by lack of blood flow.
- Lipid-lowering agents (e.g., lovastatin, atorvastatin, simvastatin, and pravastatin)	These drugs reduce serum cholesterol levels and decrease inflammation in vessel walls. There is increasing evidence, especially in individuals with diabetes mellitus, that a small amount of antihyperlipidemic agent is useful in preventing cardiac complications and stroke.
- Antihypertensive agents (e.g., angiotensin-converting enzyme inhibitors, beta-blockers, diuretics, or calcium channel blockers)	Controlling both systolic and diastolic hypertension is important in patients with peripheral arterial disease. Increased blood pressures promote further arterial wall damage, plaque formation, and rupture.
Explain surgical intervention if one has been scheduled.	For patients who have tissue loss, rest pain, or disabling claudication, surgical intervention may be necessary to open the occluded vessel or bypass the vessel to improve distal circulation.
- Endarterectomy	This involves removal of the atheromatous obstruction via arterial incision.
- Distal revascularization	This surgical procedure bypasses the obstructed segment by suturing an autogenous vein or graft proximally and distally to the obstruction. In larger arteries, such as the aorta, graft material is either Dacron or Gore-Tex, while in the distal circulation autogenous veins are best.

Continued

INTERVENTIONS	RATIONALES
- Percutaneous transluminal angioplasty (PTA or PTLA)	This procedure may be used to treat focal arterial obstruction and works best in a large artery with a short lesion. A balloon-tipped catheter is inserted through the artery to the area of occlusion. The balloon is gradually inflated to ablate the obstruction.
- Stent	During an arteriogram, a hollow tube is positioned and deployed within a stenosed vessel to stretch and improve blood flow. A variety of designs, materials, and deployment techniques have been developed. Combined with angioplasty, a stent may provide longer patency of the vessel. Stents are used in renal, mesenteric, carotid, and iliac arteries.
Assess peripheral pulses and involved extremity for the six Ps. Report significant findings.	Sensory changes usually precede other symptoms of ischemia, that is, pain, loss of two-point discrimination, and paresthesias. Such findings should be reported promptly for timely intervention. **Note:** Some health care centers document pulses as A (absent), D (requires Doppler), W (weak), N (normal), or B (bounding).
If necessary, use Doppler ultrasonic probe to check pulses, holding probe to the skin at a 45-degree angle to the blood vessel. Record presence or absence of pulsations, as well as rate, character, frequency, and intensity of sounds.	Doppler probes are capable of evaluating amount of blood flow in arteries in which pulses are difficult to palpate. Optimally, pulsatile blood flow will be heard. In the presence of normal blood flow, wavelike, whooshing sounds will be heard.
To prevent pressure on tissue, use a foot cradle or foam protectors to keep sheets and blankets off legs and feet.	These devices keep sources of pressure away from sensitive lower extremities.
Monitor blood pressure (BP). Report to health care provider any significant increase or decrease greater than 15-20 mm Hg, or as directed.	BP is another indicator of peripheral perfusion pressure. An increase in BP may interrupt the surgical site; decreased BP may cause graft occlusion.
For the first 48-72 hr after surgery (or as directed), prevent acute joint flexion in the presence of a graft.	Joint flexion can impede blood flow and hence perfusion. Mild foot elevation or light Ace-wrapping may help ease hyperemia of the extremity.
In the absence of acute cardiac or renal failure, encourage adequate fluid intake.	Adequate fluid intake enhances perfusion; inadequate fluid intake can lead to dehydration and poor perfusion.

••• **Related NIC and NOC labels:** *NIC:* Circulatory Care: Arterial Insufficiency; Positioning *NOC:* Tissue Perfusion: Peripheral

ADDITIONAL NURSING DIAGNOSES/ PROBLEMS:

"Perioperative Care"   p. 45

✓ PATIENT-FAMILY TEACHING AND DISCHARGE PLANNING

When providing patient-family teaching, focus on sensory information, avoid giving excessive information, and initiate a visiting nurse referral for necessary follow-up teaching. Include verbal and written information about the following:

✓ Exercise program as prescribed by health care provider; importance of rest periods if claudication occurs.

✓ Skin and foot care.

✓ Medications, including drug name, purpose, dosage, schedule, precautions, and potential side effects. Also discuss drug-drug, food-drug, and herb-drug interactions.

✓ Referral to a smoking/tobacco cessation program in your area if appropriate.

Cardiac and Noncardiac Shock 17 (Circulatory Failure)

OVERVIEW/PATHOPHYSIOLOGY

A shock state exists when tissue perfusion decreases to the point of cellular metabolic dysfunction. Shock is classified according to the causative event.

Hypovolemic shock: Occurs when volume in the intravascular space is inadequate and cannot meet the metabolic needs of tissues, as with severe hemorrhage or dehydration.

Cardiogenic shock: Occurs when cardiac failure results in decreased tissue perfusion, as in *severe* myocardial infarction (MI) in which more than 40% of heart muscle has been affected.

Distributive shock conditions: Characterized by displacement of a significant amount of vascular volume. The three types are neurogenic shock, anaphylactic shock, and septic shock.

Neurogenic shock: Occurs when a neurologic event (e.g., spinal cord injury) causes loss of sympathetic tone, resulting in massive vasodilation and decreased perfusion pressures.

Anaphylactic shock: Caused by a severe systemic response to an allergen (foreign protein), resulting in massive vasodilation, increased capillary permeability, decreased perfusion, decreased venous return, and subsequent decreased cardiac output.

Septic shock: Occurs when bacterial toxins cause an overwhelming systemic infection.

Regardless of the cause, shock results in cellular hypoxia secondary to decreased perfusion and ultimately in cellular, tissue, and organ dysfunction. A prolonged shock state can result in death; therefore early recognition and intervention are essential.

HEALTH CARE SETTING

Critical care unit (e.g., cardiogenic shock in coronary care unit; distributive shock in medical intensive care unit [ICU])

ASSESSMENT

Early signs and symptoms: Cool, pale, and clammy skin; decreased pulse strength; dry and pale mucous membranes; restlessness; hyperventilation; anxiety; nausea; thirst; weakness.

Physical assessment: Rapid HR; decreased SBP and increased DBP secondary to catecholamine (sympathetic nervous system [SNS]) response.

Late signs and symptoms: Decreased urinary output, hypothermia, drowsiness, diaphoresis, confusion, and lethargy, all of which can progress to a comatose state.

Physical assessment: Thready, rapid HR; low or decreasing BP, usually with SBP less than 90 mm Hg; rapid and possibly irregular RR.

DIAGNOSTIC TESTS

Diagnosis is usually based on presenting symptoms and clinical signs.

ABG values: May reveal metabolic acidosis or respiratory alkalosis (bicarbonate [HCO_3^-] less than 22 mEq/L and pH less than 7.40) caused by anaerobic metabolism.

Serial measurement of urinary output: Less than 30 ml/hr (0.5 ml/kg/hr) indicates decreased perfusion and decreased renal function.

BUN and creatinine: Increase with decreased renal perfusion.

Serum electrolyte levels: Identify renal complications and metabolic dysfunction as evidenced by hyperkalemia and hypernatremia.

For septic shock

Cultures of blood, sputum, wound, and urine: To identify causative organism.

WBC count: Elevated in the presence of infection.

For hypovolemic shock

CVP: A reading less than 5 cm H_2O suggests hypovolemia.

CBC: Hct and Hgb will be decreased because of decreased blood volume or falsely elevated in severe dehydration.

For anaphylactic shock

WBC count: Will reveal increased eosinophils, a type of granulocyte that appears in the presence of allergic reaction.

Nursing Diagnosis:

Ineffective Tissue Perfusion: Peripheral, Cardiopulmonary, Cerebral, and Renal

related to decreased circulating blood volume

Desired Outcome: Within 1-2 hr of treatment, patient has adequate perfusion as evidenced by peripheral pulse amplitude more than 2+ on a 0-4+ scale; brisk capillary refill (less than 2 sec); SBP greater than 90 mm Hg; Spo_2 greater than 90%; MAP 70-100 mm Hg; CVP at least 5 cm H_2O; HR regular and 100 bpm or less; no significant change in mental status; orientation to person, place, and time; and urine output at least 30 ml/hr (0.5 ml/kg/hr).

INTERVENTIONS	RATIONALES
Assess and document peripheral perfusion status. Report significant findings.	Decreased peripheral perfusion is an early sign of decreased cardiac output and shock. Significant findings include coolness and pallor of the extremities, decreased amplitude of pulses, and delayed capillary refill.
Monitor blood pressure (BP) at frequent intervals; be alert to readings more than 20 mm Hg below patient's normal range or to other indicators of hypotension, such as dizziness, altered mentation, or decreased urinary output.	Decreased systolic blood pressure (SBP) of greater than 20 mm Hg below patient's normal range necessitates immediate intervention to avoid irreversible organ damage due to poor perfusion.
If hypotension is present, place patient in a supine position.	This position promotes venous return. BP must be at least 80/60 mm Hg for adequate coronary and renal artery perfusion.
Monitor central venous pressure (CVP) (if line is inserted).	CVP will show adequacy of venous return and blood volume; 5-10 cm H_2O usually is considered an adequate range. Values near zero can indicate hypovolemia, especially when associated with decreased urinary output, vasoconstriction, and increased heart rate (HR).
Be alert to restlessness, confusion, mental status changes, and decreased level of consciousness (LOC). Intervene to keep patient safe, and reorient as indicated.	These are indicators of decreased cerebral perfusion, which could result in injury to patient due to disorientation.
Avoid use of sedatives or tranquilizers.	LOC can be altered by these medications, and tissue hypoperfusion makes absorption unpredictable.
Monitor for the presence of chest pain and an irregular HR. Report significant findings.	These are indicators of decreased coronary artery perfusion and should be reported for prompt intervention.
Monitor urinary output hourly. Notify health care provider if it is less than 30 ml/hr (0.5 ml/kg/hr) in the presence of adequate intake. Check weight daily for evidence of gain.	Decreased urinary output is a sign of decreased cardiac output and decreased renal perfusion. Weight gain may be a signal of fluid retention, which can occur with decreased renal perfusion.
Monitor laboratory results for elevated blood urea nitrogen (BUN) and creatinine levels; report increases.	BUN more than 20 mg/dl and creatinine more than 1.5 mg/dl are signals of decreased renal perfusion.
Monitor serum electrolyte values for evidence of imbalances, particularly of Na$^+$ and K$^+$. Be alert to clinical signs of hyperkalemia, such as muscle weakness, hyporeflexia, and irregular HR, and to clinical signs of hypernatremia, such as fluid retention and edema.	Hypernatremia (Na$^+$ level greater than 147 mEq/L) and hyperkalemia (K$^+$ level greater than 5.0 mEq/L) may be signs of renal and metabolic complications of shock as a result of decreased renal perfusion and the kidneys' inability to regulate electrolytes.
Administer fluids and medications as prescribed and according to type of shock, patient's clinical situation, and hemodynamic interventions as follows:	Interventions are determined by clinical presentation and severity of the shock state. Patients are transferred to ICU for invasive hemodynamic monitoring with pulmonary artery catheter and use of vasoactive IV drips to improve tissue perfusion.
For Cardiogenic Shock	
Vascular support	To reduce cardiac workload.
Intraaortic balloon counterpulsation	To augment perfusion pressures.
Ventricular assist devices	To bypass or assist the ventricles, lowering myocardial oxygen requirements, reducing cardiac stress, and permitting cardiac muscle rest.

Continued

INTERVENTIONS	RATIONALES
Fluid administration or diuretics.	To optimize blood volume. Fluids probably will be limited to prevent overload (the heart is not able to handle the volume already in the intravascular space), yet dehydration must be avoided. Decreasing preload (fluids) may be the treatment of choice to take the workload off the heart. An indwelling catheter should be inserted for accurate output measurement.

Pharmacotherapy

Inotropes (e.g., dopamine)	To increase cardiac contractility.
Antidysrhythmics	To control irregular, rapid heart rate.
Morphine	To relieve severe chest pain and reduce preload and afterload.
Vasodilators (e.g., nitroprusside, nitroglycerin)	To increase peripheral perfusion and reduce afterload vasoconstriction caused by vasopressors.
Osmotic diuretics	To increase renal blood flow.
O_2 support	To increase O_2 availability to the tissues.
Monitor for and correct acidosis and electrolyte imbalances.	Electrolyte imbalances and acidosis are life-threatening and need immediate correction.
	Correction likely will include oxygen therapy, fluid resuscitation, and replacement or excretion of electrolytes.

For Anaphylactic Shock
Pharmacotherapy

Epinephrine (0.5 ml, 1:1000 in 10 ml saline):	To promote vasoconstriction and decrease the allergic response by counteracting vasodilation caused by histamine release.
Bronchodilators	To relieve bronchospasm.
Antihistamines	To prevent relapse and relieve urticaria.
Hydrocortisone	For its anti-inflammatory effects.
Vasopressors	May be necessary for reversing shock state.
O_2 and airway support: As needed	To increase oxygen availability to the tissues.
Albumin	Sometimes used to increase vascular volume.
Ringer's solution	Often used as an isotonic solution to replace electrolytes and ions lost with bleeding.

For Septic Shock

Antibiotic therapy	Initial therapy is broad spectrum. Once the causative organism is identified, specific antibiotic therapy can be initiated.
Fluid administration	To maintain adequate vascular volume.
Vasoactive drugs (e.g., norepinephrine, dopamine)	May be required to reverse vasodilation and maintain perfusion.
Positive inotropic drugs	To augment cardiac contractility.

For Hypovolemic Shock

Control of volume loss	If possible, depending on location and cause.
Blood transfusion	To increase O_2 delivery at the tissue level when more than 2 L of blood has been lost. Often a combination of packed red blood cells (RBCs) and a crystalloid solution is administered.
Albumin	Sometimes used to increase vascular volume.
Ringer's solution	Often used as an isotonic solution to replace electrolytes and ions lost with bleeding.
	Caution: Very rapid infusion of fluids may precipitate pulmonary edema.

••• **Related NIC and NOC labels:** *NIC:* Circulatory Precautions: Shock Management: Cardiac; Fluid Management; Vital Signs Monitoring; Blood Products Administration; Fluid Monitoring; Shock Prevention; Hypovolemia Management; Fluid Resuscitation; Laboratory Data Interpretation; Intravenous Therapy; Electrolyte Management; Neurologic Monitoring; Positioning *NOC:* Tissue Perfusion: Abdominal Organs; Tissue Perfusion: Peripheral; Electrolyte & Acid-Base Balance; Circulation Status; Tissue Perfusion: Cerebral; Tissue Perfusion: Cardiac; Tissue Perfusion: Pulmonary

Nursing Diagnosis:

Impaired Gas Exchange

related to altered oxygen supply secondary to decreased respiratory muscle function occurring with altered metabolism

Desired Outcome: Within 1-2 hr of intervention, patient has adequate gas exchange as evidenced by SpO_2 greater than 92%; PaO_2 at least 80 mm Hg; $PaCO_2$ 45 mm Hg or less; pH at or near 7.35; presence of eupnea; and orientation to person, place, and time.

INTERVENTIONS	RATIONALES
Monitor arterial blood gas (ABG) results. Report significant findings.	The presence of hypoxemia (decreased PaO_2), hypercapnia (increased $PaCO_2$), and acidosis (decreased pH, increased $PaCO_2$) are signs of decreased gas exchange; medical intervention is needed.
Monitor SpO_2. Report significant findings.	Readings of 92% or less are indicators of decreased oxygenation; oxygen therapy is required.
Monitor respirations q30min; note and report presence of tachypnea or dyspnea.	Fast or labored breaths may signal respiratory distress and possibly respiratory failure and the need for supplemental oxygen or other respiratory intervention. Tachypnea and dyspnea also may be signs of pain, anxiety, or infection and should be evaluated accordingly.
Be alert to mental status changes, restlessness, irritability, and confusion.	Often these are symptoms of hypoxia.
Teach patient to breathe slowly and deeply in through the nose and out through the mouth.	These actions slow the respiratory cycle for better alveolar gas exchange.
Ensure patient has a patent airway; suction secretions as needed.	This intervention promotes gas exchange.
Administer O_2 as prescribed; deliver O_2 with humidity.	These interventions increase oxygen supply and help prevent its convective drying effects on oral and nasal mucosa.

••• **Related NIC and NOC labels:** *NIC:* Acid-Base Monitoring; Acid-Base Management; Laboratory Data Interpretation; Respiratory Monitoring; Oxygen Therapy; Airway Suctioning *NOC:* Tissue Perfusion: Pulmonary; Respiratory Status: Ventilation; Respiratory Status: Gas Exchange

ADDITIONAL NURSING DIAGNOSES/ PROBLEMS:

"Psychosocial Support"	p. 73
"Psychosocial Support for the Patient's Family and Significant Other"	p. 87

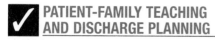

PATIENT-FAMILY TEACHING AND DISCHARGE PLANNING

For interventions, see discussion of patient's primary diagnosis.

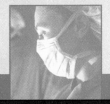

Cardiac Surgery 18

OVERVIEW/PATHOPHYSIOLOGY

Surgical intervention may be necessary to treat acquired or congenital heart disease. *Coronary artery bypass grafting (CABG)* is done to treat blocked coronary arteries. A portion of the saphenous vein, internal mammary artery, gastroepiploic artery, or radial artery is excised and anastomosed to coronary arteries, thereby revascularizing the affected myocardium. *Valve repair* or *replacement*, another type of cardiac surgery, is performed for patients with valvular stenosis or valvular incompetence of the mitral, tricuspid, pulmonary, or aortic valve. Some patients may require replacement of the aortic arch and aortic valve because of an aortic aneurysm. Cardiac surgery is also performed to correct heart defects that are either acquired or congenital, such as ventricular aneurysm, ventricular or atrial-septal defects, transposition of the great vessels, and tetralogy of Fallot. *Heart transplantation* may be considered for some patients diagnosed with end-stage cardiac disease; however the national shortage of acceptable donor organs remains a problem. Many patients waiting for heart transplants will undergo surgery to receive a ventricular assist device, which will serve as a bridge to transplant. *Combined heart-lung transplantation* is performed for patients with end-stage disease affecting both organs. Immunosuppressive treatment to prevent organ rejection after heart transplantation is similar to that of patients who receive a renal transplant. See "Care of the Renal Transplant Recipient," p. 239.

Many patients undergoing cardiac surgery may have temporary epicardial pacing wires in place. These wires are placed on the heart at the time of surgery and pulled through the chest wall where they can be attached to a temporary pacemaker. They are used for temporary pacing postoperatively if needed for bradycardia. When they are no longer needed, they are removed by nurses or other health care providers who have demonstrated technical proficiency.

HEALTH CARE SETTING

Under normal circumstances, patients are admitted to hospital on day of surgery.

After surgery, most patients are in an intensive care unit (ICU) for 24 hr and then transferred to a step-down unit for 3-5 days, although heart transplant patients have a longer stay.

Nursing Diagnosis:

Deficient Knowledge:

Diagnosis, surgical procedure, preoperative routine, and postoperative course

Desired Outcome: Before surgery, patient verbalizes knowledge about the diagnosis, surgical procedure, and preoperative and postoperative regimens.

INTERVENTIONS	RATIONALES
Assess patient's health care literacy (language, reading, comprehension). Assess culture and culturally specific information needs.	This assessment helps ensure that information is presented in a manner that is culturally and educationally appropriate.
Assess patient's level of knowledge about the diagnosis and surgical procedure, and provide information where necessary. Encourage questions, and allow time for verbalization of concerns and fears.	Some patients may be knowledgeable and others may not. Some find detailed explanations helpful; others prefer brief and simple explanations. The amount of information given should depend on the patient, enabling an individualized teaching plan.
When appropriate, provide orientation to the ICU and equipment that will be used postoperatively.	Patient's familiarity with the unit and equipment optimally will promote compliance and minimize stress.

Continued

INTERVENTIONS	RATIONALES
Provide instructions for and demonstrate deep breathing and coughing; ask patient to give a return demonstration.	Deep breathing and coughing are essential postoperative techniques that reinflate the lungs after heart-lung bypass and help prevent atelectasis and pneumonia.
Reassure patient that postoperative discomfort will be relieved with medication.	This information likely will reduce anxiety about postoperative pain.
	Note: Pain after a midline sternotomy (usual incision with cardiac surgery) usually is less than that with conventional thoracotomy because the somatic nerves are not divided by the surgical incision.
Advise patient that in the immediate postoperative period, speaking will be impossible but that other means of communication (e.g., nodding, writing) will be available.	An endotracheal tube that will assist with breathing will prevent speech. Knowledge that alternative methods will be employed will reassure patient and prepare him or her for their use.
Review and demonstrate sternal precautions with patient.	Sternal precautions include how to get in and out of bed and chair without using upper extremities; not lifting, pushing, or pulling more than 5-10 lb with each upper extremity for a period of 4-6 wk; and not driving a car for the same period of time.

••• **Related NIC and NOC labels:** *NIC:* Preparatory Sensory Information; Teaching: Procedure/Treatment; Anxiety Reduction; Learning Facilitation; Teaching: Disease Process *NOC:* Knowledge: Treatment Procedures

Nursing Diagnosis:

Activity Intolerance

related to generalized weakness and bedrest secondary to cardiac surgery

Desired Outcome: By a minimum of 24 hr before hospital discharge, patient rates perceived exertion at 3 or less on a 0-10 scale and exhibits cardiac tolerance to activity after cardiac surgery as evidenced by HR 110 bpm or less, SBP within 20 mm Hg of resting SBP, and RR 20 breaths/min or less with normal depth and pattern (eupnea).

INTERVENTIONS	RATIONALES
Ask patient to rate perceived exertion (RPE) during activity, and monitor for evidence of activity intolerance. Notify health care provider of significant findings.	An RPE of greater than 3, along with cool, diaphoretic skin, is a signal to stop the activity and notify health care provider. See **Risk for Activity Intolerance** in "Prolonged Bedrest," p. 61 for a discussion of RPE.
Monitor vital signs at frequent intervals, and be alert to any changes. Notify health care provider of significant findings.	Hypotension, tachycardia, crackles (rales), tachypnea, and diminished amplitude of peripheral pulses are signs of cardiac complications and should be reported promptly for timely intervention.
Monitor blood pressure (BP) and note a decrease greater than 20 mm Hg from resting systolic blood pressure (SBP).	A 20 mm Hg or greater decrease in BP may signify blood volume loss due to bleeding or dehydration, which may compromise organ perfusion.
Facilitate coordination of health care providers to provide rest periods between care activities and thus decrease cardiac workload.	Ninety minutes of uninterrupted rest helps decrease cardiac workload. An increased cardiac workload is likely if too many activities are performed without concomitant rest.
Assist with exercises, depending on tolerance and prescribed activity limitations. As prescribed, initiate physical therapy (PT).	Exercise and PT increase activity tolerance.
See **Risk for Activity Intolerance,** p. 61, and **Risk for Disuse Syndrome,** p. 63, for a discussion of in-bed exercises.	

••• **Related NIC and NOC labels:** *NIC:* Energy Management; Exercise Promotion; Cardiac Care: Rehabilitative; Medication Management *NOC:* Energy Conservation; Activity Tolerance

ADDITIONAL NURSING DIAGNOSES/ PROBLEMS:

"Perioperative Care" for **Risk for Infection**   p. 54

"Prolonged Bedrest" for **Ineffective Tissue**   p. 65
    Perfusion: Peripheral

"Pulmonary Embolus" for **Ineffective Protection**   p. 139
    related to risk of prolonged bleeding or hemor-
    rhage secondary to anticoagulation therapy

"Coronary Artery Disease" for **Health-Seeking**   p. 172
    Behaviors: Relaxation technique effective for
    stress reduction

Ineffective Tissue Perfusion: Renal   p. 175

✔ PATIENT-FAMILY TEACHING AND DISCHARGE PLANNING

When providing patient-family teaching, focus on sensory information, avoid giving excessive information, and initiate a visiting nurse referral for necessary follow-up teaching. Include written information with verbal reinforcement and time for questions about the following:

✓ Medications, including drug name, dosage, schedule, purpose, precautions, and potential side effects. Also discuss drug-drug, herb-drug, and food-drug interactions.

✓ Untoward symptoms requiring medical attention for patients taking warfarin, such as bleeding from the nose (epistaxis) or gums, hemoptysis, hematemesis, hematuria, melena, hematochezia, menometrorrhagia, and excessive bruising. In addition, stress the following: take warfarin at the same time every day, notify health care provider if any signs of bleeding occur, avoid over-the-counter and herbal medications unless approved by health care provider, carry a medical alert bracelet or card, avoid constrictive or restrictive clothing, and use a soft-bristled toothbrush and electric razor.

✓ Maintenance of low sodium and low-cholesterol diet. Encourage patients to use food labels to determine sodium, fat, and cholesterol content of foods.

✓ Importance of pacing activities at home and allowing frequent rest periods.

✓ Technique for assessing radial pulse, temperature, and weight, if these indicators require monitoring at home, and reporting significant changes to health care provider.

✓ Telephone number of nurse available to discuss concerns and questions or clarify unclear instructions.

✓ Importance of follow-up visits with health care provider; confirm date and time of next appointment.

✓ Signs and symptoms that necessitate immediate medical attention: edema, chest pain, dyspnea, shortness of breath, weight gain, and decrease in exercise tolerance.

✓ Activity restrictions (e.g., no heavy lifting, pushing, or pulling anything heavier than 5-10 lb with upper extremities for at least 4-6 wk); prescribed exercise program; and resumption of sexual activity, work, and driving a car, as directed.

✓ Care of incision site; importance of assessing for signs of infection, such as drainage, swelling, fever, persistent redness, and local warmth and tenderness.

✓ Referral to a cardiac rehabilitation program.

✓ Discussion of patient's home environment and potential need for changes or adaptations (e.g., too many steps to climb, activities of daily living that are too strenuous).

✓ Introduction to local American Heart Association activities. Either provide the address or telephone number for the local chapter or encourage patient to contact the following.

- American Heart Association at *www.americanheart. org*
- For patients awaiting heart transplantation, as appropriate: The United Network for Organ Sharing at *www.unos.org*

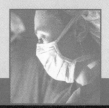

Coronary Artery Disease 19

OVERVIEW/PATHOPHYSIOLOGY

Coronary artery disease (CAD) is the leading cause of death in the United States, affecting more than 13 million Americans. The coronary arteries supply the myocardial muscle with oxygen and the nutrients necessary for optimal function. In CAD, the arteries are narrowed or obstructed, potentially resulting in cardiac muscle death. Atherosclerotic lesions, arterial spasm, platelet aggregation, and thrombus formation all may cause obstruction. The most common symptom of CAD is angina, which is the result of decreased blood flow and insufficient oxygen supply to the heart muscle.

Acute coronary syndrome (ACS) refers to an imbalance between myocardial oxygen supply and demand secondary to an acute plaque disruption or erosion. ACS is an umbrella term that includes unstable angina (USA), non–ST-elevation myocardial infarction (NSTEMI), and ST-segment elevation myocardial infarction (STEMI).

USA is defined as an increase in severity, frequency, or intensity of anginal pain or a new onset of prolonged rest angina. This definition is based largely on clinical presentation. NSTEMI is defined by clinical presentation of chest pain with an elevation in cardiac biomarkers and electrocardiograph (ECG) changes that may include T-wave inversion or ST-segment depression but no ST-segment elevation. Diagnosis of STEMI is based on elevated cardiac biomarkers plus ST-segment elevation on ECG signifying ischemia. Of the three, STEMI is the most serious and life-threatening.

Time is of the essence in determining the treatment plan. All patients presenting to the emergency department (ED) with STEMI are considered high-priority triage cases. Primary angioplasty is widely viewed as therapy of choice for reperfusion in acute myocardial infarction (AMI). However, not all acute care hospitals in the United States have availability for percutaneous coronary intervention (PCI). Because time is so critical in patients presenting with STEMI, a decision must be made by the ED physician to proceed with either fibrinolytic therapy or primary PCI within 10 min of presentation. The goal for door-to-needle time is within 30 min and door-to-balloon time within 90 min. Initiating thrombolysis within 70 min of symptom onset is key to reducing mortality and morbidity. If catheterization laboratory facilities for primary intervention are not available within this "golden hour," fibrinolytics are administered until transport can be arranged.

HEALTH CARE SETTING

Primary care, acute care, coronary care unit

ASSESSMENT

Signs and symptoms: Chest pain, substernal pressure and burning, and pain that radiates to the jaw, shoulder, or arm are the most common symptoms of CAD. Weakness, diaphoresis, nausea, vomiting, shortness of breath, and acute anxiety also can occur. Heart rate (HR) may be abnormally slow (bradycardia), especially in right coronary artery (RCA) infarct, or it may be rapid (tachycardia). Stable or progressively worsening angina occurs when myocardial demand for O_2 is more than the supply, such as during exercise. Pain usually is described as a feeling of pressure or as a crushing or burning substernal pain that radiates down one or both arms. It can be felt also in the neck, cheeks, and teeth. Usually it is relieved by discontinuation of exercise or administration of nitroglycerin (NTG).

Physical assessment: Acute syndromes may include the physical findings of anxiety, hypertension, tachycardia, tachypnea, and dynamic ECG changes. Severe hypotension may occur in shock states. Temperature elevations can occur secondary to the inflammatory process. Intensity of S_1 and S_2 heart sounds may be decreased. Pulmonary congestion may occur if ventricular failure is present, and S_3 and S_4 sounds may be auscultated.

History and risk factors: Family history, increasing age, male gender, smoking, low high-density-lipoprotein (HDL) values, hypercholesterolemia, diabetes mellitus, hypertension. Obesity, glucose intolerance, and a sedentary, stressful lifestyle also contribute to increased risk. Chest pain often occurs with exertion.

DIAGNOSTIC TESTS

ECG: Usually normal unless a myocardial infarction (MI) has occurred or the individual is experiencing angina at the time of the test. If ECG is performed during chest pain, characteristic changes may include ST-segment elevation or depression greater than 0.05 mV in leads over the area of ischemia. The presence of a bundle branch block also can be determined on ECG as well as dysrhythmias. Serial ECGs are done in patients with ACS to identify area and extent of the infarct.

Cardiac biomarkers: CPK, CK-MB, and troponin are proteins released in response to ischemia or MI. Troponin may not be elevated on initial presentation. Serial enzymes q8h for 24 hr are recommended for accurate assessment of myocardial damage.

C-reactive protein: If elevated from normal range of 0.03-1.1 mg/dl, signals that coronary artery plaques are inflammatory and patient is at higher likelihood of an acute coronary event.

Echocardiogram: Assesses ventricular function, chamber size, valvular function, ejection fraction, wall motion, and hemodynamic measurements. Heart muscle damage may alter ventricular function, wall motion, and hemodynamic pressures. The part of the heart that moves weakly may have been damaged during a heart attack or may be receiving too little oxygen.

Chest x-ray examination: Usually normal unless heart failure is present.

Total lipid panel: Obtained at some point during patient's evaluation and treatment to assess for hyperlipidemia, a risk factor in CAD. Low HDL (value less than 40 mg/dl) and high low-density-lipoprotein (LDL) (value greater than 100 mg/dl) are linked to atherosclerotic heart disease.

Stress tests: Over the past two decades, stress testing with concurrent imaging of the heart has become a standard means of evaluation. Stress tests typically are prescribed to assess coronary artery flow.

Exercise treadmill test: To determine amount of exercise-induced ischemia, hemodynamic response, and ECG changes with exercise. Significant findings include 1 mm or more ST-segment depression or elevation, dysrhythmias, or a sudden decrease in blood pressure (BP).

Stress echocardiogram: Typically performed using either a treadmill or bicycle. Echocardiograms are obtained before and immediately after exercise. A stress-induced imbalance in the myocardial supply/demand ratio will produce myocardial ischemia and regional wall motion abnormality. Stress echocardiography is particularly useful for identifying CAD in patients with multivessel disease.

Dobutamine stress echocardiogram: Dobutamine is used as a stress agent in combination with an echocardiogram for patients who cannot exercise.

Cardiac nuclear imaging modalities

Myocardial perfusion imaging

- Detection of CAD is found by differential blood flow through the left ventricular myocardium. Normal blood flow and normal tracer uptake are seen with unobstructed coronary arteries; diminished flow and diminished tracer uptake are found with coronary stenosis. A perfusion abnormality will be present in an area of MI.

- Commonly used radiopharmaceutical agents are thallium-201 and technetium-99m sestamibi. Adenosine and dipyridamole are pharmacologic stress agents used in combination with a radiopharmaceutical agent if patient is unable to exercise or fails to reach 85% of age-predicted maximum heart rate (HR).

- Single photon emission computed tomography (SPECT) is used to develop three-dimensional views of cardiac processes and cellular level metabolism by viewing the heart from several different angles and using tomography methods to reconstruct the image. SPECT enables clearer resolution of myocardial ischemia and better quantification of cardiac damage.

Radionuclide angiography: Used to evaluate left and right ventricular ejection fraction (EF), left ventricular volume, and regional wall motion. The first-pass technique is a fast acquisition of myocardial images. Gated pool ejection or multiple-gated acquisition (MUGA) scan permits calculation of the amount of blood ejected with ventricular contraction and is used for risk stratification of patients after MI or with CAD.

CT: May be helpful in differentiating AMI from aortic dissection in patients with severe, tearing back pain and associated dyspnea and/or syncope.

Ambulatory monitoring: A 24-hr ECG monitoring (Holter monitor) can show activity-induced ST-segment changes or ischemia-induced dysrhythmias.

Coronary arteriography via cardiac catheterization: The gold standard of diagnostic testing for CAD. Arterial lesions (plaque) are located and the amount of occlusion determined. During this test, feasibility for coronary artery bypass grafting (CABG) or angioplasty is determined. For details, see "Cardiac Surgery," p. 161.

Intravascular ultrasound: To assess degree of atherosclerosis during coronary angiogram. A flexible catheter with a miniature transducer at the tip is threaded from an arteriotomy (commonly femoral) retrograde to the coronary arteries to provide information on the interior of the coronary arteries. Ultrasound is used to create a cross-sectional image of the three layers of the arterial wall and its lumen.

Nursing Diagnosis:

Acute Pain (Angina)

related to decreased oxygen supply to the myocardium

Desired Outcomes: Within 30 min of onset of pain, patient's subjective perception of angina decreases, as documented by a pain scale. Objective indicators, such as grimacing and diaphoresis, are absent or decreased.

INTERVENTIONS	RATIONALES
Assess location, character, and severity of pain. Record severity on a subjective 0 (no pain) to 10 (worst pain) scale.	This assessment monitors degree, character, precipitator, and trend of pain for initial check and subsequent comparisons.
Record amount of NTG or morphine sulphate needed to relieve each episode, the factor or event that precipitated pain, and alleviating factors. Document angina relief obtained, using pain scale.	IV NTG drip should be increased in increments of 10 mcg if pain persists. Systolic blood pressure (SBP) should be maintained at 90 mm Hg or higher until pain is relieved to avoid worsening ischemia secondary to hypotension. IV morphine sulfate is added in small increments (2 mg).
Keep sublingual NTG within reach of patient, and explain that it is to be administered as soon as angina begins, repeating q5min × 3 if necessary.	NTG increases microcirculation, perfusion to the myocardium, and venous dilation. Venous dilation causes pooling in the periphery so that less blood comes back to the right side of the heart, which in turn lowers O_2 demand.
If pain is unrelieved or returns very quickly after the patient is discharged, advise emergency medical treatment.	
Obtain ECG as prescribed.	ECG assesses for ischemia, as evidenced by dynamic ST- or T-wave changes, evidence of new Q waves, or left bundle branch block.
Stay with patient and provide reassurance during periods of angina.	These measures reduce anxiety, which might otherwise worsen the angina.
Monitor HR and BP during episodes of chest pain. Be alert to and report significant findings.	Increases in HR and changes in SBP greater than 20 mm Hg from baseline signal increased myocardial O_2 demands and necessitate prompt medical intervention.
Monitor for presence of headache and hypotension after administering NTG.	These are side effects of NTG as a result of vasodilation.
Keep patient recumbent with head of bed (HOB) elevated no higher than 30 degrees during angina and NTG administration.	This position minimizes potential for headache/hypotension by enabling better blood return to the heart and head.
Administer O_2 as prescribed.	Hypoxia is common because of the decreased perfusion and adds stress to the compromised myocardium.
Deliver O_2 with humidity.	Humidity helps prevent oxygen's convective drying effects on oral and nasal mucosa.
Emphasize to patient importance of immediately reporting angina to health care team.	Early treatment decreases morbidity and mortality.
Instruct patient to avoid activities and factors known to cause stress.	Stress may precipitate angina.
Discuss value of relaxation techniques, including tapes, soothing music, biofeedback, meditation, or yoga. See **Health-Seeking Behaviors,** later.	Relaxation helps reduce stress and anxiety, which otherwise may precipitate angina.
Administer beta-blockers (e.g., metoprolol, atenolol, carvedilol) as prescribed.	These drugs block beta stimulation to the sinoatrial (S-A) node and myocardium. Heart rate, blood pressure, and contractility are decreased, subsequently reducing workload of the heart and myocardial oxygen demand, ultimately improving myocardial oxygenation. Metoprolol may be administered IV as initial treatment.
Administer long-acting nitrates (isosorbide preparations) and/or topical nitrates as prescribed.	Nitrates are given for anginal prophylaxis via vasodilation, lowering of BP, and decreasing O_2 demand.
Administer angiotensin-converting enzyme (ACE) inhibitor (e.g., enalapril, captopril, quinapril, ramipril) as prescribed.	ACE inhibitors reduce BP, down-regulate the renin-angiotensin aldosterone system (RAAS), and improve long-term survival.
Administer calcium channel blockers (e.g., nifedipine, diltiazem) as prescribed.	Calcium channel blockers decrease coronary artery vasospasm, a potential cause of ischemia and subsequent angina. They also cause the vessels to open, increasing blood flow to the heart.

Continued

INTERVENTIONS	RATIONALES
Administer aspirin as prescribed.	Aspirin reduces the ability of the blood to clot, which may prevent obstruction of the coronary arteries.
Administer antihyperlipidemic agents (e.g., atorvastatin, rosuvastatin) as prescribed.	These agents, also known as "statin" drugs, are used to reduce hyperlipidemia and can stabilize plaque.

••• **Related NIC and NOC labels:** *NIC:* Medication Management; Pain Management; Biofeedback; Emotional Support; Meditation Facilitation; Presence; Simple Relaxation Therapy; Anxiety Reduction; Music Therapy; Oxygen Therapy; Progressive Muscle Relaxation *NOC:* Comfort Level; Pain Control

Nursing Diagnosis:

Activity Intolerance

related to generalized weakness and imbalance between oxygen supply and demand secondary to tissue ischemia (MI)

Desired Outcome: During activity, patient rates perceived exertion at 3 or less on a 0-10 scale and exhibits cardiac tolerance to activity as evidenced by RR 20 breaths/min or less, HR 120 bpm or less (or within 20 bpm of resting HR), SBP within 20 mm Hg of patient's resting SBP, and absence of chest pain and new dysrhythmias.

INTERVENTIONS	RATIONALES
Observe for and report increasing frequency of angina, angina that occurs at rest, angina that is unrelieved by NTG, or decreased exercise tolerance without angina.	This assessment detects evidence of imbalance between oxygen supply and demand and hence potential activity intolerance.
	The four classifications of angina as follows:
	Class I: Angina occurs only with strenuous activity.
	Class II: Angina occurs with moderate activity such as walking quickly or climbing stairs, walking uphill, or walking at a normal pace more than two blocks or one flight of stairs.
	Class III: Angina occurs with mild activity such as climbing one flight of stairs or walking level for one to two blocks.
	Class IV: Angina occurs with any physical activity and may be present at rest.
Assess patient's response to activity and report significant findings.	Chest pain, increase in HR (greater than 20 bpm), change in SBP (20 mm Hg over or under resting BP), excessive fatigue, and shortness of breath are signs of activity intolerance that should be reported promptly for timely intervention.
Ask patient to rate perceived exertion (RPE). See p. 61 for details.	RPE higher than 3 is a signal to stop the activity.
Assist patient with recognizing and limiting activities that increase O$_2$ demands, such as exercise and anxiety.	This information helps patient recognize and ultimately control factors that increase ischemia.
Administer O$_2$ as prescribed for angina episodes.	This measure increases oxygen supply to the myocardium.
Deliver O$_2$ with humidity.	Humidity helps prevent oxygen's convective drying effects on oral and nasal mucosa.
Have patient perform range-of-motion (ROM) exercises, depending on tolerance and prescribed activity limitations.	Cardiac intolerance to activity can be further aggravated by prolonged bedrest.
Consult health care provider about in-bed exercises and activities that can be performed by patient as the condition improves.	This intervention enables progressive pacing toward patient's optimal activity potential.
For further interventions, see "Prolonged Bedrest," **Risk for Activity Intolerance**, p. 61, and **Risk for Disuse Syndrome**, p. 63.	

••• **Related NIC and NOC labels:** *NIC:* Energy Management; Exercise Promotion; Cardiac Care: Rehabilitative; Teaching: Prescribed Activity/Exercise; Oxygen Therapy *NOC:* Activity Tolerance; Energy Conservation

Nursing Diagnosis:

Imbalanced Nutrition:

More than body requirements of calories, sodium, or fats

Desired Outcome: Within the 24-hr period before hospital discharge, patient demonstrates knowledge of the dietary regimen by planning a 3-day menu that includes and excludes appropriate foods.

INTERVENTIONS	RATIONALES
If patient is over ideal body weight, explain that a low-calorie diet is necessary.	Being overweight is a risk factor for CAD and puts more workload on the heart.
Discuss ways to decrease dietary intake of saturated (animal) fats and increase intake of polyunsaturated (vegetable oil) fats.	Reducing dietary saturated fat is effective in lowering risk of heart and blood vessel disease in many individuals.
Teach patient to limit dietary intake of cholesterol to less than 300 mg/day. Encourage use of food labels to determine cholesterol content of foods.	Reducing cholesterol intake is effective in lowering risk of heart and blood vessel disease in many individuals.
Teach patient to limit dietary intake of refined/processed sugar.	Refined sugars are empty calories that can convert to fat stores.
Teach patient to limit dietary intake of sodium chloride (NaCl) to less than 4 g/day (mild restriction). Encourage use of food labels to determine sodium content of foods.	Increased sodium intake can lead to water retention by the kidneys. This increased fluid/vascular volume puts more work on the heart.
Instruct patient and significant other in use of "Nutrition Facts" (federally mandated public information on all food product labels).	This information reveals the amount of calories, total fat, saturated fat, cholesterol, and sodium in foods. Patient should be especially aware of the serving size listed for respective nutrients (i.e., a serving size listed as 4 oz on a package containing 12 oz would mean patient would get 3 times the amount of each ingredient if patient eats the entire contents of the container!).
Encourage intake of fresh fruits, natural (unrefined or unprocessed) carbohydrates, fish, poultry, legumes, fresh vegetables, and grains.	These food groups ensure a healthy, balanced diet.

••• **Related NIC and NOC labels:** *NIC:* Weight Reduction Assistance; Nutrition Management; Nutritional Counseling; Teaching: Prescribed Diet *NOC:* Weight Control; Nutritional Status: Nutrient Intake

Nursing Diagnosis:

Deficient Knowledge:

Purpose, precautions, and side effects of nitrates

Desired Outcome: Within the 24-hr period before hospital discharge, patient verbalizes understanding of the purpose, precautions, and side effects of the prescribed medication.

INTERVENTIONS	RATIONALES
Assess patient's health care literacy (language, reading, comprehension). Assess culture and culturally specific information needs.	This assessment helps ensure that information is presented in a manner that is culturally and educationally appropriate.
Teach patient the purpose of the prescribed nitrate (isosorbide, NTG).	These drugs are given during angina to increase microcirculation, venous dilation, and blood to the myocardium, which should decrease angina. A patient who is knowledgeable about the purpose of this drug will be more likely to adhere to the therapeutic regimen.
Instruct patient to report to health care provider or staff the presence of a headache associated with nitrates.	The vasodilation effect of nitrates can result in transient headaches, in which case the health care provider may alter the dose of the isosorbide. Tylenol may be recommended for treatment of headache if not contraindicated.

Continued

INTERVENTIONS	RATIONALES
Teach patient to assume a recumbent position with HOB slightly elevated if a headache occurs.	This position may reduce pain by enabling better blood return to the heart and head.
Instruct patient to rise slowly from a sitting or lying position and to remain by chair or bed for 1 min after standing to be assured he or she is not going to experience orthostatic changes.	Vasodilation from nitrates also may decrease BP, which can result in orthostatic hypotension and result in injury to the patient.

●●● **Related NIC and NOC labels:** *NIC:* Teaching: Prescribed Medication *NOC:* Knowledge: Medication

Nursing Diagnosis:

Deficient Knowledge:

Purpose, precautions, and side effects of beta-blockers

Desired outcome: Within the 24-hr period before hospital discharge, patient verbalizes understanding of the purpose, precautions, and side effects of beta-blockers.

INTERVENTIONS	RATIONALES
Teach patient the purpose of beta-blockers.	These drugs block beta stimulation to the S-A node and myocardium. HR and contractility are decreased, subsequently decreasing workload of the heart. As well, they decrease myocardial oxygen demand, thereby improving myocardial oxygenation. A patient who is knowledgeable about the purpose of this drug will be more likely to adhere to therapy.
Instruct patient to be alert to depression, fatigue, dizziness, erythematous rash, respiratory distress, and sexual dysfunction. Explain importance of notifying health care provider promptly if these side effects occur.	These are side effects of beta-blockers.
Explain that weight gain and peripheral and sacral edema can occur. Teach patient how to assess for edema and importance of reporting signs and symptoms promptly if they occur.	Weight gain and peripheral and sacral edema can occur as side effects of this drug and should be reported promptly for timely intervention.
Explain that BP and HR are assessed before administration of beta-blockers.	These drugs can cause hypotension and excessive slowing of the heart.
Caution patient not to omit or abruptly stop taking beta-blockers.	Stopping this drug abruptly may result in rebound tachycardia, potentially causing angina or MI.

●●● **Related NIC and NOC labels:** *NIC:* Teaching: Prescribed Medication *NOC:* Knowledge: Medication

Nursing Diagnosis:

Deficient Knowledge:

Disease process and lifestyle implications of CAD

Desired Outcome: Within the 24-hr period before hospital discharge, patient verbalizes knowledge about the disease process of CAD and concomitant lifestyle implications.

INTERVENTIONS	RATIONALES
Teach patient about CAD, including pathophysiologic processes of cardiac ischemia, angina, and infarction.	Increasing patient's knowledge of health status optimally will promote adherence to the treatment regimen.
Assist with identifying risk factors for CAD and risk factor modification.	Risk factor identification optimally will result in risk factor modification, including: - Diet low in cholesterol and saturated fat - Smoking cessation - Regular activity/exercise program - Weight loss (if appropriate)
Discuss symptoms that necessitate medical attention.	Progression to unstable angina, loss of consciousness, decreased exercise tolerance, angina unrelieved by NTG, increasing frequency of angina, and need to increase the number of NTG tablets to relieve angina are symptoms that necessitate medical attention to prevent MI.
Discuss guidelines for sexual activity.	Viagra cannot be taken with NTG because an acute MI could occur. Resting before intercourse, finding a comfortable position, taking prophylactic NTG, and postponing intercourse for 1-1½ hr after a heavy meal are valid guidelines that help minimize oxygen demand on the heart.
Discuss the rationale for antihyperlipidemic therapy with patient, which may include the following:	
HMG-CoA reductase inhibitors (e.g., lovastatin, simvastatin, fluvastatin, pravastatin, atorvastatin)	These agents inhibit the enzyme involved in early cholesterol formation, thereby reducing total cholesterol levels, including LDL and triglycerides, while increasing HDL.
Nicotinic acid (niacin)	This vitamin lowers triglyceride and LDL levels while raising HDL levels.
Fibric acid derivatives (e.g., gemfibrozil, fenofibrate)	These agents lower triglycerides and raise HDL.
Bile acid sequestrant resins (e.g., cholestyramine, colestipol)	These bind with bile acids in the intestine and remove LDL and cholesterol from the blood.
Discuss procedures such as cardiac catheterization, percutaneous coronary intervention (PCI), and CABG, if appropriate.	PCI is a procedure that improves coronary blood flow by using a balloon inflation catheter to rupture plaque and dilate the artery. It is performed in the cardiac catheterization laboratory under local anesthesia and with mild sedation, enabling patient to be awake and interact with the health care team. PCI is a common alternative to bypass surgery for individuals with discrete lesions. Balloon angioplasty traditionally is followed by stent placement. Following the procedure, patients routinely are placed on antiplatelet agents (e.g., ASA and Plavix) to reduce risk of in-stent restenosis post-PCI. Additionally, drug-eluting stents are now available, which further reduce risk of restenosis. An anti-restenotic drug contained within the polymer of these stents is released over a period of time to modify the healing response that would result in restenosis. Complications of PCI include bleeding, vascular injury, infection, MI, stroke, contrast-induced nephropathy, allergic reaction to medications or contrast, and death. Cardiac catheterization is discussed later in this section and CABG is discussed in "Cardiac Surgery," p. 161.

••• **Related NIC and NOC labels:** *NIC:* Teaching: Disease Process; Discharge Planning; Teaching: Prescribed Diet; Teaching: Prescribed Activity/Exercise; Teaching: Procedure/Treatment *NOC:* Knowledge: Disease Process; Knowledge: Illness Care; Knowledge: Treatment/Procedures; Knowledge: Treatment Regimen

Nursing Diagnosis:

Health-Seeking Behaviors:

Relaxation technique effective for stress reduction

Desired Outcome: Patient reports subjective relief of stress after using relaxation technique.

INTERVENTIONS	RATIONALES
Discuss importance of relaxation for patients with CAD.	Relaxation decreases nervous system tone (sympathetic), energy requirements, and O_2 consumption. A knowledgeable patient is more likely to adhere to this and other techniques that promote relaxation.
Speaking slowly and softly, give patient the following guidelines:	This technique promotes relaxation, decreases energy requirements, and can be used easily by anyone.
1. Find a comfortable position. Close your eyes.	
2. Begin by concentrating on your feet and toes; tighten the muscles in your feet and toes, and hold this tightness for a count of three. Now slowly relax your feet and toes. Feel or imagine the tension flowing out of your feet and toes. Now concentrate on your lower legs. Tense the muscles of your lower legs for a count of three. Now slowly release this tightness and feel the tension drain from your lower legs. Continue with this purposeful tightening and relaxation with each successive major body part, moving up the body, until finally you reach your facial muscles. When you reach your face, tighten the muscles of your face for a count of three. When you relax the muscles in your face, take a deep breath and exhale. As you breathe out, imagine that you are blowing all the tension of your body out and away from you, leaving you totally relaxed and calm.	
3. Now breathe through your nose. Concentrate on feeling the air move in and out. As you exhale, say the word "one" silently to yourself. Again continue feeling the air move in and out of your lungs. Continue for approximately 20 min.	
4. Try to clear your mind of worries; be passive. Let relaxation occur. If distractions appear, gently push them away. Continue breathing through your nose, repeating "one" silently.	
Encourage patient to practice this technique 2-3 times/day or whenever feeling stressed or tense.	Although this technique may feel strange at first, it becomes easier and more effective with each practice.
Suggest that patient play baroque or new age music during this relaxation exercise.	This type of music, played softly, is known to help many individuals achieve an even greater state of relaxation.

••• **Related NIC and NOC labels**: *NIC:* Health Education *NOC:* Health Promoting Behavior

For patients undergoing cardiac catheterization

Nursing Diagnosis:

Deficient Knowledge:

Catheterization procedure and postcatheterization regimen

Desired Outcome: Before the procedure, patient verbalizes knowledge about cardiac catheterization and the postcatheterization plan of care.

INTERVENTIONS	RATIONALES
Assess patient's health care literacy (language, reading, comprehension). Assess culture and culturally specific information needs.	This assessment helps ensure that information is presented in a manner that is culturally and educationally appropriate.
Assess patient's knowledge about the catheterization procedure. As appropriate, reinforce health care provider's explanation, and answer any questions or concerns. If possible, arrange for an orientation visit to catheterization laboratory before the procedure.	Knowledge about a procedure and familiarization with rooms and equipment may help reduce anxiety.
Before cardiac catheterization, have patient practice techniques that will be used during procedure.	Valsalva's maneuver, coughing, and deep breathing will be required during the cardiac catheterization, and many people are unfamiliar with proper technique.
Explain the postcatheterization regimen and caution that flexing the insertion site is contraindicated.	After the procedure bedrest will be required and vital signs, circulation, and insertion site will be checked at frequent intervals to ensure integrity. Flexing the insertion site (arm or groin) is contraindicated to prevent bleeding.
Stress importance of promptly reporting signs and symptoms of concern.	Groin, leg, or back pain; dizziness; chest pain; or shortness of breath may signal hemorrhage or embolization of the stent. Prompt reporting enables rapid intervention.

••• **Related NIC and NOC Labels:** *NIC:* Preparatory Sensory Information; Teaching: Procedure/Treatment; Teaching: Psychomotor Skill; Learning Readiness Enhancement; Anxiety Reduction; Culture Brokerage *NOC:* Knowledge: Treatment/Procedure

Nursing Diagnosis:

Ineffective Tissue Perfusion: Cardiopulmonary, Peripheral, and Cerebral

related to interrupted arterial flow secondary to catheterization procedure

Desired Outcome: Within 1 hr after procedure, patient has adequate perfusion as evidenced by HR regular and within 20 bpm of baseline HR; apical/radial pulse equality; BP within 20 mm Hg of baseline BP; peripheral pulse amplitude greater than 2+ on a 0-4+ scale; warmth and normal color in the extremities; no significant change in mental status; and orientation to person, place, and time.

INTERVENTIONS	RATIONALES
Monitor BP q15min until stable on 3 successive checks, q2h for the next 12 hr, and q4h for 24 hr unless otherwise indicated.	These assessments monitor BP trend.
If SBP drops 20 mm Hg or more below previous recordings, lower HOB and notify health care provider.	A drop in BP could signify acute bleeding or shock. Lowering the HOB assists perfusion to the heart and brain.
Note: If insertion site was the antecubital space, measure BP in unaffected arm.	This measure prevents bleeding or blood vessel injury.
Be alert to and report cool extremities, decreased amplitude of peripheral pulses, cyanosis, changes in mental status, decreased level of consciousness, and shortness of breath.	These are indicators of decreased perfusion.
Monitor HR, and notify health care provider if dysrhythmias occur. If patient is not on a cardiac monitor, auscultate apical and radial pulses with every BP check and report irregularities or apical/radial discrepancies.	Dysrhythmias and apical/radial discrepancies may be signs of cardiac ischemia.
If the femoral artery was the insertion site, maintain HOB at no greater than a 30-degree elevation.	This measure prevents acute hip joint flexion, which could compromise arterial flow.

••• **Related NIC and NOC labels:** *NIC:* Cardiac Care: Acute; Dysrhythmia Management; Shock Management: Cardiac; Circulatory Precautions; Vital Signs Management; Lower Extremity Monitoring; Shock Prevention; Bleeding Reduction; Respiratory Monitoring; Cerebral Perfusion Promotion; Neurologic Monitoring; Positioning; Circulatory Care: Arterial Insufficiency *NOC:* Cardiac Pump Effectiveness; Circulation Status; Tissue Perfusion: Cardiac; Tissue Perfusion: Pulmonary; Vital Signs; Cognition; Tissue Perfusion: Cerebral; Tissue Perfusion: Peripheral

Nursing Diagnosis:

Risk for Deficient Fluid Volume

related to hemorrhage caused by arterial puncture and/or osmotic diuresis from the dye

Desired Outcomes: Patient remains normovolemic as evidenced by HR 100 bpm or less; BP 90/60 mm Hg or greater (or within 20 mm Hg of baseline range); no significant change in mental status; and orientation to person, place, and time. The dressing is dry, and there is no swelling at the puncture site.

INTERVENTIONS	RATIONALES
Be alert to and report a decrease in BP, increase in HR, and decreasing LOC.	These are indicators of hemorrhage and/or shock. Rapid reporting enables prompt intervention.
Inspect dressing on groin or antecubital space at frequent intervals.	This measure detects presence of frank bleeding or hematoma formation (fluctuating swelling), which would necessitate prompt intervention.
Be alert to diminished amplitude or absence of distal pulses, delayed capillary refill, coolness of the extremities, and pallor.	These signs of decreased peripheral perfusion may signal embolization or hemorrhagic shock.
Caution patient about flexing elbow or hip more than 30 degrees for 6-8 hr, or as prescribed.	These restrictions minimize risk of bleeding and circulation compromise.
If bleeding occurs, maintain pressure at insertion site as prescribed, usually 1 inch proximal to puncture site or introducer insertion site.	Pressure stabilizes bleeding. Typically this is done with a pressure dressing or a 2-5-lb sandbag.

••• **Related NIC and NOC labels:** *NIC:* Vital Signs Monitoring; Bleeding Precautions; Bleeding Reduction; Cardiac Care: Acute; Hemorrhage Control; Shock Prevention; Surveillance *NOC:* Fluid Balance

Nursing Diagnosis:

Ineffective Tissue Perfusion: Peripheral (or risk for same)

related to interrupted arterial flow in the involved limb secondary to embolization

Desired Outcome: Patient has adequate perfusion in the involved limb as evidenced by peripheral pulse amplitude greater than 2+ on a 0-4+ scale; normal color, sensation, and temperature; and brisk capillary refill (less than 2 sec).

INTERVENTIONS	RATIONALES
Assess peripheral perfusion by palpating peripheral pulses q15min for 30 min, then q30min for 1 hr, then hourly for 2 hr, or per protocol.	Prompt recognition of a diminished or absent pulse is essential to prevent limb damage.
Monitor for and report faintness or absence of pulse; coolness of extremity; mottling; decreased capillary refill; cyanosis; and complaints of numbness, tingling, and pain at insertion site. Instruct patient to report any of these indicators promptly.	These are signs of embolization in the involved limb. Prompt recognition will result in rapid intervention.
If there is no evidence of an embolus or thrombus formation, instruct patient to move fingers or toes and rotate wrist or ankle.	These measures promote circulation in the involved limbs.
Ensure that patient maintains bedrest for 4-6 hr or as prescribed.	Bedrest or immobility enables the puncture site to stabilize, thereby avoiding bleeding.

••• **Related NIC and NOC labels:** *NIC:* Circulatory Care: Arterial Insufficiency; Embolus Precautions; Circulatory Precautions; Lower Extremity Monitoring; Exercise Promotion *NOC:* Tissue Perfusion: Peripheral

Nursing Diagnosis:

Ineffective Tissue Perfusion: Renal (or risk for same)

related to interrupted blood flow secondary to decreased cardiac output or reaction to contrast dye

Desired Outcome: Patient has adequate renal perfusion as evidenced by a stable BUN/creatinine, urinary output of at least 30 ml/hr (0.5 ml/kg/hr), specific gravity less than 1.030, good skin turgor, and moist mucous membranes.

INTERVENTIONS	RATIONALES
Monitor for indicators of dehydration, such as poor skin turgor, dry mucous membranes, and high urine specific gravity (1.030 or more).	Contrast dye for cardiac catheterization may cause osmotic diuresis.
Monitor intake and output. Notify health care provider if urinary output is less than 30 ml/hr (0.5 ml/kg/hr) in the presence of adequate intake.	This assessment determines if urine output is sufficient. A fall in urinary output is a sign of dehydration or renal insufficiency.
Monitor blood urea nitrogen (BUN) and creatinine daily.	A rise in these renal markers may signify renal insufficiency or acute renal failure. See "Laboratory Tests Discussed in This Manual: Normal Values," p.791, for optimal values.
If urinary output is insufficient despite adequate intake, restrict fluids.	This measure helps prevent fluid overload.
Be alert to and report crackles (rales) on auscultation of lung fields, distended neck veins, and shortness of breath.	These signs are other indicators of fluid overload.
Notify health care provider about significant findings.	Prompt detection and reporting enable rapid intervention.
If patient does not exhibit signs of cardiac or renal failure, encourage daily intake of 2-3 L of fluids, or as prescribed.	Increasing hydration helps flush contrast dye out of the system more quickly.

●●● **Related NIC and NOC labels:** *NIC:* Fluid Monitoring; Laboratory Data Interpretation; Fluid Management; Bedside Laboratory Testing; Hypervolemia Management; Hypovolemia Management; Vital Signs Monitoring *NOC:* Circulation Status; Fluid Balance

ADDITIONAL NURSING DIAGNOSES/PROBLEMS:

"Psychosocial Support"	p. 73
"Psychosocial Support for the Patient's Family and Significant Other"	p. 87
"Pulmonary Embolus" for **Ineffective Protection** related to risk of prolonged bleeding or hemorrhage secondary to anticoagulation therapy	p. 139
"Cardiac Surgery" for a discussion of CABG	p. 161
"Dysrhythmias and Conduction Disturbances"	p. 177

✓ PATIENT-FAMILY TEACHING AND DISCHARGE PLANNING

When providing patient-family teaching, focus on sensory information, avoid giving excessive information, and initiate a visiting nurse referral for necessary follow-up teaching. Include verbal and written information about the following:

✓ Medications, including drug name, dosage, purpose, schedule, precautions, and potential side effects. Also discuss drug-drug, food-drug, and herb-drug interactions. Explain the potential for headache and dizziness after NTG administration. Caution patient about using NTG more frequently than prescribed and notifying health care provider if three tablets do not relieve angina.

✓ Importance of reducing or eliminating intake of caffeine, which causes vasoconstriction and increases HR.

✓ Dietary changes: low saturated fat, low sodium, low cholesterol, and need for weight loss if appropriate. Encourage use of food labels to determine caloric, cholesterol, fat, and sodium content of foods.

✓ Pulse monitoring: how to self-measure pulse, including parameters for target heart rates and limits.

✓ Prescribed exercise program and importance of maintaining a regular exercise schedule, with referral to a cardiac rehabilitation program, in which individualized exercise programs are outlined for the patient.

✓ Signs and symptoms necessitating immediate medical attention, including chest pain unrelieved by NTG, decreased exercise tolerance, increasing shortness of breath, increased leg edema or pain (postcatheterization), and loss of consciousness.

✓ Activity and dietary limitations as prescribed.

✓ Importance of follow-up with health care provider; confirm date and time of next appointment.

✓ Elimination of smoking and tobacco use. Refer patient to a "stop smoking" program as appropriate. The following free brochures outline ways to help patients stop smoking:

- *How to Help Your Patients Stop Using Tobacco: A National Cancer Institute Manual for the Oral Health Team*, from the Smoking and Tobacco Control Program of the National Cancer Institute.
- *Clinical Practice Guideline: A Quick Reference Guide for Smoking Cessation Specialists*, from the Agency for Health Care Policy and Research (AHCPR).

✓ Importance of involvement and support of significant others in patient's lifestyle changes.

✓ Importance of getting BP checked at regular intervals (at least monthly if patient is hypertensive).

✓ Importance of avoiding strenuous activity for at least 1 hr after meals to help prevent excessive O_2 demands.

✓ Importance of reporting to health care provider any change in pattern or frequency of angina.

✓ Availability of community and medical support, such as American Heart Association at *www.americanheart.org*.

Dysrhythmias and Conduction Disturbances 20

OVERVIEW/PATHOPHYSIOLOGY

Dysrhythmias are abnormal rhythms of the heart's electrical system. They can originate in any part of the conduction system, such as the sinus node, atrium, atrioventricular (A-V) node, His-Purkinje system, bundle branches, and ventricular tissue. Although a variety of diseases may cause dysrhythmias, the most common are coronary artery disease (CAD) and myocardial infarction (MI). Other causes may include electrolyte imbalance, changes in oxygenation, and drug toxicity. Cardiac dysrhythmias may result from the following mechanisms:

Disturbances in automaticity: May involve an increase or decrease in automaticity in the sinus node (e.g., sinus tachycardia or sinus bradycardia). Premature beats may arise via this mechanism from the atria, junction, or ventricles. Abnormal rhythms, such as atrial or ventricular tachycardia, also may occur.

Disturbances in conductivity: Conduction may be too rapid, as in conditions caused by an accessory pathway (e.g., Wolff-Parkinson-White syndrome), or too slow (e.g., A-V block). Reentry is a situation in which a stimulus reexcites a conduction pathway through which it already has passed. Once started, this impulse may circulate repeatedly. For reentry to occur, there must be two different pathways for conduction: one with slowed conduction and one with unidirectional block.

Combinations of altered automaticity and conductivity: Observed when several dysrhythmias are noted, for example, a first-degree A-V block (disturbance in conductivity) and premature atrial contractions (disturbance in automaticity).

HEALTH CARE SETTING

Primary care with possible hospitalization in coronary care unit (CCU) resulting from complications

ASSESSMENT

Signs and symptoms: Can vary on a continuum from absence of symptoms to complete cardiopulmonary collapse. General indicators include alterations in level of consciousness (LOC), vertigo, syncope, seizures, weakness, fatigue, activity intolerance, shortness of breath, dyspnea on exertion, chest pain, palpitations, sensation of "skipped beats," anxiety, and restlessness.

Physical assessment: Increases or decreases in heart rate (HR), blood pressure (BP), and respiration rate (RR); dusky color or pallor; crackles (rales); cool skin; decreased urine output; weakened and paradoxical pulse and abnormal heart sounds (e.g., paradoxical splitting of S_1 and S_2).

ECG results: Some findings seen with various dysrhythmias include abnormalities in rate such as sinus bradycardia or sinus tachycardia, irregular rhythm such as atrial fibrillation, extra beats such as premature atrial contractions (PACs) and premature junctional contractions (PJCs), wide and bizarre-looking beats such as premature ventricular contractions (PVCs) and ventricular tachycardia (VT), a fibrillating baseline such as ventricular fibrillation (VF), and a straight line as with asystole.

History and risk factors: CAD, recent MI, electrolyte disturbances, substance abuse, drug toxicity, obesity, diabetes mellitus, obstructive sleep apnea, advanced age, genetic factors, thyroid problems, certain medications and supplements, and hypertension.

DIAGNOSTIC TESTS

12-lead ECG: To detect dysrhythmias and identify possible cause.

Serum electrolyte levels: To identify electrolyte abnormalities that can precipitate dysrhythmias. The most common are potassium and magnesium abnormalities.

Drug levels: To identify toxicities (e.g., of digoxin, quinidine, procainamide, aminophylline) that can precipitate dysrhythmias, or to determine substance abuse that can affect heart rate and rhythm, such as cocaine.

Ambulatory monitoring (e.g., Holter monitor or cardiac event recorder): To identify subtle dysrhythmias, associate abnormal rhythms by means of patient's symptoms, and assess response to exercise.

Electrophysiologic study: Invasive test in which two to three catheters are placed into the heart, giving it a pacing stimulus at varying sites and of varying voltages. The test determines origin of dysrhythmia, inducibility, and effectiveness of drug therapy in dysrhythmia suppression.

Exercise stress testing: Used in conjunction with Holter monitoring to detect advanced grades of PVCs (those caused by ischemia) and to guide therapy. During the test, electrocardiogram (ECG) and BP readings are taken while patient walks on a treadmill or pedals a stationary bicycle; response to a constant or increasing workload is observed. The test continues until patient reaches target heart rate or symptoms such as chest pain, severe fatigue, dysrhythmias, or abnormal BP occur.

Oximetry or ABG values: To document trend of hypoxemia.

Nursing Diagnosis:

Decreased Cardiac Output

related to altered rate, rhythm, or conduction or negative inotropic changes secondary to cardiac disease

Desired Outcome: Within 1 hr of treatment/intervention, patient has adequate cardiac output as evidenced by BP 90/60 mm Hg or higher, HR 60-100 bpm, and normal sinus rhythm on ECG.

INTERVENTIONS	RATIONALES
Monitor patient's heart rhythm continuously.	This assessment will reveal whether dysrhythmias occur or increase in occurrence.
Note BP and symptoms if dysrhythmias occur.	Signs of decreased cardiac output include decreased BP and symptoms such as unrelieved and prolonged palpitations, chest pain, shortness of breath, weakened and rapid pulse (more than 150 bpm), sensation of skipped beats, palpitations, dizziness, and syncope.
Report significant findings to health care provider.	Decreased cardiac output should be reported promptly for timely intervention.
If symptoms of decreased cardiac output occur, prepare to transfer patient to CCU.	Patient likely will be transferred to CCU for specialized and intensive care and monitoring.
Document dysrhythmias with rhythm strip, using a 12-lead ECG as necessary.	This assessment will identify dysrhythmias and their general trend.
Monitor patient's laboratory data, particularly electrolyte and digoxin levels.	Serum potassium levels less than 3.5 mEq/L or more than 5.0 mEq/L can cause dysrhythmias. Digoxin toxicity may cause heart block or dysrhythmias.
Administer antidysrhythmic agents as prescribed; note patient's response to therapy based on action of the following classifications:	
Class IA: sodium channel blockers; quinidine, procainamide, disopyramide	Decreases depolarization moderately and prolongs repolarization
Class IB: sodium channel blockers; phenytoin, mexiletine, tocainide	Decreases depolarization and shortens repolarization
Class IC: sodium channel blockers; encainide, flecainide, propafenone	Significantly decreases depolarization with minimal effect on repolarization
Class II: Beta-blockers; propranolol, metoprolol, atenolol, acebutolol	Slows sinus automaticity, slows conduction via A-V node, controls ventricular response to supraventricular tachycardias, and shortens the action potential of Purkinje fibers
Class III: potassium channel blockers; bretylium, amiodarone, sotalol	Increases the action potential and refractory period of Purkinje fibers, increases ventricular fibrillation threshold, restores injured myocardial cell electrophysiology toward normal, and suppresses reentrant dysrhythmias
Class IV: calcium channel blockers; verapamil, diltiazem, nifedipine	Depresses automaticity in the S-A and A-V nodes, blocks the slow calcium current in the A-V junctional tissue, reduces conduction via the A-V node, and is useful in treating tachydysrhythmias because of A-V junction reentry. This class of drugs also vasodilates.
Monitor corrected QT interval (QTc) when initiating drugs known to cause QT prolongation (e.g., sotalol, propafenone, dofetilide, flecainide).	When QTc is prolonged, it can increase risk of dysrhythmias. QTc equals QT (in seconds) divided by the square root of the R to R interval (in seconds).

Continued

INTERVENTIONS	RATIONALES
Provide O_2 as prescribed.	O_2 may be beneficial if dysrhythmias are related to ischemia.
Deliver O_2 with humidity.	Humidity helps prevent oxygen's drying effects on oral and nasal mucosa.
Maintain a quiet environment, and administer pain medications promptly.	Both stress and pain can increase sympathetic tone and cause dysrhythmias.
If life-threatening dysrhythmias occur, initiate emergency procedures and cardiopulmonary resuscitation (as indicated by advanced cardiac life support [ACLS] protocol).	This action provides circulation to vital organs and restores heart to normal or viable rhythm.
When dysrhythmias occur, stay with patient; provide support and reassurance while performing assessments and administering treatment.	This action reduces stress and provides comfort, which optimally will decrease dysrhythmias.

●●● **Related NIC and NOC labels:** *NIC:* Dysrhythmia Management; Cardiac Care: Acute; Electrolyte Monitoring; Vital Signs Monitoring; Medication Administration; Emergency Care *NOC:* Cardiac Pump Effectiveness; Vital Signs Status

Nursing Diagnosis:

Deficient Knowledge:

Mechanism by which dysrhythmias occur and lifestyle implications

Desired Outcome: Within the 24-hr period before hospital discharge, patient and significant other verbalize knowledge about causes of dysrhythmias and implications for patient's lifestyle modifications.

INTERVENTIONS	RATIONALES
Assess patient's health care literacy (language, reading, comprehension). Assess culture and culturally specific information needs.	This assessment helps ensure that information is presented in a manner that is culturally and educationally appropriate.
Discuss causal mechanisms for dysrhythmias, including resulting symptoms. Use a heart model or diagrams as necessary.	This information increases patient's knowledge about health status. Visual aids augment understanding of verbal information. A knowledgeable patient is more likely to adhere to the therapeutic regimen.
Teach signs and symptoms of dysrhythmias that necessitate medical attention.	Indicators such as unrelieved and prolonged palpitations, chest pain, shortness of breath, rapid pulse (more than 150 bpm), dizziness, and syncope are serious and should be reported promptly for timely intervention.
Teach patient and significant other how to check pulse rate for a full minute.	Checking pulse rate for a full minute ensures a better average of rate and rhythm than if it were measured for 15 seconds and multiplied by 4.
Teach patient and significant other about medications that will be taken after hospital discharge, including drug name, purpose, dosage, schedule, precautions, and potential side effects. Also discuss drug-drug, food-drug, and herb-drug interactions.	The more knowledgeable the patient is, the more likely he or she is to adhere to therapy and report side effects and complications promptly for timely intervention.
Stress that patient will be taking long-term antidysrhythmic therapy and that it could be life threatening to stop or skip these medications without health care provider involvement.	Stopping or skipping these drugs may decrease blood levels effective for dysrhythmia suppression.
Advise patient and significant other about availability of support groups and counseling; provide appropriate community referrals. Explain that anxiety and fear, along with periodic feelings of denial, depression, anger, and confusion, are normal following this experience.	Patients who survive sudden cardiac arrest may experience nightmares or other sleep disturbances at home.
Stress importance of leading a normal and productive life. If patient is going on vacation, advise taking along sufficient medication and investigating health care facilities in the vacation area.	This concept may be difficult to implement for patients who fear breakthrough of life-threatening dysrhythmias and alter their lives accordingly.
Advise patient and significant other to take cardiopulmonary resuscitation classes; provide addresses for community programs.	Emergency life-saving procedures may be necessary in the future.

Continued

INTERVENTIONS	RATIONALES
Teach importance of follow-up care; confirm date and time of next appointment if known. Explain that outpatient Holter monitoring is performed periodically.	Medical follow-up is important for ongoing assessment and management of cardiac dysrhythmias.
Explain dietary restrictions that individuals with recurrent dysrhythmias should follow. Discuss need for reduced intake of products containing caffeine, including coffee, tea, chocolate, and colas.	Caffeine is a stimulant that can cause abnormal heart rhythms.
Provide instruction for a general low-cholesterol diet. Encourage patient to use food labels to determine cholesterol content of foods.	There is an overlap between dysrhythmias and CAD, often necessitating a low-cholesterol diet that decreases hyperlipidemia.
As indicated, teach patient relaxation techniques, such as those found on p. 172.	Such techniques enable patient to reduce stress and decrease sympathetic tone. In some types of dysrhythmias, stress can increase incidence of occurrence.

If Patient Has Had an Implantable Cardioverter-Defibrillator (ICD) Inserted, Teach the Following:

INTERVENTIONS	RATIONALES
The ICD is programmed to deliver the electrical stimulus at a predetermined rate and/or after assessing morphology of the ECG. First- and second-generation ICDs provide for only cardioversion or defibrillation; third-generation ICDs also provide overdrive pacing and backup ventricular pacing.	ICD is recommended for patients who have survived an episode of sudden cardiac death (cardiac arrest), patients with CAD who have had a cardiac arrest, and those in whom conventional antidysrhythmic therapy has failed.
The ICD will have a pulse generator.	The pulse generator is powered by lithium batteries and surgically inserted (in the operating room [OR] or catheterization laboratory) into a "pocket" formed in the pectoral area. Leads are tunneled beneath the skin from the pocket to the subclavian vein through which they are advanced to the right ventricle.
Postoperative complications include atelectasis, pneumonia, seroma at the generator "pocket," pneumothorax, and thrombosis. Lead migration and lead fracture are the two most common structural problems. Interference from unipolar pacemakers and "myopotentials" (electrical interference) are common mechanical complications.	Patient should be informed of these complications and structural problems in order to report them promptly for timely intervention.
Some procedures interfere with and may change programming of the device. In addition, the ICD may "see" these procedures as a dysrhythmia and shock the patient.	ICDs may need to be deactivated during surgical procedures, use of electrocautery, and magnetic resonance imaging.
Patient should keep a pocket card on hand with all relevant ICD data on it.	This card ensures that medical information is available at all times in case a medical event occurs.
Explain importance of follow-up care; confirm date and time of next appointment if known.	Follow-up care helps ensure proper functioning of the device. Outpatient Holter monitoring also may be performed periodically.
If indicated, teach patient about left ventricular aneurysmectomy and infarctectomy.	Surgical excision of possible focal spots of ventricular dysrhythmias may be indicated, depending on etiology and severity of disease.

••• Related NIC and NOC labels: *NIC:* Teaching: Disease Process; Teaching: Individual; Discharge Planning; Teaching: Prescribed Medication; Teaching: Procedure/Treatment; Teaching: Psychomotor Skills *NOC:* Knowledge: Disease Process; Knowledge: Illness Care; Knowledge: Treatment Procedures; Knowledge: Medication; Knowledge: Diet; Knowledge: Prescribed Activity

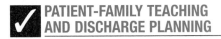

**PATIENT-FAMILY TEACHING
AND DISCHARGE PLANNING**

See patient's primary diagnosis.

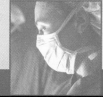
Heart Failure 21

OVERVIEW/PATHOPHYSIOLOGY

Heart failure (HF) is a complex clinical syndrome in which the heart is unable to pump sufficient blood to meet the body's metabolic demands. It is caused by any structural or functional cardiac disorder that impairs the ventricle's ability to fill with or eject blood. HF is a chronic condition that is prone to acute exacerbations (termed *acute decompensated heart failure* [ADHF]). In most cases of ADHF, severe volume overload and pulmonary edema are present. Acute pulmonary edema is an emergency situation in which hydrostatic pressure in the pulmonary vessels is greater than the vascular colloid osmotic pressure that holds fluid in the vessels. As a result, fluid floods the alveoli. When the alveoli contain fluid, their ability to participate in gas exchange is reduced and hypoxia occurs. HF usually is a result of either systolic (previously known as left-sided heart failure) or diastolic (previously known as right-sided heart failure) cardiac dysfunction or a combination of both.

Systolic dysfunction: Ventricular dilation and impaired ventricular contraction occur because of myocardial muscle injury or abnormality (see dilated cardiomyopathy, below). The initial injury or stressor to the heart muscle results in impaired cardiac output. This triggers a cascade of compensatory mechanisms, which together contribute to development and progression of HF.

Increased neurohormonal activation: Activation of the sympathetic nervous system (SNS) and renin-angiotensin system (RAS) stimulates catecholamines and other neurohormones, causing increases in HR and blood pressure (BP), systemic vasoconstriction, decreased renal perfusion, and sodium and fluid retention in an effort to increase cardiac output.

Hemodynamic alterations: Increase in left ventricular end-diastolic volume/pressure (preload) and thickening and elongation of the myofibrils (stretch) initially result in increased force of contraction (Frank-Starling law). The rise in myocardial oxygen demand further stimulates the neurohormonal response. Increases in preload and afterload (because of increased systemic resistance) add to left ventricular workload and cause excessive "stretch" of the myofibrils, thereby impairing ventricular contraction.

Remodeling: The above mechanisms eventually lead to hypertrophy (enlargement and thickening of the left ventricular [LV] wall). The heart becomes more spherical (dilated) in shape because of lengthening of the myofibrils, cell slippage, fibrosis, and myocyte death. These progressive changes in size, shape, and structure of the heart muscle are termed *remodeling*.

The structural, hemodynamic, and neurohormonal alterations cause progressive deterioration in systolic function associated with decreased left ventricular ejection fraction (LVEF), increased intracardiac pressures, impaired valvular function, decreased forward flow to vital organs and tissues, and increased pulmonary pressures. This results in pulmonary (left-sided failure) and hepatic (right-sided failure) congestion, edema, renal impairment, and impaired oxygenation and metabolism. Ventricular and atrial dysrhythmias are common because of structural changes to the myocytes and increased myocardial oxygen demand and are a major cause of mortality for this population.

Diastolic dysfunction: The ventricle becomes noncompliant and unable to accommodate increased preload and afterload (or decreased preload). These patients may have symptoms of HF because of volume overload without a reduction in systolic function as seen in individuals with longstanding hypertension, coronary artery disease (CAD), and hypertrophic and restrictive cardiomyopathies (see below).

Cardiomyopathies: HF commonly occurs in the presence of an underlying cardiomyopathy (disorder of the heart muscle). Cardiomyopathies are classified according to underlying cause and abnormality in structure and function.

• ***Dilated cardiomyopathy:*** Most prevalent type, characterized by enlargement of one (usually left) or both ventricles and impaired contraction (systolic dysfunction). The most common form is ischemic cardiomyopathy caused by severe coronary (ischemic) heart disease and/or myocardial infarction. Dilated cardiomyopathy (DCM) also occurs secondary to hypertension, valvular heart disease, diabetes mellitus (DM), cardiotoxins, genetic causes, and metabolic, infectious, or systemic diseases. DCM is termed *idiopathic* when the cause cannot be identified. See "Systolic dysfunction," earlier, for additional information.

• ***Hypertrophic cardiomyopathy:*** Characterized by an abnormally enlarged left ventricle but without a concomitant increase in cavity size. Filling is restricted and may be associated with left ventricular outflow tract obstruction. Cardiac function can remain normal for varying periods before decompensation occurs. Symptoms are varied and include HF symptoms, chest pain, palpitations, dizziness, near-syncope, or syncope. Patients may be prone to ventricular dysrhythmias.

Although it is theorized that hypertrophic cardiomyopathy has a strong hereditary link, etiology is unknown.

• *Restrictive cardiomyopathy:* Least common in Western countries, it is characterized by inadequate compliance causing restriction of diastolic filling.

Other causes of heart failure

HF or acute pulmonary edema can occur secondary to other conditions that place excessive demands on cardiac output, such as hypertensive crisis, tachycardia due to hyperthyroidism, dysrhythmias, severe anemia, faulty heart valves, congenital heart defects, dysrhythmias, cardiomyopathy, myocarditis, trauma, infection, volume overload (i.e., caused by IV fluids, postoperative fluid shifts), pregnancy, and conditions that affect capillary permeability. In these cases, treatment/correction of the underlying cause is essential and may result in normalization or improvement of cardiac function.

Severe pulmonary diseases, including COPD, pulmonary hypertension, and obstructive sleep apnea (OSA) can lead to diastolic heart failure (cor pulmonale). This is less likely to be reversible. Poorly compensated pulmonary disease, upper respiratory infection, and pneumonia can exacerbate all types of HF and need to be treated aggressively.

HEALTH CARE SETTING

Primary care with possible hospitalization, including intensive care unit (ICU), resulting from complications. **Note:** Eighty percent of HF admissions are due to preventable factors.

ASSESSMENT

General

Signs and symptoms: Dyspnea on exertion (DOE) or at rest, fatigue, decreased exercise tolerance, weakness, orthopnea (unable to lie flat; may need to sleep on pillows or sitting in a chair), paroxysmal nocturnal dyspnea, wheezing, cough, cyanosis, irregular or rapid HR, sudden weight gain from fluid retention, lower extremity edema, abdominal distention, nausea, early satiety, and nocturia. Associated indicators include chest/anginal pains, palpitations, near-syncope, syncope, and falls. *Low-output symptoms* include positional lightheadedness, weakness, mental status changes, and decreased urine output.

Physical assessment: Decreased or elevated BP, dysrhythmias, tachycardia, tachypnea, increased venous pulsations, pulsus alternans (alternating strong and weak heart beats), increased central venous pressure (CVP), jugular venous distention, crackles (rales), wheezes, decreased breath sounds, cardiac gallop and/or murmur, hepatomegaly, ascites, and pitting edema in dependent areas (lower extremities, sacrum).

History/risk factors: CAD, hypertension, DM, OSA or other pulmonary disease, recent IV fluid infusions, surgery, pregnancy, recent/current infectious illness, pneumonia, nonadherence to medication or diet regimen, obesity, hypercholesterolemia, and recent nonsteroidal antiinflammatory drug or COX-2 inhibitor use. In addition, see "Other causes of heart failure," earlier.

Acute decompensated heart failure

Signs and symptoms: Typified by marked severity of HF symptoms and deterioration of one or more NYHA functional classes. Pulmonary edema and cardiogenic shock (see p. 157) may be present, and, in more severe cases, renal dysfunction.

Acute pulmonary edema

Signs and symptoms: Extreme dyspnea, anxiety, restlessness, frothy and blood-tinged sputum, severe orthopnea, and paroxysmal nocturnal dyspnea. Patient exhibits "air hunger" and may thrash about and describe a sensation of drowning.

Physical assessment: Crackles (rales), wheezing, decreased breath sounds, tachycardia, tachypnea, engorged neck veins, and cardiac gallop/murmur.

DIAGNOSTIC TESTS

Chest x-ray examination: May show cardiomegaly, engorged pulmonary vasculature, "Kerley-B lines" suggestive of HF, and pleural or pericardial effusions.

ECG: Changes may indicate CAD, acute myocardial ischemia, left ventricular hypertrophy (widened QRS), conduction defects, and dysrhythmias.

Left ventricular ejection fraction: Percentage of blood ejected from the left ventricle during systole. Normal LVEF is 50%-70%. In systolic dysfunction, it is reduced. LVEF less than 35% is associated with increased risk for mortality-related HF and dysrhythmias. In hypertrophic cardiomyopathy, LVEF may be greater than 70%. LVEF assessment can be measured during echocardiogram, LV gram, magnetic resonance imaging (MRI), or radionuclide studies (multiple-gated acquisition scan, nuclear stress test [see below]).

Echocardiography: Most commonly used means of evaluating ventricular function. It assesses left- and right-sided systolic function, LVEF, degree of ventricular dilation, wall thickness, abnormal wall and septal motion, valvular function, estimated pulmonary pressure, presence of thrombus, restriction, outflow tract obstruction, and pericardial effusion. Diastolic dysfunction may be evident. Tissue Doppler/three-dimensional echocardiography may reveal degree of ventricular synchrony and utility of cardiac resynchronization therapy.

Cardiac catheterization: Rules out underlying ischemic heart disease and assesses hemodynamics (left- and right-sided filling pressures, cardiac output, and systemic and pulmonary vascular resistance).

Left ventriculography: Provides assessment of LV function and LVEF.

Endomyocardial biopsy: May be obtained during right heart catheterization. Usually it is reserved for severe, refractory HF in nonelderly patients to assist in identifying pathologic agent and reversible causes.

Radionuclide stress test, stress echocardiogram: To assess for underlying ischemic heart disease and reversible or fixed ischemic defects.

Pulmonary function tests: Useful in differentiating causes of shortness of breath and other HF symptoms. Pulmonary function tests (PFTs) may reveal underlying chronic obstructive pulmonary disease (COPD) or reactive airways disease (asthma).

Oximetry/ABG values: Will reveal hypoxemia. Desaturations may be noted with activity. Overnight (sleep) oximetry may reveal OSA.

Serum BUN, creatinine: Elevated in renal insufficiency and chronic kidney disease due to low cardiac output and hypotension, possibly related to treatment with diuretics, angiotensin-converting enzyme (ACE) inhibitors, angiotensin receptor blockers (ARBs), or aldosterone antagonists.

Serum electrolytes: May reveal hyperkalemia due to renal dysfunction or ACE inhibitor/ARB or aldosterone antagonist use. Hypokalemia may occur as a result of diuretic use. The presence of hyponatremia is a poor prognostic indicator in advanced HF.

Serum enzymes: Mild elevation in cardiac troponins (with normal CK) are not uncommon in patients with chronic HF or chronic kidney disease. Cardiac troponin elevation in the presence of elevated CK may indicate acute coronary syndrome.

Liver function tests, including serum aspartate aminotransferase and serum bilirubin: May be elevated in patients with hepatic congestion.

Brain natriuretic peptide: Released from the ventricles in response to wall stress. This test is useful in differentiating HF from other causes of dyspnea, including pulmonary disease. Negative brain natriuretic peptide (BNP) (less than 100 pg/ml) suggests non-HF etiology. When used in conjunction with standard clinical assessment, elevated BNP may support diagnosis of HF and evaluate patient's response to treatment.

Digoxin level: The goal in HF is a level less than 1.0 ng/ml. Hypokalemia and impaired renal function can predispose patient to digoxin toxicity.

CBC: May reveal decreased hemoglobin (Hgb) and hematocrit (Hct) in the presence of anemia.

Thyroid-stimulating hormone level: To rule out hyperthyroidism or hypothyroidism, either of which may contribute to HF and dysrhythmias.

Nursing Diagnosis:

Impaired Gas Exchange

related to alveolar-capillary membrane changes secondary to fluid accumulation in the alveoli

Desired Outcome: Within 30 min of treatment/intervention, patient has adequate gas exchange as evidenced by normal breath sounds and skin color, presence of eupnea, HR 100 bpm or less, Pao_2 80 mm Hg or higher, and $Paco_2$ 45 mm Hg or less.

INTERVENTIONS	RATIONALES
Auscultate lung fields for breath sounds.	The presence of crackles (rales) may signal alveolar fluid congestion and systolic dysfunctional (left-sided) heart failure.
Monitor oximetry and arterial blood gas (ABG) values and report significant findings.	Oximetry of 92% or less and the presence of hypoxemia (decreased Pao_2) and hypercapnia (increased $Paco_2$) signify decreased oxygenation.
Be alert to and report increased respiratory rate (RR), mental status changes, gasping for air, cyanosis, or rapid heart rate (HR).	These are signs of increasing respiratory distress that should be reported promptly for timely intervention.
Assist patient into high Fowler's position with head of bed (HOB) up 90 degrees.	This position decreases work of breathing, reduces cardiac workload, and promotes gas exchange.
Teach patient to take slow, deep breaths. Administer O_2 as prescribed.	Taking deep breaths increases oxygenation to the myocardium and improves prognosis. Hypoxia adds stress to the already distressed myocardium.
Deliver oxygen with humidity.	In ADHF/pulmonary edema, high-flow O_2 may be given either by non-rebreathing mask, positive airway pressure devices, or endotracheal intubation and mechanical ventilation. Once stabilized, O_2 is titrated to keep pulse oximetry readings higher than 92%.
	Humidity helps prevent oxygen's convective drying effects on oral and nasal mucosa.
Administer diuretics as prescribed.	Diuretics promote normovolemia by controlling fluid accumulation and reducing blood volume. Fluid overload decreases perfusion in the lungs, causing hypoxemia.

Continued

INTERVENTIONS	RATIONALES
Monitor K+ levels.	There is potential for hypokalemia (K+ less than 3.5 mEq/L) in patients taking some diuretics, such as furosemide and metolazone.
Administer vasodilators as prescribed.	Vasodilators increase venous capacitance (venous dilation) and decrease pulmonary congestion, which will improve gas exchange.
	Hydralazine is an oral vasodilator and afterload reducer. It is used in combination with nitrates in patients who are ACE inhibitor/ARB intolerant because of renal dysfunction. It improves mortality and HF symptoms to a lesser degree than ACE inhibitors and can cause reflex tachycardia.
	Nitrates are coronary vasodilators used in conjunction with hydralazine (see above). They are also used in ischemic heart disease as anti-anginal drugs.
	ACE inhibitors (enalapril, lisinopril, benazepril, captopril, quinapril, ramipril) suppress effects of the renin-angiotensin-system by reducing angiotensin II and causing decreased aldosterone secretion. These drugs lower BP and reduce preload and afterload, decreasing work of the left ventricle.
	Angiotensin II receptor antagonists (ARBs—losartan, valsartan, candesartan) are used for patients who do not tolerate ACE inhibitors because of cough caused by bradykinin release.
As indicated, have emergency equipment (e.g., airway, manual resuscitation bag) available and functional.	Patients with severely decompensated heart failure may suffer cardiac arrest.
As indicated, prepare to transfer patient to ICU.	Patient may require invasive and/or closer monitoring.

••• **Related NIC and NOC labels:** *NIC:* Acid-Base Monitoring; Electrolyte Monitoring; Fluid Management; Respiratory Monitoring; Vital Signs Monitoring; Ventilation Assistance; Positioning; Laboratory Data Interpretation; Airway Management; Oxygen Therapy *NOC:* Electrolyte and Acid-Base Balance; Respiratory Status: Gas Exchange

Nursing Diagnosis:

Excess Fluid Volume

related to compromised regulatory mechanisms secondary to decreased cardiac output

Desired Outcomes: Within 1 hr of intervention/treatment, patient demonstrates less shortness of breath and has output greater than intake on I&O monitoring. Within 1 day of treatment/intervention, edema is 1+ or less on a 0-4+ scale. Weight becomes stable within 2-3 days.

INTERVENTIONS	RATIONALES
Closely monitor intake and output (I&O), including insensible losses from diaphoresis and respirations.	Decreasing urinary output can signal decreased cardiac output, which decreases renal blood flow.
Assess daily morning weight; report steady gains.	This assessment assists in early identification of fluid retention, enabling titration of diuretics.
Assess for edema (interstitial fluids), especially in dependent areas such as ankles and sacrum.	The presence of weight gain and edema is a key determinate of fluid retention. If diligent assessment is maintained and early intervention is practiced, the occurrence of rehospitalization can be decreased dramatically.
Assess respiratory system for indicators of fluid extravasation, such as crackles (rales) or pink-tinged, frothy sputum.	These are signs of fluid volume excess and systolic dysfunction (left-sided) heart failure.
Monitor for jugular vein distention, peripheral edema, and ascites.	These are other indicators of fluid overload.

Continued

INTERVENTIONS	RATIONALES
Monitor laboratory results for increased urinary specific gravity, decreased Hct, increased urine osmolality, hyponatremia, and hypochloremia.	These findings are indicators of fluid retention.
Monitor IV rate of flow. Use an infusion control device.	These measures help prevent volume overload during IV infusion.
Unless contraindicated, provide ice chips or ice pops. Record amount on I&O record. Provide frequent mouth care to reduce dry mucous membranes.	These measures help patient control thirst while providing minimal amounts of fluid. **Note:** Some care centers advocate small amounts of room-temperature water instead because it may relieve thirst better.
Administer diuretics as prescribed, and record patient's response.	Diuretics promote normovolemia by controlling fluid accumulation and reducing blood volume. *Loop diuretics* (furosemide, bumetanide, torsemide): These agents promote excretion of water and sodium, reduce preload, and prevent fluid retention. In ADHF, these diuretics are administered via IV bolus or in drip form until stabilization occurs. These drugs can cause neurohormonal activation and aggravate preexisting renal dysfunction or hypokalemia. *Thiazide diuretics* (hydrochlorothiazide, metolazone): Hydrochlorothiazide may be used for mild fluid retention. Metolazone is a potent drug that, when given ½ hr before loop diuretics, markedly potentiates diuresis and therefore is reserved for more severe volume overload in ADHF or late-stage HF. Hyponatremia, hypokalemia, and worsening of renal function may occur and necessitate careful assessment.
Administer morphine sulfate if prescribed.	Morphine induces vasodilation and decreases venous return to the heart.
Teach patients and families about the importance of adhering to a low-sodium diet.	Hypernatremia can promote excess fluid retention. A 2-g per day sodium diet is recommended for most patients.

••• **Related NIC and NOC labels**: *NIC:* Fluid/Electrolyte Management; Fluid Monitoring; Hypervolemia Management; Laboratory Data Interpretation; Nutrition Management; Vital Signs Monitoring; Cardiac Care: Acute; Respiratory Monitoring *NOC:* Fluid Balance; Electrolyte & Acid-Base Balance

Nursing Diagnosis:

Ineffective Tissue Perfusion: Cardiopulmonary, Peripheral, and Cerebral

related to interrupted blood flow secondary to decreased cardiac output

Desired Outcome: Within 2 hr of intervention/treatment, patient has adequate tissue perfusion as evidenced by BP within 20 mm Hg of baseline BP; HR 100 bpm or less with regular rhythm; RR 20 breaths/min or less with normal depth and pattern (eupnea); brisk capillary refill (less than 2 sec); and significant improvement in mental status or orientation to person, place, and time.

INTERVENTIONS	RATIONALES
Monitor BP q15min or more frequently if unstable. Be alert to decreases greater than 20 mm Hg over patient's baseline or associated changes such as dizziness and altered mentation.	Hypotension is a side effect of many heart failure drugs, as well as a consequence of aggressive diuresis. Careful monitoring is essential to avoid decreased perfusion to vital organs.
Check pulse rate q15-30min. Monitor for irregularities, increased HR, or skipped beats.	These signs can signal decompensation and decreased function of the heart.
Monitor for cool extremities, pallor, and diaphoresis.	These signs are indicators of peripheral vasoconstriction (from SNS compensation).

Continued

INTERVENTIONS	RATIONALES
Report any of these changes immediately to health care provider.	These changes may be life-threatening.
Evaluate capillary refill.	Optimally, pink color should return within 1-2 sec after applying pressure to nail beds.
Monitor for restlessness, anxiety, mental status changes, confusion, lethargy, stupor, and coma. Institute safety precautions accordingly.	These are indicators of decreased cerebral perfusion and hypoxia, and should be addressed promptly for timely intervention.
Administer inotropic drugs and vasodilators as prescribed. Monitor effects closely. Be alert to problems such as hypotension and irregular heartbeats.	IV inotropic drugs (dobutamine, dopamine, milrinone) increase strength of contractions and are reserved for use in ADHF-associated low-cardiac output and cardiogenic shock until patient is stabilized. They may be used longer term in advanced stage HF as a bridge to transplantation or for palliation of symptoms. Use may be associated with increased mortality and ventricular dysrhythmias. Administration of inotropic drugs may require transfer to coronary care unit (CCU) to monitor for hemodynamic effects and dysrhythmias.
	IV vasodilators (nitroglycerine [NTG], nitroprusside, nesiritide) are used in ADHF to decrease cardiac workload by reducing ventricular filling pressures and SVR (afterload). These drugs are avoided in low-output HF, cardiogenic shock, and in SBP less than 90 mm Hg.
	- *Nesiritide:* Balanced arterial and venous vasodilator. This drug can alleviate acute dyspnea and reduce pulmonary capillary wedge pressure (PCWP) within the first 30 min of therapy. It promotes diuresis and natriuresis but does not replace need for diuretic therapy. It improves cardiac output by off-loading the heart and decreases neurohormonal activation. It does not require CCU monitoring.
	- *NTG:* Arterial and venous vasodilator. It also reduces PCWP and may require CCU monitoring. Because of tachyphylaxis (tolerance), patients may need escalating doses to achieve desired effect.
	- *Nitroprusside:* Potent arterial and venous vasodilator and afterload reducer. It must be administered in CCU because of the need for hemodynamic monitoring.
	- *Morphine sulfate:* A coronary vasodilator that may be given in ADHF or acute pulmonary edema to decrease anxiety and work of breathing and to relieve angina if ischemic heart disease is present.

••• **Related NIC and NOC labels:** *NIC:* Cardiac Care: Acute; Dysrhythmia Management; Hemodynamic Regulation; Shock Management: Cardiac; Shock Management: Cardiac; Emergency Care; Invasive Hemodynamic Monitoring; Vital Signs Monitoring; Medication Administration: Intravenous (IV); Medication Management; Lower Extremity Monitoring; Neurologic Monitoring; Technology Management *NOC:* Cardiac Pump Effectiveness; Circulation Status; Tissue Perfusion: Cardiac; Vital Signs; Tissue Perfusion: Peripheral; Tissue Perfusion: Cerebral

Nursing Diagnosis:

Decreased Cardiac Output

related to negative inotropic changes in the heart (decreased cardiac contractility) secondary to cardiac muscle changes

Desired Outcomes: By at least the 24 hr before hospital discharge, patient exhibits adequate cardiac output as evidenced by SBP at least 90 mm Hg, HR 100 bpm or less, urinary output at least 30 ml/hr (0.5 ml/kg/hr), stable weight, eupnea, normal breath sounds, and edema 1+ or less on a 0-4+ scale. By at least 48 hr before hospital discharge, patient is free of new dysrhythmias, does not exhibit significant changes in mental status, and remains oriented to person, place, and time.

INTERVENTIONS	RATIONALES
Assess for and document jugular venous distention, extra heart sound such as S3, changes in mental status or level of consciousness, cool extremities, hypotension, tachycardia, and tachypnea.	These are indicators of decreased cardiac output, which should be reported promptly for timely intervention.
Also monitor for adventitious breath sounds and shortness of breath.	Dyspnea, crackles, and shortness of breath signal fluid accumulation in the lungs and may be a direct indicator of ventricular failure and decreased cardiac output. Cardiac output decreases as heart failure progresses.
Keep accurate I&O records; weigh patient daily.	Decreasing urine output and weight gain can occur as a result of decreased cardiac contractility, which can cause decreased renal perfusion and fluid retention.
Monitor for peripheral (sacral, pedal) edema.	This edema can occur with diastolic dysfunction (right-sided) heart failure/myocardial infarction.
Assist with activities of daily living and facilitate coordination of health care providers, allowing 90 min for undisturbed rest. If necessary, limit visitors.	Rest decreases cardiac workload.
Administer medications as prescribed, such as beta-blockers, calcium channel blockers, and antidysrhythmic agents.	*Beta-blockers* (metoprolol XL) and *alpha/beta-adrenergic blockers* (carvedilol): Block effects of SNS and toxic effects of neurohormones on the myocardium. These drugs decrease HR and BP, thereby decreasing cardiac workload.
	Calcium channel blockers: May be used in diastolic HF to assist with relaxation and filling and reduce outflow tract obstruction (hypertrophic cardiomyopathy). Except for amlodipine or felodipine, calcium channel blockers are avoided in LV systolic dysfunction because they decrease cardiac contractility.
	Amiodarone is an example of an *antidysrhythmic* given for patients with HF.
Explain the potential for dysrhythmia management under the guidance of an electrophysiologist/cardiologist.	Dysrhythmias have become a major factor in quality-of-life issues and rehospitalization in patients with heart failure. Many of these patients require an implantable cardioverter-defibrillator (ICD) because of repeated life-threatening episodes of ventricular tachycardia from an irritable myocardium. Patients with ventricular asynchrony, as seen in bundle branch blocks, may benefit from a biventricular pacer. Pacing each ventricle in synchrony may result in better cardiac output.
Assist patient into position of comfort, usually semi-Fowler's position (HOB up 30-45 degrees).	This position decreases work of breathing and reduces cardiac workload.

••• **Related NIC and NOC labels:** *NIC:* Cardiac Care: Acute; Fluid Management; Vital Signs Monitoring; Emergency Care *NOC:* Cardiac Pump Effectiveness; Tissue Perfusion: Abdominal Organs; Tissue Perfusion: Peripheral: Vital Signs Status

Nursing Diagnosis:

Activity Intolerance

related to imbalance between oxygen supply and demand secondary to decrease in cardiac muscle contractility

Desired Outcome: During activity, patient rates perceived exertion at 3 or less on a 0-10 scale and exhibits cardiac tolerance to activity as evidenced by RR 20 breaths/min or less, SBP within 20 mm Hg of resting range, HR within 20 bpm of resting HR, and absence of chest pain and new dysrhythmias.

INTERVENTIONS	RATIONALES
Monitor patient's physiologic response to activity and report significant findings.	Chest pain, new dysrhythmias, increased shortness of breath, HR increased greater than 20 bpm over resting HR, and SBP greater than 20 mm Hg over resting SBP are significant findings of decreased cardiac output or cardiac failure that can manifest during activity.
Ask patient to rate perceived exertion (RPE) (see p. 62 for a description).	Optimally, patients should not experience RPE of more than 3. If this happens, intensity of the activity should be decreased and its frequency increased until RPE of 3 or less is achieved.
Monitor BP and other vital signs q4h, and report significant findings.	Findings such as irregular HR, HR greater than 100 bpm, or decreasing BP may be signs of cardiac ischemia.
Before hospital discharge teach patient self-measurement of HR for gauging exercise tolerance.	An HR that is too high increases myocardial O_2 demand; an HR that is too low may cause more ischemia. Patients should use an exertion scale and a pain scale to gauge exercise tolerance and ensure that HR is less than 20 bpm over baseline or as prescribed by health care provider.
Observe for and report oliguria, decreasing BP, decreased mentation, and dizziness.	These are signs of acute decreased cardiac output.
Assess peripheral pulses, distal extremity skin color, and urinary output. Report significant findings.	This assessment reveals integrity of peripheral perfusion. Changes such as decreased amplitude of pulses, pallor or cyanosis, and decreased urinary output are significant findings that should be reported for timely intervention.
In the presence of acute decreased cardiac output, ensure that patient's needs are met (e.g., by keeping water at the bedside and urinal or commode nearby, maintaining a quiet environment, and limiting visitors as necessary).	These measures promote adequate rest, prevent activity intolerance, and decreases cardiac workload.
Facilitate coordination of health care providers to provide rest periods between care activities. Allow 90 min for undisturbed rest.	Rest helps decrease cardiac workload.
Administer O_2 as prescribed.	Increasing oxygen supply to the myocardium promotes activity tolerance.
Assist with passive and some active or assistive range-of-motion and other exercises, depending on patient's tolerance and prescribed limitations.	Exercise prevents complications to joints and tissue caused by prolonged immobility.
Also discuss with health care provider patient's potential participation in an exercise program after hospital discharge.	Progressive monitored exercise for patients with heart failure can improve quality of life, activity tolerance, heart function, and disease outcomes.

••• **Related NIC and NOC labels:** *NIC:* Energy Management; Cardiac Care: Rehabilitative; Environmental Management; Exercise Therapy; Joint Mobility; Self-Care Assistance *NOC:* Activity Tolerance; Energy Conservation; Self-Care: Activities of Daily Living

Nursing Diagnosis:

Fear

related to potentially life-threatening situation

Desired Outcome: Within the 24 hr of this diagnosis, patient communicates fears and concerns and relates attainment of increasing physical and psychological comfort.

INTERVENTIONS	RATIONALES
Acknowledge patient's fears and provide opportunities for patient and significant other to express their feelings. Be reassuring and supportive.	Acknowledging feelings encourages communication and hence reduces fear. Empathy lessens a sense of isolation and fear.
Help make patient as comfortable as possible with prompt pain relief and positioning, typically high Fowler's position (HOB up 90 degrees).	Comfort measures may decrease the physiologic event that is contributing to the fear.
Keep environment as calm and quiet as possible.	This measure prevents or reduces the sensory overload that may contribute to patient's fear.
Explain all treatment modalities, especially those that may be uncomfortable (e.g., O_2 face mask and rotating tourniquets).	Increasing patient's knowledge level about therapies and procedures reduces/eliminates fear of the unknown and affords a sense of control.
Remain with patient if possible, providing emotional support for both patient and significant other.	Many individuals benefit from the support of others and find that it reduces their stress/fear level.
For further interventions, see "Psychosocial Support" for **Fear,** p. 76.	

••• Related NIC and NOC labels: *NIC:* Anxiety Reduction; Active Listening; Coping Enhancement; Presence; Support System Enhancement; Support Group *NOC:* Anxiety Control; Fear Control

Nursing Diagnosis:

Deficient Knowledge:

Purpose, precautions, and side effects of diuretic therapy

Desired Outcome: Within the 24-hr period before hospital discharge, patient verbalizes knowledge of the precautions and side effects of diuretic therapy.

INTERVENTIONS	RATIONALES
Assess patient's health care literacy (language, reading, comprehension). Assess culture and culturally specific information needs.	This assessment helps ensure that information is presented in a manner that is culturally and educationally appropriate.
Teach the purpose of the prescribed diuretic.	These drugs control fluid accumulation and reduce blood volume. Patients who are knowledgeable about their drug's purpose are more likely to adhere to the therapeutic regimen.
Depending on type of diuretic used, teach patient to report signs and symptoms of the following:	A knowledgeable patient will know how to monitor for and report symptoms that necessitate medical attention.
Hypokalemia: Anorexia, irregular pulse, nausea, apathy, and muscle cramps.	Use of furosemide and metolazone, potassium-wasting diuretics, can cause these symptoms.
Hyperkalemia: Muscle weakness, hyporeflexia, and irregular HR.	Use of amiloride and spironolactone, potassium-sparing diuretics, can cause these symptoms.
Hyponatremia: Fatigue, weakness, and edema (caused by fluid extravasation).	Use of bumetanide, a diuretic that promotes excretion of NaCl, may cause these symptoms.
For patients on long-term diuretic therapy, explain importance of follow-up monitoring of blood levels of potassium and sodium.	Although the most common electrolyte problem with diuretic use is hypokalemia, the potential for hyperkalemia and electrolyte imbalance of sodium continues with long-term therapy.
For patients receiving potassium-wasting diuretics (e.g., furosemide), teach need to consume supplemental high-potassium foods.	Foods high in potassium content, such as apricots, bananas, oranges, and raisins will help replenish potassium lost via diuretics.
As appropriate, instruct patient to use care when rising from a sitting or recumbent position.	There is potential for injury from orthostatic hypotension, which can occur with diuretic use because of diuresis.

••• Related NIC and NOC labels: *NIC:* Teaching: Prescribed Medication *NOC:* Knowledge: Medication

Nursing Diagnosis:

Deficient Knowledge:

Purpose, precautions, and side effects of digoxin therapy

Desired Outcome: Within the 24-hr period before hospital discharge, patient verbalizes understanding of the purpose, precautions, and side effects associated with digoxin therapy.

INTERVENTIONS	RATIONALES
Assess patient's health care literacy (language, reading, comprehension). Assess culture and culturally specific information needs.	This assessment helps ensure that information is presented in a manner that is culturally and educationally appropriate.
Teach the purpose of digoxin therapy.	Digoxin slows conduction through the atrioventricular (A-V) node and increases strength of contractility. Although not a first-line drug as originally believed for heart failure patients, it is used for dysrhythmia management when atrial fibrillation coexists, or to improve symptoms in class III-IV heart failure patients. A patient who is knowledgeable about the purpose of digoxin will be more likely to adhere to the therapy.
Teach technique and importance of assessing HR before taking digoxin.	Although patients should obtain HR parameters from their health care providers, digoxin is usually withheld when HR is less than 60 bpm (unless patient's usual HR is less than 60 bpm).
Teach patient to hold dose if there is 20 bpm or greater change from his or her normal rate and to notify health care provider if he or she has omitted a dose because of a slow or significantly changed HR.	Such a change may signal that patient is receiving too much medication and a dose adjustment may be necessary if a slowing of the HR persists.
Explain that serum potassium levels are monitored routinely.	Low levels of potassium can potentiate digoxin toxicity.
Explain that apical HR and peripheral pulses are assessed for irregularity.	Irregularity may signal presence of dysrhythmias (e.g., heart block), which is associated with digoxin toxicity.
Teach patient to be alert to nausea, vomiting, anorexia, headache, diarrhea, blurred vision, yellow-haze vision, and mental confusion. Explain importance of reporting signs and symptoms promptly to health care provider or staff if they occur.	These are other indicators of digoxin toxicity that necessitate prompt medical attention for timely intervention.

••• **Related NIC and NOC labels:** *NIC:* Teaching: Prescribed Medication *NOC:* Knowledge: Medication

Nursing Diagnosis:

Deficient Knowledge:

Precautions and side effects of vasodilators

Desired Outcome: Within the 24-hr period before hospital discharge, patient verbalizes knowledge of the purpose, precautions, and side effects of vasodilators.

INTERVENTIONS	RATIONALES
Assess patient's health care literacy (language, reading, comprehension). Assess culture and culturally specific information needs.	This assessment helps ensure that information is presented in a manner that is culturally and educationally appropriate.
Teach the purpose of this drug.	See discussion with **Impaired Gas Exchange,** earlier.
Explain that a headache can occur after administration of a vasodilator.	Headache can occur because of dilation of the cranial vessels or from orthostatic hypotension.
Suggest that lying down will help alleviate pain.	A supine position may help alleviate the pain by increasing blood flow to the heart and head, although blood flow to the head may worsen the headache. Pain medication and decreased dosage of the vasodilator may be necessary.
Teach importance of assessment for weight gain and signs of peripheral or sacral edema.	A possible side effect of vasodilator therapy is a decrease in venous return to the right side of the heart with subsequent accumulation in the periphery.
For patients on long-term ACE inhibitor therapy, explain importance of follow-up monitoring of blood levels of serum creatinine.	ACE inhibitors may cause kidney damage, resulting in decreased creatinine clearance. If this occurs, the patient may need to be taken off the drug.
For patients receiving ACE inhibitors, teach importance of using care when rising from a sitting or recumbent position.	There is potential for injury caused by orthostatic hypotension, a potential side effect of ACE inhibitors.
Teach patient receiving ACE inhibitors the technique for and importance of assessing BP before taking medication. Explain that it is possible to purchase automatic BP machines from local pharmacies and if necessary to seek reimbursement or funding information from a social worker.	Vasodilators can cause an excessive reduction in BP. Although patients should obtain BP parameters from health care providers, ACE inhibitors are usually withheld when BP is less than 110/60 mm Hg.
Teach patient to notify health care provider if he or she has omitted a dose because of a low or significantly changed BP.	It may be necessary to lower the dose or change the drug.

••• **Related NIC and NOC labels:** *NIC:* Teaching: Prescribed Medication *NOC:* Knowledge: Medication

ADDITIONAL NURSING DIAGNOSES/ PROBLEMS:

"Prolonged Bedrest"	p. 61
"Psychosocial Support"	p. 73
"Coronary Artery Disease" for **Imbalanced Nutrition: More Than Body Requirements**	p. 169
"Dysrhythmias and Conduction Disturbances" Patients with heart failure may require an ICD.	p. 177

✓ PATIENT-FAMILY TEACHING AND DISCHARGE PLANNING

When providing patient-family teaching, focus on sensory information, avoid giving excessive information, and initiate a visiting nurse referral for necessary follow-up teaching. Include verbal and written information about the following:

✓ Medications, including drug name, purpose, dosage, schedule, precautions, and potential side effects. Also discuss drug-drug, food-drug, and herb-drug interactions.

✓ Signs and symptoms that necessitate immediate medical attention: dyspnea, decreased exercise tolerance, alterations in pulse rate/rhythm, loss of consciousness (caused by dysrhythmias or decreased cardiac output), oliguria, and weight gain of greater than 2-3 lb in 24 hr or 3-5 lb in 48 hr.

✓ Reinforcement that heart failure/cardiomyopathy is a chronic disease requiring lifetime treatment.

✓ Importance of abstaining from alcohol, which increases cardiac muscle deterioration. Importance of a low-sodium diet to prevent undue fluid retention.

✓ Need for physical support from family and outside agencies as disease progresses.

✓ Availability of community and medical support, such as American Heart Association at *www.americanheart.org*.

Hypertension 22

OVERVIEW/PATHOPHYSIOLOGY

The incidence of hypertension among adults in the United States is 29%-31%, affecting 58 to 65 million persons. One half of individuals older than 65 years of age are affected by hypertension. Risk factors include heredity, race (incidence is higher in African Americans), high salt intake, renal disease, obesity, excessive alcohol intake, and some endocrine disorders (e.g., Cushing's disease, pheochromocytoma).

Complications of this disease include increased incidence of transient ischemic attack/stroke, retinopathy, coronary artery disease, heart failure, aortic aneurysm, and renal failure.

The seventh report of the Joint National Committee (JNC VII) defines hypertension as follows (based on the average of two or more properly measured readings at each of two or more visits after an initial screen):

- Normal blood pressure: SBP less than 120 mm Hg and DBP less than 80 mm Hg
- Prehypertension: SBP 120-139 mm Hg or DBP 80-89 mm Hg
- Hypertension
  - Stage 1: SBP 140-159 mm Hg or DBP 90-99 mm Hg
  - Stage 2: SBP 160 mm Hg or greater or DBP 100 mm Hg or greater

HEALTH CARE SETTING

Primary care or cardiology clinic setting most commonly; patients with severe hypertension may require acute hospitalization

Nursing Diagnosis:

Deficient Knowledge:

Need for frequent BP checks and adherence to antihypertensive therapy and lifestyle changes

Desired Outcome: Patient verbalizes knowledge of the importance of frequent BP checks and adhering to antihypertensive therapy and lifestyle changes.

INTERVENTIONS	RATIONALES
Teach importance of getting blood pressure (BP) checked at frequent intervals and adhering to prescribed medication therapy.	This measure will confirm if BP is within acceptable parameters. The goal of treatment is a BP less than 120/80 mm Hg or less than 120/70 mm Hg if diabetes or renal disease is present.
	The seventh Joint National Committee (JNC VII) recommends initiating therapy in uncomplicated hypertensive patients with a low-dose thiazide diuretic (e.g., 12.5 to 25 mg of hydrochlorothiazide). This drug improves outcomes, has few side effects, and is low in cost. Second-line drug therapy includes adding an angiotensin-converting enzyme inhibitor, ARB (angiotensin-renin blocker), beta-blocker, or calcium channel blocker.

Continued

INTERVENTIONS	RATIONALES
Provide teaching guidelines on importance of exercise, stress reduction, weight loss (if appropriate), and 2 g/day sodium diet. Review with patient how to read food labels and choose low sodium foods.	Treatment for this disease includes promotion of lifestyle modification, which can lower BP significantly if adhered to.
Caution patient about importance of seeking medical evaluation if BP reading is greater than 200/100 mm Hg or less than 90/60 mm Hg, or if headache, dizziness, or blurred vision occurs.	Severe hypertension or hypotension can be life threatening, compromising perfusion to vital organs.

●●● **Related NIC and NOC labels:** *NIC:* Anxiety Reduction; Behavior Modification; Teaching: Disease Process; Teaching: Prescribed Activity/ Exercise; Teaching: Prescribed Diet; Teaching: Prescribed Medication; Weight Management *NOC:* Knowledge: Cardiac Disease Management; Knowledge: Treatment Regimen

ADDITIONAL NURSING DIAGNOSES/ PROBLEMS:

"Psychosocial Support"	p. 73
"Coronary Artery Disease" for **Imbalanced Nutrition: More Than Body Requirements**	p. 169
Deficient Knowledge: Purpose, precautions, and side effects of beta-blockers	p. 170
Health-Seeking Behaviors: Relaxation technique effective for stress reduction	p. 172

✓ PATIENT-FAMILY TEACHING AND DISCHARGE PLANNING

When providing patient-family teaching, focus on sensory information, avoid giving excessive information, and initiate a visiting nurse referral for necessary follow-up teaching. Include verbal and written information about the following:

✓ Medications, including drug name, purpose, dosage, schedule, precautions, and potential side effects. Also discuss drug-drug, food-drug, and herb-drug interactions.

✓ Signs and symptoms that necessitate immediate medical attention: elevated or decreased BP readings (greater than 200/100 mm Hg or less than 90/60 mm Hg), headache, dizziness, blurred vision, chest pain, dyspnea, or syncope.

✓ Reinforcement that hypertension is a chronic disease requiring lifetime treatment.

✓ Importance of abstaining from excessive salt or alcohol intake, which increases blood pressure.

✓ Need for physical support from family and outside agencies.

✓ Self-blood pressure evaluation if indicated. Monitoring machines are available in local department stores and pharmacies. Remind patient that evaluation of BP should be done while seated, ideally at the same time each day, and recorded.

✓ Availability of community and medical support such as the American Heart Association at *www.americanheart.org*.

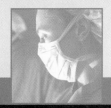

Pulmonary Hypertension 23

OVERVIEW/PATHOPHYSIOLOGY

As blood passes through the pulmonary vasculature, it exchanges CO_2 and particulate matter for O_2. Normally the pulmonary vascular bed offers little resistance to blood flow, but when resistance occurs, pulmonary pressures rise and pulmonary hypertension results. Pulmonary hypertension can be primary (rare), which has a poor prognosis and affects primarily young and middle-age women; or it can be secondary (most common), which often responds to therapy and is found in a variety of medical conditions. The cause of primary pulmonary hypertension (PPH) is unknown. It may be familial and has been linked to the bone morphogenetic protein receptor 2 (BMPR2). The underlying cause of secondary pulmonary hypertension often is chronic hypoxia, which can result from increased pulmonary blood flow from a ventricular or atrial shunt, left ventricular failure, chronic obstructive pulmonary disease (COPD) or sleep apnea, pulmonary embolus, interstitial lung disease, human immunodeficiency virus (HIV) infection, collagen vascular disorders such as scleroderma or lupus, portal hypertension due to liver disease, or any physiologic occurrence that increases pulmonary vascular resistance or constriction of the vessels in the pulmonary tree.

HEALTH CARE SETTING

Primary care with possible hospitalization in a medical-surgical unit resulting from complications or in a special center for heart-lung transplantation

ASSESSMENT

Acute indicators: Exertional dyspnea and fatigue (the most common presenting symptoms), eventually progressing to dyspnea at rest. Syncope, precordial chest pain, and palpitations can occur because of low cardiac output or hypoxia.

Chronic indicators: Signs of right or left ventricular failure as a result of right ventricular enlargement and eventual fluid overload.

Right ventricular failure: Peripheral edema, increased venous pressure and pulsations, liver engorgement, distended neck veins.

Left ventricular failure: Dyspnea; shortness of breath, particularly on exertion; decreased blood pressure (BP); oliguria; orthopnea; anorexia.

Physical assessment: Cyanosis from decreased cardiac output with subsequent systemic vasoconstriction and ventilation-perfusion mismatch, systolic murmur caused by tricuspid regurgitation or pulmonary stenosis, diastolic murmur caused by pulmonary valvular incompetence, accentuated S_2 heart sound, possible S_3 or S_4 heart sound, and a parasternal heave caused by right ventricular enlargement.

DIAGNOSTIC TESTS

Chest x-ray examination: Will show enlargement of the pulmonary artery and right atrium and ventricle. Pulmonary vasculature may appear engorged.

Echocardiography: Valuable for showing increased right ventricular dimension, thickened right ventricular wall, and possible tricuspid or pulmonary valve dysfunction. This test indirectly measures pulmonary artery systolic pressure.

Radionuclide imaging: Equilibrium-gated blood pool imaging and thallium imaging assess function of the right ventricle.

CT: Evaluates diameter of the main pulmonary arteries, which is helpful in evaluating severity of disease. High-resolution computerized axial tomography (CT) can confirm the presence of interstitial lung disease. Spiral CT is more specific in evaluating pulmonary embolus.

Right heart catheterization: Necessary to confirm pulmonary hypertension. It also provides helpful information regarding severity of the disease and establishing prognosis. Pulmonary vascular resistance will be very high, and pulmonary artery and right ventricular pressures can approach or equal systemic arterial pressures. Vasodilator challenge is often performed to assess reactivity and guide treatment. Adenosine, epoprostenol, and nitric oxide typically are used.

Pulmonary perfusion scintigraphy (perfusion scan): A noninvasive way to assess pulmonary blood flow. This study involves IV injection of serum albumin tagged with trace amounts of a radioisotope, most often technetium. The particles pass through the circulation and lodge in the pulmonary vascular bed. Subsequent scanning reveals concentrations of particles in areas of adequate pulmonary blood flow. Scan is normal in PPH. Abnormal scan suggests presence of thromboembolic pulmonary hypertension.

ECG results: Will show evidence of right atrial enlargement and right ventricular enlargement (evidenced by right axis deviation, right bundle branch block, tall and peaked P waves, and large R waves in V_1) secondary to the increased pressure needed to force blood through the hypertensive pulmonary vascular bed.

Pulmonary function test: Results are usually normal, although some individuals will have increased residual volume, reduced maximum voluntary ventilation, and decreased vital capacity.

Sleep study: Confirms diagnosis of sleep apnea as etiology for secondary pulmonary hypertension.

Exercise testing: Symptom-limited stress test or 6-min walk test can help assess severity of symptoms and guide response to treatment.

ABG analysis: May show low $Paco_2$ and high pH, which occur with hyperventilation, or increased $Paco_2$ with decreased gas exchange.

Oximetry: May show decreased O_2 saturation (e.g., 92% or less).

Blood tests to rule out secondary causes of pulmonary hypertension: Anti-nuclear antibody, rheumatoid arthritis, erythrocyte sedimentation rate (tests for collagen vascular disorders), HIV, and thyroid-stimulating hormone (thyroid abnormalities commonly coexist with pulmonary hypertension).

CBC: Polycythemia can occur in the presence of chronic hypoxemia as a result of compensation.

Liver function tests: May be abnormal if venous congestion is significant. Examples include increased aspartate aminotransferase (AST), alanine aminotransferase (ALT), and bilirubin.

Nursing Diagnosis:

Impaired Gas Exchange

related to altered blood flow secondary to pulmonary capillary constriction

Desired Outcome: Patient has improved gas exchange by at least 24 hr before hospital discharge, as evidenced by O_2 saturation greater than 92% (90% or greater for patients with COPD) and Pao_2 80 mm Hg or higher.

INTERVENTIONS	RATIONALES
Monitor for and document low O_2 saturation; report O_2 saturation 92% or less to health care provider.	This assessment detects low O_2 saturation, which may signal need for oxygen supplementation.
Monitor arterial blood gas (ABG) results. Report significant findings to health care provider.	This assessment detects signs of hypoventilation (decreased Pao_2, increased $Paco_2$, and decreased pH), which can signal respiratory failure, or hyperventilation (low $Paco_2$ and high pH), which can occur with anxiety or respiratory distress. Hypoxemia is the key gas deficit seen with pulmonary vascular vasoconstriction. Blood flow through the lungs is impaired, making it difficult to exchange O_2 for CO_2. O_2 becomes low (hypoxemia) and CO_2 becomes high (hypercarbia). Hypercarbia causes a change in pH to the acid side. Although initially respiratory in origin, hypoxemia eventually results in metabolic acidosis because of lactic acid production. Values outside of normal or acceptable range should be reported promptly for timely intervention.
Auscultate lung fields to assess lung sounds q4-8h, or more frequently as indicated.	This assessment detects adventitious sounds (especially rales), which can occur with fluid overload.
Assess respiratory rate (RR), pattern, and depth; chest excursion; and use of accessory muscles of respiration q4h.	Increased RR, abdominal breathing, use of accessory muscles, and nasal flaring are signals of hypoxia and respiratory distress.
Observe for and document presence of cyanosis or skin color change.	These indicators can occur as later signs of decreased gas exchange.
Monitor mental status and report significant changes.	Changes in mental acuity or level of consciousness (LOC) may be indications of acid-base imbalance.
Assist patient into Fowler's position (HOB up 90 degrees), if possible.	This position reduces work of breathing and maximizes chest excursion.
Teach patient to take slow, deep breaths.	This promotes gas exchange.
Administer prescribed O_2 as indicated.	Oxygen treats hypoxia. It can be administered continuously or only at bedtime or with exercise when oxygen desaturation is most likely to occur. If hypoxia is severe, O_2 is administered by mask.

Continued

INTERVENTIONS

Caution: Use care when administering O_2 to patients with a history of COPD.

Deliver O_2 with humidity.

RATIONALES

High concentrations of O_2 can depress the respiratory drive in individuals with chronic CO_2 retention.

Humidity helps prevent oxygen's drying effects on oral and nasal mucosa.

••• **Related NIC and NOC labels:** *NIC:* Oxygen Therapy; Positioning; Respiratory Monitoring; Laboratory Data Interpretation; Acid-Base Management *NOC:* Respiratory Status: Gas Exchange

Nursing Diagnosis:

Activity Intolerance

related to generalized weakness and imbalance between oxygen supply and demand secondary to right and left ventricular failure

Desired Outcome: By at least 24 hr before hospital discharge, patient rates perceived exertion at 3 or less on a 0-10 scale and exhibits cardiac tolerance to activity as evidenced by RR 20 breaths/min or less, HR 20 bpm or less over resting HR, and SBP within 20 mm Hg of resting range.

INTERVENTIONS	RATIONALES
Ask patient to rate perceived exertion (RPE) during activity, and monitor for evidence of activity intolerance. For details, see **Risk for Activity Intolerance** in "Prolonged Bedrest," p. 61. Notify health care provider of significant findings.	These assessments determine if activity intolerance is present (RPE higher than 3).
Observe for and document any changes in vital signs. Monitor BP at least q4h.	Drops in BP greater than 10-20 mm Hg, which can signal decompensation of cardiac muscle, should be reported promptly for timely intervention.
Also be alert to dyspnea, shortness of breath, crackles (rales), and decreased O_2 saturation (92% or less) as determined by oximetry.	These are signs of left ventricular failure.
Measure and document intake and output and weight, reporting any steady gains or losses. Be alert to peripheral edema, both pedal and sacral; ascites; distended neck veins; and increased central venous pressure (more than 12 cm H_2O).	These are signs of right ventricular failure.
Administer diuretics, vasodilators, and calcium channel blockers as prescribed.	*Diuretics:* These are used in the presence of right-sided (diastolic dysfunction) or left-sided (systolic dysfunction) heart failure and fluid overload.
	Vasodilators: The goal of medical therapy is to decrease pulmonary artery pressure by vasodilation. Epoprostenol is a potent IV vasodilator that also inhibits platelet aggregation. It is continuously infused through a long-term venous access device. Drawbacks to this medication include significant cost and severe side effects, including rebound pulmonary hypertension if stopped abruptly. Treprostinil is another vasodilator that is administered continuously via subcutaneous infusion. Like epoprostenol, it is expensive and cannot be discontinued abruptly. Bosentan is an oral vasodilator approved for use in pulmonary hypertension.
	Calcium channel blockers: These are helpful in patients who demonstrate response to vasodilator challenge and are administered in higher doses than when they are used to treat hypertension.
Facilitate coordination of health care providers. Allow time for undisturbed rest. If necessary, limit visitors.	Rest helps decrease oxygen demand.
Keep frequently used items within patient's reach.	This measure prevents exertion as much as possible.

Continued

INTERVENTIONS	RATIONALES
Assist with maintaining prescribed activity level and progress as tolerated. If activity intolerance is observed, stop the activity and have patient rest.	These measures increase patient's activity tolerance while preventing overexertion.
Assist with range-of-motion exercises at frequent intervals. Plan progressive ambulation and exercise based on patient's tolerance and prescribed activity restrictions.	These measures help prevent complications caused by immobility while avoiding overexertion.

••• **Related NIC and NOC labels:** *NIC:* Energy Management; Medication Management; Visitation Facilitation; Exercise Promotion; Environmental Management *NOC:* Activity Tolerance; Energy Conservation; Endurance

Nursing Diagnosis:

Deficient Knowledge:

Disease process and treatment

Desired Outcome: Within the 24 hr period before hospital discharge, patient and significant other verbalize knowledge of the disease, its treatment, and measures that promote wellness.

INTERVENTIONS	RATIONALES
Assess patient's health care literacy (language, comprehension, reading). Assess culture and culturally specific information needs.	This assessment helps ensure that information is presented in a manner that is culturally and educationally appropriate.
Assess patient's level of knowledge of the disease process and its treatment.	This information enables development of an individualized teaching plan. A knowledgeable patient is more likely to adhere to the treatment.
Discuss purposes of the medications:	
Vasodilators	These ease workload of the heart by decreasing systemic resistance.
Calcium channel blockers	These "relax" the heart by decreasing coronary artery spasm.
Diuretics	These prevent fluid accumulation.
Anticoagulants (warfarin sodium)	These promote improved long-term survival by preventing thromboembolic complications.
Provide emotional support to the patient adapting to the concept of having a chronic disease.	This action reinforces need to adhere to lifetime therapy while also expressing empathy.
If the cause of pulmonary hypertension is known, reinforce explanations of the disease process and treatment.	A knowledgeable patient is more likely to adhere to the treatment regimen.
Discuss lifestyle changes that may be required.	Changes may be necessary to prevent future complications and facilitate self-control of the disease process.
Explain value of relaxation techniques, including tapes, soothing music, meditation, and biofeedback.	See "Coronary Artery Disease," **Health-Seeking Behaviors:** Relaxation technique effective for stress reduction, p. 172.
If patient smokes, provide materials that explain benefits of smoking cessation, such as pamphlets prepared by the American Heart Association (*www.americanheart.org*). Provide telephone numbers for local smoking cessation programs.	Smoking increases workload of the heart by causing vasoconstriction.
Confer with health care provider about type of exercise program that will benefit patient; provide patient teaching as indicated.	Exercise is good for vascular tone. However, increasing circulation as it relates to pulmonary hypertension will be determined by health care provider and physical therapist.
If appropriate, involve dietitian to assist patient with planning low-sodium meals.	A diet low in sodium may be necessary if signs of heart failure are present.

Continued

INTERVENTIONS	RATIONALES
Discuss treatment of causative factor, if possible.	Examples include surgical closure of arteriovenous shunts; replacement of defective valves; or treatment of sleep apnea, pulmonary embolism, or COPD.
As indicated, explain possibility of a heart-lung transplantation.	Transplantation may be considered for advanced (end-stage) pulmonary vascular disease that is not responsive to medical therapy.

••• **Related NIC and NOC labels:** *NIC:* Teaching: Disease Process; Discharge Planning; Teaching: Prescribed Medication *NOC:* Knowledge: Disease Process; Knowledge: Medication; Knowledge: Illness Care

ADDITIONAL NURSING DIAGNOSES/ PROBLEMS:

"Psychosocial Support"	p. 73
"Psychosocial Support for the Patient's Family and Significant Other"	p. 87
"Coronary Artery Disease" for **Health-Seeking Behaviors:** Relaxation technique effective for stress reduction	p. 172
"Heart Failure" for **Excess Fluid Volume**	p. 184
Deficient Knowledge: Precautions and side effects of diuretic therapy	p. 189
Deficient Knowledge: Precautions and side effects of vasodilators	p. 190

 PATIENT-FAMILY TEACHING AND DISCHARGE PLANNING

When providing patient-family teaching, focus on sensory information, avoid giving too much information, and initiate a visiting nurse referral for necessary follow-up teaching. Include verbal and written information about the following:

✓ Indicators that necessitate medical attention: decreased exercise tolerance, increasing shortness of breath or dyspnea, swelling of ankles and legs, steady weight gain.

✓ Medications, including drug name, purpose, dosage, schedule, precautions, and potential side effects. Also discuss drug-drug, food-drug, and herb-drug interactions.

✓ Elimination of smoking; refer patient to a smoking cessation program as appropriate. The following free brochures outline ways to help patients stop smoking:

- *How to Help Your Patients Stop Using Tobacco: A National Cancer Institute Manual for the Oral Health Team*, from the Smoking and Tobacco Control Program of the National Cancer Institute.
- *Clinical Practice Guideline: A Quick Reference Guide for Smoking Cessation Specialists*, from the Agency for Health Care Policy and Research (AHCPR).

For additional information see **Deficient Knowledge** on p. 198.

Venous Thrombosis/ 24
Thrombophlebitis

OVERVIEW/PATHOPHYSIOLOGY

Although venous thrombosis and thrombophlebitis are different disorders, clinically the terms are used interchangeably to refer to development of a venous thrombus or thrombi, with associated inflammation. Disturbances in the venous system can have a variety of causes and precipitating factors, including stasis of blood, hemoconcentration, venous trauma, inflammation, or hypercoagulable states. Venous stasis can occur with heart failure, shock states, immobility from prolonged bedrest, structural disorders of the veins, and immobility on the operating room table or from abdominal, pelvic, or orthopedic operative procedures. Hemoconcentration most commonly occurs with dehydration or inadequate fluid resuscitation after surgery. Vessel trauma can result from chemical irritation caused by IV solutions, direct trauma, or positioning. Hypercoagulable states can occur because of malignancies, hereditary factors, or estrogen therapy (replacement or contraception). Venous thrombosis generally occurs in the deep venous system and thrombophlebitis in the superficial system. Both most often occur in the lower extremities, and the most serious complication is embolization from the deep system causing a pulmonary embolus.

HEALTH CARE SETTING

Primary care with hospitalization resulting from complications

ASSESSMENT

Signs and symptoms: Assessments may be divided into those in the area of the thrombus (associated with inflammation) and those distal to the clot (associated with venous congestion). Over the site of thrombus, assessments include pain, tenderness, erythema, local warmth, and increased limb circumference. Distal to the area of thrombus, the extremity will be cool, pale or cyanotic, and edematous and will display prominent superficial veins. Additional findings include unilateral leg swelling, fever, and tachycardia. Sometimes the condition is clinically "silent," and the presenting sign is a pulmonary embolus (PE). (See "Pulmonary Embolus," p. 137.)

Physical assessment: A knot or bump occasionally can be felt on palpation. If patient is asymptomatic for deep vein thrombosis (DVT), pain elicited with foot dorsiflexion (Homans' sign) may be a sign of DVT, but clinical suspicion often guides further diagnostic workup.

Risk factors: Prolonged bedrest and immobility, leg trauma, recent surgery, use of oral contraceptives or hormone replacement therapy, hypercoagulable condition, obesity, varicose veins.

DIAGNOSTIC TESTS

Doppler ultrasound: Identifies changes in blood flow secondary to presence of a thrombus. Doppler venous sounds are similar to that of wind blowing and are respirophasic (wax and wane with patient's inspiration).

Duplex imaging: Use of ultrasound to assess veins for changes in flow and increased velocities when a clot is obstructing flow. Accuracy and sensitivity are good diagnostic measures for DVT.

Impedance plethysmography: Estimates blood flow using measures of resistance and normal changes that occur during pulsatile blood flow. It is highly accurate above the knee.

Plasma markers (D-dimer test): A positive plasma D-dimer test is indicative of fibrin breakdown, and further evaluation is warranted. A negative D-dimer test is helpful in excluding DVT if noninvasive testing also is negative.

Nursing Diagnosis:

Ineffective Tissue Perfusion: Peripheral and Cardiopulmonary
(or risk of same)

related to interrupted blood flow secondary to embolization from thrombus formation

Desired Outcome: Patient has adequate peripheral and cardiopulmonary perfusion as evidenced by normal extremity color, temperature, and sensation; RR 12-20 breaths/min with normal depth and pattern (eupnea); HR 100 bpm or less; BP within 20 mm Hg of baseline BP; O_2 saturation greater than 92%; and normal breath sounds.

INTERVENTIONS	RATIONALES
Be alert to and promptly report pain, erythema, increased limb girth, local warmth, distal pale skin, edema, and venous dilation. If indicators appear, maintain patient on bedrest and notify health care provider promptly.	These are early indicators of peripheral thrombus formation, which necessitate bedrest and prompt medical attention to prevent embolization.
Monitor for and immediately report sudden onset of chest pain, dyspnea, tachypnea, tachycardia, hypotension, hemoptysis, shallow respirations, crackles (rales), O_2 saturation of 92% or less, decreased breath sounds, and diaphoresis.	These are signs of PE, a life-threatening situation. If they occur, prompt medical attention is crucial.
Administer anticoagulants as prescribed.	Anticoagulants prevent propagation of a clot. Heparin is used during the acute phase, and long-term warfarin therapy is used after the acute phase. Six months of anticoagulation is recommended for a first occurrence of DVT. Low-molecular-weight heparin is administered subcutaneously, enabling outpatient management of DVT until warfarin levels are therapeutic.
	Note: Some surgeons implant a vena caval filter transvenously to provide filtration of blood from distal sites to prevent PE. This is most often used when patients cannot be anticoagulated or have had PEs while being therapeutically anticoagulated.
Double-check drip rates and doses with a colleague.	Correct dosing is essential to avoid bleeding while preventing clot formation.
Keep patient on bedrest, provide range-of-motion (ROM) exercises and apply support hose, sequential compression device, or pneumatic foot compression device as prescribed.	These measures decrease lower extremity edema and minimize risk of or prevent further DVTs.
Caution: In the presence of DVT/clot, avoid these interventions.	This restriction helps prevent embolization, although the interventions may be used on other extremities.
Maintain elevation of foot of bed.	This measure promotes venous drainage.

••• Related NIC and NOC labels: *NIC:* Bleeding Precautions; Embolus Care: Peripheral; Embolus Care: Pulmonary; Embolus Precautions; Medication Administration *NOC:* Circulation Status; Tissue Perfusion: Pulmonary; Tissue Perfusion: Peripheral

Nursing Diagnosis:

Acute Pain

related to inflammatory process caused by thrombus formation

Desired Outcomes: Within 1 hr of intervention, patient's subjective perception of pain decreases, as documented by a pain scale. Objective indicators, such as grimacing, are absent.

INTERVENTIONS	RATIONALES
Monitor patient for presence of pain. Document degree of pain, using a pain scale from 0 (no pain) to 10 (worst pain). Administer analgesics as prescribed, and document relief obtained using pain scale.	This assessment and these interventions evaluate trend of pain, determine most effective analgesic, relieve pain, and enable more accurate assessment of degree of pain relief obtained.
Ensure patient maintains bedrest during acute phase.	This measure minimizes painful engorgement and potential for embolization.
If prescribed, apply warm, moist packs. Be sure packs are warm (but not extremely so) and not allowed to cool.	Continuous moist heat may be beneficial in reducing discomfort and pain by promoting vasodilation and blood supply to the area.
Keep legs elevated when possible.	Elevation promotes venous drainage and reduces engorgement.
Avoid flexion of hips or knees.	Flexion contributes to venous stasis and discomfort.

••• **Related NIC and NOC labels:** *NIC:* Pain Management; Analgesic Administration; Positioning; Heat Application *NOC:* Comfort Level; Pain Control

Nursing Diagnosis:

Ineffective Tissue Perfusion: Peripheral (or risk for same)

related to interrupted venous flow secondary to venous engorgement or edema

Desired Outcome: Patient has adequate peripheral perfusion as evidenced by absence of discomfort and presence of normal extremity temperature, color, sensation, and motor function.

INTERVENTIONS	RATIONALES
Assess for pain and changes in skin temperature, color, and motor or sensory function. Be alert to venous engorgement (prominence) in lower extremities.	These are signs of inadequate peripheral perfusion.
Elevate patient's legs.	Elevation promotes venous drainage.
As prescribed for patients without evidence of thrombus formation, apply antiembolic hose.	These hose compress superficial veins to increase blood flow to the deeper veins.
Remove stockings for approximately 15 min q8h.	This measure enables skin inspection for evidence of irritation and decreased circulation.
In the absence of known DVT, apply sequential compression device or pneumatic foot compression device as prescribed.	These devices increase blood flow in the deep and superficial veins to prevent DVT and are often indicated for patients who are mostly immobile.
Remove these devices for 15 min q8h.	Removal enables skin inspection for evidence of irritation and decreased circulation.
Place a cloth sleeve (stockinette) beneath plastic device.	This measure prevents trapping of heat and moisture, which could irritate or harm skin.
Encourage patient to perform ankle circling and active or assisted ROM exercises of the lower extremities. Perform passive ROM exercises if patient cannot.	These exercises prevent venous stasis, which is a known cause of venous disorders.
Caution: If there are any signs of acute thrombus formation, such as calf hardness or tenderness, exercises are contraindicated. Notify health care provider.	This restriction minimizes risk of embolization.
Encourage deep breathing.	Deep breathing creates increased negative pressure in the lungs and thorax to assist in emptying of large veins.
Assess peripheral pulses regularly.	Although arterial circulation usually will not be impaired unless there is arterial disease or severe edema compressing arterial flow, regular pulse assessment will confirm presence of good arterial flow.

••• **Related NIC and NOC labels:** *NIC:* Circulatory Care: Venous Insufficiency; Circulatory Precautions; Positioning; Pneumatic Tourniquet Precautions *NOC:* Tissue Perfusion: Peripheral

Nursing Diagnosis:

Deficient Knowledge:

Disease process with venous thrombosis/thrombophlebitis and the necessary at-home treatment/management measures after hospital discharge

Desired Outcome: Before hospital discharge, patient verbalizes knowledge of the disease process and treatment/management measures that are to occur after hospital discharge.

INTERVENTIONS	RATIONALES
Assess patient's health care literacy (language, reading, comprehension). Assess culture and culturally specific education needs.	This assessment helps ensure that information is present in a manner that is culturally and educationally appropriate.
Discuss process of venous thrombosis/thrombophlebitis and ways to prevent thrombosis and discomfort.	Avoiding restrictive clothing, avoiding prolonged periods of standing, and elevating legs above heart level when sitting promote venous return and help prevent DVT while promoting comfort. In addition, regular walking and active ankle and leg ROM exercises promote venous return, strengthen leg muscles, and facilitate development of collateral vessels.
Teach signs of venous stasis ulcers.	Such indicators as redness and skin breakdown are signals of venous stasis ulcers, which necessitates medical attention before they lead to complications such as infection or even gangrene.
Stress importance of avoiding trauma to extremities and keeping skin clean and dry.	Avoiding trauma decreases risk of skin breakdown; clean and dry skin helps prevent infection that could develop in broken skin.
Instruct patient to inspect both feet each day. If necessary, suggest patient use a long-handled mirror to see bottoms of feet. Advise patient to report any open areas to health care provider.	Foot inspection will detect bruises or open wounds, inasmuch as tissues of the lower extremities are especially affected by decreased perfusion and are susceptible to injury. In addition, patients on anticoagulant therapy are at risk for bruising and bleeding. This can result in open wounds, which can lead to infection and even gangrene. Patient needs to report problems promptly for timely intervention.
Discuss prescribed exercise program.	Walking usually is considered the best exercise, although other exercises involving the lower extremities also prevent venous stasis, strengthen lower leg muscles, and help develop collateral vessels where circulation may be routed.
Teach patient how to wear antiembolic hose if prescribed.	Decreasing venous distention with these hose optimally will increase blood flow back to the heart.
Teach patient that the hose fit properly without wrinkling.	For example, some hose are worn snug over the feet and progressively less snug as they reach the knee or thigh. Such hose facilitate movement of blood forward and up, increasing blood return to the heart.
Describe indicators that necessitate medical attention.	Persistent redness, swelling, tenderness, weak or absent pulses, and ulcerations in the extremities may be signs of infection and worsening venous congestion. This needs to be reported to the health care provider promptly to avoid systemic infection and further compromise to circulation.
Encourage long-term management with elastic stockings.	This measure will help prevent sequelae associated with postphlebitic syndrome and chronic venous insufficiency.

●●● **Related NIC and NOC labels:** *NIC:* Teaching: Disease Process; Discharge Planning; Teaching: Prescribed Activity/Exercise; Teaching: Psychomotor Skill *NOC:* Knowledge: Disease Process; Knowledge: Illness Care; Knowledge: Prescribed Activity

---

ADDITIONAL NURSING DIAGNOSES/ PROBLEMS:

"Pulmonary Embolus" for **Ineffective Protection**   p. 139
related to prolonged bleeding or hemorrhage
secondary to anticoagulation therapy

✓ ## PATIENT-FAMILY TEACHING AND DISCHARGE PLANNING

When providing patient-family teaching, focus on sensory information, avoid giving excessive information, and initiate a visiting nurse referral for necessary follow-up teaching. Include verbal and written information about the following:

✓ See **Deficient Knowledge** for topics to discuss, both verbally and through written information, with patient and significant other.

✓ If patient is discharged from hospital on warfarin therapy, provide information about the following:

- As directed, see health care provider for scheduled international normalized ratio checks.
- Take warfarin at same time each day; do not skip days unless directed to by health care provider.
- Wear a medical alert bracelet.
- Avoid alcohol consumption and changes in diet (e.g., changing to a vegetarian diet), both of which can alter the body's response to warfarin.
- When making appointments with other health care providers and dentists, inform them that warfarin is being taken.
- Be alert to indicators that necessitate immediate medical attention: hematuria, hematemesis, menometrorrhagia, hematochezia, melena, epistaxis, bleeding gums, ecchymosis, hemoptysis, dizziness, and weakness.
- Avoid taking over-the-counter medications (e.g., aspirin, which also prolongs coagulation time) without consulting health care provider or nurse.
- Avoid trauma to extremities.

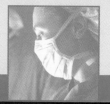

Benign Prostatic Hypertrophy 25

OVERVIEW/PATHOPHYSIOLOGY

The prostate is an encapsulated gland that surrounds the male urethra below the bladder neck and produces a thin, milky fluid during ejaculation. As a man ages, the prostate gland grows larger. Although the exact cause of enlargement is unknown, one theory is that hormonal changes affect the estrogen-androgen balance. This noncancerous enlargement is common in men older than 50 yr of age, and as many as 80% of men older than 65 yr of age are believed to have symptoms of prostatic enlargement. Treatment is given when symptoms of bladder outlet obstruction appear.

HEALTH CARE SETTING

Primary care; outpatient acute (surgical) care

ASSESSMENT

Chronic indicators: Urinary frequency, hesitancy, urgency, and dribbling or postvoid dribbling; decreased force and caliber of stream; nocturia (several times each night); hematuria. Scores on American Urological Association (AUA) questionnaire are 0-7 (mild), 8-19 (moderate), and 20-35 (severe).

Acute indicators/bladder outlet obstruction: Anuria, nausea, vomiting, severe suprapubic pain, severe and constant urgency, flank pain during micturition.

Physical assessment: Bladder distention, kettledrum sound with percussion over the distended bladder. Rectal examination reveals a smooth, firm, symmetric, and elastic enlargement of the prostate.

DIAGNOSTIC TESTS

Urinalysis: Checks for presence of white blood cells (WBCs), leukocyte esterase, WBC casts, bacteria, and microscopic hematuria.

Urine culture and sensitivity: Verifies presence of an infecting organism, identifies type of organism, and determines the organism's antibiotic sensitivities. **Note:** All urine specimens

should be sent to the laboratory immediately after they are obtained, or they should be refrigerated if this is not possible (specimens for urine culture should not be refrigerated). Urine left at room temperature has a greater potential for bacterial growth, turbidity, and alkaline pH, any of which can distort test results.

Hct and Hgb: Decreased hematocrit (Hct) and hemoglobin (Hgb) values may signal mild anemia from local bleeding.

BUN and creatinine: To evaluate renal and urinary function. **Note:** Blood urea nitrogen (BUN) can be affected by patient's hydration status, and results must be evaluated accordingly: fluid volume excess reduces BUN levels, whereas fluid volume deficit increases them. Serum creatinine may not be a reliable indicator of renal function in older adults because of decreased muscle mass and decreased glomerular filtration rate; results of this test must be evaluated along with those of urine creatinine clearance, other renal function studies, and patient's age.

Prostate-specific antigen: Elevated above normal (0-4.0 ng/ml; normal range may increase with age); correlates well with positive digital examination findings. This glycoprotein is produced only by the prostate and reflects prostate size.

Cystoscopy: Visualizes prostate gland, estimates its size, and ascertains presence of any damage to the bladder wall secondary to an enlarged prostate. **Note:** Because patients undergoing cystoscopy are susceptible to septic shock, this procedure is contraindicated in patients with acute urinary tract infection (UTI) because of the possible danger of hematogenous spread of gram-negative bacteria.

Transrectal ultrasound: Assesses prostate size and shape via a probe inserted into the rectum.

Maximal urinary flow rate: Rate less than 15 ml/sec indicates significant obstruction to flow.

Postvoid residual volume: Normal volume is less than 12 ml; higher volumes signal obstructive process.

Nursing Diagnosis:

Acute Confusion (or risk for same)

related to fluid volume deficit secondary to postsurgical bleeding/hemorrhage, fluid volume excess secondary to absorption of irrigating fluid during surgery, or cerebral hypoxia secondary to infectious process or sepsis

Desired Outcomes: Patient's mental status returns to normal for patient within 3 days of treatment. Patient exhibits no evidence of injury as a result of altered mental status.

INTERVENTIONS	RATIONALES
Assess patient's baseline level of consciousness (LOC) and mental status on admission. Ask patient to perform a three-step task.	Asking patient to perform a three-step task (e.g., "Raise your right hand, place it on your left shoulder, and then place the right hand by your side") is an effective way to evaluate baseline mental status because patient may be admitted with chronic confusion.
Test short-term memory.	Short-term memory can be tested by showing patient how to use call light, having patient return the demonstration, and then waiting 5 min before having patient demonstrate use of call light again. Inability to remember beyond 5 min indicates poor short-term memory.
Document patient's response.	Patient's baseline status can then be compared with postsurgical status for evaluation, which will help determine presence of acute confusion.
Document patient's actions in behavioral terms. Describe "confused" behavior.	This ensures that patient's current/postsurgical status is compared with his normal status.
Obtain description of prehospital functional and mental status from sources familiar with patient (e.g., patient's family, friends, personnel at nursing home or residential care facility).	The cause may be reversible.
Identify cause of acute confusion as follows:	
- Assess oximetry or request arterial blood gas values.	Low levels of oxygen can contribute to diminished mental status.
- Check serum or fingerstick glucose.	Hypoglycemia can affect mental status.
- Request current serum electrolytes and WBC count.	Imbalances in electrolytes and the presence of infection (reflected by elevated WBC count) can affect mental status.
- Assess hydration status by reviewing intake and output (I&O) records after surgery. Output should match intake.	Both excess and deficient fluid volumes can affect mental status.
- Assess legs for presence of dependent edema.	Dependent edema can signal overhydration with poor venous return, which can affect mental status.
- Assess cardiac and lung status.	Abnormal heart sounds or rhythms and presence of crackles (rales) in lung bases can signal fluid excess, which could affect mental status.
- Assess mouth for furrowed tongue and dry mucous membranes.	These signs signal fluid deficit, which can affect mental status.
- For oximetry readings 92% or less, anticipate initiation of oxygen therapy to increase oxygenation.	Patients usually require supplementary oxygen at these levels. Decreased levels of oxygen can adversely affect mental status.
- As appropriate, anticipate initiation of antibiotics in the presence of sepsis, diuretics to increase diuresis, and increased fluid intake by mouth or IV to rehydrate patient.	These interventions may help reverse acute confusion.
As appropriate, have patient wear glasses and hearing aid, or keep them close to the bedside and within patient's easy reach.	Disturbed sensory perception can contribute to confusion.
Keep patient's urinal and other commonly used items within easy reach.	Patients with short-term memory problems cannot be expected to use call light.
As indicated by mental status, check on patient frequently or every time you pass by the room.	This intervention helps ensure patient's safety.
If indicated, place patient close to nurse's station if possible. Provide environment that is nonstimulating and safe.	These measures provide a safer and less confusing environment for patient.
Provide music, but avoid use of television.	Individuals who are acutely confused regarding place and time often think action on television is happening in the room.

Continued

INTERVENTIONS	RATIONALES
Attempt to reorient patient to surroundings as needed. Keep clock and calendar at the bedside, and remind patient verbally of date and place.	These orientation measures help reduce confusion.
Encourage patient or significant other to bring items familiar to patient.	Familiar items provide a foundation for orientation and can include blankets, bedspreads, and pictures of family or pets.
If patient becomes belligerent, angry, or argumentative while you are attempting to reorient him, *stop this approach.* Do not argue with patient or patient's interpretation of the environment.	Arguing with confused patients likely will increase their belligerence. State "I can understand why you may (hear, think, see) that."
If patient displays hostile behavior or misperceives your role (e.g., nurse becomes thief, jailer), leave the room. Return in 15 min. Introduce yourself to patient as though you have never met. Begin dialogue anew.	Patients who are acutely confused have poor short-term memory and may not remember the previous encounter or that you were involved in that encounter.
If patient attempts to leave the hospital, walk with him and attempt distraction. Ask patient to tell you about his destination. For example, "That sounds like a wonderful place! Tell me about it." Keep tone pleasant and conversational. Continue walking with patient away from exits and doors around the unit. After a few minutes, attempt to guide patient back to his room.	Distraction is an effective technique with individuals who are confused.
If patient has permanent or severe cognitive impairment, check on him frequently and reorient to baseline mental status as indicated; however, do not argue with patient about his perception of reality.	Arguing can cause a cognitively impaired person to become aggressive and combative. Patients with severe cognitive impairments (e.g., Alzheimer's disease, dementia) also can experience acute confusional states (i.e., delirium) and can be returned to their baseline mental state.

••• **Related NIC and NOC labels:** *NIC*: Delirium Management; Delusion Management; Reality Orientation; Cognitive Stimulation; Cerebral Perfusion Management; Environmental Management: Safety; Fall Prevention; Neurologic Monitoring; Hypoglycemia Management; Distraction; Fluid/Electrolyte Management; Calming Technique *NOC*: Cognitive Orientation; Distorted Thought Control; Information Processing; Safety Behavior: Personal

Nursing Diagnosis:

Risk for Deficient Fluid Volume

related to postsurgical bleeding/hemorrhage

Desired Outcomes: Patient is normovolemic as evidenced by balanced I&O; HR 100 bpm or less (or within patient's normal range); BP 90/60 mm Hg or more (or within patient's normal range); RR 20 breaths/min or less; and skin that is warm, dry, and of normal color. Following instruction, patient relates actions that may result in hemorrhage of the prostatic capsule and participates in interventions to prevent them.

INTERVENTIONS	RATIONALES
On patient's return from recovery room, monitor vital signs (VS) as patient's condition warrants or per agency protocol.	These assessments evaluate trend of patient's recovery. Increasing pulse, decreasing BP, diaphoresis, pallor, and increasing respirations can occur with hemorrhage and impending shock.
Monitor and document I&O q8h. Subtract amount of fluid used with continuous bladder irrigation (CBI) from total output.	This assessment evaluates trend of patient's hydration status and assesses for postsurgical bleeding.
Monitor catheter drainage closely for first 24 hr. Watch for dark red drainage that does not lighten to reddish pink or drainage that remains thick in consistency after irrigation.	Drainage should lighten to pink or blood tinged within 24 hr after surgery. Dark red drainage that does not lighten to reddish pink or drainage that remains thick in consistency after irrigation can signal bleeding within the operative site.
Be alert to bright red, thick drainage at any time.	This drainage can occur with arterial bleeding within the operative site.

Continued

INTERVENTIONS	RATIONALES
Do not measure temperature rectally or insert tubes or enemas into rectum. Instruct patient not to strain with bowel movements or sit for long periods.	These actions can result in pressure on the prostatic capsule and may lead to hemorrhage.
Obtain prescription for and provide stool softeners or cathartics as necessary. Encourage a diet high in fiber and increased fluid intake.	These measures aid in producing soft stool and preventing straining.
Maintain traction on indwelling urethral catheter for 4-8 hr after surgery or as directed.	The surgeon may establish traction on indwelling urethral catheter in the operating room to help prevent bleeding.

Note: Urethral catheters used after prostatic surgery commonly have a large retention balloon (30 ml). |
| Also monitor patient for signs of disseminated intravascular coagulation (DIC). Report significant findings promptly if they occur. For more information, see "Disseminated Intravascular Coagulation," p. 497. | DIC can result from release of large amounts of tissue thromboplastins during a transurethral prostatectomy (TURP). Indicators of DIC include active bleeding (dark red) without clots and unusual oozing from all puncture sites. |

••• **Related NIC and NOC labels:** *NIC:* Bleeding Precautions; Fluid Monitoring; Vital Signs Monitoring; Hemorrhage Control *NOC:* Fluid Balance

Nursing Diagnosis:

Excess Fluid Volume (or risk for same)

related to absorption of irrigating fluid during surgery (TURP syndrome)

Desired Outcomes: Following surgery, patient is normovolemic as evidenced by balanced I&O (after subtraction of irrigant from total output); orientation to person, place, and time with no significant changes in mental status; BP and HR within patient's normal range; absence of dysrhythmias; and electrolyte values within normal range. Urinary output is 30 ml/hr or more.

INTERVENTIONS	RATIONALES
Monitor and record VS.	This assessment evaluates hydration status along with corresponding electrolyte status. Sudden increases in BP with corresponding decrease in HR can occur with fluid volume excess.
Monitor pulse for dysrhythmias, including irregular rate and skipped beats.	Dysrhythmias, including irregular HR and skipped beats, can signal electrolyte imbalance, which can occur as a result of the high volumes of fluid used during irritation.
Monitor and record I&O. To determine true amount of urinary output, subtract amount of irrigant (CBI) from total output.	Large amounts of fluid, commonly plain sterile water, are used to irrigate the bladder during operative cystoscopy to remove blood and tissue, thereby enabling visualization of the surgical field. Over time, this fluid may be absorbed through the bladder wall into the systemic circulation.
Report discrepancies between I&O.	Differences may signal either fluid retention or fluid loss.
Monitor patient's mental and motor status. Assess for presence of muscle twitching, seizures, and changes in mentation.	These are signs of water intoxication and electrolyte imbalance, which can occur within 24 hr after surgery because of the high volumes of fluid used in irrigation.
Monitor electrolyte values, in particular those of Na^+.	Normal range for Na^+ is 137-147 mEq/L. Values less than that signal hyponatremia, which can occur with absorption of the extra fluids and its dilutional effect.
Promptly report indications of fluid overload and electrolyte imbalance to health care provider.	This intervention ensures prompt treatment, which may include diuretics.

••• **Related NIC and NOC labels:** *NIC:* Fluid Management; Fluid Monitoring; Fluid/Electrolyte Management; Electrolyte Management: Hyponatremia; Laboratory Data Interpretation; Vital Sign Monitoring; Neurologic Monitoring *NOC:* Electrolyte & Acid/Base Balance; Fluid Balance

Nursing Diagnosis:

Acute Pain

related to bladder spasms

Desired Outcomes: Within 1 hr of intervention, patient's subjective perception of pain decreases, as documented by pain scale. Objective indicators, such as grimacing, are absent or diminished.

INTERVENTIONS	RATIONALES
Assess and document quality, location, and duration of pain. Devise a pain scale with patient, rating pain from 0 (no pain) to 10 (worst pain).	This assessment establishes a baseline, monitors trend of pain, and determines subsequent response to medication.
Medicate patient with prescribed analgesics, narcotics, and antispasmodics as appropriate; evaluate and document patient's response, using pain scale.	Suppositories (e.g., belladonna and opium [B&O] suppositories) are contraindicated because of the potential for disrupting the incision, which is close to the rectum. Oral anticholinergics, such as oxybutynin, are used as antispasmodics instead.
Instruct patient to request analgesic before pain becomes severe.	Prolonged stimulation of the pain receptors results in increased sensitivity to painful stimuli and will increase amount of drug required to relieve pain.
Provide warm blankets or heating pad to affected area.	These measures increase regional circulation and relax tense muscles.
Monitor for leakage around catheter.	Leakage can signal presence of bladder spasms.
If patient has spasms, assure him that they are normal.	Spasms can occur from irritation of the bladder mucosa or from a clot that results in backup of urine into the bladder with concomitant mucosal irritation.
Encourage fluid intake.	Adequate hydration helps prevent spasms.
If health care provider has prescribed catheter irrigation for removal of clots, follow instructions carefully.	Gentle irrigation will prevent discomfort and injury to patient.
Monitor for presence of clots in the tubing. If clots are present for patient with CBI, adjust rate of bladder irrigation to maintain light red urine (with clots). If clots inhibit flow of urine, irrigate catheter by hand according to agency or health care provider's directive.	Total output should be greater than the amount of irrigant instilled. If output equals amount of irrigant or patient complains that his bladder is full, the catheter may be clogged with clots.

••• **Related NIC and NOC labels:** *NIC:* Medication Management; Pain Management; Heat/Cold Application *NOC:* Pain Control; Comfort Level

Nursing Diagnosis:

Risk for Impaired Skin Integrity

related to wound drainage from suprapubic or retropubic prostatectomy

Desired Outcome: Patient's skin remains nonerythremic and intact.

INTERVENTIONS	RATIONALES
Monitor skin and incisional dressings frequently during first 24 hr; change or reinforce dressings as needed.	If an incision has been made into the bladder, irritation can result from prolonged contact of urine with the skin.
Use Montgomery straps or gauze net (Surginet) rather than tape to secure dressing.	These measures ensure that the dressing is secure without the damage that tape can cause to the skin.
If drainage is copious after drain removal, apply wound drainage or ostomy pouch with skin barrier over the incision.	These measures provide a barrier between the skin and drainage.
Use pouch with an antireflux valve.	This valve prevents contamination from reflux.

••• **Related NIC and NOC labels:** *NIC:* Incision Site Care; Wound Care: Drainage *NOC:* Wound Healing: Primary Intention; Tissue Integrity: Skin

Nursing Diagnosis:

Deficient Knowledge:

Postsurgical sexual function

Desired Outcome: Following intervention/patient teaching, patient discusses concerns about sexuality and relates accurate information about sexual function.

INTERVENTIONS	RATIONALES
Assess patient's level of readiness to discuss sexual function; provide opportunities for patient to discuss fears and anxieties.	This assessment enables the appropriate time to provide patient teaching and optimally will reveal patient's specific fears and anxieties.
Assure patient who has had a simple prostatectomy that ability to attain and maintain an erection is unaltered.	Retrograde ejaculation (backward flow of seminal fluid into the bladder, which is eliminated with next urination) or "dry" ejaculation will occur in most patients, but this probably will end after a few months. However, it will not affect ability to achieve orgasm.
Be aware of your own feelings about sexuality.	If you are uncomfortable discussing sexuality, request that another staff member take responsibility for discussing concerns with the patient.
As indicated, encourage continuation of counseling after hospital discharge. Confer with health care provider and social services to identify appropriate referral.	Conferring with health care provider and social services will help identify appropriate referrals.

●●● **Related NIC and NOC labels:** *NIC:* Sexual Counseling; Teaching *NOC:* Sexual Functioning

Nursing Diagnosis:

Constipation (or risk for same)

related to postsurgical discomfort or fear of exerting excess pressure on prostatic capsule

Desired Outcome: By the third to fourth postoperative day, patient relates presence of a bowel pattern that is normal for him with minimal pain or straining.

INTERVENTIONS	RATIONALES
Document presence or absence and quality of bowel sounds in all four abdominal quadrants.	A patient whose bowel sounds have not yet returned but who states that he needs to have a bowel movement during the first 24 hr after surgery may have clots in the bladder that are creating pressure on the rectum. Assess for presence of clots (see **Acute Pain,** earlier) and irrigate the catheter as indicated.
Gather baseline information on patient's normal bowel pattern and document findings.	Each patient has a bowel pattern that is normal for him.
Teach patient to avoid straining when defecating.	Straining puts excess pressure on the prostatic capsule.
Unless contraindicated, encourage patient to drink 2-3 L of fluids on the day after surgery.	Adequate hydration helps ensure a softer stool with less of a tendency to strain.
Consult health care provider and dietitian about need for increased fiber in patient's diet.	Adding bulk to stools will minimize risk of damaging the prostatic capsule by straining.
Encourage patient to ambulate and be as active as possible.	Increased activity helps promote bowel movements by increasing peristalsis.
Consult health care provider about use of stool softeners for patient during postoperative period.	Soft stool will be less painful to evacuate following surgery and will cause less straining.
See "Prolonged Bedrest" for **Constipation,** p. 67, for more information.	

●●● **Related NIC and NOC labels:** *NIC:* Bowel Management; Fluid Management; Pain Management; Nutrition Management; Exercise Promotion; Medication Administration *NOC:* Bowel Elimination; Hydration; Symptom Control

Nursing Diagnosis:

Urge Urinary Incontinence

related to urethral irritation after removal of urethral catheter

Desired Outcome: Patient reports increasing periods of time between voidings by the second postoperative day and regains normal pattern of micturition within 4-6 wk after surgery.

INTERVENTIONS	RATIONALES
Before removing urethral catheter, explain to patient that he may void in small amounts for first 12 hr after catheter removal.	Irritation from the catheter may cause patient to void in small amounts. Initially patient may void q15-30min, but the interval between voidings should increase toward a more normal pattern.
Instruct patient to save urine in a urinal for first 24 hr after surgery. Inspect each voiding for color and consistency.	First urine specimens can be dark red from passage of old blood. Each successive specimen should be lighter in color.
Note and document time and amount of each voiding.	Initially patient may void q15-30min, but the time interval between voidings should increase toward a more normal pattern.
Encourage patient to drink 2.5-3.0 L/day if not contraindicated.	Low intake leads to highly concentrated urine, which irritates the bladder and can lead to incontinence.
Before hospital discharge, inform patient that dribbling may occur for first 4-6 wk after surgery.	Dribbling occurs because of disturbance of the bladder neck and urethra during prostate removal. As muscles strengthen and healing occurs (the urethra reaches normal size and function), dribbling stops.
Teach patient Kegel exercises (see **Deficient Knowledge,** p. 214.)	These exercises improve sphincter control.

••• **Related NIC and NOC labels:** *NIC:* Urinary Elimination Management; Fluid Management; Pelvic Muscle Exercise; Teaching: Procedure/Treatment *NOC:* Urinary Continence; Urinary Elimination

Nursing Diagnosis:

Stress Urinary Incontinence

related to temporary loss of muscle tone in urethral sphincter after radical prostatectomy

Desired Outcome: Within the 24-hr period before hospital discharge, patient relates understanding of cause of the temporary incontinence and regimen that must be observed to promote bladder control.

INTERVENTIONS	RATIONALES
Explain to patient that there is a potential for urinary incontinence after prostatectomy but that it should resolve within 6 mo. Describe reason for the incontinence, using aids such as anatomic illustrations.	A knowledgeable patient likely will adhere to the therapeutic regimen. Understanding that incontinence is a possibility but that it usually resolves should be encouraging.
Encourage patient to maintain adequate fluid intake of at least 2-3 L/day (unless contraindicated by an underlying cardiac dysfunction or other disorder).	Dilute urine is less irritating to the prostatic fossa and less likely to result in incontinence.
Instruct patient to avoid caffeine-containing drinks.	These fluids irritate the bladder and have a mild diuretic effect, which would make bladder control even more difficult.
Establish a bladder routine with patient before hospital discharge.	The goal of bladder training is to reduce the number of small voidings and thereby return patient to a more normal bladder function.
	The amount of time between voidings is determined to estimate how long the patient can hold his urine.
	Patient schedules times for emptying his bladder and has a copy of the written schedule. An example initially would be q1-2h when awake and q4h at night. Then if this is successful, the patient lengthens the intervals between voidings.

Continued

INTERVENTIONS	RATIONALES
Teach patient Kegel exercises (see next nursing diagnosis).	These exercises promote sphincter control, thereby decreasing incontinence episodes.
Remind patient to discuss any incontinence problems with health care provider during follow-up examinations.	This information helps ensure that patient's needs are addressed and treated.

••• **Related NIC and NOC labels:** *NIC:* Pelvic Muscle Exercise; Bladder Training; Teaching: Individual *NOC:* Urinary Continence; Urinary Elimination

Nursing Diagnosis:

Deficient Knowledge:

Pelvic muscle (Kegel) exercise program to strengthen perineal muscles (effective for individuals with mild to moderate stress incontinence)

Desired Outcome: Within the 24-hr period following teaching, patient verbalizes and demonstrates accurate knowledge about the pelvic muscle (Kegel) exercise program.

INTERVENTIONS	RATIONALES
Explain purpose of Kegel exercises.	Kegel exercises strengthen pelvic area muscles, which will help regain bladder control.
Assist patient with identifying the correct muscle group.	A common error when attempting to perform this exercise is contracting the buttocks, quadriceps, and abdominal muscles.
Teach the exercise as follows:	
- Attempt to shut off urinary flow after beginning urination, hold for a few seconds, and then start the stream again.	This strengthens the proximal muscle. If it can be accomplished, the correct muscle group is being used.
- Contract the muscle around the anus as though to stop a bowel movement.	This strengthens the distal muscle.
- Repeat these exercises 10-20 times, qid.	These exercises must be done frequently throughout the day and for 2-9 mo before benefits are obtained.

••• **Related NIC and NOC labels:** *NIC:* Teaching: Prescribed Exercise *NOC:* Knowledge: Prescribed Activity (Exercise)

ADDITIONAL NURSING DIAGNOSES/ PROBLEMS:

"Perioperative Care"   p. 45

✓ PATIENT-FAMILY TEACHING AND DISCHARGE PLANNING

When providing patient-family teaching, focus on sensory information, avoid giving excessive information, and initiate a visiting nurse referral for necessary follow-up teaching. Include verbal and written information about the following:

✓ Medications, including drug name, purpose, dosage, schedule, precautions, and potential side effects. Also discuss drug-drug, herb-drug, and food-drug interactions.

✓ Necessity of reporting the following indicators of urinary tract infection (UTI) to health care provider: chills; fever; hematuria; flank, costovertebral angle, suprapubic, low back, buttock, or scrotal pain; cloudy and foul-smelling urine; frequency; urgency; dysuria; and increasing or recurring incontinence.

✓ Care of incision, if appropriate, including cleansing, dressing changes, and bathing. Advise patient to be aware of indicators of infection: persistent redness, increasing pain, edema, increased warmth along incision, or purulent or increased drainage.

✓ Care of catheters or drains if patient is discharged with them.

✓ Daily fluid requirement of at least 2-3 L/day in nonrestricted patients.

✓ Importance of increasing dietary fiber or taking stool softeners to soften stools. This will minimize risk of damage to the prostatic capsule by preventing straining with bowel movements. Caution patient to avoid using suppositories or enemas for treatment of constipation.

✓ Use of a sofa, reclining chair, or footstool to promote venous drainage from legs and to distribute weight on perineum, not the rectum.

✓ Avoiding the following activities for the period prescribed by health care provider: sitting for long periods, heavy lifting (more than 10 lb), and sexual intercourse.

✓ Kegel exercises to help regain urinary sphincter control for postoperative dribbling. See **Deficient Knowledge** on p. 214.

Chronic Kidney Disease 26

OVERVIEW/PATHOPHYSIOLOGY

Chronic kidney disease (CKD) is a progressive, irreversible loss of kidney function that develops over days to years. Aggressive management of hypertension and diabetes mellitus (DM) and avoidance of nephrotoxic agents may slow progression of CKD; however loss of glomerular filtration is irreversible, and eventually CKD can progress to end-stage renal disease (ESRD), at which time renal replacement therapy (dialysis or transplantation) is required to sustain life. Before ESRD, the individual with CKD can lead a relatively normal life managed by diet and medications. The length of this period varies, depending on the cause of renal disease and patient's level of renal function at the time of diagnosis.

Of the many causes of CKD, some of the most common are DM, hypertension, glomerulonephritis (GN), long-term exposure to certain classes of medications (e.g., nonsteroidal antiinflammatories), or metals (e.g., gold therapy, lead), and polycystic kidney disease. Regardless of the cause, clinical presentation of CKD, particularly as the individual approaches ESRD, is similar. Retention of metabolic end products and accompanying fluid and electrolyte imbalances adversely affect all body systems. Alterations in neuromuscular, cardiovascular, and gastrointestinal (GI) function are common. Renal osteodystrophy and anemia are early and common complications, with alterations being seen when the glomerular filtration rate (GFR) decreases to 60 ml/min. The collective manifestations of CKD are termed *uremia*.

HEALTH CARE SETTING

Primary care with possible hospitalization resulting from complications or during ESRD

ASSESSMENT

Fluid volume abnormalities: Crackles (rales), hypertension, edema, oliguria, anuria.

Electrolyte disturbances: Muscle weakness, dysrhythmias, pruritus, neuromuscular irritability, tetany.

Metabolic acidosis: Deep respirations, lethargy, headache.

Uremia—retention of metabolic wastes: Weakness, malaise, anorexia, dry and discolored skin, peripheral neuropathy, irritability, clouded thinking, ammonia odor to breath, metallic taste in mouth, nausea, vomiting. **Note:** Uremia adversely affects all body systems.

POTENTIAL ACUTE COMPLICATIONS

Heart failure: Crackles (rales), dyspnea, orthopnea.

Pericarditis: Heart pain, elevated temperature, presence of pericardial friction or rub on auscultation.

Cardiac tamponade: Hypotension, distant heart sounds, pulsus paradoxus (exaggerated inspiratory drop in systolic blood pressure [SBP]).

Physical assessment: Pallor, dry and discolored skin, edema (peripheral, periorbital, sacral); fluid overload, crackles and elevated blood pressure (BP) may be present.

History: GN; DM; polycystic kidney disease; hypertension; systemic lupus erythematosus; chronic pyelonephritis; and analgesic abuse, especially the combination of phenacetin and aspirin.

DIAGNOSTIC TESTS

GFR: May be calculated using a mathematical formula. The MDRD (Modification of Diet in Renal Disease) GFR calculator is:

$$\text{GFR} = 170 \times (\text{plasma creatinine in mg/dl})^{-0.999} \times (\text{age})^{-0.176} \times (0.762 \text{ if female}) \times (1.180 \text{ if patient is black}) \times (\text{serum urea nitrogen in mg/dl})^{-0.170} \times (\text{albumin in g/dl})^{0.318}$$

Creatinine clearance: Measures kidney's ability to clear the blood of creatinine and approximates the GFR. Creatinine clearance decreases as renal function decreases. Dialysis is usually begun when the GFR is 12 ml/min if patient is symptomatic or the GFR is less than 6 ml/min. Creatinine clearance normally is decreased in older adults. Creatinine clearance may be measured through collection of a 24-hr urine sample or calculated using the Cockcroft-Gault equation:

$$\text{For men: CrCl} = (140 - \text{age}) \times \text{weight (in kg)}/\text{plasma creatinine (in mg/dl)} \times 72$$

$$\text{For women: CrCl} = (140 - \text{age}) \times \text{weight (in kg)}/\text{plasma creatinine (in mg/dl)} \times 85$$

Note: Failure to collect all urine specimens during the period of study will invalidate test results.

BUN and serum creatinine: Both will be elevated. **Note:** Nonrenal problems, such as dehydration or GI bleeding, also can cause the blood urea nitrogen (BUN) to increase, but there will not be a corresponding increase in creatinine.

Serum chemistries, chest and hand x-ray examinations, and nerve conduction velocity test: To assess for development and progression of uremia and its complications. **Note:** Acetylcysteine (Mucomyst) may be prescribed as a prophylactic therapy before, during, and/or after administration of IV contrast in order to reduce the risk of further insult to the kidneys or dye-mediated acute renal failure.

KUB x-ray examination: By kidney-ureter-bladder (KUB) x-ray examination, documents presence of two kidneys, changes in size or shape, and some forms of obstruction.

Intravenous pyelogram, renal ultrasound, renal biopsy, renal scan (using radionuclides), and CT scan: Additional tests for determining cause of renal insufficiency. Once patient has reached ESRD, these tests are not performed.

Nursing Diagnosis:

Activity Intolerance

related to generalized weakness secondary to anemia and uremia

Desired Outcome: Following treatment, patient rates perceived exertion at 3 or less on a 0-10 scale and exhibits improving endurance to activity as evidenced by HR 20 bpm or less over resting HR, SBP 20 mm Hg or less over or under resting SBP, and RR 20 breaths/min or less with normal depth and pattern (eupnea).

Note: Anemia is better tolerated in the uremic than in the nonuremic patient.

INTERVENTIONS	RATIONALES
Monitor patient during activity, and ask patient to rate perceived exertion (RPE) (see **Risk for Activity Intolerance,** p. 61, in "Prolonged Bedrest," for details).	This assessment evaluates the degree of activity intolerance. Optimally RPE should be at 3 or less on a 0-10 scale.
Notify health care provider of increased weakness, fatigue, dyspnea, chest pain, or further decreases in hematocrit (Hct).	This action enables rapid treatment of anemia and dose adjustment of epoetin alfa, which induces erythrocyte production and reticulocyte production in the bone marrow. Low levels of Hgb and Hct may result in angina. Shortness of breath and shortness of breath on exertion in the long-term contribute to the development of ventricular hypertrophy, increasing the risk of morbidity from cardiovascular disease (CVD), the most significant cause of death in CKD patients. Conversely, high levels of Hgb may result in hypertension and increased thrombosis.
Administer oral or parenteral iron if prescribed.	Iron deficiency anemia is common in CKD patients. In addition, iron is required for epoetin alfa to make new red blood cells. Thus, effectiveness of epoetin alfa requires that patients maintain their iron stores. **Note:** Anaphylaxis is a possible complication of IV iron administration, most commonly during the first dose.
For patients receiving oral iron, monitor for signs and symptoms of constipation.	Constipation is a common side effect of oral iron. See **Constipation** in "Prolonged Bedrest," p. 67.
Administer epoetin alfa, if prescribed.	Current clinical practice guidelines recommend that epoetin alfa (Epogen) be started when Hgb decreases below 10 g/dl. Target Hgb for patients receiving epoetin alfa is 11.5 g/dl (or a range of 11.0-12.0 g/dl). Epoetin alfa may be contraindicated in patients with uncontrolled hypertension or sensitivity to human albumin.
Gently mix container; use only one dose per vial (do not reenter used vials; discard unused portions).	Shaking may denature the glycoprotein.

Continued

INTERVENTIONS	RATIONALES
Monitor for increasing hypertension, dyspnea, chest pain, seizures, calf pain, erythema, swelling, severe headache, and seizures.	These are potential untoward effects of epoetin alfa therapy. Dose adjustment or discontinuation may be necessary. Patients with uncontrolled hypertension should not be started on Epogen therapy until their hypertension is controlled. Blood pressure must be closely monitored in all patients during initiation of therapy. Hypertension may occur as a side effect of Epogen therapy during the period in which Hct levels are rapidly rising, even in nonhypertensive patients. Headaches may accompany the rise in blood pressure. Epogen has also been associated with increased thrombosis. Patients should be monitored for evidence of thrombotic events (i.e., symptoms of myocardial infarction [MI], deep vein thrombosis [DVT], stroke, transient ischemic attack [TIA], or clotting of the vascular access in hemodialysis patients), and those symptoms should be reported immediately to the health care provider. Epogen should be used with caution in patients with a known seizure history. There is an increased risk of seizures in chronic renal failure patients within the first 3 months of Epogen therapy.
Coordinate laboratory studies.	This intervention minimizes blood drawing. CKD patients are already at risk for anemia.
Monitor for and report evidence of occult blood and blood loss.	Blood loss can cause anemia.
Provide and encourage optimal nutrition and consider referral to a renal dietitian.	Protein and phosphorus are initially restricted to slow progression of CKD and prevent early development of renal osteodystrophy. (*Renal osteodystrophy* is a collective term for changes in the bone structure of patients with CKD, resulting most often in rapid bone turnover. These changes result from a combination of hyperphosphatemia, hypocalcemia, stimulation of parathyroid hormone, and alterations in the kidney's ability to convert vitamin D to its active form.) Carbohydrates are increased for patients on protein-restricted diets to ensure adequate caloric intake, thereby preventing tissue catabolism, which would contribute to buildup of nitrogenous wastes. As patient approaches ESRD, sodium intake is limited to reduce thirst and fluid retention, K^+ intake is limited because of the kidneys' decreased ability to excrete this ion, and protein may be further restricted to limit production of nitrogenous wastes. For patients on protein-restricted diets, protein intake should be restricted to sources primarily of high biologic value. Over-restriction of protein may lead to malnutrition; therefore referral to a renal dietitian is recommended to ensure adequate intake.
Do not administer ferrous sulfate at the same time as antacids.	To maximize absorption of ferrous sulfate, antacids or calcium carbonate medications are given at least 1 hr before or after ferrous sulfate.
Assist with identifying activities that increase fatigue and adjusting those activities accordingly.	It is important to minimize fatigue while attempting to promote tolerance to activity.
Assist with activities of daily living (ADL) while encouraging maximum independence to tolerance. Establish realistic, progressive exercises and activity goals that are designed to increase endurance. Ensure that they are within patient's prescribed limitations. Examples are found in **Risk for Activity Intolerance,** p. 61, and **Risk for Disuse Syndrome,** p. 63, in "Prolonged Bedrest."	Same as above.
Administer packed red blood cells as prescribed.	This measure treats severe or symptomatic anemia.

●●● **Related NIC and NOC labels:** *NIC:* Energy Management; Nutrition Management: Medication Management *NOC:* Activity Tolerance; Endurance; Energy Conservation; Self-Care: Activities of Daily Living (ADL)

Nursing Diagnosis:

Imbalanced Nutrition: Less Than Body Requirements

related to nausea, vomiting, anorexia, and dietary restrictions

Desired Outcome: Within 2 days of admission, patient has stable weight and demonstrates normal intake of food within restrictions, as indicated.

INTERVENTIONS	RATIONALES
See also **Imbalanced Nutrition: Less Than Body Requirements** in "Acute Renal Failure," p. 236.	
In addition:	
Administer multivitamins and folic acid, if prescribed.	Anorexia and nausea and vomiting may occur with increased anorexia. Vitamin supplementation assists with ensuring that patients maintain adequate nutrition. **Note:** Use of over-the-counter multivitamins is contraindicated in CKD patients because some vitamin levels (e.g., of vitamin A) may be toxic. Multivitamins for patients on dialysis are specially formulated (e.g., Nephro-Vite, Dialyvite).
Monitor for proteinuria, and refer to dietitian if excessive protein losses and/or low serum albumin is noted.	Proteinuria results in malnutrition. Patients with poor nutritional status at the start of dialysis have increased risk of mortality.

••• **Related NIC and NOC labels:** *NIC:* Nutrition Management; Nutrition Monitoring; Weight Gain Assistance *NOC:* Nutitional Status: Food Intake

Nursing Diagnosis:

Impaired Skin Integrity

related to pruritus and dry skin secondary to uremia, hyperphosphatemia (if severe), and edema

Desired Outcome: Patient's skin remains intact and free of erythema and abrasions.

INTERVENTIONS	RATIONALES
Monitor for presence/degree of pruritus.	Pruritus is common in patients with uremia and occurs when accumulating nitrogenous wastes begin to be excreted through the skin, causing frequent and intense itching with scratching. Pruritus also may result from prolonged hyperphosphatemia.
Encourage use of phosphate binders and reduction of dietary phosphorus if elevated phosphorus level is a problem.	Pruritus often decreases with a reduction in BUN and improved phosphorus control. Phosphate binders are medications that, when taken with food, bind dietary phosphorous and prevent GI absorption. Calcium carbonate, sevelamer hydrochloride, aluminum hydroxide, and calcium acetate are common phosphate binders.
Note: Administer phosphate binders while food is present in the stomach.	Prolonged elevation of serum phosphorous and/or calcium absorption from ingestion of phosphate binders on an empty stomach results in an increased calcium-phosphorous product (serum calcium × serum phosphorous). When this product exceeds a level of 55 (normal product is approximately 40), phosphorous binds with calcium, and the resulting calcium-phosphate complex is deposited in soft tissues of the body. Deposition of these complexes in the skin produces necrotic patches. In addition, elevation in calcium-phosphate product is associated with increased risk of death, aortic calcification, mitral valve calcification, and coronary artery calcification.
If necessary, administer prescribed antihistamines.	Antihistamines help control itching.
Keep patient's fingernails short.	If patient is unable to control scratching, short fingernails will cause less damage.
Instruct patient to monitor scratches for evidence of infection and to seek early medical attention if signs and symptoms of infection appear.	Uremia retards wound healing; nonintact skin can lead to infection.

Continued

INTERVENTIONS	RATIONALES
Encourage use of skin emollients and soaps with high fat content. Advise patient to bathe every other day and to apply skin lotion immediately upon exiting bath/shower.	Uremic skin is often dry and scaly because of reduction in oil gland activity. Patients should avoid harsh soaps, soaps or skin products containing alcohol, and excessive bathing.
Advise patient and significant others that easy bruising can occur.	Patients with uremia are at increased risk for bruising because of clotting abnormalities and capillary fragility.
Provide scheduled skin care and position changes for patients with edema.	These measures decrease risk of skin/tissue damage resulting from decreased perfusion and increased pressure.

••• **Related NIC and NOC labels:** *NIC:* Skin Care: Topical Treatments; Positioning; Medication Management; Nutrition Management *NOC:* Tissue Integrity: Skin & Mucous Membranes

Nursing Diagnosis:

Deficient Knowledge:

Need for frequent BP checks and adherence to antihypertensive therapy and the potential for change in insulin requirements for individuals who have DM

Desired Outcomes: Within the 24-hr period before hospital discharge, patient verbalizes knowledge about importance of frequent BP checks and adherence to antihypertensive therapy. Patients with DM verbalize knowledge about the potential for change in insulin requirements.

INTERVENTIONS	RATIONALES
Assess patient's health care literacy (language, reading, comprehension). Assess culture and culturally specific information needs.	This assessment helps ensure that information is presented in a manner that is culturally and educationally appropriate.
Teach importance of getting BP checked at frequent intervals and adhering to prescribed antihypertensive therapy.	Patients with CKD may experience hypertension because of fluid overload, excess renin secretion, or arteriosclerotic disease. Control of hypertension may slow progression of chronic renal insufficiency and decrease risk of cardiovascular disease.
Teach patient about antihypertensive medications, including drug name, purpose, dosage, schedule precautions, and potential side effects. Also discuss drug-drug, herb-drug, and food-drug interactions.	These medications control BP, slow progression of CKD, and/or reduce proteinuria/microalbuminuria. Angiotensin-converting enzyme (ACE) inhibitors and angiotensin receptor blockers (ARBs) are considered first-line drugs for management of patients with CKD and coexisting diabetes, proteinuria, and/or microalbuminuria. Additional antihypertensives are often added in the following order to achieve a target BP of less than 130/80 mm Hg: diuretic, then beta-blocker or calcium channel blocker. Patients may require up to four antihypertensives to control BP adequately. Because increased release of angiotensin may occur with renal pathology, some patients require bilateral nephrectomies to control excessive hypertension.
Teach patient importance of a target BP of less than 130/80 mm Hg.	This knowledge will help the patient keep BP within optimal levels.
Teach patients with DM that insulin requirements often decrease as renal function decreases.	Anorexia or nausea/vomiting, which occur with uremia, may decrease dietary consumption and thereby decrease insulin requirements.
Instruct these patients to be alert to weakness, blurred vision, and headache.	These symptoms are indicators of hypoglycemia, which can occur as insulin requirements decrease.
Teach patients on ACE inhibitors or ARBs the importance of medical follow-up.	Follow-up is important for monitoring GFR, potassium levels, and hypotension. Hypotension and cough are common side effects. ACE inhibitors and ARBs may increase serum potassium and decrease GFR. Angioedema is a potential side effect.
Teach patients receiving diuretics the importance of medical follow-up.	Follow-up enables monitoring for volume depletion, decreased GFR, and electrolyte abnormalities. Use of diuretics can result in dehydration and hypokalemia and may hasten loss of renal function.

Continued

INTERVENTIONS	RATIONALES
Teach patient that restriction of sodium to less than 2.4 g/day is recommended. Consider referral to a dietitian.	These measures help manage hypertension and slow progression of CKD.
Teach that weight loss should be considered if body mass index is greater than 25 kg/m^2. Refer to a dietitian as indicated.	Obesity increases hypertension, resulting in progression of CKD and increased mortality rates due to CVD.
Teach importance of limiting alcohol intake to less than 2 drinks/day for men, and less than 1 drink/day for women.	Excessive alcohol intake may increase the risk of malnutrition, hypertension, and CVD resulting in progression of CKD and increased mortality.
Counsel patient on smoking cessation if applicable.	CVD is the leading cause of death in CKD patients. Smoking increases the risk of CVD and arteriosclerosis.
Teach benefits of exercise and physical activity.	Thirty minutes of physical activity of moderate intensity most days of the week is recommended for hypertension management in patients with CKD. Management of hypertension may slow progression of CKD.

• • • Related NIC and NOC labels: *NIC:* Teaching: Prescribed Medications; Teaching: Procedure *NOC:* Knowledge: Treatment Procedure; Knowledge: Medication

ADDITIONAL NURSING DIAGNOSES/ PROBLEMS:

"Prolonged Bedrest" for **Constipation** related to changes in dietary intake, immobility, and oral iron supplementation	p. 67
"Psychosocial Support" for **Disturbed Body Image** related to changes in body parts or function or presence of dialysis catheters	p. 80
"Care of the Patient Undergoing Hemodialysis"	p. 223
"Care of the Patient Undergoing Peritoneal Dialysis"	p. 227

✓ **PATIENT-FAMILY TEACHING AND DISCHARGE PLANNING**

When providing patient-family teaching, focus on sensory information, avoid giving excessive information, and initiate a visiting nurse referral for necessary follow-up teaching. Include verbal and written information about the following:

✓ Medications, including drug name, purpose, dosage, schedule, precautions, and potential side effects. Also discuss drug-drug, herb-drug, and food-drug interactions.

✓ For patients not on dialysis but requiring epoetin alfa, teach patient and/or significant other preparation of the medication and subcutaneous injections. Demonstrate how to gently mix the container (shaking may denature the glycoprotein); use only one dose per vial (do not reenter used vials, discard unused portions). Instruct patient and/or significant other to store epoetin alfa in refrigerator but not to allow it to freeze. Teach importance of monitoring for and rapidly reporting to health care provider any of the following: dyspnea, chest pain, seizures, and severe headache.

✓ Diet, including fact sheet listing foods that are to be restricted or limited. Inform patient that diet and fluid restrictions may be altered as renal function decreases. Provide sample menus, and have patient demonstrate understanding by preparing 3-day menus that incorporate dietary restrictions.

✓ Care and observation of dialysis access if patient has one (see next two care plans).

✓ Signs and symptoms that necessitate medical attention: irregular pulse, fever, unusual shortness of breath or edema, sudden change in urine output, and unusual muscle weakness.

✓ Need for continued medical follow-up; confirm date and time of next health care provider appointment.

✓ Importance of avoiding infections and seeking treatment promptly should one develop. Teach indicators of frequently encountered infections, including upper respiratory infection (URI), urinary tract infection (UTI), impetigo, and otitis media. For details, see **Risk for Infection,** p. 239, in "Care of the Renal Transplant Recipient."

✓ Telephone numbers to call in case questions or concerns arise about therapy or disease after discharge. Additional general information can be obtained by contacting the following:

- National Kidney and Urologic Diseases Information Clearinghouse at *www.kidney.niddk.nih.gov*
- National Kidney Foundation at *www.kidney.org*

✓ For patient with or approaching ESRD, provide data concerning various treatment options and support groups. The local chapter of the National Kidney Foundation can be helpful in identifying support groups and organizations in the area. Patient and significant others should meet with renal dietitian and social worker before discharge.

✓ Coordinate discharge planning and teaching with dialysis unit or facility. If possible, have patient visit dialysis unit before discharge.

✓ For individuals with ESRD, teach importance of coordinating all medical care through their nephrologist and alerting all medical and dental personnel to ESRD status because of increased risk of infection and need to adjust medication dosages. In addition, dentists may want to premedicate ESRD patients with antibiotics before dental work and avoid scheduling dental work on the day of dialysis because of heparinization that is used with dialytic therapy.

Care of the Patient Undergoing Hemodialysis 27

OVERVIEW/PATHOPHYSIOLOGY

During hemodialysis, blood is removed via a special vascular access, heparinized, pumped through an artificial kidney (dialyzer), and then returned to patient's circulation. Hemodialysis is a temporary, acute procedure performed as needed, or it is performed long term 2-4 times/wk for 3-5 hr each treatment.

Indications for hemodialysis: Acute renal failure or acute episodes of renal insufficiency that cannot be managed by diet, medications, and fluid restriction; end-stage renal disease (ESRD); drug overdose; hyperkalemia; fluid overload; and metabolic acidosis.

Continuous venovenous hemodiafiltration (CVVHD): A double-lumen catheter is placed in a large vein and blood is pumped from the vein, through the dialysis circuit, passing through the hemofilter and returning to the patient's circulation via a venous access. Ultrafiltrate (fluid, metabolic wastes, and electrolytes) drains from the hemofilter into a collection device.

HEALTH CARE SETTING

Dialysis center, with possible hospitalization in an acute care setting during initiation of therapy

Use of CVVHD is currently limited to patients in critical care settings because it requires continuous monitoring.

Components of Hemodialysis

Artificial kidney (dialyzer): Composed of a blood compartment and dialysate compartment, separated by a semipermeable membrane that allows diffusion of solutes and filtration of water. Protein and bacteria do not cross the artificial membrane.

Dialysate: Electrolyte solution similar in composition to normal plasma. Each of the constituents may be varied according to patient need. The most commonly altered component is K^+ and bicarbonate. Glucose may be added to prevent sudden drops in serum osmolality and serum glucose during dialysis.

Vascular access: Necessary to provide a blood flow rate of 300-500 ml/min for an effective dialysis. Vascular access sites may include an arteriovenous fistula, arteriovenous graft, internal jugular catheters (right side preferred), femoral vein catheters, or subclavian catheters.

Nursing Diagnosis:

Risk for Imbalanced Fluid Volume

related to excessive fluid removal from dialysis, or related to compromised regulatory mechanism resulting in fluid retention secondary to renal failure

Desired Outcomes: Postdialysis patient is normovolemic as evidenced by stable weight, RR 12-20 breaths/min with normal depth and pattern (eupnea), CVP 5-12 cm H_2O, HR and BP within patient's normal range, and absence of abnormal breath sounds and abnormal bleeding. After instruction, patient relates signs and symptoms of fluid volume excess and deficit.

INTERVENTIONS	RATIONALES
Monitor intake and output (I&O) and daily weight as indicators of fluid status.	Intake greater than output and steady weight gain indicate retained fluid. In addition, patient's weight is an important guideline for determining quantity of fluid that needs to be removed during dialysis.
Weigh patient at the same time each day, using same scale and with patient wearing same amount of clothing (or with same items on the bed if using a bed scale).	Consistency in weighing patient is important to ensure a measurement that is as precise as possible.
Instruct patient and staff to monitor for edema, hypertension, crackles (rales), tachycardia, distended neck veins, shortness of breath, and increased central venous pressure (CVP).	These are indicators of fluid volume excess. Dependent edema likely will be detected in the legs or feet of patients who are ambulatory, whereas the sacral area will be edematous in those who are on bedrest. Periorbital edema also may result from excessive fluid overload. Jugular veins are likely to be distended with head of bed (HOB) elevated 45 degrees owing to increased intravascular volume if patient has excessive fluid volume. Crackles and shortness of breath can occur as a result of fluid volume overload. Low serum albumin decreases colloid osmotic pressure, allowing fluid to leak into the extravascular space. Low serum albumin also may contribute to generalized edema and pulmonary edema. Hypertension, tachycardia, and increased CVP may result from sodium and fluid retention.
After dialysis, observe for and report hypotension, decreased CVP, tachycardia, and complaints of dizziness or lightheadedness. Describe signs and symptoms to patient, and explain importance of reporting them promptly if they occur.	These are indicators of fluid volume deficit, which may result from rapid or excessive fluid losses during dialysis. It should be noted that patients with uremia may not develop compensatory tachycardia owing to autonomic neuropathy, which can occur with uremia. **Note:** Antihypertensive medications usually are held before and during dialysis to help prevent hypotension during dialysis. Clarify medication prescriptions with health care provider.
Monitor for postdialysis bleeding (needle sites, incisions).	This bleeding can occur because of use of heparin during dialysis.
Alert patient to potential for bleeding from these areas.	If these signs and symptoms occur, patient will be able to report them promptly to staff or health care provider for timely intervention.
Do not give IM injection for at least 1 hr after dialysis.	Avoiding IM injections for this amount of time prevents hematoma formation.
Test all stools for presence of blood. Report significant findings.	Gastrointestinal (GI) bleeding is common in patients with renal failure, especially after heparinization.

••• **Related NIC and NOC labels:** *NIC:* Fluid Monitoring; Hemodialysis Therapy; Bleeding Precautions *NOC:* Fluid Balance; Hydration

Nursing Diagnosis:

Risk for Deficient Fluid Volume

related to bleeding/hemorrhage that can occur with vascular access puncture or disconnection

Risk for Ineffective Tissue Perfusion: Peripheral

related to interrupted blood flow that can occur with clotting in the vascular access

Risk for Infection

related to invasive procedure (creation of vascular access for hemodialysis)

Desired Outcomes: Patient's vascular access remains intact and connected, and patient is normovolemic (see description in **Risk for Imbalanced Fluid Volume**). Patient has adequate tissue perfusion as evidenced by normal skin temperature and color and brisk capillary refill (less than 2 sec) distal to the vascular access. Patient's access is patent as evidenced by presence of thrill with palpation and bruit with auscultation of fistula or graft. Patient is free of infection as evidenced by normothermia and absence of erythema, local warmth, exudate, swelling, and tenderness at access site.

INTERVENTIONS	RATIONALES
After surgical creation of the vascular access, assess for patency, auscultate for bruit, and palpate for thrill.	These assessments reveal whether the patient's vascular access is patent. A bruit is a hissing sound that is made when blood moves through the access. A thrill is a vibration felt when placing hand over the access, denoting blood flow.
Report complaints of severe or unrelieved pain, numbness, and tingling of the area of vascular access or extremity distal to the access.	These indicators can signal impaired tissue perfusion caused by occlusion of the vascular access.
Be alert to postoperative swelling along graft or fistula or area around the shunt; elevate extremity accordingly.	Postoperative swelling along the graft or fistula or area around the shunt is expected and will diminish with extremity elevation.
Notify health care provider if extremity distal to the vascular access becomes cool or swollen, has decreased capillary refill, or has decreased pulse or is discolored.	These problems can indicate hypoxia as a result of reduced blood supply to the extremity (called *steal syndrome*).
Follow the three principles of nursing care common to all types of vascular access: (1) prevent bleeding, (2) prevent clotting, and (3) prevent infection. Never use the vascular access for instillation of IV medications or blood letting. Monitor it closely, and handle it with care.	The vascular access is the patient's lifeline, and it must be monitored closely to ensure maintenance of patency and prevention of infection.
Explain monitoring and care procedures to patient.	A knowledgeable patient is more likely to adhere to these principles.
Vascular accesses include the following:	
Subclavian or femoral lines	External, temporary catheters inserted into a large vein.
1. Anchor catheter securely because it might not be sutured in. Tape all connections. Keep clamps at bedside in case line becomes disconnected. If the line is removed or accidentally pulled out, apply firm pressure to site for at least 10 min.	These measures prevent bleeding.
Caution: If an air embolus occurs:	
a. Immediately clamp the line.	An air embolus can occur if a subclavian line accidentally becomes pulled out or disconnected.
b. Turn patient onto a left-side-lying position.	This position helps prevent air from blocking the pulmonary artery.
c. Lower HOB into Trendelenburg position. Administer 100% oxygen by mask, and obtain vital signs. Notify health care provider *stat*!	This position increases intrathoracic pressure, which will decrease the flow of inspiratory air into the vein.
2. Allow only the dialysis staff to access the line.	Improper heparin flushing increases risk of clotting. Accessing the line for nondialysis treatments increases risk of infection.
3. Monitor for and report presence of erythema, local warmth, exudate, swelling, and tenderness at exit site.	These are indicators of infection. Dressing changes and cultures of any drainage should be performed only by dialysis staff. If a dressing loosens, it needs to be reinforced and the dialysis unit contacted to perform the dressing change.
Fistula or graft	Internal, permanent connection between an artery and a vein, or the insertion of an internal graft that is joined to an artery and vein. Grafts can be straight or U-shaped. Grafts and fistulas are most commonly located in the arm but may be placed in the thigh.
1. Inspect needle puncture sites. If bleeding occurs, apply just enough pressure over the site to stop it. Release the pressure and check for bleeding q5-10min.	These measures inspect for and intervene in the event of postdialysis bleeding.
2. Place a sign above HOB indicating extremity in which the fistula or graft has been placed, and stating not to take blood pressure (BP), start an IV, or draw blood from affected limb. Ensure that this information is clearly documented on the Kardex. Caution patient to avoid tight clothing, jewelry, name bands, or restraint on affected extremity.	These procedures and precautions help prevent blood clotting in the vascular access.

Continued

INTERVENTIONS	RATIONALES
3. Palpate for thrill and auscultate for bruit at least every shift and after hypotensive episodes. Notify health care provider *stat* if bruit or thrill has changed significantly or is absent.	These assessments determine whether the vascular access is patent.
4. Observe for and report presence of erythema, local warmth, swelling, exudate, and unusual tenderness at graft, fistula, or shunt site.	These are indicators of infection. Dressing changes and cultures of any drainage should only be performed by dialysis staff. If a dressing loosens, it needs to be reinforced and the dialysis unit contacted to perform the dressing change.

••• **Related NIC and NOC labels:** *NIC:* Circulatory Care Neurologic Monitoring; Positioning; Specimen Management; Incision Site Care; Infection Protection; Bleeding Precautions *NOC:* Sensory Function: Cutaneous; Tissue Integrity: Skin and Mucous Membranes; Infection Status; Wound Healing: Primary Intention; Fluid Balance

PATIENT-FAMILY TEACHING AND DISCHARGE PLANNING

When providing patient-family teaching, focus on sensory information, avoid giving excessive information, and initiate a visiting nurse referral if indicated for follow-up teaching. Include verbal and written information about the following:

✓ Medications, including drug name, purpose, dosage, schedule, drug-drug and food-drug interactions, precautions, and potential side effects.

✓ Diet and fluid restrictions: Include fact sheets that list foods to limit or restrict. Review fluid restrictions. Provide sample menus with examples of how dietary restrictions may be incorporated into daily meals. Have patient demonstrate understanding of dietary restrictions by preparing 3-day menus.

✓ Care of fistula or graft to prevent/detect bleeding, clotting, and infection.

✓ Need for and importance of monitoring daily weights, I&O, and monitoring of BP at home, if necessary.

✓ Importance of continued medical follow-up; confirm date and time of next health care provider and hemodialysis appointments.

✓ Signs and symptoms that necessitate medical attention: increased weight gain, unusual shortness of breath, edema, dizziness or fainting, fever, increased hypertension, redness around access site, decrease in bruit or thrill (fistulas, graft), prolonged bleeding from fistula or graft, discoloration or coldness distal to fistula or graft, accidental pulling on subclavian line.

✓ Telephone numbers to call in case questions or concerns arise about therapy or disease after discharge. Additional general information can be obtained by contacting:

- National Kidney and Urologic Diseases Information Clearinghouse at *www.kidney.niddk.nih.gov*
- National Kidney Foundation at *www.kidney.org*

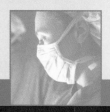

Care of the Patient Undergoing Peritoneal Dialysis 28

OVERVIEW/PATHOPHYSIOLOGY

Peritoneal dialysis uses the peritoneum as the dialysis membrane. Dialysate is instilled into the peritoneal cavity via a catheter surgically placed in the abdominal wall. Once the dialysate is within the abdominal cavity, movement of solutes and fluid occurs between the patient's capillary blood and the dialysate. At set intervals, the peritoneal cavity is drained and new dialysate is instilled.

Indications for dialysis: Acute renal failure or acute episodes of renal insufficiency that cannot be managed by diet, medications, and fluid restriction; end-stage renal disease (ESRD); drug overdose; hyperkalemia; fluid overload; and metabolic acidosis.

Components of Dialysis

Catheter: Silastic tube that is either implanted using general anesthesia as a surgical procedure for patients who will have long-term treatment or is inserted using local anesthetic at the bedside for short-term dialysis.

Dialysate: Sterile electrolyte solution similar in composition to normal plasma. The electrolyte composition of the dialysate can be adjusted according to individual need. Glucose is added to the dialysate in varying concentrations to remove excess body fluid via osmosis. **Note:** Some glucose crosses the peritoneal membrane and enters the patient's blood. Patients with diabetes mellitus may require additional insulin. Observe for and report indicators of hyperglycemia (e.g., complaints of thirst, changes in sensorium). Insulin and other medications may be added directly to the dialysate by dialysis nurses.

Types of Dialysis

Intermittent peritoneal dialysis (IPD): Patient is dialyzed for periods of 8-10 hr, 4-5 times/wk. A predetermined amount of dialysate (usually 2 L) is instilled for a set length of time (usually 20-30 min). It is then allowed to drain by gravity, and the process is repeated. IPD can be performed manually with individual bags or mechanically using a proportioning machine or cycler. The patient is restricted to a chair or bed. IPD can be performed also as an acute, temporary procedure. Continuous hourly exchanges are performed for 48-72 hr. The patient is restricted to bed.

Continuous ambulatory peritoneal dialysis (CAPD): Using sterile technique, the patient attaches a new bag of dialysate to the peritoneal catheter, allows the dialysate to drain out, and then allows new dialysate to drain in. The patient then clamps the catheter and places a new cap on the tubing using sterile technique. This process is repeated q4-6h (8 hr at night), 7 days/wk. CAPD is used primarily for ESRD.

Continuous cycling peritoneal dialysis (CCPD): This is a combination of IPD and CAPD. A cycler performs three dialysate exchanges at night. In the morning a fourth exchange is instilled and left in the peritoneal cavity for the entire day. At the end of the day, the fourth exchange is allowed to drain out and the process is repeated. The patient is ambulatory by day and restricted to bed at night. CCPD is commonly done every night.

HEALTH CARE SETTING

For IPD: Dialysis center; acute care if patient has complications
For CAPD and CCPD: Home setting; acute care if patient has complications

<u>Nursing Diagnosis:</u>

Risk for Infection

related to risk factors associated with an invasive procedure (direct access of the catheter to the peritoneum)

Desired Outcomes: Patient is free of infection as evidenced by normothermia and absence of the following: abdominal pain, cloudy outflow, nausea, malaise, erythema, edema, increased local warmth, drainage, and tenderness at the exit site. Before hospital discharge, patient verbalizes signs and symptoms of infection and need for sterile technique for bag, tubing, and dressing changes.

INTERVENTIONS	RATIONALES
Monitor for and report indications of peritonitis (see "Peritonitis", p. 481).	The most common complication of peritoneal dialysis is peritonitis. Indicators include fever, abdominal pain, distention, abdominal wall rigidity, rebound tenderness, cloudy outflow, nausea, and malaise.
Maintain sterile technique when adding medications to dialysate.	To minimize risk of peritonitis and other infections, the dialysate must remain sterile because it is instilled directly into the body.
Follow agency policy for care of catheter exit site.	Exit site infections may lead to development of peritonitis.
Observe for and report redness, local warmth, edema, drainage, or tenderness at exit site. Culture any exudate, and report results to health care provider.	These are signs of infection at the exit site.
Report to health care provider if dialysate leaks around catheter exit site.	This leakage can signal an obstruction or need for another purse-string suture around catheter site. Leakage around the exit site has been associated with increased risk of tunnel infections, exit site infections, and peritonitis. Organisms may track through subcutaneous tissue into the peritoneum, causing infection.
Instruct patient in the preceding interventions and observations if peritoneal dialysis will be performed after hospital discharge.	An informed patient likely will adhere to infection prevention interventions and know when to report untoward signs to health care provider.

••• **Related NIC and NOC labels:** *NIC:* Infection Protection; Incision Site Care; Specimen Management *NOC:* Infection Status

<u>Nursing Diagnosis:</u>

Risk for Imbalanced Fluid Volume

related to hypertonicity of the dialysate or inadequate exchange

Desired Outcomes: Postdialysis the patient is normovolemic as evidenced by balanced I&O, stable weight, good skin turgor, CVP 5-12 cm H_2O, RR 12-20 breaths/min with normal depth and pattern (eupnea), and BP and HR within patient's normal range. The volume of dialysate outflow equals or exceeds inflow.

INTERVENTIONS	RATIONALES
Monitor for and report hypertension, dyspnea, tachycardia, distended neck veins, or increased central venous pressure (CVP).	These are indicators of fluid overload.
Also be alert to incomplete dialysate returns.	Fluid retention can occur because of catheter complications that prevent adequate outflow, a severely scarred peritoneum that prevents adequate exchange, or inadequate dialysis prescriptions. Accurate measurement and recording of outflow are critical to detect these problems promptly.

Continued

INTERVENTIONS	RATIONALES
In the presence of outflow problems, monitor for the following: *Full color:* Use stool softeners, high-fiber diet, laxatives, or enemas if necessary. *Catheter occlusion by fibrin* (usually occurs soon after insertion): Obtain prescription to irrigate with heparinized saline. *Catheter obstruction by omentum:* Turn patient from side to side, elevate HOB or foot of bed, or apply firm pressure to the abdomen. **Note:** Notify health care provider for unresolved outflow problems.	These factors are potential causes of outflow problems, and they necessitate intervention to reverse the problem.
Monitor intake and output (I&O) and weight daily.	Patient's weight is one of the key indicators in choosing dialysis solutions. For example, a steady weight gain indicates fluid retention and may indicate a need for increased dialysis.
Weigh patient at same time each day, using same scale and with patient wearing same amount of clothing (or with same items on the bed if using a bed scale).	Weighing patient under the same conditions helps ensure accurate measurement of fluid status.
Monitor patient for respiratory distress.	Respiratory distress can occur because of compression of the diaphragm by the dialysate, especially when patient is supine.
If this occurs, elevate HOB, and notify health care provider.	Raising HOB may help alleviate this problem because the diaphragm will be less compressed by the dialysis solution. If respiratory distress continues, the dialysis nurse should be notified because drainage of the solution may alleviate diaphragmatic pressure.
Report gross bloody outflow.	Bloody outflow may appear with initial exchanges as a sign of peritonitis (see earlier nursing diagnosis). Because bloody outflow can also appear as a result of menstruation, the nurse should ask female patient if she is menstruating during assessment for signs and symptoms of peritonitis.
Observe for and report indicators of volume depletion.	Volume depletion (e.g., poor skin turgor, hypotension, tachycardia, and decreased CVP) can occur with excessive use of hypertonic dialysate and should be reported promptly for timely intervention.

••• **Related NIC and NOC labels:** *NIC:* Fluid Monitoring; Vital Signs Monitoring; Peritoneal

Nursing Diagnosis:

Imbalanced Nutrition: Less Than Body Requirements

related to protein loss in the dialysate

Desired Outcomes: At a minimum of 24 hr before hospital discharge, patient exhibits adequate nutrition as evidenced by stable weight. Patient's protein intake is 1.2-1.5 g/kg/day.

INTERVENTIONS	RATIONALES
Ensure adequate dietary intake of protein: 1.2-1.5 g/kg/day.	Protein crosses the peritoneum, and a significant amount is lost in the dialysate. An increased intake of protein is necessary to prevent excessive tissue catabolism. Protein loss increases with peritonitis.
Ensure that a dietary evaluation and teaching program are performed when patient changes from one type of dialysis to the other.	Patients undergoing peritoneal dialysis typically have fewer dietary restrictions than those on hemodialysis. Usually sodium and potassium restrictions are less for a patient receiving peritoneal dialysis than for one on hemodialysis. This is due, in part, to the fact that dialysis is provided continuously to peritoneal dialysis patients versus only 3 times/wk for those receiving hemodialysis.

Continued

INTERVENTIONS	RATIONALES
Provide lists of restricted and encouraged foods with menus that illustrate their integration into the daily diet.	This information helps ensure patient's understanding of the dietary regimen.
Request that patient plan a 3-day menu that incorporates appropriate foods and restrictions.	Asking patient to apply newly learned information via menu planning is a valid way of teaching and evaluating patient's understanding.

••• **Related NIC and NOC labels:** *NIC:* Nutrition Monitoring; Nutrition Management; Teaching: Prescribed Diet *NOC:* Nutritional Status: Nutrient Intake

ADDITIONAL NURSING DIAGNOSES/PROBLEMS:

"Prolonged Bedrest" for **Constipation** related to changes in dietary intake, immobility, and oral iron supplementation   p. 67

"Psychosocial Support" for **Disturbed Body Image** related to changes in body parts or function or presence of dialysis cathete   p. 80

✓ PATIENT-FAMILY TEACHING AND DISCHARGE PLANNING

When providing patient-family teaching, focus on sensory information, avoid giving excessive information, and initiate a visiting nurse referral if indicated for follow-up teaching. Include verbal and written information about the following:

✓ Medications, including drug name, purpose, dosage, schedule, drug-drug and food-drug interactions, precautions, and potential side effects.

✓ Diet and fluid restrictions: Include fact sheets that list foods to limit or restrict. Review fluid restrictions. Provide sample menus with examples of how dietary restrictions may be incorporated into daily meals. Have patient demonstrate understanding of dietary restrictions by preparing 3-day menus.

✓ Care and observation of exit site as per agency protocol.

✓ Need for and importance of monitoring daily weights, intake and output, and monitoring of BP at home, if necessary.

✓ Importance of continued medical follow-up; confirm date and time of next health care provider appointment.

✓ Signs and symptoms that necessitate medical attention. For example, symptoms that may indicate need for alteration in dialysis prescription: increased weight gain, unusual shortness of breath, edema, dizziness or fainting; symptoms that may indicate infection: fever, abdominal pain, redness or discharge from exit site, cloudy or decreased outflow, or nausea.

✓ Telephone numbers to call in case questions or concerns arise about therapy or disease after discharge. Additional general information can be obtained by contacting:

- National Kidney and Urologic Diseases Information Clearinghouse at *www.kidney.niddk.nih.gov*
- National Kidney Foundation at *www.kidney.org*

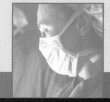

Renal Failure, Acute 29

OVERVIEW/PATHOPHYSIOLOGY

Acute renal failure (ARF) is a sudden loss of renal function as a result of reduced blood flow or glomerular injury, which may or may not be accompanied by oliguria. The kidneys lose their ability to maintain biochemical homeostasis, causing retention of metabolic wastes and dramatic alterations in fluid, electrolyte, and acid-base balance. Although alteration in renal function usually is reversible, ARF may be associated with a mortality rate of 40%-80%. Mortality varies greatly with the cause of ARF, patient's age, and co-morbid conditions.

Causes of ARF are classified according to development as prerenal, intrinsic, and postrenal. A decrease in renal function secondary to decreased renal perfusion but without renal parenchymal damage is called *prerenal failure*. Causes of prerenal failure include fluid volume deficit, shock, and decreased cardiac function. If hypoperfusion has not been prolonged, restoration of renal perfusion will restore normal renal function. A reduction in urine output because of mechanical obstruction to urine flow is called *postrenal failure*. Conditions causing postrenal failure include neurogenic bladder, tumors, and urethral strictures. Early detection of prerenal and postrenal failure is essential because, if prolonged, they can lead to parenchymal damage. Restoration of renal function in cases of postrenal failure is directly related to removal of the obstruction.

The most common cause of *intrinsic* or *intrarenal failure*, or renal failure that develops secondary to renal parenchymal damage, is acute tubular necrosis (ATN). Although typically associated with prolonged ischemia (prerenal failure) or exposure to nephrotoxins (aminoglycoside antibiotics, heavy metals, radiographic contrast media), ATN also can occur after transfusion reactions, septic abortions, or crushing injuries. Additional medications associated with the development of ARF include nonsteroidal antiinflammatory drugs (NSAIDs), angiotensin-converting enzyme (ACE) inhibitors, immuno-suppressants (e.g., cyclosporine), antineoplastics (e.g., cisplatin), and antifungals (e.g., amphotericin B). The clinical course of ATN can be divided into the following three phases: oliguric (urine output of greater than 100 ml and less than 400 ml/day, lasting approximately 7-21 days), diuretic (7-14 days), and recovery (3-12 mo). Causes of intrinsic renal failure other than ATN include acute glomerulonephritis (GN), malignant hypertension, and hepatorenal syndrome.

HEALTH CARE SETTING

Acute medical-surgical care unit

ASSESSMENT

Electrolyte disturbance: Muscle weakness and dysrhythmias.

Excess fluid volume: Oliguria, pitting edema, hypertension, pulmonary edema.

Metabolic acidosis: Kussmaul respirations (hyperventilation), lethargy, headache.

Uremia (retention of metabolic wastes): Altered mental state, anorexia, nausea, diarrhea, pale and sallow skin, purpura, decreased resistance to infection, anemia, fatigue. **Note:** Uremia adversely affects all body systems.

GI system: Nausea, vomiting, diarrhea, constipation, gastrointestinal (GI) bleeding, anorexia, abdominal distention.

Infection: Urinary tract infection, septicemia, pulmonary infections, peritonitis.

Physical assessment: Pallor, edema (peripheral, periorbital, sacral), jugular vein distention, crackles (rales), and elevated blood pressure (BP) in patient who has fluid overload.

History of: Exposure to nephrotoxic substances, recent blood transfusion, prolonged hypotensive episodes or decreased renal perfusion, sepsis, administration of radiolucent contrast media, or prostatic hypertrophy.

DIAGNOSTIC TESTS

Creatinine clearance: Measures kidney's ability to clear the blood of creatinine and approximates the glomerular filtration rate. It will decrease as renal function decreases. Creatinine clearance is normally decreased in older persons. **Note:** Failure to collect all urine during the period of study can invalidate the test.

BUN and serum creatinine: Assess progression and management of ARF. Although both blood urea nitrogen (BUN) and creatinine will increase as renal function decreases, creatinine is a better indicator of renal function because it is not affected by diet, hydration, or tissue catabolism.

Urinalysis: Can provide information about cause and location of renal disease as reflected by abnormal urinary sediment (renal tubular cells and cell casts).

Urinary osmolality and urinary sodium levels: To rule out renal perfusion problems (prerenal). In ATN, the kidney loses its ability to adjust urine concentration and conserve

231

sodium, producing urine Na^+ level greater than 40 mEq/L (in prerenal azotemia the urine Na^+ is less than 20 mEq/L).

Note: All urine samples should be sent to the laboratory immediately after collection or should be refrigerated if this is not possible. Urine left at room temperature has greater potential for bacterial growth, turbidity, and alkalinity, any of which can distort the reading.

Renal ultrasound: Provides information about renal anatomy and pelvic structures, evaluates renal masses, and detects obstruction and hydronephrosis. Because no IV contrast agent is used, this procedure limits risk of further compromise to renal function.

Renal scan: Provides information about perfusion and function of the kidneys.

CT scan: Identifies dilation of renal calices in obstructive processes.

Retrograde urography: Assesses for postrenal causes (i.e., obstruction).

Nursing Diagnosis:

Risk for Infection: With Risk Factors Associated with Uremia

Desired Outcome: Patient is free of infection as evidenced by normothermia; WBC count 11,000/mm^3 or less; urine that is clear and of normal odor; normal breath sounds; eupnea; and absence of erythema, warmth, tenderness, swelling, and drainage at the catheter or IV access sites.

Note: One of the primary causes of death in ARF is sepsis.

INTERVENTIONS	RATIONALES
Monitor temperature and secretions for indicators of infection.	Even minor increases in temperature can be significant because uremia masks the febrile response and inhibits the body's ability to fight infection.
Use meticulous sterile technique when changing dressings or manipulating venous catheters, IV lines, or indwelling catheters.	These measures prevent infection via spread of pathogens.
Avoid long-term use of indwelling urinary catheters. Whenever possible, use intermittent catheterization instead.	Indwelling urinary catheters are a common source of infection.
Provide oral hygiene and skin care at frequent intervals.	Intact skin and oral mucous membranes are barriers to infection.
Use emollients and gentle soap.	These measures prevent drying and cracking of skin, which could lead to breakdown and infection.
Rinse off all soap when bathing patient.	Soap residue may further irritate skin and affects its integrity.

••• **Related NIC and NOC labels:** *NIC:* Infection Control; Infection Prevention *NOC:* Infection Status; Immune Status

Nursing Diagnosis:

Ineffective Protection

related to neurosensory, musculoskeletal, and cardiac changes secondary to uremia, electrolyte imbalance, and metabolic acidosis

Desired Outcomes: After treatment, patient verbalizes orientation to person, place, and time and is free of injury caused by neurosensory, musculoskeletal, or cardiac disturbances. Within the 24-hr period before hospital discharge, patient verbalizes signs and symptoms of electrolyte imbalance and metabolic acidosis and importance of reporting them promptly should they occur.

INTERVENTIONS	RATIONALES
Assess for and alert patient to indicators of alterations in fluid, electrolyte, and acid-base balance.	In ARF, the kidneys lose the ability to maintain biochemical homeostasis, causing retention of metabolic wastes and dramatic alterations in fluid, electrolyte, and acid-base balance. The following may occur:
	Hypokalemia: Muscle weakness, lethargy, dysrhythmias, abdominal distention, and nausea and vomiting (secondary to ileus). It may occur during the diuretic phase because of urinary potassium losses.
	Hyperkalemia: Muscle cramps, dysrhythmias, muscle weakness, and peaked T waves on electrocardiogram. Hyperkalemia is a common and potentially fatal complication of ARF during the oliguric phase. It may occur if the kidney is unable to excrete potassium ions into the urine.
	Caution: A normal serum K^+ level is necessary for normal cardiac function.
	Hypocalcemia: Neuromuscular irritability, for example, positive Trousseau's sign (carpopedal spasm) and Chvostek's sign (facial muscle spasm), and paresthesias. Hypocalcemia may occur because of increased serum phosphate (there is a reciprocal relationship between calcium and phosphorus—as one rises, the other decreases).
	Hyperphosphatemia: Although usually asymptomatic, may cause bone or joint pain, painful/itchy skin lesions. Serum phosphorus may increase because of a decreased ability of the kidneys to excrete this ion.
	Uremia: Anorexia, nausea, metallic taste in the mouth, irritability, confusion, lethargy, restlessness, and itching. Uremic symptoms result from increased BUN as the kidney loses its ability to excrete nitrogenous wastes.
	Metabolic acidosis: Rapid, deep respirations; confusion. A buildup of hydrogen ions occurs in the serum because of the kidneys' inability to buffer and secrete this ion.
Avoid giving patient foods high in potassium.	This restriction helps patient's potassium levels return to more normal levels. Salt substitutes also contain potassium and should be avoided along with apricots, avocados, bananas, cantaloupe, carrots, cauliflower, chocolate, dried beans and peas, dried fruit, mushrooms, nuts, oranges, peanuts, potatoes, prune juice, pumpkins, spinach, sweet potatoes, Swiss chard, tomatoes, and watermelon.
Maintain adequate nutritional intake (especially calories).	If caloric intake is inadequate, body protein will be used for energy, resulting in increased end products of protein metabolism (i.e., nitrogenous wastes). A high-carbohydrate diet helps minimize tissue catabolism and production of nitrogenous wastes.
Prevent infections.	This measure minimizes tissue catabolism by controlling fevers. See **Risk for Infection,** earlier.
Avoid or use with caution the following medications: NSAIDs, ACE inhibitors, and potassium-sparing diuretics.	These medications may cause an increase in serum potassium.
	Note: Soon after renal disease is initially diagnosed, ACE inhibitors may be prescribed for their renal protective effects. However, after chronic kidney disease has developed, ACE inhibitors may be contraindicated because of risk of hyperkalemia and their potential to increase rate of progression to end-stage renal disease (ESRD).
Prepare patient for possibility of altered taste and smell.	These sense alterations may occur with uremia as a result of toxin buildup due to inability of the kidney to excrete nitrogenous waste.
Avoid use of magnesium-containing medications.	Patients with renal failure are at risk for increased magnesium levels because of decreased urinary excretion of dietary magnesium. Patients using magnesium-containing antacids such as Maalox typically are switched to aluminum hydroxide preparations such as ALternaGEL or Amphojel. Milk of Magnesia should be substituted with another, non–magnesium-containing laxative such as casanthranol.

Continued

INTERVENTIONS	RATIONALES
Administer aluminum hydroxide or calcium antacids as prescribed. Experiment with different brands, or try capsules for patients who refuse certain liquid antacids.	These agents are administered to control hyperphosphatemia. Phosphate binders vary in their aluminum or calcium content, however, and one may not be exchanged for another without first ensuring that patient is receiving the same amount of elemental aluminum or calcium. **Note:** Aluminum-containing phosphate binders should not be used long term because of their potential to cause bone damage.
Administer other medications as prescribed:	
- Diuretics	These drugs are used in nonoliguric ARF for fluid removal. For example, furosemide (Lasix) (100-200 mg) or mannitol (12.5 g) may be given early in ARF to limit or prevent development of oliguria.
- Antihypertensives	These drugs are used to control BP in the presence of underlying illness, fluid overload, sodium retention, or stimulation of the renin-angiotensin system in patients with renal ischemia.
- Cation exchange resins (Kayexalate)	These resins are used to control hyperkalemia. Kayexalate is most effectively administered orally, but it may be administered as an enema. The resin acts in the intestinal tract via exchange of sodium ions (from the Kayexalate) for potassium ions. Kayexalate is usually administered with sorbitol to prevent constipation and fecal impaction. **Note:** Severe hyperkalemia may be treated also with *IV sodium bicarbonate,* which shifts potassium into the cells temporarily, or *glucose and insulin.* Insulin also helps move potassium into the cells, and glucose helps prevent dangerous hypoglycemia, which could result from the insulin. *IV calcium* is given to reverse the cardiac effects of life-threatening hyperkalemia.
- Calcium or vitamin D supplements	These supplements are given to patients with hypocalcemia.
- Sodium bicarbonate	This is given to treat metabolic acidosis when serum bicarbonate level is less than 15 mmol/L. It is used cautiously in patients with hypocalcemia, edema, or sodium retention. Rapidly rising serum pH may result in muscle spasms in patients with hypocalcemia.
- Vitamins B and C	These vitamins replace losses if patient is on dialysis.
Assure patient and significant other that irritability, restlessness, and altered thinking are temporary and will improve with treatment.	Reassurance may help allay added anxiety.
Display calendars and request that significant others bring radios and familiar objects.	These measures will help orient patient to person, place, and time.
Ensure safety measures (e.g., padded side rails, airway) for patients who are confused or severely hypocalcemic. For patients who exhibit signs of hyperkalemia, have emergency supplies (e.g., manual resuscitator bag, crash cart, emergency drug tray) available.	These measures are for patient's protection until electrolyte disturbance is reversed.

••• **Related NIC and NOC labels:** *NIC:* Cerebral Profusion Promotion; Neurologic Monitoring *NOC:* Neurologic Status: Consciousness

Nursing Diagnosis:

Excess Fluid Volume

related to compromised regulatory mechanisms secondary to renal dysfunction: *Oliguric phase*

Desired Outcome: Patient adheres to prescribed fluid restrictions and becomes normovolemic as evidenced by decreasing or stable weight, normal breath sounds, edema 1+ or less on a 0-4+ scale, CVP 12 cm H_2O or less, and BP and HR within patient's normal range.

INTERVENTIONS	**RATIONALES**
Closely monitor and document intake and output (I&O).	This assessment detects trend of fluid volume, particularly decreasing urinary output when compared to intake. Patients with ARF may/may not develop oliguria. Urine volume does not necessarily reflect renal function in patients with ARF. For example, in postrenal failure, large volumes of urine may be associated with relief of obstruction. In ARF, the kidneys lose their ability to maintain biochemical homeostasis. This causes retention of metabolic wastes and dramatic alterations in fluid, electrolyte, and acid-base balance. For details about likely electrolyte imbalances and metabolic acidosis, see **Ineffective Protection,** p. 232.
Monitor weight daily.	The patient likely will lose 0.5 kg/day if not eating; a sudden weight gain suggests excessive fluid volume.
Weigh patient at the same time each day, using same scale and with patient wearing same amount of clothing.	This ensures that weight measurements are performed under the same conditions with each assessment, thereby facilitating more precise measurements.
Monitor for edema, hypertension, crackles (rales), tachycardia, distended neck veins, shortness of breath, and increased central venous pressure (CVP).	These signs are indicators of fluid volume excess. In ARF, dependent edema likely will be detected in the legs or feet of patients who are ambulatory, whereas the sacral area will be edematous in those who are on bedrest. Periorbital edema may also result from excessive fluid overload. Jugular veins are likely to be distended with head of bed elevated 45 degrees owing to increased intravascular volume if patient has excessive fluid volume. Crackles and shortness of breath can occur as a result of pulmonary fluid volume overload. Low serum albumin decreases colloid osmotic pressure, allowing fluid to leak into the extravascular space. Low serum albumin also may contribute to generalized edema and pulmonary edema.
	Hypertension, tachycardia, and increased CVP may result from sodium and fluid retention. Decreased renal perfusion also may activate the renin-angiotensin system, exacerbating these symptoms.
Carefully adhere to prescribed fluid restriction.	This measure helps patient return to normovolemia. Fluids usually are restricted on the basis of "replace losses + 400 ml/24 hr." Insensible fluid losses are only partially replaced to offset water formed during the metabolism of proteins, carbohydrates, and fats.
Provide oral hygiene at frequent intervals, and offer fluids in the form of ice chips or ice pops. Spread allotted fluids evenly over a 24-hr period, and record amount given. Instruct patient and significant others about need for fluid restriction.	These interventions minimize thirst during fluid restriction. Hard candies also may be given to decrease thirst.
	Note: Patients nourished via total parenteral nutrition are at increased risk for fluid overload because of the necessary fluid volume involved and its hypertonicity.
Monitor results of BUN, serum creatinine, and creatinine clearance tests.	Although both BUN and creatinine will increase as renal function and renal excretion decrease, creatinine is a better indicator of renal function because it is not affected by diet, hydration, or tissue catabolism. Creatinine clearance measures the ability of the kidney to clear the blood of creatinine and approximates the glomerular filtration rate. It will decrease as renal function decreases. **Note:** Creatinine clearance is normally decreased in older persons.
Administer medications that promote diuresis as prescribed.	Control of fluid overload in ARF may include use of large doses of furosemide in nonoliguric patients to induce diuresis.
Arrange for or administer renal dialysis as prescribed. For more information, see "Hemodialysis," p. 223, or "Peritoneal Dialysis," p. 227, as indicated.	Hemodialysis treatments remove excess fluid through the process of ultrafiltration (removal of fluids using pressure). Peritoneal dialysis removes fluid via osmotic pressures across the peritoneal membrane. The present trend is to use dialysis early in ARF. It is done q1-3days (but may be done continuously in critical care). Prophylactic use of dialysis has reduced the incidence of complications and rate of death in patients with ARF.

••• **Related NIC and NOC labels:** *NIC:* Fluid Management; Fluid Monitoring; Fluid & Electrolyte Management; Hypervolemia Management *NOC:* Fluid Balance; Electrolyte & Acid-Base Balance

Nursing Diagnosis:

Risk for Deficient Fluid Volume

related to active loss secondary to excessive urinary output: *Diuretic phase*

Desired Outcome: Patient remains normovolemic as evidenced by stable weight, balanced I&O, good skin turgor, CVP 5 cm H_2O or greater, and BP and HR within patient's normal range.

INTERVENTIONS	RATIONALES
Closely monitor and document I&O.	This assessment detects trend of fluid volume. Following relief of the obstruction in patients with postrenal failure, postobstructive diuresis may occur if the kidney is unable to concentrate the urine. Consequently, large volumes of solute and fluid may be lost (8-20 L/day of urinary losses), resulting in volume depletion.
Monitor weight daily.	A weight loss of 0.5 kg/day or more may reflect excessive volume loss.
Weigh patient at the same time each day, using same scale and with patient wearing same amount of clothing.	When weight is measured under the same conditions, more precise measurements can be anticipated.
Monitor patient for complaints of lightheadedness, poor skin turgor, hypotension, postural hypotension, tachycardia, and decreased CVP.	These are indicators of volume depletion, which may result from loss of intravascular volume caused by urinary fluid losses.
As prescribed, encourage fluids in dehydrated patient.	This intervention promotes rehydration and prevents life-threatening electrolyte abnormalities caused by the large-volume urinary and solute losses.
Report significant findings to health care provider.	Although renal function usually can be reversed, there is a mortality rate of 40%-80% associated with ARF, depending on cause and patient's age and comorbid conditions.

••• **Related NIC and NOC labels:** *NIC:* Fluid Management; Fluid Monitoring; Hypovolemia Management *NOC:* Fluid Balance; Hydration

Nursing Diagnosis:

Imbalanced Nutrition: Less Than Body Requirements

related to nausea, vomiting, anorexia, and dietary restrictions

Desired Outcome: Within 2 days of admission, patient has stable weight and demonstrates normal intake of food within restrictions, as indicated.

INTERVENTIONS	RATIONALES
Alert health care providers to untoward GI symptoms, and monitor BUN levels.	The presence of nausea, vomiting, and anorexia may signal increased uremia. BUN levels 80-100 mg/dl usually require dialytic therapy.
Provide frequent, small meals in a pleasant atmosphere, especially controlling unpleasant odors.	Smaller, more frequent meals are usually better tolerated than larger meals.
Administer prescribed antiemetics as necessary. Instruct patient to request medication before discomfort becomes severe.	Antiemetics (e.g., hydroxyzine, ondansetron, prochlorperazine, and promethazine) are given to reduce nausea, which is better controlled when it is treated early.
Coordinate meal planning and dietary teaching with patient, significant others, and renal dietitian.	Dietary restriction may include reduced protein, sodium, potassium, phosphorus, and fluid intake.
Provide fact sheets that list foods to restrict.	Protein is limited to minimize retention of nitrogenous wastes. Sodium is limited to prevent thirst and fluid retention. Potassium and phosphorus are limited because of the kidney's decreased ability to excrete them.

Continued

INTERVENTIONS	RATIONALES
Demonstrate with sample menus examples of how dietary restrictions may be incorporated into daily meals.	Sample menus show patient how to apply this new knowledge.
Provide oral hygiene at frequent intervals.	Oral hygiene decreases metallic taste in the mouth associated with uremia.

••• **Related NIC and NOC labels:** *NIC:* Nutrition Management; Nutrition Monitoring; Weight Gain Assistance *NOC:* Nutritional Status: Food Intake

ADDITIONAL NURSING DIAGNOSES/ PROBLEMS:

"Prolonged Bedrest" for **Constipation** related to less than adequate fluid or dietary intake and bulk, immobility, lack of privacy, positional restrictions, and use of narcotic analgesics	p. 67
"Care of the Patient Undergoing Hemodialysis"	p. 223
"Care of the Patient Undergoing Peritoneal Dialysis"	p. 227

✔ PATIENT-FAMILY TEACHING AND DISCHARGE PLANNING

When providing patient-family teaching, focus on sensory information, avoid giving excessive information, and initiate a visiting nurse referral for necessary follow-up teaching. Include verbal and written information about the following:

✓ Medications: Include drug name, purpose, dosage, schedule, precautions, and potential side effects. Also discuss drug-drug, herb-drug, and food-drug interactions.

✓ Diet: Include fact sheets that list foods to restrict. Provide sample menus with examples of how dietary restrictions may be incorporated into daily meals.

✓ Care and observation of dialysis access if patient is being discharged with one.

✓ Importance of continued medical follow-up of renal function.

✓ Signs and symptoms of potential complications. These should include **Excess Fluid Volume,** p. 234; electrolyte imbalance (see **Ineffective Protection,** p. 232); indicators of infection (see **Risk for Infection,** p. 232); and bleeding (especially from the GI tract for patients who are uremic).

✓ Telephone numbers to call in case questions or concerns arise about therapy or disease after discharge. Additional general information can be obtained by contacting the following:

- National Kidney and Urologic Diseases Information Clearinghouse at *www.kidney.niddk.nih.gov*
- National Kidney Foundation at *www.kidney.org*

If patient requires dialysis after discharge, coordinate discharge planning with dialysis unit staff.

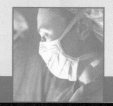

Care of the Renal 30
Transplant Recipient

OVERVIEW/PATHOPHYSIOLOGY

Individuals with end-stage renal disease (ESRD) have several treatment modalities from which to choose—hemodialysis, peritoneal dialysis, no treatment, and renal transplantation. Diabetes is the leading cause of renal failure in the United States, and there is an increasing number of simultaneous kidney-pancreas transplants. In order for a solid organ transplant to survive, patients need to take immunosuppressive medications for the life of the graft. Renal transplantation is not a cure for renal failure, and it can only be done in Medicare-approved facilities. There are several types of donors for renal transplant patients: deceased (formerly cadaveric), living related, living unrelated, voluntary nondirected, and kidney-paired donors. Postoperatively, patients are sent to specialized units where nephrology nurses monitor them on an hourly basis for the first 24-36 hr. Subsequent admissions may occur at any hospital for treatment of a rejection episode, infection, medication complication, or unrelated illness. Rejection is the major complication of renal transplantation. Long-term complications occur secondary to use of immunosuppressive agents and include infection, hypertension, cardiovascular disease, chronic liver disease, bone demineralization, cataracts, gastrointestinal (GI) hemorrhage, and cancer.

HEALTH CARE SETTING

Transplant center; acute care surgical unit or critical care unit for complications or rejection

Immunosuppression

With the exception of identical twin donors, all transplant recipients must take drugs that suppress their immune system to prevent graft rejection. Each transplant center has a drug protocol outlining which combination of medications will be given to each patient. **Note:** A complete list of patient's medications, including herbal remedies, should be included on patient's chart. Some herbs interfere with absorption of immunosuppressive medications, causing patients to have lower levels of medications in their systems and potentially resulting in episodes of graft rejection and/or loss of the graft. Check the herbal PDR if unsure about interactions.

Rejection

Acute: May begin weeks to 1 year after surgery; potentially reversible; treated with increased immunosuppression.

Chronic: Usually classified as starting 1 year after transplant; irreversible; managed conservatively with diet and antihypertensive agents until dialysis is required.

Indicators of rejection: Oliguria, tenderness over graft site (located in iliac fossa), sudden weight gain (2-3 lb/day), fever, malaise, hypertension, and increased blood urea nitrogen (BUN) and serum creatinine. In addition, hyperglycemia will develop with combined kidney-pancreas transplants.

Nursing Diagnosis:
Risk for Infection

related to invasive procedures, exposure to infected individuals, and immunosuppression

Desired Outcomes: Patient is free of infection as evidenced by normothermia; HR 100 bpm or less (or within patient's normal range); RR 12-20 bpm with normal depth and pattern; and absence of erythema, edema, increased local warmth, tenderness, or purulent drainage at wounds or catheter exit sites. Patient is free of signs and symptoms of oral, esophageal, respiratory, GI, genitourinary, and cutaneous infections. Patient verbalizes indicators of infection and importance of reporting them promptly to health care provider or staff.

INTERVENTIONS	RATIONALES
When caring for these patients, increase your sensitivity to *any* indicator of infection as a cue to increase depth and frequency of assessments for infection.	Transplant recipients are taking large doses of immunosuppressive agents, and their immune response and thus response to infectious agents will be muted. Infections therefore are potentially life threatening in an individual who is immunosuppressed.
Be especially sensitive to low-grade temperature elevation, fever, and unexplained tachycardia.	These are indicators that might signal infection in a transplant recipient.
Instruct patient to be alert to signs and symptoms of commonly encountered infections and importance of reporting them promptly.	Infections and their indicators include *urinary tract infection* (UTI)—cloudy and malodorous urine; dysuria, frequency, and urgency; pain in the suprapubic area, buttock, thighs, labia, or scrotum; *upper respiratory tract infection* (URI)—productive cough, malodorous, purulent, colored, and copious secretions, chest pain or heaviness; *pharyngitis*—painful swallowing; *otitis media*—malaise, earache; *impetigo*—inflamed or draining areas on the skin.
	Prompt reporting of these indicators is essential because infections can be life threatening in a patient undergoing immunosuppression.
Monitor for indicators of cytomegalovirus (CMV), including fever, malaise, fatigue, and muscle aches.	CMV is a common infectious agent among these patients. Other infectious complications include *Legionella pneumophila;* cutaneous herpes simplex (shingles); varicella zoster (chickenpox); Epstein-Barr virus (EBV); oral, esophageal, deep fungal or mycotic pseudoaneurysm caused by *Candida;* and *Pneumocystis jiroveci* (formerly called *Pneumocystis carinii*).
Teach patient to avoid exposure to individuals known to have infections and to wash hands frequently.	Washing hands consistently is a proven method of removing pathogens from the skin that could otherwise cause infection and is especially important in patients whose immune systems are compromised.
Discuss use of prophylactic antibiotics for any minor invasive procedures.	Prophylactic antibiotics reduce infection risk, which can occur in even minor procedures. Some health care providers encourage antibiotics for any minor invasive procedures, including dental cleaning.
Use sterile technique with all invasive procedures and dressing changes.	Following sterile technique reduces the possibility of infection, which is increased with invasive procedures into the body and involving nonintact skin.
Teach patient to avoid working in soil for the first 6 months after transplantation.	This restriction minimizes the risk of acquiring aspergillus infection.
As indicated, advise patient to quit smoking; provide smoking cessation literature.	Smoking increases susceptibility to respiratory infection because it damages protective mechanisms such as cilia in the lungs. Smoking also causes detrimental changes to blood pressure (BP), heart rate (HR), cholesterol levels, and clotting factors.

●●● **Related NIC and NOC labels:** *NIC:* Infection Control; Communicable Disease Management; Vital Signs Monitoring; Health Education
NOC: Infection Status; Immune Status

Nursing Diagnosis:

Deficient Knowledge:

Signs and symptoms of rejection, side effects of immunosuppressive agents, transplantation complications, and importance of protecting existing hemodialysis vascular access

Desired Outcome: Within the 24-hr period before hospital discharge, patient verbalizes knowledge of signs and symptoms of rejection, side effects of immunosuppressive therapy, complications of transplantation, and importance of protecting the hemodialysis vascular access.

INTERVENTIONS	RATIONALES
Assess patient's health care literacy (language, reading, comprehension). Assess culture and culturally specific information needs.	This assessment helps ensure that information is presented in a manner that is culturally and educationally appropriate.

Continued

INTERVENTIONS	RATIONALES
Explain importance of renal function monitoring: intake and output, daily weight, and BUN and serum creatinine values.	These tests evaluate kidney status and guide the therapeutic drug regimen and treatment plan: as renal function decreases, BUN and creatinine values will increase.
Teach patient the signs and symptoms of rejection.	Signs and symptoms of rejection necessitate prompt intervention to save the kidney. These include oliguria, tenderness over transplanted kidney (located in iliac fossa), sudden weight gain (2-3 lb), fever, malaise, hypertension, and increased BUN (greater than 20 mg/dl) and serum creatinine (greater than 1.5 mg/dl). In addition, patient may have body aches, swelling in legs or hands, and temperature greater than 100° F.
Instruct patients to weigh themselves at same time each day, using same scale and wearing same amount of clothing. Provide a notebook in which to record daily vital signs (VS) and weight measurements. Remind patients to bring the notebook to all outpatient visits and to report abnormal values promptly should they occur.	These assessments monitor the trend of VS and weight measurements. Using same standards daily ensures accuracy with weight measurements.
Teach patients that if a rejection episode occurs, they will be removed from their antirejection medications and started on other agents until their creatinine level drops below 3 mg/dl.	Agents such as OKT3 and antithymocyte globulin are substitute antirejection medications that are less nephrotoxic. OKT3 requires a chest x-ray study to ensure no pulmonary edema occurs during administration and patients will need VS monitored q4h to assess for temperature elevation after administration. Patients taking antithymocyte globulin require premedication to prevent possible anaphylaxis.
Explain importance of serial white blood cell (WBC) and platelet count monitoring.	Significant decreases in WBC and platelet counts can be a side effect of immunosuppressive agents, and therefore serial monitoring is essential.
Teach signs and symptoms of GI bleeding and importance of reporting them promptly if they occur.	GI bleeding is a potential side effect of immunosuppressive agents and can be life threatening if it is excessive. Prompt reporting of the onset of these symptoms (e.g., tarry stools, "coffee-ground" emesis, orthostatic changes, dizziness, tachycardia, increasing fatigue and weakness) enables health care provider to adjust medications or add medications such as antacids and H_2-receptor blockers to treat cause of the bleeding.
Teach patient and/or significant others how to measure BP, and provide guidelines for values that would necessitate notification of health care provider or staff member.	In a patient who has undergone renal transplantation, hypertension may develop for a variety of reasons, including cyclosporine or steroid use, rejection, or renal artery stenosis. In addition, patient may have had hypertension before the transplant. A value that would necessitate notification of the health care provider is BP 20% above or below patient's "normal" BP. This value and parameters for calling health care provider are generally agreed on before patient leaves the hospital.
For patients with a patent fistula or graft (hemodialysis vascular access), explain that taking BP, drawing blood, and starting IVs are contraindicated in the vascular access arm and therefore patient should warn others about these contraindications.	Patient will need the fistula, shunt, or graft if a return to dialysis is indicated, and therefore it must be handled carefully.
Stress need for continued medical evaluation of the transplant.	Continued evaluation will confirm that the kidney is working properly and patient is not undergoing rejection.
Verify patient's knowledge of immunosuppressive medication precautions and dosages.	A knowledgeable patient is likely to participate more effectively in the therapeutic regimen.
	Azathioprine: Dosage is adjusted or held based on patient's WBC count.
	Prednisone: Some patients may become steroid-induced diabetics due to use.
	Cyclosporine: Although most commonly given as a capsule, if liquid oral form is required, a glass container and metal spoon are used; it is mixed with orange juice or chocolate milk to make it more palatable; the solution must not be allowed to stand; and it must not be mixed with grapefruit juice. Grapefruit juice has been known to potentiate medication and could cause nephrotoxicity and/or loss of graft function.

••• **Related NIC and NOC labels:** *NIC:* Teaching: Prescribed Medications; Teaching: Individual *NOC:* Knowledge: Treatment Regimen

✓ PATIENT-FAMILY TEACHING AND DISCHARGE PLANNING

When providing patient-family teaching, focus on sensory information, avoid giving excessive information, and make appropriate referrals (e.g., visiting or home health nurse, community health resources) for follow-up teaching. Include verbal and written information about the following:

✓ Medications, including name, dosage, purpose, schedule, precautions, drug-drug and food-drug interactions, and potential side effects. Provide guidelines for how to cope with medication side effects.

✓ Measures for preventing infection, including incision care. Stress to patient that infections can be life threatening because of immunosuppression.

✓ Prescribed diet and activity level progression.

✓ Community resources for emotional and financial support.

✓ Importance of follow-up care to ensure long-term viability of transplanted kidney.

✓ Telephone numbers to call in case problems or questions arise after discharge from care facility.

✓ Internet resources:
- United Network for Organ Sharing at *www.unos.org*
- National Kidney Disease Education Program at *www.nkdep.nih.gov*
- National Kidney Foundation at *www.kidney.org*
- International Transplant Nurses Society at *www.transweb.org/itns*
- Transplant Recipients International Organization (TRIO) at *www.trioweb.org*

Also see discussions in **Deficient Knowledge:** Signs and symptoms of rejection, side effects of immunosuppressive agents, transplantation complications, and importance of protecting the existing hemodialysis vascular access, earlier.

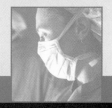

Ureteral Calculi 31

OVERVIEW/PATHOPHYSIOLOGY

Ureteral calculi (stones) constitute the third most common urologic condition after urinary tract infections (UTIs) and pathologic conditions of the prostate. Although the cause of stones is unknown in 50% of reported cases, it is believed that they originate in the kidney and are passed through the kidney to the ureter. About 90% of all stones pass from the ureter into the bladder and out of the urinary system spontaneously.

HEALTH CARE SETTING

Primary care; may require hospitalization for complications or surgery

ASSESSMENT

Signs and symptoms: Pain that is sharp, sudden, and intense or dull and aching; located in the flank area; and often radiating toward the groin. Pain may be intermittent (colic) as the stone moves along the ureter and may subside when it enters the bladder. Nausea, vomiting, diarrhea, abdominal pain, and paralytic ileus may occur. Patient may experience urgency and frequency, void in small amounts, and have hematuria. Fever may indicate an infected stone or secondary UTI.

Physical assessment: Pallor, diaphoresis, tachycardia, and tachypnea may be observed. Costovertebral angle (CVA) tenderness and guarding may be present. Bowel sounds may be absent secondary to ileus, and the abdomen may be distended and tympanic. The patient will be restless and unable to find a position of comfort.

History of: Sedentary lifestyle; residence in geographic area in which water supply is high in stone-forming minerals; vitamin A deficiency; vitamin D excess; hereditary cystinuria; inflammatory bowel disease; recurrent UTIs; prolonged periods of immobilization; gout or prophylactic therapy with allopurinol; use of indinavir sulfate, a protease inhibitor used in patients with human immunodeficiency virus (HIV) infection; decreased fluid intake; hyperparathyroidism; sarcoidosis; and familial history of calculi or renal disease such as renal tubular acidosis.

DIAGNOSTIC TESTS

Serum tests: To assess calcium levels greater than 5.3 mEq/L, phosphorus levels greater than 2.6 mEq/L, and uric acid levels greater than 7.5 mg/dl, which have been implicated in stone formation.

BUN and creatinine tests: To evaluate renal-urinary function. Abnormalities are reflected by high blood urea nitrogen (BUN) and serum creatinine and low urine creatinine levels. **Note:** Be aware that BUN levels are affected by fluid volume excess and deficit. Volume excess will reduce BUN levels, whereas volume deficit will increase levels. For the older adult, serum creatinine level may not be a reliable measure of renal function because of reduced muscle mass and a decreased glomerular filtration rate (GFR). These tests must be evaluated based on an adjustment for the patient's age and hydration status and in comparison with other renal-urinary tests.

Urinalysis: To provide baseline data on urinary system functioning, detect metabolic disease, and assess for the presence of UTI. A cloudy or hazy appearance; foul odor; pH greater than 8.0; and presence of red blood cells, leukocyte esterase, white blood cells (WBCs), and WBC casts signal UTI. A pH less than 5 is associated with uric acid calculi, whereas a pH of 7.5 or greater may signal presence of urea-splitting organisms (responsible for magnesium-ammonium-phosphate or struvite calculi).

Urine culture: To determine type of bacteria present in the genitourinary tract. To avoid contamination, a midstream specimen should be collected.

24-hr urine collection: To test for high levels of uric acid, cystine, calcium, magnesium, oxalate, calcium, phosphorus, or creatinine. A second 24-hour urine collection may be done after the patient has been on a diet restricted in sodium, oxalate, and calcium.

Note: All urine samples should be sent to the laboratory immediately after they are obtained or refrigerated if this is not possible (specimens for culture are not refrigerated). Urine left at room temperature has greater potential for bacterial growth, turbidity, and alkaline pH, any of which can distort the reading.

CT scan with or without injection of contrast medium: To distinguish cysts, tumors, calculi, and other masses and determine presence of ureteral dilation and bladder distention.

Excretory urogram/intravenous pyelogram (IVP): Used to visualize kidneys, renal pelvis, ureters, and bladder. It can identify size of the stone and presence and severity of the obstruction. This test also outlines nonradiopaque stones within the ureters. Nonradiopaque stones (e.g., uric acid calculi) are seen as radiolucent defects in the contrast media.

Renal ultrasound: To identify ureteral dilation and presence of stones in the ureters.

Nursing Diagnosis:

Acute Pain

related to presence of a calculus or the surgical procedure to remove it

Desired Outcomes: Patient's subjective perception of pain decreases within 1 hr of intervention, as documented by a pain scale. Objective indicators, such as grimacing, are absent or diminished.

INTERVENTIONS	RATIONALES
Assess and document quality, location, intensity, and duration of pain. Devise a pain scale with patient that ranges from 0 (no pain) to 10 (worst pain).	This assessment evaluates intensity and trend of pain and subsequent relief obtained.
Notify health care provider of sudden and/or severe pain.	This is a sign that a stone is passing through the ureter.
Notify health care provider of a sudden cessation of pain. Strain all urine for solid matter, and send to laboratory for analysis.	This can signal passage of the stone.
Medicate patient with prescribed analgesics, narcotics, and antispasmodics; evaluate and document response based on pain scale.	Conservative therapy may consist of a trial of analgesia, dissolution agents, and normal fluid intake to 1500-2000 ml/day. Dissolution agents such as orange juice alkalinize urine and work to shrink stones so that they can pass through the ureter.
	Note: Morphine increases ureteral peristalsis, which aids in stone passage, but ureteral peristalsis can increase pain.
Encourage patient to request medication before discomfort becomes severe.	Pain is easier to manage when it is treated before it gets too severe because prolonged stimulation of pain receptors increases sensitivity to painful stimuli and increases amount of drug required to relieve pain.
Administer antiemetics (e.g., hydroxyzine, ondansetron, prochlorperazine, promethazine) as prescribed.	These agents promote comfort from nausea and vomiting.
Provide warm blankets or heating pad to affected area, or supply warm baths.	These measures increase regional circulation and relax tense muscles.
Provide back rubs.	Back rubs are especially helpful for postoperative patients who were in the lithotomy position during surgery.
See "Pain," p. 39, for other interventions.	

••• **Related NIC and NOC labels:** *NIC:* Medication Management; Pain Management; Simple Massage; Heat Application *NOC:* Comfort Level; Pain Control; Pain Level

Nursing Diagnosis:

Impaired Urinary Elimination: Dysuria, Urgency, Frequency

related to obstruction caused by the ureteral calculus

Desired Outcomes: Patient relates return of a normal voiding pattern within 2 days. Patient demonstrates ability to record I&O and strain urine for stones.

INTERVENTIONS	RATIONALES
Determine and document patient's normal voiding pattern.	This assessment establishes a baseline for subsequent assessment.
Monitor quality and color of urine.	Optimally, urine is straw colored and clear and has a characteristic odor. Dark urine is often indicative of dehydration, and blood-tinged urine can result from rupture of ureteral capillaries as the calculus passes through the ureter.
In patients for whom fluids are not restricted, encourage fluid intake of at least 2-3 L/day.	Increased hydration helps flush the calculus through the ureter into the bladder and out through the system.

Continued

INTERVENTIONS	RATIONALES
Record accurate intake and output (I&O); teach patient how to record I&O.	Output that is less than input could signal an obstruction. Patient should participate in I&O documentation to ensure that all output and intake is being recorded.
Strain all urine for evidence of solid matter; teach patient the procedure.	This intervention can detect passage of stones.
Send any solid matter to the laboratory for analysis.	The laboratory will test for high levels of uric acid, cystine, oxalate, calcium, or phosphorus, which would signal presence and type of stones.

••• **Related NIC and NOC labels:** *NIC:* Fluid Management; Urinary Elimination Management *NOC:* Urinary Continence; Urinary Elimination

Nursing Diagnosis:

Impaired Urinary Elimination

related to obstruction or postsurgical positional problems of the ureteral catheter

Desired Outcome: Following intervention, patient has output from the ureteral catheter and is free of spasms or flank pain, which could signal obstruction or displacement.

INTERVENTIONS	RATIONALES
If patient has more than one catheter, label one *right* and the other *left*; keep all drainage records separate.	Occasionally, patients return from surgery with ureteral catheters. Ureteral catheters, also known as *stents*, are positioned postoperatively to enable healing and promote ureteral patency in the presence of edema. If patient has two ureteral catheters, separate output records are used to identify how each ureter is functioning.
Monitor output from ureteral catheter.	The amount will vary with each patient and will depend on catheter dimension.
If drainage is scanty or absent, milk catheter and tubing gently. If this fails, notify health care provider.	This action will help dislodge the obstruction.
Caution: Never irrigate catheter without specific health care provider instructions to do so. If irrigation is prescribed, use gentle pressure and sterile technique. Always aspirate with sterile syringe before instillation. Use another sterile syringe to insert instillation amounts 3 ml or less.	There is potential for ureteral damage and infection during irrigation caused by overdistention and/or introduction of pathogens.
Explain to patient that semi-Fowler's and side-lying positions are acceptable but that Fowler's position should be avoided.	Fowler's position should be avoided because sutures are seldom used and gravity can cause the catheter to move into the bladder. Typically patient will require bedrest if the ureteral catheter is indwelling.
Carefully monitor urethral catheter for movement, and ensure that it is securely attached to patient.	Ureteral catheters are often attached to the urethral catheter after placement in the ureters. The urethral catheter should be monitored to detect movement and to ensure that it is securely attached to patient.
Note: After ureteral catheters have been removed (usually simultaneously with urethral catheter), monitor for flank pain, CVA tenderness, nausea, and vomiting.	These are indicators of ureteral obstruction, which necessitates prompt intervention.

••• **Related NIC and NOC labels:** *NIC:* Tube Care: Urinary *NOC:* Urinary Elimination

Nursing Diagnosis:

Risk for Impaired Skin Integrity

related to wound drainage after ureterolithotomy or procedures entering the ureter

Desired Outcome: Patient's skin surrounding wound site remains nonerythremic and intact.

INTERVENTIONS	RATIONALES
Monitor incisional dressings frequently during first 24 hr, and change or reinforce as needed. Note and document odor, consistency, and color of drainage.	Immediately after surgery, drainage may be red. Flank approaches to the ureter require muscle-splitting incisions and result in significant post-operative oozing of blood. Because drainage will also include urine leaking from the entered ureter, excoriation can result from prolonged contact of urine with the skin.
Use Montgomery straps or net wraps (e.g., Surginet) rather than tape to secure dressing.	This intervention facilitates frequent dressing changes without harming the skin with tape removal.
If drainage is copious after drain removal, apply wound drainage or ostomy pouch with a skin barrier over the incision.	These measures prevent contact of wound drainage with the skin.
Use a pouch with an antireflux valve.	This valve prevents contamination from reflux.

••• **Related NIC and NOC labels:** *NIC:* Skin Surveillance; Skin Care: Topical Treatments; Wound Care; Incision Site Care
NOC: Tissue Integrity: Skin and Mucous Membranes; Wound Healing: Primary Intention

Nursing Diagnosis:

Deficient Knowledge:

Dietary regimen and its relationship to calculus formation

Desired Outcome: Within the 24-hr period before hospital discharge, patient verbalizes knowledge about foods and liquids to limit in order to prevent stone formation and demonstrates this knowledge by planning a 3-day menu that excludes or limits these foods.

INTERVENTIONS	RATIONALES
Assess patient's knowledge about diet and its relationship to stone formation.	This assessment will reveal patient's baseline knowledge, which will enable formulation of an individualized teaching plan.
Advise nonrestricted patient to maintain a urine output of at least 2-3 L/day.	Increasing urine output reduces saturation of stone-forming solutes.
Teach patient to maintain adequate hydration of at least 2-3 L/day, especially after meals and exercise.	Good hydration after meals and exercise is important because patient's solute load is highest at these times.
Caution: Patients with cardiac, liver, or renal disease require special fluid intake instructions from their health care provider.	These patients likely will need some degree of fluid restriction to prevent fluid overload.
Teach technique for measuring urine specific gravity via a hydrometer.	In order to minimize stone formation, specific gravity should remain less than 1.010.
As appropriate, provide the following information.	
For uric acid stones:	
- Limit intake of foods such as lean meat, legumes, whole grains. Limit protein intake to 1 g/kg/day.	These foods are high in purines, which can lead to formation of uric acid stones.
- Explain that allopurinol or sodium bicarbonate may be given.	These agents reduce uric acid production or alkalinize the urine, keeping pH at 6.5 or higher.
For calcium stones:	
- Limit intake of foods such as milk, cheese, green leafy vegetables, yogurt.	These foods are high in calcium content.
- Limit sodium intake.	A low-sodium diet helps reduce intestinal absorption of calcium.
- Limit intake of refined carbohydrates and animal proteins.	These foods can cause hypercalciuria.
- Encourage foods high in natural fiber content (e.g., bran, prunes, apples).	These foods provide phytic acid, which binds dietary calcium.
- Explain that sodium cellulose phosphate, 5 g, may be given three times a day, before each meal. It should be used cautiously in post-menopausal women at risk for osteoporosis.	Sodium cellulose phosphate, when used with calcium-restricted diet, reduces risk of stone formation by binding with intestinal calcium and thus increasing excretion of calcium.

Continued

INTERVENTIONS	RATIONALES
- Explain that orthophosphates (potassium acid phosphate and disodium and dipotassium phosphates) or thiazides also may be given for calcium stones.	These agents decrease urinary excretion of citrate and pyrophosphate and thus inhibit stone formation.
For oxalate stones:	
- Limit intake of foods such as chocolate, caffeine-containing drinks (including instant and decaffeinated coffees), beets, spinach, rhubarb, berries, draft beer, and nuts such as almonds, walnuts, pecans, and cashews.	These foods are high in oxalate content.
- Explain that large doses of pyridoxine may help with certain types of oxalate stones, and cholestyramine, 4 g four times daily, may be prescribed.	These agents bind with oxalate enterally.
- Explain that vitamin C supplements should be avoided.	As much as half of the vitamin C is converted to oxalic acid.
Ask patient to plan a 3-day menu that includes or excludes appropriate foods.	This will demonstrate patient's level of understanding of the prescribed diet and areas in which teaching should be reinforced. This effort by patient also will reinforce learning.

••• **Related NIC and NOC labels:** *NIC:* Teaching: Prescribed Diet; Teaching: Prescribed Medications *NOC:* Knowledge: Diet; Knowledge: Medications.

ADDITIONAL NURSING DIAGNOSES/ PROBLEMS:

"Perioperative Care"	p. 45

PATIENT-FAMILY TEACHING AND DISCHARGE PLANNING

When providing patient-family teaching, focus on sensory information, avoid giving excessive information, and initiate a visiting nurse referral for necessary follow-up teaching. Include verbal and written information about the following:

✓ Medications, including drug name, purpose, dosage, schedule, precautions, and potential side effects. Also discuss drug-drug, herb-drug, and food-drug interactions.

✓ Indicators of UTI that necessitate medical attention: chills; fever; hematuria; flank, CVA, suprapubic, low back, buttock, scrotal, or labial pain; cloudy and foul-smelling urine; increased frequency, urgency; dysuria; and increasing or recurring incontinence.

✓ Care of incision, including cleansing and dressing. Teach patient signs and symptoms of local infection, including redness, swelling, local warmth, tenderness, and purulent drainage.

✓ Care of drains or catheters if patient is discharged with them.

✓ Importance of daily fluid intake of at least 2-3 L/day in nonrestricted patients.

✓ Dietary changes as specified by health care provider. Include fact sheets that list foods to restrict or add to the diet. Provide sample menus with examples of how dietary restrictions and requirements may be incorporated into daily meals.

✓ Activity restrictions as directed for patient who has had surgery: avoid lifting heavy objects (more than 10 lb) for the first 6 wk, be alert to fatigue, get maximum rest, increase activities gradually to tolerance.

✓ Use of Nitrazine paper to assess pH of urine. Desired pH will be determined by type of stone formation to which patient is prone. Instructions for use are on Nitrazine container.

✓ Importance of walking or other exercise to decrease risk of stone formation.

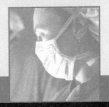

Urinary Diversions 32

OVERVIEW/PATHOPHYSIOLOGY

When the bladder must be bypassed or is removed, a urinary diversion is created. Urinary diversions most commonly are created for individuals with bladder cancer. However, malignancies of the prostate, urethra, vagina, uterus, or cervix may require creation of a urinary diversion if anterior, posterior, or total pelvic exenteration must be done. Individuals with severe, nonmalignant urinary problems, such as radiation or interstitial cystitis, or urinary incontinence that cannot be managed conservatively also are candidates for urinary diversion. Although most urinary diversions are permanent, some act as a temporary bypass of urine, and undiversion can be performed if the patient's condition changes.

The urinary stream may be diverted at multiple points: the renal pelvis (pyelostomy or nephrostomy), the ureter (ureterostomy), the bladder (vesicostomy), or via an intestinal "conduit." Vesicostomies are most commonly performed in children as a temporary diversion. While construction of a small bowel pouch (Kock procedure) or ileocolonic pouch (Indiana or Mainz procedure) is still the most common type of urinary diversion, the neobladder or orthotopic bladder is becoming the standard of definitive care. All these procedures reconstruct a new bladder from intestinal segments, resulting in a more normal urinary pattern. In addition, because males have an external urinary sphincter that can be left in place when the bladder is removed, men may undergo attachment of a reconstructed bladder to the urethra, which will enable urination without the use of catheterization. However, there is a 5%-10% risk of urethral reoccurrence of neoplasm with this procedure.

Continent urinary diversions: All continent urinary diversions are constructed with the following three components: a reservoir or reconstructed bladder, a continence mechanism, and an antireflux mechanism.

Orthotopic neobladder: This surgery involves use of the small intestine or small bowel–large bowel combination to create a low-pressure spherical reservoir that attaches to the patient's urinary sphincter. Additionally, a cystoprostatectomy is performed in men and a urethral-preserving anterior exenteration is performed in women. Similar to the Mainz and Kock techniques, the created "bladder" has the characteristics of low pressure, adequate volume, and control of urination without leakage or residual urine. The patient can sense a full bladder and urinate without catheterization. Normal continence is the goal for this procedure.

Indiana and Kock pouches: Both the Indiana and Kock pouches use the ileum to create a pouch and an antireflux valve. These types of continent urostomies require the patient to perform catheterizations to remove urine from the pouch.

Intestinal (ileal conduit): Any segment of bowel may be used to create a passageway for urine but the ileum conduit is most commonly used. A 15- to 20-cm section of ileum is resected from the intestine to form a passageway for the urine. The proximal end is closed, and the distal end is brought out through the abdomen, forming a stoma. The ureters are resected from the bladder and anastomosed to the ileal segment. The intestine is reanastomosed to the ileal segment. The intestine is reanastomosed, and therefore bowel function is unaffected. Occasionally, the jejunum is used for the conduit. However, jejunal-conduit syndrome (hyperkalemia, hyponatremia, hypochloremia) often occurs.

HEALTH CARE SETTING

Surgical unit; primary care

Nursing Diagnosis:

Anxiety

related to threat to self-concept, interaction patterns, or health status secondary to urinary diversion surgery

Desired Outcome: Before surgery, patient communicates fears and concerns, relates attainment of increased psychologic and physical comfort, and exhibits a coping environment.

INTERVENTIONS	RATIONALES
Assess patient's perception of his or her impending surgery and resulting body function changes. Listen actively.	This assessment provides an opportunity for patient to express anxieties about the upcoming surgery and for the nurse to evaluate the response. For example, "You seem very concerned about next week's surgery." Anger, denial, withdrawal, and demanding behaviors may be coping responses.
Acknowledge patient's concerns.	This will help focus attention on anxieties and concerns so that they can be dealt with.
Provide brief, basic information regarding physiology of the procedure and equipment that will be used after surgery, including tubes and drains.	Knowledge is one of the best means of decreasing anxiety.
Show patient pouches that will be used after surgery. Assure patient that the pouch usually cannot be seen through clothing and that it is odor resistant.	Patient may worry that others will be able to see and smell the pouch.
For patient about to undergo a continent urostomy procedure of Kock or Indiana pouch, explain that a pouching system may be needed for a short time after surgery. Reassure patient that teaching about accessing the continent urostomy will be done in the surgeon's office or by the home care nurse.	This intervention likely will decrease anxiety by reassuring patient that he or she will be taught necessary skills.
Discuss postsurgical activities of daily living with patient.	This information decreases anxiety that such ADL as showers, baths, and swimming can continue and that diet is not affected after the early postoperative period.
As appropriate, ask patient what information has been relayed by the surgeon about sexual implications of the surgery.	Patient may be very anxious about sexual implications of this surgery but afraid to ask. Asking this question will help establish an open relationship between patient and nurse. For example, some males undergoing radical cystectomy with urinary diversion may become impotent, but recent surgical advances have enabled preservation of potency for others. The pelvic plexus, which innervates the corpora cavernosa (allowing penile erection) may be damaged permanently as a result of autonomic nerve damage. However, sensation and orgasm are mediated by the pudendal nerve (sensorimotor) and are not affected.
Arrange for a visit by the enterostomal (ET) nurse during the preoperative period. Collaborate with surgeon, ET nurse, and patient to identify and mark the most appropriate site for the stoma.	Showing patient the actual spot for placement may help alleviate anxiety by reinforcing that impact on lifestyle and body image will be minimal.

••• **Related NIC and NOC labels:** *NIC:* Anxiety Reduction; Active Listening; Emotional Support; Teaching: Preoperative Sensory Information *NOC:* Anxiety Control: Coping

Nursing Diagnosis:

Impaired Urinary Elimination

related to postoperative use of ureteral stents, catheters, or drains and to urinary diversion surgery

Desired Outcome: Patient's urinary output is 30 ml/hr or greater; urine is clear and straw-colored with normal, characteristic odor.

INTERVENTIONS	RATIONALES
Monitor intake and output, and record total amount of urine output from urinary diversion for the first 24 hr postoperatively. Differentiate and record separately amounts from all drains, stents, and catheters. Notify health care provider of an output less than 60 ml during a 2-hr period.	This assessment checks for discrepancies between intake and output. In the presence of adequate intake a decreased output can signal a ureteral obstruction, a leak in one of the anastomotic sites, or impending renal failure.

Continued

INTERVENTIONS	RATIONALES
	Ureterostomy: Urine is drained via the stoma and/or ureteral stents.
	Intestinal conduit: Urine is drained via the stoma. Patient also may have ureteral stents and/or conduit catheter/stent in the early postoperative period to stabilize ureterointestinal anastomoses and maintain drainage from the conduit during early postoperative edema.
	Continent urinary diversions or reservoirs: The Kock urostomy usually has a reservoir catheter and also may have ureteral stents. The Indiana (ileocecal) reservoir usually has ureteral stents exiting from the stoma, through which most of the urine drains, and may have a reservoir catheter exiting from a stab wound, which serves as an overflow catheter. The neobladder has a urethral catheter in place that will drain urine, which initially will be light red to pink in color with mucus but should clear in 24-48 hr. This catheter generally remains in place for 21 days to ensure adequate healing of the anastomosis.
Also assess for flank pain, costovertebral angle (CVA) tenderness, nausea, vomiting, and anuria.	These are other indicators of ureteral obstruction.
Monitor functioning of ureteral stents.	Ureteral stents, which exit from the stoma into the pouch, maintain ureteral patency and assist in healing of the anastomosis. Stents may become blocked with mucus, but as long as urine is draining adequately around the stent and the volume of output is adequate, this is not a problem. Right stents usually are cut at a 90-degree angle, and left stents are cut at a 45-degree angle. Each usually produces approximately the same amount of urine, although the amount produced by each is not important as long as each drains adequately and total drainage from all sources is 30 ml/hr or greater. Urine is usually red to pink for the first 24-48 hr and becomes straw-colored by the third postoperative day. Absent or lessening amounts of urine may indicate a blocked stent or problems with the ureter.
Monitor functioning of stoma catheters.	Expect output from stoma catheter to include pink or light red urine with mucus and small red clots for the first 24 hr. Urine should become amber colored with occasional clots within 3 postoperative days. Mucus production will continue but should decrease in volume.
	In continent urinary diversions, a catheter is placed in the reservoir to prevent distention and promote healing of suture lines. This new reservoir (i.e., resected intestine) exudes large amounts of mucus, necessitating catheter irrigation with 30-50 ml of normal saline, which is instilled gently and allowed to empty via gravity.
Monitor functioning of drains.	Any urinary diversion may have Penrose drains or closed drainage systems in place to facilitate healing of the ureterointestinal anastomosis. Drainage from these systems may be light red to pink for the first 24 hr and then lighten to amber and decrease in amount. Excessive lymph fluid and urine can be removed via these drains to reduce pressure on anastomotic suture lines. In a continent urinary diversion, an increase in drainage after amounts have been low might signal an anastomotic leak, which necessitates notification of health care provider.
Monitor drainage from Foley catheter or urethral drain (if present). Note color, consistency, and volume of drainage, which may be red to pink with mucus.	Patients who have had a cystectomy may have a urethral drain, whereas those with a partial cystectomy will have an indwelling catheter in place.
Report sudden increase or decrease in drainage to health care provider.	A sudden increase would occur with hemorrhage; a sudden decrease can signal blockage that can lead to infection or, with partial cystectomy, hydronephrosis.
Encourage an intake of at least 2-3 L/day in the nonrestricted patient.	Increased hydration keeps the urinary tract well irrigated and helps prevent infection that could be caused by urinary stasis.

••• **Related NIC and NOC labels:** *NIC:* Tube Care: Urinary; Urinary Catheterization *NOC:* Urinary Elimination

Nursing Diagnosis:

Risk for Infection

related to an invasive surgical procedure and risk of ascending bacteriuria with urinary diversion

Desired Outcome: Patient is free of infection as evidenced by normothermia; WBC count 11,000/mm^3 or less; and absence of purulent or excessive drainage, erythema, edema, warmth, and tenderness along the incision.

INTERVENTIONS	RATIONALES
Monitor patient's temperature q4h during first 24-48 hr after surgery. Notify health care provider of fever (temperature greater than 101° F).	Elevated temperature is a sign that the body is mounting a defense against infection.
Inspect dressing frequently after surgery. Change dressing when it becomes wet, using sterile technique. Use extra care to prevent disruption of drains.	Infection is most likely to become evident after the first 72 hr. The presence of purulent or excessive drainage on the dressing signals infection and the need to notify health care provider promptly for timely intervention.
Note condition of the incision.	Erythema, tenderness, local warmth, edema, and purulent or excessive drainage are indicators of infection at the incision line.
Monitor and record character of urine at least q8h.	Urine should be yellow or pink tinged during the first 24-48 hr after surgery. Mucus particles are normal in urine of patients with ileal conduits and continent urinary diversions because of the nature of the bowel segment used. Cloudy urine, however, is abnormal and can signal infection.
Assess for flank or CVA pain, malodorous urine, chills, and fever.	These are indicators of urinary tract infection (UTI).
Note position of the stoma relative to the incision. If they are close together, apply pouch first to avoid overlap of the pouch with the suture line, which can increase risk of infection.	Overlapping of the pouch with the suture line increases risk of infection.
If necessary, cut pouch down on one side or place it at an angle.	This measure prevents contact of the pouch with drainage, which may loosen adhesive.
Wash your hands before and after caring for patient.	This intervention helps prevent contamination and cross-contamination.
Do not irrigate indwelling urethral catheters of patients with cystectomies.	Patients with cystectomies without anastomosis to the urethra may have an indwelling urethral catheter to drain serosanguineous fluid from the peritoneal cavity. Irrigation of this catheter can result in peritonitis.
Encourage fluid intake of at least 2-3 L/day.	Increased hydration helps flush urine through the urinary tract, removing mucus shreds, and preventing stasis that could result in infection.

••• **Related NIC and NOC labels:** *NIC:* Infection Control: Intraoperative; Incision Site Care; Skin Surveillance; Wound Care: Closed Drainage; Tube Care: Urinary *NOC:* Infection Status; Wound Healing: Primary Intention

Nursing Diagnosis:

Ineffective Protection

related to neurosensory, musculoskeletal, and cardiac changes secondary to hyperchloremic metabolic acidosis with hypokalemia

Desired Outcomes: Patient verbalizes orientation to person, place, and time (within patient's normal range) and remains free of injury caused by neurosensory, musculoskeletal, and cardiac changes. Electrolytes remain within normal limits.

INTERVENTIONS	RATIONALE
For patients with ileal conduits, assess for nausea and changes in level of consciousness (LOC) and muscle tone, and irregular heart rate (HR).	Changes in neurosensory, musculoskeletal, and cardiac status are indicators of hypokalemia and metabolic acidosis that can occur secondary to the presence of Na^+ and Cl^- from the urine in the ileal segment, which results in compensatory loss of K^+ and HCO_3^-.
Monitor serum electrolyte studies.	K^+ less than 3.5 mEq signals hypokalemia, and HCO_3^- less than 7.40 signals metabolic acidosis.
If patient displays confused behavior or exhibits signs of motor dysfunction, keep bed in lowest position and raise side rails. If convulsions appear imminent, pad side rails. Notify health care provider of significant findings.	These are standard safety precautions for patients who have confusion or motor dysfunction.
Encourage oral intake as directed, and assess fluid balance.	Maintaining fluid balance will help ameliorate acid-base and electrolyte imbalances.
If patient is hypokalemic and allowed to eat, encourage foods high in potassium.	Foods high in potassium, such as potatoes, prune juice, pumpkin, spinach, sweet potatoes, Swiss chard, tomatoes, and watermelon will help reverse hypokalemia.
	The health care provider may prescribe IV fluids with potassium supplements to prevent or treat hypokalemia.
Encourage patient to ambulate by second day after surgery.	Mobility will help prevent urinary stasis, which increases risk of electrolyte problems.

●●● **Related NIC and NOC labels:** *NIC:* Seizure Precautions; Vital Signs Monitoring: Neurologic Monitoring *NOC:* Neurologic Status: Consciousness

Nursing Diagnosis:

Risk for Impaired Skin Integrity

related to presence of urine or sensitivity to appliance material

Desired Outcome: Patient's peristomal skin remains nonerythematous and intact.

INTERVENTIONS	RATIONALE
For patient with significant allergy history, patch-test the skin for a 24-hr period, at least 24 hr before surgery. If erythema, swelling, bleb formation, itching, weeping, or other indicators of tape allergy occur, document type of tape that caused the reaction and note on cover of chart, "Allergic to _____ tape." Place allergy armband on patient.	This assessment evaluates for and documents allergies to different tapes that might be used on the postoperative appliance.
Inspect integrity of peristomal skin with each wafer change. Question patient about itching or burning under the wafer. Change wafer routinely (per agency or surgeon preference) or immediately if leakage is suspected.	Itching or burning can signal leakage of pouch under the wafer. If the seal between the adhesive backing of the wafer and skin becomes compromised, leaking onto the peristomal skin can occur.
	Note: All pouches must be attached to a wafer and pouches are never placed directly over a stoma. The wafer covers the skin surrounding the stoma (peristomal skin). Pouches may come already attached to a wafer (one-piece system) or come separately (two-piece system).
Teach patient how often to change the wafer and/or pouch if a one-piece system is used.	Routine wafer/pouch change is every 4-7 days. This schedule provides the consistency that usually avoids surprise leakage problems.
Teach patient to monitor skin for leakage and odor.	Leakage and odor indicate that the wafer and/or pouch must be changed.
Teach patient to report signs of rash to health care provider	A rash can occur with a yeast infection and will require a topical medication for treatment.
Assess stoma, pouch, and skin for crystalline deposits.	These deposits are signals of alkaline urine, which can compromise skin integrity if exposure occurs.

Continued

INTERVENTIONS	RATIONALE
In the presence of alkaline urine, teach the following: drink fluids that leave acid ash in the urine, such as cranberry juice, or take ascorbic acid in a dose consistent with patient's size.	These actions help decrease urine pH, which will improve peristomal skin condition.
When changing wafer, measure stoma with a measuring guide and ensure that skin barrier opening is cut to the exact size of stoma.	
For a patient using a two-piece system or pouch with a wafer:	
Size the wafer to fit snugly around stoma. For pouch placement, size pouch to clear stoma by at least ⅛ inch.	These measures protect peristomal area from maceration caused by pooling of urine on the skin.
For a patient using a one-piece "adhesive only" pouch:	
If pouch has an antireflux valve, size the pouch to clear stoma and any peristomal creases.	This helps ensure that the pouch adheres to a flat, dry surface. An antireflux valve prevents pooling of urine on skin.
If pouch does not have an antireflux valve, size pouch so that it clears the stoma by ⅛ inch.	This will help prevent stomal trauma while minimizing amount of exposed skin.
Use a copolymer film sealant wipe on peristomal skin before applying wafer or adhesive only pouch and wafer system.	This will provide a moisture barrier and reduce epidermal trauma when wafer is removed.
Wash peristomal skin with water or a special cleansing solution marketed by ostomy supply companies. Dry skin thoroughly before applying skin barrier, wafer, and pouch.	Other products can dry out the skin, which would increase risk of irritation and infection.
When changing pouch or wafer, instruct patient to hold a gauze pad or clean small towel on (but not in) stoma.	This will absorb urine and keep skin dry.
After applying pouch, connect it to bedside drainage system if patient is on bedrest. When patient is no longer on bedrest, empty pouch when it is one-third to one-half full, opening spigot on bottom of pouch and draining urine into patient's measuring container.	These interventions facilitate drainage of urine.
Do not allow pouch to become too full. Instruct patient accordingly.	An overly full pouch could break the seal of the wafer with patient's skin.
Teach patient to treat peristomal irritation as follows after hospital discharge:	
Dry skin with a hair dryer on cool setting.	This eliminates necessity of wiping skin, which would increase the irritation.
Dust peristomal skin with karaya powder or spread Stomahesive paste.	These agents absorb moisture.
If desired, blot skin with water or a sealant wipe or copolymer protectant that seals in the powder.	These agents provide a moisture barrier.
Use a porous tape if tape is required.	Porous tape prevents trapping of moisture.
Notify health care provider or wound, ostomy, and continence (WOC)/ET nurse of any severe or nonresponsive skin problems.	These problems call for skilled interventions.

••• **Related NIC and NOC labels:** *NIC:* Skin Surveillance; Incision Site Care; Ostomy Care; Skin Care: Topical Treatments
NOC: Tissue Integrity: Skin and Mucous Membranes

Nursing Diagnosis:

Ineffective Tissue Perfusion: Stomal (or risk for same)

related to altered circulation

Desired Outcomes: Patient's stoma is pink or bright red and shiny. The stoma of a cutaneous urostomy is raised, moist, and red.

INTERVENTIONS

INTERVENTIONS	RATIONALES
Inspect stoma at least q8h and as indicated. Report significant findings promptly.	The stoma of an ileal conduit will be edematous and should be pink or red with a shiny appearance. The stoma formed by a cutaneous urostomy is usually raised during the first few weeks after surgery, red, and moist. A stoma that is dusky or cyanotic is indicative of insufficient blood supply and impending necrosis and must be reported to health care provider for immediate intervention.
Also assess degree of swelling. For patients with ileal conduit, evaluate stomal height and plan accordingly (see **Risk for Impaired Skin Integrity**, p. 253).	The stoma should shrink considerably over the first 6-8 wk and less significantly over the next year. The stoma formed by a cutaneous ureterostomy is usually raised during the first few weeks after surgery, red in color, and moist.

●●● **Related NIC and NOC labels:** *NIC:* Pressure Management; Skin Surveillance *NOC:* Tissue Integrity: Skin and Mucous Membrane

Nursing Diagnosis:

Deficient Knowledge:

Self-care regarding urinary diversion

Desired Outcome: Patient or significant other demonstrates proper care of stoma and urinary diversion before hospital discharge.

INTERVENTIONS	RATIONALES
Assess patient's health care literacy (language, reading, comprehension). Assess culture and culturally specific information needs.	This assessment helps ensure that information is presented in a manner that is culturally and educationally appropriate.
Also assess patient's or significant other's readiness to participate in care.	A well-thought out teaching plan is useless if patient is unable or unwilling to understand/learn it.
Involve ET or WOC nurse in patient teaching if available.	An ET or WOC nurse is specially trained and skilled in teaching urinary diversion care.
Assist patient with organizing the equipment and materials that are needed to accomplish home care.	Usually patient is discharged with disposable pouching systems. Most of these patients continue using disposable systems for the long term. Those who will use reusable systems usually are not fitted for 6-8 wk after surgery.
Teach how to remove and reapply pouch; how to empty it; and how to use gravity drainage system at night, including procedures for rinsing and cleansing drainage system.	These are the basic skills the patient will need in order to accomplish self-care after hospital discharge.
Teach signs and symptoms of UTI, peristomal skin breakdown, and appropriate therapeutic responses, including maintenance of an acidic urine (if not contraindicated), importance of adequate fluid intake, and techniques for checking urine pH (which should be assessed weekly). Explain that urine pH should remain at 6.0 or less.	Persons with urinary diversion have a higher incidence of UTI than the general public, so it is important to keep their urinary pH acidic. If it is greater than 6.0, advise patient to increase fluid intake and, with health care provider approval, to increase vitamin C intake to 500-1000 mg/day, which will increase urine acidity.
Teach patient with continent urinary diversion the technique for reservoir catheter irrigation.	In continent urinary diversions, a catheter is placed in the reservoir to prevent distention and promote healing of suture lines. This new reservoir (i.e., resected intestine) exudes large amounts of mucus, necessitating catheter irrigation with 30-50 ml of normal saline, which is instilled gently and allowed to empty via gravity.
Teach patient with continent urinary diversion with urethral anastomosis signals of the urge to void.	Feelings of vague abdominal discomfort and abdominal pressure or cramping are sensations of the need to void.
Instruct patient with continent urinary diversion with urethral anastomosis about the procedure to void.	Relaxing the perineal muscles and employing Valsalva's maneuver help empty the diversion.
Emphasize importance of follow-up visits, particularly for patients with continent urinary diversions.	Follow-up visits, particularly for patients with continent urinary diversions who will be taught how to catheterize the reservoir and use a small dressing over the stoma rather than an appliance, help ensure that patient can manipulate pouch and facilitate follow-up for questions.

Continued

INTERVENTIONS	RATIONALES
Provide a list of ostomy support groups and ET nurses in the area.	Referrals such as this will assist the patient after hospital discharge.
Provide patient with enough equipment and materials for the first week after hospital discharge.	The first postoperative visit is usually 1 wk after hospital discharge.
Remind patient of the importance of proper cleansing of ostomy appliances.	This knowledge will help patient reduce risk of bacterial growth and UTI after hospital discharge.

••• **Related NIC and NOC labels:** *NIC:* Teaching: Individual; Teaching: Procedure *NOC:* Knowledge: Illness Care

ADDITIONAL NURSING DIAGNOSES/ PROBLEMS:

"Cancer Care"	p. 1
"Perioperative Care"	p. 45
"Fecal Diversions" for **Disturbed Body Image**	p. 459

✓ PATIENT-FAMILY TEACHING AND DISCHARGE PLANNING

When providing patient-family teaching, focus on sensory information, avoid giving excessive information, and initiate a visiting nurse referral for necessary follow-up teaching. Include verbal and written information about the following:

✓ Medications, including drug name, dosage, schedule, precautions, and potential side effects. Also discuss drug-drug, herb-drug, and food-drug interactions.

✓ Indicators that necessitate medical intervention: fever or chills; nausea or vomiting; abdominal pain, cramping, or distention; cloudy or malodorous urine; incisional drainage, edema, local warmth, pain, or redness; peristomal skin irritation; or abnormal changes in stoma shape or color from the normal bright and shiny red.

✓ Maintenance of fluid intake of at least 2-3 L/day to maintain adequate kidney function.

✓ Importance of keeping urinary pH acidic. Individuals with urinary diversions have a higher incidence of urinary tract infection (UTI) than the general public; therefore it is important to keep their urinary pH acidic. Because many fruits and vegetables tend to make urine alkaline, the patient should drink cranberry juice rather than orange juice or other citrus juices or take vitamin C daily. (Check with health care provider first.)

✓ Care of stoma and application of urostomy appliances. Patient should be proficient in application technique before hospital discharge.

✓ Care of urostomy appliances. Remind patient that proper cleansing will reduce risk of bacterial growth, which would contaminate urine and increase risk of UTI.

✓ Importance of follow-up care with health care provider and ET nurse. Confirm date and time of next appointment.

✓ Telephone numbers to call in case questions or concerns arise about therapy after discharge. In addition, many cities have local support groups. Information for these patients can be obtained by contacting the following:

- United Ostomy Association at *www.uoa.org*
- American Cancer Society at *www.cancer.org*
- National Cancer Institute Information Service (CIS) at *www.cis.nci.nih.gov*

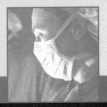

Urinary Tract Obstruction 33

OVERVIEW/PATHOPHYSIOLOGY

Urinary tract obstruction usually is the result of blockage from pelvic tumors, calculi, and urethral strictures. Additional causes include neoplasms, benign prostatic hypertrophy, ureteral or urethral trauma, inflammation of the urinary tract, pregnancy, and pelvic or colonic surgery in which ureteral damage has occurred. Obstructions can occur suddenly or slowly, over weeks to months. They can occur anywhere along the urinary tract, but the most common sites are the ureteropelvic and ureterovesical junctions, bladder neck, and urethral meatus. The obstruction acts like a dam, blocking passage of urine. Muscles in the area contract to push urine around the obstruction, and structures behind the obstruction begin to dilate. The smaller the site of obstruction, the greater the damage. Obstructions in the lower urinary structures, such as the bladder neck or urethra, can lead to urinary retention and urinary tract infection (UTI). Obstructions in the upper urinary tract can lead to bilateral involvement of the ureters and kidneys, leading to hydronephrosis, renal insufficiency, and kidney destruction. Hydrostatic pressure increases, and filtration and concentration processes in the tubules and glomerulus are compromised.

HEALTH CARE SETTING

Primary care and acute care

ASSESSMENT

Signs and symptoms: Anuria, nausea, vomiting, local abdominal tenderness, hesitancy, straining to start a stream, dribbling, decreased caliber and force of urinary stream, hematuria, oliguria, and uremia. Pain may be sharp and intense or dull and aching; localized or referred (e.g., flank, low back, buttock, scrotal, labial pain).

Physical assessment: Bladder distention and "kettle drum" sound over bladder with percussion (absent if obstruction is above the bladder) and mass in flank area, abdomen, pelvis, or rectum.

History of: Recent fever (possibly caused by the obstruction), hypertensive episodes (caused by increased renin production from the body's attempt to increase renal blood flow).

DIAGNOSTIC TESTS

Serum K^+ and Na^+ levels: To determine renal function. Normal range for K^+ is 3.5-5.0 mEq/L; normal range for Na^+ is 137-147 mEq/L.

BUN and creatinine: To evaluate renal-urinary status. Normally, their values are elevated with decreased renal-urinary function. **Note:** These values must be considered based on patient's age and hydration status. For the older adult, serum creatinine level may not be a reliable indicator because of decreased muscle mass and a decreased glomerular filtration rate. Hydration status can affect blood urea nitrogen (BUN): fluid volume excess can result in reduced values, whereas volume deficit can cause higher values.

Urinalysis: To provide baseline data on functioning of the urinary system, detect metabolic disease, and assess for presence of UTI. A cloudy, hazy appearance; foul odor; pH greater than 8.0; and presence of red blood cells, leukocyte esterase, white blood cells (WBCs), and WBC casts are signals of UTI.

Urine culture: To determine type of bacteria present in the genitourinary tract. To minimize contamination, a sample should be obtained from midstream collection.

Hgb and Hct: To assess for anemia, which may be related to decreased renal secretion of erythropoietin.

KUB radiography: To identify size, shape, and position of the kidneys, ureters, and bladder (KUB) and abnormalities such as tumors, calculi, or malformations.

Imaging studies: A variety of imaging studies may be used to identify area and cause of obstructions:

- Excretory urography/intravenous pyelography: To evaluate cause of urinary dysfunction by visualizing the kidneys, renal pelvis, ureters, and bladder.
- Antegrade urography: Involves placement of percutaneous needle or nephrostomy tube through which radiopaque contrast is injected. Antegrade urography is indicated when the kidney does not concentrate or excrete IV dye.
- Retrograde urography: Radiopaque dye is injected through ureteral catheters placed during cystoscopy.
- Cystogram: Radiopaque dye is instilled via cystoscope or catheter. This enables visualization of the bladder and evaluation of the vesicoureteral reflex.
- Computerized axial tomography (CT) scans: To identify degree and location of obstruction, as well as cause in many situations.

Maximal urinary flow rate: Less than 15 ml/sec indicates significant obstruction to flow.

Postvoid residual volume: Normal is less than 12 ml. Higher volume signals obstructive process.

Cystoscopy: To determine degree of bladder outlet obstruction and facilitate visualization of any tumors or masses.

Ultrasonography: To reveal areas of ureteral dilation or distention from retained urine.

Nursing Diagnosis:

Risk for Deficient Fluid Volume

related to postobstructive diuresis

Desired Outcomes: Patient is normovolemic as evidenced by HR 100 bpm or less (or within patient's normal range); BP 90/60 mm Hg or greater (or within patient's normal range); RR 20 breaths/min or less; no significant changes in mental status; and orientation to person, place, and time (within patient's normal range). Within 2 days after bladder decompression, output approximates input, patient's urinary output is normal for patient (or 30-60 ml/hr or greater), and weight becomes stable.

INTERVENTIONS	RATIONALES
Using sterile technique, insert a urinary catheter.	Catheterization will drain patient's bladder of the urine whose passage has been obstructed.
Monitor patient carefully during catheterization; clamp the catheter if patient complains of abdominal pain or has a symptomatic drop in systolic blood pressure of 20 mm Hg or greater.	Although research has demonstrated that rapid bladder decompression of greater than 750-1000 ml does not result in shock syndrome as previously believed, this assessment/action could determine presence of an electrolyte imbalance as a result of postobsructive diuresis.
Monitor intake and output hourly for 4 hr and then q2h for 4 hr after bladder decompression.	This assessment monitors for postobstructive diuresis.
Notify health care provider if output exceeds 200 ml/hr or 2 L over an 8-hr period.	This can signal postobstructive diuresis, which can lead to major electrolyte imbalance. If this occurs, anticipate initiation of IV infusion.
Monitor vital signs for decreasing blood pressure (BP), changes in level of consciousness or mentation, tachycardia, tachypnea, thready pulse.	These are signs of shock.
Anticipate need for urine specimens for analysis of electrolytes and osmolality and blood specimens for analysis of electrolytes.	Postobstructive diuresis can lead to major electrolyte imbalance.
Monitor for and report the following:	
- Abdominal cramps, lethargy, dysrhythmias.	These are signs of hypokalemia.
- Diarrhea, colic, irritability, nausea, muscle cramps, weakness, irregular apical or radial pulses.	These are signs of hyperkalemia.
- Muscle weakness and cramps, complaints of tingling in fingers, positive Trousseau's and Chvostek's signs.	These are signs of hypocalcemia.
- Excessive itching.	These are signs of hyperphosphatemia.
Monitor mentation, noting signs of disorientation.	Disorientation can occur with electrolyte disturbance.
Weigh patient daily using same scale and at same time of day (e.g., before breakfast).	Weight fluctuations of 2-4 lb (0.9-1.8 kg) normally occur in a patient who is undergoing diuresis. Losses greater than this can result in dehydration and electrolyte imbalances.
	Weighing patient in a consistent manner and under the same conditions helps ensure more precise measurements.

●●● **Related NIC and NOC labels:** *NIC:* Electrolyte Management; Electrolyte Monitoring; Laboratory Data Interpretation; Vital Signs Monitoring; Shock Prevention; Intravenous (IV) Insertion *NOC:* Electrolyte and Acid-Base Balance; Fluid Balance; Hydration

Nursing Diagnosis:

Acute Pain

related to bladder spasms

Desired Outcomes: Within 1 hr of intervention, patient's subjective perception of discomfort decreases, as documented by a pain scale. Objective indicators, such as grimacing, are absent or diminished.

INTERVENTIONS	RATIONALES
Assess for and document complaints of pain in suprapubic or urethral area. Devise a pain scale with patient, rating pain from 0 (no pain) to 10 (worst pain).	This assessment establishes a baseline for subsequent assessment and evaluates degree of pain relief obtained. Spasms occur frequently with obstruction.
Medicate with antispasmodics or analgesics such as oxybutynin and flavoxate as prescribed. Document pain relief obtained, using pain scale.	These medications relieve spasms and pain.
If patient is losing urine around the catheter and has a distended bladder (with or without bladder spasms), check catheter and drainage tubing for evidence of obstruction. Inspect for kinks and obstructions in drainage tubing, compress and roll catheter gently between fingers to assess for gritty matter within catheter, milk drainage tubing to release obstructions, or instruct patient to turn from side to side. Obtain prescription for catheter irrigation if these measures fail to relieve the obstruction.	These assessments detect and manage obstructions in the catheter and tubing that may be contributing to spasms.
In nonrestricted patients, encourage intake of fluids to at least 2-3 L/day to help reduce frequency of spasms.	Increased hydration reduces the frequency of spasms. IV fluid therapy may be indicated for acutely ill, dehydrated patient, or to increase fluids in patients with calculi.
Teach nonpharmacologic methods of pain relief, such as guided imagery, relaxation techniques, and distraction. See relaxation technique described in "Coronary Artery Disease," **Health-Seeking Behaviors,** p. 172.	These pain relief techniques augment pharmacologic interventions.

••• Related NIC and NOC labels: *NIC:* Medication Management; Pain Management; Distraction; Progressive Relaxation Therapy; Simple Guided Imagery *NOC:* Comfort Level; Pain Control; Pain Level

ADDITIONAL NURSING DIAGNOSES/ PROBLEMS:

"Perioperative Care"	p. 45
"Ureteral Calculi" for **Risk for Impaired Skin Integrity** related to wound drainage	p. 245

✓ PATIENT-FAMILY TEACHING AND DISCHARGE PLANNING

When providing patient-family teaching, focus on sensory information, avoid giving excessive information, and initiate a visiting nurse referral for necessary follow-up teaching. Include verbal and written information about the following:

✓ Medications, including drug name, dosage, purpose, schedule, precautions, and potential side effects. Also discuss drug-drug, herb-drug, and food-drug interactions.

✓ Indicators that signal recurrent obstruction and require prompt medical attention: pain, fever, decreased urinary output.

✓ Activity restrictions as directed for patient who has had surgery: avoid lifting heavy objects (more than 10 lb) for first 6 wk, be alert to fatigue, get maximum rest, increase activities gradually to tolerance.

✓ Care of drains or catheters if patient is discharged with them; care of surgical incision if present.

✓ Indicators of wound infection: persistent redness, local warmth, tenderness, drainage, swelling, and fever.

✓ Indicators of UTI that necessitate medical attention: chills; fever; hematuria; flank, costovertebral angle, suprapubic, low back, buttock, scrotal, or labial pain; cloudy and foul-smelling urine; increased frequency, urgency; dysuria; and increasing or recurring incontinence.

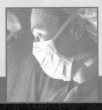

General Care of Patients 34 with Neurologic Disorders

Nursing Diagnosis:

Decreased Intracranial Adaptive Capacity

related to altered blood flow with risk of increased intracranial pressure (IICP) and herniation secondary to positional factors, increased intrathoracic or intraabdominal pressure, fluid volume excess, hyperthermia, or discomfort secondary to brain injury

Desired Outcome: Patient is free of symptoms of IICP and herniation as evidenced by stable or improving Glasgow Coma Scale score; stable or improving sensorimotor functioning; BP within patient's normal range; HR 60-100 bpm; pulse pressure 30-40 mm Hg (difference between SBP and DBP); orientation to person, place, and time; normal vision; bilaterally equal and normoreactive pupils; RR 12-20 breaths/min with normal depth and pattern (eupnea); normal gag, corneal, and swallowing reflexes; and absence of headache, nausea, nuchal rigidity, posturing, and seizure activity.

INTERVENTIONS	RATIONALES
Monitor for and report any of the following indicators of IICP or impending/occurring herniation:	Increased cranial pressure (ICP) is the pressure exerted by brain tissue, cerebrospinal fluid (CSF), and cerebral blood volume within the rigid, unyielding skull. An increase in any one of these components without a corresponding decrease in another will increase ICP. Normal ICP is 0-10 mm Hg; IICP is greater than 15 mm Hg. Cerebral perfusion pressure (CPP) is the difference between mean arterial pressure and ICP. As ICP rises, CPP may decrease. Normal CPP is 70-100 mm Hg. If CPP falls below 40-60 mm Hg, ischemia occurs. When CPP falls to 0, cerebral blood flow ceases. Cerebral edema and IICP usually peak 2-3 days after injury and then decrease over 1-2 wk.
Early indicators of IICP: Declining Glasgow Coma Scale score, alterations in level of consciousness (LOC) ranging from irritability, restlessness, and confusion to lethargy; possible onset of or worsening of headache; beginning pupillary dysfunction, such as sluggishness; visual disturbances, such as diplopia or blurred vision; onset of or increase in sensorimotor changes or deficits, such as weakness; onset of or worsening of nausea.	The single most important indicator of early IICP is a change in LOC.
Late indicators of IICP: Continuing decline in Glasgow Coma Scale score; continued deterioration in LOC leading to stupor and coma; projectile vomiting; hemiplegia; posturing; widening pulse pressure, decreased heart rate (HR), and increased systolic blood pressure (SBP); Cheyne-Stokes breathing or other respiratory irregularity; pupillary changes, such as oval-shaped, inequality, dilation, and nonreactivity to light; papilledema; and impaired brainstem reflexes (corneal, gag, swallowing).	Late indicators of IICP signal impending or actual herniation and are generally related to brainstem compression and disruption of cranial nerves and vital centers.

Continued

INTERVENTIONS	RATIONALES
Brain herniation: Deep coma, fixed and dilated pupils (first unilateral and then bilateral), posturing progressing to bilateral flaccidity, lost brainstem reflexes, and continuing deterioration in vital signs (VS) and respirations.	Brain herniation occurs when IICP causes displacement of brain tissue from one cranial compartment to another.
If changes occur, prepare for possible transfer of patient to intensive care unit (ICU).	Insertion of ICP sensors for continuous ICP monitoring, continuous bed-side cerebral blood flow (CBF) monitoring (e.g. continuous transcranial Doppler), CSF ventricular drainage, vasopressor usage (e.g., dopamine), intubation, mechanical ventilation, propofol sedation, neuromuscular blocking, or barbiturate coma therapy may be necessary. Continuous cardiac monitoring for dysrhythmias also will be done. Intensive insulin therapy may be needed to maintain normal serum glucose values (80-100 mg/dl). Testing (e.g., computerized axial tomography [CT]) may be done, but lumbar puncture [LP] is contraindicated or used with caution in the presence of IICP.
Institute preventive measures for patients at risk for IICP. These include ensuring a patent airway, delivering O_2 as prescribed, and may include intubation and mechanical ventilation as necessary. Monitor arterial blood gas (ABG) or pulse oximetry values.	Preventing hypoxia necessitates maintaining oxygen saturation at 92% or greater. Therefore it is important to preoxygenate before suctioning and limit suctioning to 10 sec. Prevention of CO_2 retention (and the resulting respiratory acidosis) is essential for preventing vasodilation of cerebral arteries, which can lead to cerebral edema.
Be aware that CBF measurements, continuous jugular venous oxygen saturation (SjO_2), and brain tissue oxygenation ($PbtO_2$) should be considered to monitor for effectiveness (i.e., decreased IICP without decreased cerebral oxygen delivery) if hyperventilation is used as a treatment.	Mechanical hyperventilation, by lowering cerebral $Paco_2$, results in an alkalosis, which causes cerebral vasoconstriction resulting in decreased CBF and ICP. The vasoconstriction also may cause decreased cerebral oxygen delivery, which could increase injury by increasing cerebral ischemia. Hyperventilation (e.g., with Ambubag or if ventilated to keep $Paco_2$ to 30-35 mm Hg) is now generally used only in cases of acute deterioration as a "quick fix" until other interventions can be instituted (e.g., mannitol) or in cases in which IICP is refractory and responds to nothing else.
Maintain head and neck alignment to avoid hyperextension, flexion, or rotation, ensuring that tracheostomy, endotracheal tube ties, or O_2 tubing does not compress the jugular vein, and avoiding Trendelenburg position for any reason.	These measures promote venous blood return to the heart to reduce cerebral congestion.
Ensure that pillows under patient's head are flat.	This measure maintains head in a neutral rather than flexed position, thereby preventing backup of jugular venous outflow.
Keep head of bed (HOB) at whatever level optimizes CPP.	CPP needs to be at least 70 mm Hg or as prescribed to prevent ischemia. Without monitoring equipment, having the HOB at 30 degrees is considered safe and effective in promoting venous drainage and lowering ICP as long as patient is not hypovolemic, which could threaten CPP.
Take precautions against increased intraabdominal and intrathoracic pressure in the following ways:	
- Teach patient to exhale when turning or during activity.	This action reduces intrathoracic pressure.
- Provide passive range-of-motion (ROM) exercises rather than allow active or assistive exercises.	This prevents increases in intraabdominal and intrathoracic pressures that could raise ICP.
- Administer prescribed stool softeners or laxatives; avoid enemas and suppositories.	These measures prevent straining at stool, which would increase intraabdominal and intracranial pressures.
- Instruct patient not to move self in bed; to allow only passive turning; and use a pull sheet and avoid pushing against foot of bed or pulling against side rails. Avoid footboards; use high-top tennis shoes with toes removed to level of the metatarsal heads instead.	Movements involving pushing would increase intraabdominal and intrathoracic pressures.
- Assist patient with sitting up and turning.	This action prevents increases in intraabdominal and intrathoracic pressures.
- Instruct patient to avoid coughing and sneezing or, if unavoidable, to do so with an open mouth; provide antitussive for cough as prescribed and antiemetic for vomiting.	As above.

Continued

INTERVENTIONS	RATIONALES
- Instruct patient to avoid hip flexion. Do not place patient in a prone position.	These positions increase intraabdominal pressure.
- Avoid using restraints.	Straining against restraints increases ICP.
- Rather than have patient perform Valsalva's maneuver to prevent an air embolism during insertion of a central venous catheter, health care provider should use a syringe to aspirate air from the catheter lumen.	Valsalva's maneuver increases intraabdominal and intrathoracic pressures.
Administer IV fluids with an infusion control device to prevent fluid overload. Keep accurate intake and output (I&O) records. (Patient usually has an indwelling urinary catheter.)	Isotonic or hypertonic IV fluids are given to maintain normovolemia and balanced electrolyte status. Fluid restrictions are avoided because resulting increased blood viscosity and decreased volume may lead to hypotension, thereby decreasing CPP.
When administering additional IV fluids (e.g., IV drugs) avoid using D_5W.	D_5W's hypotonicity can increase cerebral edema and hyperglycemia, which have been associated with inferior neurologic outcomes.
Help maintain patient's body temperature within normal limits by giving prescribed antipyretics, regulating temperature of the environment, limiting use of blankets, keeping patient's trunk warm to prevent shivering, and administering tepid sponge baths or using hypothermia blanket or convection cooling units to reduce fever.	Hypothalamic dysfunction from swelling or injury may cause hyperthermia. In turn, fever increases metabolic requirements (10% for each 1° C) and aggravates hypoxia.
When using a hypothermia blanket, wrap the patient's extremities in blankets or towels, and if prescribed, administer chlorpromazine.	Both measures prevent shivering, which would increase ICP. Mild (e.g., 35° C) hypothermia treatment also may be attempted to minimize metabolic needs of the brain if ICP is increased.
Administer prescribed osmotic (e.g., mannitol) and loop diuretics (e.g., furosemide).	These agents reduce cerebral edema and blood volume, thereby lowering ICP.
Administer blood pressure (BP) medications as prescribed.	These medications keep BP within prescribed limits that will promote optimal CBF without increasing cerebral edema. Hypotension is particularly detrimental inasmuch as it directly affects CBF. Hypertension may be allowed or treated first with drugs such as labetalol. Vasoactive drugs such as nitroprusside may worsen cerebral edema via vasodilation.
Administer prescribed analgesics promptly and as necessary.	Pain can increase ICP. Barbiturates and opioids usually are contraindicated because of the potential for masking the signs of IICP and causing respiratory depression. However, intubated, restless patients are usually sedated. A continuous propofol or midazolam drip has been demonstrated to decrease IICP. Lidocaine is sometimes used to block coughing before suctioning an endotracheal tube.
Administer antiepilepsy drugs (AEDs) as prescribed.	AEDs prevent or control seizures, which would increase cerebral metabolism, hypoxia, and CO_2 retention, which in turn would increase cerebral edema and ICP.
Monitor bladder drainage tubes for obstruction or kinks.	A distended bladder can increase ICP.
Provide a quiet and soothing environment. Control noise and other environmental stimuli. Speak softly, use a gentle touch, and avoid jarring the bed. Try to limit painful procedures; avoid tension on tubes (e.g., urinary catheter); and consider limiting pain-stimulation testing. Avoid unnecessary touch (e.g., leave BP cuff in place for frequent VS; use automatic recycling BP monitoring devices); and talk softly, explaining procedures before touching to avoid startling patient. Try to avoid situations in which the patient may become emotionally upset. Do not say anything in the presence of the patient that you would not say if he or she were awake. Limit visitors as necessary.	A quiet and soothing environment optimally will help keep BP and other pressures within therapeutic limits. Family discussions should take place outside the room.
Encourage significant other to speak quietly to patient. If possible, arrange for patient to listen to soft favorite music with earphones.	Hearing a familiar voice or listening to soft music may promote relaxation and decrease ICP.
Individualize care to ensure rest periods and optimal spacing of activities; avoid turning, suctioning, and taking VS all at one time. Plan activities and treatments accordingly so that patient can sleep undisturbed as often as possible.	Multiple procedures and nursing care activities can increase ICP. For example, rousing patients from sleep has been shown to increase ICP.

Continued

INTERVENTIONS	RATIONALES
Administer mild sedatives (e.g., diphenhydramine) or antianxiety agents (haloperidol, lorazepam, midazolam) as prescribed to restless/agitated patient. Attempt to identify and relieve cause (e.g., overstimulation, pain) before medicating.	These measures decrease restlessness or decrease/control agitation that may increase ICP.
Administer skeletal muscle relaxants (e.g., propofol, atracurium, pancuronium) as prescribed. (This therapy requires intubation and ventilation.)	These agents decrease the skeletal muscle tension that is seen with abnormal flexion and extension posturing, which can increase ICP. Bispectral index technology (BIS) may be used to guide administration of these drugs for sedation and neuromuscular blockade. BIS translates information from the electroencephalogram (EEG) into a single number that represents each patient's LOC. This number ranges from 100 (indicating an awake patient) to zero (indicating the absence of brain activity).

••• **Related NIC and NOC labels:** *NIC:* Cerebral Edema Management; Cerebral Perfusion Promotion; Intracranial Pressure (ICP) Monitoring; Neurologic Monitoring; Fluid Management; Fluid Monitoring; Medication Administration; Positioning: Neurologic; Vital Signs Monitoring; Seizure Precautions; Anxiety Reduction *NOC:* Neurological Status; Neurological Status: Consciousness

Nursing Diagnosis:

Risk for Infection

related to inadequate primary defenses secondary to ventilator intubation in patients with such neurologic disorders as Guillain-Barré, bacterial meningitis, spinal cord injury, traumatic brain injury, and stroke

Desired Outcome: Patient exhibits reduced incidence/absence of ventilator-associated pneumonia as evidenced by normothermia, white blood cell count 11,000/mm³ or less, sputum clear to whitish in color, lungs clear to auscultation, RR 14-20 breaths/min, and oxygen saturation 92% or more.

INTERVENTIONS	RATIONALES
Ensure the ventilator bundle discussed in the following interventions has been implemented on any patient who is mechanically ventilated.	This bundle is a series of interventions that, when implemented together (rather than individually), is associated with decreased incidence of ventilator-associated pneumonia (VAP). VAP is a leading cause of prolonged hospital stay and death.
Monitor lung sounds, sputum characteristics, respiratory rate (RR), heart rate (HR), temperature, oximetry, ABG values, chest x-ray, and complete blood count (CBC). Report abnormal changes to health care provider.	Monitoring for and reporting early indicators of infection will enable early intervention and treatment.
Elevate HOB, preferably to 30 degrees.	This position reduces risk of aspirating gastric contents by moving them away from the diaphragm, making ventilation easier. This position may be contraindicated in some patients.
On a daily basis, attempt "sedation vacations" per facility protocol or as prescribed, and assess and document neurologic status and readiness to extubate. For example, "Patient awake, breathing at a sufficient rate and depth of breaths to maintain oxygenation, is able to cough and protect airway, and has adequate ABG values." Note prior documentation as a basis of comparison (e.g., improvement or deterioration) and notify care provider as appropriate (e.g., if patient does not wake or respond despite sedation being turned off).	These measures promote early extubation and minimize sedation. A "sedation vacation" involves reducing sedation until patient is awake and can follow simple commands or becomes agitated. During this "awake" time, a weaning trial may be done to test patient's ability to breathe spontaneously. The patient's unsedated neurologic status also can be tested. If sedation is reinstated, it can be titrated to the minimal amount needed to achieve a calm, relaxed state. Decreasing sedation reduces the amount of time spent on mechanical ventilation and therefore the risk of ventilator-acquired pneumonia.

Continued

INTERVENTIONS

INTERVENTIONS	RATIONALES
Ensure a closed endotracheal suction system, ideally one that allows for continuous subglottic secretion drainage.	A closed system reduces risk of contamination. A system that also allows for continuous subglottic secretion drainage will further reduce contamination of the lower airway by removing stagnant oropharyngeal secretions above the cuff that might otherwise be aspirated.
When possible, use oral tubes rather than nasal tubes.	Oral tubes reduce risk of sinusitis and aspiration of infected secretions.
Provide oral hygiene q2h, possibly including use of a dental oral antibiotic rinse (e.g., chlorhexidine gluconate washes).	Oral hygiene reduces oral bacterial flora, which could be aspirated. Swabs and toothbrushes with built in suction catheter capability may facilitate oral care.
As prescribed, implement other components that may be included in the bundle.	Many agencies also include peptic ulcer disease prophylaxis (to reduce miniaspiration of acid secretions) and deep vein thrombosis prophylaxis.

••• **Related NIC and NOC labels:** *NIC:* Infection Prevention; Laboratory Data Interpretation; Medication Management; Respiratory Monitoring; Vital Signs Monitoring; Airway Management; Artificial Airway Management; Aspiration Precautions; Oral Health Maintenance; Tube Care *NOC:* Infection Severity

Nursing Diagnosis:

Risk for Falls

related to weakness, difficulties with balance, or unsteady gait secondary to sensorimotor deficit

Desired Outcomes: Patient is free of trauma caused by gait unsteadiness. Before hospital discharge, patient demonstrates proficiency with assistive devices if appropriate.

INTERVENTIONS	RATIONALES
Evaluate gait and assess for weakness, difficulty with balance, tremors, spasticity, or paralysis.	These are indicators of motor deficits that could lead to falls.
Document baseline assessments.	Documentation helps ensure that changes in status can be detected and interventions made promptly to help prevent falls.
Incorporate a fall risk assessment tool into patient's plan of care. Include appropriate interventions, specific-to-patient lifting/transferring/mobilization aids and techniques, and appropriate amount of assistance. Update as appropriate with changes in patient status.	Assessment and documentation of patient's fall risk via an armband, identifying wall placard, and/or care plan provides added insurance in helping prevent injury to patient resulting from falls.
Assist patient as needed when unsteady gait, weakness, or paralysis is noted. Instruct patient to ask or call for assistance with ambulation. Frequently check on patients who may forget to call for assistance. Stand on patient's weak side to assist with balance and support. Use transfer belt for safety. Instruct patient to use stronger side for gripping railing when stair climbing or using a cane.	These measures minimize risk of falls by providing assistance and surveillance.
Orient patient to new surroundings. Keep necessary items (including water, snacks, phone, call light) within easy reach.	These measures minimize risk of falls as a result of strange environment, unfamiliarity with such items as call light, and need to walk to get them.
Assess patient's ability to use these items.	Patients who are very weak or partially paralyzed may require a tap bell or specially adapted call light.
Maintain an uncluttered environment with unobstructed walkways. Ensure adequate lighting at night (e.g., provide a night light) to help prevent falls in the dark. In addition, keep side rails up and bed in its lowest position with bed brakes on.	These measures promote safety by ensuring better sensory acuity.
Encourage patient to use any needed hearing aids and corrective lenses when ambulating.	These measures minimize risk of tripping, falls in the dark, or injury from falling out of bed.

Continued

INTERVENTIONS	RATIONALES
For unsteady, weak, or partially paralyzed patient, encourage use of low-heel, nonskid, supportive shoes for walking. Teach use of a wide-based gait.	These measures minimize risk of falls in patients with special needs.
Instruct patient to note foot placement when ambulating or transferring.	This action ensures that the foot is flat and in a position of support before patient ambulates and transfers.
Teach, reinforce, and encourage use of assistive device, such as a cane, walker, or crutches.	These devices provide added stability.
Teach exercises that strengthen arm and shoulder muscles for using walkers and crutches. Teach safe use of transfer or sliding boards. Teach patients in wheelchairs how and when to lock and unlock wheels.	These actions promote added stability and safety.
Demonstrate how to secure and support weak or paralyzed arms.	These actions help prevent subluxation and injury from falling into wheelchair spokes or wheels.
Suggest that patients with poor sitting balance may need a seat or chest belt, H-straps for leg positioning, and a wheelchair with an anti-tip device.	Such devices likely will prevent patients with poor sitting balance from falling or tipping the wheelchair.
Teach patient to maintain sitting position before assuming standing position for ambulating.	Maintaining this position for a few minutes gives patient time to get feet flat and under self for balance and minimizes any dizziness that may occur because of rapid position changes.
Monitor spasticity, antispasmodic medications, and their effect on physical function.	Uncontrolled or severe spasms may cause falls, whereas mild to moderate spasms can be useful in activities of daily living (ADL) and transfers if patient learns to control and trigger them.
Review with patient and significant other potential safety needs at home.	Such measures include safety appliances (wall, bath, toilet grab rails; elevated toilet seat; nonslip surface in bathtub or shower). Loose rugs should be removed to prevent slipping and falling. Temperatures on hot water heaters should be turned down to prevent scalding in the event of a fall in the shower or tub. Furniture in the home may need to be moved to provide clear, safe pathways that avoid sharp corners on furniture, glass cabinets, or large windows patient could fall against. Strategically placed additional lighting also may be needed. Edges of steps in the home may require taping with brightly colored strips to provide sufficient contrast so that edges can be recognized and more safely negotiated. Beds should be modified to prevent rolling. Activity should be balanced with rest periods because fatigue tends to increase unsteadiness and potential for falls. Ramps may need to be used instead of stairs.
Seek referral for physical therapist (PT) as appropriate.	Patient may have special needs that cannot be met by nursing staff.

••• **Related NIC and NOC labels:** *NIC:* Fall Prevention; Surveillance: Safety; Environmental Management: Safety; Home Maintenance Assistance; Area Restriction; Risk Identification *NOC:* Safety Status: Falls Occurrence; Safety Status: Physical Injury

Nursing Diagnosis:

Risk for Aspiration

related to facial and throat muscle weakness, depressed gag or cough reflex, impaired swallowing, or decreased LOC

Desired Outcomes: Patient is free of the signs of aspiration as evidenced by RR 12-20 breaths/min with normal depth and pattern (eupnea), O_2 saturation greater than 92%, normal color, normal breath sounds, normothermia, and absence of adventitious breath sounds. Following instruction and on an ongoing basis, patient or significant other relates measures that prevent aspiration.

INTERVENTIONS	RATIONALES
Assess lung sounds before and after patient eats, effectiveness of patient's cough, and quality, amount, and color of sputum.	New onset of crackles or wheezing can signal aspiration. Patients with a weak cough are at risk for aspiration. An increase in quantity or color change of sputum may indicate an infection from aspiration.
Keep HOB elevated after meals or assist patient into a right side-lying position.	This position facilitates flow of ingested food and fluids by gravity from the greater stomach curve to the pylorus, thereby minimizing potential for regurgitation and aspiration.
If indicated, consult health care provider about use of an upper gastrointestinal (GI) stimulant (e.g., metoclopramide).	Metoclopramide stimulates upper GI tract motility and gastric emptying, which also decreases potential for regurgitation.
Provide oral hygiene after meals.	Oral hygiene removes food particles that could be aspirated.
Assess the mouth frequently, and suction prn.	These actions assess for particles or secretions that could be aspirated and removes them.
If patient has nausea or vomiting or has secretions, turn on one side.	This position facilitates drainage and prevents their aspiration.
Anticipate need for artificial airway if secretions cannot be cleared. Teach significant other the Heimlich maneuver.	These measures help ensure a patent airway.
For general interventions, see this nursing diagnosis in "Older Adult Care," p. 96.	

••• **Related NIC and NOC labels:** *NIC:* Aspiration Precautions; Vomiting Management; Airway Suctioning; Artificial Airway Management; Positioning; Respiratory Monitoring *NOC:* Aspiration Control

Nursing Diagnosis:

Impaired Swallowing

related to neuromuscular impairment (e.g., decreased or absent gag reflex, decreased strength or excursion of muscles involved in mastication, perceptual impairment, facial paralysis)

Desired Outcome: Before oral foods and fluids are reintroduced, patient exhibits ability to swallow safely without aspirating.

INTERVENTIONS	RATIONALES
Assess for factors that affect ability to swallow safely, including LOC, gag and cough reflexes, and strength and symmetry of tongue, lip, and facial muscles.	This assessment determines if swallowing deficits are present that necessitate aspiration precautions.
Monitor for coughing, regurgitation of food and fluid through the nares, drooling, food oozing from the lips, food trapped in buccal spaces, and development of a weak, "wet," or hoarse voice during or after eating.	These are signs of impaired swallowing.
Check swallow reflex by first asking patient to swallow own saliva. Place a finger gently on top of larynx. If the larynx elevates with the attempt, next ask patient to swallow 3-5 ml of plain water. Document your findings.	Inability to swallow own saliva or small amount of water and presence of a stationary larynx during attempt to swallow signal loss of the swallowing reflex.
Caution: Presence of the cough reflex is essential for patient to relearn swallowing safely.	The cough reflex protects against aspiration and if delayed may signal silent aspiration.
Obtain a referral to a speech therapist for patients with a swallowing dysfunction.	The act of swallowing is complex, and interventions vary according to the phase of swallowing that is dysfunctional. Video fluoroscopy may be used to evaluate swallowing, and some patients with swallowing dysfunction are referred to speech therapists for evaluation.
Encourage patient to practice any prescribed exercises.	Exercises such as tongue and jaw ROM; sound phonation such as "gah-gah-gah" to promote elevation of the soft palate; puckering lips; and sticking the tongue out to touch the nose, chin, cheeks may be prescribed to facilitate swallowing ability.

Continued

INTERVENTIONS	RATIONALES
Recognize that a nasogastric (NG) tube may hinder patient's ability to re-learn to swallow.	NG tubes may desensitize and impair reflexive response to food bolus stimulus.
Alert health care provider to your findings.	Parenteral nutrition may be necessary for patients who cannot chew or swallow effectively or safely.
Keep suction equipment and a manual resuscitation bag with face mask at patient's bedside. Suction secretions in patient's mouth as necessary.	This equipment enables immediate intervention in the event aspiration occurs.
Ensure that patient is alert and responsive to verbal stimuli before attempting to swallow. Provide a rest period before meals or swallowing attempts.	Patients who are drowsy, inattentive, or fatigued have difficulty cooperating and are at risk of aspirating.
Initiate swallowing attempts with plain water (see earlier). Progressively add easy-to-swallow food and liquids as patient's ability to swallow improves. Determine which foods and liquids are easiest for patient to swallow.	Generally, semisolid foods of medium consistency, such as puddings, hot cereals, and casseroles, tend to be easiest to swallow. Thicker liquids, such as nectars, tend to be better tolerated than thin liquids.
If indicated/prescribed, add commercially available powders (e.g., Thicket) to liquids.	Thickening foods increases their viscosity and makes them more easily swallowed. Gravy or sauce added to dry foods often facilitates swallowing as well.
Avoid giving peanut butter, chocolate, or milk.	Foods such as these may stick in the patient's throat or produce mucus.
Avoid nuts, hard candies, or popcorn.	These foods may be aspirated.
Reduce stimuli in the room (e.g., turn off television, lower radio volume, minimize conversation, and limit disruptions from phone calls). Caution patient not to talk while eating.	These measures help patient focus on swallowing.
If patient must remain in bed, use high Fowler's position if possible. Support shoulders and neck with pillows.	Most patients swallow best when in an upright position. Sitting in a straight-back chair with feet on the floor is ideal.
Ensure that patient's head is erect and flexed forward slightly, with chin at the midline and pointing toward chest (i.e., the "chin tuck").	This head position minimizes the risk that food will go into the airway by forcing the trachea to close and the esophagus to open. In addition, stroking the anterior neck lightly may help some patients swallow.
Maintain patient in an upright position for at least 30-60 min after eating.	This position helps prevent regurgitation and aspiration by facilitating flow of foods and fluids by gravity from the stomach to the pylorus.
Teach patient to break down the act of chewing and swallowing into the following steps.	Taking patient through these steps promotes concentration and focus, which will help ensure optimal swallowing.
- Take small bites or sips (approximately 5 ml each).	
- Place food on tongue.	
- Use tongue to transfer food so that it is directly under teeth on unaffected side of the mouth.	
- Chew food thoroughly.	
- Move food to middle of tongue and hold it there.	
- Flex neck and tuck chin against chest.	
- Hold the breath and think about swallowing.	
- Without breathing, raise tongue to roof of mouth and swallow.	
- Swallow several times if necessary.	
- When mouth is empty, raise chin and clear throat or cough purposefully once or twice.	
Start with small amounts of food or liquid. Feed slowly.	For optimum safety, each bite should not exceed 5 ml (1 tsp).
Ensure that each previous bite has been swallowed. Check mouth for pockets of food. After every few bites of solid food, provide a liquid to help clear the mouth.	Food may become pocketed in the affected side of the mouth, which could result in aspiration.
Avoid using a syringe.	The force of the fluid in the syringe, if sprayed, may cause aspiration.
Avoid use of drinking straws.	The act of sucking may add to the complexity of swallowing and allow too much liquid to enter the mouth, thereby increasing the risk of aspiration.

Continued

INTERVENTIONS	RATIONALES
Tear a piece out of a Styrofoam cup to make a space for the nose so that patient can drink with neck flexed.	Having the neck in a flexed position minimizes risk that food will go into the airway by forcing the trachea to close and the esophagus to open.
Teach patient who has food pockets in the buccal spaces to periodically sweep mouth with tongue or finger or to clean these areas with a napkin. Explain that applying external pressure to cheek with a finger will help remove a trapped food bolus.	These actions help prevent aspiration of food particles, stomatitis, and tooth decay.
Teach patient who has a weak or paralyzed side to place food on side of the face patient can control.	Tilting head toward stronger side will allow gravity to help keep food or liquid on side of the mouth patient can manipulate. However, some patients may find that rotating head to the weak side will close the damaged side of the pharynx and facilitate more effective swallowing.
Serve only warm or cool foods to individuals with loss of oral sensation.	Patients with loss of oral sensation may be unable to identify foods or fluids of tepid temperature with tongue or oral mucosa. Verbal cues and use of a mirror may help ensure that these patients keep their mouths clear after swallowing.
To facilitate movement of food in some patients, encourage repeated swallowing attempts. Evaluate patient's swallowing ability at different times of the day. Reschedule mealtimes to times when patient has improved swallowing, or, as appropriate, discuss with health care provider the possibility of changing dose schedule of patient's anti-parkinsonian medication.	Patients with a rigid tongue (e.g., with parkinsonism) have difficulty getting the tongue to move a bolus of food into the pharynx for swallowing.
If decreased salivation is contributing to patient's swallowing difficulties, perform one of the following before feeding: swab patient's mouth with a lemon-glycerin sponge; have patient suck on a tart-flavored hard candy, dill pickle, or lemon slice; teach patient to move tongue in a circular motion against inside of cheek; or use artificial saliva.	These actions stimulate salivation, which optimally will contribute to effective swallowing.
Moisten food with melted butter, broth or other soup, or gravy. Dip dry foods such as toast into coffee or other liquid.	These actions moisten and soften food when salivation is decreased.
Rinse patient's mouth as needed.	This intervention removes particles and lubricates the mouth.
Investigate medications patient is taking for potential side effect of decreased salivation.	Drugs such as antiparkinsonian medications or those with extrapyramidal side effects may result in decreased salivation.
Consult with health care provider regarding use of tablets, capsules, and liquids for patients with swallowing difficulties. Check with pharmacist to confirm that crushing a tablet or opening a capsule does not adversely affect its absorption or duration (i.e., slow-release medications should not be crushed).	Tablets or capsules may be swallowed more easily when added to foods such as puddings or ice cream. Crushed tablets or opened capsules also mix easily into these types of foods. Liquid forms of medications also may be available through the pharmacy.
Teach significant other the Heimlich or abdominal thrust maneuver.	This information helps ensure that he or she can intervene in the event of patient's choking.

●●● **Related NIC and NOC labels:** *NIC:* Aspiration Precautions; Airway Management; Airway Suctioning; Positioning; Risk Identification; Swallowing Therapy; Cough Enhancement; Referral *NOC:* Aspiration Control; Swallowing Status

Nursing Diagnosis:

Risk for Injury

related to impaired pain, touch, and temperature sensations secondary to sensory deficit or decreased LOC

Desired Outcomes: Patient is free of symptoms of injury caused by impaired pain, touch, and temperature sensations. Before hospital discharge, patient and significant other identify factors that increase the potential for injury.

INTERVENTIONS	RATIONALES
Assess for decreased or absent vision and impaired temperature and pain sensation.	These sensory deficits could result in patient injury.
Document baseline neurologic and physical assessments.	These assessments enable rapid detection of deteriorating status so that changes can be detected and responded to promptly, thereby helping prevent injury.
Avoid use of heating pads. Encourage use of sunscreen when outside. Do not serve scalding hot foods and beverages.	These measures protect patient from exposure to hot items and sun that can burn the skin.
Always check temperature of heating devices and bath water before patient is exposed to them. Teach patient and significant other about these precautions.	Patient's tactile senses are altered and would not recognize if water or device is too hot.
Inspect skin twice daily for evidence of irritation. Teach coherent patient to perform self-inspection, and provide mirror for inspecting posterior aspects of the body.	Patient is not able to feel skin irritation.
Use emollient lotions liberally on patient's skin.	These lotions keep skin soft and pliable and less likely to break down.
Teach patient to inspect placement of limbs with altered sensation.	This helps ensure that limbs are in a safe and supported position and avoids placing ankles directly on top of each other.
Pad wheelchair seat, preferably with a gel pad.	Padding evenly distributes patient's weight and decreases pressure areas that could result in skin breakdown.
Teach patient to change position q15-30min by lifting self and shifting position side to side and forward to backward. Encourage frequent turning while in bed and, if tolerated and not contraindicated, periodic movement into prone position.	Changing positions and turning promote circulation and prevent pressure ulcers. Patient likely will not sense the need to do this and therefore should do it on a scheduled basis. Spending time in the prone position with hips extended helps prevent hip flexion contractures.
Have patient lift, not drag, self during transfers.	This action prevents shearing damage to skin.
Avoid injecting more than 1 ml into a flaccid muscle. If possible, give injections only in muscles with tone.	Injections into muscles with tone will enable better absorption with less risk of sterile abscess formation.

••• **Related NIC and NOC labels:** *NIC:* Peripheral Sensation Management; Skin Surveillance; Cutaneous Stimulation; Positioning; Pressure Management *NOC:* Sensory Function: Cutaneous

<u>Nursing Diagnosis:</u>

Impaired Tissue Integrity: Corneal

related to irritation secondary to diminished blink reflex or inability to close the eyes

Desired Outcome: Patient's corneas remain clear and intact.

INTERVENTIONS	RATIONALES
If patient has a diminished blink reflex or is stuporous or comatose, assess eyes for irritation or presence of foreign objects.	Indicators of corneal irritation include red, itchy, scratchy, or painful eye; sensation of foreign object in eye; scleral edema; blurred vision; or mucus discharge.
Instill prescribed eye drops or ointment. Instruct coherent patients to make a conscious effort to blink eyes several times each minute. Apply eye patches or warm, sterile compresses over closed eyes.	These actions provide corneal lubrication and prevent corneal irritation. Normally, blinking occurs every 5-6 sec.
If the eyes cannot be completely closed, use caution in applying eye shield or taping eyes shut. Consider use of moisture chambers (plastic eye bubbles), protective glasses, soft contacts, or humidifiers.	Semiconscious patients may open eyes underneath the shield or tape and injure their corneas.
For chronic eye closure problems, consider use of special springs or weights on upper lids. Surgical closure (tarsorrhaphy) also may be necessary.	These measures help ensure closure of the eyelid.

Continued

INTERVENTIONS	RATIONALES
Teach patient to avoid exposing eyes to talc or baby powder, wind, cold air, smoke, dust, sand, or bright sunlight. Instruct patient not to rub eyes. Advise patient to wear glasses to protect against wind and dust and to wear tight-fitting goggles when swimming.	These are irritants that could harm patient's corneas.

••• **Related NIC and NOC labels:** *NIC:* Eye Care; Medication Administration: Eye *NOC:* Tissue Integrity: Skin and Mucous Membranes

Nursing Diagnosis:

Risk for Deficient Fluid Volume

related to facial and throat muscle weakness, depressed gag or cough reflex, impaired swallowing, or decreased LOC affecting access to and intake of fluids

Desired Outcome: Patient is normovolemic as evidenced by balanced I&O, stable weight, good skin turgor, moist mucous membranes, BP within patient's normal range, HR 100 bpm or less, normothermia, and urinary output at least 30 ml/hr with a specific gravity 1.030 or less.

INTERVENTIONS	RATIONALES
Assess gag reflex, alertness, and ability to cough and swallow before offering fluids.	These assessments demonstrate if patient has intact swallowing and gag reflexes, can cough, and is alert and therefore can safely ingest fluids.
Keep suction equipment at bedside if indicated.	This enables immediate intervention in the event of aspiration.
Monitor I&O. Involve patient or significant other with keeping fluid intake records. Perform daily weights if patient is at risk for sudden fluid shifts or imbalances.	Patients with neurologic deficits may have difficulty attaining adequate fluid intake. Involving patient and significant other in record keeping optimally will keep them aware of the need for increased oral intake and influence their participation in fluid intake accordingly.
Alert health care provider to a significant I&O imbalance.	This imbalance may signal need for enteral or IV therapy to prevent dehydration.
Assess for and teach patient and significant other such indicators as thirst, poor skin turgor, decreased BP, increased pulse rate, dry skin and mucous membranes, increased body temperature, concentrated urine (specific gravity more than 1.030), and decreased urinary output.	These are indicators of dehydration. Conditions such as fever and diarrhea increase fluid loss and risk of dehydration. A knowledgeable person is more likely to report these indicators promptly for timely intervention and will understand the need to increase fluid intake during conditions that promote dehydration.
Evaluate fluid preferences (type and temperature). Offer fluids q1-2h. Establish a fluid goal. For nonrestricted patients, encourage a fluid intake of at least 2-3 L/day.	Patients, especially if fatigued, will be more prone to consume preferred fluids in small volumes at frequent intervals. A fluid intake of 2-3 L/day will keep patient well hydrated. Renal and cardiac patients may have fluid restrictions.
Feed or assist very weak or paralyzed patients.	Such measures help ensure that fluid goals are met.
Instruct patient to flex head slightly forward.	Flexing the head forward closes the airway and helps prevent aspiration.
Begin with small amounts of liquid. Instruct patient to sip rather than gulp fluids. Do not hurry patient.	Sipping small amounts tests and promotes patient's ability to swallow the fluid without choking.
For patient at risk for aspiration, use thickened fluids. Maintain appropriate upright position while patient is eating/drinking and for at least 1½ hr after the meal.	Thickened liquids form a cohesive bolus that can be swallowed more readily. Gravity aids swallowing, and staying upright decreases risk of aspiration.
Provide periods of rest.	Rest prevents fatigue, which can contribute to decreased oral intake.
Provide oral care as needed.	Oral care promotes taste perception and prevents stomatitis, which otherwise may decrease oral intake
If appropriate, provide assistive devices (e.g., plastic, unbreakable, special-handled, spill-proof cups or straws).	These devices promote independence, which is likely to increase fluid consumption. The individual who is paralyzed (e.g., with spinal cord injury [SCI]) may be able to drink independently via extra-long tubing or straw connected to a water pitcher.

Continued

INTERVENTIONS	RATIONALES
Teach patient with hemiparalysis or hemiparesis to tilt head toward unaffected side.	Fluids will drain by gravity to the side of the face and throat over which patient has control.
For patients with chewing or swallowing difficulties, see interventions under **Impaired Swallowing**, p. 267.	

••• **Related NIC and NOC labels:** *NIC:* Fluid Management; Fluid Monitoring; Vital Signs Monitoring; Bedside Laboratory Testing; Enteral Tube Feeding; Total Parenteral Nutrition Administration; Intravenous Therapy; Oral Health Restoration; Swallowing Therapy; Self-Care Assistance: Feeding *NOC:* Fluid Balance; Nutritional Status: Food and Fluid Intake

Nursing Diagnosis:

Imbalanced Nutrition: Less Than Body Requirements

related to inability to ingest food secondary to chewing and swallowing deficits, fatigue, weakness, paresis, paralysis, visual neglect, or decreased LOC

Desired Outcome: Patient has adequate nutrition as evidenced by maintenance of or return to baseline body weight by hospital discharge.

INTERVENTIONS	RATIONALES
Assess alertness, ability to cough and swallow, and gag reflexes before all meals. Keep suction equipment at bedside if indicated.	Deficits found during this assessment signal that patient is at risk for aspiration, which in turn could lead to imbalanced nutrition.
Assess for type of diet that can be eaten safely. Request soft, semisolid, or chopped foods as indicated.	Although a pureed diet may be needed eventually, pureed food can be unappealing and may have a negative impact on self-concept as well as decrease patient's intake.
Reduce stimuli in the room (e.g., turn off TV or radio). Minimize conversation and other disruptions such as phone calls. If patient wears glasses, put them on patient; ensure adequate lighting. As needed, redirect patient's attention to eating.	These measures help patient focus on eating.
Provide analgesics, if appropriate, before meals.	Pain relief helps ensure that patient is comfortable and can concentrate on eating.
Evaluate food preferences and offer small, frequent servings of nutritious food. Consider cultural or religious factors that may affect patient eating when evaluating food preferences. Encourage significant other to bring in patient's favorite foods if not contraindicated. Plan meals for times when patient is rested; use a warming tray or microwave oven to keep food warm and appetizing until patient is able to eat. Serve cold foods while they are cold.	Optimally, these measures will promote eating.
Provide oral care before feeding. Clean and insert dentures before each meal, and ensure that they fit properly.	Oral care and good dentition promote comfort and patient's ability to taste and chew.
Encourage liquid nutritional supplements. Try different methods to make them more palatable (e.g., making a milkshake, serving over ice, or diluting with carbonated beverages).	Making supplements more appetizing may promote intake.
Cut up foods, unwrap silverware, and otherwise prepare food tray.	This assistance helps ensure that patient with a weak or paralyzed arm can manage the tray one-handed.
For patient with visual neglect, place food within unaffected visual field. Return during meal to make sure patient has eaten from both sides of the plate. Turn plate around so that any remaining food is in patient's visual field.	These actions help ensure that patient eats all or most of the food on the plate.

Continued

INTERVENTIONS	RATIONALES
Feed or assist very weak or paralyzed patients. If not contraindicated, position patient in a chair or elevate HOB as high as possible. Ensure that patient's head is flexed slightly forward. Begin with small amounts of food. Encourage chewing food on unaffected side. Do not hurry patient. Be sure that each bite is completely swallowed before giving another. Encourage patient with hemiplegia to consciously sweep paralyzed side of mouth with the tongue to clear it.	Raising HOB helps prevent aspiration by promoting drainage into the stomach and through the pylorus. Assisting patient also helps conserve his or her energy and provides social interaction, which may promote eating. Flexing the head slightly forward closes the airway.
If appropriate, provide assistive devices such as built-up utensil handles, broad-handled spoons, spill-proof cups, rocker knife for cutting, wrist or hand splints with clamps to hold utensils, stabilized plates, and sectioned plates.	Assistive devices promote self-feeding and independence.
Provide materials for oral hygiene after meals. Give oral care to patients unable to do so for themselves.	Oral care minimizes risk of aspiration of food particles. Good oral hygiene will also help maintain integrity of mucous membranes to minimize risk of stomatitis, which otherwise may prevent adequate oral intake.
Document your assessment of patient's appetite. Weigh patient regularly (at least weekly) to assess for loss or gain. If indicated, notify health care provider of potential need for high-protein or high-calorie supplements.	Trend of patient's weight is a good indicator of nutritional status. Calculation of weight enables determination of percentage below ideal weight for patient's height and frame.
Obtain dietitian consultation. For additional information, see "Providing Nutritional Support," p. 565.	The patient may need enteral or parenteral nutrition.
For weak, debilitated, or partially paralyzed patient, assess support systems, such as family or friends, who can assist patient with meals. Consider referral to an organization that will deliver a daily meal to patient's home.	These actions help ensure patient's optimum nutritional status.
If appropriate for patient's diagnosis (e.g., multiple sclerosis [MS]) consider referral to a speech pathologist.	This specialist will teach exercises that enhance ability to swallow.
For patient with visual problems, assess ability to see food. Identify utensils and foods, and describe their location. Arrange foods in an established pattern.	These measures promote patient's independence with eating. Poor vision has been associated with lower caloric intake.
For patient with diplopia, consider patching one eye.	Patching one eye may enable better vision.
For patient with chewing or swallowing difficulties, see interventions in **Impaired Swallowing**, p. 267.	

••• **Related NIC and NOC labels:** *NIC:* Nutrition Management; Weight Gain Assistance; Self-Care Assistance: Feeding; Sustenance Support; Nutrition Therapy; Swallowing Therapy *NOC:* Nutritional Status: Food and Fluid Intake

Nursing Diagnosis:

Acute Pain

related to spasms, headache, and photophobia secondary to neurologic dysfunction

Desired Outcomes: Within 1 hr of intervention, patient's subjective perception of discomfort decreases, as documented by a pain scale. Objective indicators, such as grimacing, are absent or diminished.

INTERVENTIONS	RATIONALES
Assess characteristics (e.g., quality, severity, location, onset, duration, precipitating factors) of patient's pain or spasms. Devise a pain scale with patient, and document discomfort on a scale of 0 (no pain) to 10 (worst pain). Determine patient's acceptable pain level and ways of coping with and relieving pain.	These assessments demonstrate degree and type of discomfort, trend of the discomfort, and relief obtained after interventions. A graphic pain scale using facial expression may be used for patients who cannot use a numeric scale.

Continued

INTERVENTIONS	RATIONALES
Respond immediately to patient's complaints of pain. Administer analgesics and antispasmodics as prescribed. Consider scheduling doses of analgesia. Document effectiveness of the medication, using pain scale, approximately 30 min after administration. Monitor for untoward effects. Consult health care provider if dose or interval change seems necessary.	Prolonged stimulation of pain receptors results in increased sensitivity to painful stimuli and will increase the amount of drug required to relieve pain.
Teach patient and significant other about importance of timing the pain medication.	Providing this information helps ensure that analgesia is taken before pain becomes too severe and before major moves.
Teach patient about relationship between anxiety and pain, as well as other factors that enhance pain and spasms (e.g., staying in one position for too long, fatigue, chilling).	This information gives patient control over some causes of pain.
Instruct patient and significant other in use of nonpharmacologic pain management techniques. See also **Health-Seeking Behaviors:** Relaxation technique effective for stress reduction, p. 172.	Such techniques as repositioning; ROM; supporting painful extremity or part; back rubs, acupressure, massage, warm baths, and other tactile distraction; auditory distraction such as listening to soothing music; visual distraction such as television; heat applications such as warm blankets or moist compresses; cold applications such as ice massage; guided imagery; breathing exercises; relaxation tapes and techniques; biofeedback; and a transcutaneous electrical nerve stimulation (TENS) device may be effective when used to supplement pharmacologic treatment. These methods also promote a sense of focus and self-control.
Encourage rest periods. Try to provide uninterrupted sleep time at night.	Fatigue tends to exacerbate the pain experience. Pain may result in fatigue, which in turn may cause exaggerated pain and further exhaustion.
If patient has photophobia, provide a quiet and dark environment. Close the door and curtains, provide sunglasses, and avoid use of artificial lights whenever possible.	These actions eliminate painful light sources for patients with photophobia.
Recognize that pain in the SCI patient often is poorly localized and may be referred.	In the SCI patient, intrascapular pain may be from the stomach, duodenum, or gallbladder. Umbilical pain may be from the appendix. Testicular or inner thigh pain may be from the kidneys (e.g., with pyelonephritis).
Evaluate SCI patient for tachycardia, restlessness, urinary incontinence when it was previously controlled, and fever.	These are signs of infection or inflammatory processes that may or may not result in discomfort in the SCI patient but should be reported promptly for timely intervention.
If patient's present complaint of pain varies significantly from previous pain or if interventions are ineffective, notify health care provider.	These situations may signal a new or acute problem and should be reported promptly for timely intervention.

••• **Related NIC and NOC labels:** *NIC:* Medication Management; Documentation; Pain Management; Environmental Management: Comfort; Simple Relaxation Therapy; Sleep Enhancement; Biofeedback; Cutaneous Stimulation; Distraction; Heat/Cold Application; Simple Guided Imagery; Transcutaneous Electrical Nerve Stimulation *NOC:* Pain Control; Pain: Disruptive Effects

Nursing Diagnosis:

Risk for Imbalanced Body Temperature

related to illness or trauma affecting temperature regulation and inability or decreased ability to perspire, shiver, or vasoconstrict

Desired Outcome: Following intervention(s), patient is normothermic with core temperatures between 36.5° and 37.7° C (97.8° and 100° F).

INTERVENTIONS	RATIONALES
Monitor rectal, tympanic, or bladder core temperature q4h or, if patient is in spinal shock, q2h.	Infection and hypothalamic dysfunction as a result of cerebral insult (trauma, edema) are two common causes of hyperthermia. Rapid development of spinal lesions (e.g., in SCI) breaks the connection between the hypothalamus and sympathetic nervous system (SNS), causing an inability to adapt to environmental temperature. In spinal cord shock, temperatures tend to lower toward the ambient temperature. Inability to vasoconstrict and shiver makes heat conservation difficult; inability to perspire prevents normal cooling.

Caution: Steroids may mask fever or infection. |
Be alert to impaired ability to think, disorientation, confusion, drowsiness, apathy, and reduced HR and RR. Monitor for complaints of being too cold, goose bumps (piloerection), and cool skin (in SCI patients, above level of injury).	These are signs of hypothermia.
Monitor for flushed face, malaise, rash, respiratory distress, tachycardia, weakness, headache, and irritability. Monitor for complaints of being too warm, sweating, or hot and dry skin (in SCI patients, above level of injury).	These are signs of hyperthermia.
Be alert to parched mouth, furrowed tongue, dry lips, poor skin turgor, decreased urine output, increased concentration of urine (specific gravity greater than 1.030), and weak, fast pulse.	These are signs of dehydration that can occur as a result of hyperthermia.
For hyperthermia: Maintain a cool room temperature (20° C [68° F]). Provide a fan or air conditioning. Remove excess bedding and cover patient with a thin sheet. Give tepid sponge baths. Place cool, wet cloths at patient's head, neck, axilla, and groin. Administer antipyretic agent as prescribed. Use a padded hypothermia blanket (wrap hands and feet in towels or blankets to prevent shivering) or convection cooling device if prescribed. Provide cool drinks. Evaluate for potential infectious cause.	These are measures that help prevent overheating.
For hypothermia: Increase environmental temperature. Protect patient from drafts. Provide warm drinks. Provide extra blankets. Provide warming (hyperthermia) blanket or convection warming device.	These are measures that help increase body temperature.
Keep feverish patient dry. Change bed linens after diaphoresis. Provide careful skin care when patient is on a hypothermia or hyperthermia blanket.	These actions prevent skin irritation and potential loss of skin integrity that could result from hyperthermia and diaphoresis.
Monitor I&O and maintain adequate hydration. Unless contraindicated, encourage increased fluid intake in febrile patients (e.g., more than 3000 ml/day).	Insensible water loss from fever should be a consideration when monitoring I&O because it may affect total hydration.
Increase caloric intake.	Patients with fever have increased metabolic needs.

●●● Related NIC and NOC labels: *NIC:* Temperature Regulation; Environmental Management; Fever Treatment; Fluid Management; Bathing; Environmental Management: Comfort Heat/Cold Application; Vital Signs Monitoring *NOC:* Thermoregulation

Nursing Diagnosis:

Impaired Verbal Communication

related to facial/throat muscle weakness, intubation, or tracheostomy

Desired Outcome: Following intervention and on an ongoing basis, patient communicates effectively, either verbally or nonverbally, and relates decreasing frustration with communication.

INTERVENTIONS	RATIONALES
Assess patient's ability to speak, read, write, and comprehend.	This assessment helps determine patient's communication abilities and interventions that would promote them.
If appropriate, obtain referral to a speech therapist or pathologist. Encourage patient to perform exercises that increase ability to control facial muscles and tongue.	These actions assist patient in strengthening muscles used in speech. Such exercises may include holding a sound for 5 sec; singing the scale; reading aloud; and extending tongue and trying to touch chin, nose, or cheek.
Provide a supportive and relaxed environment for patient who is unable to form words or sentences or who is unable to speak clearly or appropriately. Provide enough time for patient to articulate. Ask patient to repeat unclear words. Observe for nonverbal cues; watch patient's lips closely. Do not interrupt or finish sentences. Anticipate needs and phrase questions to allow simple answers, such as "yes" or "no."	Patient likely will be frustrated over inability to communicate. Maintaining a calm, positive, reassuring attitude and continuing to speak to patient using normal volume (unless patient's hearing is impaired) will help ease frustrations.
Maintain eye contact.	This will help patient maintain focus.
If patient is unable to speak, provide language board, alphabet cards, picture or letter-number board, flash cards, pad and pencil. Other systems use eye blinks, tongue clicks, or hand squeezes; bell signal taps; or gestures such as hand signals, head nods, pantomime, or pointing. Use communication board for urgent situations.	These are alternative methods of communication.
Document method of communication used.	Documentation helps ensure that other health care team members use the same method(s).
If patient's voice is weak and difficult to hear, reduce environmental noise.	This will enhance listener's ability to hear and comprehend patient's words.
Suggest that patient take a deep breath before speaking; provide a voice amplifier if appropriate.	These measures project patient's voice.
Encourage patient to organize thoughts and plan what he or she will say before speaking. Encourage patient to express ideas in short, simple phrases or sentences.	These measures help make efficient use of voice strength or breath the patient does have.
Remind patient to speak slowly, exaggerate pronunciation, and use facial expressions.	Patient may have a flat affect in both pronunciation and facial expression. Exaggerating both may make patient's conversation more engaging.
If patient has swallowing difficulties that result in accumulation of saliva, suction mouth.	Suctioning will promote clearer speech.
If indicated, massage facial and neck muscles before patient attempts to communicate.	Massage promotes clearer speech in patient with muscle rigidity or spasm.
If patient has a tracheostomy, ensure that a tap bell is within reach.	Tap bell sounds give patient the means to communicate and increase a sense of self-control and safety.
Teach patient with a temporary tracheostomy that ability to speak will return.	This provides reassurance about future ability to communicate.
For patient with permanent tracheostomy, discuss learning alternate communication systems.	Alternate communication systems include sign language or esophageal speech, in which fenestrated tubes or covering tracheostomy tube opening with a finger will enable speech.
Establish a method of calling for assistance, and make sure that patient knows how to use it. Keep calling device where patient can activate it (e.g., place call bell on nonparalyzed side). Depending on deficit, use a tap bell for weak patient, a pillow pad call light (triggered by arm or head movement), or a sip and puff device (triggered by mouth).	These measures ensure that patients of varying abilities will be able to call for assistance.
Encourage patient with ability to write to keep a diary or write letters. If patient has a weak writing arm, evaluate need for a splint or other device that will enable patient to hold a pen or pencil.	These measures provide patient with a means of ventilating feelings and expressing concerns. Felt-tip markers are useful because they require minimal pressure for writing. Large-barrel pens may be easier for grasping and writing. Patient may be able to type. For patient able to speak, a computer voice recognition program may facilitate written and e-mail communication.

●●● **Related NIC and NOC labels:** *NIC:* Active Listening; Communication Enhancement: Speech Deficit; Anxiety Reduction
NOC: Communication Ability; Communication: Expressive Ability

Nursing Diagnosis:

Constipation

related to inability to chew and swallow a high-roughage diet, side effects of medications, immobility, and spinal cord involvement

Desired Outcome: Within 2-3 days of intervention, patient passes soft, formed stools and regains and maintains his or her normal bowel pattern.

INTERVENTIONS	RATIONALES
Teach patients with chewing and swallowing difficulties that consuming 1 or 2 servings of applesauce with added bran, prune juice, or cooked bran cereal each day may be effective. Otherwise encourage use of natural fiber laxatives such as psyllium (e.g., Metamucil).	Although a high-roughage diet is ideal for patient who is immobilized or on prolonged bedrest, individuals with chewing and swallowing difficulties may be unable to consume such a diet.
Encourage/promote a bowel elimination program. Keep a call bell within patient's reach.	Elements that may be included in a successful bowel elimination program include the following: setting a regular time of day for attempting a bowel movement, preferably 30 min after eating a meal or drinking a hot beverage; using a commode instead of a bedpan for more natural positioning during elimination; using a medicated suppository 15-30 min before a scheduled attempt; bearing down by contracting abdominal muscles or applying manual pressure to abdomen to help increase intraabdominal pressure; and drinking 4 oz of prune juice nightly.
As indicated, include abdominal and pelvic exercises in patient's morning and evening routine.	For more detail, see **Risk for Activity Intolerance,** p. 61, in "Prolonged Bedrest."
Assess patient's sitting balance and ability to assume a normal toileting position, and intervene accordingly.	This will help ensure patient's safety while on the commode.
Caution: Spinal cord injury (SCI) patients with involvement at T8 and above should use extreme caution if using an enema or suppository. If either measure is unavoidable, use large amounts of anesthetic jelly in the rectum.	Either measure can precipitate life-threatening autonomic dysreflexia (AD). Using anesthetic jelly reduces that risk.
In addition, instruct patient at risk of IICP not to bear down with bowel movements.	This action can cause increased intraabdominal pressure, which in turn increases ICP. See **Decreased Intracranial Adaptive Capacity,** earlier.
Unless contraindicated, encourage fluid intake to at least 2500 ml/day or more, including liberal amounts of fresh fruit juices.	Adequate fluid intake helps prevent hard, dry stools that are difficult to evacuate.
If indicated by patient's diagnosis (e.g., MS), provide instructions for anal digital stimulation.	This action promotes reflex bowel evacuation.
Caution: This intervention is contraindicated for SCI patients with involvement at T8 or above.	It can precipitate life-threatening AD.
For other interventions, see **Constipation**, p. 67, in "Prolonged Bedrest."	

••• **Related NIC and NOC labels:** *NIC:* Bowel Management; Constipation/Impaction Management; Fluid Management; Medication Management; Self-Care Assistance: Toileting; Nutrition Management *NOC:* Bowel Elimination; Hydration; Symptom Control

Nursing Diagnosis:

Self-Care Deficit: Bathing/Hygiene, Dressing/Grooming, Feeding, Toileting

related to spasticity, tremors, weakness, paresis, paralysis, or decreasing LOC secondary to sensorimotor deficits

Desired Outcome: At least 24 hr before hospital discharge, patient performs care activities independently and demonstrates ability to use adaptive devices for successful completion of ADL. (Totally dependent patient expresses satisfaction with activities that are completed for him or her.)

INTERVENTIONS	RATIONALES
Assess patient's ability to perform ADL.	This assessment demonstrates performance barriers and degree to which patient needs assistance with completing ADL. These data will enable development of an individualized care plan.
As appropriate, demonstrate use of adaptive devices, such as long- or broad-handled combs; long-handled pickup sticks, brushes, and eating utensils; dressing sticks; stocking helpers, Velcro fasteners; elastic waste bands; nonspill cups; and stabilized plates. Also consider electric toothbrush and electric razor.	Adaptive devices may assist patient in maintaining independent care. For example, a flexor-hinge splint or universal cuff may aid in brushing teeth and combing hair.
Set short-range, realistic goals with patient. Acknowledge progress. Encourage continued effort and involvement (e.g., in selection of meals, clothing).	These actions help decrease frustration and improve learning.
Provide care to totally dependent patient. Assist those who are not totally dependent according to degree of disability. Encourage patient to perform self-care to the maximum ability as defined by patient. Encourage autonomy.	Promoting autonomy and positive self-image helps prevent learned helplessness.
Allow sufficient time for task performance; do not hurry patient. Involve significant other with care activities if he or she is comfortable doing so. Ask for patient's input in planning schedules. Supervise activity until patient can safely perform task without help.	Preserving energy by providing sufficient time for the task increases activity to tolerance.
Encourage use of electronically controlled wheelchair and other technical advances (e.g., environmental control system).	These devices help improve mobility and enable independent operation of electronic devices such as lights, radio, door openers, and window shade openers.
Provide privacy and a nondistracting environment. Place patient's belongings within reach. Set out items needed to complete self-care tasks in the order they are to be used. Apply any needed adaptive devices such as hand splints.	These actions convey respect, simplify the task, and increase patient's motivation.
Encourage patient to wear any prescribed corrective eye lenses or hearing aids.	Enhanced vision and hearing may increase patient's participation in self-care.
Provide prescribed analgesics to relieve pain.	Pain can hinder self-care.
Provide a rest period before self-care activity, or plan activity for a time when patient is rested.	Fatigue reduces self-care ability.
Encourage patient or significant other to buy shoes without laces; long-handled shoe horns; front opening garments; wide-legged pants; and clothing that is loose-fitting with enlarged arm holes, front fasteners, zipper pulls, elastic waist bands, or Velcro closures. Avoid items with small buttons or tight buttonholes. Lay out clothing in the order it will be put on. Advise patient to sit while dressing. Suggest that use of a dressing stick may help to pull up pants or retrieve clothing.	These products and devices facilitate dressing and undressing.
Place stool in shower.	A stool will help patients for whom sitting down will enhance self-care with bathing.
Explain that bathrooms should have nonslip mats and grab bars.	These mats and bars promote safety in self care by preventing falls.
Suggest use of a handheld showerhead and a long-handled bath sponge or a washer mitt with a pocket that holds soap.	These devices and products facilitate autonomy in bathing.
Provide commode chair, elevated toilet seat, or male or female urinal.	These chairs, seats, and urinals promote self-care with elimination.
Teach self-transfer techniques.	These techniques enable patient to get to commode or toilet independently.
Keep call light within patient's reach. Instruct patient to call as early as possible.	Calling early provides time for staff to respond and patient will not have to rush because of urgency.
Offer toileting reminders q2h, after meals, and before bedtime.	Toileting schedules convey the message that continence is valued, optimally reducing episodes of incontinence.
Suggest use of a long-handled grasper that can hold tissues or washcloth for perineal care.	Some patients with limited hand or arm mobility may have difficulty with perineal care after elimination.

Continued

INTERVENTIONS	RATIONALES
For patient with hemiparesis or hemiparalysis, teach use of stronger or unaffected hand and arm for dressing, eating, bathing, and grooming. Instruct patient to dress weaker side first.	These measures simplify tasks and conserve energy.
For patient with visual field deficit, avoid placing items on blind side. Encourage patient to scan environment for needed items by turning head.	These measures enable visualization of the task at hand.
Suggest use of splints, weighted utensils, or wrist weights for patients with tremors. Teach patient to rest head against a high-backed chair.	Adaptive devices increase speed and safety of self-care and decrease exertion. Resting head against a high-backed chair may reduce head tremors.
Obtain referral for occupational therapist (OT) if indicated.	This referral will help determine best method for performing activities.
Provide consistent caregiver and ADL routine for patients with cognitive deficits.	Individuals with cognitive defects need simple visual or verbal cues, increased gesture use, demonstration, reminders of next step, and gentle repetition.
If indicated, teach patient self-catheterization, or teach technique to caregiver.	At-home intermittent catheterization usually is done with clean (not sterile) technique and equipment. The catheter is washed after use in warm, soapy water; rinsed; and placed in a clean plastic sack. Catheter insertion guides are available commercially for females with limited upper arm mobility. Crusted catheters are soaked in a solution of half distilled vinegar and half water.
Teach patient to monitor and notify health professional of cloudy, foul-smelling, or bloody urine; urine with sediment; chills or fever; pain in lower back or abdomen; or a red or swollen urethral meatus.	These are indicators of urinary tract infection (UTI), which necessitates timely intervention.
Discuss, as appropriate, modifying home environment.	Modifying home environment (e.g., with extended sinks, grab bars, lower closet hooks, wheelchair-accessible shower, modified phones, lowered mirrors, and lever door handles that operate with reduced hand pressure) likely will promote independence and performance of ADL at home.
Listen and provide opportunities for patient to express self, and communicate that it is normal to have negative feelings about changes in autonomy. Discuss with health care team ways to provide consistent and positive encouragement and strategies that increase independence progressively. Suggest a local support group.	Frustration can be decreased and coping skills increased when an individual expresses feelings in a supportive environment.

••• **Related NIC and NOC labels:** *NIC:* Self-Care Assistance: Bathing/Hygiene, Dressing/Grooming, Feeding, Toileting; Energy Management; Self-Responsibility Enhancement *NOC:* Self-Care: Activities of Daily Living

Nursing Diagnosis:

Self-Care Deficit: Oral Hygiene

related to sensorimotor deficit or decreased LOC

Desired Outcome: Before hospital discharge, patient or significant other demonstrates ability to perform patient's oral care.

INTERVENTIONS	RATIONALES
Assess patient's ability to perform mouth care.	This assessment enables identification of performance barriers (e.g., sensorimotor or cognitive deficits).
If patient has decreased LOC or is at risk for aspiration, remove dentures and store them in a water-filled denture cup.	This action protects and prevents loss of dentures.
If patient cannot perform mouth care, clean teeth, tongue, and mouth at least twice daily with a soft-bristled toothbrush and nonabrasive toothpaste.	This intervention promotes oral hygiene and prevents accumulation of bacteria that can cause oral inflammation.

Continued

INTERVENTIONS	RATIONALES
If patient is unconscious or at risk for aspiration, turn to a side-lying position. Swab mouth and teeth with sponge-tipped applicator (Toothette) moistened with diluted (half strength) mouthwash solution, and irrigate mouth with a large syringe. If patient cannot self-manage secretions, use only a small amount of liquid for irrigation each time, and, using a suction catheter or Yankauer tonsil suction tip, remove secretions.	These measures provide effective oral cleansing while preventing aspiration of oral solutions.
Perform this oral hygiene regimen at least q4h. As appropriate, teach procedure to significant other.	Good oral hygiene helps prevent stomatitis and tooth decay and reduces risk of infections caused by an oral mucous membrane that is not intact.
Make toothbrush adaptations for patients with physical disabilities.	*For patients with limited hand mobility:* Enlarge toothbrush handle by covering it with a sponge hair roller or aluminum foil (attaching with an elastic band) or by attaching a bicycle handle grip with plaster of Paris.
	For patients with limited arm mobility: Extend toothbrush handle by overlapping another handle or rod over it and taping them together.

••• **Related NIC and NOC labels:** *NIC:* Self-Care Assistance: Bathing/Hygiene; Oral Health Maintenance; Teaching: Individual; Oral Health Promotion; Oral Health Restoration *NOC:* Self-Care Hygiene

Nursing Diagnosis:

Disturbed Sensory Perception: Visual

related to diplopia secondary to neurologic deficit

Desired Outcome: Immediately following intervention, patient verbalizes that vision has improved.

INTERVENTIONS	RATIONALES
Assess for diplopia.	Diplopia may occur in neurologic patients resulting from dysfunction of cranial nerves III, IV, and VI.
If patient has diplopia, provide an eye patch or eyeglasses with a frosted lens. Alternate eye patch q4h.	This is a temporary measure for eliminating diplopia.
Orient patient to the environment as needed.	Orientation will promote safety and help prevent falls resulting from visual deficit.
Advise patient of availability of "talking books" (tapes) and large-type reading materials.	It would be difficult for patients with diplopia to read books with smaller print.
Place a sign over patient's bed that indicates patient's visual impairment.	This communicates to health care staff and visitors that patient may require visual assistance.
Teach patient that depth perception will be altered and to use visual cues and scanning.	This information will help prevent injury from bumping into things.

••• **Related NIC and NOC labels:** *NIC:* Environmental Management; Surveillance: Safety; Communication Enhancement: Visual Deficit; Fall Prevention *NOC:* Sensory Function: Vision; Vision Compensation: Behavior

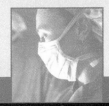

Bacterial Meningitis 35

OVERVIEW/PATHOPHYSIOLOGY

Bacterial meningitis is an infection that results in inflammation of the meningeal membranes covering the brain and spinal cord. Bacteria in the subarachnoid space multiply and cause an inflammatory reaction of the pia and arachnoid meninges. Purulent exudate is produced, and inflammation and infection spread quickly through the cerebrospinal fluid (CSF) that circulates around the brain and spinal cord. Bacteria and exudate can create vascular congestion, plugging the arachnoid villi. This obstruction of CSF flow and decreased reabsorption of CSF can lead to hydrocephalus, increased intracranial pressure (IICP), brain herniation, and death.

Meningitis generally is transmitted in one of four ways: (1) via airborne droplets or contact with oral secretions from infected individuals; (2) from direct contamination (e.g., from a penetrating skull wound; a skull fracture, often basilar, causing a tear in the dura; lumbar puncture (LP); ventricular shunt; or surgical procedure); (3) via the bloodstream (e.g., pneumonia, endocarditis); or (4) from direct contact with an infectious process that invades the meningeal membranes, as can occur with osteomyelitis, sinusitis, otitis media, mastoiditis, or brain abscess. In adults, pneumonococcal meningitis, caused by *Streptococcus pneumoniae*, is the most common bacterial meningitis. Meningococcal meningitis, caused by *Neisseria meningitidis*, is the next leading cause. This organism can cause adrenal hemorrhage and insufficiency, leading to vascular collapse and death. Myocarditis also can occur. *Listeria monocytogenes* is being seen more frequently, especially in immune compromised people and in the extremely young or old. Outbreaks have been associated with consumption of contaminated dairy or undercooked fish, chicken, and meat. Any bacteria can cause meningitis, and some forms of meningitis, such as that caused by *Staphylococcus aureus*, can be difficult to treat because of their resistance to antibiotic therapy. Adhesions and fibrotic changes in the arachnoid layer and subspace may cause obstruction or reabsorption problems with CSF, resulting in hydrocephalus.

HEALTH CARE SETTING

Acute care setting

ASSESSMENT

Cardinal signs: Headache, fever, stiff neck, change in mental status.

Infection: Fever, chills, malaise.

IICP and herniation: Decreased level of consciousness (LOC) (irritability, drowsiness, stupor, coma), nausea and vomiting, decreasing Glasgow Coma Scale score, vital sign (VS) changes (increased blood pressure [BP], decreased heart rate [HR], widening pulse pressure), changes in respiratory pattern, decreased pupillary reaction to light, pupillary dilation or inequality, severe headache.

Meningeal irritation: Back stiffness and pain, headache, nuchal rigidity.

Other: Generalized seizures and photophobia. In the presence of *Haemophilus influenzae*, deafness or joint pain may occur.

PHYSICAL ASSESSMENT

- Positive Brudzinski's sign may be elicited because of meningeal irritation: when the neck is passively flexed forward, both legs flex involuntarily at the hip and knee.
- Positive Kernig's sign also may be found: when the thigh is flexed 90 degrees at the hip, the individual cannot extend the leg completely without pain.
- In the presence of meningococcal meningitis, a pink, macular rash; petechiae; ecchymoses; purpura; and increased deep tendon reflexes (DTRs) may occur. The rash signals septicemia and is associated with a 40% mortality rate, even with appropriate antibiotics. The rash can progress to gangrenous necrosis and may need débridement or even amputation.

DIAGNOSTIC TESTS

LP, CSF analysis, and Gram stain and culture: To identify causative organism. Glucose is generally decreased, and protein increased. Increased total lactate dehydrogenase (LDH) in CSF is a consistent finding. Presence or absence of C-reactive protein (CRP) in the CSF can differentiate between bacterial (positive for CRP) and nonbacterial (negative for CRP) meningitis. Typically, CSF will be cloudy or milky because of increased white blood cells (WBCs); CSF pressure will be increased because of the inflammation and exudate, causing an obstruction in outflow of CSF from the arachnoid villi. This test, in the presence of IICP, can cause brain herniation. If CSF pressure is elevated, check neurologic status and VS at frequent intervals for signs of brain herniation (decreased LOC; pupillary changes such as dilation, inequality, or decreased reaction; irregular respirations; hemiparesis).

Culture and sensitivity testing of blood, sputum, urine, and other body secretions: To identify infective organism and/or its source and determine appropriate antibiotic.

Coagglutination tests: To detect microbial antigens in CSF and enable identification of the causative organism. Generally coagglutination tests have replaced counterimmunoelectrophoresis because results are obtainable much more rapidly.

Polymerase chain reaction: To analyze DNA in peripheral blood or CSF to identify causative infectious agents.

Radioimmunoassay, latex particle agglutination, or enzyme-linked immunosorbent assay: To detect microbial antigens in the CSF to identify causative organism.

Petechial skin scraping: For Gram stain analysis of bacteria.

Sinus, skull, and chest x-ray examinations: Taken after treatment is started to rule out sinusitis, pneumonia, and cranial osteomyelitis.

CT scan with contrast: To rule out hydrocephalus or mass lesions such as brain abscess and detect exudate in CSF spaces.

MRI: To rule out hydrocephalus or mass lesion and detect exudate in CSF spaces.

Nursing Diagnosis:

Deficient Knowledge:

Rationale and procedure for Transmission-Based Precautions: Droplet

Desired Outcome: Before visitation, patient and significant other verbalize knowledge about the rationale for Transmission-Based Precautions: Droplet, and comply with prescribed restrictions and precautionary measures.

INTERVENTIONS	RATIONALES
For patients with meningitis caused by *H. influenzae* or *N. meningitidis*, explain method of disease transmission via respiratory droplets generated by patient when coughing, sneezing, or talking or during performance of cough-inducing procedures (e.g., suctioning) and by contact with oral secretions and rationale for private room and droplet precautions.	Patients with *N. meningitidis*, with *H. influenzae*, or in whom the causative organism is in doubt require observation with Transmission-Based Precautions: Droplet, for 24 hr after initiation of appropriate antibiotic therapy. Patient should be placed in a private room if possible. If private room is not available, infected patient may be placed in a room with another patient who is at low risk for adverse outcome if transmission occurs, ensuring that patients are physically separated (i.e., more than 3 ft) from each other.
Provide instructions for covering mouth before coughing or sneezing and properly disposing of tissue (Respiratory Hygiene/Cough Etiquette).	Infection may be spread by contact with respiratory droplets or oral secretions. Masks should be worn for close patient contact (e.g., within 3 ft), along with adherence to Standard Precautions (see p. 783).
Instruct patients with Transmission-Based Precautions: Droplet, to stay in their room. If they must leave the room for a procedure or test, explain that a mask must be worn to protect others from contact with respiratory droplets.	As above.
For individuals in contact with patient, explain importance of wearing a surgical mask and using good handwashing technique. Gloves should be worn when handling any body fluid, especially oral secretions. For more information, see Appendix A, "Infection Prevention and Control," p. 783.	As above.
Reassure patient that Transmission-Based Precautions: Droplet are temporary.	These precautions will be discontinued once patient has been taking the appropriate antibiotic for at least 24 hr.
Instruct individuals in contact with patient that if symptoms of meningitis develop (e.g., headache, fever, neck stiffness, photophobia, change in mental status), they should report immediately to their health care provider.	This measure helps ensure prompt treatment. Mortality rate is high (70%-100%) in persons in whom meningitis is left untreated. However, in individuals in whom diagnosis and antibiotic treatment are established early, prognosis is good, and complete neurologic recovery is possible.

••• **Related NIC and NOC labels:** *NIC:* Teaching: Procedure/Treatment; Teaching: Disease Process; Infection Protection; Infection Control
NOC: Knowledge: Illness Care; Knowledge: Infection Control

Nursing Diagnosis:

Acute Pain

related to headache, photophobia, and neck stiffness secondary to meningitis

Desired Outcomes: Within 1-2 hr of intervention, patient's subjective perception of discomfort decreases, as documented by pain scale. Objective indicators, such as grimacing, are absent or diminished.

INTERVENTIONS	RATIONALES
Provide a quiet environment, darkened room or sunglasses, and restrict visitors as necessary.	These measures reduce noise and help prevent photophobia.
Promote bedrest and assist with ADL as needed.	These measures decrease movement that may cause pain.
Apply ice bag to head or cool cloth to eyes.	These actions help diminish headache.
Support patient in a position of comfort. Keep neck in alignment during position changes.	Many persons with meningitis are comforted in a position with head in extension and body slightly curled. Head of bed (HOB) elevated to 30 degrees also may help.
Provide gentle passive range of motion (ROM) and massage to neck and shoulder joints and muscles. If patient is afebrile, apply moist heat to neck and back.	These measures help relieve stiffness, promote muscle relaxation, and decrease pain.
Keep communication simple and direct, using a soft, calm tone of voice. Avoid needless stimulation. Consolidate activities. Loosen constricting bed clothing. Avoid restraining patient. Reduce stimulation to the minimal amount needed to accomplish required activity.	Patients tend to be hyperirritable with hyperalgesia. Sounds are loud, and even gentle touching may startle patient.
Administer medications as prescribed.	Analgesics (e.g., acetaminophen, codeine) are given to relieve headache, myalgia, and other pain.
	Antipyretics (e.g., acetaminophen) are given for control of fever to reduce cerebral metabolism.
	Mild sedatives (e.g., diphenhydramine) are given to promote rest.
For other interventions see **Acute Pain** in "General Care of Patients with Neurologic Disorders," p. 273.	

••• **Related NIC and NOC labels:** *NIC:* Medication Administration; Environmental Management: Comfort; Pain Management; Positioning; Heat/Cold Application; Simple Massage *NOC:* Comfort Level; Pain Control Pain: Disruptive Effects

Nursing Diagnosis:

Deficient Knowledge:

Side effects and precautions for the prescribed antibiotics

Desired Outcome: Before beginning medication regimen, patient and significant other verbalize knowledge about potential side effects and precautions for prescribed antibiotics.

INTERVENTIONS	RATIONALES
Assess patient's and significant others' health care literacy (language, reading, comprehension). Assess culture and culturally specific information needs.	This assessment helps ensure that information is presented in a manner that is culturally and educationally appropriate.
Teach patient about the prescribed antibiotic.	Because treatment cannot be delayed until culture results are known, high doses of parenteral antibiotics are started immediately, based on Gram stain results. The antibiotic must penetrate the blood-brain barrier into the CSF. Adjustments in therapy can be made after coagglutination test, Counter immunoelectrophoresis (CIE), and culture and sensitivity test results are available. Antibiotics may include the following (usually in combination): penicillin G, ampicillin, cefotaxime, ceftriaxone, ceftazidime, chloramphenicol, gentamicin, and vancomycin.
As appropriate, teach patient that sometimes intrathecal (i.e., in the subarachnoid space) antibiotics are used.	Intrathecal antibiotics may be used if it is believed that systemic antibiotics alone will not be curative in the presence of particular bacteria (e.g., *Pseudomonas, Enterobacter, Staphylococcus*).
Explain significance of giving glucocorticosteroid (e.g., dexamethasone).	Ideally it is given before or at same time as first dose of antibiotics and then on an ongoing basis to reduce inflammation caused by toxic byproducts released by bacterial cells as they are killed by antibiotics. In children, this therapy can reduce hearing loss caused by *Haemophilus influenzae.*
Explain purpose of CRP replacement therapy (e.g., drotrecogin alfa [activated]) if it is used.	This antisepsis agent improves outcomes in septic meningococcal meningitis and purpura fulminans.
For close contacts of patient, explain importance of taking prophylactic antibiotic, including prescribed dose and schedule and symptoms to report.	Usually rifampin is administered. Other antibiotics, such as ciprofloxacin, ceftriaxone, chloramphenicol, sulfadiazine, or minocycline, may be used as well. It is important that all contacts be notified as soon as possible for treatment and known signs and symptoms of meningitis to report to health care provider (e.g., headache, fever, stiff neck, change in mental state).
Explain that rifampin should be taken 1 hr before meals.	This ensures maximum absorption.
Emphasize purpose of taking rifampin and its potential side effects.	Rifampin is taken as a preventive measure against meningitis. Potential side effects such as nausea, vomiting, diarrhea, orange urine, headache, and dizziness can occur.
Explain precautions when taking rifampin.	Persons taking this drug should avoid wearing contact lenses because the drug will permanently color them orange. In addition, rifampin reduces effectiveness of oral contraceptives and is contraindicated during pregnancy. Contacts who are taking rifampin also should report onset of jaundice (yellow skin or sclera), allergic reactions, and persistence of gastrointestinal side effects.

••• **Related NIC and NOC labels:** *NIC:* Teaching: Prescribed Medication *NOC:* Knowledge: Medication

ADDITIONAL NURSING DIAGNOSES/ PROBLEMS:

"Prolonged Bedrest" — p. 61

"Psychosocial Support" — p. 73

"Psychosocial Support for the Patient's Family and Significant Other" — p. 87

"Older Adult Care" for **Risk for Aspiration** — p. 96

"Cardiac and Noncardiac Shock" for patients who are in septic shock — p. 157

Decreased Intracranial Adaptive Capacity — p. 261

"General Care of Patients with Neurologic Disorders" for **Risk for Falls** related to unsteady gait — p. 265

Impaired Swallowing — p. 267

Risk for Injury related to impaired pain, touch, and temperature sensations — p. 269

Impaired Tissue Integrity: Corneal — p. 270

Risk for Deficient Fluid Volume — p. 271

Imbalanced Nutrition: Less Than Body Requirements — p. 272

Risk for Imbalanced Body Temperature — p. 274

Self-Care Deficit — p. 277

Constipation — p. 277

"Seizures and Epilepsy" for **Risk for Trauma** related to oral, musculoskeletal, and airway vulnerability secondary to seizure activity — p. 325

"Traumatic Brain Injury" for **Excess Fluid Volume** secondary to SIADH — p. 366

Deficient Knowledge: Ventricular Shunt procedure — p. 370

"Disseminated Intravascular Coagulation" for patients with or at risk for this condition — p. 497

"Pressure Ulcers" for patients who are immobile — p. 562

"Providing Nutritional Support" for patients needing nutritional support — p. 565

For patients on mechanical ventilation, see:

"Pneumonia" for **Risk of Infection** related to inadequate primary defenses — p. 127

"General Concepts of Patients with Neurologic Disorders" for **Risk for Infection** related to inadequate primary defenses — p. 264

✓ PATIENT-FAMILY TEACHING AND DISCHARGE PLANNING

The extent of teaching and discharge planning will depend on whether the patient has any residual damage. When providing patient-family teaching, focus on sensory information, avoid giving excessive information, and initiate a visiting nurse referral for necessary follow-up teaching. Include verbal and written information about the following:

✓ Referrals to community resources, such as public health nurse, visiting nurses association, community support groups, social workers, psychologic therapy, vocational rehabilitation agency, home health agencies, and extended and skilled care facilities.

✓ Medications, including drug name, purpose, dosage, schedule, precautions, and potential side effects for patient's medications, as well as those for the prophylactic antibiotics taken by family and significant other. Also discuss drug-drug, herb-drug, and food-drug interactions. Close contacts taking prophylactic antibiotics should know signs and symptoms to report to health care provider (e.g., headache, fever, neck stiffness).

✓ Vaccination: A pneumococcal vaccine is available to help protect against meningitis and other infections caused by *Streptococcus pneumoniae*. *N. meningitidis* has several subgroup strains. For people at increased risk (e.g., travelers to countries with endemic infections), a meningococcal vaccine (group A, C, Y, W135) is available although it does not confer 100% protection. Centers for Disease Control and Prevention recommends this meningococcal vaccine for children 11-12 years of age, adolescents at high school entry, and college freshmen living in dormitories. The most common *N. meningitidis* in the United States is from Group B, and work is progressing on a Group B vaccine. *H. influenzae* Group B vaccine should be incorporated as part of all routine childhood inoculations.

✓ For patients with residual neurologic deficits, teach the following as appropriate: exercises that promote muscle strength and mobility; measures for preventing contractures and skin breakdown; transfer techniques and proper body mechanics; safety measures if patient has decreased pain and sensation or visual disturbances; use of assistive devices; indications of constipation, urinary retention, or UTI; bowel and bladder training programs; self-catheterization technique or care of indwelling catheters; and seizure precautions if indicated.

✓ Obtain additional information from the following: Meningitis Foundation of America, Inc., at *www.musa.org*.

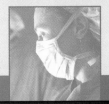

Guillain-Barré Syndrome 36

OVERVIEW/PATHOPHYSIOLOGY

Guillain-Barré syndrome (GBS) is a rapidly progressing poly-neuritis of unknown cause. An inflammatory process enables lymphocytes to enter perivascular spaces and destroy the myelin sheath covering peripheral or cranial nerves. Posterior (sensory) and anterior (motor) nerve roots can be affected because of this segmental demyelinization, and individuals may experience both sensory and motor losses. There is relative sparing of the axon. Respiratory insufficiency may occur in as many as half of affected individuals. Life-threatening respiratory muscle weakness can develop as rapidly as 24-72 hr after onset of initial symptoms. In about 25% of cases, motor weakness progresses to total paralysis.

Peak severity of symptoms usually occurs within 1-3 wk after onset of symptoms. A plateau stage follows that usually lasts 1-2 wk. The recovery stage starts with a return of function as remyelinization occurs, but it may take months to years for a full recovery. Fifteen percent of patients have full neurologic recovery, and another 65% have mild deficits that do not interfere with activities of daily living (ADL). Eighty percent to 90% of patients either recover completely or have only minor residual weakness or abnormal sensations, such as numbness or tingling. Of GBS patients, 5%-10% may have permanent severe disability. Deficits are the result of axonal nerve degeneration.

GBS may follow a recent viral illness, such as upper respiratory infection (URI) or gastroenteritis, rabies or influenza vaccination, lupus erythematosus, or Hodgkin's disease or other malignant process. Although the exact cause of GBS is unknown, it is believed to be an autoimmune response to a viral infection. *Campylobacter jejuni* enteritis has been identified as a trigger for GBS in more than 26% of cases. Cytomegalovirus also has been implicated.

HEALTH CARE SETTING

The patient is likely to be in acute care (intensive care unit [ICU]) when the neurologic deficit is progressing and in an acute rehabilitation setting during the recovery phase.

ASSESSMENT

Progressive weakness and areflexia are the most common indicators. Typically, numbness and weakness begin in the legs and ascend symmetrically upward, progressing to the arms and facial nerves. Ascending GBS is most common, but descending GBS,

in which cranial nerves are affected first and weakness progresses downward with rapid respiratory involvement, also can occur. Variants of GBS include primarily a motor component, and another called Miller Fisher syndrome is characterized by abnormal muscle coordination, paralysis of eye muscles, and absence of tendon reflexes. Peak severity usually occurs within 10-14 days of onset. GBS does not affect level of consciousness (LOC), cognitive function, or pupillary function.

Anterior (motor) nerve root involvement: Weakness or flaccid paralysis that can progress to tetraplegia. Respiratory muscle involvement can be life threatening. There is loss of reflexes, muscle tension, and tone, but muscle atrophy usually does not occur.

Autonomic nervous system involvement: Sinus tachycardia, bradycardia, hypertension, hypotension, cardiac dysrhythmias, facial flushing, diaphoresis, inability to perspire, loss of sphincter control, urinary retention, adynamic ileus, syndrome of inappropriate antidiuretic hormone secretion, and increased pulmonary secretions may occur. Autonomic nervous system (ANS) involvement may occur unexpectedly and can be life threatening, but usually it does not persist for longer than 2 wk.

Cranial nerve involvement: Inability to chew, swallow, speak, or close the eyes.

Posterior (sensory) nerve root involvement: Presence of paresthesias, such as numbness and tingling, which usually are minor compared with the degree of motor loss. Ascending sensory loss often precedes motor loss. Muscle cramping, tenderness, or pain may occur.

Physical assessment: Symmetric motor weakness, impaired position and vibration sense, hypoactive or absent deep tendon reflexes, hypotonia in affected muscles, and decreased ventilatory capacity.

DIAGNOSTIC TESTS

Diagnostic tests are performed to rule out other diseases, such as acute poliomyelitis. Diagnosis of GBS is based on clinical presentation, history of recent viral illness, and cerebrospinal fluid (CSF) findings.

Lumbar puncture and CSF analysis: About 7 days after initial symptoms, elevated protein (especially IgG) without an increase in white blood cell (WBC) count may be present. Although CSF pressure usually is normal, in severe disease it may be elevated.

Electromyography: Reveals slowed nerve conduction velocities soon after paralysis appears because of demyelination. Denervation potentials appear later.

Serum CBC: Will show presence of leukocytosis early in illness, possibly as a result of the inflammatory process associated with demyelination.

Evoked potentials (auditory, visual, brainstem): May be used to distinguish GBS from other neuropathologic conditions.

Nursing Diagnosis:

Ineffective Breathing Pattern

related to neuromuscular weakness or paralysis of the facial, throat, and respiratory muscles (severity of symptoms peaks around wk 1-3)

Desired Outcome: Deterioration in patient's breathing pattern (e.g., Pao_2 less than 80 mm Hg, vital capacity less than 800-1000 ml [or less than 10-12 ml/kg], tidal volume less than 75% of predicted value, or O_2 saturation 92% or less via oximetry) is detected and reported promptly, resulting in immediate and effective medical treatment.

INTERVENTIONS	RATIONALES
Test for ascending loss of sensation by touching patient lightly with a pin or fingers at frequent intervals (hourly or more frequently initially). Assess from the level of the iliac crest upward toward the shoulders. Measure the highest level at which decreased sensation occurs.	Decreased sensation often precedes motor weakness; therefore, if it ascends to the level of the T8 dermatome, anticipate that intercostal muscles (used with respirations) soon will be impaired.
Check patient for the presence of arm drift and inability to shrug the shoulders. Alert health care provider to significant findings.	Shoulder weakness is present if patient cannot shrug shoulders. Arm drift is present if one arm pronates or drifts down or out from its original position. Arm drift is detected in the following way: have patient hold both arms out in front of the body, level with the shoulders and with palms up; instruct patient to close eyes while holding this position. These findings need to be reported promptly because they are known to precede respiratory dysfunction.
Monitor patient's ability to take fluids orally. Assess patient q8h and before oral intake for cough reflexes, gag reflexes, and difficulty swallowing. Assist with oral intake accordingly.	These assessments detect changes or difficulties that may indicate ascending paralysis. Impaired swallowing and cough and gag reflexes likely will necessitate parenteral feedings to prevent aspiration until reflexes return to normal.
Monitor patient's respiratory rate, rhythm, and depth. Observe for changes in mental status, LOC, and orientation. Auscultate for diminished breath sounds.	Accessory muscle use, nasal flaring, dyspnea, shallow respirations, diminished breath sounds, and apnea are signs of respiratory deterioration that necessitate prompt notification of the health provider for rapid intervention.
Observe for changes in mental status, LOC, and orientation.	These changes may signal reduced oxygenation to the brain as a result of ineffective breathing pattern.
Monitor patient for breathlessness while speaking. To assess for breathlessness, ask patient to take a deep breath and slowly count as high as possible on one breath. Alert health care provider to significant findings.	A reduced ability to count to a higher number before breathlessness occurs may signal grossly reduced ventilatory function.
Monitor effectiveness of breathing by checking serial vital capacity results on pulmonary function tests.	If vital capacity is less than 800-1000 ml or is rapidly trending downward or if patient exhibits signs of hypoxia such as tachycardia, increasing restlessness, mental dullness, cyanosis, decreased pulse oximetry readings, or difficulty handling secretions, these findings must be reported immediately to health care provider to prevent further deterioration in status. Vital capacity initially is measured q2-4h and then more frequently if deterioration is present.
Monitor arterial blood gas levels and pulse oximetry.	These assessments detect hypoxia or hypercapnia ($Paco_2$ more than 45 mm Hg), a signal of hypoventilation. Pao_2 less than 80 mm Hg or O_2 saturation 92% or less usually signals need for supplemental oxygen.

Continued

INTERVENTIONS	RATIONALES
Raise head of bed.	This position promotes optimal chest excursion by taking pressure of abdominal organs off the lungs, which may increase oxygenation.
Encourage coughing and deep breathing to the best of patient's ability.	These actions mobilize and enable expectoration of secretions to optimize breathing pattern. This position also will reduce aspiration risk.
Prepare patient emotionally for life-saving procedures or for the eventual transfer to ICU or transition care unit for closer monitoring.	The patient may require tracheostomy, endotracheal intubation, or mechanical ventilation to support respiratory function.
For other interventions, see **Risk for Aspiration** in "Older Adult Care," p. 96.	

••• **Related NIC and NOC labels:** *NIC:* Respiratory Monitoring; Ventilation Assistance; Aspiration Precautions; Mechanical Ventilation; Oxygen Therapy; Positioning; Acid-Base Monitoring *NOC:* Respiratory Status: Ventilation

Nursing Diagnosis:

Ineffective Tissue Perfusion: Cardiopulmonary and Cerebral (or risk for same)

related to interrupted sympathetic outflow with concomitant BP fluctuations secondary to autonomic dysfunction

Desired Outcomes: Patient has optimal cardiopulmonary and cerebral tissue perfusion as evidenced by SBP at least 90 mm Hg and less than 160 mm Hg, no significant mental status changes, and orientation to person, place, and time. BP fluctuations, if they occur, are detected and reported promptly.

INTERVENTIONS	RATIONALES
Monitor blood pressure (BP), noting wide fluctuations; report significant findings to health care provider.	Changes in BP that result in severe hypotension or hypertension may occur because of unopposed sympathetic outflow or loss of outflow to the peripheral nervous system, causing changes in vascular tone. Health care provider may prescribe a short-acting vasoactive agent for persistent hypotension or hypertension. Phenoxybenzamine may be used to treat paroxysmal hypertension, headache, sweating, anxiety, and fever.
Monitor carefully for changes in heart rate (HR) and BP during activities such as coughing, suctioning, position changes, or straining at stool.	These are events that can trigger BP changes.
For patients with hypotension or postural hypotension, see **Ineffective Tissue Perfusion: Cardiopulmonary and Cerebral,** p. 338, in "Spinal Cord Injury."	

••• **Related NIC and NOC labels:** *NIC:* Medication Administration; Dysrhythmia Management; Emergency Care; Fluid Management; Intravenous Therapy; Vital Signs Monitoring; Neurologic Monitoring; Hypovolemia Management *NOC:* Tissue Perfusion: Cardiac; Tissue Perfusion: Pulmonary; Tissue Perfusion: Cerebral

Nursing Diagnosis:

Imbalanced Nutrition: Less Than Body Requirements

related to adynamic ileus

Desired Outcome: Patient has adequate nutrition as evidenced by maintenance of baseline body weight.

INTERVENTIONS	RATIONALES
Auscultate abdominal sounds, noting presence, absence, or changes from baseline that may signal onset of ileus. Notify health care provider of significant findings.	Abdominal distention or tenderness, nausea and vomiting, and absence of stool output are signals of the onset of ileus, which can occur in the presence of ANS involvement. Also, GBS has been associated with *Campylobacter jejuni,* an infection that manifests as gastroenteritis. These findings should be reported for timely intervention.
Provide a high-fiber diet as prescribed.	Fiber provides bulk, which helps prevent constipation.
Initiate gastric, gastrostomy, or parenteral feedings as prescribed.	Patients with adynamic ileus generally require gastric decompression with a nasogastric tube. If patient cannot chew or swallow effectively because of cranial nerve involvement, gastric, gastrostomy, or parenteral feedings may be initiated. Patient is advanced to a solid diet upon return of gag reflex and swallowing ability. See "Providing Nutritional Support," p. 565.
For general interventions, see **Imbalanced Nutrition**, p. 272, in "General Care of Patients with Neurologic Disorders."	

••• Related NIC and NOC labels: *NIC:* Nutrition Management; Nutrition Monitoring; Enteral Tube Feeding; Total Parenteral Nutrition Administration; Weight Gain Assistance *NOC:* Nutritional Status: Nutrient Intake; Nutritional Status: Food and Fluid Intake

Nursing Diagnosis:

Anxiety

related to threat to biologic integrity and loss of control

Desired Outcome: Within 24 hr of this diagnosis, patient expresses concern regarding changes in life events, states anxiety is lessened or under control, and exhibits fewer symptoms of increased anxiety (e.g., less apprehension, decreased tension).

INTERVENTIONS	RATIONALES
For patients with progressing neurologic deficit, arrange for transfer to a room close to nurses' station.	This action will help alleviate the anxiety of being suddenly incapacitated and helpless.
Be sure call light is within easy reach, and frequently assess patient's ability to use it.	These measures that promote patient's safety also will help allay anxiety.
Provide continuity of patient care through assignment of staff and use of care plan.	Familiarity may help reduce anxiety.
Perform assessments at frequent intervals, letting patient know you are there. Provide care in a calm and reassuring manner.	Calm begets calm. Frequent assessments also reassure patient that he or she is being watched out for.
Allow time for patient to ventilate concerns; provide realistic feedback regarding what patient may experience. Determine past effective coping behaviors.	Unexpressed concerns can contribute to frustration and stress. Information helps reduce anxiety caused by a lack of knowledge. Knowing past effective coping behaviors facilitates problem solving for ways in which these behaviors, or others, may prove useful in current situation.
For other interventions, see **Anxiety**, p. 74, and **Fear**, p. 76, in "Psychosocial Support."	

••• Related NIC and NOC labels: *NIC:* Anxiety Reduction; Active Listening; Calming Technique; Coping Enhancement; Presence; Environmental Management *NOC:* Anxiety Control

Nursing Diagnosis:

Deficient Knowledge:

Therapeutic plasma exchange procedure

Desired Outcome: Before scheduled date of each procedure, patient verbalizes accurate information about the plasma exchange procedure.

INTERVENTIONS	RATIONALES
Assess patient's health care literacy (language, reading, comprehension). Assess culture and culturally specific information needs.	This assessment helps ensure that information is presented in a manner that is culturally and educationally appropriate.
Before the plasma exchange procedure, patient's health care provider explains the reason for the procedure, its risks, and anticipated benefits or outcome, and obtains a signed consent. Determine patient's level of understanding of health care provider's explanation.	This assessment provides an opportunity to clarify or reinforce information accordingly. Alternatives to plasma exchange include IV immunoglobulins, which may be given soon (1-5 days) after symptom onset to positively affect antibody response, or immunoadsorption therapy as an alternative to plasmapheresis for antibody removal. Informed consent is needed for invasive procedures.
Notify health care provider if patient is taking angiotensin-converting enzyme (ACE) inhibitor medication.	ACE inhibitor use is associated with flushing, hypotension, abdominal cramping, and other gastrointestinal symptoms while on plasmapheresis. These medications usually are held for 24 hr before the procedure to avoid these problems.
Determine patient's experience with plasmapheresis, positive or negative effects, and nature of any fears or concerns. Document and communicate this information to other caregivers.	This will clarify the nurse's understanding of the patient's perspective, which in turn will enable further information gathering and clarification, optimally decreasing patient's fears and concerns.
Explain in words patient can understand the goal of plasma exchange.	The procedure is similar to hemodialysis. Blood is removed from patient and separated into its components. Patient's plasma is discarded; other blood components (e.g., red blood cells, WBCs, platelets) are saved and returned to patient with donor plasma or replacement fluid. Multiple exchanges over a period of weeks can be expected.
Explain that if started within 1-2 wk of GBS symptoms, the exchange process seems to decrease disease duration and severity.	Antibodies to patient's peripheral and cranial nerve tissue are reduced by removal of the blood's plasma portion, which contains the circulating antibodies.
Answer any questions regarding these complications accordingly.	Although the following complications are rare, patient is at risk during this procedure: deficient fluid volume, hypotension, fluid overload, hypokalemia (from dilution with albumin replacement), hypocalcemia (from free calcium binding to the citrate used during the procedure), cardiac dysrhythmias (from electrolyte shifts), clotting disorders (from decreased clotting factors with plasma removal), anemia, phlebitis, infection, hypothermia, and air embolism.
If the antecubital site is used, place a sign alerting others to avoid using this site for routine laboratory blood draws.	This procedure requires good blood flow, and the access site must be preserved for plasma exchange. Central or femoral access may be needed for sufficient blood flow.
Explain that patient can expect the procedure to take 2-4 hr, although it may take considerably longer.	The length of time will depend on condition of patient's veins, blood flow, and hematocrit level.
Explain that patient can expect preprocedure and postprocedure blood work.	Blood will be assessed for clotting factors and electrolyte level, particularly of potassium and calcium, which can be reduced during this exchange procedure.
Explain that weight and vital signs (VS) will be taken before and after the procedure, with frequent VS checks during the procedure.	Hypotension and shift in fluid volume are possible.
Advise that calcium gluconate or potassium may be administered.	These agents will correct electrolyte imbalances.
Encourage patient to report any unusual feelings or symptoms during plasma exchange.	Unusual feelings or symptoms may include chills, fever, hives, sweating, or lightheadedness, which may signal reaction to donor plasma.
	Thirst, faintness, or dizziness can occur with hypotension or hypovolemia. Patients should take oral fluids during the procedure if possible.
	Numbness or tingling around lips or in the hands, arms, and legs; muscle twitching; cramping; or tetany can occur with hypocalcemia.
	Fatigue, nausea, weakness, or cramping may signal hypokalemia.

Continued

INTERVENTIONS	RATIONALES
Inform patient that medications (e.g., plasma-bound drugs) may be held until after the procedure.	Medications otherwise would be removed from the blood during the plasma exchange.
If patients do not have a urinary catheter, remind them to void before and during the procedure, if necessary.	This measure prevents the mild hypotension caused by a full bladder
Explain that intake and output will be monitored closely during the procedure.	Decreased urine output may signal hypovolemia.
Explain that patient's temperature will be checked during the procedure and warm blankets will be provided.	These measures assess for and prevent hypothermia.
Explain that patient probably will feel fatigued 1-2 days after the procedure. Encourage extra rest, high-protein diet, and milk products during this time.	Fatigue could result from decreased plasma protein level that occurs during the exchange.
Teach patient to monitor IV access site for warmth, redness, swelling, or drainage, and to report significant findings.	These are signs of local infection.
Teach patient to monitor for signs of bruising or bleeding. Caution patient about avoiding cutting self or bumping into objects and to sustain pressure over cuts. Inform patient that black, tarry stools usually signal presence of blood and should be reported.	The anticoagulant citrate dextrose is used in the extracorporeal machine circuitry to prevent clotting. This may cause excessive bleeding at the access site. A pressure dressing may be kept in place over the access site for 2-4 hr after the procedure.

••• Related NIC and NOC labels: *NIC:* Preparatory Sensory Information; Teaching: Procedure/Treatment; Learning Readiness Enhancement *NOC:* Knowledge: Treatment Procedure

Nursing Diagnosis:

Acute Pain

related to muscle tenderness; hypersensitivity to touch; or discomfort in shoulders, thighs, and back

Desired Outcomes: Within 1-2 hr of intervention, patient's subjective perception of discomfort decreases, as documented by pain scale. Objective indicators, such as grimacing, are absent or diminished.

INTERVENTIONS	RATIONALES
For patients with hypersensitivity, assess amount of touch that can be tolerated and incorporate this information into patient's plan of care.	This assessment facilitates development of an individualized plan of care and helps ensure that patient is not touched more than necessary by all staff members.
For patients with muscle tenderness, consider use of massage, moist heat packs, cold application, or warm baths.	These measures may be very soothing for tender muscles.
Reposition patient at frequent intervals.	Repositioning will help decrease muscle tension and fatigue. Some individuals find that a supine "frog-leg" position is particularly comfortable.
Provide passive range of motion and advise gentle stretching.	These measures reduce joint stiffness.
Administer pain medications as prescribed.	Opioids are often the most effective means of pain control, and a continuous morphine drip may be needed. Other medications that may be used to relieve uncomfortable paresthesias include anticonvulsants such as gabapentin and carbamazepine and tricyclics such as amitriptyline.
For other interventions, see **Acute Pain**, p. 273, in "General Care of Patients with Neurologic Disorders."	

••• Related NIC and NOC labels: *NIC:* Pain Management; Heat/Cold Applications; Medication Administration; Positioning; Simple Massage *NOC:* Pain Level

ADDITIONAL NURSING DIAGNOSES/ PROBLEMS:

"Prolonged Bedrest" for **Risk for Disuse Syndrome** related to paralysis, mechanical immobilization, prescribed immobilization, severe pain or altered LOC — p. 63

Ineffective Tissue Perfusion: Peripheral related to interrupted venous flow secondary to prolonged mobility — p. 65

"Psychosocial Support," particularly for **Disturbed Sleep Pattern** related to environmental changes, illness, therapeutic regimen, pain, immobility, psychologic stress or hypoxia — p. 73

"Psychosocial Support for the Patient's Family and Significant Other" — p. 87

"Dysrhythmias and Conduction Disturbances" for **Decreased Cardiac Output** related to altered rate, rhythm, or conductive changes — p. 178

"Heart Failure" for **Decreased Cardiac Output** related to negative inotropic changes — p. 187

"General Care of Patients with Neurologic Disorders" for **Risk for Falls** related to unsteady gait — p. 265

Impaired Swallowing — p. 267

Risk for Injury related to impaired pain, touch, and temperature sensations — p. 269

Impaired Tissue Integrity: Corneal — p. 270

Risk for Deficient Fluid Volume — p. 271

Imbalanced Body Temperature, Risk for — p. 274

Impaired Verbal Communication — p. 275

Self-Care Deficit — p. 277

Constipation — p. 277

"Spinal Cord Injury" for **Ineffective Tissue Perfusion: Cardiopulmonary and Cerebral** related to relative hypovolemia secondary to decreased vasomotor tone — p. 338

"Diabetes Insipidus" for related discussions — p. 373

"Syndrome of Inappropriate Antidiuretic Hormone" — p. 415

"Peptic Ulcers" for related discussions — p. 477

"Managing Wound Care" for **Impaired Tissue Integrity** (or risk for same) related to potential for excessive external pressure, friction, and shear — p. 563

For patients on mechanical ventilation, see

"Pneumonia" for **Risk for Infection** related to inadequate primary defenses — p. 127

"General Care of Patients with Neurologic Disorders" for **Risk for Infection** related to inadequate primary defenses — p. 264

✓ PATIENT-FAMILY TEACHING AND DISCHARGE PLANNING

Most patients with GBS eventually recover fully, but because the recovery period can be prolonged, the patient often goes home with some degree of neurologic deficit. Discharge planning and teaching will vary according to the degree of disability. When providing patient-family teaching, focus on sensory information, avoid giving excessive information, and initiate a visiting nurse referral for necessary follow-up teaching. Include verbal and written information about the following:

✓ Disease process, expected improvement, and importance of continuing in rehabilitation or physical therapy (PT) program to promote as full a recovery as possible.

✓ Safety measures relative to decreased sensorimotor deficit.

✓ Exercises that promote muscle strength and mobility, measures for preventing contractures and skin breakdown, transfer techniques and proper body mechanics, and use of assistive devices.

✓ Indications of constipation, urinary retention, or urinary tract infection; implementation of bowel and bladder training programs; and, if appropriate, care of indwelling catheters or self-catheterization technique.

✓ Indications of URI; measures for preventing regurgitation, aspiration, and respiratory infection.

✓ Medications, including drug name, purpose, dosage, schedule, precautions, and potential side effects. Also discuss drug-drug, herb-drug, and food-drug interactions.

✓ Importance of follow-up care, including visits to health care provider, PT, and occupational therapy.

✓ Referrals to community resources such as public health nurse, visiting nurse association, community support groups, social workers, psychologic therapy, home health agencies, and extended and skilled care facilities. Additional general information can be obtained by contacting the Guillain-Barré Syndrome Foundation International at *www.guillain-barre.com* or at *www.gbsfi.com*.

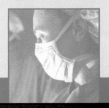

Intervertebral Disk Disease 37

OVERVIEW/PATHOPHYSIOLOGY

The intervertebral disk is a semifluid-filled fibrous capsule that facilitates movement of the spine and acts as a shock absorber. The disk's ability to withstand stressors is not unlimited and diminishes with aging. Pressure on the disk eventually may force elastic material from the center of the disk, called the *nucleus pulposus*, to break (herniate) through the fibrous rim of the disk, called the *annulus*. Herniation usually occurs posteriorly because the posterior longitudinal ligament is inherently weaker than the anterior longitudinal ligament. The bulging or rupture (protrusion or extrusion) of an intervertebral disk causes its typical symptoms by pressing on and irritating the spinal nerve roots or spinal cord itself. Herniated nucleus pulposus usually is the result of injury or a series of insults to the vertebral column from lifting or twisting. When the disk ruptures without a known discrete injury, it is believed to be caused by degenerative changes. Deterioration usually occurs suddenly with rupture, but it may happen gradually, with symptoms appearing months or years after the initial injury. Almost all herniated disks occur in the lumbar spine, with 90% of the problems occurring at L4-5 and L5-S1. The spinal cord ends around L1, so lumbar herniated disks impinge on spinal nerves, which are more resilient than actual spinal cord tissue. The spinal nerves usually bounce back and function normally once the problem is relieved. Cervical disk problems most often occur at C5-6 and C6-7, and generally are caused by degenerative changes or trauma, such as whiplash or hyperextension. Cervical herniations may compress spinal nerves or impinge on the spinal cord itself. A genetic mutation (COL 9 AZ gene) also can cause some disk disease. Thoracic disk problems are rare because of the rigid structure of the thoracic spine.

Herniated disks account for about 4% of back pain. Most back pain is related to muscle and ligament strain. Spondylolisthesis (slippage between two vertebrae) and degenerative changes such as stenosis; osteophyte (e.g., bone spur) formation, which can cause spinal nerve root compression; osteoporosis, which can lead to compression fractures; and osteoarthritis of the facet joints are other causes of non-disk back pain. Neoplasm and infection also can be sources of back pain.

HEALTH CARE SETTING

Primary care or acute care

ASSESSMENT

General indicators: Onset can be sudden, with intense unilateral pain or with pain that is dull, diffuse, deep, and aching. Symptoms vary according to level of injury and nerves involved. Usually, pain is increased with movement or activities that increase intraabdominal or intrathoracic pressure, such as sneezing, coughing, and straining. Often pain is improved by lying down. **Note:** Immediate medical attention is essential if there is any weakness or paralysis, extreme sensory loss, or altered bowel or bladder function, which indicate spinal cord compression in the lumbar back (e.g., cauda equina syndrome) and need for emergency decompression surgery. Indicators of cervical spinal cord compression (and need for early surgical treatment) include balance problems, unsteadiness when standing with eyes closed (Romberg's sign), hyperreflexes, and generalized numbness in feet and legs.

Cervical disk disease: Pain or numbness in upper extremities, shoulders, thorax, occipital area, or back of the head or neck. Pain can radiate down the forearms and into hands and fingers. Interscapular aching or suboccipital headaches are commonly associated with cervical disk disease. Usually the neck has restricted mobility, and there can be cervical muscle spasm and loss of normal cervical lordosis. Patients may have upper extremity muscle weakness with diminished biceps or triceps reflexes.

Lumbar disk disease: Pain in the lumbosacral area with possible radiculopathy (sciatica) to the buttock, down the posterior surface of the thigh and calf, and to the lateral border of the foot and toes. Sensory distribution for the L5 nerve root is the medial portion of the foot and the great toe, whereas sensory distribution for S1 is the lateral aspect of the foot, fifth toe, and sole of the foot. Often mobility is altered, as evidenced by decreased ability to stand upright, listing to one side, asymmetric gait, limited ability to flex forward, and restricted side movement caused by pain and muscle spasms. The individual walks cautiously, bearing little weight on the affected side, and often finds sitting or climbing stairs particularly painful. Reflex muscle spasms can cause bulging of the back with concomitant flattening of the lumbar curve and possible scoliosis at the level of the affected disk. Usually patellar and Achilles tendon reflexes are depressed due to nerve impingement. Sciatica usually is associated with intervertebral disk herniation.

Physical assessment: Possible findings include depressed reflexes, muscle atrophy, paresthesias (described as "pins and needles"), or anesthesia (numbness) in the dermatome of the involved nerves. The following tests are two of several that are performed to confirm presence of lumbar disk disease.

Straight leg raise test: Examiner extends and raises patient's leg. The test is positive if patient has pain on the posterior aspect of the leg. People without injury usually can have a leg raised to 90 degrees without significant discomfort.

Sciatic nerve test: Examiner extends and raises patient's leg until pain is elicited and then lowers the leg to a comfortable level. The examiner then dorsiflexes the foot to stretch the sciatic nerve. If this causes pain, the test is positive for sciatic nerve involvement.

Risk factors: Repetitive bending or lifting involving a twisting motion, continuous vibration, smoking, poor physical condition (especially weak abdominal muscles), poor posture, obesity, above-average height, osteoporosis, prolonged sitting, depression, severe scoliosis, spondylolisthesis, or genetic predisposition.

DIAGNOSTIC TESTS

In the absence of serious symptoms, diagnostic testing may not be done until 3 mo have passed and symptoms persist (90% of back pain resolves in less than 1 mo). Diagnostic testing should be done for pain that is constant, severe, unrelieved by rest or position, and is not calmed by antiinflammatory medication inasmuch as these symptoms may indicate presence of neoplasm or infection. Thoracic back pain also should be investigated because it may be caused by medical problems (e.g., aortic aneurysm).

MRI scan: May reveal a disk impinging on the spinal cord or nerve root, or may show a related pathologic condition, such as a tumor or spondylosis. A magnetic resonance (MR)

neurogram helps image nerves after they leave the spinal column and can show compressions as they travel through the spinal foramina. MR myelogram helps view the cerebral spinal fluid sac without having to use a needle puncture. MR imaging (MRI) has replaced computerized axial tomography (CT) scan and myelogram as the test of choice in diagnosing herniated nucleus pulposus and is considered the "gold standard."

CT scan of the spine: May reveal disk protrusion/prolapse or a related pathologic condition, such as a bone spur, tumor, spondylosis, or spinal stenosis.

X-ray examination of the spine: May show narrowing of the vertebral interspaces in affected areas, loss of spine curvature, bone spur formation, and spondylosis.

Diskography: Identifies degenerated or extruded disks or annulus tear by means of contrast medium injected into the disk space using fluoroscopy. Often it is done in combination with CT and may differentiate between disk infection and rupture.

Myelogram: May show characteristic deformity and filling defect or a related pathologic condition; it is usually done in conjunction with a CT scan.

Electromyography: May show denervation patterns of specific nerve roots to indicate level and site of injury.

Evoked potential studies: For example, somatosensory studies may show slowed conduction due to nerve root compromise and can localize specific nerve root.

LABORATORY TESTS

Serum alkaline and acid phosphatase, glucose, calcium, erythrocyte sedimentation rate (ESR), and white blood cell count may rule out metabolic bone disease, metastatic tumors, diabetic mononeuritis, and disk space infection.

Nursing Diagnosis:

Health-Seeking Behaviors:

Proper body mechanics and other measures that prevent back injury

Desired Outcome: Within the treatment session (outpatient) or within the 24-hr period before hospital discharge, patient verbalizes knowledge of measures that prevent back injury and demonstrates proper body mechanics.

INTERVENTIONS	RATIONALES
Teach patient proper body mechanics: - Stand and sit straight with chin and head up and pelvis and back straight; avoid slouching. - Bend at knees and hips (squat) rather than at the waist, keeping back straight (not stooping forward). - When carrying objects, hold them close to the body, avoiding twisting when lifting or reaching. Spread feet for a wider base of support. Lift with legs, not the back. - Turn using entire body. - Do not strain to reach things. If an object is overhead, raise yourself to its level, or move things out of the way if they are obstructing the object.	Using proper body mechanics avoids movements such as twisting, lifting with the back, and straining to reach that can cause back injury.

Continued

INTERVENTIONS	RATIONALES
- Avoid lifting anything heavier than 10-20 lb.	
- Encourage use of long-handled pickup sticks to pick up small objects.	
- Have patient demonstrate proper body mechanics, if possible, before hospital discharge.	
Teach about the following measures for keeping body in alignment:	Keeping the body in proper alignment avoids strain on the back, thereby helping to prevent recurring back injury.
- Sit close to pedals when driving a car, and use a seat belt and firm back rest to support the back.	
- Support feet on a footstool when sitting so that knees are elevated to hip level or higher.	
- Obtain a firm mattress or bed board; use a flat pillow when sleeping to avoid strain on neck, arms, and shoulders; sleep in a side-lying position with knees bent or in a supine position with knees and legs supported on pillows; avoid sleeping in a prone position.	
- Avoid reaching or stretching to pick up objects.	
- Avoid sitting on furniture that does not support back.	
Encourage patient to achieve and/or maintain proper weight for age, height, and gender; continue exercise program prescribed by health care provider; use thoracic and abdominal muscles when lifting; when standing for any length of time, stand with one foot on a step stool; sit in a firm chair for support.	Being overweight or obese can cause back strain and alteration in the center of balance, which can result in back pain and pressure. Exercise strengthens abdominal, thoracic, and back muscles. Using thoracic and abdominal muscles when lifting keeps a significant portion of weight off vertebral disks. Standing with one foot on a step stool helps relieve sciatica. Sitting in a firm chair provides support to the back.
Teach rationale and procedure for Williams' back exercises:	
Pelvic tilt: Tighten stomach and buttock muscles, and tilt the pelvis while keeping the lower spine flat against the floor; that is, the hips and buttocks are kept on the floor.	*Pelvic tilt*: To strengthen abdominal muscles.
Knee-to-chest raise: Start with a pelvic tilt. Raise each knee individually to the chest and return to the starting position. Then raise each knee individually to the chest and hold them there (both knees on chest together).	*Knee-to-chest raise*: To help make a stiff back limber.
Nose-to-knee touch: Raise knee to the chest, and then pull knee to chest with hands. Raise head, and try to touch nose to knee. Keep lower back flat on floor.	*Nose-to-knee touch*: To stretch hip muscles and strengthen abdominal muscles.
Half sit-ups: Slowly raise head and neck to top of chest. Reach both hands forward to knees, and hold for a count of 5. Repeat, keeping lower back flat on floor.	*Half sit-ups*: To strengthen abdomen and back.
Instruct patient to wear supportive shoes with a low or moderate heel height for walking.	This measure helps maintain proper alignment of back and hips.
Encourage smoking cessation.	Smoking causes vasoconstriction thus reducing circulation to disks.
Teach the following technique for sitting up at the bedside from a supine position:	This technique prevents strain on the back and promotes good body alignment.
Logroll to side, then raise to sitting position by pushing against mattress with hands while swinging legs over side of bed. Instruct patient to maintain alignment of the back during procedure.	
Caution patient that pain is the signal to stop or change an activity or position.	This precaution helps prevent additional back injury.
Encourage patient to continue with a regular exercise and stretching program, including physical therapy (PT) as indicated, walking, and exercising in water.	PT and a graded exercise program are initiated after acute symptoms subside and are the mainstay of therapy for low back pain. Exercise strengthens abdominal, thoracic, and back muscles to help prevent subsequent back injury. High-impact activities such as running may be limited until the injury is well healed.
Teach patient that the following indicators necessitate medical attention: increased sensory loss, increased motor loss/weakness, and loss of bowel and bladder function.	These indicators signal disk herniation, which necessitates timely intervention to prevent further damage.

••• **Related NIC and NOC labels:** *NIC:* Health Education; Exercise Promotion; Weight Management *NOC:* Health Promoting Behavior

Nursing Diagnosis:

Deficient Knowledge:

Pain control measures

Desired Outcome: Following instruction within outpatient treatment session or within the 24-hr period before hospital discharge, patient verbalizes knowledge about pain control measures and demonstrates ability to initiate these measures when appropriate.

INTERVENTIONS	RATIONALES
Teach methods of controlling pain and their individual applications.	Methods include distraction, use of counterirritants, massage, hydrotherapy, aquatherapy, acupressure, dorsal column stimulation, use of transcutaneous electrical nerve stimulation, behavior modification, relaxation techniques, hypnosis, music therapy, imagery, biofeedback, and diathermy. Whole body vibration exercise and spinal manipulation may be considered for uncomplicated back problems with no radiculopathy.
	In addition, applying intermittent heat may reduce muscle spasm, whereas icing may prevent further inflammatory swelling and provide some topical anesthesia. Icing should be done frequently, especially for the first 24-48 hr after surgery, and is often recommended after exercise. Continuous low-level heat wrap therapy reduces pain and improves function. Heat may be applied via warm/hot showers or heating pads. Cold can be achieved by freezing water in a paper cup, tearing off top of cup to expose the ice, and massaging in a circular motion, using remaining portion of cup as a handle. A bag of frozen peas or corn may be used to apply continuous cold to lower back. With any of these methods, a layer of cloth should be used so that ice does not touch the skin. A 20-min application of cold 4-6 times per day is recommended.
Suggest patient use a stool to rest affected leg when standing.	This measure will help relieve sciatica.
Advise patient to sit in a straight-back chair that is high enough to get out of easily, including toilet seats that are raised.	Higher seats facilitate ease of movement in and out of chairs and provide comfort. Straddling a straight-back chair and resting arms on the chair back is comfortable for many individuals.
Encourage use of a moderately firm to firm mattress and extra pillows as needed for positioning.	These measures support normal lumbar curvature. Some patients find the normal bed height too low and use blocks to raise it to a more comfortable height.
Instruct patient on bedrest to roll rather than lift off bedpan.	This action prevents straining of the back. The patient may find a fracture bedpan more comfortable than a regular bedpan.
Caution patient to avoid sudden twisting or turning movements. Explain importance of logrolling when moving from side to side.	These measures prevent movements that could induce further back injury. Orthotics (e.g., splints, braces, girdles, cervical collars) also may be used to limit motion of the vertebral column. Temporary use of a back brace or corset may enable earlier return to activity with lumbar disk disease. Generally, long-term use of braces is discouraged because it prohibits development of necessary supporting musculature.
Advise patient to avoid staying in one position too long, fatigue, chilling, and anxiety.	These factors can cause back spasms.
Suggest lying on side with knees bent or lying supine with knees supported on pillows. Advise patient that a small pillow supporting the nape of the neck may be helpful with cervical pain. Teach patient to avoid prolonged periods of sitting, which stress the back.	These measures promote spinal comfort.
If appropriate, teach patient to apply a heating pad to the back for 15-30 min before getting out of bed in the morning.	Heat will help allay stiffness and discomfort after a night in bed. Heating pads should be used only for short intervals and only if patient's temperature sensations are intact.
Remind patient to place a towel or cloth between heating pad and skin.	This measure will help prevent burns.

Continued

INTERVENTIONS	RATIONALES
Encourage patient to rest when tired or stressed and not to exercise when in pain.	Tired muscles are more susceptible to injury. Usually patient resumes normal activity as soon as possible, but pain is an indicator to limit the offending activity.
Instruct in use of cervical traction if prescribed.	Although infrequently prescribed, it may be used to help a cervical disk that has been bulging to slip back into place and unload the neck muscles and ligaments. Traditional method is a neck/head harness attached to a pulley and weight. A device for home use may include an inflatable collar that expands to push the head away from the shoulders.
Encourage a high-bulk diet, adequate or increased fluids, and stool softeners.	These measures prevent constipation, which would cause straining and pain.
Teach purpose and potential side effects of the following medications for acute pain:	
- Analgesics (e.g., acetaminophen and tramadol, and opiate combinations such as hydrocodone and acetaminophen or oxycodone and acetaminophen)	Sufficient medication is given to achieve pain relief or adequate pain reduction.
- Nonsteroidal antiinflammatory drugs (NSAIDs) and salicylates	These medications reduce inflammation and relieve pain. Dosing usually is scheduled initially to obtain a sustained antiinflammatory effect. Side effects include blood thinning and gastric irritation, and kidneys may be affected if these drugs are taken for a long time.
- Misoprostol or stomach protectants such as sucralfate or ranitidine	These agents may be considered to reduce gastric irritation caused by stress, medications, and steroids (if used).
- Muscle relaxants (e.g., cyclobenzaprine , carisoprodol, methocarbamol, diazepam)	These medications decrease muscle spasms, thereby reducing pain. Common side effects are drowsiness, fatigue, dizziness, dry mouth, and gastrointestinal (GI) upset.
- Corticosteroids (e.g., dexamethasone)	Steroids may be given for a short period to reduce cord edema, if present, but use is controversial.
Teach patient about the following medications used for chronic pain:	
- Analgesics (e.g., NSAIDs, tramadol, gabapentin, amitriptyline)	Nonnarcotic analgesia such as NSAIDs is used for chronic pain. Tramadol, a centrally acting analgesic, may be used long-term, especially for older adults. Tricyclic antidepressants (e.g., amitriptyline, desipramine, doxepin) also may help with chronic pain. Anticonvulsants such as gabapentin, carbamazepine, phenytoin, and levetracetam help with neuropathic pain caused by nerve injury.
- Local injection of anesthetic (lidocaine or bupivacaine) and/or cortisone into epidural spaces, facet joints, sacroiliac joint, or trigger points	These medications reduce pain and muscle spasms and increase function.
- Botulinum toxin injection into paravertebral regions	This injection relieves pain, probably through decreased muscle spasm, and improves function for 3-8 wk.
Teach patient about the following techniques that may be effective in controlling chronic pain:	
- Souchard's global postural reeducation (GPR)	This French physical therapy technique has been effective in restoring function and relieving long-term chronic pain. It consists of a series of maneuvers in which patient is in supine, sitting, and standing positions and involves stretching the paraspinal muscles and those of the abdominal wall so that joints are relieved of the compression that is typically the source of pain.
- Percutaneous electrical nerve stimulation	This device uses acupuncture-like needle probes positioned in soft tissue and/or muscles to stimulate peripheral sensory nerves to relieve persistent back pain.
- Implantable epidural spinal cord stimulator	This stimulator may be used to aid in the control of chronic pain when all other measures (e.g., PT, medications, surgery) have failed.

••• **Related NIC and NOC labels:** *NIC:* Teaching: Procedure/Treatment; Teaching: Psychomotor Skill; Health Education; Behavior Modification
NOC: Knowledge: Treatment Procedures; Knowledge: Health Behaviors

Nursing Diagnosis:

Deficient Knowledge:

Diskectomy with laminectomy or fusion procedure

Desired Outcomes: Before surgery, patient verbalizes knowledge about the surgical procedure, preoperative routine, and postoperative regimen. Patient demonstrates activities and exercises correctly.

INTERVENTIONS	RATIONALES
For general interventions, see this nursing diagnosis in "Perioperative Care," p. 45.	Surgery is performed without delay if signs of spinal cord compression are present, such as significant motor or sensory loss or loss of sphincter control. Otherwise, surgery is considered only after symptoms fail to respond to conservative therapy.
Instruct patient to expect surgical team to confirm verbally and then mark the correct spinal level and correct side (e.g., anterior, posterior, right, left) of the surgical site.	These confirmations ensure that the appropriate surgery will be performed.
Reinforce surgeon's explanation about the following:	
- Microdiskectomy	The herniated portion of the disk and small parts of the lamina are removed, using microsurgical techniques. Patient usually is out of bed the first day and may be released as an outpatient or discharged the next day.
- Diskectomy with laminectomy	An incision is made, enabling removal of part of the vertebra (laminectomy) so that the disk's herniated portion can be removed (diskectomy). If multiple intervertebral disk spaces are explored, a wound drain may be present after surgery.
- Percutaneous lumbar disk removal	Ultrasonic nucleotome cannula or fiberoptic arthroscopic cannula can be inserted into the intervertebral space via fluoroscopy to enable fragmentation of the disk and its aspiration. A laser may be used to aid in disk excision. This is a relatively less-invasive method of relieving pain from herniated disk, is done under local anesthesia, and may be performed on an outpatient basis.
- Spinal fusion	Fusion may be indicated for patients with recurrent low back or neck pain, spondylolisthesis, subluxation of the vertebrae, or with multilevel disease. Bone chips are harvested from the iliac crest or tibia and placed between vertebrae in the prepared area of the unstable spine to fuse and stabilize the area.
	Internal fixation (e.g., rods, wiring, pedicle screws, lateral mass screws, fusion cages, interbody implants, bone rings, and plates) may be necessary to provide added stability until the fusion has healed fully. If the patient's own bone quality or quantity is inadequate, allograft (e.g., cadaver) bone or use of a recombinant human osteogenic protein preparation ("bone putty") as a bone graft substitute or supplement may be considered.
- Intradiskal electrothermal treatment (IDET)	IDET employs a probe that uses electricity to heat and shrink collagen tissue within the annulus wall to seal up painful tears. After healing, the disk toughens and desensitizes.
- Total intervertebral disk replacement with artificial disks such as the Charité	This procedure may help reduce need for spinal fusions and avoid premature degeneration at adjacent levels of the spine.
- Diskoplasty	This procedure reduces or reshapes a bulging disk via a small puncture, threading a probe into the center of the disc, and using a laser or radiofrequency to remove/evaporate the disk's center.

Continued

INTERVENTIONS	RATIONALES
Teach technique for deep breathing. Also teach patient use of incentive spirometry.	Deep breathing and incentive spirometry are performed immediately after surgery to help expand the alveoli and aid in mobilizing lung secretions. Coughing may be contraindicated in the immediate postoperative period to prevent disruption of the fusion or surgical repair.
Document baseline and serial neurovascular checks, including color, capillary refill, pulse, warmth, muscle strength, movement, and sensation.	Vital signs and neurologic status are evaluated at frequent intervals after surgery and compared with baseline to monitor trend.
Teach the following signs and symptoms and importance of reporting them promptly: paresthesias, weakness, paralysis, radiculopathy, and changes in bowel or bladder function.	These indicators of impairment necessitate immediate attention by health care staff because they signal presence of autonomic stimulation—signs of cord compression caused by bleeding or hematoma formation.
Teach the following signs and symptoms and importance of reporting them promptly: increased HR, thirst, faintness, or dizziness.	These are signs, along with decreased blood pressure, of hypovolemia and may occur because of blood loss. Patients undergoing fusion lose more blood during surgery than do those undergoing laminectomy.
Explain that the surgical dressing will be inspected for excess drainage or oozing at frequent intervals and that a closed wound drainage device may be present for 1-3 days postoperatively with a fusion procedure.	Bleeding with a laminectomy usually is minimal. Patients with a fusion may have slight bloody oozing postoperatively. Serous drainage usually is checked with a glucose reagent strip. Presence of glucose is a signal of cerebrospinal fluid (CSF) leakage. Bulging in the area of the wound may also signal CSF leakage or hematoma formation and should be reported promptly.
Advise that dressings will be inspected for increased drainage after patient has been up, and lumbar dressings will be checked after each bedpan use. Inform patient undergoing fusions that he or she will have a second dressing at the donor site.	Wet or contaminated dressings require prompt changing to prevent infection.
Instruct patient to report any nausea or vomiting.	This helps ensure that antiemetics are given promptly. Vomiting could cause increased intraspinal pressure, which would result in pain.
Explain that patient will be monitored for bowel and bladder dysfunction after the procedure.	Nerve injury during surgery can contribute to paralytic ileus. The abdomen will be checked for bowel sounds and distention. Patient may be asked to void within 8 hr of the procedure to check for urinary retention.
Caution patient to avoid straining at stool.	Straining could cause increased intraspinal pressure, which would result in pain. Stool softeners may be given for that purpose.
Explain that fever may occur during first few days postoperatively but that this does not necessarily signal an infection.	Early fever may be caused by drainage and contamination of CSF. Patient will be assessed for other indicators of infection, such as heat, redness, irritation, swelling, or drainage at wound site.
Instruct patient to report headache, neck stiffness, or photophobia.	These are possible signs of meningeal irritation.
Inform patient that pain may take days or weeks to resolve and does not indicate that surgery was unsuccessful.	Postoperative pain or tingling (paresthesia) often is caused by nerve root irritation and edema. Spasms are common on the third or fourth postoperative day and should not discourage patient.
Teach patient to request medication for pain as needed and not let pain get out of control. Instruct in use of 0-10 pain scale.	Pain is easier to manage before it becomes severe. Prolonged stimulation of pain receptors results in increased sensitivity to painful stimuli and will increase the amount of analgesic required to relieve pain. Patients who have had a fusion may expect significant pain from bone graft donor site (commonly the iliac crest). The donor site may have extra padding. Muscle relaxants may be prescribed to supplement pain control. Patient-controlled analgesia (PCA) and NSAIDs also may be used for postoperative pain control. Use of the pain scale enables more accurate assessment of relief obtained.

Continued

INTERVENTIONS	RATIONALES
Explain that in the immediate postoperative period patient will follow the surgeon's activity restrictions and that new techniques and stabilization devices may enable earlier mobilization (some same day) and fewer activity restrictions.	Patients may be required to lie supine for several hours to minimize possibility of wound hematoma formation. After this period, head of bead (HOB) of laminectomy patients usually can be raised to 20 degrees to facilitate eating and bedpan use. Patients undergoing spinal fusion may be kept flat and on bedrest longer than patients with laminectomies. Activity progression for spinal fusion patients is usually more cautious and slower than for laminectomy patients. Best practice regarding trapeze use is to restrict it during the initial 24-48 hr following lumbar and cervical procedures and avoid its use after thoracic procedures because of the torque and weight strain trapeze use can have on the spine.
Teach patient the following logroll technique for turning: Position a pillow between legs, cross arms across chest while turning, and contract long back muscles to maintain shoulders and pelvis in straight alignment. Explain that, initially, patient will be assisted in this procedure.	Only the logroll method is used for turning. This method stabilizes the spine and maintains alignment to enable healing and prevent dislodgement of the bone graft if fusion is done. A turning sheet and sufficient help are used when logrolling patient.
Teach patient the following technique for getting out of bed: logroll to side, splint back, and rise to a sitting position by pushing against mattress while swinging legs over side of bed.	This technique facilitates ease of getting out of bed and prevents disruption of the bone graft for fusion patients.
Explain that initially patient will be helped to a sitting position and should not push against mattress. Teach patient with cervical laminectomy not to pull self up with arms. When assisting patients with cervical laminectomy to a sitting position, caution them not to put their arms on nurse's shoulders.	While in hospital with an electric bed, the HOB may be raised to facilitate a sitting position. These restrictions prevent neck flexion, extension, and hyperextension and strain on the operative site and incision. Pillows can be used to support arms for comfort.
Explain that antiembolism hose and possibly sequential compression devices (SCDs) will be applied after surgery.	These garments and devices promote venous return and prevent thrombus formation while patient is on bedrest. SCDs or hose should be worn until amount of time out of bed ambulating is equal to amount of time in bed.
Teach techniques for ankle circling and calf pumping.	These techniques promote leg circulation.
Teach patient to report calf pain, tenderness, or warmth.	These are signs of deep vein thrombosis.
Advise patient that health care provider will prescribe certain postoperative activity restrictions.	Sitting is commonly restricted or allowed for only limited, prescribed periods in a straight-back chair.
Teach patient not to sit for long periods on edge of mattress.	A mattress does not provide enough support to the spine.
Explain that weakness, dizziness, and lightheadedness may occur on a first walk.	These problems may occur secondary to orthostatic hypotension. For management, see discussion in **Ineffective Tissue Perfusion: Cerebral**, p. 66, in "Prolonged Bedrest."
Explain that patient will be encouraged to walk progressively longer distances.	This action will promote endurance.
Instruct patient to avoid stretching, twisting, flexing, or jarring spine. Explain that the spine should be kept aligned and in a neutral position and that lifting and pulling/pushing objects are to be avoided.	These restrictions help prevent vertebral collapse, shifting of bone graft, or a bleeding episode.
If patient is scheduled for cervical laminectomy or fusion, caution not to pull with arms on objects such as side rails and avoid twisting, flexion, and extensions of the neck.	These restrictions prevent torque and strain on the spine that could cause misalignment.
Explain that a cervical collar may be worn postoperatively.	The collar aids in immobilizing the cervical spine.
Teach use of braces or corsets if prescribed.	Persons undergoing a fusion procedure often wear a supportive brace or corset for 3 mo or less to keep operative site immobile so that the graft will heal and not dislodge. Braces should be applied while in bed.
Explain importance of wearing cotton underwear under brace, powdering skin lightly with cornstarch, or providing additional padding under braces.	These measures help protect skin from irritation. Skin should be inspected daily for irritation or breakdown.

Continued

INTERVENTIONS / RATIONALES

INTERVENTIONS	RATIONALES
Explain that driving or riding in car (may be restricted 6-8 wk up to several mo), sexual activity, lifting and carrying objects, tub bathing (generally, soaking incision is avoided until about 1 wk after sutures are out), going up and down stairs, amount of time to spend in and out of bed, back exercises, and expected time away from work will be discussed by health care provider before discharge.	These guidelines and activity restrictions promote patient safety and an uneventful recovery once he or she is at home.
Explain that patient should call health care provider for symptoms such as increased weakness and numbness or change in bowel or bladder function.	These are indicators of spinal cord or nerve compression.
Teach importance of reporting the following to health care provider: swelling, discharge, drainage, persistent redness, local warmth, fever, and pain.	These signs and symptoms of postoperative wound infection require timely intervention.
Caution patient to keep the incision dry and open to the air.	Moisture can promote infection. Wet dressings should be changed promptly. After 24-48 hr, the incision is usually undressed to promote "air" drying.

••• **Related NIC and NOC labels:** *NIC:* Preparatory Sensory Information; Teaching: Procedure/Treatment; Teaching: Psychomotor Skill; Anxiety Reduction; Teaching: Preoperative; Teaching: Prescribed Activity/Exercise *NOC:* Knowledge: Treatment Regimen; Knowledge: Treatment Procedures

Nursing Diagnosis:

Impaired Swallowing (or risk for same)

related to postoperative edema or hematoma formation secondary to anterior cervical fusion

Desired Outcome: Patient regains uncompromised swallowing ability (usually by the third postoperative day) as evidenced by normal breath sounds and absence of food in the oral cavity or choking/coughing.

INTERVENTIONS	RATIONALES
As part of preoperative teaching, instruct patient in potential for difficulty with swallowing or managing secretions after anterior cervical fusion and need to report these problems promptly.	Postoperative edema or bleeding causing difficulty with swallowing is related to retraction of the trachea and esophagus during surgery to gain access to the disk. An informed individual likely will report postoperative difficulties with swallowing promptly for timely intervention.
Explain that a soft diet and throat lozenges may be prescribed for 2-3 days postoperatively.	A sore throat can be expected after this surgery due to surgical manipulation and/or endotracheal tube.
Monitor for edema of face or neck or tracheal compression or deviation that could compromise respiratory function. Monitor for complaints of excessive pressure in the neck or severe, uncontrolled incisional pain. Promptly report significant findings.	These indicators may be signs of hematoma or bleeding at the operative site that could cause airway compromise and therefore necessitate immediate intervention.
Listen for hoarseness. Encourage voice rest and facilitate alternative communication (e.g., provide storyboards, pen and pencil, flash cards).	Hoarseness can indicate laryngeal nerve irritation and signal ineffective cough or swallowing difficulty and necessitate choking and aspiration precautions. For most patients with hoarseness, the voice usually will return to normal as inflammation around the laryngeal nerve subsides.
Report immediately any respiratory distress, stridor, inability to speak, worsening hoarseness, or voice change.	These may be signs of aspiration, laryngeal nerve involvement/irritation, or increased edema or hematoma formation affecting the laryngeal nerve and vocal cords, any of which can be life-threatening and necessitate immediate intervention.

Continued

INTERVENTIONS	RATIONALES
Monitor for and report diminished breath sounds compared with patient's normal or preoperative status.	Diminished breath sounds could signal that aspiration has occurred and may result in pneumonia.
As indicated, monitor oximetry as a quantitative measure of systemic oxygenation.	Values 92% or less may signal need for supplemental oxygen.
Monitor closed suction devices, and recharge suction device/chamber as indicated.	Recharging the closed suction device facilitates wound drainage.
Check for gag and swallowing reflexes before oral intake.	Absence of gag and swallowing reflexes indicates that patient cannot begin oral intake. A postoperative diet with clear fluids and progression to more solid foods may begin only after patient demonstrates ability to ingest fluids safely.
Position patient in Fowler's position, or semi-Fowler's position at minimum, when initiating fluid intake.	These positions minimize risk of aspiration by promoting movement of fluids by gravity to the stomach and into the pylorus.
If not prohibited by surgery, encourage use of chin tuck to lessen potential for aspiration.	A chin tuck forces the trachea to close and the esophagus to open, thereby decreasing risk of aspiration.
Also see **Risk for Aspiration**, p. 96, in "Older Adult Care."	

••• **Related NIC and NOC labels:** *NIC:* Aspiration Precautions; Positioning; Risk Identification; Feeding *NOC:* Aspiration Control; Swallowing Status: Oral Phase

ADDITIONAL NURSING DIAGNOSES/ PROBLEMS:

"Perioperative Care" for related nursing diagnoses and interventions	p. 45
"Prolonged Bedrest"	p. 61
"General Care of Patients with Neurologic Disorders" for **Risk for Injury** related to impaired pain, touch, and temperature sensation	p. 269
"Pressure Ulcers"	p. 562

PATIENT-FAMILY TEACHING AND DISCHARGE PLANNING

When providing patient-family teaching, focus on sensory information, avoid giving excessive information, and initiate a visiting nurse referral for necessary follow-up teaching. Include verbal and written information about the following:

✓ Prescribed exercise regimen, including rationale for each exercise, technique for performing the exercise, number of repetitions of each, and frequency of exercise periods. If possible, ensure that patient demonstrates understanding of exercise regimen and proper body mechanics before hospital discharge.

✓ Wound incision care. Indicators of postoperative wound infection that necessitate medical attention include swelling, discharge, persistent redness, local warmth, fever, and pain.

✓ Review of use and application of cervical collar for patients who have had a cervical fusion and importance of wearing collar at all times.

✓ Use and care of a brace or immobilizer if appropriate.

✓ Medications, including drug name, rationale, dosage, schedule, precautions, and potential side effects. Also discuss drug-drug, herb-drug, and food-drug interactions.

✓ Anticonstipation routine, which should be initiated during hospitalization.

✓ Pain control measures.

✓ Telephone number of a resource person in case questions arise after hospital discharge.

✓ Postsurgical activity restrictions as directed by health care provider. These may affect the following: driving and riding in a car, returning to work, sexual activity, lifting and carrying, tub bathing, going up and down steps, and amount of time spent in or out of bed.

✓ Signs and symptoms of worsening neurologic function and the importance of notifying health care provider immediately if they develop. These include numbness, weakness, paralysis, and bowel and bladder dysfunction.

✓ Additional general information, which can be obtained by contacting *www.spine-health.com*.

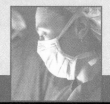

Multiple Sclerosis 38

OVERVIEW/PATHOPHYSIOLOGY

Multiple sclerosis (MS) is an inflammatory disorder causing scattered and sporadic demyelinization of the central nervous system (CNS). Myelin permits nerve impulses to travel quickly through the nerve pathways of the CNS. In response to the inflammation, the myelin nerve sheaths scar, degenerate, or separate from the axon cylinders. This demyelinization interrupts electrical nerve transmission and causes the wide variety of symptoms associated with MS. As less severe inflammation resolves, myelin function may regenerate, enabling electric nerve impulse transmission to be restored. If the inflammation is severe and causes irreversible destruction of myelin or axon degeneration, involved areas are replaced by dense glial scar tissue that forms patchy areas of sclerotic plaque, which permanently damage conductive pathways of the CNS. Axon nerve fibers may degenerate. Deficits present after 3 mo usually are permanent.

The course of MS is highly variable, with several general categories of progression. Motor or coordination symptoms from onset and/or frequent attacks during the first 2 yr of the disease usually indicate a poor outlook. In the benign form of MS (10% of patients), attacks are few and mild. Complete or nearly complete clearing of symptoms occurs with little or no disability. At least initially, most patients (70%-80%) have the relapsing-remitting form characterized by episodes of neurologic impairment ("attacks," exacerbations), followed by complete or nearly complete recovery and stability with no disease progression (remission). Typically, an increasing number of symptoms occur with each exacerbation, with less complete clearing of symptoms and with deficits becoming cumulative. Over time, the relapsing-remitting form usually transitions to the secondary progressive form in which neurologic impairment progresses continuously with or without superimposed relapses. A small portion of patients (10%-20%) initially begin with the primary progressive form, characterized by gradual ongoing accumulation of symptoms and deficits, with absence of clear-cut exacerbations and remissions. The progressive relapsing form (5%) is characterized by a progressive disease course from onset, with clear acute exacerbations. Progression continues during the periods between disease exacerbations. In the most severe cases of acute MS, significant disability may occur in weeks or months.

HEALTH CARE SETTING

Primary care or long-term care, with possible hospitalization resulting from complications

ASSESSMENT

Onset of MS can be extremely rapid, or it can be insidious with exacerbations and remissions. Signs and symptoms vary widely, depending on site and extent of demyelinization, and can change from day to day. Usually early symptoms are mild, including fatigue, weakness, heaviness, clumsiness, numbness, and tingling. Optic neuritis or visual problems often are the first symptoms.

Damage to motor nerve tracts: Weakness, paralysis, and spasticity. Fatigue is common. Diplopia may occur secondary to ocular muscle involvement.

Damage to cerebellar or brainstem regions: Intention tremor, nystagmus, or other tremors; incoordination, ataxia; and weakness of facial and throat muscles resulting in difficulty chewing, dysphagia, and dysarthria. Slurred speech often occurs early, whereas scanning speech (slow speech with pauses between syllables) is usually seen in later stages.

Damage to sensory nerve tracts: Often, only sensory symptoms occur in the beginning and may include decreased perception of pain, touch, and temperature; paresthesias such as numbness and tingling or "pins and needles"; decrease or loss of proprioception; and decrease or loss of vibratory sense. Optic neuritis is a common early symptom, potentially causing partial or total loss of vision, visual clouding or shimmering, and pain with eye movement.

Damage to cerebral cortex (especially frontal lobes): Mood swings, inappropriate affect, euphoria, apathy, irritability, depression, hyperexcitability, and poor memory, judgment, foresight and planning, and abstract reasoning. There is often trouble with word finding and difficulty with concentration, attention, and processing or learning new information.

Damage to motor and sensory control centers: Urinary frequency, urgency, or retention; urinary and fecal incontinence; constipation.

Sacral cord lesions: Impotence; diminished sensations that result in inhibited sexual response.

Physical assessment: Liermitte's sign may be present, in which an electrical sensation runs down the back and legs during neck flexion. Ophthalmoscopic inspection may reveal temporal pallor of optic disks. Reflex assessment may show increased deep tendon reflexes (DTRs) and diminished abdominal skin and cremasteric reflexes.

History/risk factors: Although the cause of MS is unknown, it is generally believed to result from an environmental insult to the body, such as an earlier viral infection that triggers an autoimmune response in a predisposed individual. MS is most common among people who have lived in cool, temperate climates before puberty. African Americans have half the incidence of white Americans. More females than males are affected (not quite 2:1). Onset is usually 10-50 yr of age with peak onset at 20-40 yr of age. It is 15-20 times more common among siblings of individuals with the disease than in the general population, suggesting a possible genetic susceptibility. Exacerbations may be fewer during pregnancy but increase immediately postpartum. Heat and fever tend to aggravate symptoms.

DIAGNOSTIC TESTS

Note: MS is sometimes called the "great masquerader." Diagnosis of MS usually is made after other neurologic disorders with similar symptoms have been ruled out (when the patient has experienced two or more exacerbations of neurologic symptoms) and when the patient has two or more areas of demyelination or plaque formation throughout the CNS, as demonstrated by diagnostic tests such as magnetic resonance imaging (MRI) and evoked potential (EP) studies, or by the patient's clinical symptoms.

MRI scan: Reveals presence of plaques and demyelination in the CNS. This is the test of choice when MS is suspected. Expanding MRI technology is becoming ever more sensitive and capable of identifying current sites of inflammation and demyelination and showing changes associated with disease progression. T1-weighted MRI may show hypointense lesions (black holes), which correlates with axonal loss and indicates old lesions. T2-weighted MRI can show old and new lesions and is used to follow response to treatment. Gadolinium enhancement shows areas of active demyelination. MRI diffusion tensor imaging and MR spectroscopy frequently reveal involvement of otherwise normal-appearing white matter. Magnetization transfer imaging may show indirect evidence of axonal loss. MR spectroscopy can measure decline in a brain chemical called N-acetylaspartate (NAA) as a marker of axonal damage and appears to predict disease severity. Functional MRI (fMRI) can show new lesions. Fluid attenuated inversion recovery (FLAIR) is also used for detecting cerebral lesions, and short tau inversion recovery (STIR) is useful in detecting demyelination.

EP studies: May be slow or absent because of interference of nerve transmission from demyelination or plaque formation. Visual EP studies are particularly useful because optic neuritis is so common.

Lumbar puncture and CSF analysis: Evaluates cerebrospinal fluid (CSF) levels of oligoclonal bands and free kappa chains of immunoglobulin G (IgG), protein, gamma globulin, myelin basic protein, and lymphocytes, any of which may be elevated in the presence of MS. During acute MS attacks, destruction of the myelin sheath releases myelin basic protein into the CSF. A serum blood test to detect antimyelin antibodies also is being developed. Oligoclonal bands of IgG are seen in 85%-95% of patients with MS. This and the finding of free kappa chains in the CSF support a diagnosis of MS.

CT scan: Demonstrates presence of plaques and rules out mass lesions. This technique is less effective than MRI in detecting areas of plaque and demyelination.

Electroencephalogram: Shows abnormal slowing in one third of patients with MS because of altered nerve conduction.

Positron emission tomography: May show altered locations and patterns of cerebral glucose metabolism. This test usually is available only at research centers.

Nursing Diagnosis:

Deficient Knowledge:

Factors that aggravate and exacerbate MS symptoms

Desired Outcome: By day 3 (or before hospital discharge), patient and significant other verbalize factors that exacerbate, prevent, and ameliorate symptoms of MS.

INTERVENTIONS	RATIONALES
Assess patient's health care literacy (language, reading, comprehension). Assess culture and culturally specific information needs.	This assessment helps ensure that materials are presented in a manner that is culturally and educationally appropriate.
Inform patient and significant other to avoid heat, both external (hot weather, bath) and internal (fever).	Heat tends to aggravate weakness, pain, and other symptoms of MS.
Teach preventive measures, such as avoiding hot baths or showers and using acetaminophen or aspirin to reduce fever, if present.	Coolants and antipyretics aid in reducing body temperature.

Continued

INTERVENTIONS	RATIONALES
Also instruct patient in use of fans or air conditioning, chilled drinks, cool showers, and cool cloths.	High humidity with heat is especially problematic.
Caution patient to avoid exposure to persons known to have infections of any kind.	Infection often precedes exacerbations. Patients should receive immunizations and instructions in importance of and proper technique for hand washing.
Teach indicators of common infections and importance of seeking prompt medical treatment in case they occur. Instruct patient to check body temperature periodically for fever and indications that a urinary tract infection (UTI) has reached the kidneys (e.g., costovertebral angle tenderness, chills, flank pain). In addition, teach patient to monitor for increased frequency, urgency, or incontinence and to check urine for changes in odor or presence of cloudiness or blood.	A person with MS is especially susceptible to UTI because of urinary retention. Because of the disease process, patients may not feel any pain with urination and therefore need to be alert to other signs of UTI. See "Care of the Renal Transplant Recipient," p. 239-240, for a discussion of common infections.
Teach relationship between stress and fatigue to the exacerbations. Encourage patient to reduce factors that cause stress. Encourage use of stress reduction techniques such as progressive relaxation, self-coaching, and guided imagery.	Avoiding stress and fatigue may prevent exacerbations. See **Health-Seeking Behaviors**: Relaxation Technique Effective for Stress Reduction, p. 172.
If patient is depressed, suggest that he or she discuss use of antidepressants (e.g., amitriptyline, fluoxetine, sertraline) with health care provider.	Depression caused by cerebral lesions can contribute to sense of fatigue. These antidepressants may be given for both their anxiety-reducing and muscle relaxant effects, which may help with spasms and tremors.
Encourage patient to get sufficient rest, stop activity short of fatigue, schedule activity and rest periods, and conserve energy in activities of daily living (ADL).	Patient can conserve energy during ADL by sitting while getting dressed, rather than standing; sliding heavy objects along work surfaces, rather than lifting them; using a wheeled cart to transport items; having work surfaces at the proper height; and using assistive devices and delegating.
Suggest that patient ask health care provider about antifatigue medications.	Antifatigue drugs (e.g., amantadine, fluoxetine, modafinil) relieve fatigue associated with MS. See "Parkinsonism," p. 318, for side effects and precautions when using amantadine. Fatigue is the most common complaint and does not correlate with level of disability.
Encourage patient to plan each day, break projects into smaller tasks, distribute tasks throughout the day, rest before difficult tasks, take planned recovery time after tasks, identify priorities, and eliminate nonessential activities.	Conserving energy and decreasing fatigue are effective strategies for decreasing exacerbations.
Provide information about birth control measures to female patients who desire counseling.	There may be a decreased relapse rate during pregnancy but increased exacerbations postpartum. Those planning a pregnancy should consult and work with their health care providers before pregnancy.
As appropriate, reassure patient and significant other that most persons with MS do not become severely disabled.	Optic neuritis is common with damage to sensory nerve tracts and can be particularly frightening, but usually remits. Blindness occurs rarely.
Encourage continued activity and normal lifestyle even when limitations are necessary.	Deconditioning can be reduced with a planned exercise program that can be incorporated into a scheduled activity/rest plan.

••• **Related NIC and NOC labels:** *NIC:* Teaching: Disease Process; Learning Facilitation; Teaching: Prescribed Activity/Exercise; Infection Control; Energy Management *NOC:* Knowledge: Disease Process; Knowledge: Illness Care; Knowledge: Infection Control; Knowledge: Prescribed Activity

Nursing Diagnosis:

Deficient Knowledge:

Precautions and potential side effects of prescribed medications

Desired Outcome: By day 3 (or before hospital or clinic discharge), patient verbalizes accurate information about the prescribed medications.

INTERVENTIONS	RATIONALES
Provide verbal instructions and language-appropriate written handouts that describe name, purpose, dose, and schedule of the prescribed medications. Also discuss drug-drug, herb-drug, and food-drug interactions.	A well-informed patient is likely to follow the prescribed medication regimen, recognize side effects, and report those that necessitate prompt attention.
Give patients taking *glatiramer injections* this additional information:	Glatiramer injections may be prescribed to reduce frequency of relapses in relapsing-remitting MS. It is a synthetic copy of myelin basic protein and is believed to act as a "decoy" to spare the patient's myelin from immune system attack.
- Self-limiting reaction of chest tightness, palpitation, flushing, panic, and anxiousness may occur and last 30 sec to 30 min after injection. Injection site reaction (redness, swelling, pain) is also common.	These are common side effects.
- Notify health care provider of injection site redness, ongoing chest pain, shortness of breath, or dizziness.	These are side effects that warrant medical attention.
- Importance of refrigerating medication.	Refrigeration ensures its potency.
- Administer it subcutaneously only.	Muscle stiffness may occur via IM route.
- Rotate injection site daily.	Pain at injection site is common.
Teach the following for patients taking *interferon injection.*	Interferon β-1b and β-1a may be prescribed for patients with relapsing-remitting MS to reduce the rate of exacerbation and aid in stabilizing clinical status by moderating the immune response.
- Apply ice before injections; cortisone creams and rotating sites may help.	These measures help reduce skin inflammation, redness, and irritation from the injection.
- Postinjection fever, chills, headache, muscle aches and pains, and malaise can be managed with analgesics such as acetaminophen and antihistamines such as diphenhydramine.	Flulike symptoms are common following injection.
- Fatigue, diarrhea, abdominal pain, nausea, vomiting, joint aches, back pain, and dizziness also can occur.	These are other common side effects.
- Depression or suicidal thoughts can occur.	These are potential side effects that need to be reported for prompt intervention.
- Patient needs to have periodic assessments of blood counts and liver function.	Mild anemia, thrombocytopenia, and elevated liver transaminase levels (AST, ALT) may occur.
For patients taking *prednisone,* provide additional instructions for the following and reinforce importance of reporting all side effects to health care provider:	Prednisone may be prescribed during an exacerbation and for optic neuritis in an attempt to reduce symptoms by decreasing inflammation and associated edema of the myelin, thereby hastening onset of remission.
- Take the medication with food, milk, or buffering agents; avoiding aspirin, indomethacin, caffeine, or other gastrointestinal (GI) irritants while taking this medication.	These measures help prevent stomach upset and gastric irritation. In addition to antacids, histamine H2-receptor blockers may be prescribed to prevent gastric ulcer.
- Taper rather than abruptly stop the drug when it is discontinued.	This helps maintain the body's own cortisone sources. Abrupt discontinuation may result in adrenal crisis.
- Be alert to and report symptoms of potassium deficiency, such as anorexia, nausea, and muscle weakness and to eat foods high in potassium.	Hypokalemia is a common side effect of steroid use. Potassium supplements also may be prescribed.
- Eat a diet low in sodium and monitor for and report unusual weight gain or swelling of extremities.	A low-sodium diet minimizes the potential for fluid retention, which is a common occurrence with steroids.
	Diuretics may be prescribed to reduce fluid retention.
- Measure blood pressure daily.	Hypertension is another side effect. Home blood pressure kits are available at most drug stores. Antihypertensives may be prescribed.
- Monitor glucose for hyperglycemia, report elevations, and as indicated, control glucose level with diet, oral agents, or insulin.	Hyperglycemia is a side effect of steroid use.
- Monitor for and report tarry stools.	Tarry stools may signal occult blood, which can occur because of gastric ulcers, a common side effect of steroid use.

Continued

INTERVENTIONS	RATIONALES
- Monitor injuries and report wounds that are slow in healing.	Steroids can impair wound healing.
- Avoid contact with persons known to have infections. Monitor for and report fever, prolonged sore throat, and colds or other infections.	Steroids can mask infections, making them appear less severe; therefore follow up with care provider is important.
- Monitor for and report mood changes.	Antipsychotropic agents may be prescribed to help with mood changes associated with steroid use.
If patient is taking *baclofen* or *dantrolene,* provide additional instructions for the following:	These drugs may be given to decrease spasticity. Severe spasticity may be treated with IM injections of botulinum toxin or intrathecal baclofen administered continually via a surgically implanted pump. Dantrolene causes muscle weakness and usually is reserved for nonambulatory patients.
- Importance of taking the medication with food, milk, or a buffering agent.	This reduces gastric upset or nausea.
- Although drowsiness is usually transient, patient should avoid activities that require alertness until the effect of the drug on the CNS is known. The patient also should avoid alcohol intake because of its additive CNS depression effects.	These are standard safety precautions.
- Advise caution during initial transfers/ambulation.	Weak patients may not be able to tolerate the loss of spasticity that may be permitting them to bear weight.
- Baclofen never should be stopped abruptly.	Baclofen can lower the seizure threshold and should be used cautiously in susceptible patients.
- Individuals with diabetes mellitus may need an insulin dose adjustment.	Baclofen may raise blood glucose levels.
- Patients taking dantrolene should monitor for and report fever, jaundice, dark urine, clay-colored stools, and itching.	These symptoms signal hepatitis, a potential side effect of this drug.
- Patients taking dantrolene should report severe diarrhea, avoid exposure to the sun, and use sunscreens if exposure is unavoidable.	Dantrolene may cause diarrhea and photosensitivity.
If *bethanechol chloride* has been prescribed, provide additional instructions for the following:	Bethanechol chloride is a smooth muscle stimulant that helps prevent urinary retention.
- There is potential for hypotension, diarrhea, abdominal cramps, urinary urgency, and bronchoconstriction.	These are common side effects.
- Importance of taking the drug on an empty stomach.	This helps prevent nausea and vomiting.
- Notifying health care provider if lightheadedness occurs.	This is a sign of hypotension.
- Seeking medical attention if an asthmatic attack occurs.	This is a possible side effect.
- Caution patient to make position changes slowly and in stages.	Orthostatic hypotension is possible.
If patient is taking *propantheline bromide* or *tolterodine,* provide additional instructions for the following:	These drugs are smooth muscle relaxants that decrease bladder spasms and urinary frequency and urgency.
- Measures for remaining cool in hot or humid weather.	Heat stroke can develop while taking the medication because of decreased sweating.
- Importance of notifying health care provider immediately if urinary retention or overflow incontinence occurs.	These are conditions that necessitate prompt intervention.
- If the patient can chew and swallow effectively, suggest use of sugarless gum, hard candy, or artificial saliva products.	These products may reduce mouth dryness.
- Importance of slow position changes and monitoring for dizziness.	Postural hypotension may occur when the drug is first started.
- Monitor for constipation.	See **Constipation,** p. 277.
- Monitor for and report blurred vision, palpitations, and tachycardia.	These are other common side effects.
For patient taking *mitoxantrone,* teach the following:	This drug has received approval of the Food and Drug Administration for secondary-progressive or worsening MS as an immunosuppressive, but it is recommended only for aggressive disease.

Continued

INTERVENTIONS	RATIONALES
- Patient will be evaluated for normal cardiac function before starting the drug and will need periodic cardiac monitoring to ensure that there are no toxic cardiac effects. Patient should report swelling of feet and lower legs and shortness of breath.	Cardiac toxicity is a possible side effect.
- Medication has a lifetime cumulative dose restriction.	This restriction limits toxicities.
- Avoid people with infections as well as live virus vaccinations. Report signs of infection to health care provider (e.g., fever, chills, cough, hoarseness, lower back or side pain, and painful or difficult urination). Also report mouth or lip sores, black tarry stools, and stomach pains. Expect both white blood cell (WBC) and liver function tests. Patient also should report any jaundice.	This medication can decrease WBCs and thus risk of infection is increased. Liver toxicity is another possible side effect.
- Other side effects include nausea, temporary hair loss, and menstrual changes. After taking medication, urine may be blue-green in color for about 24 hr. The medication also may cause diarrhea, which should be reported if it continues.	These side effects generally do not require medical follow-up.

••• **Related NIC and NOC labels:** *NIC:* Teaching: Prescribed Medication *NOC:* Knowledge: Medication

Nursing Diagnosis:

Chronic Pain (and spasms)

related to motor and sensory nerve tract damage

Desired Outcomes: Within 1-2 hr of intervention, patient's subjective evaluation of pain and spasms improves, as documented by pain scale. Objective indicators, such as grimacing, are absent or reduced.

INTERVENTIONS	RATIONALES
Maintain a comfortable room temperature. Advise patient to keep environment cool in warm weather and avoid hot baths or showers.	Heat tends to aggravate MS symptoms.
Provide passive, assisted, or active range of motion q2h and periodic stretching exercises. Teach these exercises to patient and significant other, and encourage their performance several times daily. Explain that sleeping in a prone position may help decrease flexor spasm of the hips and knees and that splints or cones for hands with elastic bands may help control hand spasms.	These interventions reduce muscle tightness and spasms, maintain joint function, and prevent contractures. Physical therapy (PT), occupational therapy (OT), and assistive devices or braces may be prescribed to maintain mobility and independence with ADL. Placing weights on the affected limbs may help with mild tremors.
Administer antispasmodics as prescribed.	See discussion of baclofen and dantrolene, earlier.
Administer tranquilizers (e.g., diazepam) as prescribed.	These medications may be given for both their anxiety-reducing and muscle relaxant effects, which may help spasms and tremors.
Administer analgesics (e.g., acetaminophen) and neuropathic pain medications as prescribed.	Neuropathic pain medications include anticonvulsants such as carbamazepine, gabapentin, topiramate, lamotrigine (see "Seizures and Epilepsy," p. 328, for side effects/precautions), and tricyclic antidepressants (e.g., amitriptyline or imipramine). Uncontrolled pain may require nerve blocks or surgical intervention.
For other interventions, see "General Care of Patients with Neurologic Disorders," **Acute Pain**, p. 273.	

••• **Related NIC and NOC labels:** *NIC:* Pain Management; Exercise Promotion; Stretching; Exercise Promotion: Joint Mobility *NOC:* Pain Control

ADDITIONAL NURSING DIAGNOSES/PROBLEMS:

"Cancer Care," for patients undergoing immunosuppressive drug or radiation therapy — p. 1

"Prolonged Bedrest," for patients who are immobile — p. 61

"Psychosocial Support" — p. 73

"Older Adult Care," for **Risk for Aspiration** — p. 96

"General Care of Patients with Neurologic Disorders" for **Risk for Falls** related to unsteady gait — p. 265

Impaired Swallowing — p. 267

Risk for Injury related to impaired pain, touch, and temperature sensations — p. 269

Impaired Tissue Integrity: Corneal — p. 270

Risk for Deficient Fluid Volume related to decreased intake — p. 271

Imbalanced Nutrition: Less Than Body Requirements — p. 272

Impaired Verbal Communication — p. 275

Self-Care Deficit related to spasticity, tremors, weakness, paresis, paralysis, or decreasing LOC secondary to sensorimotor deficits — p. 277

Constipation — p. 277

Disturbed Sensory Perception: Visual — p. 280

"Guillain-Barré Syndrome" for **Deficient Knowledge**: Therapeutic plasma exchange procedure, for patients undergoing plasmapheresis — p. 291

Ineffective Tissue Perfusion: Peripheral and Cardiopulmonary related to interrupted blood flow (venous stasis) with corresponding risk of thrombophlebitis and pulmonary emboli (PE) secondary to immobility — p. 338

Urinary Retention or **Reflex Urinary Incontinence** — p. 339

"Spinal Cord Injury" for **Constipation** — p. 342

Risk for Disuse Syndrome — p. 343

Sexual Dysfunction — p. 346

"Pressure Ulcers" — p. 562

"Providing Nutritional Support," for patients with impaired nutrition — p. 565

✔ PATIENT-FAMILY TEACHING AND DISCHARGE PLANNING

The patient with MS may have a wide variety of symptoms that cause disability, ranging from mild to severe. When providing patient-family teaching, focus on sensory information, avoid giving excessive information, and initiate a visiting nurse referral for necessary follow-up teaching. Include verbal and written information about the following:

✓ Remission/exacerbation aspects of the disease process and progression. Explain effects of demyelinization on sensory and motor function and factors that aggravate symptoms. Generally, treatment is symptomatic and supportive. Various treatments slow the rate of exacerbation or hasten recovery from an exacerbation, but the general course of the disease process has not been positively affected.

✓ Safety measures relative to decreased sensation, visual disturbances, and motor deficits.

✓ Medications, including drug name, purpose, dosage, frequency, precautions, and potential side effects. Also discuss drug-drug, herb-drug, and food-drug interactions.

✓ Exercises that promote muscle strength and mobility, measures for preventing contractures and skin breakdown, transfer techniques and proper body mechanics, and use of assistive devices and other measures to minimize neurologic deficits.

✓ Measures for relieving pain, muscle spasms, or other discomfort.

✓ Indications of constipation, urinary retention, or UTI; implementation of bowel and bladder training programs; and self-catheterization technique or care of indwelling urinary catheters.

✓ Indications of upper respiratory infection (URI); implementation of measures that help prevent regurgitation, aspiration, and respiratory infection.

✓ Measures for managing fatigue.

✓ Measures for fall prevention.

✓ Dietary adjustments that may be appropriate for neurologic deficit (e.g., soft, semisolid foods for patients with chewing difficulties or a high-fiber diet for patients experiencing constipation).

✓ Importance of follow-up care, including visits to health care provider, PT, and OT, as well as speech, sexual, or psychologic counseling to help patient and significant other adapt to the disability and deal with emotions and feelings that are either a direct or an indirect result of the disease process.

✓ Referrals to community resources, such as local and national Multiple Sclerosis Society chapters, public health nurse, visiting nurse association, community support groups, social workers, psychologists, vocational rehabilitation agencies, home health agencies, extended and skilled care facilities, and financial counseling. Additional general information can be obtained by contacting the following organizations:

- National Multiple Sclerosis Society at *www.nmss.org*
- Multiple Sclerosis Foundation at *www.msfacts.org*
- Multiple Sclerosis Association of America at *www.msaa.com*

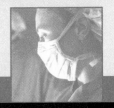

Parkinsonism 39

OVERVIEW/PATHOPHYSIOLOGY

Parkinson's disease (PD) is a slowly progressive degenerative disorder of the central nervous system (CNS) affecting the brain centers that regulate movement and balance. For unknown reasons, cell death occurs in the substantia nigra of the midbrain. When healthy, the substantia nigra projects dopaminergic neurons into the corpus striatum and releases the neurotransmitter dopamine in that area. Degeneration of these neurons leads to an abnormally low concentration of dopamine in the basal ganglia. The basal ganglia control muscle tone and voluntary motor movement via a balance between two main neurotransmitters, dopamine and acetylcholine. The deficit of dopamine, which has an inhibitory effect, allows the relative excess of acetylcholine. The excitatory effect of acetylcholine causes overactivity of the basal ganglia, which interferes with normal muscle tone and control of smooth, purposeful movement, causing the characteristic symptoms of PD: muscle rigidity, tremors, and slowness of movement. Nerve cell loss in the substantia nigra and accumulation of Lewy bodies in the brainstem and pigmented areas of the brain are the pathologic hallmarks of PD. Lewy bodies are tiny abnormal spherical alpha-synuclein protein deposits that accumulate inside the damaged nerve cells and disrupt the brain's normal functioning. Symptoms start when cell loss reaches about 80%.

Approximately 1% of all individuals older than 60 yr have this disease. PD is usually progressive, and death can result from aspiration pneumonia or choking. *Neuroleptic malignant syndrome*, a medical emergency, is usually precipitated by failure to take the prescribed medications. *Acute akinesia*, sometimes referred to as *parkinsonian crisis*, is another medical emergency and seems associated with infections or surgical procedures.

HEALTH CARE SETTING

Primary care with possible acute care hospitalization resulting from complications as the disease progresses

ASSESSMENT

Initially, symptoms are mild and include stiffness or slight hand tremors. They gradually increase and can become disabling. Cardinal features are tremors, rigidity, and bradykinesia that start on one side and over time become bilateral.

Clinical features most suggestive of idiopathic PD include unilateral onset, presence of resting tremor, and a clear-cut response to treatment with L-dopa. Assessment findings vary in degree and are highly individualized. PD is sometimes categorized as either tremor-dominant type or postural instability and gait disturbance (PIGD)-dominant type.

Tremors: Increase when the limb is at rest and completely supported against gravity, and stop with voluntary movement and during sleep (nonintentional "resting" tremor). "Pill-rolling" tremor of the hands and "to-and-fro" tremor of the head are typical.

Bradykinesia: Slowness, stiffness, and difficulty initiating movement. Patients may have a masklike, blank facial expression; "unblinking" stare; difficulty chewing and swallowing; drooling caused by decreased frequency of swallowing; and a high-pitched, monotone, weak voice. Speech may be slow and slurred. The patient also has loss of automatic associated movements, such as the normal arm-swing movement when walking unless making a conscious effort and episodes of "freezing." Handwriting becomes progressively smaller, cramped, and tremulous.

Increased muscle rigidity: Limb muscles become rigid on passive motion. Typically, this rigidity results in jerky ("cogwheel") motions or steady resistance to all movement ("lead-pipe" rigidity).

Loss of postural reflexes: Causes the typical stooped, forward-leaning, shuffling, propulsive gait with short, rapidly accelerating steps; stumbling; and difficulty maintaining or regaining balance, which makes the individual prone to stumbling and falling. Abnormal gait in which the body is bent backward (retropulsion) also may be present.

Autonomic: Excessive diaphoresis, seborrhea, postural hypotension, decreased libido, hypomotility of the gastrointestinal (GI) tract (causing constipation), and urinary hesitancy. Vision may blur as a result of lost accommodation.

Mental health/psychiatric: Dementia (e.g., forgetfulness, irritability, paranoia, hallucinations) is commonly associated with PD. However, not all patients develop impaired intellectual and mental functioning. Mental status testing may be complicated by the patient's movement disorder. Some patients may experience akathisia, a condition of motor restlessness in which there is a compelling need to walk about constantly. Depression is common. Psychosis is often drug-induced.

Neuroleptic malignant syndrome: The classic triad of symptoms includes fever (100%), rigidity (90%), and cognitive changes (e.g., drowsiness, confusion progressing to stupor and coma). Other symptoms include tremor, tachypnea, diaphoresis, and occasionally dystonia and chorea. Symptoms are associated with discontinuation or reduction in dopaminergic medications. This sudden and severe increase in muscle rigidity can cause inability to swallow or maintain a patent airway.

Acute akinesia: This sudden decrease in motor performance or inability to move ("frozen") lasts for more than 48 hr and is transiently unresponsive to dopaminergic rescue medication (e.g., apomorphine) or increases in dopaminergic medications. Triggering factors include infections, surgery, fractures, GI disease, and drug manipulations.

Oculogyric crisis: Fixation of eyes in one position, generally upward, sometimes for several hours. This is relatively rare.

Physical assessment: Usually a positive blink reflex is elicited by tapping a finger between the patient's eyebrows. Blinking may occur 5-10 times/min instead of the normal 20 times/min. A positive palmomental (palm-chin) reflex can be elicited (muscles of the chin and corner of mouth contract when the patient's palm is stroked). Diminished postural reflexes are present on neurologic examination; however, there is risk of injury with this test because patients may quickly lose balance and fall.

History/risk factors: PD has many possible causes. Metabolic causes such as hypothyroidism need to be ruled out. Long-term therapy with large doses of medications, such as haloperidol, phenothiazines, metoclopramide, methyldopa, reserpine, or chlorpromazine can produce extrapyramidal side effects known as pseudoparkinsonism. If caused by these medications, symptoms will disappear when the drug is discontinued. The recreational drug "ecstasy" and an improperly synthesized heroin-like substance, 1-methyl-4-phenyl-1,2,3,6-tetrahydropyridine (MPTP), also have induced parkinsonism. Other causes include toxins (e.g., heavy metals, pesticides, lacquer thinner, and carbon monoxide), cerebrovascular disease, head injury (especially repeated injury), and viral encephalitis. Living in a rural area is associated with increased PD risk, while nicotine intake is associated with decreased PD risk. The vast majority of cases of PD occur without an apparent or known cause, although genetic susceptibility is believed to play a role. Genetic factors appear to be more predominant when the disease begins before the age of 45-50, with the most common known forms of hereditary parkinsonism caused by mutations in the parkin gene (PARK2) and alpha-synuclein gene.

Unified PD rating scale: May be used as a standardized assessment tool and includes evaluation of self-reported disability (i.e., inability to perform activities of daily living) as well as clinical scoring by a health care provider.

Hoehn and Yahr stage scale: Simple and popular scale that establishes PD severity. The different stages of disease are classified from I (mild) to V (severe).

DIAGNOSTIC TESTS

Diagnosis usually is made on the basis of physical assessment and characteristic symptoms and after other neurologic problems have been ruled out.

Positron emission tomography: May reveal areas of decreased dopamine metabolism via use of the labeled dopamine-transporter amino acids 6-^{18}å-fluoro-b-dopa (F-DOPA, used for diagnosis in Europe) or 18F-fluorodeoxyglucose (FDG) used with PET imaging.

Urinalysis for dopamine metabolites: May reveal decreased dopamine level, which supports the diagnosis.

Lumbar puncture with CSF analysis: Cerebrospinal fluid (CSF) is analyzed for specific proteins and chemicals that are leaked from the brain in PD and that cannot be measured in blood. Abnormalities of a protein called apha-synuclein are found in PD and may serve as a disease marker and be used to monitor disease progression.

Single photon emission computed tomography: Reveals how a radioisotope-tagged drug accumulates in the brain. It may be useful in detecting PD and gauging disease progress.

Tremor studies: Serial measurements of functional activity will show decreased performance.

Cineradiographic study of swallowing: May show abnormal pattern and delayed relaxation of cricopharyngeal muscles.

Electroencephalogram: Often shows such abnormalities as diffuse, nonspecific slowing of theta waves, which are slow, high-amplitude waves present during sleep but abnormal in awake adults.

Nursing Diagnosis:

Risk for Falls

related to unsteady gait secondary to bradykinesia, tremors, and rigidity

Desired Outcome: Following instruction, patient demonstrates safe and effective ambulatory techniques and preventive measures against falls and remains free of trauma.

INTERVENTIONS	RATIONALES
During ambulation, encourage patient to deliberately swing arms and raise feet.	These actions assist gait, thereby helping to prevent falls.
Advise patient to step over imaginary object or line, practice taking long steps, and avoid shuffling.	This will help raise feet higher and increase stride, which will help prevent falls.
Have patient practice movements that are especially difficult (e.g., turning). Teach patient to walk in a wide arc ("U-turn") rather than pivot when turning.	These actions prevent crossing of one leg over the other and causing a fall.
Teach head and neck exercises.	These exercises promote good posture, which in turn helps the gait.
Remind patient repeatedly to maintain upright posture and look up, not down, especially when walking.	This is particularly important for patients with bifocal glasses inasmuch as a stooped posture promotes looking down through the reading portion of the bifocal lens where distant items are blurred.
Advise patient to stop or consciously slow down periodically. Teach patient to concentrate on listening to feet as they touch the floor and to count cadence to prevent too fast a gait.	This will slow the walking speed, which is less likely to result in falls.
Encourage patient to lift toes and to walk with heels touching floor first.	This action keeps soles of feet flat on the floor, which is less likely to cause tripping.
Remind patient to maintain a wide-based gait.	This gait improves balance.
Provide a clear pathway while patient is walking. Teach patient to avoid crowds, scatter rugs, uneven surfaces, fast turns, narrow doorways, and obstructions.	These actions minimize risk of tripping and falling.
Encourage patient to perform range of motion and stretching exercises daily.	Exercising promotes flexibility, strength, gait, and balance, thereby decreasing risk of falls. Routine exercises, along with prescribed medications, may prevent or delay disability.
Advise patient to wear leather-soled or smooth-soled shoes but to test shoes to ensure they are not too slippery.	Rubber-soled or crepe-soled shoes tend to catch on floors, especially carpeted floors, and may cause falls.
Encourage patient not to hurry or rush.	Hurrying may precipitate falls.
Encourage males to keep a urinal at bedside. A commode at bedside may be helpful for females.	Slowness of gait and inability to get to the bathroom fast enough may cause incontinence or falls in an effort to get there.
Ask physical therapy department to suggest exercises that improve balance.	Tai chi, for example, uses slow, graceful movements to relax and strengthen muscles and joints and may be encouraged as an option for some patients.
For other interventions, see **Risk for Falls**, p. 265, in "General Care of Patients with Neurologic Disorders."	

••• **Related NIC and NOC labels:** *NIC:* Fall Prevention; Surveillance: Safety; Environmental Management: Safety; Home Maintenance Assistance; Risk Identification; Teaching: Prescribed Activity/Exercise *NOC:* Safety Status: Falls Occurrence

Nursing Diagnosis:

Impaired Physical Mobility

related to difficulty initiating movement

Desired Outcome: Following instruction, patient demonstrates measures that enhance ability to initiate desired movement.

INTERVENTIONS	RATIONALES
Teach patient measures that may help initiate movement.	Patients with PD often have difficulty initiating movement because their disease affects the brain centers that regulate movement and balance. Rocking from side to side may help initiate leg movement. Marching in place a few steps before resuming forward motion also may be helpful. Other measures include relaxing back on heels and raising toes; tapping hip of the leg to be moved; bending at knees and straightening up; raising arms in a sudden, short motion; or humming a marching tune.
If feet remain "glued" to the floor despite these measures, suggest that patient think of something else for a few moments and then try again.	It might help also to try changing directions (e.g., move sideways if going forward is impossible).
Teach patient to get out of a chair by getting to edge of seat, placing hands on arm supports, bending forward slightly, moving feet back, and then rhythmically rocking in the chair a few times before trying to get up.	The deficit of dopamine, which has an inhibitory effect, allows the relative excess of acetylcholine. The excitatory effect of acetylcholine causes overactivity of the basal ganglia, which interferes with normal muscle tone and the control of smooth, purposeful movement, causing the characteristic symptoms of PD: muscle rigidity, tremors, and slowness of movement. These combined problems make it difficult to get out of a chair.
Advise patient to sit in chairs with backs and arms and to purchase elevated toilet seats or sidebars in the bathroom.	These items will assist with rising from a sitting position and help prevent falls.
Teach measures that may help with getting out of bed: rocking to a sitting position, placing blocks under legs of head of bed to elevate it, and tying a rope or sheet to foot of bed to help patient pull to a sitting position.	See discussion with getting out of a chair, above.
Teach patient and significant others to recognize situations that can cause freezing episodes.	"Freezing" is variable and can fluctuate with stress or emotional state. For example, attempting two movements simultaneously, such as trying to change direction quickly while walking can cause freezing. Distracting environmental, visual, or auditory stimuli also can precipitate a freezing episode. Doorways; narrow passages; or a change in floor color, texture, or slope can pose problems for many patients.
Provide a referral to an organization such as Canine Partners as indicated.	Specially trained dogs (e.g., Canine Partners) can help patients walk and get up after a fall and are trained to help break a "freeze" by tapping on patient's foot.
Suggest that sexual relations be planned for when the prescribed drug is working to good effect and the person is rested. Being flexible about time; experimenting with positions; use of manual, oral, and vibrator stimulation; and use of sildenafil have proved beneficial.	PD makes it more difficult to move, which can affect intimacy.

••• Related NIC and NOC labels: *NIC:* Positioning; Teaching: Psychomotor Skill; Self-Care Assistance; Teaching: Prescribed Activity/Exercise; Body Mechanics Promotion; Fall Prevention *NOC:* Transfer Performance; Mobility Level

Nursing Diagnosis:

Deficient Knowledge:

Side effects of and precautionary measures for taking anti-Parkinson medications

Desired Outcome: Following instruction and before hospital discharge, patient and significant other verbalize knowledge about side effects of and necessary precautionary measures for taking anti-Parkinson medications.

Note: Teach patient and significant other to report adverse side effects promptly because many side effects are dose related and can be controlled by a dosage adjustment.

INTERVENTIONS	RATIONALES

Side Effects Common to Most Anti-Parkinson Medications

Stress importance of taking medication on schedule and not forgetting a dose.	Missing a dose may adversely affect mobility. Patient and health care provider can adjust dose schedule so that medication peaks at mealtime or at times when patient needs mobility most.
Teach patient or significant other how to premeasure doses in segmented or separate containers labeled with date and time of dose.	This assists patients having difficulty with self-medication.
Teach patient to take non–levodopa-containing medications with meals.	This will decrease the potential for nausea. If an antiemetic is needed for nausea, trimethobenzamide or domperidone may be prescribed. Promethazine, however, is avoided because it can worsen PD symptoms.
Encourage patient with anorexia to eat frequent small, nutritious snacks and meals.	Eating smaller meals rather than three larger meals is usually better tolerated in patients who are anorexic.
Advise patient to elevate head of bed and make position changes slowly and in stages. Teach patient to dangle legs a few minutes before standing. Antiembolism hose may help as well. Advise avoiding dehydration in warm weather by increasing fluid intake. Give tips for reducing morning orthostatic hypotension, including not limiting late evening fluid intake and keeping a glass of water at the bedside at night so it is available to drink in the morning before getting up. Encourage males to urinate from a sitting rather than standing position if possible. Provide a bedside commode for female patients. Suggest increasing dietary salt intake.	These measures counteract orthostatic hypotension, which is a potential side effect of these drugs. Fludrocortisone or midodrine may be prescribed to prevent or reduce orthostatic hypotension.
Teach patient to report dizziness to health care provider.	Medication adjustment may be needed.
Advise use of sugarless chewing gum or hard candy, frequent mouth rinses with water, or artificial saliva products.	These measures ease dry mouth, a common side effect of these medications, and help maintain integrity of oral mucous membrane. In the presence of drooling, however, an anticholinergic such as hyoscyamine or glycopyrrolate; a beneficial side effect is a reduction in secretions.
Advise patient to report any urinary hesitancy or incontinence.	Either may signal urinary retention. Individuals taking anticholinergics may find that voiding before taking medication eliminates this problem.
Teach patient how to counteract constipation. For interventions, see **Constipation**, p. 67, in "Prolonged Bedrest."	Constipation is a common problem with these medications. Laxative and stool softeners as well as reduction in anticholinergic medications may help. If anorectal dysfunction is causing constipation, botulinum toxin injection into the puborectalis muscle may correct it.
Teach patient to report mental status changes to health care provider promptly.	Many of these drugs can cause or aggravate changes in mental status such as confusion; mental slowness or dullness; and even agitation, paranoia, and hallucinations. Health care provider may adjust dose. Atypical antipsychotic agents such as quetiapine, olanzapine, and clozapine may be prescribed to decrease psychotic symptoms. Haloperidol may make PD symptoms worse and is therefore avoided.
Teach patient to report feelings of depression to health care provider promptly.	Depression can be a side effect of some drugs as well as a normal response to disability. Counseling or psychotherapy may help patient and significant other adapt to the disability and deal with emotions and feelings such as depression that are either a direct or an indirect result of the disease process or drug therapy. Antidepressants (e.g., fluoxetine, sertraline, paroxetine, venlafaxine, amitriptyline) may be prescribed to treat depression as well as help some PD symptoms (may help to block reabsorption of dopamine and have some anticholinergic properties). Occasionally, electroconvulsive therapy is used for persistent and serious depression.
Implement safety measures for patient with vision problems: orient to surroundings, identify self when entering room, keep walkways unobstructed, and encourage patient to ask for assistance when ambulating.	Blurred vision is a side effect of many anti-Parkinson drugs.
Teach measures that promote sleep. See **Disturbed Sleep Pattern**, p. 73.	Insomnia is a side effect of many of these drugs. Reducing the evening dose may help promote sleep. Modafinil may be prescribed to reduce daytime sleepiness.

Continued

INTERVENTIONS	RATIONALES
Side Effects Specific to Dopamine Replacement Therapy (Levodopa)	Levodopa, the metabolic precursor of dopamine, crosses the blood-brain barrier and restores dopamine levels in the extrapyramidal centers in the brain. Before levodopa crosses the blood-brain barrier, much of it is converted into dopamine by the peripheral metabolism (GI tract and liver), causing many of the drug's side effects. Dopamine is given in increasing amounts until symptoms are reduced or patient's tolerance to side effects is reached. It may be used as initial therapy or later when other medications can no longer control symptoms.
Teach patient that levodopa should be taken with a full glass of water on an empty stomach.	This measure facilitates absorption. Timing of medication 20-30 min before meals will aid nutrition by improving mobility and movement.
Teach patient to avoid vitamin preparations or fortified cereals that contain pyridoxine (vitamin B₆).	Pyridoxine reduces effectiveness of levodopa. Intake of foods high in pyridoxine, such as wheat germ, whole grain cereals, legumes, and liver, may be limited.
Teach patient that a dietary intake high in protein may interfere with effectiveness of levodopa.	Although diet should meet recommended daily allowance of protein (i.e., 0.8 g/kg body weight/day), patient should avoid excessive amounts of meat, eggs, dairy products, and legumes. If prescribed, dietary supplementation with l-tryptophan needs to be calculated into total protein allotment. If possible, protein intake should be shifted to evening meals to minimize interaction with levodopa.
Instruct patient to report muscle twitching or spasmodic winking.	These are early signs of overdose.
Explain signs and symptoms of neuroleptic malignant syndrome and acute akinesia (see Assessment). Teach patient that to avoid neuroleptic malignant syndrome, it is necessary to take levodopa as scheduled and not to stop this medication abruptly.	There is need for immediate medical intervention with these crises because respiratory and cardiac support may be necessary. In neuroleptic malignant syndrome, the dopaminergic drug needs to be restarted immediately and measures taken to treat fever and renal dysfunction. In acute akinesia, the triggering cause must be found and treated.
Explain signs of on-off response, wearing-off, other complications of therapy, interventions, and importance of working with health care provider on fine-tuning medication regimen.	Many of the problems with dopamine replacement therapy are related to fluctuating blood levels. Dose redistribution, adding a dopamine agonist or catechol O-methyltransferase (COMT) inhibitor, and use of medication preparations in extended-release forms, transdermal forms (as they are developed and become available), or continuous infusion forms (enteral) should help prevent these problems.
	On-off response: A rapid fluctuation or change in patient's condition. The individual is "on" one moment, in a state of relative mobility, and "off" the next, in a state of complete or nearly complete immobility. Although the cause is uncertain, it is believed that it is related to fluctuating dopamine blood levels in the brain.
	"End-of-dose" wearing-off phenomenon: Return of symptoms (bradykinesis, tremors, rigidity) before next dose is given.
	Other complications: Choreiform or involuntary, spasmodic, jerking movements (e.g., facial grimacing, tongue protrusion, restlessness) and vivid dreaming. Dose reduction may help these side effects.
Teach patient and significant other to monitor for behavioral changes.	Severe depression with suicidal overtones can be caused by this drug and should be reported immediately. The health care provider may prescribe a dose reduction.
Explain that patient's medication may cause dark-colored urine and sweat.	Knowing what to expect may eliminate anxiety if these problems occur.
Caution patient to avoid alcohol.	Alcohol impairs effectiveness of levodopa.
Explain importance of medical follow-up while taking this drug.	Follow-up monitors for and manages such problems as increased intraocular pressure and changes in glucose control.
Side Effects Specific to Antiviral Agent (e.g., amantadine)	Although this drug is less effective than levodopa, it has fewer severe side effects. It may be used as initial therapy or as an adjunct. Effects diminish in a few months; therefore this drug may be used intermittently.
Teach patient to take this drug early in the day.	This may prevent insomnia, which is one of its side effects.

Continued

INTERVENTIONS	RATIONALES
Teach patient and significant other to monitor for and report any short-ness of breath, peripheral edema, significant weight gain, or change in mental status.	These signs often signal heart failure, a possible side effect of this drug.
Instruct patient not to stop taking this medication abruptly.	Doing so may precipitate parkinsonian crisis.
Teach patient to report a change in skin coloration if it occurs, but reassure that the condition is more cosmetic than serious.	A diffuse, rose-colored mottling of the skin, usually confined to lower extremi-ties, may develop. The condition may subside with continued therapy and will disappear in a few weeks to months after the drug is discontinued. Exposure to cold or standing may make color more prominent.
Instruct patient to monitor and promptly report to health care provider a loss of seizure control.	Patients with history of seizures may have an increase in the number of seizures.
Caution patient to avoid alcohol and CNS depressants.	These agents potentiate effects of amantadine.
Explain that most side effects of amantadine are dose related.	Many side effects can be controlled by an adjustment in dosage.
Side Effects Specific to Dopamine Agonist (e.g., pramipexole, ropinirole, bromocriptine, pergolide, and ropinirole, cabergoline, apomorphine)	These drugs are administered with a concomitant reduction of dopamine replacement dosage. They may be used to reduce levodopa-induced dyskinesia (such as involuntary movements) and the frequency of "on-off" responses.
Caution patient to avoid alcohol when taking this medication.	Alcohol tolerance will be lessened.
Teach patient to avoid exposure to cold and to report onset of finger or toe pallor.	Bromocriptine can cause digital vasospasm.
Teach patient taking bromocriptine, cabergoline, and pergolide to have regular follow-up evaluation of lungs.	These drugs have been associated with pulmonary fibrosis.
Teach patient taking pergolide to have regular follow-up evaluations to monitor the heart.	Pergolide has potential for promoting cardiac valve problems.
Teach patient that changing the medication should help with gambling problems if they occur.	Dopamine agonist therapy has been associated with potentially revers-ible pathological gambling. Pramipexole is the medication predomi-nantly implicated.
Caution patient taking pramipexole against driving or using machinery while on this drug to avoid accidents.	Pramipexole is associated with abrupt onset of somnolence without warning.
Teach patient that despite its name, apomorphine does not contain mor-phine and is not addictive. Explain that an antiemetic (e.g., trimetho-benzamide) needs to be taken before taking apomorphine, ideally on a prophylaxis basis 3 days before initiation of therapy.	Apomorphine is a dopamine agonist given subcutaneously as a "rescue" drug for acute, intermittent treatment of hypomobility ("off" episodes). It frequently causes severe nausea and vomiting, although tolerance usually develops after about 8 wk. Dizziness or postural hypotension can occur.
Teach patient to implement safety precautions when taking apomorphine.	
Explain that the following can occur with apomorphine: injection site re-actions including bruising, itching, and lumps that typically resolve on their own. Yawning, dyskinesia, somnolence, rhinorrhea, hallucination, and extremity edema also can occur.	These are common side effects.
Explain that erections in men can occur spontaneously with apomorphine and should be reported to health care provider if they last longer than 3-4 hr.	This side effect of apomorphine may be beneficial for selected patients. A sublingual form of apomorphine for erectile dysfunction is being used and may provide an alternative to sildenafil. A transdermal form is also being developed.
Side Effects Specific to Anticholinergic Medications (e.g., trihexyphenidyl, benztropine mesylate, ethopropa-zine, cycrimine, procyclidine, biperiden)	These drugs are often used in conjunction with dopamine replacement therapy but may be used alone if patient's symptoms are mild or if patient cannot tolerate levodopa. They may improve tremors and ri-gidity but often do little for bradykinesia or balance problems.
Explain that patient should avoid strenuous exercise and keep cool dur-ing summer to avoid heat stroke.	This medication may decrease perspiration.
Teach patient not to stop taking this medication abruptly.	Doing so can result in parkinsonian crisis.
Teach patient to monitor for tachycardia or palpitation and to report ei-ther condition.	Many side effects such as these can be controlled by an adjustment in dosage.
Teach patient and significant others to monitor for memory dysfunction and confusion and urinary hesitancy and retention (especially in older males) and to report symptoms to health care provider.	As above.

Continued

INTERVENTIONS	RATIONALES
Side Effects Specific to Monoamine Oxidase (MAO) Type B Inhibitor (e.g., selegiline, lazabemide)	This drug is used as an early intervention or as an adjunct with levodopa to inhibit the breakdown of levodopa, resulting in less fluctuation in blood levels.
Stress importance of taking this medication only in prescribed dose and following dietary modifications to reduce intake of tyramine-containing foods.	Selegiline and lazabemide administered in the recommended dose of 10 mg/day or less do not cause the hypertensive crisis that can occur when tyramine-containing foods (e.g., cheese, red wine, beer, yogurt) are eaten. Dosages greater than 10 mg/day may result in hypertension if these foods are eaten.
Suggest avoidance of meperidine and other opioids.	At recommended doses, no drug interactions have been noted. However, fatal drug interactions have occurred with patients taking other non-selective MAO inhibitors and could conceivably occur if higher-than-recommended doses are taken.
Teach patient to take the drug early in the day.	This may help prevent insomnia, a potential side effect.
Side Effects Specific to COMT Inhibitor (e.g., entacapone)	This drug reduces levodopa degradation in the GI tract, kidneys, and liver to minimize fluctuation in serum levels.
Teach patient that this medication might cause urine discoloration (brownish orange) but it is not clinically important.	An informed patient is not likely to become anxious if urine discoloration occurs.
Explain that hallucinations, increased dyskinesia, persistent nausea, abdominal pain, and diarrhea should be reported promptly.	Many side effects are dose related and can be controlled by adjustment in dosage.

••• **Related NIC and NOC labels:** *NIC:* Teaching: Prescribed Medication *NOC:* Knowledge: Medication

Nursing Diagnosis:

Health-Seeking Behaviors:

Facial and tongue exercises that enhance verbal communication and help prevent choking

Desired Outcome: Following demonstration and within the 24-hr period before hospital discharge, patient demonstrates facial and tongue exercises and states the rationale for their use.

INTERVENTIONS	RATIONALES
Explain that special exercises can help strengthen and control facial and tongue muscles, which in turn will improve verbal communication and help prevent choking. Refer patient to a speech pathologist to design and individualize a speech program.	Routine exercises of facial and tongue muscles, along with prescribed medications, may prevent or delay disability.
Teach exercises that will improve verbal communication and help prevent choking. Have patient return the demonstration.	Teaching, followed by return demonstration, is an effective way of helping patient understand and retain knowledge. Teaching patient how to hold a sound for 5 sec; sing the scale; recite the alphabet and days of the week; practice vowel breaths (ah, oh, oo) and nonsense syllables (ma, me, mi, pull, pill, pie), read aloud, and extend the tongue and try to touch the chin, nose, and cheek will help improve verbal communication skills and prevent choking.
Encourage patient to practice increasing voice volume. Suggest that patient read newspapers out loud and determine how many words can be said in one breath before volume decreases. Advise that voice should vary from soft to loud.	This exercise will help combat monotone speech while promoting speech quality and understandability. This may be accomplished by having patient take a deep breath before speaking, open mouth to let sound come out more, use shorter sentences, exaggerate sound of every syllable, speak louder than others may think necessary, and use a tape recorder for feedback. Patient should practice reading or reciting out loud, focusing on breathing, and using a strong voice.
Teach patient to raise voice with a question and lower it with an answer.	These actions improve speech understandability.

Continued

INTERVENTIONS	RATIONALES
Teach tongue exercises: stick out tongue as far as possible and hold; move tongue slowly from corner to corner; stretch tongue to nose and then chin and then cheek; stick out tongue and put it back in the mouth as quickly as possible; move tongue in circles as quickly as possible.	These exercises will improve articulation.
Teach patient to open and close mouth slowly and then quickly; close lips and press tightly; stretch lips in a wide smile and hold; then pucker lips and hold.	These are effective lip and jaw exercises for improving articulation.
Advise patient to practice in front of a mirror.	This will enable patient to see and evaluate lip and tongue movement.
Provide a written handout that lists and describes the preceding exercises. Encourage patient to perform them hourly while awake.	These measures reinforce patient's knowledge.
Teach importance of stating feelings verbally. Encourage use of a mirror to practice expressing emotions such as happiness and displeasure.	Monotone speech and lack of facial expression impede nonverbal communication.
Advise patients to face the people to whom they are speaking and speak for themselves and not let others speak for them.	Individuals who have difficulty speaking often remain quiet and let others talk for them.

••• **Related NIC and NOC labels:** *NIC:* Health Education; Self-Modification Assistance; Exercise Promotion *NOC:* Health Promoting Behavior

Nursing Diagnosis:

Deficient Knowledge:

Deep brain stimulation

Desired Outcome: Following the explanation, patient verbalizes accurate understanding of the deep brain stimulation procedure and general follow-up care.

INTERVENTIONS	RATIONALES
Explain that the neurostimulator is an implantable pulse generator powered by a small battery that is implanted subcutaneously near the clavicle. The stimulation parameter is set to optimize symptom management with minimum adverse effects.	Deep brain electrostimulation is used preferentially over ablative procedures (e.g., stereotactic pallidotomy) because it has the same effect without actually destroying parts of the brain. Stimulation of the thalamus helps with tremors. Globus pallidus stimulation works better in controlling rigidity and balance and reduces medication side effects, leading to better drug tolerance, but it does not actually reduce the amount of medication given. Stimulation of the subthalamic nucleus (STN) helps with all parkinsonian symptoms and enables a reduction in medication. STN is the preferred target for deep brain stimulation. The patient switches stimulation on/off with a magnet.
Explain that health care provider follow-up is essential.	Adverse effects may include paraesthesia, muscle contractions, double vision, and mood disturbances, all of which are usually transient. It is seldom possible to alleviate completely all PD symptoms with the stimulator alone. Therefore medication may be needed and adjustments made for the first few months.
Advise that the sudden appearance of additional parkinsonian symptoms may be the only indicator of battery failure.	There are handheld devices that enable determination of the on/off status of the neurostimulator as well as battery charge status.
Advise that turning the neurostimulator off at night to conserve the battery is not recommended.	Some symptoms, such as rigidity, respond only to continuous stimulation.
Explain that ineffective stimulation may signal incorrect lead placement, poor anchoring, and drifting of leads.	This may necessitate removal for accurate repositioning of the electrodes.
Teach that adverse effects resulting from stimulation of nearby structures are corrected by reducing the amount of stimulation.	These include tingling of the head or hand, depression, slurred speech, loss of balance or muscle tone, and double vision. Patient should see health care provider for adjustments.

Continued

INTERVENTIONS	RATIONALES
Explain that excessive STN stimulation may cause disabling dyskinesia.	This would be a valid reason for turning off the device until reprogramming can be performed.
Caution patient that some devices, such as theft detectors and screening devices found in airports, department stores, and public libraries can cause the neurostimulator to switch on or off. Ultrasonic dental equipment and electrocautery also may affect the device.	Usually, this only causes an uncomfortable sensation. However, symptoms could worsen suddenly. Patient always should carry the identification card given with the device and use it to request assistance to bypass those devices. Computers and cellular phones do not interfere with the device.
Caution that patient should avoid activities that may result in blunt trauma to the implanted device area.	This will help prevent loss of function of implant generator or leads.
Caution patients they cannot undergo chest or thoracic magnetic resonance imaging (MRI) scan because of possible movement of the leads or diathermy (shortwave or microwave).	MRI scan can heat up the wires and leads, resulting in serious injury or death.
Instruct in use of magnet to activate and deactivate the stimulator.	Magnet may damage televisions, credit cards, and computer disks and therefore should be kept at least 1 foot away from these items.

●●● **Related NIC and NOC labels**: *NIC:* Teaching: Procedure/Treatment; Teaching: Individual *NOC:* Knowledge: Treatment Procedure

ADDITIONAL NURSING DIAGNOSES/ PROBLEMS:

"Perioperative Care" for patients undergoing surgery   p. 45

"Prolonged Bedrest" for patients with varying degrees of immobility   p. 61

"Psychosocial Support"   p. 73

"Psychosocial Support for the Patient's Family and Significant Other"   p. 87

"Older Adult Care" for **Risk for Aspiration**   p. 96

Impaired Swallowing   p. 267

"General Care of Patients with Neurologic Disorders" for **Impaired Tissue Integrity:** Corneal   p. 270

Risk for Deficient Fluid Volume   p. 271

Imbalanced Nutrition   p. 272

Impaired Verbal Communication   p. 275

Self-Care Deficit   p. 277

Constipation   p. 277

"Pressure Ulcers"   p. 562

✓ PATIENT-FAMILY TEACHING AND DISCHARGE PLANNING

When providing patient-family teaching, focus on sensory information, avoid giving excessive information, and initiate a visiting nurse referral for necessary follow-up teaching. Include verbal and written information about the following:

✓ Referrals to community resources, such as local and national Parkinson's Society chapters, public health nurse, visiting nurses association, community support groups, social workers, psychologic therapy, vocational rehabilitation agency, home health agencies, and extended and skilled care facilities. Additional general information can be obtained by contacting the following organizations:

- The American Parkinson Disease Association, Inc., at *www.apdaparkinson.com*
- Parkinson's Disease Foundation, Inc., at *www.pdf.org*
- National Parkinson Foundation, Inc., at *www.parkinson.org*

✓ Importance of avoiding certain medications that can worsen extrapyramidal symptoms. Examples include phenothiazines, prochlorperazine, metoclopramide, chlorpromazine, methyldopas, tetrabenazine, haloperidol, and reserpine. An exception is ethopropazine, which is a phenothiazine derivative that does not increase extrapyramidal effects and is used to treat PD symptoms.

✓ Speech therapy tips for communication related to dysarthria and for swallowing precautions.

✓ Related safety measures and fall prevention for patients with bradykinesia, muscle rigidity, and tremors.

✓ Emphasis that disability may be prevented or delayed through exercises and medications.

✓ Evaluation of home environment and tips for home accident prevention.

✓ Measures to prevent or lessen postural hypotension.

✓ Signs and symptoms of neuroleptic malignant and acute akinesia and the need for immediate medical attention.

✓ For other interventions, see "Patient-Family Teaching and Discharge Planning" (third through tenth entries only), in "Multiple Sclerosis," p. 311.

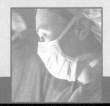

Seizures and Epilepsy 40

OVERVIEW/PATHOPHYSIOLOGY

Seizures result from an abnormal, uncontrolled electrical discharge from the neurons of the cerebral cortex in response to a stimulus. If the activity is localized in one portion of the brain, the individual will have a partial seizure, but when it is widespread and diffuse, a generalized seizure occurs. Symptoms vary widely, depending on the involved area of the cerebral cortex. Seizures are generally manifested as an alteration in sensation, behavior, movement, perception, or consciousness lasting from seconds to several minutes. A seizure can be an isolated incident that may not recur once the underlying cause is corrected (e.g., fever, alcohol withdrawal). *Epilepsy* is the term used for recurrent, unprovoked seizures.

Seizure threshold refers to the amount of stimulation needed to cause neural activity. Although anyone can have a seizure if the stimulus is sufficient, the seizure threshold is lowered in some individuals and this may result in spontaneous seizures. Potential causes for lowered seizure threshold include congenital defects; craniocerebral trauma, particularly that from a penetrating wound; subarachnoid hemorrhage; stroke; intracranial tumors; infections, such as meningitis or encephalitis; exposure to toxins, such as lead; hypoxia; alcohol or other drug withdrawal; and metabolic and endocrine disorders, such as hypoglycemia, hypocalcemia, uremia, hypoparathyroidism, excessive hydration, and fever. Phenothiazine, tricyclic antidepressants, and alcohol usage increase risk of seizure by lowering the seizure threshold. For susceptible individuals, triggers may include emotional tension or stress; physical stimulation, such as loud music, bright flashing lights, and some videos; lack of sleep or food; fatigue; menses or pregnancy; and excessive drug/alcohol use. If a trigger stimulus is identified, the individual has what is termed *reflex epilepsy*.

Although a seizure itself generally is not fatal, individuals can be injured by hitting their heads or breaking bones if they lose consciousness and fall to the ground. Seizure activity increases cerebral O_2 consumption by 60% and cerebral blood flow by 250%. Instances of prolonged and repeated generalized seizures, *status epilepticus (SE)*, can be life threatening because apnea, hypoxia, acidosis, cerebral edema, dysrhythmias, and cardiovascular collapse can occur.

HEALTH CARE SETTING

Primary care with possible hospitalization for complications of therapy, continuous diagnostic video electroencephalogram (EEG) monitoring during pharmacologic or surgical interventions, or intensive care unit (ICU) for SE

ASSESSMENT

It is important to obtain an accurate description of seizure characteristics and duration, as well as any antecedent events, precipitating factors, and postictal phase. There are many clinical types of seizures, but the following are the most serious or common.

Generalized tonic-clonic (grand mal): Caused by bilateral electrical activity, usually symmetrical from onset, and always involves loss of consciousness. A possible prodromal phase of increased irritability, tension, mood changes, or headache may precede the seizure by hours or days. Patients may experience an aura (a sensory warning, such as a sound, odor, or flash of light) immediately preceding the seizure by seconds or minutes. The seizure usually does not last more than 2-5 min and includes the following phases:

- *Tonic (rigid/contracted muscles /extended limbs):* Often lasts only 15 sec, usually subsiding in less than 1 min. Symptoms include loss of consciousness, clenched jaws (potential for tongue to be bitten), apnea (may hear a cry as air is forced out of the lungs), and cyanosis. The patient may be incontinent, and pupils may dilate and become nonreactive to light.
- *Clonic (rhythmic contraction and relaxation of extremities and muscles):* May subside in 30 sec but can last 2-4 min. Eyes roll upward, and excessive salivation results in foaming at the mouth. During this phase, the potential is greatest for biting the tongue.
- *Postictal:* The first few minutes after the seizure, the individual may be limp and nonresponsive. Pupils begin to react to light and return to their normal size. After about 5 min, patients may be sleepy, semiconscious, confused, unable to speak clearly, and uncoordinated; have a headache; complain of muscle aches; and have no recollection of the seizure event. This phase usually lasts less than 15 min. Temporary weakness, dysphasia, or hemianopia lasting up to 24 hr after the seizure may be experienced.

Generalized absence (petit mal): Patient has momentary loss of awareness and consciousness with abrupt cessation of voluntary muscle activity. Patient may appear to be daydreaming with a vacant stare and may experience facial, eyelid, or hand twitching. Patient usually does not lose general body muscle tone and so does not fall. The individual resumes previous activity when the seizure ends. There is usually no memory of the seizure, and patients may have difficulty reorienting after the seizure event. This type of seizure can last 1-10 sec, may occur up to 100 times/day, and usually resolves by puberty.

Generalized myoclonic: Sudden, very brief contraction or jerking of muscles or muscle groups. Individuals may have a very brief, momentary loss of consciousness with some postictal confusion.

Partial simple motor (focal motor seizures): An irritative focus located in the motor cortex of the frontal lobe causes clonic movement in a particular part of the body, such as the hands or face. If the seizure activity spreads or marches in an orderly fashion to an adjacent area (e.g., hands to arms to shoulders), the seizure is termed a *focal motor seizure with jacksonian march.* The seizure usually lasts several seconds to minutes. There is no loss of consciousness. Other simple, partial seizures include those with somatosensory symptoms (e.g., smells, sounds), autonomic symptoms (e.g., tachycardia, tachypnea, diaphoresis, goose bumps [piloerection], pallor, flushing), or psychic symptoms (e.g., fear, déjà vu).

Partial complex seizure (psychomotor, "temporal lobe"): Generally lasts 1-4 min and involves impaired consciousness and a postictal state of confusion lasting several minutes. However, the individual does not fall to the ground, is able to interact with the environment, exhibits purposeful but inappropriate movements or behavior, and has no memory of the event. The individual will perform such automatisms as lip smacking, chewing, facial grimacing, picking, or swallowing movements. These patients may experience and remember various sensory or emotional hallucinations or sensations that occur immediately before the seizure, such as smells; ringing or hissing sounds; or feelings of déjà vu, fear, or pleasure.

Status epilepticus: State of continuous seizure activity lasting more than 5 min or two or more recurring seizures in which the individual does not completely recover baseline neurologic functioning between seizures. Individuals who suddenly stop taking their antiepilepsy medication are likely to develop this condition. Other common causes are drug withdrawal (e.g., alcohol, sedatives) and fever. This is a medical emergency, especially with tonic-clonic seizures, resulting in such potential complications as cerebral anoxia and edema, aspiration, rhabdomyolysis, hyperthermia, and exhaustion. Brain injury may occur in 20-30 min, and irreversible damage may occur in 60 min. Death may ensue. SE can occur in the absence of movement. The patient does not regain consciousness. This nonconvulsive SE may not be life threatening, but it can cause brain damage and will require continuous EEG monitoring. Expect patients in SE to be transferred to ICU.

Other classifications: Seizures also can be classified according to epileptic syndrome (e.g., generalized epilepsies, idiopathic with age-related onset). Establishing the correct diagnosis of seizure type and, when possible, epilepsy syndrome, will help tailor effective antiepilepsy drugs (AEDs) and treatment.

DIAGNOSTIC TESTS

Because a variety of problems can precipitate seizures, testing may be extensive. Common tests for initial workup include the following:

Laboratory tests: To rule out metabolic causes, such as hypoglycemia, hyponatremia, or hypocalcemia; kidney and liver problems; toxicology screens; and AED level.

EEG—both sleeping and awake: To reveal abnormal patterns of electrical activity, particularly with such stimuli as flashing lights or hyperventilation. Ambulatory EEGs may record brain activity for 48-72 hr, and 24-hr continuous EEG monitoring with video recording may show association of brain activity with the observed seizure. Generalized tonic-clonic seizures show up as high, fast-voltage spikes in all leads. A normal EEG does not rule out seizures.

MRI scan: To show structural lesions causing seizures; also may reveal a space-occupying lesion such as a tumor or hematoma. Fast fluid-attenuated inversion-recovery (FLAIR) magnetic resonance imaging (MRI) may be particularly sensitive in finding tumors.

Positron emission tomography: To check for areas of cerebral glucose hypometabolism that correlate with the irritative seizure-causing focus. This test is useful in partial seizures but is available only in a few centers.

CT scan: To check for presence of a space-occupying lesion, such as a tumor or hematoma.

Skull x-ray examination: To reveal fractures, tumors, calcifications, or congenital anomalies (pineal shift, ventricular deformity).

Lumbar puncture and cerebrospinal fluid analysis: If infection such as meningitis is suspected. It also can rule out increased intracranial pressure and determine brain levels of gamma-aminobutyric acid.

New diagnostic technologies and combining of technologies: Have aided in localizing epileptic activity more precisely. Some of these include the following:

- *Functional MRI (fMRI):* Enables direct observation of cerebral blood flow (CBF) changes associated with cognitive, sensory, and motor processes and generally has replaced the intracarotid sodium amytal (Wada's) test to determine hemispheric dominance and function.
- *Simultaneous EEG-correlated functional MRI (EEG/fMRI):* During this test, blood oxygen level–dependent MRI focal changes match up to changes in blood flow.
- *Subtraction ictal and postictal imaging SPECT co-registered on MRI:* To assess focal changes in cerebral perfusion, which may identify eleptogenic areas.
- *Magnetic source imaging:* Magnetoencephalography [MEG] information is superimposed on a co-recorded MRI scan for a noninvasive functional/anatomic imaging technique.

- *EEG dipole source modeling:* Data from EEG and MEG are taken to locate origin of epileptic paroxysm.
- *Methohexital suppression test:* Can distinguish the primary focus in temporal lobe epilepsy with multifocal discharges.
- *Optical imaging:* Noninvasive tool to analyze seizure activity by measuring dynamic changes in blood flow and oxygen during epileptic activity.

- *Invasive intracranial EEG monitoring:* Depth electrodes are placed in brain tissue, and a subdural "grid" is applied directly to the cortical surface to evaluate deep epileptic sources.

Nursing Diagnosis:

Risk for Trauma

related to oral, musculoskeletal, and airway vulnerability secondary to seizure activity

Desired Outcomes: Patient exhibits no signs of oral or musculoskeletal tissue injury or airway compromise after the seizure. Before hospital discharge, patient's significant other verbalizes knowledge of actions necessary during seizure activity.

INTERVENTIONS	RATIONALES
Seizure precautions	
Pad side rails with blankets or pillows. Keep side rails up and bed in its lowest position when patient is in bed. Keep bed, wheelchair, or stretcher brakes locked.	These actions promote safety and protect the patient from trauma in case a seizure occurs.
Tape a soft rubber oral airway to the bedside. Remove wooden tongue depressors (if used, they may splinter). Keep suction and oxygen equipment readily available.	These measures enable a patent airway, prevent hypoxia, and protect patient from trauma in case a seizure occurs.
Consider a saline lock for IV access for high-risk patient.	Some AEDs must be administered IV, especially as a loading dose or in case of sustained seizure activity.
Use electronic tympanic thermometers for patients at high risk for seizure. If only breakable thermometers are available, take temperature via axillary or rectal route.	Glass or other breakable oral thermometers should be avoided when taking patient's temperature because of the harm they could cause patient if they break.
Caution patients to lie down and push call button if they experience prodromal or aural warning. Keep call light within reach.	Prodromal or aural warnings precede seizures in many patients.
Encourage patient to empty mouth of dentures or foreign objects.	This helps prevent choking in case a seizure occurs.
Do not allow unsupervised smoking.	This restriction prevents fire damage to patient and surroundings if a seizure occurs.
Evaluate need for and provide protective headgear as indicated.	This protects patient's head in case of a seizure.
During the seizure	
Remain with patient and stay calm. Observe for, record, and report type, duration, and characteristics of seizure activity and any postseizure response.	Seizure activity should be documented in detail to aid in management and differentiation of seizure type and identification of triggering factors. This should include, as appropriate, precipitating event, aura, initial location and progression, automatisms, type and duration of movement, changes in level of consciousness, eye movement (e.g., deviation, nystagmus), pupil size and reaction, bowel and bladder incontinence, head deviation, tongue deviation, or teeth clenching.
Prevent or break the fall and ease patient to floor if seizure occurs while patient is out of bed.	These actions promote patient's physical safety.
Keep patient in bed if seizure occurs while there, and lower head of bed to a flat position.	Flattening patient's position reduces risk of falling out of bed during seizure activity.
If patient's jaws are clenched, do not force an object between the teeth.	Forcing objects into patient's mouth can break teeth or lacerate oral mucous membranes.
If able to do so safely and without damage to oral tissue, insert an airway.	An airway will serve as a bite block to prevent lip and tongue laceration.
As an alternative to an airway, use a rolled washcloth.	A rolled washcloth will help prevent lip and tongue biting.

Continued

INTERVENTIONS	RATIONALES
Never put your fingers in patient's mouth.	Patient may bite your fingers.
Be sure patient's head position does not occlude airway. Remove from environment objects (e.g., chairs) that patient may strike. Pad floors to protect patient's arms and legs. Remove patient's glasses.	These measures protect patient's airway from occlusion and body from injury during the seizure. A towel folded flat or hands may be used to cushion the head from striking the ground.
Do not restrain patient but rather guide patient's movements gently.	This action helps prevent injury caused by flailing.
Roll patient into a side-lying position. Use head-tilt/chin-lift maneuver. Provide O_2 and suction as needed.	This promotes drainage of secretions, maintains a patent airway, and prevents hypoxia.
Loosen tight clothing, collar, or belt.	This prevents trauma/hypoxia caused by constrictive clothing.
Maintain patient's privacy. Clear nonessential people from the room.	Seizures likely are embarrassing for the patient.
Administer antiepilepsy drugs as prescribed.	IV administration of prescribed AED can shorten length and prevent reoccurrence of seizures.

After the seizure

Determine if patient has had SE: that is, the seizure is continuous (longer than 5 min), longer than patient's usual length of time by 1 or 2 min, or patient has two or more seizures without recovering baseline neurologic functioning between seizures.	This condition is life threatening and can cause cerebral anoxia and edema, aspiration, hyperthermia, and exhaustion. Anticipate transfer to ICU but do not delay initial interventions, including administration of prescribed IV lorazepam or diazepam.
Reassure and gently reorient patient. Check neurologic status and vital signs (VS).	During the postictal period that follows the seizure, patient will need to be reoriented and reassured because some memory lapse will have occurred during the event.
Ask patient if an aura preceded seizure activity. Record this information and postictal characteristics.	An aura is a sensory warning such as a sound, odor, or flash of light. It can be used in the future to warn patient of an impending seizure.
Provide a quiet, calm environment. Keep talk simple and to a minimum. Speak slowly and with pauses between sentences.	Sounds and stimuli can be confusing to the awakening patient. Repetition may be necessary if patient is confused.
Use room light that is behind, not above, patient.	This prevents additional seizures triggered by the light and promotes patient comfort.
Do not offer food or drink until patient is fully awake.	This prevents vomiting/aspiration.
Check patient's tongue for lacerations and body for injuries. Monitor for weakness or paralysis, dysphasia, or visual disturbances.	These are potential occurrences during a seizure.
Monitor urine for red or cola color.	Rhabdomyolysis or myoglobinuria may occur from muscle trauma.
If patient vomited during the seizure, notify health care provider.	This is a sign that aspiration can occur with subsequent seizures.
Check fingerstick blood glucose.	Hypoglycemia is a potential metabolic cause of the seizure.
Obtain serum laboratory tests as prescribed.	Electrolyte disorders such as hyponatremia and hypocalcemia can trigger a seizure.
Stay with patient for 15-20 min postseizure.	Sudden unexplained death in epileptic patients is not well understood, but it may be related to central respiratory apnea that can occur with a seizure.
Provide significant other with verbal and written information for the preceding interventions.	Significant other is likely to be in patient's presence during subsequent seizures. If well informed, he or she will be able to protect patient from trauma and life-threatening complications.

If SE has occurred:

Implement the ABCs: Assess airway, breathing, and circulation. Initiate O_2 therapy, oral airway suctioning, and intubation as needed.	These actions help maintain the airway and prevent hypoxia.
Place patient in a side-lying position.	Positioning on the side reduces aspiration risk in case of vomiting.
Monitor VS, pulse oximetry, heart rhythm, and arterial blood gas values.	This assessment enables early detection of hypoxia, dysrhythmias, and overall hemodynamics.
Obtain IV access.	IV access ensures administration of fluids and medications.
Assess blood glucose (fingerstick) and administer IV glucose (and thiamine) as appropriate.	This will reverse hypoglycemia, a potential cause of the seizure. If alcohol withdrawal is suspected or a possibility, thiamine should be given before dextrose to protect against an exacerbation of Wernicke's encephalopathy.

Continued

INTERVENTIONS	RATIONALES
As indicated, draw blood for serum laboratory studies.	Hypoglycemia and electrolyte (e.g., hyponatremia, hypocalcemia, hypomagnesia) or metabolic imbalances (kidney, liver) may be causing seizures. Serum drug screens are performed to assess serum AED level and determine presence of alcohol or other drugs that may be causing the seizures.
Ensure priority administration of IV lorazepam or diazepam within 3-10 min.	Initially the drug is given as a slow bolus. Sublingual lorazepam or rectal diazepam gel may be given if there is no IV access. If the seizure stops, this may be the extent of the interventions if patient is already on AEDs.
Ensure priority administration of IV fosphenytoin (loading dose).	This drug is given if patient is not already on AEDs or if the seizure continues.
Administer loading dose of fosphenytoin no faster than 150 mg phenytoin equivalents/min.	This prevents hypotension caused by faster loading doses.
Administer IV phenobarbital if prescribed.	Phenobarbital is prescribed if diazepam and phenytoin are unsuccessful or if patient is allergic to other drugs.
Monitor for signs of respiratory depression.	This is a possible side effect of phenobarbital.

••• **Related NIC and NOC labels:** *NIC:* Environmental Management: Safety; Fall Prevention; Home Maintenance Assistance; Vital Signs Monitoring; Seizure Precautions *NOC:* Safety Status: Physical Injury

Nursing Diagnosis:

Deficient Knowledge:

Life-threatening environmental factors and preventive measures for seizures

Desired Outcomes: Before hospital discharge, patient verbalizes accurate information about measures that may prevent seizures and environmental factors that can be life threatening in the presence of seizures. Patient exhibits health care measures that reflect this knowledge.

INTERVENTIONS	RATIONALES
Assess knowledge of measures that can prevent seizures and environmental hazards that can be life threatening in the presence of seizure activity. Provide or clarify information as indicated.	This assessment enables nurse to provide or clarify information as indicated and facilitates development of an individualized teaching plan.
Advise patient to check into state regulations about automobile operation.	Most states require 3 months to 2 seizure-free years before an individual can obtain a driver's license.
Caution patient to refrain from operating heavy or dangerous equipment, swimming, climbing excessive heights, and possibly even tub bathing until he or she is seizure free for amount of time specified by health care provider.	These restrictions prevent injury that can result while performing these activities in case a seizure occurs.
Teach patient never to swim alone regardless of amount of time he or she has been seizure free.	This makes rescue easier if a seizure occurs. Patient should swim only in shallow water and in the company of a strong swimmer.
Advise patient to turn temperature of hot water heaters down.	This prevents scalding if a seizure occurs in the shower.
Encourage stress management, progressive relaxation techniques, and diaphragmatic respiratory training.	These measures help control emotional stress and hyperventilation, which can trigger seizures.
Advise patient that some activities, such as climbing or bicycle riding, require careful risk/benefit evaluation.	The patient who decides to ride a bike should wear a helmet and avoid heavy traffic. Contact sports should be avoided.
Encourage vocational assessment and counseling.	The patient's epilepsy may place others at risk in some occupations, such as bus driver or airline pilot.
Advise female patients that seizure activity may change (increase or decrease) during menses or pregnancy (especially at 3-4 months' gestation).	Tonic-clonic seizures have caused fetal death. AEDs are associated with birth defects; however, 90% of women have normal pregnancies and healthy children.

Continued

INTERVENTIONS	RATIONALES
Provide birth control information if requested.	Oral contraceptive effectiveness may be reduced by many AEDs. Intrauterine devices or other methods may be needed. When seizures in women worsen with hormonal changes, suppressing ovulation with medication may be recommended. Women wanting to get pregnant should consult with their health care provider. Monotherapy is preferred. They should be taking folate acid and receive vitamin K during the last 2-4 wk of pregnancy before delivery to avoid neonatal hemorrhage.
Teach that use of stimulants (e.g., caffeine) and depressants (e.g., alcohol) should be avoided.	Their use can change the seizure threshold, and withdrawal from stimulants and depressants can increase likelihood of seizures.
Teach that getting adequate amounts of rest, avoiding physical and emotional stress, maintaining a nutritious and balanced diet and hydration status, and avoiding certain stimuli may help prevent seizure activity.	These are measures that may help prevent seizures. Meals should be spaced throughout the day to prevent hypoglycemia. Overhydration may precipitate seizure activity. Stimuli such as flashing lights, video or computer games, or loud music appear to trigger seizures, and patient should avoid environments that are likely to have these stimuli. Poorly adjusted TVs may trigger seizures and should be fixed. Patients should monitor for and treat fever early during an illness.
Encourage individuals who have seizures that occur without warning to avoid chewing gum or sucking on lozenges.	They may be aspirated during a seizure.
Encourage patient to wear a medical alert bracelet or similar identification or to carry a medical information card.	They provide information to health care professionals if patient is unable to.

••• **Related NIC and NOC labels:** *NIC:* Teaching: Disease Process; Learning Readiness Enhancement; Teaching: Individual; Risk Identification; Health Education; Behavior Modification *NOC:* Knowledge: Disease Process; Knowledge: Health Behaviors; Knowledge: Personal Safety

Nursing Diagnosis:

Deficient Knowledge:

Purpose, precautions, and side effects of AEDs

Desired Outcome: Before hospital discharge, patient verbalizes accurate knowledge about the prescribed AED.

INTERVENTIONS	RATIONALES
Stress importance of taking prescribed AED regularly and on schedule, and not discontinuing medication without health care provider guidance.	Missing a scheduled dose can precipitate a seizure several days later. Stress that abrupt withdrawal of any AED can precipitate seizures and that discontinuing these medications is the most common cause of SE.
Assist patients in finding methods that will help them remember to take their medication and monitor their drug supply to avoid running out.	AEDs may be necessary for duration of patient's life. Medications cannot be taken "as-needed," and lack of seizures does not mean the drug is unnecessary.
Explain concept of drug half-life and steady blood levels.	It is important to maintain a therapeutic blood level of the AED to manage seizures.
Caution patients to consult health care provider before changing from a trade name to a generic medication and to avoid abrupt withdrawal.	Drugs differ in amount of time they remain in the body and reach peak activity, and there may be differences in bioavailability. Drugs are usually withdrawn slowly over 1-2 weeks rather than abruptly stopped, which could result in seizures.
Stress importance of informing health care provider about side effects and keeping appointments for periodic laboratory work.	Laboratory tests will reveal whether blood levels of AEDs are therapeutic. Many side effects are dose related, and medication can be adjusted based on AED blood levels and symptoms.
Teach patient to report immediately any bruising, bleeding, jaundice, or rash.	Many AEDs can cause blood dyscrasias or liver damage.

Continued

INTERVENTIONS | ## RATIONALES

INTERVENTIONS	RATIONALES
Supplement with vitamin K, vitamin D, and folic acid if prescribed.	Certain AEDs, such as phenytoin, decrease absorption of folic acid and metabolism of vitamins D and K, which can lead to deficiencies. For pregnant women, folic acid supplementation is critical to prevent birth defects. Vitamin K may be given to pregnant women 1 mo before and during delivery to prevent neonatal hemorrhage.
Teach patient that grapefruit juice should be avoided.	It can inhibit hepatic metabolism of many AEDs and affect drug level.
Advise that calcium supplementation should not be taken within about 2 hr of AEDs.	AEDs taken at the same time as calcium supplements may decrease absorption and effects of both medicines. Vitamin D and calcium supplementation are used to prevent osteomalacia (soft bone) associated with some AEDs such as phenytoin, valproic acid, and carbamazepine. Periodic bone density monitoring is recommended.
Advise patient to avoid activities that require alertness until central nervous system (CNS) response to the medication has been determined.	AEDs may make people drowsy. Splitting the dose or giving main dose at bedtime may help.
Teach patient to take the drug with food or large amounts of liquid.	Nausea and vomiting are common side effects of most AEDs.
Advise patients taking valproic acid, topiramate, and zonisamide not to chew the medication.	These AEDs may irritate oral mucous membrane.
Advise patients taking valproic acid that this drug may produce a false-positive test for urine ketones.	It is important for patients, especially those with diabetes, to know this because ketone assessment is one aspect of managing their diabetes.
Advise patient that any visual changes or pain should be reported immediately.	With valproic acid, a visual change may signal ocular toxicity. With topiramate, blurred vision or difficulty seeing may indicate glaucoma. Patients on vigabatrin must have periodic visual field testing because irreversible damage to the retina can occur. Prompt reporting and timely intervention may preserve vision.
Instruct patient to notify health care provider if a significant weight gain or weight loss occurs.	A change in dose or scheduling may be necessary.
Teach patient to avoid alcoholic beverages and over-the-counter (OTC) medications containing alcohol.	Long-term alcohol use stimulates the body to metabolize phenytoin more quickly, thus lowering the seizure threshold because of decreased plasma phenytoin levels.
Caution patients taking phenobarbital or primidone to avoid alcohol.	Alcohol potentiates the CNS depressant effects of these drugs.
Caution patient to avoid OTC medications.	AEDs are potentiated or inhibited by many other drugs, including aspirin and antihistamines, and may affect potency of other medications as well.
Instruct patient to report uncoordinated movement (ataxia), diplopia, nystagmus, and dizziness.	These are other side effects common to AEDs that may necessitate drug, dosage, or schedule change.
Teach patients who take carbamazepine, ethosuximide, or zonisamide to report immediately fever, mouth ulcers, sore throat, peripheral edema, dark urine, bruising, or bleeding.	These are possible side effects that may necessitate drug, dose, or schedule change.
Advise patients taking phenytoin to perform frequent oral hygiene with gum massage and gentle flossing and brush teeth 3-4 times/day with a soft toothbrush. Teach patient to report immediately any measles-like rash.	Phenytoin can cause gingival hypertrophy and rash.
Caution patients taking phenytoin that there are two types of this drug and neither should be substituted for the other.	It is important not to confuse extended-release phenytoin (e.g., Dilantin Kapseal) with prompt-release phenytoin (e.g., Dilantin). Doing so may cause dangerous underdose or overdose.
Caution that generic phenytoin should not be substituted for Dilantin Kapseal.	Dilantin Kapseal is absorbed more slowly and is longer acting.
Monitor for increased body hair with phenytoin.	Hair removal creams can be used if increased hair is a problem.
Monitor for hyperglycemia with phenytoin.	Phenytoin blocks the release of insulin, which may cause increased blood sugar levels. Persons with diabetes in particular may need adjustments in their diabetic medications.

Continued

INTERVENTIONS	RATIONALES
Encourage patient to keep a drug and seizure chart diary.	This will help detect trend of seizures, which will enable health care provider to determine if current treatment is at a therapeutic level.
	Patients with intractable seizures that are not controlled by medication, excision, ablation of known epileptogenic areas (e.g., scar removal), or cortical resection (e.g., temporal lobectomy or corpus callostomy) may undergo certain procedures in an attempt to obtain seizure control. One example is multiple subpial transections consisting of horizontal cuts to prevent spread of the seizure impulse. Implanted vagus nerve stimulation (VNS) may have an anticonvulsant effect on partial seizures. Surgical procedures require a craniotomy (see "Traumatic Brain Injury," p. 367).

••• **Related NIC and NOC labels:** *NIC:* Teaching: Prescribed Medication; Medication Management *NOC:* Knowledge: Medication

Nursing Diagnosis:

Noncompliance: Therapy

related to denial of the illness or perceived negative consequences of the treatment regimen secondary to social stigma, negative side effects of antiepilepsy medications, or difficulty with making necessary lifestyle changes

Desired Outcome: Before hospital discharge, patient verbalizes knowledge about the disease process and treatment plan, acknowledges consequences of continued nonadhering behavior, explains the experience that caused altering of the prescribed behavior, describes appropriate treatment of side effects or appropriate alternatives, and exhibits health care measures that reflect this knowledge, following an agreed-on plan of care.

INTERVENTIONS	RATIONALES
Assess patient's understanding of the disease process, medical management, and treatment plan. Explain or clarify information as indicated.	This assessment enables nurse to explain or clarify information as indicated and facilitates development of an individualized care plan that promotes adherence.
Assess for causes of nonadherence, such as financial constraints, inconvenience, forgetfulness or memory problems, medication side effects, misunderstanding of instructions, or difficulty making significant lifestyle changes or following medication schedule.	Once causes are identified, the nurse can then focus the care plan accordingly.
Explain drug half-life and concept of a steady blood level. Explain importance of health care provider guidance if medication is stopped for any reason. Instruct and provide written instructions for patient on how to contact health care provider and importance of health care provider and laboratory follow-up. Explain what to do if a dose is missed and how to refill a prescription if medication is lost or depleted.	Intermittent medication use may be informal experimentation or an effort to gain control. Explanation of consequences of nonadherence helps ensure awareness that stopping medications can be life threatening (e.g., cause SE).
Promote patient's expression of feelings (e.g., dependence, powerlessness, embarrassment, being different). In addition, evaluate patient's perception of effectiveness or ineffectiveness of treatment.	This will help clarify patient's perception of vulnerability to the disease process and signs of denial of the illness.
Confront myths and stigmas. Provide realistic assessment of risks, and counter misconceptions.	This will help determine if a value, cultural conflict, or spiritual conflict is causing nonadherence.
Discuss methods of dealing with common problems, such as obtaining insurance and job or workplace discrimination.	Helping to eliminate barriers and problems optimally will promote adherence.

Continued

INTERVENTIONS	RATIONALES
Assess patient's support systems.	This will help determine if a family disruption pattern (whether or not it is caused by patient's illness) is making adherence difficult and "not worth it."
After the reason for nonadherence is found, intervene accordingly. If it appears that changing medical treatment plan (e.g., in scheduling medications) may promote adherence, discuss this possibility with health care provider. Provide patient with information about interventions that can minimize drug side effects (e.g., taking drug with food or large amounts of liquid to minimize gastric distress).	All may help facilitate adherence.
Encourage involvement with support systems such as local epilepsy centers and national organizations.	Many people appreciate the support of others with the same condition. Feeling less alone and supported by others may promote adherence.
If indicated, suggest counseling or psychotherapy.	This may help patients with poor self-concept or coping difficulties related to the diagnosis that may be a cause of the nonadherence.

••• **Related NIC and NOC labels:** *NIC:* Patient Counseling; Behavior Modification; Learning Facilitation; Support System Enhancement; Teaching: Disease Process; Family Involvement Promotion; Coping Enhancement; Family Support *NOC:* Compliance Behavior; Adherence Behavior

---

ADDITIONAL NURSING DIAGNOSES/ PROBLEMS:

"Psychosocial Support" for **Ineffective Coping** and   p. 76
  Disturbed Body Image

"Psychosocial Support for the Patient's Family and   p. 88
  Significant Other" for **Interrupted Family
  Processes**

 PATIENT-FAMILY TEACHING AND DISCHARGE PLANNING

When providing patient-family teaching, focus on sensory information, avoid giving excessive information, and initiate a visiting nurse referral for necessary follow-up teaching. Include verbal and written information about the following:

✓ Reinforcement of knowledge of disease process, pathophysiology, symptoms, and precipitating or aggravating factors.

✓ Medications, including drug name, purpose, dosage, schedule, precautions, and potential side effects. Also discuss drug-drug, herb-drug, and food-drug interactions and importance of adhering to medication routine. Some herbs (ginkgo, valerian root, evening primrose, ephedra) may be proconvulsant and should be avoided. Supplements such as taurine, selenium, and vitamin D and Asian herbs such as Saiko-keishi mixture are being investigated for possible benefit.

✓ Importance of follow-up care and keeping medical appointments. Stress that use of AEDs necessitates periodic monitoring of blood levels to ensure therapeutic medication levels and assessment for side effects. Instruct patient to keep emergency contact numbers for health care provider.

✓ Seizure first aid. An uncomplicated convulsive seizure in an individual known to have epilepsy is not necessarily a medical emergency. On average, these people can continue about their business after a rest period. An ambulance should be called or medical attention sought if the seizure happens in water; if the individual is injured, pregnant, or diabetic; if the seizure lasts longer than 5 min; if a second seizure starts; if consciousness does not begin to return; or if there is any question the seizure may have been caused by something other than epilepsy.

✓ Environmental factors that can be life threatening in the presence of seizures, measures that may help prevent seizures, and safety interventions during seizures. Review state and local laws that apply to individuals with seizure disorders. Review home and personal safety tips.

✓ Employment or vocational counseling as needed. Discuss need to avoid overprotection and maintain, as possible, normal work and recreation. Review or provide information regarding the Americans with Disabilities Act.

✓ Risks of using AEDs during pregnancy. Provide birth control information or genetic counseling referral as requested.

✓ Benefits of joining local support groups. Provide the following addresses as appropriate:
- Epilepsy Foundation at *www.efa.org*
- *www.epilepsy.com*
- Epilepsy Information Page: National Institute of Neurological Disorders and Stroke at *www.ninds.nih.gov/disorders/epilepsy/epilepsy.htm*
- Antiepileptic Drug Pregnancy Registry at *www.aedpregnancyregistry.org*
- American Epilepsy Society at *www.aesnet.org*

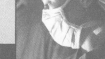

Spinal Cord Injury 41

OVERVIEW/PATHOPHYSIOLOGY

Spinal cord injuries (SCIs) are caused by vertebral fractures or dislocations that sever, lacerate, stretch, or compress the spinal cord and interrupt neuronal function and transmission of nerve impulses. Concussive trauma can cause damage from bruising, swelling, and inflammation. When blood supply to the spinal cord is interrupted, the spinal cord swells in response, and this, along with hemorrhage, can cause additional compression, ischemia, and compromised function. Neurologic deficits resulting from compression may be reversible if the resulting edema and ischemia do not lead to spinal cord degeneration and necrosis. Common causes of injury include motor vehicle accidents, diving or other sporting accidents, falls, and gunshot wounds. SCIs are classified in a number of different ways according to type (open, closed), cause (concussion, contusion, laceration, transection), site (level of spinal cord involved), mechanism of injury (compression, hyperflexion, hyperextension, rotational, penetrating), stability, and degree of spinal cord function loss (complete, incomplete), or syndromes (central cord, Brown-Séquard [lateral], anterior cord, conus medullaris, cauda equina, and posterior cord). A *spinal cord concussion* involves a transient loss of cord function caused by a traumatic event, resulting in immediate flaccid paralysis that resolves completely in a matter of minutes or hours.

Prognosis: Any evidence of voluntary motor function, sensory function, or sacral sensation below the level of injury (lowest level in which motor function and sensation remain intact) indicates an incomplete SCI, with potential for partial or complete recovery. After an acute injury, the spinal cord usually goes into a condition called *spinal shock,* in which there can be total loss of spinal cord function below the level of injury. During spinal shock there is no reflex activity. Resolution of spinal shock with return of reflexes usually occurs within 1-2 wk, but may take 6 mo or more. If there is no evidence of returning motor function after local reflexes have returned, the spinal cord is considered irreversibly damaged. Generally, SCI does not cause immediate death unless it is at C1 through C3, which results in respiratory muscle paralysis. Individuals who survive these injuries require a ventilator for the rest of their lives. If the injury occurs at C4, respiratory difficulties may result in death, although some individuals who have survived the initial injury have been successfully weaned from the ventilator. Injuries

below C4 also can be life threatening because of ascending cord edema, which can cause respiratory muscle paralysis. Immediately after injury, common complications that require treatment include hypotension (systolic blood pressure [SBP] less than 80 mm Hg), bradycardia, paralytic ileus, urinary retention, pneumonia, and stress ulcers. Other long-term, life-threatening complications of SCI include autonomic dysreflexia (AD), pneumonia, decubitus ulcers, sepsis, urinary calculi, and urinary tract infection (UTI).

HEALTH CARE SETTING

Acute care, subacute care, rehabilitation center

ASSESSMENT

There are a variety of neurologic assessment and functional outcome scales, including the American Spinal Injury Association (ASIA) Impairment scale in which the following are described:

- A Complete: No motor or sensory function is preserved in sacral segment S4-S5.
- B Incomplete: No motor but some sensory function is preserved below the neurologic level and includes the sacral segment S4-S5.
- C Incomplete: Motor function is preserved below the neurologic level, and more than half of key muscles below the neurologic level have a muscle grade less than 3 (unable to lift against gravity).
- D Incomplete: Motor function is preserved below the neurologic level, and more than half of key muscles below the neurologic level have a muscle grade of 3 or more (can lift against gravity).
- E Normal: Motor and sensory functions are normal.

Acute indicators: Loss of sensation, weakness, or paralysis below level of injury, localized pain or tenderness over site of injury, headache, hypothermia or hyperthermia, and alterations in bowel and bladder function.

Cervical injury: Possible alterations in level of consciousness (LOC); weakness or paralysis in all four extremities (*tetraparesis* or *tetraplegia,* previously termed *quadriparesis* or *quadriplegia*); and paralysis of respiratory muscles or signs of respiratory problems, such as flaring nostrils and use of accessory muscles for respirations. Any cervical injury can result in low body temperature (to 96° F [35.5° C]), slowed pulse rate (less than 60 bpm) caused by vagal stimulation of the heart, hypotension (SBP less than 80 mm Hg) caused by vasodilation, and decreased peristalsis.

Thoracic and lumbar injuries: Paraparesis/paraplegia or altered sensation in the legs; hand and arm involvement in upper thoracic injuries.

Acute spinal shock: Can last from 2 days to 4-6 mo but usually resolves in 1-2 wk. Spinal shock results from loss of sympathetic nerve outflow and reflex function in all segments below level of injury. Indicators depend on injury severity and include total loss of spinal cord function, loss of skin sensation, flaccid paralysis or absence of reflexes below level of injury, paralytic ileus and constipation secondary to atonic bowel, bladder distention secondary to atonic bladder, bradycardia, low/falling blood pressure (BP) secondary to loss of vasomotor tone and decreased venous return, and anhidrosis (absence of sweating and loss of temperature regulation) below level of injury. Autonomic instability is more dramatic in higher (e.g., cervical) lesions. Resolution of spinal shock is indicated by return of both the bulbocavernosus reflex (slight muscle contraction when glans penis is squeezed or urinary catheter is pulled, causing scrotal retraction) and the anal reflex (anal puckering on digital examination or gentle scratching around the anus). Remaining reflexes may take weeks to return.

Chronic indicators: As spinal shock resolves, muscle tone, reflexes, and some function may return, depending on severity and level of injury. Return of reflexes usually results in muscle spasticity. Chronic autonomic dysfunction may be manifested as fever; mild hypotension; anhidrosis; and alterations in bowel, bladder, and sexual function. Chronic neural pain may occur after SCI and tends to occur as either diffuse pain below level of injury or pain adjacent to level of injury. Injuries at or below L1 may result in permanent flaccid paralysis. Orthostatic hypotension is more typical of lesions above T7.

UMN involvement: Upper motor neurons (UMNs) are nerve cell bodies that originate in high levels of the central nervous system (CNS) and transmit impulses from the brain down the spinal cord. Injury interrupts this impulse transmission, causing muscle or organ dysfunction below level of injury. However, because the injury does not interrupt reflex arcs coming from those muscles or organs to the spinal cord, hypertonic reflexes, clonus paralysis, and spastic paralysis are seen. The patient will have a positive Babinski's reflex.

LMN involvement: Lower motor neurons (LMNs) are anterior horn cell bodies that originate in the spinal cord. LMNs transmit nerve impulses to muscles and organs and are involved in reflex arcs that control involuntary responses. Damage to LMNs will abolish voluntary and reflex responses of muscles and organs, resulting in flaccid paralysis, hypotonia, atrophy, and muscle fibrillations and fasciculations. The patient will have an absent Babinski's reflex. The spinal cord ends at the T12-L1 level. Below that level, a bundle of nerve roots from the spinal cord, called the *cauda equina*, fills the spinal canal. Injuries at or below L1 that damage nerve fiber after it leaves the spinal cord result in flaccid paralysis because of interrupted reflex arc activity.

Bowel and bladder dysfunction: Usually conscious sensation of the need to void or defecate is lost. UMN bowel and bladder involvement results in reflex incontinence. Flaccid LMN bladder involvement causes urinary retention with overflow incontinence. Flaccid LMN bowel involvement causes fecal retention/impaction.

Sexual dysfunction: Degree of dysfunction varies according to degree of completeness and whether injury is UMN or LMN. Males with complete UMN injuries have a loss of psychogenic erection but may have reflex erections. Ejaculation rates with complete UMN injuries are as low as 4%. Females have a loss of psychogenic lubrication but may have reflex lubrication. With complete LMN injuries, about 25% of males will have psychogenic erections but none will have reflex erections. About 50% of both sexes (by questionnaire) say they can experience orgasm regardless of injury level (possibly through other erogenous zones). Incomplete injuries will result in better sexual functioning that may include both erections and ejaculations.

Autonomic dysreflexia: Also known as autonomic hyperreflexia, autonomic dysreflexia (AD) is the exaggerated and unopposed sympathetic response to noxious stimuli below the SCI lesion and can be life threatening as reflex activity returns. AD is seen most commonly in patients with injuries at or above T6, but it has been reported with injuries as low as T8. Signs and symptoms include gross hypertension (BP more than 20 mm Hg above baseline, but BP can be as high as 240-300/150 mm Hg), pounding headache, blurred vision, bradycardia, nausea, and nasal congestion. Above level of injury, flushing and sweating may occur. Below level of injury, piloerection (goose bumps) and skin pallor, which signal vasoconstriction, may be present. Seizures, subarachnoid hemorrhage, stroke, or retinal hemorrhage also may occur.

PHYSICAL ASSESSMENT

Acute (spinal shock): Absence of deep tendon reflexes (DTRs) below level of injury; absence of cremasteric reflex (scratching or light stroking of inner thigh for male patients causes testicle on that side to elevate) for T12 and L1 injuries; absence of penile or anal sphincter reflex.

Chronic: Generally, increased DTRs occur if the spinal cord lesion is of the UMN type.

DIAGNOSTIC TESTS

Complete spine immobilization with a rigid cervical collar and backboard or other firm surface is essential until diagnostic tests rule out injury.

X-ray examination of spine: To delineate fracture, deformity, displacement of vertebrae, and soft tissue masses such as hematomas.

MRI scan: To reveal changes in spinal cord and surrounding soft tissue. Magnetic resonance imaging (MRI) scan evaluation is preferred and considered the "gold" standard for evaluation of degree of injury in patients who can tolerate it.

CT scan: To reveal changes in the spinal cord, vertebrae, and soft tissue surrounding the spine.

ABG/pulmonary function tests: To assess effectiveness of respirations and detect need for O_2 or mechanical ventilation.

Myelography: To show blockage or disruption of the spinal canal and used if other diagnostic examinations are inconclusive. Radiopaque dye is injected into the subarachnoid space of the spine, using a lumbar or cervical puncture.

Cystometry/urodynamic evaluation: To assess bladder capacity and function after resolution of spinal shock for the best type of bladder training program.

Pulmonary fluoroscopy: To evaluate degree of diaphragm movement and effectiveness in individuals with high cervical injuries.

Evoked potential studies (e.g., somatosensory): To help locate level of spinal cord lesion by evaluating integrity of anatomic pathways and connections of the nervous system. Stimulation of a peripheral nerve triggers a discrete electrical response along a neurologic pathway to the brain. Response or lack of response to stimulation is measured in this test.

DVT studies (e.g., venogram, duplex Doppler ultrasound, impedence plethysmography): To monitor for development of deep vein thrombosis (DVT).

Nursing Diagnosis:

Autonomic Dysreflexia (or risk for same)

related to exaggerated unopposed autonomic response to noxious stimuli for individuals with SCI at or above T6

Desired Outcomes: On an ongoing basis, patient is free of AD symptoms as evidenced by BP within patient's baseline range, HR 60-100 bpm, and absence of headache and other clinical indicators of AD. Following instruction, patient and significant other verbalize factors that cause AD, treatment and prevention, and when immediate emergency treatment is indicated.

INTERVENTIONS	RATIONALES
Monitor for indicators of AD, including hypertension (BP more than 20 mm Hg above baseline, but may go as high as 240-300/150 mm Hg), pounding headache, bradycardia, blurred vision, nausea, nasal congestion, flushing and sweating above the level of injury, and pilo-erection (goose bumps) or pallor below level of injury.	AD is a medical emergency that can occur after spinal shock resolution in patients with injuries at or above T6, but cases have been reported in patients with injuries as low as T8.
Remove antiembolism hose.	This enables assessment of the lower extremities. See discussion of "Skin" in this nursing diagnosis.
If AD is suspected, raise head of bed (HOB) immediately to 90 degrees or assist patient into a sitting position.	These actions lower patient's BP and decrease venous return. Seizures, subarachnoid hemorrhage, myocardial infarction (MI), stroke, or retinal hemorrhage can occur if severe hypertensive episode continues.
Call for someone to notify health care provider; stay with patient, and systematically search to identify and relieve the noxious stimulus. Speed is essential.	The noxious stimulus (e.g., distended bladder) must be found and alleviated as quickly as possible in order to remove the stimulus triggering AD.
Monitor BP q3-5min during hypertensive episode.	This assesses trend of the BP.
Remain calm and supportive of patient and significant other.	They will be very anxious.
Assess the following sites for causes, and implement measures for removing the noxious stimulus.	
Bladder: Distention, UTI, calculus and other obstructions, bladder spasms, catheterization, or bladder irrigations performed too quickly or with too cold a liquid.	Problems with the bladder are the most likely cause of AD.
Do not use Credé's method for a distended bladder.	The increased bladder pressure could further stimulate the reflex and worsen the condition.
Catheterize patient (ideally using anesthetic jelly) if there is a possibility or question of bladder distention. Consult health care provider *stat.*	Bladder distention is a potential cause of AD and requires immediate intervention. Anesthetic jelly prevents skin stimulation, which could trigger AD.
If a catheter is already in place, check tubing for kinks and lower drainage bag. For obstruction, such as sediment in tubing, slowly irrigate catheter as indicated, using 30 ml or less of normal saline. If catheter patency is uncertain, recatheterize patient using anesthetic jelly.	These interventions enable checking for catheter tube patency. Obstruction is a potential cause of AD.

Continued

INTERVENTIONS

INTERVENTIONS	RATIONALES
If the bladder is not distended, check for cloudy urine, hematuria, and positive laboratory or x-ray examination results.	These are signs of UTI and/or urinary calculi—two potential causes of AD.
Obtain urine specimen.	Culture and sensitivity studies will show if UTI, a potential cause of AD, is present.
Instill tetracaine or lidocaine into the bladder if prescribed.	These agents will reduce bladder excitability.
Institute preventive measures as prescribed to prevent UTI and urinary calculi.	Future episodes may be caused by these factors.
Bowel: Constipation, impaction, insertion of suppository or enema, or rectal examination.	Problems with the bowel are the second most likely cause of AD. A good bowel regimen is a key factor in preventing the noxious stimuli that constipation may cause.
Do not attempt rectal examination without first anesthetizing the rectal sphincter and anal canal with anesthetic jelly.	Anesthetic jelly prevents skin stimulation, which could trigger AD.
Use large amounts of anesthetic jelly in anus and rectum before disimpacting bowel to remove potential stimulus.	Bowel impaction is a potential cause of AD.
Wait 5 minutes and check BP before disimpacting.	A lowered BP is a sign that anesthetic jelly has become effective.
Skin: Pressure, infection, injury, heat, pain, or cold.	These are possible causes of AD. A good skin integrity program is another key factor in preventing these noxious stimuli.
Loosen clothing and remove antiembolism hose, leg bandages, abdominal binder, or constrictive sheets as appropriate.	Pressure on the skin is a potential cause of AD.
For male patients, check for pressure source on penis, scrotum, or testicles and remove pressure if present.	
Check skin surface below level of injury. Monitor for presence of a pressure area or sore, infection, laceration, rash, sunburn, ingrown toenail, or infected area, or check skin for contact with a hard object. If indicated, apply a topical anesthetic.	Skin infection, pain, and injury are potential causes of AD.
Observe for and remove source of heat or cold (e.g., ice pack, heating pad).	Topical heat or cold are two potential causes of AD.
Turn patient on side and ensure that bed linen is free of wrinkles. Consider adhering to a more frequent turning schedule.	These measures relieve other possible sources of pressure.
Additional causes: Surgical manipulation, incisional pain, sexual activity, menstrual cramps, labor, vaginal infection, or intra-abdominal problems such as appendicitis.	
Administer antihypertensive agents such as nifedipine (oral, sublingual), nitroglycerin (sublingual, spray, or topical ointment), hydralazine, diazoxide, terazosin, or phenoxybenzamine as prescribed.	These medications lower patient's blood pressure.
Check for use of sildenafil, an erectile dysfunction medication, before giving nitroglycerin.	Sildenafil is contraindicated for people who are taking nitrates (e.g., nitroglycerin) because of the additive hypotensive effect.
Administer mecamylamine, prazosin, or clonidine if prescribed for recurrent AD.	These medications reduce severity of recurrent episodes.
On resolution of the crisis, answer patient's and significant other's questions about AD. Discuss signs and symptoms, treatment, and methods of prevention.	Prevention is the best way to deal with AD. A bowel regimen and skin integrity program are key factors in preventing the noxious stimuli that constipation and pressure areas may cause.
Encourage patient to wear a medical alert bracelet or tag.	These items inform health care providers of patient's condition in case the patient is unable to do so during AD.
Encourage keeping an AD kit on hand that includes a glove, lubricant jelly, straight catheter, electronic BP machine, and alert card.	This kit will help relieve and monitor this medical emergency when it occurs.

●●● **Related NIC and NOC labels:** *NIC:* Dysreflexia Management; Neurologic Monitoring; Vital Signs Monitoring; Anxiety Reduction; Emergency Care; Infection Control; Medication Administration; Positioning; Surveillance: Safety; Temperature Regulation; Urinary Elimination Management; Bowel Management; Heat Exposure Treatment; Infection Protection; Skin Surveillance; Urinary Catheterization *NOC:* Neurological Status: Autonomic; Symptom Severity; Vital Signs Status

Nursing Diagnosis:

Ineffective Airway Clearance

related to neuromuscular paralysis/weakness or restriction of chest expansion secondary to halo vest obstruction

Desired Outcome: Following intervention, patient has a clear airway as evidenced by RR of 12-20 breaths/min with normal depth and pattern (eupnea) and absence of adventitious breath sounds.

INTERVENTIONS	RATIONALES
Monitor ventilation capability by checking vital capacity, tidal volume, and pulmonary function tests. Monitor serial arterial blood gas (ABG) values and/or pulse oximetry readings.	If vital capacity is less than 1 L or if patient exhibits signs of hypoxia (Pao_2 less than 80 mm Hg, O_2 saturation 92% or less, tachycardia, increased restlessness, mental status changes or dullness, cyanosis), health care provider should be notified immediately.
Monitor for increasing difficulty with secretions, coughing, respiratory difficulties, bradycardia, fluctuating BP, and increased motor and sensory losses at a higher level than baseline findings.	These signs may signal ascending cord edema secondary to effects of contusion or bleeding. If present, patient may require increased respiratory support.
Monitor for loss of previous ability to bend arms at the elbows (C5-6) or shrug shoulders (C3-4). If these findings are noted, notify health care provider immediately.	Changes from baseline or previous assessment may signal problems such as contusion, compression, bleeding, or damage to blood supply, and they necessitate prompt intervention.
Keep patient's head in neutral position, and suction as necessary. Be aware that suctioning may cause severe bradycardia in the patient with autonomic dysfunction. If indicated, prepare patient for a tracheostomy, endotracheal intubation, and/or mechanical ventilation to support respiratory function. If appropriate, arrange for transfer to intensive care unit for continuous monitoring.	These actions maintain a patent airway and support respiratory function. Patients with injuries above C5 are intubated and put on a ventilator. Nasal intubation or tracheostomy may be used to prevent neck extension (and thus further damage) during intubation.
	An implanted phrenic nerve stimulator (e.g., diaphragm pacer) eventually may be inserted to enable selected patients on ventilators to be off the ventilator for short periods.
If patient is wearing halo vest traction, assess respiratory status at least q4h or more frequently as indicated.	This action ascertains whether the vest is restricting chest expansion.
Monitor ability to swallow for patient in halo traction.	Inability to swallow may indicate improper position of neck and chin or changes in cranial nerve function caused by cranial pin compression or irritation.
Teach use of incentive spirometry.	Spirometry promotes adequate ventilation and assesses quality of patient's inspiratory abilities.
Be alert to shortness of breath, hemoptysis, tachycardia, sudden shoulder pain, and diminished breath sounds.	These are indicators of pulmonary embolus (PE), which can occur because of impaired ventilation, altered vascular tone, and decreased mobility. Pain may or may not be present with PE, depending on level of SCI. Sudden shoulder pain may be referred pain from PE.
If patient's cough is ineffective, implement the following technique, known as *assisted coughing*: place the heel of your hand under patient's diaphragm (below xiphoid process and above navel). Have patient take several deep breaths, hold a deep breath, and then cough. As patient exhales forcibly, quickly push up into the diaphragm to assist in producing a more forceful cough.	This technique enables production of a more forceful cough. Assisted coughing may be contraindicated in patients with spinal instability.
	An insufflation-exsufflation cough machine may be used to deliver breaths to patient in order to produce a more effective mechanically assisted cough.
Instruct patient regarding intermittent positive pressure breathing and chest physiotherapy, if prescribed.	These therapies prevent and treat atelectasis. Respiratory therapy is ongoing past the acute stage. Noninvasive positive pressure ventilation may be used with some patients.
Feed patients in Stryker frames, Foster beds, or similar mechanical beds in prone position. Raise stable patients in halo traction to high Fowler's position if it is not contraindicated.	These actions minimize potential for aspiration.
For additional information, see **Risk for Aspiration**, p. 96, in "Older Adult Care."	

••• **Related NIC and NOC labels:** *NIC:* Airway Management; Respiratory Monitoring; Vital Signs Monitoring; Ventilation Assistance; Airway Suctioning; Aspiration Precautions; Positioning; Cough Enhancement; Artificial Airway Management; Mechanical Ventilation; Laboratory Data Interpretation *NOC:* Respiratory Status: Ventilation; Respiratory Status: Gas Exchange; Respiratory Status: Airway Patency; Aspiration Control

Nursing Diagnosis:

Ineffective Tissue Perfusion: Cardiopulmonary and Cerebral

related to relative hypovolemia secondary to decreased vasomotor tone with SCI

Desired Outcomes: By at least 24 hr before hospital discharge (or as soon as vasomotor tone improves), patient has adequate cardiopulmonary and cerebral tissue perfusion as evidenced by SBP 90 mm Hg or higher and orientation to person, place, and time. For a minimum of 48 hr before hospital discharge, patient is free of dysrhythmias.

INTERVENTIONS	RATIONALES
Monitor for hypotension (drop in SBP more than 20 mm Hg, SBP less than 90 mm Hg), lightheadedness, dizziness, fainting, and confusion.	Low/falling BP can occur secondary to loss of vasomotor tone and decreased venous return.
Monitor heart rate (HR) and rhythm. Document dysrhythmias.	Sinus tachycardia/bradycardia may develop because of impaired sympathetic innervation or unopposed vagal stimulation. Atropine may be prescribed for symptomatic bradycardia.
Monitor intake and output.	Adequate hydration and elimination are necessary to maintain stable hemodynamics.
Give prescribed IV fluids cautiously.	Impaired vascular tone can make the patient sensitive to small increases in circulating volume. Intravascular volume expanders or vasopressors (e.g., dopamine) may be required for hypotension.
Implement measures that prevent episodes of decreased cardiac output caused by postural hypotension.	Decreased cardiac output compromises cerebral and peripheral circulation. Postural hypotension is seen frequently in SCI, but it can be prevented and managed.
Change position slowly.	This helps prevent postural hypotension.
Perform range-of-motion (ROM) exercises q2h. Prevent patient's legs from crossing, especially when in a dependent position.	This prevents venous pooling and contractures.
If indicated, ensure that patients with SCI at higher levels, especially above T6, wear abdominal binder in addition to antiembolic hose, leg wraps, and sequential compression devices or pneumatic foot pumps.	This helps prevent venous pooling. These individuals are prone to more severe hypotensive reactions, even with minor changes such as raising HOB.
Work with physical therapist to implement a gradual sitting program that will help patient progress from a supine to an upright position.	The goal is to increase patient's ability to sit upright while avoiding adverse effects, such as hypertension, dizziness, and fainting. This may include a bed that can rotate gradually from a horizontal position to a vertical position or a chair that has multiple positions progressing from flat to sitting.
Administer salt tablets and fludrocortisone as prescribed if nonmedication methods are ineffective.	These agents prevent orthostatic hypotension.
For additional information, see **Ineffective Tissue Perfusion: Cerebral** in "Prolonged Bedrest," p. 66.	

••• **Related NIC and NOC labels:** *NIC:* Cardiac Care: Acute Dysrhythmia Management; Fluid Management; Vital Signs Monitoring; Hypovolemia Management; Neurologic Monitoring; Cerebral Perfusion Promotion; Positioning *NOC:* Cardiac Pump Effectiveness; Tissue Perfusion: Cardiac; Tissue Perfusion: Pulmonary; Vital Signs Status; Tissue Perfusion: Cerebral

Nursing Diagnosis:

Ineffective Tissue Perfusion: Peripheral and Cardiopulmonary

related to interrupted blood flow (venous stasis) with corresponding risk of thrombophlebitis and PE secondary to immobility and decreased vasomotor tone

Desired Outcome: For at least 24 hr before hospital discharge and on an ongoing basis, patient has adequate peripheral and cardiopulmonary tissue perfusion as evidenced by absence of heat, erythema, and swelling in calves and thighs; HR 100 bpm or less; RR 20 breaths/min or less with normal depth and pattern (eupnea); and Pao_2 80 mm Hg or more or O_2 saturation greater than 92%.

INTERVENTIONS	RATIONALES
Monitor for erythema, warmth, decreased pulses, and swelling over area of inflammation and venous dilation, coolness, paleness, and edema distal to thrombus.	These are indicators of thrombophlebitis.
Measure calves and thighs daily while patient is supine or before activity, and monitor for increased circumference.	An increase of 1.5 cm or more in 1 day is significant, as is calf diameter greater than 3 cm larger than opposite calf.
Recognize that low-grade fever may be a more reliable signal of thrombophlebitis than pain. Notify health care provider about significant findings.	The presence of pain or tenderness depends on level of SCI.
Protect patient's legs from injury during transfers and turning, and position them so they do not cross. Avoid IM injections in the legs, and do not massage the legs.	SCI patients are prone to DVT, which can occur in the lower extremities because of immobility and changes in vascular tone.
Provide ROM to legs qid. If not contraindicated, place patient in Trendelenburg position for 15 min q2h, or elevate legs 10-15 degrees.	These measures promote venous drainage.
Monitor for tachycardia, shortness of breath, hemoptysis, decrease in Pao_2, O_2 saturation 92% or less, and decreased or adventitious breath sounds. Notify health care provider about significant findings.	All are indicators of PE. Presence of pain depends on level of injury. Sudden shoulder pain may represent referred pain from PE.
Consult health care provider about use of antiembolism hose, sequential compression devices, pneumatic foot pumps, or prophylactic pharmacotherapy (e.g., acetylsalicylic acid [ASA], warfarin, low-molecular-weight or low-dose heparin).	These measures help prevent PE.
If indicated, explain use of a vena cava filter.	This filter helps prevent emboli from reaching the lungs in the presence of DVT or PE.
For other interventions, see **Ineffective Tissue Perfusion: Peripheral** in "Prolonged Bedrest," p. 65.	

●●● **Related NIC and NOC labels:** *NIC:* Embolus Precautions; Vital Signs Monitoring; Circulatory Care: Venous Insufficiency; Respiratory Monitoring; Circulatory Care: Arterial Insufficiency; Embolus Care: Pulmonary *NOC:* Tissue Perfusion: Cardiac; Tissue Perfusion: Pulmonary; Tissue Perfusion: Cerebral

Nursing Diagnosis:

Urinary Retention or Reflex Urinary Incontinence

related to neurologic impairment (spasticity or flaccidity occurring with SCI)

Desired Outcomes: Patient has urinary output without incontinence. Patient empties bladder with residual volumes of less than 50 ml by time of discharge. Following instruction, patient demonstrates triggering mechanism and gains some control over voiding.

INTERVENTIONS	RATIONALES
General guidelines for individuals with bladder dysfunction	
If intermittent catheterization is used and episodes of incontinence occur or more than 500 ml of urine is obtained, catheterize patient more often.	Bladder dysfunction is complicated and should be assessed by cystometric testing to determine the best type of bladder program. Initially during acute spinal shock, patient will have an indwelling urinary catheter or scheduled intermittent catheterizations. As spinal reflexes return, intermittent catheterization or other bladder emptying technique is used. Indwelling catheters are avoided because of potential for UTI.
Teach patient and significant other procedure for intermittent catheterization, care of indwelling catheters, and indicators of UTI (e.g., fever, chills, cloudy and/or foul-smelling urine, malaise, anorexia, restlessness, increased frequency or urgency, incontinence).	This teaching helps ensure readiness for self- or assisted-care upon discharge from care facility.
Teach patient and significant other that habit/bladder scheduling program consists of gradually increasing time between catheterizations or periodically clamping indwelling catheters.	The goal is a gradual increase in bladder tone. When the bladder can hold 300-400 ml of urine, measures to stimulate voiding are attempted. Bladder ultrasound may be used to determine fullness and aid in retraining.
Make sure patient takes fluids at evenly spaced intervals throughout the day.	This promotes adequate hydration and increased bladder tone.
Restrict fluids before bedtime.	This helps prevent nighttime incontinence. Alcohol and caffeine-containing foods and beverages (e.g., cola, chocolate, coffee, tea) have a diuretic effect and may cause incontinence. In addition, caffeine-containing products may increase bladder spasms and reflex incontinence.
Instruct patients using bladder-emptying techniques to void at least q3h.	Maintaining a regular schedule prevents bladder distention. A wristwatch with timer alarm or an alarm clock can help patient maintain this schedule.
To obtain postvoid residual urine, catheterize patient after an attempt to empty bladder.	Residual amounts greater than 100 ml usually indicate need for return to a scheduled intermittent catheterization program.
Monitor response to measures that promote bladder training and continence, and obtain urinary specialist consult as appropriate.	Urinary diversion may be considered for patients whose bladders cannot be retrained. Artificial urinary sphincter or continent vesicotomy may be used to promote bladder continence. An external sphincterectomy may be done to reduce sphincter resistance, thereby producing continuous bladder emptying.
Guidelines for patients with UMN-involved spastic reflex bladder	
Explain to these patients that eventually they may be able to empty the bladder automatically and therefore may not require catheterization.	Lesions above conus medullaris (located at the lower two levels of the thoracic region where the cord begins to taper) generally leave the S2, S3, and S4 spinal cord nerve segments intact. If this spinal reflex arc is intact, the patient will have UMN-involved bladder, resulting in a spastic bladder. This bladder has tone and occasional bladder contractions and periodically will empty on its own, resulting in reflex incontinence. The UMN-involved bladder is "trainable" with techniques that stimulate reflex voiding.
Teach tapping of the suprapubic area with fingers, gently pulling pubic hair, digitally stretching anal sphincter, stroking glans penis, stroking inner thigh, lightly punching abdominal area just proximal to inguinal ligaments, or using a hand-held vibration device against the lower abdomen. Advise patient to perform selected technique for 2-3 min or until a good urine stream has started. Explain that patient should wait 1 min before trying another stimulation technique.	These techniques stimulate the voiding reflex.

Continued

INTERVENTIONS	RATIONALES
	The following techniques stimulate the voiding reflex and should be taught to patient accordingly. Be aware that stimulating reflex trigger zones accidentally may result in incontinence. Incontinence briefs will help control accidents.
	Bladder tapping: Patient positions self in a half-sitting position. Tapping is performed over the suprapubic area, and the patient may shift the site of stimulation within that area to find the most effective site. Tapping is performed rapidly (7-8 times/sec) with one hand for approximately 50 single taps. Patient continues tapping until a good stream starts. Explain that when the stream stops, patient should wait about 1 min and repeat tapping until bladder is empty. One or two tapping attempts without response indicate that no more urine will be expelled.
	Anal stretch technique (contraindicated in individuals with lesions at T8 or above because of the potential for AD): Patient positions self on commode or toilet, leans forward on thighs, and inserts 1 or 2 lubricated fingers into anus to anal sphincter. Patient then spreads the anal sphincter gently by spreading fingers apart or pulling in a posterior direction. Patient maintains stretching position, takes a deep breath, and holds breath while bearing down to void. Patient relaxes and repeats until bladder is empty.
Avoid plastic or rubber sheets.	They trap heat and moisture, promoting skin breakdown.
Administer baclofen if it is prescribed.	Baclofen may be prescribed because it tends to promote more complete emptying of the bladder by reducing tone of external urinary sphincter.
Guidelines for patients with LMN-involved flaccid bladders	
Teach patient that increasing intraabdominal pressure can overcome sphincter pressure, which may empty the bladder. Explain that this may be contraindicated, however, depending on risk of ureteral reflux.	Lesions below the conus medullaris (T12) may injure S2, S3, and S4 nerve segments, which will disrupt the reflex arc, causing LMN-involved flaccid bladder. This bladder has no tone and will distend until it overflows, resulting in overflow incontinence.
	Bladder-emptying techniques (e.g., straining, Valsalva's maneuver) to increase intraabdominal pressure are controversial and generally not encouraged because of potential for reflux past the vesicoureteral junction, thus increasing potential for ascending UTIs.
Explain that patient may be able to empty bladder manually well enough to avoid catheterization.	Need for catheterization can be determined by checking residual urine volume.
If Credé's method is prescribed, teach the technique to patient.	Credé's method is another technique for increasing intraabdominal pressure. It is performed as follows: The ulnar surface of the hand is placed horizontally along or just below umbilicus; while patient bears down with abdominal muscles, the hand is pressed downward and toward the bladder in a kneading motion until urination is initiated. This is continued for 30 sec or until urination ceases. The patient then waits a few minutes and repeats the procedure to ensure complete emptying of the bladder.
Suggest alternative measures if patient's bladder cannot be trained to empty completely.	Intermittent catheterization or external collection devices usually are indicated, and patient may be a candidate for an artificial inflatable sphincter device or urinary diversion.

••• Related NIC and NOC labels: *NIC:* Urinary Elimination Management; Urinary Retention Care; Fluid Management; Self-Care Assistance: Toileting; Urinary Catheterization: Intermittent; Urinary Bladder Training; Urinary Habit Training *NOC:* Urinary Elimination

<u>**Nursing Diagnosis:**</u>

Constipation or Fecal Impaction

related to immobility and decreased peristalsis, atonic bowel, and loss of sensation and voluntary sphincter control secondary to sensorimotor deficit

Desired Outcome: Patient has bowel movements that are soft and formed every 1-3 days or within patient's preinjury pattern.

INTERVENTIONS	RATIONALES
Assess patient's bowel function by auscultating for bowel sounds; inspecting for presence of abdominal distention; and monitoring for nausea, vomiting, and fecal impaction. Notify health care provider of significant findings.	During acute phase of spinal shock, which usually resolves in 1-6 wk, constipation and paralytic ileus are common.
Manage a flaccid bowel with increased intraabdominal pressure technique (see below), manual disimpaction, and small-volume enemas.	Lesions below the conus medullaris (T12) may injure S3, S4, and S5 nerve segments, resulting in disruption of the reflex arc and causing LMN flaccid bowel and loss of anal tone.
Administer small-volume enemas only. In the presence of fecal impaction, gentle manual removal or a small cleansing enema may be prescribed.	The atonic intestine distends easily, and therefore only small volumes are recommended.
Avoid long-term use of enemas.	Enemas may disrupt normal flora and affect peristalsis and sphincter tone.
For UMN reflex bowel, once bowel activity returns, teach patient to attempt bowel movement 30 min after a meal or warm drink.	This regimen will allow patient's gastrocolic and duodenocolic mass peristalsis reflexes to assist with evacuation. Lesions above the conus medullaris (located at the lower two levels of the thoracic region where the cord begins to taper) generally leave S3, S4, and S5 spinal cord nerve segments intact. If this spinal reflex arc is intact, patient will have UMN bowel and be capable of stimulating (training) reflex evacuation of the bowel.
In addition, teach patient to sit, bear down, bend forward, or apply manual pressure to the abdomen. If allowed, provide a bedside commode. Check patient's ability to maintain balance on a commode. If patient is bedridden, turn patient onto side and use a pad rather than a bedpan to catch bowel movement.	These measures promote bowel movements by increasing intraabdominal pressure. An abdominal belt may be used if patient is unable to strain at stool. Massaging abdomen in a clockwise, circular motion also may help promote bowel evacuation. A prescribed, medicated suppository may be used if necessary.
For patients with injuries at T8 or above, promote adequate fluid intake (more than 2500 ml/day) and use of stool softeners and high-fiber diet.	These measures facilitate bowel evacuation by adding bulk and moisture to the stool.
Use suppositories and enemas only when essential and with extreme caution. Use anesthetic jelly liberally when performing a rectal examination or inserting a suppository or an enema.	Their use can precipitate AD. Anesthetic jelly prevents skin stimulation, which could otherwise trigger AD.
For patients with hand mobility (who are not at risk for AD), teach technique for suppository insertion and digital stimulation of the anus.	These measures promote reflex bowel evacuation. Suppository inserters and rectal stimulation devices are available for patients with limited hand mobility.
For digital stimulation, teach patient to insert lubricated finger about 1½-2½ inches into rectum and gently rotate in a slow circular motion, gently stretching sphincter, for about 30 sec (but no longer than 1 min at a time) until the internal sphincter relaxes. Restart circular motion if sphincter tightens and remove finger if bowel movement begins. Stop if sphincter spasms are felt or if signs of AD occur. Repeat q5-10min several times until adequate evacuation occurs. If unsuccessful after 20-30 min of stimulation, insert a suppository.	Digital stimulation stretches and relaxes the internal sphincter to facilitate bowel movement.
Teach patient to keep fingernails cut short.	This helps prevent injury to the rectal mucosa.
For other interventions, see **Constipation** in "Prolonged Bedrest," p. 67.	

••• **For Related NIC and NOC labels:** *NIC:* Bowel Management; Constipation/Impaction Management; Fluid Management; Medication Management; Nutrition Management; Self-Care Assistance: Toileting *NOC:* Bowel Elimination

Nursing Diagnosis:

Risk for Disuse Syndrome

related to paralysis, immobilization, or spasticity secondary to SCI

Desired Outcomes: After stabilization of the injury, patient exhibits complete ROM of all joints. By time of discharge, patient demonstrates measures that enhance mobility, reduce spasms, and prevent complications.

INTERVENTIONS	RATIONALES
Once injury is stabilized, assist patient with position changes on a regular schedule.	This action alternates sites of pressure relief and decreases risk of contracture formation. For example, a prone position, if not contraindicated, helps prevent sacral decubiti and hip contractures.
For patients with spasticity, use hand splints or cones, keeping fingers extended.	These devices assist with maintaining a functional grasp.
If patient has spasticity, fit him or her with splints or high-top tennis shoes that are cut off at the toes so that each shoe ends just proximal to the metatarsal head.	This helps prevent foot contractures for patients with spasticity. These shoes help keep feet dorsiflexed but prevent contact of balls of feet with a hard surface, which can cause spasticity.
Avoid footboards for these patients.	The hard surface may trigger spasticity and promote plantar flexion.
Teach patient that some factors that trigger spasms are cold temperatures, anxiety, fatigue, emotional distress, infections, bowel or bladder distention, ulcers, pain, tight clothing, and lying too long in one position.	Controlling these factors may reduce number of spasms experienced.
Teach patients with spasticity techniques such as proper positioning, ROM, and daily sustained stretching exercises.	Steady, continuous, directional stretching several times daily is especially important because it may decrease spasticity for several hours. Cooling and icing techniques, heat, vibration therapy, and transcutaneous electrical nerve stimulation of spastic muscles also may be helpful.
When touch is necessary, do it in a firm, gentle, steady manner. Teach caregivers that touch may need to be limited.	Tactile stimulation may trigger spasms.
Administer prescribed muscle relaxants (e.g., diazepam) and antispasmodics (e.g., baclofen, tizanidine, or dantrolene).	These medications decrease spasms. More severe spasticity may be treated with IM injections of botulinum toxin. Dantrolene causes muscle weakness so it is generally reserved for patients on bedrest. Intrathecal baclofen involves use of a programmable implanted pump to deliver a continuous dose of baclofen into the spinal canal sheath to control spasticity. Intrathecal baclofen must not be abruptly stopped because doing so may cause seizures and hallucinations.
Encourage participation in PT or occupational therapy program.	A therapy program is ongoing throughout the patient's rehabilitation. Passive ROM is started on all joints. After the injury is stabilized, an aggressive rehabilitation program is initiated, including muscle strengthening and conditioning exercises to develop alternative muscle groups needed for independence; a sitting program; massage; instruction in adaptive devices, equipment, and transfer techniques as appropriate; and instruction in orthotics and braces or splints to prevent contractures. Patients with sacral injuries have the potential to walk and should be instructed in use of braces, crutches, or cane as appropriate. Functional electrical stimulation of paralyzed muscles assists some paraplegic patients with walking.
Monitor effectiveness of measures for spasticity.	Tenotomy, myotomy, peripheral neurectomy, and rhizotomy are some of the surgical approaches that may be used to treat spasticity that cannot be managed by medications or more conservative measures such as stretching or ROM.

Continued

INTERVENTIONS	RATIONALES
Monitor for pain, swelling, warmth, and decreased ROM function around joints, especially the hips.	These indicators may signal heterotopic ossification (HO), which is the abnormal formation of true bone within the extraskeletal soft tissues. Etidronate; nonsteroidal antiinflammatories, such as indomethacin; ROM exercises; and external beam radiation are prevention therapies. Once HO has formed, resection usually is necessary.
For additional interventions, see **Risk for Disuse Syndrome**, p. 63, in "Prolonged Bedrest."	

••• **Related NIC and NOC labels:** *NIC:* Exercise Promotion: Stretching; Positioning; Teaching: Prescribed Activity/Exercise; Pressure Ulcer Prevention   *NOC:* Immobility Consequences: Physiological

Nursing Diagnosis:

Risk for Injury

related to incorrect neck position, irritation of cranial nerves, and impaired lateral vision secondary to presence of halo vest traction as well as lack of access for external cardiac compression

Desired Outcome: At time of discharge (and ongoing during use of halo traction), patient exhibits no adverse changes in motor, sensory, or cranial nerve function and is free of symptoms of injury caused by impaired vision.

INTERVENTIONS	RATIONALES
Assess position of patient's neck in relation to the body. Alert health care provider to presence of flexion or hyperextension.	To ensure proper alignment and optimal healing, patient's neck should be in a neutral position.
Assess any difficulty with swallowing.	Swallowing difficulty may signal improper position of neck and chin.
Keep a torque screwdriver in a secure place.	This ensures that health care provider can readily adjust tension on bars to return patient's neck position to neutral.
Evaluate degree of sensation and movement of upper extremities, and assess cranial nerve function. Notify health care provider of sudden changes in motor, sensory, or cranial nerve function (e.g., weakness, paresthesias, ptosis, difficulty chewing or swallowing).	Changes in cranial nerve function can occur if cranial pins compress or irritate a nerve. **Note:** Jaw pain may occur when chewing is attempted, and this needs to be differentiated from cranial nerve problems. A diet of soft foods, cut into small pieces, will help jaw pain.
Assess pins, bolts, and vest structure for looseness at least daily. Notify health care provider if pins or vest become loose or dislodged.	Clicking sounds may signal a loose pin, and if this occurs, it will be necessary to stabilize patient's head to prevent misalignment.
Never use superstructure of halo traction in turning or moving patient. Avoid putting pillows under support bars when patient is lying down (e.g., to sleep).	This could result in misalignment of patient's affected area.
Instruct patient to avoid pulling clothes over top of halo apparatus but rather to step into clothes and pull them up over feet and legs. Advise patient to buy strapless bras, tube tops, or clothes that are several sizes too large, or to modify neck openings (e.g., with Velcro closures, ties).	These measures help prevent loosening of pins.
Avoid loosening a buckle without health care provider's directive.	The device must be worn correctly to maintain alignment, prevent skin breakdown, and prevent nerve injury. Buckle holes or straps should be marked so that they are always cinched correctly to appropriate snugness.
If patient is ambulatory, teach him or her to walk initially with assistance of two people and how to survey environment while walking, either by using a mirror, by turning eyes to their extreme lateral positions, or by turning entire body.	The halo vest impairs lateral vision.

Continued

INTERVENTIONS	RATIONALES
If indicated, suggest use of a cane.	A cane will help determine height of curbs and detect unseen objects or uneven walking surfaces.
Explain that trunk flexibility is limited and that achieving balance can be difficult. Teach patient that bending over can be hazardous.	The vest's weight is top-heavy. Ambulating with a walker initially may help patient learn to adjust. Abdominal- and back-strengthening exercises may aid balance and walking.
Advise patient to walk only in low-heeled shoes, use long-handled assistive devices to reach or pick up objects, and realize that extra space allowance may be needed when passing through doorways and to avoid bumping into objects.	These measures prevent falls and other injuries caused by wearing the vest.
Advise that a shower chair that rolls usually can fit over a toilet seat, providing an extra 3-6 inches in height.	This is the best method to promote safety and avoid straining to raise and lower body onto toilet seat.
To get out of bed, teach patient to roll onto his or her side at edge of bed and then drop legs over side of bed while pushing up trunk sideways.	This technique promotes good alignment and body mechanics to prevent injury.
Recommend backing into car seat with body bent forward when getting into a car.	This prevents hitting pins and device on car doorframe.
Caution patient against driving.	Patient will have limited field of vision when wearing the vest.
Teach patient to use high tables and swivel chairs at home.	A high table will help bring objects into view and a swivel chair will permit easier visualization of the environment.
Explain that patient will need assistance of another person to shampoo hair safely.	This promotes safety and helps prevent falling if water spills on the floor.
Advise that shampooing a short haircut is easiest, and hair should be blown dry.	Toweling hair may loosen pins.
Teach caregivers and significant other how to release vest in an emergency such as need for external cardiac compression.	Most vests have side straps that, when released, enable vest to be opened to midline. If a wrench is required, it should be kept with jacket (e.g., attached with Velcro).

••• **Related NIC and NOC labels:** *NIC:* Fall Prevention; Surveillance: Safety; Emergency Care; Environmental Management: Safety
NOC: Safety Status: Physical Injury

Nursing Diagnosis:

Risk for Impaired Skin Integrity and/or Impaired Tissue Integrity

related to altered circulation and mechanical factors secondary to presence of halo vest traction or tongs

Desired Outcome: At time of discharge and on an ongoing basis, patient's skin is non-erythremic and unbroken; tissue underlying and surrounding the halo vest blanches appropriately.

INTERVENTIONS	RATIONALES
Inspect skin around vest edges for erythema and other signs of irritation. Keep skin dry.	These are signs of impaired circulation caused by the vest. Skin is kept dry to prevent irritation.
Gently massage nonerythematous areas routinely.	Massage promotes circulation and helps prevent breakdown.
Teach skin inspection, which may require use of a mirror, flashlight, or another person.	For timely intervention, patient should alert medical personnel if breakdown, sensitive spots, odor, dirty vest liner, or loose pins are present.
Investigate complaints of discomfort or uncomfortable fit. Pad vest as needed until it can be properly adjusted or trimmed by health care provider. Protect vest from moisture and soiling.	A finger should be able to fit between vest and patient's skin. Weight loss or gain can affect fit.
Be alert to foul odor from in or around cast openings and to serosanguineous drainage on a pillowcase slipped through the vest from one side to another.	A foul odor can signal pressure necrosis beneath the vest, and serosanguineous drainage may indicate an area of skin breakdown.

Continued

INTERVENTIONS	RATIONALES
Instruct/assist patient with changing body position q2h. Support vest while patient is in bed, and use logroll technique with sufficient help.	Changing positions promotes circulation and prevents skin and tissue breakdown by alternating sites of pressure relief.
Use soft padding. Use a small pillow under the head at sleep time.	Padding helps prevent pressure on prominent body areas such as forehead or shoulder and a small pillow promotes comfort and support for the neck.
Wash skin under the vest with soap and warm water.	Usually, releasing one vest belt at a time as patient is lying down is allowed for washing.
Avoid use of lotion and powder under vest.	These products can cake under the vest.
Replace soiled linens promptly. Dry perspiration with hair dryer on a cool setting.	These actions prevent skin irritation and breakdown caused by moisture.
Inspect under both sides of vest for redness, swelling, bruising, or chafing. Close the open side and repeat on the opposite side.	If a rash appears, patient may be allergic to vest's lining. A synthetic liner, knitted body stockinette, or T-shirt may correct this problem.
In the event of skin breakdown, keep skin cleansed, dried, and covered with a transparent dressing. Notify health care provider, wound, ostomy, continence/enterostomal (WOC/ET) nurse, and orthotist accordingly.	At the first sign of skin breakdown, a WOC/ET nurse can implement a wound care regimen. An orthotist can make a brace adjustment to prevent further breakdown.
Place rubber corks over tips of halo device.	This will diminish annoying sound vibrations if the apparatus is bumped and prevent lacerations from sharp edges.
Check tong placement (e.g., Crutchfield, Vinke, Gardner-Wells) at least daily.	If slippage has occurred, patient's head should be immobilized with a sandbag and health care provider notified promptly to prevent misalignment of neck. Pain may signal erosion of bone and displacement into muscle.
Check drainage from tong sites for presence of cerebrospinal fluid (CSF) (see p. 365).	The presence of CSF indicates tong has penetrated through the skull, and risk of meningitis and neurologic damage is possible.
Ensure that tong traction weights are hanging freely.	This helps ensure that traction is maintained as prescribed.
For a discussion of pin care, see "Fractures," p. 520, for **Deficient Knowledge:** Function of external fixation, pin care, and signs and symptoms of pin site infection.	

••• Related NIC and NOC labels: *NIC:* Pressure Management; Circulatory Precautions; Positioning; Simple Massage; Traction/Immobilization Care; Skin Surveillance; Skin Care: Topical Treatments; Pressure Ulcer Prevention *NOC:* Immobility Consequences: Physiological; Tissue Integrity: Skin & Mucous Membranes

Nursing Diagnosis:

Sexual Dysfunction

related to altered body function secondary to SCI

Desired Outcome: Within the 24-hr period before hospital discharge, patient discusses concerns about sexuality and verbalizes knowledge of alternative methods of sexual expression.

INTERVENTIONS	RATIONALES
Evaluate your own feelings about sexuality. Refer patient to someone (e.g., knowledgeable staff member, professional sexual therapy counselor) who can address patient's sexual concerns if you are uncomfortable discussing these issues or unable to answer specific concerns and questions.	Nurses may not be able to answer all the patient's questions or may be uncomfortable discussing sexual issues. The nurse's discomfort would add to patient's discomfort.
Provide a supportive, nonjudgmental environment that gives patient permission to have and freely express sexual concerns. Elicit patient's knowledge, concerns, and questions.	Sexuality can be discussed as it relates to an erection that occurs during a bath or to objective findings noted during physical assessment.

Continued

INTERVENTIONS	RATIONALES
Expect acting-out behavior related to patient's sexuality.	This is a normal response to anxiety about sexual response and progno- sis. Such behaviors may include asking personal questions, sexual jokes or innuendoes, self-deprecating remarks, or flirting with staff.
Provide information about normal sexual response and changes caused by SCI.	Sexual functioning may be different but still possible with SCI. The gen- eral rule for men is the higher the lesion, the greater the chance of retaining the ability to have an erection (but with a lesser chance of ejaculation). Women may have problems with lubrication, and orgasm may be difficult to achieve because of decreased sensation. Women may also have a transient loss of ovulation; however, ovulation usu- ally returns, and women can become pregnant and deliver vaginally.

Sperm quality decreases in men after SCI, but they may still be capable of fathering a child naturally. Use of electroejaculation via electrical stimulation in the area of the prostate to obtain sperm, in utero in- semination, in vitro fertilization, or intracytoplasmic sperm injection have improved fertility. |
Provide information about birth control and oral contraception for women who desire it.	Uterine contractions of labor in women with SCI lesion at T8 or above may cause AD. Oral contraceptives may be contraindicated because of risk of thrombophlebitis.
Provide specific suggestions that may provide gratification including oral- genital sex, digital stimulation, vibrator stimulation, cuddling, mutual masturbation, anal eroticism, and massage. Provide specific sugges- tions for managing common problems including decreasing fluid in- take 2-3 hr before sexual encounter, emptying bladder and bowels (if necessary) before a sexual encounter, (for men) folding back indwell- ing catheter along the penis and holding it in place with a condom, (for women) taping catheter to the abdomen and leaving it in place, taking a warm bath before sexual activity to reduce spasticity, plan- ning sexual activity for a time of day in which both partners are rested, experimenting with a variety of positions, and applying topical anesthetics to areas that are hypersensitive to touch.	Sexual activity may seem impossible to the SCI patient. These and the suggestions that follow may provide gratification and facilitate the act. Oral medications such as sildenafil generally have replaced other erectile dysfunction medications such as suppositories, penile injec- tions, and topical applications. Patients with erections lasting longer than 4 hours should seek medical attention. Sublingual and nasally administered apomorphine (used in Europe and awaiting Food and Drug Administration approval in the United States) also may help ob- tain a long-lasting erection. Erection assistive techniques and devices (e.g., vacuum suction pump, penile prosthesis or implant) may help men with SCI attain erections.
Explain that water-soluble lubricants are useful, if needed, but that petroleum-based lubricants should be avoided.	Petroleum-based lubricants can cause UTI.
Explain that adductor spasms in women may pose a barrier but can be overcome if a rear entry is acceptable. Suggest that prolonged fore- play with stroking and light massage may also relax muscles. If AD occurs during sexual activity, suggest that patient consult health care provider about preventive measures (e.g., taking a ganglionic block- ing agent before having sexual intercourse or applying topical anesthetic).	These are guidelines for managing less common problems that can oc- cur during a sexual encounter.
Suggest that patient's partner be included in discussion about sexual concerns.	Explaining the physical condition caused by SCI and preparing the part- ner for scars, lack of muscle tone, atrophy, and presence of a cathe- ter will provide the partner with an opportunity to discuss sexual concerns.
For additional interventions, see **Ineffective Sexuality Pattern** in "Prolonged Bedrest," p. 70.	

••• **Related NIC and NOC labels:** *NIC:* Sexual Counseling; Self-Esteem Enhancement; Teaching: Sexuality; Energy Management
NOC: Sexual Functioning

ADDITIONAL NURSING DIAGNOSES/ PROBLEMS:

"Perioperative Care" for individuals undergoing surgery   p. 45

"Prolonged Bedrest" for patients with varying degrees of immobility   p. 61

"Psychosocial Support"   p. 73

"Psychosocial Support for the Patient's Family and Significant Other"   p. 87

"Ureteral Calculi" for nursing diagnoses for the prevention and treatment of renal or ureteral calculi   p. 243

"General Care of Patients with Neurologic Disorders" for **Risk for Falls** related to unsteady gait   p. 265

Risk for Injury related to impaired pain, touch, and temperature sensations   p. 269

Risk for Deficient Fluid Volume   p. 271

Imbalanced Nutrition: Less Than Body Requirements   p. 272

Acute Pain   p. 273

Self-Care Deficit   p. 277

"Intervertebral Disk Disease" for **Deficient Knowledge:** Diskectomy with laminectomy or fusion procedure   p. 300

Impaired Swallowing, for patients undergoing diskectomy with laminectomy or spinal fusion   p. 303

"Multiple Sclerosis" for **Deficient Knowledge:** Precautions and potential side effects of prescribed medications   p. 307

For patients on mechanical ventilation, see the following:

"Pneumonia" for **Risk of Infection** related to inadequate primary defenses   p. 127

"General Care of Patients with Neurologic Disorders" for **Risk for Infection** related to inadequate primary defenses   p. 264

✔ PATIENT-FAMILY TEACHING AND DISCHARGE PLANNING

When providing patient-family teaching, focus on sensory information, avoid giving excessive information, and initiate a visiting nurse referral for necessary follow-up teaching. Include verbal and written information about the following:

✓ Spinal cord functioning and the effects trauma has on how the body works.

✓ Referrals to community resources, such as public health nurse, visiting nurses association, community support groups, social workers, psychologic therapy, vocational rehabilitation agency, home health agencies, and extended and skilled care facilities. Additional general information can be obtained by contacting the following organizations:

- National Spinal Cord Injury Association at *www.spinalcord.org*
- Christopher Reeve Paralysis Foundation at *www.spinalcord.org*
- Paralyzed Veterans of American at *www.pva.org*
- Cure Paralysis Now at *www.cureparalysis.org*
- Rehabilitation Research Center at *www.tbi-sci.org*
- Paralinks at *www.paralinks.net*
- DisABILITY Information and Resources at *www.makoa.org*

✓ Safety measures relative to decreased sensation, motor deficits, orthostatic hypotension and symptoms, preventive measures, and interventions for AD.

✓ Use and care of a brace or immobilizer, medical equipment, and mobility aids as appropriate.

✓ What patient can expect if transferred to rehabilitation center.

✓ Techniques and devices for performing activities of daily living, including bathing, grooming, turning, feeding, and other self-care activities to patient's maximum potential. The patient may need a home accessibility evaluation and a driving evaluation and training.

✓ Indicators of ureteral calculi and dietary measures to prevent their formation (see p. 243).

✓ Indicators of DVT and measures to prevent it (see p. 201).

✓ Importance of participation in counseling and psychotherapy to help patient and significant other adjust to the disability. This should include addressing of sexual functioning and vocational rehabilitation.

✓ For additional information, see teaching and discharge planning interventions (the fourth through tenth entries only) as appropriate in "Multiple Sclerosis," p. 311.

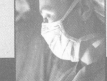

Stroke 42

OVERVIEW/PATHOPHYSIOLOGY

A stroke (previously known as cerebrovascular accident, or CVA) is the sudden disruption of O_2 supply to the brain or rupture in one or more of the blood vessels that supply the brain. *Ischemic stroke* has three main mechanisms: thrombosis, embolism, and systemic hypoperfusion. Thrombosis or embolism results in a blockage of blood supply to the brain tissue. The resulting ischemia, if prolonged, causes brain tissue necrosis (infarction), cerebral edema, and increased intracranial pressure (IICP). Most thrombotic strokes are caused by blockage of large vessels as a result of atherosclerosis. Thrombi in small penetrating arteries result in "lacunar" strokes. Most embolic strokes are cardiogenic and the result of emboli produced from valve disease or during atrial fibrillation of the heart. Ischemic stroke caused by systemic hypoperfusion usually is the result of decreased cerebral blood flow owing to circulatory failure. Circulatory failure results from too little blood, too low blood pressure (BP), or failure of the heart to pump blood adequately. Hypoxia from any cause also can produce this syndrome.

A *transient ischemic attack (TIA)*, which is a temporary (less than 24 hr) neurologic deficit that resolves completely without permanent damage, occurs when the artery cannot deliver enough blood to meet the O_2 requirement of the brain. However, restoration of blood flow is timely enough to make the ischemia (and deficits) transient, thereby avoiding infarction and permanent damage. TIAs usually are associated with thrombosis but may be caused by any of the ischemic mechanisms just mentioned. TIAs may precede a permanent ischemic stroke by hours, days, months, or years. TIAs are a warning sign, and treatment may prevent a stroke. Most TIAs last an average of 5-10 min, although some can last longer than an hour. A *reversible ischemic neurologic deficit (RIND)* lasts longer than 24 hr but otherwise is similar to a TIA.

Hemorrhagic stroke causes neural tissue destruction because of the infiltration and accumulation of blood. Ischemia and infarction may occur distal to the hemorrhage because of interrupted blood supply. Although a cerebral hemorrhage usually results from hypertension or an aneurysm, trauma also can cause hemorrhagic stroke. Bleeding may spread into the brain tissue itself, causing an intracerebral hemorrhage, or into the subarachnoid space. Usually there is a large rise in ICP with a hemorrhagic stroke because of cerebral edema and the mass effect of blood.

A stroke may be classified as a *progressive stroke in evolution*, in which deficits continue to worsen over time, or as a *completed stroke*, in which maximum deficit has been acquired and has persisted for longer than 24 hr. Progressive strokes usually are the result of thrombus formation and often take 1-3 days to become "completed." Embolic strokes typically have sudden onset with maximal deficits. *Stroke syndromes* classically have been described according to distribution of the vessels (middle cerebral artery, anterior cerebral artery, posterior cerebral artery, vertebral, basilar) that supply particular regions of the brain and will have typical assessment findings. Stroke is the third most common cause of death and the most common cause of neurologic disability. Half the survivors are left permanently disabled or experience another stroke. Improvement may continue for 1-2 yr, but deficits at 6 mo usually are considered permanent.

A *brain attack*, also sometimes called a *code stroke* or *stroke alert*, is a sudden event and medical emergency with the same urgency as a heart attack. If the stroke is ischemic and the patient qualifies, "time-is-tissue" and the sooner the patient can be treated, the better the outcome. For appropriate patients, treatment with recombinant tissue plasminogen activator (rt-PA) needs to occur within 3 hr of symptom onset. To achieve this, all people should be educated to recognize warning signs of stroke and immediately call 911. Rapid transport to a hospital, preferably a stroke center, should occur, with the emergency medical technician starting the medical history, especially the time of symptom onset, and alerting the hospital before arrival so the stroke team (if available) can be assembled. Upon arrival at the hospital door, the time-to-treatment goal is 60 min and is further broken down into subgoals:

Time from arrival at hospital door to:
- Evaluation by physician—10 min
- Neurologic expert and "stroke team" (if available) contacted—15 min
- Head computerized axial tomography (CT) or magnetic resonance imaging (MRI) scan completed; other data (e.g., laboratory values) collected—25 min
- Interpretation of CT or MRI scan completed; decision to treat based upon data, contraindications—45 min
- Start of treatment (e.g., rtPA) in appropriate patients—60 min

Intraarterial rtPA, available at some research centers, may extend the window of opportunity to 6 hr. Thrombolytic therapy reverses symptoms of stroke by dissolving the clot(s) causing the ischemia before actual cell death. Use of a mechanical blood clot retrieval device (e.g., MERCI) may extend this time window further.

Stroke care can be differentiated into these basic types: thrombolytic ischemic stroke care, nonthrombolytic ischemic stroke care (including TIAs), and hemorrhagic stroke care. Care differences center mostly around BP management and use of anticoagulant and antiplatelet agents. Most hospitals, especially stroke centers, have protocols for stroke management.

HEALTH CARE SETTING

Critical care unit, step-down unit, acute rehabilitation unit, outpatient rehabilitation program

ASSESSMENT

Note: Because of the narrow 3-hr window that may reverse permanent neurologic damage, it is critical to teach patients not to ignore symptoms and to call 911 without delay for the following:

- Sudden numbness or weakness of the face, arm, or leg, especially on one side of the body
- Sudden confusion, trouble speaking or understanding
- Sudden trouble seeing in one or both eyes
- Sudden trouble walking, dizziness, loss of balance or coordination
- Sudden, severe headache with no known cause

A history to determine time of symptom onset is critical inasmuch as this may determine eligibility for treatment. Time of onset is when patient was last known to be "normal," so if patient woke up after sleeping with symptoms, time of onset would be when the patient went to bed "normal" and not when he or she woke up symptomatic.

General findings: Classically, symptoms appear on the side of the body opposite the damaged site. For example, a stroke in the left hemisphere of the brain will produce symptoms in the right arm and leg. However, when the stroke affects the cranial nerves, symptoms of cranial nerve deficit will appear on the same side as the site of injury. Similarly, an obstruction of an anterior cerebral artery can produce bilateral symptoms, as will severe bleeding or multiple emboli. Hemiplegia is fairly common. Initially, patient usually has flaccid paralysis. As spinal cord depression resolves, more normal tone is seen and hyperactive reflexes occur.

Signs and symptoms: Vary with the size and site of injury and may improve in 2-3 days as the cerebral edema decreases. Changes in mentation, including apathy, irritability, disorientation, memory loss, withdrawal, drowsiness, stupor, or coma; bowel and bladder incontinence; numbness or loss of sensation; weakness or paralysis on part or one side of the body; aphasia; headache; neck stiffness and rigidity; vomiting; seizures; dizziness or syncope; ataxia; and fever may occur. A brain stem infarct leaving the patient completely paralyzed with intact cortical function is called *locked-in syndrome.* With

cranial nerve involvement, visual disturbances include diplopia, blindness, and hemianopia. Inequality or fixation of the pupils, nystagmus, tinnitus, and difficulty chewing and swallowing also occur.

Physical assessment: Papilledema, arteriosclerotic retinal changes, or hemorrhagic retinal areas on ophthalmic examination. Hyperactive deep tendon reflexes (DTRs), decreased superficial reflexes, and positive Babinski's sign also may be present. To check for Babinski's response, stroke the lateral aspect of the sole of the foot (from the heel to the ball of the foot) with a hard object. Dorsiflexion of the great toe with fanning of the other toes is a positive sign. Positive Kernig's or Brudzinski's sign (see "Bacterial Meningitis," p. 281) indicates meningeal irritation.

TIA: Typical symptoms include temporary episodes of slurred speech, weakness, numbness or tingling, blindness in one eye, blurred or double vision, dizziness or ataxia, and confusion.

Risk factors: TIAs; hypertension; atherosclerosis; high serum cholesterol or triglycerides; high homocysteine levels; diabetes mellitus; gout; smoking; obesity; cardiac valve diseases, such as those that may result from rheumatic fever, valve prosthesis, and atrial fibrillation; cardiac surgery; blood dyscrasias; anticoagulant therapy; neck vessel trauma; oral contraceptive use; cocaine or methamphetamine use; family predisposition for arteriovenous malformation (AVM); aneurysm; advanced age; or previous stroke.

Assessment scales (e.g., GCS and NIHSS): The Glasgow Coma Scale (GCS) is helpful for quickly assessing level of consciousness (LOC). The National Institutes of Health Stroke Scale (NIHSS) not only assesses LOC but also assesses deficits and provides a standardized approach to neurologic examinations. An NIHSS total score of 0-1 is normal; 1-4 is a minor stroke; 5-15 is a moderate stroke; 15-20 is a moderately severe stroke; and more than 20 is a severe stroke. The NIHSS score also strongly predicts likelihood of recovery, with higher scores resulting in more disability and poorer outcomes. Use of thrombolytics (e.g., rtPA) is considered appropriate for ischemic stroke if the total score is more than 4-6 and there is sustained, nonimproving deficit. NIHSS is used for assessing effects of thrombolytic therapy and should, at minimum, be done initially as a baseline, 2 hr post treatment, 24 hr post onset of symptoms, and 7-10 days after symptom onset. The complete scale with instructions can be obtained from *http://www.strokecenter.org.*

DIAGNOSTIC TESTS

Selection, sequence, and urgency of the following tests will be determined by the patient's history and symptoms. For example, a patient whose symptoms have resolved from a TIA will have a different set or sequence of tests compared to the patient who is in coma. Since usage of rtPA is time limited, speed is essential in determining type of stroke (ischemic vs. hemorrhagic) and other contraindications to rtPA. Obtaining computerized axial tomography (CT) scan to determine type of stroke is a top priority along with laboratory tests to assess for contraindications.

CT scan: To reveal site of infarction, hematoma, and shift of brain structures. CT scan is of particular value in identifying blood released early during hemorrhagic strokes. CT scan is the test of choice for unstable patients. Generally, identifying ischemic areas is difficult until they start to necrose at around 48-72 hr. Xenon-enhanced CT may be done to study cerebral blood flow; CT angiography may be performed to evaluate blood vessels.

MRI scan: To reveal site of infarction, hematoma, shift of brain structure, and cerebral edema. MRI diffusion and perfusion weighted studies are of particular value in identifying ischemic strokes early and in differentiating between acute and chronic lesions. Other MR techniques include MR angiography to evaluate vessels and MR spectrography.

Laboratory tests: Certain tests (e.g., serum electrolytes, complete blood count including differential and platelet count, prothrombin time with international normalized ratio, and partial thromboplastin time) should be done immediately to assess for contraindications such as hypoglycemia or clotting abnormalities if patient is a candidate for thrombolytic therapy. Other tests will be done depending on patient (e.g., toxicology screen, pregnancy test, blood culture and erythrocyte sedimentation rate for endocarditis or vasculitis process, hemoglobin HbAIC for diabetics). Lipid panel, C-reactive protein, and homocysteine levels also may be obtained.

Electrocardiogram: To evaluate for atrial fibrillation and myocardial ischemia.

Phonoangiography/Doppler ultrasonography: To identify presence of bruits if the carotid blood vessels are partially occluded. B-mode imaging and duplex scanning also may be done to evaluate the carotids to detect occlusive disease. Dimensional ultrasound improves three-dimensional visualization and includes the potential for quantitative monitoring of plaque volume changes in all three directions—circumferential, length, and thickness.

Transcranial Doppler ultrasound: To provide information (noninvasively) about pressure and flow in the intracranial arteries.

Swallowing examination/videofluoroscopy: All patients should be screened for dysphagia. Videofluoroscopy identifies problem or pathology, determines most appropriate treatment, and enables teaching of proper swallowing technique. This test is not performed for individuals known to aspirate saliva because it involves swallowing a barium-containing liquid, semisolid, and/or solid.

Positron emission tomography: To provide information on cerebral metabolism and blood flow characteristics. This test is useful in identifying ischemic stroke by showing areas of reduced glucose metabolism.

Single photon emission CT: To identify cerebral blood flow.

Electroencephalograph: To show abnormal nerve impulse transmission and indicate amount of brain wave activity present.

Lumbar puncture and CSF analysis: Not done routinely, especially in the presence of IICP, but may reveal increase in cerebrospinal fluid (CSF) pressure; clear to bloody CSF, depending on stroke type; and presence of infection or other nonvascular cause for bleeding. CSF glutamic oxaloacetic transaminase (GOT) will be increased for 10 days after injury. Blood in the CSF signals that a subarachnoid hemorrhage has occurred.

Cerebral and carotid angiography: If surgery is contemplated, this procedure is done to pinpoint site of rupture or occlusion and identify collateral blood circulation, aneurysms, or AVM.

Digital subtraction angiography: To visualize cerebral blood flow and detect vascular abnormalities, such as stenosis, aneurysm, and hematomas.

Echocardiography (e.g., transthoracic and transesophageal): To evaluate valvular heart structures for thrombus and myocardial walls for mural thrombi that may provide a source of emboli.

Evoked response test: Provides measurement of the brain's ability to process and react to different sensory stimuli. Responses from these sensory stimuli can indicate abnormal areas in the brain.

Electronystagmography: Evaluates patients who have dizziness, vertigo, or balance dysfunction and provides objective assessment of oculomotor and vestibular systems.

Nursing Diagnosis:

Impaired Physical Mobility

related to neuromuscular impairment with limited use of upper and/or lower limbs secondary to stroke

Desired Outcome: By at least 24 hr before hospital discharge, patient and significant other demonstrate techniques that promote ambulating and transferring.

INTERVENTIONS	RATIONALES
Assess for subluxation of the shoulder (e.g., shoulder pain and tenderness, swelling, decreased range of motion [ROM], altered appearance of bony prominences).	Shoulder subluxation occurs when weight of the affected arm is unable to be supported by the weakened shoulder muscles causing separation of the shoulder joint.
Never pull on the affected arm. Guide upper extremity movement from the scapula and not from the arm; use a lift sheet to reposition in bed. Ensure that the arm has a firm support surface when patient is sitting.	These measures help prevent subluxation. When in bed the shoulder should be positioned slightly forward to counteract shoulder rotation. The affected arm should be placed in external rotation when the patient is supine or lying on affected side.
Teach methods for turning and moving, using stronger extremity to move weaker extremity.	For example, to move affected leg in bed or when changing from a lying to a sitting position, slide unaffected foot under affected ankle to lift, support, and bring affected leg along in the desired movement.
Encourage patient to make a conscious attempt to look at extremities and check position before moving.	These are safety measures to prevent falling. For example, remind patient to make a conscious effort to lift and then extend foot when ambulating.
Instruct patient with impaired sense of balance to compensate by leaning toward stronger side.	The tendency is to lean toward weaker or paralyzed side. For example, patient may need to be reminded to keep body weight forward over feet when standing.
Recommend wearing well-fitting shoes.	Slippers, for example, tend to slide.
Prevent shoulder-hand syndrome with regular, gentle joint ROM exercises and proper arm positioning. Never place arm under the body. When patient is in bed, place arm on abdomen or pillow for support. Encourage repeated shoulder movement, elevation of the arm above cardiac level, and regular fist clenching and reclenching.	Shoulder-hand syndrome is a neurovascular condition characterized by pain, edema, and skin and muscle atrophy caused by impairment of the circulatory pumping action of the upper extremity.
Protect impaired arm with a sling.	The sling will support the arm and shoulder when patient is out of bed.
Position patient in correct alignment, and provide a pillow or lapboard for support. Encourage active/passive ROM to improve muscle tone.	These measures will help maintain anatomic position.
Teach and implement the following: - Encourage weight bearing on patient's stronger side. - Instruct patient to pivot on stronger side and use stronger arm for support. - Teach patient that transferring toward unaffected side is generally easiest and safest. - Instruct patient to place unaffected side closest to bed or chair to which he or she wishes to transfer. - Explain that when transferring, affected leg should be under patient with foot flat on the ground. - Position a braced chair or locked wheelchair close to patient's stronger side.	These are general principles to follow when transferring patients with impaired physical mobility. These transfer principles emphasize using the stronger or unaffected side to help support patient for safe transfers to reduce the risk of falling.
- If patient requires assistance from staff member, teach patient not to support self by pulling on or placing hands around assistant's neck.	Staff members should use their own knees and feet to brace feet and knees of patients who are very weak.
Obtain PT and OT referrals as appropriate. Reinforce special mobilization techniques (e.g., Bobath, constraint-induced movement therapy, PNF) per patient's individualized rehabilitation program.	These techniques may vary from the general principles mentioned. For example, Bobath focuses on use of affected side in mobility training so that patient tries to bear weight on affected side and move toward affected side to relearn normal movement patterns and position. Constraint-induced (CI) movement therapy involves restraining the functioning arm to induce "rewiring of the brain," thereby improving amount and quality of functional movement.

••• **Related NIC and NOC labels:** *NIC:* Exercise Therapy: Ambulation; Body Mechanics Promotion; Fall Prevention; Exercise Promotion
NOC: Ambulation: Walking; Ambulation: Wheelchair; Joint Movement: Active; Mobility Level; Transfer Performance

Nursing Diagnosis:

Impaired Verbal Communication

related to aphasia secondary to cerebrovascular insult

Desired Outcome: At least 24 hr before hospital discharge, patient demonstrates improved self-expression and relates decreased frustration with communication.

INTERVENTIONS	RATIONALES
Evaluate nature and severity of patient's aphasia. When doing so, avoid giving nonverbal cues. Assess patient's ability to speak clearly without slurring words, use words appropriately, point or look toward a specific object, follow simple directions, understand yes/no questions, understand complex questions, repeat both simple and complex words, repeat sentences, name objects that are shown, demonstrate or relate purpose or action of objects, fulfill written requests, write requests, and read. When evaluating for aphasia, be aware that patient may be responding to nonverbal cues and may understand less than you think. Document this assessment with simple descriptions and specific examples of aphasia symptoms. Use it as the basis for a communication plan.	Aphasia is the partial or complete inability to use or comprehend language and symbols and may occur with dominant (left) hemisphere damage. It is not the result of impaired hearing or intelligence. There are many different types of aphasia. Generally the patient has a combination of types that vary in severity. Fluent aphasia (e.g., Wernicke's, sensory, or receptive aphasia) is characterized by inability to recognize or comprehend spoken words. It is as if a foreign language were being spoken or the patient has word deafness. The patient often is good at responding to nonverbal cues. In nonfluent aphasia (e.g., Broca's, motor, or expressive aphasia) the ability to understand and comprehend language is retained but the patient has difficulty expressing words or naming objects. Gestures, groans, swearing, or nonsense words may be used.
Ask patient to repeat unclear words by speaking slowly in short phrases. If this is unsuccessful, ask patient to use another word or give a nonverbal clue.	Do not pretend you understand if you do not. Say so. Nonverbal cues, pointing, flash cards of basic needs, pantomime, paper/pen, spelling, or picture board, may help communication.
Obtain referral to a speech therapist or pathologist as needed. Provide therapist with a list of words that would enhance patient's independence and/or care. In addition, ask for tips that will help improve communication with patient.	Patient may need expertise of a specialist to facilitate ability to communicate.
When communicating with patient, try to reduce distractions in the environment, such as television or others' conversations.	This focuses patient's attention on communication.
Ensure that patient is well rested.	Fatigue affects ability to communicate.
Communicate with patient as much as possible. Use gestures, facial expressions, and pantomime to supplement and reinforce your message. Give short, simple directions, and repeat as needed to ensure understanding. Use concrete terms (e.g., "water" instead of "fluid" or "leg" instead of "limb"). If patient does not understand after repetition, try different words.	These are general principles for patients who may not recognize or comprehend the spoken word. Other suggestions include the following: face patient and establish eye contact, speak slowly and clearly, give patient time to process your communication and answer, keep messages short and simple, stay with one clearly defined subject, avoid questions with multiple choices but rather phrase questions so that they can be answered "yes" or "no," and use same words each time you repeat a statement or question (e.g., "pill" vs. "medication" and "bathroom" vs. "toilet").
When helping patient regain use of symbolic language, start with nouns first and progress to more complex statements as indicated, using verbs, pronouns, and adjectives.	Progression from simple to complex helps facilitate comprehension. For continuity, it is a good plan to keep at the bedside a record of words to be used (e.g., "pill" rather than "medication").
Treat patient as an adult. Be respectful.	It is not necessary to raise the volume of your voice unless patient is hard of hearing.
When patient has difficulty expressing words or naming objects, encourage patient to repeat words after you. Begin with simple words such as "yes" or "no," and progress to others, such as "cup." Progress to more complex statements as indicated.	These measures enable practice in verbal expression.
Listen and respond to patient's communication efforts. If patient makes an error, do not criticize patient's effort but rather compliment it by saying, "That was a good try." Praise accomplishments.	Otherwise patient may give up.
Be prepared for labile emotions. Do not react negatively to emotional displays. Address and acknowledge patient's frustration over the inability to communicate. Maintain a calm and positive attitude.	These patients become frustrated and emotional when faced with their impaired speech.

Continued

INTERVENTIONS	RATIONALES
When improvement is noted, let patient complete your sentence (e.g., "This is a _____"). Keep a list of words patient can say, and add to list as appropriate. Avoid finishing patient's sentences.	This list then can be used when formulating questions patient is known to be able to answer.
Avoid labeling patient as "belligerent" or "confused" when the problem is aphasia and frustration. Listen for errors in conversation, and provide feedback.	Patients who have lost ability to monitor their verbal output may not produce sensible language but may think they are making sense and not understand why others do not comprehend or respond appropriately to them.
Avoid instructing patient to "wait 5 min" because this may not be meaningful.	Patients who have lost ability to recognize number symbols or relationships will have difficulty understanding time concepts or telling time.
Point to an object and clearly state its name. Watch signals patient gives you.	This facilitates practice in receiving word images.
Bring patient with nondominant (right) hemisphere damage back to the subject by saying, "Let's go back to what we were talking about."	Patients with nondominant (right) hemisphere damage often have no difficulty speaking; however, they may use excessive detail, give irrelevant information, and get off on a tangent. These patients tend to respond better to verbal, rather than nonverbal, encouragement.
Observe for nonverbal cues, and anticipate patient's needs. Allow time to listen if patient speaks slowly.	This validates patient's message without rushing him or her, which would cause frustration.
Ensure that the call light is available and patient knows how to use it.	The call light is the first step in communicating a need for assistance.
For additional interventions for patients with dysarthria, see **Impaired Verbal Communication** in "General Care of Patients with Neurologic Disorders," p. 275.	Dysarthria can complicate aphasia.

••• Related NIC and NOC labels: *NIC:* Communication Enhancement: Speech Deficit; Active Listening; Anxiety Reduction *NOC:* Communication Ability; Communication: Expressive Ability

Nursing Diagnosis:

Unilateral Neglect

related to disturbed perceptual ability secondary to neurologic insult

Desired Outcome: Following intervention and on an ongoing basis, patient scans the environment and responds to stimuli on affected side.

INTERVENTIONS	RATIONALES
Assess patient's ability to recognize objects to right or left of his or her visual midline; perceive body parts as his or her own; perceive pain, touch, and temperature sensations; judge distances; orient self to changes in the environment; differentiate left from right; maintain posture sense; and identify objects by sight, hearing, or touch. Document specific deficits.	This assessment enables nurse to develop a plan of care individualized for the patient.

Neglect of and inattention to stimuli on affected side occur more often with right hemisphere injury. Neglect cannot be totally explained on the basis of loss of physical senses (e.g., both ears are used in hearing, but with auditory neglect, patient may ignore conversation or noises that occur on affected side). |
Arrange environment by keeping necessary objects, such as call light, on patient's unaffected side.	This will facilitate performance of activities of daily living (ADL).
Perform activities on unaffected side unless you are specifically attempting to stimulate the patient's neglected side.	Communicating and performing activities on patient's unaffected side will engage and be less confusing to patient.
If you must approach affected side, announce yourself first.	This announcement avoids startling patient.
Inform significant other about patient's deficit and compensatory interventions.	This enables significant other to be an informed participant in patient's care plan.

Continued

INTERVENTIONS	RATIONALES
Visual Neglect:	Patient does not turn head to see all parts of an object. For example, patient may read only half of a page or eat from only one side of plate.
Continuously cue patient to the environment. Initially place patient's unaffected side toward most active part of room, but as compensation occurs, reverse this. As patient begins to compensate, place additional items out of his or her visual field, thereby gradually increasing stimuli on affected side.	While communicating with patient, physically move across patient's visual boundary and stand on that side to shift patient's attention to neglected side; encourage patient to turn head past the midline and scan entire environment, especially while ambulating to prevent injury from falls or bumping into things. Place patient's food on neglected side, encouraging patient to look to neglected side and name the food before eating.
Self-Neglect:	Patient does not perceive arm or leg as being a part of the body. For example, when combing or brushing hair, patient attends to only one (unaffected) side of the head. Inadequate self-care and injury may occur.
Periodically refer to patient's body parts on neglected side. Encourage patient to touch or massage and look at affected side and make a conscious effort to care for neglected body parts first when performing ADL.	This promotes patient's self-recognition. For example, have patient use unaffected arm to perform ROM on affected side and provide a mirror so patient can watch self while shaving and brushing teeth and hair.
Encourage consciously monitoring affected side for position and checking for exposure to sharp objects, irritants, and hot or cold items.	This helps prevent contractures and skin breakdown or injury. For example, position arm on bedside table or wheelchair lap board with hand or arm past the midline, where patient can see it.
Provide structured tactile stimulation on affected side.	Stimulate with warm washcloth, cold ice chip, rough or soft-surfaced cloth, or similar item.
When patient is in bed or sitting up in a chair, provide side rails and restraints.	These are necessary safety measures because patient is unaware of the affected side and may attempt to get up.
Auditory Neglect:	Patient ignores individuals who approach and speak from affected side but communicates with those who approach or speak from unaffected side.
Move across auditory boundary while speaking, and continue speaking from patient's neglected side to bring patient's attention to that area.	This stimulates patient's attention to the affected side.

••• **Related NIC and NOC labels**: *NIC:* Unilateral Neglect Management: Body Image Enhancement; Positioning; Self-Care Assistance; Touch; Exercise Promotion; Fall Prevention; Environmental Management: Safety *NOC:* Body Image; Body Positioning: Self-Initiated; Self-Care: Activities of Daily Living

Nursing Diagnosis:

Disturbed Sensory Perception

related to altered sensory reception, transmission, and/or integration secondary to neurologic damage

Desired Outcome: Following intervention and on an ongoing basis, patient interacts appropriately with his or her environment and does not exhibit evidence of injury caused by sensory/perceptual deficit.

INTERVENTIONS	RATIONALES
Remind patients who have a dominant (left) hemisphere injury to scan their environment.	These patients may lack or have decreased pain sensation and position sense and have visual field deficit on the right side of the body. They may need reminders to scan their environment but usually do not exhibit unilateral neglect.
Give short, simple messages or questions and step-by-step directions. Keep conversation on a concrete level (e.g., say "water," not "fluid"; "leg," not "limb").	These individuals may have poor abstract thinking skills. They tend to be slow, cautious, and disorganized when approaching an unfamiliar problem and benefit from frequent, accurate, and immediate feedback on performance. They may respond well to nonverbal encouragement, such as a pat on the back.

Continued

INTERVENTIONS	RATIONALES
Enable patient to touch items (e.g., washcloth, comb) while caretaker names them.	Patient may have difficulty recognizing items by sight alone and therefore may benefit from touching items.
Encourage patients with nondominant (right) hemisphere injury to slow down and check each step or task as it is completed.	Patients with nondominant (right) hemisphere injury also may have decreased pain sensation and pain sense and visual field deficit but typically are unconcerned or unaware of or deny deficits or lost abilities. They tend to be impulsive and too quick with movements. Typically, they have impaired judgment about what they can and cannot do and often overestimate their abilities. These individuals are at risk for burns, bruises, cuts, and falls and may need to be restrained from attempting unsafe activities. They also are more likely to have unilateral neglect than individuals with dominant (left) hemisphere injury (see **Unilateral Neglect,** earlier).
Be careful what you say to these patients.	If you say "ate the lion's share," patient may think someone literally ate the lion's portion of the meal.
Have patients with apraxia return your demonstration of the task or see if they are able to be talked through a task or may be able to talk themselves through a task step-by-step.	Patients with apraxia have an inability to carry out previously learned motor tasks, although they may be able to describe them in detail.
Encourage making a conscious effort to scan the rest of the environment by turning head from side to side.	Patients may have visual field deficits in which they can physically see only a portion of the normal visual field.
Intervene as follows for patients with nondominant (right) hemisphere injury:	Patient may have the following sensory perceptual alterations:
- Direct patient's attention to a particular sound (e.g., if a cat meows on the television, state that it is the sound a cat makes and point to the cat on the screen).	*Impaired ability to recognize, associate, or interpret sounds* (e.g., voice quality, animal noises, musical pieces, types of instruments).
- Provide a structured, consistent environment. Mark outer aspects of patient's shoes or tag inside sleeve of a sweater or pair of pants with "L" and "R."	*Visual-spatial misconception:* Patient may have trouble judging distance, size, position, rate of movement, form, and how parts relate to the whole. For example, patient may underestimate distances and bump into doors or confuse inside and outside of an object, such as an article of clothing. These patients may lose their place when reading or adding up numbers and therefore never complete the task.
- Assist these individuals with eating. Monitor environment for safety hazards, and remove unsafe objects such as scissors from the bedside.	*Difficulty recognizing and associating familiar objects:* Patient may not know purpose of silverware. These patients may not recognize dangerous or hazardous objects because they do not know the purpose of the object or may not recognize subtle distinctions between objects (e.g., the difference between a fork and spoon may become too subtle to detect).
- Provide these patients with a restraint or wheelchair belt for support.	*Inability to orient self in space:* They may not know if they are standing, sitting, or leaning.
- Teach patient to concentrate on body parts (e.g., by watching feet carefully while walking). Provide a mirror to help them adjust.	*Misconception of own body and body parts:* These patients may not perceive their foot or arm as being a part of their body.
- Keep patient's environment simple to reduce sensory overload and enable concentration on visual cues. Remove distracting stimuli.	*Impaired ability to recognize objects by means of senses of hearing, vibration, or touch:* These patients rely more on visual cues.
- Verbally express what you are feeling (e.g., "I am smiling because I am happy to see you").	*Trouble recognizing emotional cues:* Patient may not be able to tell from voice, tone, words, or expression when others are happy, sad, or angry.

••• **Related NIC and NOC labels:** *NIC:* Body Image Enhancement; Self-Awareness Enhancement; Self-Care Assistance; Cognitive Stimulation; Environmental Management; Positioning; Surveillance: Safety *NOC:* Body Image; Cognitive Orientation

Nursing Diagnosis:

Deficient Knowledge:

Carotid endarterectomy or carotid angioplasty/stent procedure

Desired Outcome: Before surgery, patient verbalizes understanding of the carotid endarterectomy procedure, including the purpose, risks, expected benefits or outcome, and
postsurgical care.

INTERVENTIONS	RATIONALES
After health care provider has explained the procedure to the patient, determine patient's level of understanding and facility with language; employ an interpreter or language-appropriate written materials; and reinforce or clarify information as needed.	This enables development of an individualized teaching plan in the pre-operative stage that patient understands.
Obtain baseline neurologic and cranial nerve function test results.	These assessments will be the basis of comparison postoperatively.
For patient undergoing carotid endarterectomy	
As indicated, explain the procedure.	Carotid endarterectomy is removal of plaque in the obstructed artery to increase blood supply to the brain.
Describe the following postsurgical assessments:	
- There will be monitoring of vital signs (VS) and neurologic status at least hourly.	Pupils will be checked with a light and hands and legs will be tested for weakness and equality.
- Patient may be asked to swallow, move the tongue, smile, speak, and shrug shoulders to determine facial drooping, tongue weakness, hoarseness, speech difficulty, dysphagia, shoulder weakness, or loss of facial sensation.	Deficits in these abilities are signs of cranial nerve impairment. Stretching of the cranial nerves during surgery can occur, causing edema, and may leave a temporary deficit.
- Patient will be asked to report any numbness, tingling, or weakness.	These signs may indicate carotid occlusion.
- Superficial temporal and facial pulses will be palpated for strength, quality, and symmetry.	This will evaluate patency of the external carotid artery.
- There will be periodic assessments of the neck for edema, hematoma, bleeding, or tracheal deviation from midline. Patient should report immediately any respiratory distress, difficulty managing secretions, or sensation of neck tightness.	Any bleeding or excess edema at the surgical site can cause neck edema, which can deviate the trachea and compromise the airway. This can result in an emergent situation that necessitates airway management and surgical evacuation of the hematoma.
- Pulse oximetry may be continuously monitored and O_2 will most likely be supplied, even without respiratory distress or airway compromise.	Manipulation of the carotid sinus may cause temporary loss of normal physiologic response to hypoxia.
- Frequent blood pressure (BP) checks may be performed and patient may need vasoactive medications. Patient will be monitored for orthostatic hypotension when first getting up.	Temporary carotid sinus dysfunction may cause BP problems (usually hypertension). Vasoactive drugs may be given to keep SBP within a specified range (usually 100-150 mm Hg) to maintain cerebral perfusion while preventing disruption of graft or sutures as well as hyperperfusion syndrome.
Keep head of bed (HOB) in prescribed position (flat or elevated) and patient positioned off the operative side.	HOB may be elevated to promote wound drainage, particularly if a closed suction drain is left in place. (A closed drainage system with suction may be left in the neck for a day.) Positioning also enables visibility of wound site and promotes comfort.
If prescribed, keep ice packs on the incision.	Ice will reduce edema and pain.
Administer anticoagulant/antiplatelet therapy as prescribed.	Anticoagulant/antiplatelet therapy (e.g., aspirin, warfarin) may be instituted for 3-6 mo after the procedure and may continue longer, depending on patient's needs.
Include home instructions for the following: incision care (wash gently with soap and water), signs of infection (incision red, swollen, and painful; drainage, fever greater than 100.5° F, activity restrictions (no heavy lifting, no driving while neck turning is uncomfortable), and changes in neurologic status (alterations in speech, swallowing, vision, and numbness or weakness in arm or leg, especially on opposite side).	Following these instructions will decrease risk of infection and promote patient's physiologic safety.

Continued

INTERVENTIONS	RATIONALES
For patients undergoing carotid angioplasty and stenting	
Teach patient about angioplasty and stenting.	Angioplasty is the opening of a stenosed artery via a slender catheter that is passed through the narrow spot with balloon inflation to open up the obstruction. A stent, which will physically hold the newly unblocked vessel open, also may be placed.
Explain that frequent VS and neurology checks (as described previously) will be performed.	Cranial nerve problems are less frequent with this procedure because nerves have not been stretched, but they still will be included in the neurologic examination.
BP medications may be given to keep BP within specified parameters.	Temporary carotid sinus dysfunction may cause BP problems (usually hypertension), but this is less common than with endarterectomy. Maintaining systolic BP at less than 150 mm Hg may prevent hyperperfusion syndrome.
Advise patient that groin and distal pulses will be monitored for bleeding and patency.	The femoral artery is the usual vessel accessed.
Explain that HOB is usually elevated.	This position may help prevent headache.
Advise that patients are usually discharged the next day and go home on anticoagulants such as aspirin or ticlopidine.	Anticoagulants will help prevent clots forming in the stent and angioplasty area.

••• **Related NIC and NOC labels:** *NIC:* Preparatory Sensory Information; Teaching: Procedure/Treatment *NOC:* Knowledge: Treatment Procedures

ADDITIONAL NURSING DIAGNOSES/PROBLEMS:

"Prolonged Bedrest," for nursing diagnoses and interventions related to immobility (adjust interventions accordingly if patient has IICP or is at risk for this problem)   p. 61

"Psychosocial Support"   p. 73

"Psychosocial Support for the Patient's Family and Significant Other"   p. 87

"Older Adult Care" for **Risk for Aspiration**   p. 96

"Pulmonary Embolus" for **Ineffective Protection** related to risk of prolonged bleeding or hemorrhage secondary to anticoagulant therapy   p. 139

"General Care of Patients with Neurologic Disorders" for **Decreased Intracranial Adaptive Capacity**   p. 261

Impaired Swallowing   p. 267

Risk for Injury related to impaired pain, touch, and temperature sensations   p. 269

Impaired Tissue Integrity: Corneal   p. 270

Risk for Deficient Fluid Volume   p. 271

Imbalanced Nutrition: Less Than Body Requirements   p. 272

Constipation   p. 277

Self-Care Deficit   p. 277

ADDITIONAL NURSING DIAGNOSES/PROBLEMS—cont'd

Self-Care Deficit: Oral hygiene   p. 279

Disturbed Sensory Perception: Visual   p. 280

"Seizures and Epilepsy"   p. 323

"Traumatic Brain Injury" for **Excess Fluid Volume**   p. 366

Deficient Knowledge: Craniotomy procedure   p. 367

"Diabetes Insipidus" for patients with this disorder or who are at risk   p. 373

"Syndrome of Inappropriate Antidiuretic Hormone"   p. 415

"Peptic Ulcers"   p. 477

"Pressure Ulcers"   p. 562

For patients on mechanical ventilation, see the following:

"Pneumonia" for **Risk for Infection** related to inadequate primary defenses   p. 127

"General Care of Patients with Neurologic Disorders" for **Risk for Infection** related to inadequate primary defenses   p. 264

✓ PATIENT-FAMILY TEACHING AND DISCHARGE PLANNING

When providing patient-family teaching, focus on sensory information, avoid giving excessive information, and initiate a visiting nurse referral for necessary follow-up teaching. Include verbal and written information about the following:

✓ Symptoms that necessitate prompt attention: sudden weakness, numbness (especially on one side of the body), vision loss or dimming, trouble talking or understanding speech, unexplained dizziness, unsteadiness, or severe headache. To help families remember, teach the "FAST" acronym whereby "F" = face (have patient smile, look for weakness/numbness), "A" = arms (check for arm drift/strength/numbness), "S" = speech (have patient say simple sentence and watch for slurred or difficulty speaking/understanding, and "T" = Time (call 911 if any of these is present because "time is tissue").

✓ Interventions for safe swallowing and aspiration prevention.

✓ Importance of minimizing or treating the following risk factors: diabetes mellitus, hypertension, high cholesterol, high sodium intake, obesity, inactivity, smoking, prolonged bedrest, and stressful lifestyle.

✓ Interventions that increase effective communication in the presence of aphasia or dysarthria. Additional patient information can be obtained by contacting the National Aphasia Association at *www.aphasia.org*.

✓ Referrals to the following as appropriate: public health nurse, visiting nurses association, psychologic therapy, vocational rehabilitation agency, home health agencies, and extended and skilled care facilities.

✓ For patient information pamphlets, contact the National Institute of Neurological Disorders and Stroke (NINDS) at *www.ninds.nih.gov*.

✓ Additional general information can be obtained by contacting the following organizations:
- American Stroke Association at *www.strokeassociation.org*
- Stroke Information directory at *www.stroke-info.com*.
- Stroke Center at *www.strokecenter.org*
- On being struck by stroke *www.strokesurvivor.org*

See Also: Teaching and discharge planning (third through tenth entries only) under "Multiple Sclerosis," p. 311.

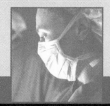

Traumatic Brain Injury 43

OVERVIEW/PATHOPHYSIOLOGY

Traumatic brain injury (TBI) can cause varying degrees of damage to the skull and brain tissue. Primary injuries occur at the time of impact and include skull fracture, concussion, contusion, scalp laceration, brain tissue laceration, and tear or rupture of cerebral vessels. Secondary problems that arise soon after and are the result of the primary injury include hemorrhage and hematoma formation from tear or rupture of vessels, ischemia from interrupted blood flow, cerebral swelling and edema, infection (e.g., meningitis or abscess), and increased intracranial pressure (IICP) or herniation, any of which can interrupt neuronal function. These secondary injuries or events increase the extent of initial injury and result in poorer recovery and higher risk of death. Cervical neck injuries are commonly associated with TBIs. Because of the potential for spinal cord injury, all TBI patients should be assumed to have cervical neck injury until it is conclusively ruled out by cervical spine x-ray examination.

Most TBIs result from direct impact to the head. Depending on force and angle of impact, the brain may suffer injury directly under the point of impact (coup) or in the region opposite the point of impact (contrecoup) because of brain rebound action within the skull, or tissue tearing or shearing may occur elsewhere because of the rotational action of the brain within the cranial vault. TBI may be classified by location, severity, extent, or mechanism (contact, acceleration, deceleration, rotational). Common causes include motor vehicle accidents; falls; and sports-related injuries, such as those occurring in football or boxing. Acts of violence, such as gunshot or stab wounds, often result in missile or impalement TBIs.

HEALTH CARE SETTING

Acute care (trauma center, intensive care); rehabilitation unit

ASSESSMENT

The Glasgow Coma Scale (GCS) standardizes observations for objective assessment of a patient's level of consciousness (LOC). GCS 13-15 is mild, 9-12 is moderate, and 3-8 is severe. This or some other objective scale should be used to prevent confusion with terminology and to quickly detect changes or trends in patient's LOC. LOC is the most sensitive indicator of overall brain function.

Concussion: Mild diffuse TBI in which there is temporary, reversible neurologic impairment may involve loss of consciousness and possible amnesia of the event. No damage to brain structure is visible on computerized axial tomography (CT) scan or magnetic resonance imaging (MRI) examination.

TBI concussions have been given the following grades:
- Grade I: No loss of consciousness
  - Transient confusion
  - Symptoms resolve in less than 15 min
- Grade II: No loss of consciousness
  - Transient confusion
  - Symptoms last more than 15 min
  - If symptoms last more than 1 wk, imaging may be needed
- Grade III: Any loss of consciousness

After concussion, patients may have headache, dizziness, nausea, lethargy, difficulty focusing, and irritability, especially to bright lights or loud noises. Although full recovery usually occurs in a few days, a postconcussion syndrome with headache; dizziness; irritability; emotional lability; lethargy; sleep disturbance; and decreased attention, judgment, concentration, and memory abilities may continue for several weeks or months.

Diffuse axonal injury: Diffuse brain injury caused by stretching and tearing of the neuronal projections because of a rotational, shearing type of injury. Diffuse microscopic damage occurs. No distinct focal lesion, such as infarction, ischemia, contusion, or intracerebral bleeding, is noted, but patients have an immediate and prolonged unconsciousness of at least 6-hr duration. CT scan may show small hemorrhagic areas in the corpus callosum, cerebral edema, and small midline ventricles. Brainstem injury may be associated with diffuse axonal injury (DAI), resulting in autonomic dysfunction. *Mild DAI* is coma lasting 6-24 hr with patient beginning to follow commands by 24 hr. Full recovery is expected. *Moderate DAI* is coma lasting longer than 24 hr but without prominent brainstem signs. *Severe DAI* is prolonged coma with prominent brainstem signs, such as decortication or decerebration, and usually predicts severe disability, possible vegetative state, or death.

Contusion: Bruising of brain tissue, which produces a longer-lasting neurologic deficit than concussion. Size and severity of bruising vary widely, and the bruise or a small, diffuse venous hemorrhage usually is visible on CT scan. Traumatic amnesia often occurs, causing loss of memory not only of the trauma, but also of events occurring before the incident. Loss of consciousness is common, and it is generally more prolonged than that with concussion. Changes in behavior, such as agitation or confusion, can last for several hours to days. Headache, nausea, lethargy, motor paralysis, paresis, and possibly seizures can occur as well. Depending on extent of damage, there is potential for either full recovery or permanent neurologic deficit, such as seizures, paralysis, paresis, or even coma and death.

Brain laceration: Actual tearing of the brain's cortical surface, resulting in direct mechanical disruption of neural function and causing focal deficits. Blood vessel tearing causes hemorrhage, resulting in contusion, edema, or hematoma formation. Seizures often occur as well. Brain lacerations usually result from depressed skull fractures, penetrating injuries, missile or impalement injuries, or rotational shearing injury within the skull. Shock waves from a bullet's high energy produce additional damage. A knife or other impalement object should be supported and left in the wound to control bleeding until it can be removed during surgery. Contusions and lacerations often are found together. The consequences of a laceration usually are more serious than those with a contusion because of the increased severity of trauma.

Skull fracture: Can be *closed* (simple, with skin intact) or *open* (compound), depending on whether the scalp is torn, thereby exposing the skull to the outside environment. Skull fractures are further classified as *linear* (hairline), *comminuted* (fragmented, splintered), or *depressed* (pushed inward toward the brain tissue). A blow forceful enough to break the skull is capable of causing significant brain tissue damage, and therefore close observation is essential. With a penetrating wound or basilar fracture (see below), there is potential for cerebrospinal fluid (CSF) leakage, meningitis, encephalitis, brain abscess, cellulitis, or osteomyelitis.

- *Basilar fractures:* Fractures of the base of the skull do not show up easily on skull/cervical x-ray examination. Indicators include blood from the nose, throat, ears; serous or serosanguineous drainage from the nose (rhinorrhea), throat, ears (otorrhea), eyes; Battle's sign (bruising noted behind the ear); "raccoon's eyes" (bruising around eyes in the absence of eye injury); and bleeding behind the tympanum (eardrum) noted on otoscopic examination. Glucose in serous drainage signals the presence of CSF. CSF leakage indicates a tear in the dura, making the patient particularly susceptible to meningitis. Basilar fractures may damage the internal carotid artery and cranial nerves. Hearing loss also may occur.

- *Temporal fractures:* May result in deafness or facial paralysis.

- *Occipital fractures:* May cause visual field and gait disturbances.

- *Sphenoidal fractures:* May disrupt the optic nerve, possibly causing blindness.

Rupture of cerebral blood vessels

- *Epidural (extradural) hematoma or hemorrhage:* Usually, bleeding between the dura mater (outer meninges) and skull causes hematoma formation. This creates pressure on the underlying brain and produces a local mass effect, causing IICP and shifting of tissue, which leads to brainstem compression and herniation. Indicators are primarily those of IICP: altered LOC, headache, vomiting, unilateral pupil dilation (on same side as the lesion), and possibly hemiparesis. Although some individuals never regain consciousness, most patients lose consciousness for a short period immediately after injury, regain consciousness, and have a lucid period lasting a few hours or 1-2 days. However, because arterial bleeding causes a rapid rise in intracranial pressure (ICP), a rapid decrease in LOC often ensues. The bleeding site often is the middle meningeal artery or vein because of temporal bone fracture. These patients are at risk for brainstem herniation. A unilateral dilated fixed pupil is a sign of impending herniation and is a neurosurgical emergency. Patients should not be left alone because respiratory arrest may occur at any time.

- *Subdural hematoma or hemorrhage:* Accumulation of venous blood between the dura mater (outer meninges) and arachnoid membrane (middle meninges) that is not reabsorbed. Hematoma formation creates pressure on the underlying brain and produces a local mass effect, causing IICP and shifting of tissue, leading to brainstem compression and herniation. This type of hematoma is classified as acute, subacute, or chronic depending on how quickly indicators arise. In acute subdural hematomas, indicators appear within 24-48 hr, resulting from focal neurologic deficit (hemiparesis, pupillary dilation) and IICP (decreased LOC, falling GCS score, nausea, vomiting, headache). When indicators occur 2-14 days later, the hematoma is considered subacute. When indicators occur more than 2 wk later, it is considered chronic. Early indicators can include headache, progressive personality changes, decreased intellectual functioning, slowness, confusion, and drowsiness. Later indicators may include unilateral weakness or paralysis, loss of consciousness, and occasionally seizures. Patients with cerebral atrophy (e.g., older persons, long-term alcohol users) are more prone to subdural hematoma formation.

- *Intracerebral hemorrhage:* Arterial or venous bleeding into the brain's white matter. Signs of IICP may develop early if the bleeding causes a rapidly expanding space-occupying lesion. If the bleeding is slower, signs of IICP can take 36-72 hr to develop. Indicators depend on hematoma location and size and can include altered LOC, headache, aphasia, hemiparesis, hemiplegia, hemisensory deficits, pupillary changes, and loss of consciousness.

- *Subarachnoid hemorrhage:* Bleeding into the subarachnoid space below the arachnoid membrane (middle meninges) and above the pia mater (inner meninges next to brain). The patient often has a severe headache. Other general indicators include vomiting, restlessness, seizures, and loss of consciousness. Signs of meningeal irritation include nuchal rigidity and positive Kernig's and Brudzinski's signs (see p. 281). This patient may be a candidate for a shunt because of hemorrhagic interference with CSF circulation and reabsorption and is at particular risk of cerebral vasospasm.

Indicators of IICP

- *Early indicators:* Alteration in LOC ranging from irritability, restlessness, and confusion to lethargy; possible onset or worsening of headache; beginning pupillary dysfunction, such as sluggishness; visual disturbances, such as diplopia or blurred vision; onset of or increase in sensorimotor changes or deficits, such as weakness; onset or worsening of nausea.
- *Late indicators:* Continued deterioration of LOC leading to stupor and coma; projectile vomiting; hemiplegia; posturing; alterations in vital signs (VS) (typically increased systolic blood pressure [SBP], widening pulse pressure, decreased pulse rate); respiratory irregularities, such as Cheyne-Stokes breathing; pupillary changes, such as inequality, dilation, and nonreactivity to light; papilledema; and impaired brainstem reflexes (corneal, gag, swallowing).

Note: The single most important early indicator of IICP is a change in LOC. Late indicators of IICP usually signal impending or occurring brainstem herniation. Signs generally are related to brainstem compression and disruption of cranial nerves and vital centers. Hypotension and tachycardia in the absence of explainable causes, such as hypovolemia, usually are seen as a terminal event in TBI. IICP usually peaks around 72 hr after initial insult and then gradually subsides over 2-3 wk.

Brain herniation: Brain herniation occurs when IICP causes displacement of brain tissue from one intracranial compartment to another, resulting in compression, destruction, and laceration of brain tissue. See late indicators of IICP for signs of impending or initial herniation. In the presence of actual brain herniation, patient is in a deep coma, pupils become fixed and dilated bilaterally, posturing may progress to bilateral flaccidity, brainstem reflexes generally are lost, and respirations and VS deteriorate and may cease.

Brain death: Criteria for determining brain death are not universally agreed upon. Check state and institutional guidelines. General criteria include absent brainstem reflexes (e.g., apnea, pupils nonreactive to light, no corneal reflex, no oculovestibular reflex to ice water calorics), absent cortical activity (e.g., several flat electroencephalogram [EEG] tracings spaced over time), and coma irreversibility continued over a specific timeframe (e.g., 24 hr). Brainstem auditory evoked responses and cerebral blood flow studies (e.g., transcranial Doppler, angiography, brain scan with a cerebral perfusion agent) also may be used to help confirm brain death.

DIAGNOSTIC TESTS

Cervical spine and skull x-ray examinations: To locate neck and skull fractures. Because of the close association between TBIs and spinal or vertebral injuries, cervical immobilization is essential until cervical x-ray examination rules out fracture and potential SCI.

CT scan: Used with acute injury to identify type, location, and extent of injury, such as accumulation of blood or a shift of midline structure caused by IICP.

MRI scan: To identify type, location, and extent of injury. Although not usually performed in acute, unstable patients, this test is the study of choice for subacute or chronic TBI. It is superior to CT scan for detecting isodense chronic subdural hematomas or evaluating contusions and shearing injuries, especially in the brainstem area. MRI techniques such as fluid attenuated inversion recovery (FLAIR) are particularly sensitive to detecting DAI and small hemorrhages.

Cerebral blood flow studies (transcranial Doppler, xenon inhalation enhanced CT): To determine focal areas of low blood flow or spasm, possibly indicating ischemic areas, by noninvasively measuring cerebral blood flow velocities.

EEG: To reveal abnormal electrical activity indicating neuronal damage caused by ischemia or hemorrhage. EEG may be used to establish brain death in conjunction with other tests and may be done serially to assess development of pathologic waves.

Evoked potentials: To evaluate integrity of the anatomic pathways and connections of the brain. Stimulation of a sense organ, such as an ear, triggers a discrete electrical response (i.e., evoked potential) along a neurologic pathway to the brain. Measurement of the brain's response to auditory, visual, and/or somatosensory stimulation also aids in predicting neurologic outcome.

Positron emission tomography: To evaluate tissue metabolism of glucose and oxygen.

Single photon emission CT: To determine low cerebral blood flow and areas at risk for ischemic tissue perfusion.

Infrared spectroscopy: To continuously and noninvasively assess cerebral O_2 saturation.

Cerebral angiography: To reveal presence of a hematoma and status of blood vessels secondary to rupture or compression. Angiography usually is performed only if CT scan or MRI scan is unavailable or to evaluate possible carotid or vertebral artery dissection.

Cisternogram: To identify dural tear site with basilar skull fracture.

CSF analysis: To evaluate for infection, if indicators are present.

Nursing Diagnosis:

Deficient Knowledge:

Caretaker's responsibilities for observing patient who is sent home with a concussion

Desired Outcomes: Following instruction, caretaker verbalizes knowledge about the observation regimen. Caretaker returns patient to the hospital if neurologic deficits are noted.

INTERVENTIONS	RATIONALES
Assess caretaker's health care literacy (language, reading, comprehension). Assess culture and culturally specific information needs.	This assessment helps ensure that materials are presented in a manner that is culturally and educationally appropriate.
Give the following instructions:	
- Do not give patient anything stronger than acetaminophen to relieve headache.	A possible exception is codeine for pain control. Otherwise, opioids and other medications that alter mentation are avoided because they can mask neurologic indicators of IICP and cause respiratory depression. Aspirin is usually contraindicated because it can prolong bleeding if it occurs.
- Assess patient at least q1-2h for first 24 hr as follows: awaken patient; ask patient's name, location, and caretaker's name; monitor for twitching or seizure activity.	This information gives caretaker the necessary information for returning patient to the hospital. To wit, caretaker should return patient to the hospital immediately if patient becomes increasingly difficult to awaken; cannot answer questions appropriately; cannot answer at all; becomes confused, restless, or agitated; develops slurred speech; develops twitching or seizures; develops or reports worsening headache or nausea/vomiting; has visual disturbances (e.g., blurred or double vision); develops weakness, numbness, or clumsiness or has difficulty walking; has clear or bloody drainage from nose or ear; or develops a stiff neck.
- Ensure that patient rests and eats lightly for first day or so after concussion or until he or she feels well.	Nausea and vomiting occur with increased ICP.
- Over the next 2-3 days, caution patient to avoid alcohol, driving, contact sports, swimming, using power tools, and taking medication for headache or nausea without calling health care provider.	These restrictions help ensure patient's safety. There is potential for neurologic deterioration at this time. For this reason, patient should return to a full schedule slowly.
Inform patient and significant other that some individuals may have postconcussion syndrome. Explain importance of reporting these problems to health care provider, especially if they worsen.	Some individuals may continue to have headaches, dizziness, or lethargy for several weeks or months after a concussion. Patient also may experience sleep disturbance, difficulty concentrating, poor memory, irritability, emotional lability, difficulty with judgment or abstract thinking, and may be very distractible with hypersensitivity to noise and light. These problems should be reported promptly for timely evaluation and intervention. Additional testing may be done to ensure other processes (e.g., chronic subdural hematoma) are not occurring, and medications may be prescribed to help with some symptoms (e.g., pain, sleep problems).

●●● **Related NIC and NOC labels:** *NIC:* Teaching: Procedure/Treatment; Teaching: Prescribed Medication; Teaching: Prescribed Diet; Teaching: Disease Process *NOC:* Knowledge: Treatment Regimen

Nursing Diagnosis:

Risk for Infection

related to inadequate primary defenses secondary to basilar skull fractures, penetrating or open TBIs, or surgical wounds

Desired Outcomes: Patient is free of symptoms of infection as evidenced by normothermia; stable or improving LOC; and absence of headache, photophobia, or neck stiffness. Patient verbalizes knowledge about signs and symptoms of infection and importance of reporting them promptly.

INTERVENTIONS	RATIONALES
Monitor injury site or surgical wounds for indicators of infection. Notify health care provider of significant findings.	Persistent erythema, local warmth, pain, hardness, and purulent drainage are indicators of localized infection that can occur as a result of loss of skin integrity.
Be alert to indicators of meningitis or encephalitis.	Meningitis or encephalitis (fever, chills, malaise, back stiffness and pain, nuchal rigidity, photophobia, seizures, ataxia, sensorimotor deficits) can occur after a penetrating, open TBI, or cerebral surgical wound. For more detail, see "Bacterial Meningitis," p. 281.
When examining scalp lacerations and assessing for foreign bodies or palpable fractures, wear sterile gloves and follow sterile technique. Cleanse area gently, and cover scalp wounds with sterile dressings.	These measures reduce possibility of infection, which can be serious if the TBI has created a breach directly into the nervous system.
Document drainage and its amount, color, and odor.	If patient has clear or bloody drainage from the nose, throat, or ears, it should be assumed patient has a dural tear with CSF leakage until proven otherwise and health care provider should be notified accordingly. Complaints of a salty taste or frequent swallowing may signal CSF dripping down the back of the throat. Bending forward may produce nasal drainage that can be tested for CSF.
Inspect dressing and pillowcases for a halo ring (blood encircled by a yellowish stain).	A halo ring may indicate CSF drainage.
Test clear drainage with a glucose reagent strip. Drainage may be sent to laboratory to test for Cl⁻.	The presence of glucose and Cl^- (CSF Cl^- is greater than serum Cl^-) in nonsanguineous drainage indicates that the drainage is CSF rather than mucus or saliva.
If CSF leakage occurs, do not clean ears or nose unless prescribed by health care provider. Position patient so that fluids can drain. Place a sterile pad over affected ear or under nose to catch drainage, but do not pack them. Change dressings when they become damp, using sterile technique.	These measures prevent introducing bacteria into the nervous system from the breach created by the TBI.
If not contraindicated, place patient in semi-Fowler's position.	This position helps reduce cerebral congestion and edema and promotes venous drainage.
With CSF leakage or possible basilar fracture, avoid nasal suction.	Nasal suction could introduce bacteria into the nervous system.
Instruct patient to avoid Valsalva's maneuver, straining with bowel movement, and vigorous coughing. Caution patient not to blow nose, sneeze, or sniff in nasal drainage.	These actions could tear the dura and increase CSF flow.
Be aware that if the gastric tube is placed nasally, the health care provider usually performs the intubation.	Nasogastric (NG) tubes have been known to enter the fracture site and curl up into patient's cranial vault during insertion attempts. **Note:** The tube for gastric decompression may be placed through the mouth for patients with basilar skull fractures to avoid passing the tube via the nose through the fracture area and into the brain.
Check tube placement, preferably by x-ray examination, before applying suction. Visually check back of patient's throat for NG tube to help confirm placement.	These measures help confirm the tube's proper placement and avoid causing harm to patient.
As prescribed, keep individuals with basilar skull fractures flat in bed and on complete bedrest.	This position helps decrease pressure and amount of CSF draining from a dural tear.
Administer antibiotics as prescribed.	Patients are given antibiotics to prevent infection and observed for healing and sealing of the dural tear within 7-10 days.
Teach patient that a CSF leak will be a source of infection until healed or repaired and that most CSF leaks from dural tears heal themselves in 5-10 days.	If a CSF leak does not heal, serial lumbar punctures or a lumbar subarachnoid drain may be needed to drain CSF, reduce CSF pressure, and promote healing. Acetazolamide or dexamethasone may be given to decrease CSF production. Radionuclide-labeled materials may be injected into the subarachnoid space and pledgets placed in the nose and ears to find the site of the CSF leak. A blood patch may be used. Surgical repair (e.g., duraplasty) may be required if other methods prove ineffective. Basilar fractures are a common site of CSF leaks and make surgical repair difficult because of location inaccessibility.

Continued

INTERVENTIONS	RATIONALES
For patients with a lumbar drain, explain that they will be on bedrest with head of bed (HOB) elevated up to 15-20 degrees. Teach patient to call for assistance and not to cough, sneeze, or strain. Explain that patient's vital signs and neurological checks will be monitored for any deterioration and patient should call for problems such as new onset weakness, numbness, difficult swallowing, and headache.	Deterioration of neurologic signs may indicate possible meningitis (see p. 281) or a pneumocranium resulting from too-rapid drainage of CSF, which causes air to siphon in through the dural tear, creating an intracranial mass effect. If neurologic signs deteriorate, care provider should be called promptly. Clamping the lumbar drain tubing and placing patient in a flat or in a slight Trendelenburg position with supplemental O_2, will promote absorption of intracranial air.
Explain that glucose may be closely monitored and kept under strict control.	Hyperglycemia is associated with poorer outcomes, including higher infection rates. Intensive insulin therapy may be used during the acute phase when patients are in intensive care unit (ICU), with insulin drips and frequent monitoring to keep glucose at less than 110 mg/dl. After stabilization, sliding scale or rainbow coverage to keep glucose at less than 150 mg/dl is usually instituted.

••• **Related NIC and NOC labels:** *NIC:* Infection Prevention; Wound Care; Tube Care: Gastrointestinal; Tube Care: Lumbar Drain *NOC:* Infection Status; Wound Care: Primary Intention

Nursing Diagnosis:

Excess Fluid Volume

related to compromised regulatory mechanisms with increased antidiuretic hormone (ADH) and increased renal resorption secondary to syndrome of inappropriate ADH secretion (SIADH)

Desired Outcome: By hospital discharge (or within 3 days of injury), patient is normovolemic as evidenced by stable weight; balanced I&O; urinary output 30 ml/hr or more; urine specific gravity 1.010-1.030; BP within patient's baseline limits; absence of fingerprint edema over the sternum; and orientation to person, place, and time.

INTERVENTIONS	RATIONALES
Differentiate between SIADH and cerebral salt wasting (CSW) syndrome, whose treatments are different.	While both syndromes involve hyponatremia (Na^+ less than 137 mEq/L), SIADH results in hypervolemia and CSW results in hypovolemia. In CSW syndrome, the kidneys are unable to conserve sodium, and a true serum hyponatremia occurs with decreased plasma volume, weight loss, high blood urea nitrogen level, decreased serum osmolality, and hypernatriuria. CSW is treated with fluid replacement (IV normal saline), volume expanders, salt tablets, and occasionally fludrocortisone to inhibit Na^+ excretion and induce Na^+ retention. If serum sodium is very low, a hypertonic saline may be used. Usually both syndromes resolve in a week or two.
Monitor serum sodium, intake and output (I&O), and weight. Notify health care provider of significant findings.	In the presence of SIADH, a potential complication of TBI, the patient will have inappropriate urinary concentration causing excessive water retention and a dilutional hyponatremia. Expect seizure activity when serum Na^+ level drops below 118 mEq/L. Serum Na^+ level less than 115 mEq/L may result in loss of reflexes, coma, and death. Seizure activity would increase the metabolic rate in the CNS and further compromise the patient's neurologic status.
Assess for fingerprint edema over sternum.	This reflects cellular edema. Because fluid is not retained in the interstitium with SIADH, peripheral edema will not necessarily occur.
Be aware that depending on serum $Na\pm$ value, fluids may be restricted to an amount as low as 500-1000 ml/24 hr. Intervene accordingly and as prescribed.	Fluid overload can increase ICP.

Continued

INTERVENTIONS

INTERVENTIONS	RATIONALES
If indicated and prescribed, enable free use of salt or salty foods in patient's diet.	This measure helps normalize patient's Na$^+$ level.
For other interventions, see this nursing diagnosis in "Syndrome of Inappropriate Antidiuretic Hormone," p. 415.	

••• **Related NIC and NOC labels:** *NIC:* Fluid/Electrolyte Management; Electrolyte Monitoring; Laboratory Data Interpretation; Electrolyte Management: Hyponatremia *NOC:* Electrolyte & Acid-Base Balance

Nursing Diagnosis:

Acute Pain

related to headaches secondary to TBI

Desired Outcome: Within 1 hr of intervention, patient's subjective perception of pain decreases, as documented by a pain scale.

INTERVENTIONS	RATIONALES
Monitor and document duration and character of patient's pain, rating it on a scale of 0 (no pain) to 10 (worst pain). Monitor for nonverbal indicators of pain such as facial grimacing, muscle tension, guarding, restlessness, increased or decreased motor activity, irritability, anxiety, or sleep disturbance.	This assessment provides a baseline for subsequent comparison and quantifies degree of pain and pain relief obtained.
Administer analgesics as prescribed.	Patients with TBI generally do not have much pain, and it is usually relieved by analgesics, such as acetaminophen. Sometimes codeine is prescribed, but as a rule, other narcotics are contraindicated because they can mask neurologic indicators of IICP and cause respiratory depression.
Monitor for pain, swelling, warmth, and decreased ROM function around joints, especially the hips.	These signs may indicate heterotopic ossification (HO), which is abnormal formation of true bone within the extraskeletal soft tissues and can occur after a fracture. Etidronate, nonsteroidal antiinflammatory drugs, such as indomethacin, range-of-motion (ROM) exercises, and external beam radiation are prevention therapies. Once HO has formed, resection usually is necessary.
For additional interventions, see **Acute Pain,** p. 273, in "General Care of Patients with Neurologic Disorders."	

••• **Related NIC and NOC labels:** *NIC:* Pain Management; Analgesic Administration *NOC:* Comfort Level

Surgical Nursing Diagnoses in TBI

Nursing Diagnosis:

Deficient Knowledge:

Craniotomy procedure

Desired Outcome: Following the explanation, patient verbalizes accurate understanding of the craniotomy procedure, including presurgical and postsurgical care.

INTERVENTIONS	RATIONALES
After health care provider's explanation of the procedure, determine patient's level of understanding of purpose, risks, and anticipated benefits or outcome. Intervene accordingly with an interpreter, or reinforce health care provider's explanation as appropriate. Provide and review language-appropriate printed material if available.	This assessment enables development of an effective teaching plan.
	A craniotomy is a surgical opening into the skull to remove a hematoma or tumor, repair a ruptured aneurysm, apply arterial clips or wrap the involved vessel to prevent future rupture, control hemorrhage, remove bone fragment or foreign objects, debride necrotic tissue, elevate depressed fractures, or decompress the brain. Trephination ("burr" holes) may be used to evacuate hematomas or insert intracranial monitoring devices. Cranioplasty is done to repair traumatic or surgical defects in the skull.
Encourage questions and discuss fears and anxiety. Obtain informed consent.	There is the possibility of cognitive and behavioral changes related to site of surgery, which frequently diminish or disappear in 6 wk to 6 mo.
As appropriate, explain that the bone flap may be left open postoperatively.	This enables accommodation of cerebral edema and prevents compression. When the bone is removed, the procedure is called a craniectomy.
Explain that before surgery, antiseptic shampoos may be given and patient may be started on corticosteroids, such as dexamethasone, and antiepilepsy drugs.	Hair can be a major source of microorganisms. Dexamethasone may be given for cerebral edema; antiepilepsy drugs may be given prophylactically.
Explain that a baseline neurologic assessment will be performed.	This provides a basis for comparison with postoperative neurologic checks.
During immediate postoperative period, patient is in ICU. Explain the following considerations and interventions that are likely to occur:	
- VS and neurologic status will be assessed at least hourly. Emphasize importance of performing these tasks to the best of patient's ability.	Patient will be asked to perform a variety of assessment measures, including squeezing tester's hand, moving extremities, extending tongue, and answering questions.
- Changes in body image that can occur because of loss of hair, presence of a head dressing, and potential for and expected duration of facial edema.	Patient may consider use of headpiece, scarf, or wig for concerns regarding change in body image.
- Presence of sequential compression devices on legs and possibly arterial line for continuous BP monitoring as well as other devices such as ICP monitoring equipment and external ventriculostomy.	This equipment will be used to prevent thrombophlebitis and pulmonary emboli, for continuous BP monitoring, and to detect changes in ICP. Typically patients are on a cardiac monitor for 24-48 hr because dysrhythmias are not unusual after posterior fossa surgery or when blood is in CSF.
- Possible need for respiratory and airway support, including O_2, intubation, or ventilation.	Respirations will be monitored for irregularity (a sign of bleeding and brainstem compression).
- Presence of large head dressing and drains. Stress importance of not pulling or tugging on dressing or drains. Advise that patient should report a sweet or salty taste in mouth inasmuch as this may indicate a CSF leak.	Dressing and incisions will be inspected periodically for bleeding or CSF leakage, which will be reported to health care provider for prompt intervention.
- Patient is given nothing by mouth (NPO) for first 24-48 hours.	There is risk of vomiting and choking. Patient may experience a dry throat at this time and will be monitored for swallowing difficulties, which may signal cranial nerve compression from IICP.
- Possible presence of periorbital swelling.	This usually occurs within 24-48 hr of supratentorial surgery. Relief is obtained with applications of cold or warm compresses around the eyes. Having HOB raised with patient lying on nonoperative side also may help reduce edema.
- Insertion of indwelling urinary catheter.	This enables accurate measurement of I&O and monitors for potential problems such as diabetes insipidus.
- Measurement of core temperature (e.g., rectal, tympanic, bladder) at frequent intervals.	A rectal probe or bladder catheter temperature probe may be used for continuous monitoring so that fever can be evaluated and treated promptly. Oral temperatures are avoided during period cognitive function is decreased.

Continued

INTERVENTIONS	RATIONALES
Teach patient that postsurgical positioning is a key factor during recovery, as discussed in the following procedures:	Patient is maintained with HOB elevated to 30 degrees or as prescribed. Patient will be assisted with turning and usually will be kept off operative site, especially if the lesion was large. Head and neck will be kept in good alignment.
- *Supratentorial craniotomy*	HOB is kept flat or as prescribed. Sitting may increase risk of venous air embolus with posterior fossa surgery. Pressure usually is kept off operative site, especially with a craniectomy; therefore these patients are kept off their backs for 48 hr. In posterior fossa surgery, the supporting neck muscles are altered. Patient is logrolled to alternate sides, keeping head in good alignment. A soft cervical collar may be used to prevent anterior or lateral angulation of the neck. A small pillow may be used for comfort.
- *Infratentorial craniotomy (for cerebellar or brainstem surgery)*	Patient is not positioned onto operative side immediately after surgery because this could cause shifting inside the space.
- *For areas of evacuation causing large intracranial space*	Turning onto side that bone was removed is avoided. Staff will label on chart and bed the location of missing bone.
- *After craniectomy*	This may involve a gradual elevation of HOB to prevent cerebral hemorrhage. For example, HOB may be flat for 24 hr, 15 degrees for next 24 hr, 30 degrees for next 24 hr, 45 degree for next 24 hr, and then 90 degrees.
- *Ventricular shunts and chronic subdural hematomas*	HOB may be flat while the drain is in place and for 24 hr after removal to prevent air from being pulled into the subdural space.
If a subdural drain is placed:	
Explain that bedrest is usually maintained for the first 24 hr.	Bedrest enables the effects of anesthesia to wear off fully, reduces activity that may increase ICP, and helps ensures stability of vital signs.
Explain that patients having supratentorial surgery near the area of the pituitary gland or hypothalamus may develop transient diabetes insipidus (DI).	Supratentorial surgery may cause localized edema around the pituitary stalk, which could cause DI. See "Diabetes Insipidus," p. 373, for details.
Teach patients undergoing infratentorial surgery that they are likely to experience the following:	
- A longer period of bedrest.	These patients are likely to experience an extended period of dizziness and hypotension.
- Nausea, which should be reported as soon as it is noted.	This ensures that antiemetics (e.g., metoclopramide, trimethobenzamide) are given promptly.
- Swallowing difficulties, extraocular movements, or nystagmus, any of which should be reported promptly.	These problems are the result of cranial nerve edema.
Teach patient the following precautions that are taken to prevent increased intraabdominal and intrathoracic pressure: exhaling when being turned; not straining at stool; not moving self in bed, but rather letting staff members do all moving; importance of deep breathing and avoiding coughing and sneezing (if coughing and sneezing are unavoidable, they must be done with an open mouth to minimize pressure buildup); and avoiding hip flexion and lying prone.	Increased intraabdominal and intrathoracic pressures can cause IICP, which could result in brain edema and ischemia, neurologic changes, and brain herniation.
	For additional precautions against IICP, see **Decreased Intracranial Adaptive Capacity,** p. 261.
Teach patient that precautions are taken for seizures.	See **Risk for Trauma** related to oral, musculoskeletal, and airway vulnerability secondary to seizure activity, p. 325.
Teach patient wound care and indicators of infection: fever; redness; drainage from surgical site, nose, or ears; and increased headache.	Generally, a surgical cap is worn after removal of head dressing. Patient must avoid scratching wound, staples, or sutures and must keep incision dry. When sutures or staples are removed, hair can be shampooed, being careful not to scrub around incision line. Hair dryers are avoided until hair is regrown to prevent tissue damage caused by heat. For more information, see **Risk for Infection,** p. 364.

Continued

INTERVENTIONS	RATIONALES
Explain that patients undergoing acoustic neuroma excision may have nausea; hearing loss; facial weakness or paralysis; diminished or absent blinking; eye dryness; tinnitus; vertigo; headache; and occasionally swallowing, throat, taste, or voice problems.	Acoustic neuromas can wrap around cranial nerve VII, and surgery may damage this cranial nerve and cause localized edema. Other cranial nerves whose nuclei are in the brainstem also may be affected.
	Nausea and dizziness may be profound problems after surgery. Prescribed antiemetics will be given, and patient should be turned and moved slowly. Patient should be spoken to on unaffected side for best hearing, and phone and call light should be placed on that side of bed. Contralateral routing of signal hearing aids may improve hearing by directing sound from deaf ear to hearing ear via a tiny microphone and transmitter. Background music or other white noise may mask tinnitus. Awareness of tinnitus eventually should lessen. Balance exercises and walking with assistance will start compensation process by the functioning vestibular system.
For additional interventions, see **Deficient Knowledge:** Surgical Procedure, p. 45, in "Perioperative Care."	Watching television or reading may be difficult because of vertigo; listening to books on tape or the radio are good alternatives. Eye dryness, from impaired eyelid function, may require use of eye drops or ointment.

••• **Related NIC and NOC labels**: *NIC:* Preparatory Sensory Information; Teaching: Procedure/Treatment; Teaching: Psychomotor Skill; Learning Facilitation *NOC:* Knowledge: Treatment Procedures

Nursing Diagnosis:

Deficient Knowledge:

Ventricular shunt procedure

Desired Outcome: Following explanation, patient verbalizes accurate information about ventricular shunt procedure, including presurgical and postsurgical care.

INTERVENTIONS	RATIONALES
Determine patient's understanding of the procedure after health care provider's explanation, including purpose, risks, and anticipated benefits or outcome. Intervene accordingly. Also assess patient's facility with language; provide an interpreter or language-appropriate written materials as indicated.	This assessment enables development of an effective teaching plan. A ventricular puncture, or ventriculostomy, is a temporary procedure used to remove excess CSF.
As indicated, reinforce purpose of the procedure.	A ventricular shunt procedure is performed to enable permanent drainage of CSF when flow is obstructed (e.g., because of presence of a tumor or blood) through a one-way pressure gradient valve.
Explain that patient may have a cranial dressing, as well as a dressing on the neck, chest, or abdomen.	Shunt types vary but can extend from the lateral ventricle of the brain to one of the following: subarachnoid space of the spinal canal, right atrium of the heart, a large vein, or the peritoneal cavity.
Explain that it is important to avoid lying on insertion site after the procedure.	This restriction prevents pressure on the shunt mechanism, which could decrease CSF drainage.
Advise that head and neck are kept in alignment.	This prevents kinking and compression of the shunt catheter.
Explain that there is a shunt valve for controlling CSF drainage or reflux.	Most shunts have a valve that is pre-set to open at a particular pressure to permit CSF flow and does not require "pumping." There also are valves that have adjustable programmable opening pressures that are adjusted externally by using a magnet or programming device. Pumping is usually contraindicated for these new shunts, depending on manufacturer recommendations.

Continued

INTERVENTIONS	RATIONALES
Explain that the valve, which is usually located behind or above the ear and is the approximate diameter of a pencil, can be felt to empty and then refill.	Malfunction may be noted by either deterioration in neurologic status or failure of the reservoir to refill when pumped.
Reassure patient and significant other that before hospital discharge, specific instructions will be given about shunt care, recognition of shunt site infection and malfunction, and steps to take should they occur. Teach signs and symptoms of IICP (i.e., headache; change in LOC such as drowsiness, lethargy, irritability, nausea, personality changes) that should be reported to health care provider and may indicate shunt malfunction.	Kinked tubing, obstructed tubing or valve, and movement of the cannula can result in inadequate drainage of ventricles. Cannula movement also can result in abdominal viscus perforation or subdural hematoma formation. For ventriculoatrial shunts, emboli or endocarditis may occur. For ventriculoperitoneal shunts, ascites may occur.
If patient is to have an endoscopic third ventriculostomy, explain the procedure and its purpose.	This procedure may be tried as an alternative to a standard shunt in order to provide drainage of CSF in cases of obstructive hydrocephalus. A small hole or holes are made in the third ventricle to enable CSF to flow into the basal cistern for absorption.

For additional interventions, see **Risk for Infection,** p. 54, and **Deficient Knowledge:** Surgical Procedure, p. 45, in "Perioperative Care."

••• **Related NIC and NOC labels:** *NIC:* Preparatory Sensory Information; Teaching: Procedure/Treatment; Teaching: Psychomotor Skill; Learning Facilitation *NOC:* Knowledge: Treatment Procedures

ADDITIONAL NURSING DIAGNOSES/PROBLEMS:

"Perioperative Care" for patients undergoing surgical procedures — p. 45

"Prolonged Bedrest" for patients with varying degrees of immobility — p. 61

"Psychosocial Support" — p. 73

"Psychosocial Support for the Patient's Family and Significant Other" — p. 87

"General Care of Patients with Neurologic Disorders" for **Decreased Intracranial Adaptive Capacity** — p. 261

Risk for Falls — p. 265

Impaired Swallowing — p. 267

Risk for Injury related to impaired pain, touch, and temperature sensation — p. 269

Impaired Tissue Integrity: Corneal — p. 270

Risk for Deficient Fluid Volume — p. 271

Imbalanced Nutrition: Less Than Body Requirements — p. 272

Risk for Imbalanced Body Temperature — p. 274

Constipation — p. 277

Self-Care Deficit — p. 277

ADDITIONAL NURSING DIAGNOSES/PROBLEMS—cont'd:

Disturbed Sensory Perception — p. 280

"Seizures and Epilepsy" for seizure-related nursing diagnoses — p. 323

"Stroke" for **Impaired Physical Mobility** — p. 351

Impaired Verbal Communication — p. 353

Disturbed Sensory Perception — p. 355

As appropriate, see nursing diagnoses in "Diabetes Insipidus" — p. 373

"Syndrome of Antidiuretic Hormone" — p. 415

"Peptic Ulcers" — p. 477

"Managing Wound Care" for **Impaired Tissue Integrity** (or risk for same) related to excessive tissue pressure — p. 563

For patients on mechanical ventilation, see the following:

"Pneumonia" for **Risk for Infection** related to inadequate primary defenses — p. 127

"General Care of Patients with Neurologic Disorders" for **Risk for Infection** related to inadequate primary defenses — p. 264

✓ PATIENT-FAMILY TEACHING AND DISCHARGE PLANNING

The patient with TBI can have varying degrees of neurologic deficit, ranging from mild to severe. When providing patient-family teaching, focus on sensory information, avoid giving excessive information, and initiate a visiting nurse referral for necessary follow-up teaching. Include verbal and written information about the following:

✓ Referrals to community resources, such as cognitive retraining specialist, head injury rehabilitation centers, visiting nurses association, community support groups, social workers, psychologic therapy, vocational rehabilitation agency, home health agencies, and extended and skilled care facilities. Additional general information can be obtained by contacting the following organizations:

- Brain Injury Association, Inc., at *www.biausa.org*
- Brain Trauma Foundation at *www.braintrauma.org*
- The Rehabilitation and Research Center at *www.tbi-sci.org*

✓ Safety measures related to decreased sensation, visual disturbances, motor deficits, and seizure activity.

✓ Measures that promote communication in the presence of aphasia.

✓ Wound care and indicators of infection. Instruct patient to avoid scratching sutures and shampoo only after sutures are out.

✓ Indicators of ICP, which include change in LOC, lethargy, headache, nausea, and vomiting and should be reported to health care provider promptly.

✓ Measures that deal with cognitive or behavioral problems. As appropriate, include home evaluation for safety. Caution significant other that personality can change drastically after TBI. Patient may demonstrate inappropriate social behavior, inappropriate affect, hallucination, delusion, and altered sleep pattern.

✓ Cognitive rehabilitation goals (e.g., Rancho Los Amigos Hospital at *www.braininjury.com/recovery.html*) for appropriate patients to promote highest level of cognitive functioning. Family can be instructed in and participate in coma stimulation techniques (usually for short periods 2-4 times/day). In addition, suggest *http://calder.med.miami.edu/pointis/tbifam/coma2.html* for appropriate patients to increase quantity, quality, and duration of responses. Most cognitive recovery occurs in the first 6 mo.

✓ If patient had a concussion, a description of problems that may occur at home and necessitate prompt medical attention (see **Deficient Knowledge,** p. 364).

✓ For other information, see teaching and discharge planning interventions (fourth through tenth entries only) in "Multiple Sclerosis," p. 311, as appropriate.

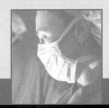

Diabetes Insipidus 44

OVERVIEW/PATHOPHYSIOLOGY

Diabetes insipidus (DI) is a condition that can result from one of several problems. *Central (neurogenic) DI* is caused by a defect in the synthesis of antidiuretic hormone (ADH) by the hypothalamus or release from the posterior pituitary. *Nephrogenic DI* results from a defect in the renal tubular response to ADH, causing impaired renal conservation of water. The primary problem is excessive output of dilute urine. Neurogenic DI may be the result of primary DI (i.e., a hypothalamic or pituitary lesion or dominant familial trait), secondary DI (following injury to the hypothalamus or pituitary stalk), or vasopressinase-induced DI, which is seen in the last trimester of pregnancy (caused by a circulating enzyme that destroys vasopressin). Nephrogenic DI either occurs as a familial X-linked trait or is associated with pyelonephritis, renal amyloidosis, Sjögren's syndrome, sickle cell anemia, myeloma, potassium depletion, or chronic hypercalcemia. A rare form of DI, termed *psychogenic diabetes insipidus*, is associated with compulsive water drinking. Another form of water consumption related DI is *dipsogenic diabetes insipidus*, caused by an abnormality in hypothalamic control of the thirst mechanism. This condition is most often idiopathic, but has been associated with chronic meningitis, granulomatous diseases, multiple sclerosis, and other widely diffuse brain diseases. Patients have severe polydipsia and polyuria. Lastly, a lack of vasopressin can develop during pregnancy, resulting is *gestagenic diabetes insipidus*. The condition may be treated with vasopressin if severe, but generally resolves 6-8 weeks following delivery.

Except for when it follows infection or trauma, DI onset is usually insidious, with progressively increasing polydipsia and polyuria. DI following trauma or infection has three phases. In the first phase, polydipsia and polyuria immediately follow the injury and last 4-5 days. In the second phase, which lasts about 6 days, the symptoms disappear. In the third phase, the patient experiences continued polydipsia and polyuria. Depending on the degree of injury, the condition can be either temporary or permanent.

DI must be differentiated from other syndromes resulting in polyuria. History, physical examination, and simple laboratory procedures assist in diagnosis. Other causes of polyuria include recent lithium or mannitol administration; renal transplantation; renal disease; hyperglycemia; hyperosmolality (early); hypercalcemia; and potassium depletion, including primary aldosteronism.

HEALTH CARE SETTING

Acute care (either medical-surgical or intensive care unit); primary care for patient who is being managed after hypophysectomy

ASSESSMENT

Signs and symptoms: Polydipsia, polyuria (2-20 L/day) with dilute urine (specific gravity less than 1.007).

Physical assessment: Usually within normal limits, but patient may show signs of dehydration if fluid intake is inadequate. Individuals with cranial injury, disease, or trauma may exhibit impairment of neurologic status, including altered level of consciousness (LOC) and sensory or motor deficits.

History of: Cranial injury, especially basilar skull fracture; meningitis; primary or metastatic brain tumor; surgery in the pituitary area; cerebral hemorrhage; encephalitis; syphilis; or tuberculosis (TB). Familial incidence rarely is a factor.

DIAGNOSTIC TESTS

Urine osmolality: Decreased (less than 200 mOsm/kg) in the presence of disease.

Specific gravity: Decreased (less than 1.007) in the presence of disease.

Serum osmolality: Increased (300 mOsm/kg or greater) in the presence of disease.

Vasopressin (DDAVP) challenge test: After administration of vasopressin subcutaneously or desmopressin by nasal spray, urine is collected q15min for 2 hr. Quantity and specific gravity are then measured. Normally, individuals will show a concentration of urine but not as pronounced as that of persons with DI; a person with kidney disease will have a lesser response to vasopressin. **Note:** One serious side effect of this test is precipitation of heart failure in susceptible individuals.

Hypertonic saline infusions: NaCl 3% solution is infused IV to assess for subsequent water conservation. Although this test seldom is necessary for diagnosis of DI, it does assist in documentation of changes in the osmotic threshold for ADH release.

Water deprivation (dehydration) test: Although less commonly used today, some health care providers do use it as a marker. Baseline measurements of body weight, serum and urine osmolalities, and urine specific gravity are obtained. Fluids are not permitted, and measurements are repeated hourly. Test is terminated when urine specific gravity exceeds

1.020 and osmolality exceeds 800 mOsm/kg (normal responses), urine specific gravity does not increase for 3 hr (a positive result), or 5% of body weight is lost. The latter is, in itself, an abnormal response, and corresponding urine osmolality will be less than 400 mOsm/kg, which is diagnostic of DI. Because the most serious side effect of this test is severe dehydration, the test should be performed early in the day so that patient can be more closely monitored. Before a firm diagnosis of DI can be made from an abnormal water deprivation test, it is also necessary to demonstrate that the kidneys can respond to vasopressin.

MRI scan of the brain: Magnetic resonance imaging (MRI) scan used to identify pituitary lesions that may have caused the DI.

Nursing Diagnosis:

Deficient Fluid Volume

related to active loss secondary to polyuria

Desired Outcome: Patient becomes normovolemic within 7 days of onset of symptoms as evidenced by stable weight, balanced intake and output (I&O), good skin turgor, moist tongue and oral mucous membrane, BP 90-140/60-100 mm Hg (or within patient's normal range), HR 60-100 bpm, urine specific gravity greater than 1.010, and CVP 2-6 mm Hg (or 5-12 cm H_2O).

INTERVENTIONS	RATIONALES
Monitor I&O, specific gravity, and vital signs (VS) hourly. Check weight daily.	Signs of hypovolemia include weight loss, inadequate fluid intake to balance output, thirst, poor skin turgor, decreased specific gravity, furrowed tongue, hypotension, and tachycardia.
If available, monitor central venous pressure (CVP).	CVP may decrease to less than 2 mm Hg in the presence of hypotension.
Immediately report the following to the health care provider: (1) urinary output more than 200 ml in each of 2 consecutive hr, (2) urinary output more than 500 ml in any 2-hr period, or (3) urine specific gravity less than 1.002.	These are signs of extreme diuresis. Diuresis may result in hypotension, hypokalemia, and dehydration leading to highly viscous blood. Patient is at increased risk of hypovolemic shock, stroke, dysrhythmias, and heart attack.
Provide unrestricted fluids: keep water pitcher full and within easy reach of patient. Explain importance of consuming as much fluid as can be tolerated.	The chief danger to patients with DI is dehydration from the inability to take in adequate fluids to balance the excessive output of urine.
Administer vasopressin and antidiuretic agents (or thiazide diuretic for patient with nephrogenic DI) as prescribed.	These measures are instituted to prevent extreme diuresis.
	Several vasopressin preparations are available, and it is important to read package insert carefully to ensure proper administration. Potential side effects of exogenous vasopressin include hypertension secondary to vasoconstriction, myocardial infarction secondary to constriction of coronary vessels, uterine cramps, and increased peristalsis of the gastrointestinal (GI) tract.
	A mild antidiuretic effect may be achieved with hydrochlorothiazide, chlorpropamide, clofibrate, carbamazepine, or other medication that increases the action or release of ADH.
	Note: Although it may seem antithetical to treat diuresis with a diuretic, one of the side effects of the thiazide diuretics is blocking of the kidneys' ability to excrete free water, which is the primary problem with DI.
For unconscious patients, administer IV fluids as prescribed. Unless otherwise directed, for every ml of urine output, deliver 1 ml of IV fluid.	To promote rehydration, lost water is replaced with IV hypotonic (e.g., 0.45% NaCl) solution. Initial replacement is rapid, necessitating close monitoring of blood pressure (BP), heart rate (HR), and urine output to prevent overhydration. IV normal saline may be used following initial fluid resuscitation.

••• Related NIC and NOC labels: *NIC:* Electrolyte Management; Fluid/Electrolyte Management; Electrolyte Monitoring; Fluid Monitoring; Intravenous (IV) Insertion; Intravenous (IV) Therapy; Laboratory Data Interpretation; Vital Signs Monitoring; Fluid Management; Hypovolemia Management; Medication Administration; Fluid Resuscitation *NOC:* Electrolyte & Acid-Base Balance; Fluid Balance

Nursing Diagnosis:

Ineffective Protection

related to potential for side effects of vasopressin

Desired Outcomes: Optimally, patient demonstrates normal mental acuity; verbalizes orientation to person, place, and time; and is free of signs of injury caused by side effects of vasopressin. As appropriate, patient or significant other demonstrates administration of coronary artery vasodilators by time of hospital discharge.

INTERVENTIONS	RATIONALES
Monitor VS and report significant changes.	Significant changes such as systolic BP (SBP) elevated more than 20 mm Hg over baseline SBP or HR increased more than 20 bpm over baseline HR are signs of vasoconstriction, which is an undesirable effect when vasopressin is used solely as an ADH.
Monitor for changes in mental status or LOC, confusion, weight gain, headache, convulsions, and coma.	These are signs of water intoxication caused by fluid retention.
If these signs develop, stop the vasopressin, restrict fluids, and notify health care provider. Institute safety measures accordingly, and reorient patient as needed.	Water intoxication causes significant dilution of circulating electrolytes, resulting in effects seen with such electrolyte disorders as hyponatremia, hypokalemia, and hypochloremia.
For older adults or persons with vascular disease, keep prescribed coronary artery vasodilators (i.e., nitroglycerin) at the bedside for use if angina occurs. Teach patient and significant other how to administer these medications.	Angina may result from coronary vasoconstriction induced by vasopressin. Vasopressin dose should be reduced if angina occurs.

••• Related NIC and NOC labels: *NIC:* Cerebral Perfusion Promotion; Environmental Management: Safety; Neurologic Monitoring; Seizure Precautions; Surveillance; Vital Signs Monitoring *NOC:* Neurological Status: Consciousness

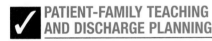

PATIENT-FAMILY TEACHING AND DISCHARGE PLANNING

When providing patient-family teaching, speak slowly and simply, avoid giving excessive information, and initiate a visiting nurse referral for necessary follow-up teaching. Include verbal and written information about the following:

✓ Importance of medical follow-up; confirm date and time of next visit to health care provider.

✓ Medications, including drug name, purpose, dosage, schedule, precautions, and potential side effects. Also discuss drug-drug, food-drug, and herb-drug interactions.

✓ Importance of seeking immediate medical attention if signs of dehydration or water intoxication occur. See **Ineffective Protection,** earlier.

✓ Recommendations for fluid replacement: guidelines on type and amount of replacement fluids prescribed for patient.

✓ Additional information available from Diabetes Insipidus Foundation, Inc., at *www.diabetesinsipidus.org.*

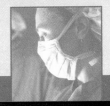

Diabetes Mellitus 45

OVERVIEW/PATHOPHYSIOLOGY

Diabetes mellitus (DM) is a disease of chronic hyperglycemia affecting more than 7% (20.8 million) of the total U.S. population. While 14 million cases are diagnosed, more than 6 million remain undiagnosed. DM may be diagnosed in up to 38% of hospitalized hyperglycemic medical patients and in 33% of hospitalized surgical patients. Prevalence has increased in a direct relationship with increasing incidence of obesity. Hispanic, Native American, and African American populations have a higher incidence than Caucasians and other groups. Metabolic, vascular, and neurologic disorders ensue from dysfunctional glucose transport into body cells. Insulin facilitates glucose transport into cells for oxidation and energy production. Food intake, glycogen breakdown, and gluconeogenesis increase the serum glucose level, which stimulates the beta islet cells of the pancreas to release needed insulin for transport of glucose from the bloodstream into the cells. At the cellular level, insulin receptors control the rate of transport of glucose into the cells. As glucose leaves the blood, serum levels return to normal (70-110 mg/dl).

Individuals with DM have impaired glucose transport because of decreased or absent insulin secretion and/or ineffective insulin receptors. Carbohydrate, fat, and protein metabolism are abnormal, and patients are unable to store glucose in the liver and muscle as glycogen, store fatty acids and triglycerides in adipose tissue, or transport amino acids into cells normally. DM is classified into the following four clinical classes as well as prediabetes:

Type 1 (5%-10%): Complete lack of effective endogenous insulin, causing hyperglycemia and ketosis resulting from beta islet cell destruction. This type is precipitated by altered immune responses, genetic factors, and environmental stressors. Certain human leukocyte antigens have been strongly associated with type 1 DM. These individuals depend on insulin for survival and prevention of life-threatening diabetic ketoacidosis (DKA).

Type 2 (90%-95%): Metabolic disorder that may range from insulin resistance with moderate insulin deficiency to a severe defect in insulin secretion with insulin resistance that results in severe hyperglycemia without ketosis. Untreated hyperglycemia can result in hyperosmolar hyperglycemic non-ketotic (HHNK) syndrome. Most individuals with type 2 diabetes are obese.

Other types: Formerly termed *secondary diabetes,* these include the following:

- *Diseases of the exocrine pancreas:* Pancreatitis, cystic fibrosis, hemochromatosis, trauma, infection, pancreatic cancer, and pancreatectomy may result in destruction of beta islet cells. All diseases except cancer generally involve extensive pancreatic destruction.
- *Drug-induced by insulin antagonists:* Many drugs impair insulin secretion, including phenytoin, steroids (hydrocortisone, dexamethasone), hormones (estrogen), IV pentamidine, nicotinic acid, thyroid hormone, thiazides, alpha-interferon, and rat poison.
- *Endocrine dysfunction/hormonal diseases:* Growth hormone, epinephrine, cortisol, and glucagons antagonize insulin and may be increased when diseases such as acromegaly, Cushing's syndrome, pheochromocytoma, or glucagonoma are present. Presence of excess antagonistic hormones results in reduced insulin action, and with somatostatinoma and aldosteronoma, insulin secretion may be reduced.
- *Genetic defects of the beta cell:* An autosomal dominant pattern results in severely impaired insulin secretion, most often characterized by hyperglycemia beginning before 25 years of age; it is also termed *maturity onset diabetes of the young.*
- *Genetic defects in insulin action:* A genetic defect manifested as abnormal insulin action is reflected by hyperinsulinemia with mild to severe hyperglycemia. Women with acanthosis nigricans and those with polycystic ovaries may have this type of insulin resistance. Leprechaunism and Rabson-Mendenhall syndrome are two pediatric syndromes in this category.
- *Infections:* Presence of several different viruses, including rubella, coxsackievirus B, cytomegalovirus (CMV), adenovirus, and mumps has resulted in beta cell destruction.
- *Uncommon immune-mediated diabetes:* Antiinsulin receptor antibodies bind to insulin receptors and can either block or increase binding of insulin, resulting in either hyperglycemia or hypoglycemia. Systemic lupus erythematosus and "stiffman" syndrome are examples of implicated disorders.
- *Other genetic syndromes:* Hyperglycemia has been linked to patients with Down's syndrome, Klinefelter's syndrome, Turner's syndrome, and Wolfram's syndrome.

Many of these "secondary" causes have recently become subclassified under type 1 and type 2 DM as possible primary causes of these diseases.

Gestational diabetes mellitus (GDM): Glucose intolerance with hyperglycemia that develops during pregnancy in approximately 4% of pregnant women, resulting in increased perinatal risk to the child and increased risk (25%) of the mother developing chronic DM during the next 10-15 yr. This type does not include *previously* diabetic pregnant women. Deterioration of glucose tolerance is considered "normal" during the third trimester of pregnancy.

Prediabetes with impaired glucose tolerance and impaired fasting glucose: Certain individuals may manifest chronic hyperglycemia without meeting other criteria for DM and are classified as having impaired glucose tolerance (IGT) or impaired fasting glucose (IFG), with fasting blood glucose levels 110 mg/dl or more but less than 126 mg/dl or 2-hr oral glucose tolerance test (OGTT) of 140 mg/dl or more but less than 200 mg/dl. These persons are at risk for developing DM and cardiovascular disease. IGT was formerly termed *borderline, chemical, latent, subclinical,* or *asymptomatic* DM. At least 20.1 million people in the United States, ages 40 to 74, have prediabetes. Some long-term damage to the body, especially heart and circulatory system, already may be occurring during prediabetes. Furthermore, if blood glucose is controlled when prediabetes is identified, development of type 2 diabetes can be prevented.

HEALTH CARE SETTING

Primary care, with possible hospitalization resulting from complications

ASSESSMENT

Metabolic signs of chronic hyperglycemia: Fatigue, weakness, weight loss, paresthesias, mild dehydration, and symptoms of hyperglycemia (polyuria, polydipsia, polyphagia). These indicators are seen in the early stages of illness.

Impending type 1 crisis (DKA): Profound dehydration and hyperglycemia, electrolyte imbalance, metabolic acidosis caused by ketosis, altered mental status, Kussmaul's respirations (paroxysmal dyspnea), acetone breath, possible hypovolemic shock (hypotension, weak and rapid pulse), abdominal pain, and possible strokelike symptoms.

Impending type 2 crisis (HHNK): Severe dehydration, hypovolemic shock (hypotension, weak and rapid pulse), severe hyperglycemia, shallow respirations, altered mental status, slight lactic acidosis or normal pH, possible strokelike symptoms.

COMPLICATIONS

Potential for acute crisis: *For type 1,* include DKA and hypoglycemia; *for Type 2,* include HHNK and hypoglycemia. All individuals with DM are at higher risk for developing cardiovascular disease. These complications should be preventable and are discussed as follows.

Long-term complications: The most important factor in delaying progression to long-term complications is stabilization of blood glucose levels to normal range.

Macroangiopathy: Patients are at higher risk for heart attack and stroke caused by vascular disease affecting the coronary arteries and larger vessels of the brain and lower extremities (peripheral vascular disease). Risk factors are hyperglycemia, hypertension, hypercholesterolemia, smoking, aging, and extended duration of DM.

Microangiopathy: Patients are at higher risk for blindness and renal failure caused by thickening of capillary basement membranes resulting in retinopathy and nephropathy. Early symptoms include increased leakage of retinal vessels and microalbuminuria.

Neuropathy: Patients are at higher risk for gastroparesis (impaired gastric emptying), lack of sensation (especially in the feet), and neurogenic bladder caused by deterioration of peripheral and autonomic nervous systems, resulting in impaired or slowed nerve transmission.

Morning hyperglycemia: Blood glucose elevation found on awakening. Causes include each of the following or a combination of the effects of their interactions.

Insufficient insulin: The most common cause of hyperglycemia before breakfast is probably inadequate levels of circulating insulin. Patient may need a higher dosage, a mixture of insulins, or longer-acting insulin.

Dawn phenomenon: Glucose remains normal until approximately 3 AM, when the effect of nocturnal growth hormone may elevate glucose in type 1 DM. It may be corrected by changing time of the evening dose of intermediate-acting insulin injection to bedtime instead of dinnertime.

Somogyi phenomenon: Patient becomes hypoglycemic during the night. Compensatory mechanisms to raise glucose levels are activated and result in overcompensation. It may be corrected by decreasing evening dose of intermediate-acting insulin and/or eating a more substantial bedtime snack.

Problems with insulin:

Insulin resistance: A problem experienced by most individuals with DM and other diseases at some point in the illness, when the daily insulin requirement to control hyperglycemia and prevent ketosis exceeds 200 U. It is characterized as one of the following anomalies:

- *Pre-receptor:* Insulin abnormal or insulin antibodies present.
- *Receptor:* Number of insulin receptors decreased or insulin binding to the receptors diminished.
- *Postreceptor:* Receptors not appropriately activated by insulin.

Local allergic reactions: Soreness, erythema, or induration at the insulin injection site within 2 hr after injection. Reactions are decreasing in frequency with the evolution of more purified insulins. Beef and beef/pork insulins are no longer commercially available in the United States. Pork insulin is used in less than 10% of patients. Use of human insulin has decreased the number of reactions significantly.

Systemic allergic reactions: With the advent of primarily human insulin and insulin analogues, systemic allergic reactions are extremely rare. The episode begins with a localized skin reaction, which evolves into generalized urticaria or ana-phylaxis. Patients must be desensitized to insulin by progression from minuscule to more normal doses over the course of 1 day, using a series of subcutaneous injections.

Lipodystrophy: Local disturbance in fat metabolism resulting in loss of fat (lipoatrophy) or development of abnormal fatty masses at the injection sites (lipohypertrophy). Lipoatrophy rarely has been seen since the development of 100 U and human source insulins. Rotation of injection sites helps prevent lipohypertrophy. Individuals experiencing lipohypertrophy should use alternate injection sites until the condition resolves.

DIAGNOSTIC TESTS

Testing for DM should be considered for persons older than 45 years old, particularly for those who are obese (body mass index greater than 25 kg/m^2). If results are normal, testing should be repeated every 3 yr. Younger obese individuals also may warrant testing, particularly if they have a first-degree relative with DM, are physically inactive, are in a high-risk ethnic group (e.g., Latino, Native American, African American, Asian American, or Pacific Islander), are hypertensive (blood pressure [BP] greater than 130/80 mm Hg), have a high-density lipoprotein (HDL) cholesterol of less than 35 mg/dl or triglycerides more than 250 mg/dl, have a history of vascular disease or other diseases associated with hyperglycemia, have a history of IFG/IGT, or have polycystic ovarian syndrome.

The World Health Organization and American Diabetes Association (ADA) define the following diagnostic criteria for DM in nonpregnant adults.

Fasting plasma glucose/blood sugar: The preferred diagnostic test, a value greater than 126 mg/dl is indicative of DM.

Fasting is defined as no calories consumed or infused for 8 hr before testing.

Oral glucose tolerance test: The 2-hr sample during the test is 200 mg/dl or more. The test is poorly reproducible and not performed often in practice. The patient is given a high glucose-containing solution and undergoes multiple blood sample testings over the following 2 hr.

Casual/random plasma glucose: Measurement is 180 mg/dl or more on at least two occasions. The blood is drawn regardless of food/beverage consumption at any time during the day.

Hemoglobin A$_{1C}$/glycosylated hemoglobin (glycohemoglobin): Normal range is 4%-7%. Individuals with DM will have values greater than 7%. This value is measured to assess control of blood glucose over a preceding 2- to 3-mo period. The larger the percentage of glycosylated Hgb, the poorer the blood glucose control. Reducing glycohemoglobin levels to less than 6% may further reduce complications. Kits are now available to monitor this value in the home.

Once the Diagnosis of Diabetes Mellitus is Made

Fasting lipid profile: If total and low-density lipoprotein (LDL) cholesterol values are elevated, triglyceride value is elevated, or HDL cholesterol level is decreased, the patient is at high risk for developing cardiovascular disease.

Urinalysis for presence of microalbuminuria, ketones, protein, and sediment: If present, may indicate early renal disease caused by hyperglycemia.

Serum creatinine: If elevated, may indicate renal disease.

12-lead ECG: If patient has symptoms of cardiovascular disease, an electrocardiogram (ECG) can identify areas of myocardial ischemia, infarction, and active injury.

Nursing Diagnosis:

Risk for Unstable Glucose Level

related to inadequate insulin production or insulin resistance that may lead to generalized vascular disease and neuropathy

Desired Outcomes: Optimally, patient has a blood glucose reading of less than 180 mg/dl at all times; fasting blood glucose readings less than 110 mg/dl; hemoglobin A$_{1C}$ level of less than 7; adequate tissue perfusion as evidenced by warmth, sensation, brisk capillary refill time (less than 2 sec), and peripheral pulses greater than 2+ on a 0-4+ scale in the extremities; BP within his or her optimal range; urinary output 30 ml/hr or more; baseline vision; good appetite; and absence of nausea and vomiting. Patient demonstrates adherence to the therapeutic regimen (essential for promoting optimal tissue perfusion).

INTERVENTIONS	RATIONALES
Check blood glucose before meals and at bedtime.	This monitors effectiveness of blood glucose control at times when patient's glucose is not increased by food being digested.
	The American Association of Clinical Endocrinologists (2003) has determined that both morbidity and mortality could be reduced for thousands of patients if hyperglycemia is diagnosed at admission and treated throughout hospitalization. Guidelines state that in critically ill patients, blood sugar level should be maintained at 80-110 mg/dl. Non–intensive care patients should be maintained at a premeal level of no more than 110 mg/dl and a maximum level of 180 mg/dl. Benefits of treatment outweigh any potential negative outcomes of low blood sugar.
Administer basal, prandial, and correction doses of insulin as prescribed.	Adherence to the therapeutic regimen is essential for promoting optimal tissue perfusion. Progression of vascular disease and neuropathy, including blindness, kidney failure, gastroparesis, heart attack, and stroke is the root cause of all complications of DM. By keeping serum glucose in a more normal range, the vascular endothelium receives better nourishment within the cells and will be less likely to deteriorate.
Encourage patient to perform regular home blood glucose monitoring.	Blood glucose is generally monitored before meals, at bedtime, and possibly during the night (3:00 AM) in order to assess whether a correction dose of short-acting insulin is needed. Self-monitoring by patients is extremely useful in reducing complications.
Check BP q4h. Alert health care provider to values outside patient's normal range. Administer antihypertensive agents as prescribed and document response.	Hypertension is commonly associated with diabetes. Careful control of BP is critical in preventing or limiting development of heart disease, stroke, retinopathy, and nephropathy.
Monitor for orthostatic hypotension after administering blood pressure medications.	Orthostatic hypotension is a potential side effect of antihypertensive agents and of autonomic neuropathy in which the patient's compensatory mechanisms may be impaired.
In addition to sensation, assess capillary refill, temperature, peripheral pulses, and color.	This assessment monitors patient's peripheral perfusion to detect macroangiopathy/PVD.
Protect patients with impaired peripheral perfusion from injury caused by sharp objects or heat (e.g., avoid use of heating pads).	Patients may experience decreased sensation in the extremities because of peripheral neuropathy.
Teach patient to avoid pressure at back of the knees by not crossing legs or "gatching" bed under the knees. Caution patient to avoid garments that constrict circulation to the extremities and lower body. For additional information see **Impaired Skin Integrity,** p. 382.	These actions could cause venous stasis and reduction in arterial perfusion in patients with macroangiopathy or impending peripheral vascular disease.
As indicated, orient patient to locations of such items as water, tissues, glasses, and call light.	This orientation provides necessary information and a safe environment for patients with diminished eyesight caused by diabetic retinopathy.
Monitor laboratory values for changes in renal function.	Laboratory values that would signal changes in renal function include increases in blood urea nitrogen (more than 20 mg/dl) and creatinine (more than 1.5 mg/dl). Approximately half of all persons with type 1 DM develop chronic kidney disease (CKD) and end-stage renal disease. Proteinuria (protein more than 8 mg/dl in a random sample of urine) or microalbuminuria are early indicators of developing CKD. (See "Chronic Kidney Disease," p. 217, for more information.)
Also monitor urine output, especially after exposure to contrast medium. Observe these patients for indicators of acute renal failure (ARF). (See "Acute Renal Failure," p. 231, for more information.)	Individuals with DM and with reduced renal function are at significant risk for dehydration and development of ARF after exposure to contrast medium. Patients who will receive contrast medium should be well hydrated and possibly receive several doses of oral acetylcysteine or an IV bicarbonate infusion to protect the kidneys from contrast-related deterioration.
Assess for changes in mentation, apprehension, erratic behavior, trembling, slurred speech, staggering gait, and seizure activity. Treat hypoglycemia as prescribed.	These are signs of hypoglycemia. Patients with hypoglycemia may experience vasodilation and diminished myocardial contractility, which decrease cerebral circulation and impair cognition.

Continued

INTERVENTIONS	RATIONALES
In addition	
Assess for the following:	Individuals with DM may experience multiple problems resulting from autonomic neuropathy.
Orthostatic hypotension:	
- Check BP while patient is lying down, sitting, and then standing. Alert health care provider to significant findings.	BP decreased from patient's normal, along with lightheadedness, dizziness, diaphoresis, pallor, tachycardia, and syncope, are signals of orthostatic hypotension. A drop in systolic BP 20 mm Hg or more signals the need to return patient to a supine position.
- Assist patients when getting up suddenly or after prolonged recumbency.	This action helps prevent falls caused by orthostatic hypotension.
Gastroparesis/impaired gastric emptying with nausea and vomiting:	Progressive autonomic neuropathy may cause a delay in gastric emptying, resulting in nausea and vomiting.
- Administer metoclopramide before meals if prescribed.	Metoclopramide is an antiemetic that also promotes gastric emptying.
- Keep a record of all stools.	Diarrhea is a potential problem in patients with DM who have autonomic neuropathy and are taking metoclopramide to increase gastrointestinal motility.
Neurogenic bladder:	
- Encourage patient to void q3-4h during the day.	Intermittent catheterization may be necessary in severe cases of neurogenic bladder secondary to autonomic neuropathy.
- Avoid use of indwelling urinary catheters.	Infection risk is increased with use of indwelling catheters.

••• **Related NIC and NOC labels:** *NIC:* Circulatory Care: Arterial Insufficiency; Circulatory Care: Venous Insufficiency; Vital Signs Monitoring; Laboratory Data Interpretation; Neurologic Monitoring; Hypovolemia Management; Nausea Management; Foot Care; Pressure Management; Skin Surveillance *NOC:* Tissue Perfusion: Cardiac; Tissue Perfusion: Cerebral; Tissue Perfusion: Abdominal Organs; Tissue Perfusion: Peripheral; Tissue Integrity: Skin and Mucous Membranes

Nursing Diagnosis:

Risk for Infection

related to chronic disease process (e.g., hyperglycemia, neurogenic bladder, poor circulation)

Desired Outcome: Patient is asymptomatic for infection as evidenced by normothermia, negative cultures, and white blood cell count 11,000/mm^3 or less.

INTERVENTIONS	RATIONALES
Monitor temperature q4h. Alert health care provider to elevations.	Infection is the most common cause of DKA. Fever can signal presence of an infection.
Maintain meticulous sterile technique when changing dressings, performing invasive procedures, or manipulating indwelling catheters.	Nonintact skin and invasive procedures and catheters place patient at risk for ingress of bacteria.
Monitor for indicators of infection, including the following:	
- Fever, chills, cough productive of sputum, crackles, rhonchi, dyspnea, inflamed pharynx, and sore throat.	These are indicators of upper respiratory infection.
- Burning or pain with urination, cloudy or malodorous urine, tachycardia, diaphoresis, nausea, vomiting, and abdominal pain.	These are indicators of urinary tract infection (UTI). Patients with DM often have a neurogenic bladder, which increases the chance of UTI due to urinary retention.
- Hypothermia, flushed skin, and hypotension.	These are indicators of systemic sepsis.
- Erythema, swelling, purulent drainage, and warmth at IV sites.	These are indicators of localized infection.
Consult health care provider about obtaining culture specimens for blood, sputum, and urine during temperature spikes or for wounds that produce purulent drainage.	Infection can be present in blood (sepsis), urine, sputum (lungs/respiratory tract), or wounds. Occult infection also can be present outside these sources.

••• **Related NIC and NOC labels:** *NIC:* Infection Control; Infection Prevention; Specimen Management; Vital Signs Monitoring; Wound Care *NOC:* Infection Status

Nursing Diagnosis:

Impaired Skin Integrity (or risk for same)

related to altered circulation and sensation secondary to peripheral neuropathy and vascular pathology

Desired Outcomes: Patient's lower extremity skin remains intact. Within the 24-hr period before hospital discharge, patient verbalizes and demonstrates knowledge of proper foot care.

INTERVENTIONS	RATIONALES
Assess integrity of the skin and evaluate reflexes of the lower extremities by checking knee and ankle deep tendon reflexes, proprioceptive sensations, two-point discrimination, and vibration sensation (using a tuning fork on the medial malleolus).	These assessments monitor presence/degree of neuropathy and vascular pathology. Although all skin is at risk, especially that on extremities and pressure points, skin on the legs is at highest risk and typically is the first to exhibit problems. If sensations are impaired, patient likely will be unable to respond appropriately to stimuli.
Monitor peripheral pulses, comparing quality bilaterally.	Peripheral pulses 2+ or less on a 0-4+ scale signal poor circulation that could compromise skin integrity.
Use foot cradle on bed, space boots for ulcerated heels, elbow protectors, and pressure-relief mattress.	These measures prevent pressure points and promote patient comfort.
Minimize patient activities and incorporate progressive passive and active exercises into daily routine. Discourage extended rest periods in same position.	These measures alleviate acute discomfort while preventing hemostasis.
Teach patient the following steps for foot care:	
- Wash feet daily with mild soap and warm water; check water temperature with water thermometer or elbow.	Patients with decreased sensation are at risk for burns if they are unaware that water temperature is too hot. Hot water and strong soaps also can promote dry skin, which can become irritated and break down.
- Inspect feet daily for presence of erythema, discoloration, or trauma, using mirrors as necessary for adequate visualization.	These are signs the skin needs vigilant assessment and preventive care. When the skin is no longer intact, the patient is at risk for infection that eventually can lead to amputation.
- Alternate between at least two pairs of properly fitted shoes.	This measure eliminates the potential for pressure points that can occur by wearing one pair only.
- Change socks or stockings daily and wear cotton or wool blends.	These measures prevent infection from moisture or dirt in contact with nonintact skin.
- Use gentle moisturizers.	These products soften and lubricate dry skin.
- Cut toenails straight across after softening them during bath. File nails with emery board.	These actions help prevent ingrown toenails, which could lead to infection.
- Do not self-treat corns or calluses; visit podiatrist regularly. Do not go barefoot indoors or outdoors.	These measures minimize risk for trauma, which could lead to infection and ultimately to amputation.
- Attend to any foot injury immediately, and seek medical attention.	This action prevents the potential complications discussed above.

••• **Related NIC and NOC labels:** *NIC:* Pressure Management; Skin Surveillance; Bathing; Foot Care; Infection Protection; Positioning; Wound Care; Bed Rest Care *NOC:* Tissue Integrity: Skin and Mucous Membranes

Nursing Diagnosis:

Deficient Knowledge:

Proper insulin administration, dietary precautions, and exercise for promoting normoglycemia

Desired Outcome: Within the 24-hr period before hospital discharge, patient verbalizes and demonstrates knowledge of proper insulin administration, symptoms and treatment of hypoglycemia, the prescribed dietary regimen, and the role of exercise in promoting normoglycemia.

INTERVENTIONS

RATIONALES

INTERVENTIONS	RATIONALES
Assess patient's health care literacy (language, reading, comprehension). Assess culture and culturally specific information needs.	This assessment helps ensure that information is presented in a manner that is culturally and educationally appropriate.
Teach patient to check expiration date on insulin vial and to avoid using it if outdated.	Insulin may lose potency if the bottle has been open for more than 30 days.
Also teach patient proper storage of insulin and importance of avoiding temperature extremes.	Extreme temperatures destroy insulin.
Teach patient to use U-100 insulin with U-100 syringes.	Although U-40 insulin and U-40 syringes are used much less frequently in the United States than in other countries, the patient must be aware there are differences in strengths of insulin suspensions, and each strength must be given using the appropriate syringe.
Explain that some intermediate- and long-acting insulins require mixing (contraindicated for intermediate/rapid). Demonstrate rolling the insulin vial between palms to mix contents.	Insulin separates when the bottle sits, and the molecules must be re-mixed to ensure appropriate concentration throughout the vial.
Explain that long-acting analogue insulins (glargine/Lantus and detemir/Levemir) work differently than older long-acting insulins and may only need to be administered once or twice daily, depending on the dose.	Long-acting insulin analogues do not have a profound peak action. Once glargine is injected and absorbed, the action is consistent over 24 hr, while the duration of action of detemir is approximately 20 hr.
Caution patient to avoid vigorous shaking.	Vigorous shaking produces air bubbles that can interfere with accurate dose measurement.
Explain that regular prandial insulin (e.g., NovoLin or HumaLin) should be injected 30 min before eating a meal; newer insulin analogues (Novo-Log, HumaLog, Apidra) may be injected immediately before or directly after eating.	Time of onset/peak of older, regular insulins is slightly delayed compared with the newer insulins. If patients are unable to finish at least half of a meal, they may be advised to hold their prandial insulin if receiving an analogue (e.g., NovoLog, HumaLog, Apidra). Because analogues can be given after a meal, dosage is more flexible than with regular human insulins, which should be injected well before eating a meal.
Explain that either making a change in insulin type or withholding a dose of insulin may be required under various circumstances.	These instances include the following: when fasting for studies or surgery, when not eating because of nausea/vomiting, or when hypoglycemic. Stress from illness or infection can increase insulin requirements (or necessitate insulin therapy for one whose condition is normally controlled with oral hypoglycemics), and increased exercise will necessitate additional food intake to prevent hypoglycemia when no change is made in insulin dose. Adjustments are always individually based and require clarification with patient's health care provider.
Provide a chart that depicts injection site rotations. Explain that injection sites should be at least 1 inch apart.	Injections in or near the same site each time may result in development of hard lumps or extra fatty deposits. Both of these problems are unsightly and make the insulin action less reliable.
Explain importance of inserting the needle perpendicular to the skin rather than at an angle.	This ensures deep subcutaneous administration of insulin. Very thin persons may need to use a 45-degree angle.
Ensure patient understands and demonstrates the technique and timing for home monitoring of blood glucose using a commercial kit.	A commercial kit provides ongoing data reflecting degree of control and may identify necessary changes in diet and medication before severe metabolic changes occur. Self-monitoring by patients is extremely useful in reducing complications, especially in type 1 DM patients who require more stringent control of serum glucose levels. Self-monitoring also enables patient's self-control and psychologic security.
Caution patient about importance of following a diet that is controlled in carbohydrates, low in fat, and high in fiber.	Adequate nutrition, consistent carbohydrates, and controlled calories are essential to maintaining normoglycemia in these individuals. A diet low in fat and high in fiber is an effective means of controlling blood fats, especially cholesterol and triglycerides. Diet is the sole method of control for many individuals with type 2 DM. Typically, three daily meals and an evening snack are prescribed. Some fat and protein should be present in all meals and snacks to slow down the elevation of postprandial blood glucose. Adding 10-15 g of fiber will slow the digestion of monosaccharides and disaccharides. For all types of diabetes, refined and simple sugars should be reduced and complex carbohydrates (breads, cereals, pasta, beans) encouraged. Exchange lists may be used for meal planning if this is preferred to carbohydrate counting.

Continued

INTERVENTIONS	RATIONALES
Teach patient how to count carbohydrates.	The "magic number" used for counting carbohydrates is 15, because 15 g of carbohydrates = one serving of carbohydrates. Many carbohydrate-controlled diets allow 4 servings of carbohydrates per meal. Complex carbohydrates are preferred to simple because they have a lower glycemic index; thus complex carbohydrates raise blood glucose more gradually than do simple carbohydrates.
For patients who experience low blood glucose at night, discuss commercially available long-acting carbohydrate sources.	Long-acting carbohydrate sources may decrease risk of nighttime low blood glucose levels.
Teach patient to be alert to changes in mentation, apprehension, erratic behavior, trembling, slurred speech, staggering gait, and seizure activity.	These are indicators of hypoglycemia.
Explain that oral hypoglycemics should be omitted several days before planned surgery. Teach patient to treat hypoglycemia as prescribed.	Hypoglycemia involving oral hypoglycemics can be severe and persistent. Monitoring must be diligent. Any condition, situation, or medication that enhances the hypoglycemic effects of these drugs requires close monitoring of blood glucose when symptoms of hypoglycemia arise. Common factors in the development of hypoglycemia are fasting for diagnostic purposes, skipping meals, unplanned increase in activity, malnourishment related to illness or nausea and vomiting, and other medication therapy (any of which adds to the hypoglycemic action of the oral hypoglycemics).
Teach patient signs, symptoms, and reasons for hyperglycemia.	Hyperglycemia can occur with increased food intake, too little insulin, decreased exercise, infection or illness, and emotional stress. Signs and symptoms of hyperglycemia (polydipsia, polyuria, polyphagia, fatigue, fruity-smelling breath) can appear within hours or even several days. Hyperglycemia will be detected during routine self-testing of blood glucose.
Explain the role that exercise has in patients with DM.	Exercise is as important as diet and insulin in treating DM. It lowers blood glucose levels, helps maintain normal cholesterol levels, and increases circulation. These effects increase the body's ability to metabolize glucose and help reduce the therapeutic dose of insulin for most patients. The exercise program must be consistent and individualized (especially for individuals with type 1 DM). Patients should be given a complete physical examination and encouraged to incorporate acceptable activities as part of their daily routine. **Note:** If blood glucose level is greater than 250 mg/dl, exercise acts as a stressor, causing blood glucose to increase rather than decrease. Patients should monitor blood glucose levels with a monitoring device before beginning an exercise program.

••• **Related NIC and NOC labels:** *NIC:* Teaching: Disease Process; Teaching: Prescribed Diet; Teaching: Prescribed Medication; Hyperglycemia Management; Hypoglycemia Management; Medication Administration: Subcutaneous; Teaching: Psychomotor Skill *NOC:* Knowledge: Diabetes Management

ADDITIONAL NURSING DIAGNOSES/ PROBLEMS:

"Psychosocial Support"	p. 73
"Atherosclerotic Arterial Occlusive Disease"	p. 151
"Amputation"	p. 509

✔ PATIENT-FAMILY TEACHING AND DISCHARGE PLANNING

Focus on sensory information, avoid giving excessive information, and initiate a visiting nurse referral for necessary follow-up teaching. Ask about existing knowledge of the disease, ability for self-management, and acceptance of the disease during initial assessment. Include verbal and written information about the following:

✓ Importance of carrying a diabetic identification card, wearing a medical alert bracelet or necklace, and having identification card outline diagnosis and emergency treatment. Contact the following organization for information: MedicAlert Foundation at *www.medicalert.org.*

✓ Recognizing warning signs of both hyperglycemia and hypoglycemia, treatment, and factors that contribute to both conditions. Emphasize importance of disclosing all alternative and complementary health practices being used because some may affect blood glucose or possibly lead to adverse drug reactions. Remind patient that stress from illness or infection can increase insulin requirements (or necessitate insulin therapy for one who is normally controlled with oral hypoglycemics) and that increased exercise will necessitate additional food intake to prevent hypoglycemia when no change is made in insulin dosage under normoglycemic conditions. Blood glucose at a level greater than 250 mg/dl at the beginning of exercise will make the exercise a stressor that elevates rather than decreases the glucose level.

✓ Drugs that cause *hyperglycemia*: estrogens, corticosteroids, thyroid preparations, beta-adrenergic agonists (many respiratory aerosols or inhalers), diuretics, phenytoin, glucagon, drugs containing sugar (e.g., cough syrup), and certain antibiotics. Drugs that cause *hypoglycemia*: salicylates, sulfonamides, tetracyclines, methyldopa, anabolic steroids, acetaminophen, monoamine oxidase (MAO) inhibitors, ethanol, haloperidol, and marijuana. Propranolol and other beta-adrenergic blocking agents may mask the signs of and inhibit recovery from hypoglycemia.

✓ Home monitoring of blood glucose using commercial kits and possibly daily urine testing for glucose and ketones, which provide ongoing data reflecting degree of control and may identify necessary changes in diet and medication before severe metabolic changes occur. These tests also provide a means for patient's self-control and psychologic security. In addition, kits for monitoring glycohemoglobin (HbA$_{1C}$) are available for home use and may assist patients in determining overall effectiveness of their diabetes management regimen. New, smaller lancets allow more frequent blood glucose testing by decreasing pain from fingersticks. Stress need for careful control of blood glucose as a means of decreasing risk of or minimizing long-term complications of DM. Encourage patient to rotate sites as much as possible to avoid possibility of injuring any one site.

✓ Importance of daily exercise, maintenance of normal body weight, and yearly medical evaluation. Explain that exercise is as important as diet in treating DM. Exercise lowers blood glucose, helps maintain normal cholesterol levels, and increases circulation. These effects increase the body's ability to metabolize glucose and help reduce the therapeutic dose of insulin for most patients. Stress that each exercise program must be individualized (especially for persons with type 1 DM) and implemented consistently. Patient should have a complete physical examination and then be encouraged to incorporate acceptable exercise activities into his or her daily routine.

✓ Review of diet that is consistent in carbohydrates, low in fat, and high in fiber as an effective means of controlling blood fats, especially cholesterol and triglycerides. Stress that diet is the sole method of control for many individuals with type 2 DM. Adequate nutrition with controlled carbohydrates and calories is essential to maintaining normoglycemia in these individuals. Patients who gained weight before developing type 2 DM are sometimes able to normalize their blood glucose by losing weight and maintaining ideal body weight.

✓ Mixing insulins properly by drawing up the regular first, followed by the intermediate- or long-acting insulin. Insulin analogues (HumaLog, NovoLog, Apidra, glargine [Lantus] and detemir [Levemir]) should not be mixed with other insulin preparations.

✓ Use of syringe magnifiers that can be used by patients with poor visual acuity. Other products that permit safe and accurate filling of syringes are also available.

✓ Rotating injection sites and injecting insulin at room temperature. Provide a chart showing possible injection sites, and describe the system for site rotation. Complications related to insulin injections, including lipodystrophy, insulin resistance, and allergic reactions, should be discussed thoroughly.

✓ Importance of daily meticulous skin, wound, and foot care.

✓ Necessity of annual eye examination for early detection and treatment of retinopathy.

✓ Scheduling dental checkups at least every 6 mo to help prevent periodontal disease, a major problem for individuals with DM. The mouth often is the primary site of origination for low-grade infections.

✓ Inserting the needle perpendicular to the skin rather than at an angle to ensure deep subcutaneous administration of insulin. Individuals who are very thin may need to use a 45-degree angle.

✓ Medications, including purpose, dosage, schedule, precautions, interactions, and potential side effects for all medications used. Also discuss drug-drug, food-drug, and herb-drug interactions.

✓ Identifying available resources for ongoing assistance and information, including nurses, dietitian, patient's health care provider, and other individuals with DM in patient care unit. Other resources include the local chapter of ADA and local library for free access to current materials on diabetes. The following is a list of resources available to patients:

- American Diabetes Association at *www.diabetes.org*
- Canadian Diabetes Association at *www.diabetes.ca*
- Juvenile Diabetes Research Foundation International at *www.jdrf.org*
- Joslin Diabetes Center at *www.joslin.org*
- National Diabetes Information Clearinghouse at *www.niddk.nih.gov/health/diabetes/ndic.htm*
- American Heart Association, National Center, at *www.americanheart.org*

- Can-Am-Care (Diabetes care store brand availability guide) at *www.canamcare.com*

The following is a list of journals available for patients.

- *Diabetes* at *www.diabetes.diabetesjournals.org*
- *Diabetes Care* at *www.care.diabetesjournals.org*
- *Diabetes Forecast* at *www.diabetes.org/diabetes-forecast. jsp?WTLPromo=HOME_1st_forecast*
- *Diabetes Health Magazine* at *www.diabeteshealth.com*
- *Diabetes Self-Management* at *www.diabetesselfmanagement.com*

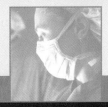

Diabetic Ketoacidosis 46

OVERVIEW/PATHOPHYSIOLOGY

Diabetic ketoacidosis (DKA) is a life-threatening condition caused by severe lack of effective insulin, resulting in major hyperglycemia and acidosis from abnormal carbohydrate, fat, and protein metabolism. The intracellular environment is unable to receive necessary glucose for oxidation and energy production without insulin to facilitate transport of glucose from the bloodstream across the cell membrane. Impairment of glucose uptake results in hyperglycemia, while the intracellular environment continues to lack necessary nutrients. Glucagon secretion increases, causing available body stores of food substances to be broken down in an attempt to provide cell nourishment. Impaired amino acid transport, protein synthesis, and protein degradation facilitate protein catabolism with a resultant increase in serum amino acids, while fat breakdown results in elevated free fatty acids (FFA) and glycerol. The liver converts the newly available amino acids, fatty acids, and glycerol into glucose (gluconeogenesis) in an attempt to provide nourishment for the cells, but instead the hyperglycemia worsens because of the lack of insulin to transport glucose into the cells. The liver also produces ketone bodies from available FFA, causing mild to severe acidosis. As ketone bodies increase in the extracellular fluid, the hydrogen ions within the ketones are exchanged with K ions from within the cells. Thus intracellular K^+ is released into the extracellular fluid and therefore to circulating fluid, where it is excreted by the kidneys into the urine. Hyperglycemia acts as an osmotic diuretic, causing severe fluid and electrolyte losses, leading to hypovolemic shock if untreated. Individuals with severe DKA may lose nearly 500 mEq of Na^+, Cl^-, and K^+, along with approximately 7 L of water in 24 hr.

HEALTH CARE SETTING

Acute care (intensive care unit)

Assessment/Diagnostic Tests			
	Diabetic Ketoacidosis	Hyperosmolar Hyperglycemic Nonketotic Syndrome	Hypoglycemia
Type of diabetes	Usually type 1	Usually type 2	
Signs, symptoms/ physical assessment	Symptoms are a result mainly of hyperglycemia, intracellular hypoglycemia, hypotension or impending hypovolemic shock, and fluid-electrolyte imbalance with possible acid-base imbalance	Same as DKA	Symptoms result from intracellular hypoglycemia and hypotension/ impending "insulin" shock (vasogenic)
Neurologic	Altered LOC (confusion, lethargy, irritability, coma); strokelike symptoms (unilateral/bilateral weakness, paralysis, numbness, paresthesia); fatigue	Same as DKA; also possible seizures and tremors	Tremors, trembling, shaking, confusion, apprehension, erratic behavior; may be same as DKA
Respiratory	Deep, rapid Kussmaul's respirations	Shallow, rapid (tachypneic) breathing	Usually rapid (tachypneic) breathing
Cardiovascular	Tachycardia, hypotension, ECG changes	Same as DKA	Same as DKA, possibly with diaphoresis
Metabolic/GI/ endocrine	Polyuria, polyphagia, polydipsia, fruity "acetone" breath, abdominal pain, weight loss, fatigue, generalized weakness, nausea, vomiting	Polyuria, polyphagia, polydipsia, fatigue, generalized weakness, nausea, vomiting	Hunger, nausea, eructation

Continued

Assessment/Diagnostic Tests

	Diabetic Ketoacidosis	Hyperosmolar Hyperglycemic Nonketotic Syndrome	Hypoglycemia
Integumentary	Dry, flushed skin; poor turgor; dry mucous membranes	Same as DKA	Cool, clammy, pale skin
VS monitoring	BP low (more than 20% below normal); HR more than 100 bpm; CVP less than 2 mm Hg (less than 5 cm H_2O); temperature normal	BP low (more than 20% below normal); HR more than 100 bpm; CVP less than 2 mm Hg (less than 5 cm H_2O); temperature possibly elevated	BP normal to low; HR more than 100 bpm; CVP usually unchanged
Diagnostic tests/ laboratory values	Values reflect dehydration/metabolic acidosis (ketosis) secondary to hyperglycemia, abnormal lipolysis, and osmotic diuresis; fluid loss 6.5 L or more	Values reflect dehydration secondary to hyperglycemia, osmotic diuresis, and possible lactic acidosis from hypoperfusion; fluid loss 9 L or more	Values reflect hypoglycemia, possibly with vasodilation owing to insulin shock
Hgb/Hct	Elevated	Same as DKA	Unchanged to slightly decreased
Serum BUN/ creatinine	Elevated	Same as DKA	Normal
Serum electrolytes	Initially elevated, then decreased	Same as DKA	Usually unchanged
Serum glucose	250-800 mg/dl (+ ketones)	400-1800 mg/dl (− ketones)	15-50 mg/dl
ABGs	pH 6.8-7.3; HCO_3^- 12-20 mEq/L; CO_2 15-25 mEq/L	pH 7.3-7.5; HCO_3^- 20-26 mEq/L; CO_2 30-40 mEq/L	pH 7.3-7.5; HCO_3^- 20-26 mEq/L; CO_2 30-40 mEq/L
Serum osmolality	300-350 mOsm/L	More than 350 mOsm/L	Less than 280 mOsm/L
Urine glucose/ acetone	Positive/positive	Positive/negative	Negative/negative
Onset	Hours to days	More than one day	Minutes to hours
History/risk factors for development of crisis	Undiagnosed DM, infections, acute pancreatitis, uremia, insulin resistance *Medications:* digitalis intoxication; omission/reduction of insulin dosage; failure to increase insulin to compensate for stress of infections; injury, emotional problems, or surgery	Undiagnosed DM; infections, especially gram-negative; acromegaly; Cushing's syndrome; thyrotoxicosis; acute pancreatitis; hyperalimentation; pancreatic carcinoma; cranial trauma/subdural hematoma; uremia, hemodialysis, peritoneal dialysis; burns, heat stroke; pneumonia; MI; stroke *Medications:* loop and thiazide diuretics (i.e., hydrochlorothiazide, chlorthalidone, furosemide); diazoxide; glucocorticoids (i.e., hydrocortisone, dexamethasone); propranolol (Inderal); phenytoin (Dilantin); sodium bicarbonate	Excessive dose of insulin; excessive dose of sulfonylureas/oral hypoglycemic agents; skipping meals; too much exercise with controlled blood glucose without extra food intake *Medications:* insulin, sulfonylureas
Mortality	10% or less	10%-25%	Less than 0.1%

ABGs, arterial blood gases; *BP*, blood pressure; *BUN*, blood urea nitrogen; *CVP*, central venous pressure; *DKA*, diabetic ketoacidosis; *DM*, diabetes mellitus; *ECG*, electrocardiogram *GI*, gastrointestinal; *Hct*, hematocrit; *Hgb*, hemoglobin; *HR*, heart rate; *LOC*, level of consciousness; *MI*, myocardial infarction; *VS*, vital signs.

Nursing Diagnosis:

Deficient Fluid Volume

related to failure of regulatory mechanisms or decreased circulating volume secondary to hyperglycemia with osmotic diuresis

Desired Outcome: Patient becomes normovolemic within 10 hr of treatment, as evidenced by BP 90/60 mm Hg or more (or within patient's normal range), HR 60-100 bpm, CVP 2-6 mm Hg (5-12 cm H_2O), good skin turgor, moist and pink mucous membranes, specific gravity less than 1.020, balanced intake and output (I&O), and urinary output 30 ml/hr or more.

INTERVENTIONS	RATIONALES
Monitor vital signs (VS) q15min until stable for 1 hr. Notify health care provider promptly of significant findings.	Hyperglycemia acts as an osmotic diuretic, causing severe fluid and electrolyte losses that can lead to hypovolemic shock if untreated. Heart rate (HR) greater than 120 bpm, blood pressure (BP) less than 90/60 or decreased 20 mm Hg or more from baseline, and central venous pressure (CVP) less than 2 mm Hg (or less than 5 cm H_2O) are signs of hypovolemia and necessitate notifying health care provider for timely intervention.
Monitor patient for poor skin turgor, dry mucous membranes, sunken and soft eyeballs, tachycardia, and orthostatic hypotension.	These are physical indicators of hypovolemia.
Weigh patient daily, and measure I&O accurately. Monitor urinary specific gravity and report findings of more than 1.020 in the presence of other indicators of dehydration. Report to health care provider if urine output is less than 30 ml/hr for 2 consecutive hr.	Decreasing urinary output may signal diminishing intravascular fluid volume or impending renal failure. Loss of weight and output that exceeds intake may signal dehydration.
Administer IV fluids as prescribed.	This ensures adequate rehydration. Usually, normal saline or 0.45% saline is administered until plasma glucose falls to 200-300 mg/dl. After that, dextrose-containing solutions usually are given to prevent rebound hypoglycemia. Initially, IV fluids are administered rapidly (i.e., 2000 ml infused during the first 2 hr of treatment and 150-250 ml/hr thereafter until BP stabilizes).
Be alert to indicators of fluid overload.	Indicators of fluid overload (jugular vein distention, dyspnea, crackles, CVP more than 6 mm Hg [more than 12 cm H_2O]) can occur with rapid infusion of fluids.
Administer insulin as prescribed.	Insulin usually is given by continuous IV infusion for rapid action and because poor tissue perfusion caused by dehydration sometimes makes the subcutaneous route less effective. Initial dose may vary from 10-25 U, or about 0.3 U/kg. Patient is maintained on 5-10 U/hr, or 0.1 U/kg/hr as a continuous infusion administered through a separate IV tubing and controlled with an infusion control device. Dosage is adjusted based on serial glucose levels and resolution of ketosis. Insulin drip should be adjusted using a formula that considers the patient's sensitivity to insulin. When formulas are used, the sensitivity number is reflected as a variable multiplier that increases with higher levels of insulin resistance. Insulin analogues (i.e., NovoLog, HumaLog) may be used in place of regular insulin to lower blood glucose levels.
Before initiating treatment, flush the tubing with at least 30 ml of the insulin-containing IV solution.	Insulin, when added to IV solutions, may be absorbed by the container and plastic tubing. Flushing the tubing ensures that maximum adsorption of the insulin by the container and tubing has occurred before it is delivered to the patient.

Continued

INTERVENTIONS	RATIONALES
Monitor laboratory results for abnormalities. Promptly report to health care provider serum K⁺ levels less than 3.5 mEq/L. Observe for clinical manifestations of the electrolyte, glucose, and acid-base imbalances associated with DKA as follows:	Before treatment there is risk of hyperkalemia from excess transport of intracellular K^+ to extracellular spaces. Na^+ and Cl^- are replaced with IV normal saline. K^+ must be monitored and corrected carefully. After initiation of treatment, K^+ returns to the intracellular compartment through accelerated transport into cells via insulin and following correction of acidosis, and therefore the patient is at risk for becoming hypokalemic. Use of phosphorus replacement is controversial, but if phosphorus levels remain low, potassium phosphate solutions can be used to assist with K^+ and phosphate replacement.

- *Hyperkalemia:* Lethargy, nausea, hyperactive bowel sounds with diarrhea, numbness or tingling in extremities, muscle weakness.
- *Hypokalemia:* Muscle weakness, hypotension, anorexia, drowsiness, hypoactive bowel sounds.
- *Hyponatremia:* Headache, malaise, muscle weakness, abdominal cramps, nausea, seizures, coma.
- *Hypophosphatemia:* Muscle weakness, progressive encephalopathy possibly leading to coma.
- *Hypomagnesemia:* Anorexia, nausea, vomiting, lethargy, weakness, personality changes, tetany, tremor or muscle fasciculations, seizures, confusion progressing to coma.
- *Hypochloremia:* Hypertonicity of muscles, tetany, depressed respirations.
- *Hypoglycemia:* Headache, impaired mentation, agitation, dizziness, nausea, pallor, tremors, tachycardia, diaphoresis.
- *Metabolic acidosis:* Lassitude, nausea, vomiting, Kussmaul's respirations, lethargy progressing to coma.

••• **Related NIC and NOC labels:** *NIC:* Fluid/Electrolyte Management; Acid-Base Management; Intravenous Therapy; Laboratory Data Interpretation; Neurologic Monitoring; Vital Signs Monitoring *NOC:* Electrolyte and Acid-Base Balance; Fluid Balance

Nursing Diagnosis:

Risk for Infection

related to inadequate secondary defenses (suppressed inflammatory response) secondary to protein depletion

Desired Outcome: Patient is free of infection as evidenced by normothermia, HR 100 bpm or less, BP within patient's normal range, WBC count 11,000/mm³ or less, and negative culture results.

INTERVENTIONS	RATIONALES
Monitor patient for evidence of infection. Monitor laboratory results for increased white blood cell (WBC) count, and culture purulent drainage as prescribed.	Infection is the most common cause of DKA in adults, whereas nonadherence to treatment regimen is more likely responsible for DKA in children and teenagers. Indicators of infection include fever, chills, pain with urination, vomiting, erythema and swelling around IV sites, and increased WBC count.
Use meticulous handwashing when caring for patient.	Patient is at increased risk for bacterial infection because of suppressed inflammatory response.
Manage invasive lines carefully. Schedule dressing changes according to agency policy.	Peripheral IV sites should be rotated q48-72h and dressings changed, depending on agency policy. Central lines should be discontinued as soon as feasible and when in place should be handled carefully.

Continued

INTERVENTIONS

INTERVENTIONS	RATIONALES
Inspect insertion sites for erythema, swelling, or purulent drainage. Document the presence of any of these indicators, and notify health care provider.	These are signs of local infection that should be reported promptly for timely intervention.
Provide good skin care.	Intact skin is a first line of defense against infection.
Use pressure-relief mattress on patient's bed.	This mattress helps prevent skin breakdown, which could lead to infection. Air circulation beds are recommended for severe skin breakdown.
Use meticulous sterile technique when caring for or inserting indwelling urinary catheters.	This minimizes the risk of bacterial entry into the body.
Note: Limit use of indwelling urethral catheters to patients who are unable to void in a bedpan or when continuous assessment of urine output is essential.	There is increased risk of infection with indwelling catheters.
Encourage hourly use of incentive spirometry while patient is awake, along with deep-breathing and coughing exercises.	Deep inhalations with incentive spirometry along with deep breathing exercises expand alveoli and aid in mobilizing secretions to the airways. Coughing further mobilizes and clears the secretions. These exercises help prevent pulmonary infection.

••• **Related NIC and NOC labels:** *NIC:* Infection Protection; Incision Site Care; Urinary Catheterization; Cough Enhancement; Tube Care: Urinary *NOC:* Infection Status

Nursing Diagnosis:

Risk for Injury

related to altered cerebral function secondary to dehydration or cerebral edema associated with DKA

Desired Outcomes: Patient verbalizes orientation to person, place, and time and does not demonstrate significant change in mental status; normal breath sounds are auscultated over patient's airway; and patient's oral cavity and musculoskeletal system remain intact and free of injury.

INTERVENTIONS	RATIONALES
Monitor patient's mental status; orientation; level of consciousness (LOC); and respiratory status, especially airway patency, at frequent intervals.	With DKA, patient's cerebral function may be altered because of dehydration or cerebral edema.
Keep an appropriate-size oral airway, manual resuscitator and mask, and supplemental oxygen at the bedside.	Increased intracranial pressure caused by cerebral edema may impinge upon the brain stem, prompting respiratory arrest. In older patients, the increased work of breathing may exceed their ability to compensate, and this can result in respiratory arrest.
Maintain bed in lowest position, keep side rails up at all times, and use soft restraints as necessary.	These measures reduce the likelihood of injury from falls resulting from patient's altered cerebral function.
Insert gastric tube in comatose patients, as prescribed. Attach gastric tube to low, intermittent suction, and assess patency q4h.	These actions decrease likelihood of aspiration.
Elevate head of bed to 45 degrees.	This elevation minimizes risk of aspiration.
Initiate seizure precautions. For details, see "Seizures and Epilepsy," p. 323.	

••• **Related NIC and NOC labels:** *NIC:* Environmental Management: Safety; Aspiration Precautions; Seizure Precautions; Positioning *NOC:* Neurological Status: Consciousness

<u>Nursing Diagnosis:</u>

Ineffective Tissue Perfusion: Peripheral
(or risk for same)

related to interrupted venous or arterial flow secondary to increased blood viscosity, increased platelet aggregation and adhesiveness, and patient immobility

Desired Outcomes: Optimally, patient has adequate peripheral perfusion as evidenced by peripheral pulses greater than 2+ on a 0-4+ scale; warm skin; brisk capillary refill (less than 2 sec); and absence of swelling, bluish discoloration, erythema, and discomfort in calves and thighs. Alternatively, if signs of altered peripheral tissue perfusion occur, they are detected and reported promptly.

INTERVENTIONS	RATIONALES
Monitor hematocrit results.	Normal values are 40%-54% (male) or 37%-47% (female). With proper fluid replacement, results should return to normal within 24-48 hr.
Assess for a falling blood urea nitrogen (BUN) value.	Normal value is 6-20 mg/dl. A falling BUN value is an indicator of improved tissue perfusion and renal function.
Assess peripheral pulses q2-4h and report significant findings.	Any decrease in amplitude or absence of pulse(s) should be reported to health care provider promptly as it would signal deep vein thrombosis (DVT) or other cause of perfusion deficit (e.g., hypovolemia, advancing peripheral vascular disease).
Be alert to erythema, pain, tenderness, warmth, and swelling over area of thrombus and bluish discoloration, paleness, coolness, and dilation of superficial veins in distal extremities, especially lower extremities.	These are indicators of DVT. For more information, see "Venous Thrombosis/Thrombophlebitis," p. 201.
Also be alert to pain, paresthesias (especially loss of sensation of light touch and two-point discrimination), cyanosis with delayed capillary refill, mottling, and coolness of the extremity.	These are indicators of arterial thrombosis, which can lead to profound limb ischemia and tissue hypoxia and eventually to tissue anoxia and death.
Report significant findings to health care provider immediately.	When untreated, limb ischemia may result in loss of limb and and/or digits.
Encourage active exercises to all extremities q2h.	Exercise increases blood flow to the tissues. Calf pumping and ankle circles should be encouraged q1h in patients susceptible to DVT.
Unless contraindicated, encourage fluid intake to more than 2500 ml/day.	Increased hydration decreases the potential for hemoconcentration, which could lead to DVT.
Apply antiembolic hose, Ace wraps, pneumatic alternating pressure stockings, or pneumatic foot pumps as prescribed.	These garments and devices promote venous return and aid in prevention of thrombosis.

••• **Related NIC and NOC labels:** *NIC:* Circulatory Care: Arterial Insufficiency; Circulatory Care: Venous Insufficiency; Circulatory Precautions; Fluid Management; Embolus Care: Peripheral; Pneumatic Tourniquet Precautions; Laboratory Data Interpretation *NOC:* Tissue Integrity: Skin and Mucous Membranes; Tissue Perfusion: Peripheral

<u>Nursing Diagnosis:</u>

Deficient Knowledge:

Cause, prevention, and treatment of DKA

Desired Outcome: Within the 24-hr period before hospital discharge, patient verbalizes understanding of the cause, prevention, and treatment of DKA.

INTERVENTIONS	RATIONALES
Assess patient's health care literacy (language, reading, comprehension). Assess culture and culturally specific information needs.	This assessment helps ensure that information is presented in a manner that is culturally and educationally appropriate.
Determine patient's knowledge about DKA and its treatment.	This will enable, as needed, further explanation of disease process of DM and DKA and common early symptoms of worsening hyperglycemia, including polyuria, polydipsia, polyphagia, dry and flushed skin, and increased irritability.
Assess patient's ability to engage in self-management of blood glucose monitoring and control. Explore whether patient psychologically accepts the disease as a significant health challenge.	This information will enable individualized teaching that will facilitate adherence to the prescribed management regimen designed to maintain normoglycemia.
Stress importance of maintaining a consistent controlled carbohydrate diet, exercise, and insulin regimen.	This regimen helps ensure optimal control of serum glucose levels and prevention of adverse physical effects of DM, such as peripheral neuropathies and increased atherosclerosis.
Explain importance of blood glucose monitoring during episodes of stress, injury, and illness. Caution that DKA necessitates professional medical management and cannot be self-treated.	Increased stress impacts metabolism of carbohydrates, fats, and proteins, causing increased blood glucose.
Discuss "sick day management" with patient, including *not* stopping insulin or skipping doses, increasing frequency of blood glucose testing to monitor more closely for hyperglycemia, and testing urine for ketones if ill or vomiting.	Testing urine ketones may be advised. Blood glucose greater than 250 mg/dl and appearance of large amounts of urine ketones should be reported to health care provider so that insulin dose can be increased.
Remind patient of importance of maintaining adequate oral fluid intake during illness despite anorexia or nausea.	Anorexia or nausea may limit food intake, but patient should make every effort to continue fluid intake to avoid dehydration, hypovolemia, and possible hypotension.
Review testing and insulin administration procedure as indicated.	Insulin or insulin analog must be taken 1-4 times/day as prescribed and lifetime insulin therapy is necessary to achieve control of blood glucose.
Teach importance of receiving prompt treatment if such indicators as dizziness, impaired mentation, irritability, pallor, and tremors occur.	These are signs of insulin or insulin analogue excess (hypoglycemia).
Conversely, caution patient to get prompt treatment if the following indicators occur: polyuria, polydipsia, polyphagia, or increasingly dry and flushed skin.	These are signs of insulin deficiency (hyperglycemia).
Explain consequences of not receiving prompt treatment.	If untreated, these conditions could lead to coma and death.
Explain importance of dietary changes as prescribed by health care provider.	Typically patient is put on a consistent carbohydrate diet composed of 60% carbohydrates, 20%-30% fats, and 12%-20% proteins. Counting carbohydrates and prescribing insulin dosage according to the amount of carbohydrates consumed is a newer strategy of blood glucose management.
Advise that fats should be polyunsaturated and proteins chosen from low-fat sources.	Reduction in saturated fat intake reduces risk of development of coronary artery and peripheral vascular disease.
Teach importance of eating three meals per day at regularly scheduled times and a bedtime snack.	Such a diet affords the best opportunity for maintaining a physiologically normal blood glucose level rather than "roller coaster" values of alternating hyperglycemia and hypoglycemia. Meals and insulin administration must be linked together, especially when insulin analogues such as HumaLog, NovoLog, or Apidra are given before meals and in conjunction with snacks. Analogues are quicker acting than regular insulins.
Explain causes for adjustments in insulin dose. Instruct patient to monitor blood glucose and urine ketone levels closely during periods of increased emotional stress and periods of increased or decreased exercise and to adjust insulin dose accordingly.	Adjustments in insulin dose include increased or decreased food or carbohydrate intake and any physical (e.g., exercise) or emotional stress. Exercise and emotional stress may increase release of glucose from the liver or increase insulin resistance.
Remind patient that alternative and complementary health strategies may alter blood glucose levels and prompt a need for adjustment of medications.	For example, certain herbal preparations can alter metabolism and may increase or decrease blood glucose. All methods used should be reported to health care provider.

Continued

INTERVENTIONS	RATIONALES
Explain that good hygiene and meticulous daily foot care are necessary to prevent infection. Stress importance of avoiding exposure to communicable diseases, and explain that the following indicators of infection necessitate prompt medical treatment: fever, chills, increased HR, diaphoresis, nausea, and vomiting. In addition, teach patient and significant other to be alert to wounds or cuts that do not heal, burning or pain with urination, and a productive cough.	Persons with diabetes are susceptible to infection because of decreased immune response.
Instruct patient to implement the following therapy when ill for any reason:	
- Do not alter insulin (NovoLin, HumuLin), insulin analogue (HumaLog, NovoLog), or oral diabetes or hyperglycemia medication dosage unless health care provider has prescribed a supplemental regimen.	Altering insulin regimen increases risk for hypoglycemia if medication dosage is increased.
- Perform blood glucose monitoring and urine ketone checks q3h, and promptly report glucose greater than 250 mg/dl and positive ketones to health care provider.	If insulin dose is decreased for persistent incidences of hypoglycemia, the blood glucose should increase to the normal range with proper dosage. The stress associated with illness alters metabolism and glucose uptake. Hyperglycemia can ensue quickly when patient becomes ill.
- Eat small, frequent meals of soft, easily digestible, nourishing foods if regular meals are not tolerated.	If carbohydrate intake falls significantly, insulin dosage may need alteration to prevent hypoglycemia. Smaller, more frequent, meals may help maintain more normal intake.
- Maintain adequate hydration, particularly if diarrhea, vomiting, or fever is persistent.	Dehydration can lead to hypovolemia, which in turn can lead to shock if left untreated.
- Use a balance of regular sodas or juices and water to ensure adequate calories yet prevent hyperosmolality caused by sugars in the beverages.	Intake of carbohydrates must be maintained unless insulin dose is altered to avoid hypoglycemia. Water must be drunk to maintain intravascular volume. There may be too much carbohydrate in juice or soda to use either as a primary source of volume.
	If carbohydrate intake is not appropriately balanced with water intake, glucose will fluctuate and patient may be at risk for hypovolemia, which can lead to shock.
Provide the following address of the ADA: American Diabetes Association at *www.diabetes.org*.	The ADA website is a source of information for pamphlets and magazines related to the disease, its complications, and appropriate treatment.

••• **Related NIC and NOC labels:** *NIC:* Teaching: Disease Process; Learning Facilitation; Learning Readiness Enhancement; Teaching: Prescribed Diet; Teaching: Prescribed Medication; Hyperglycemia Management; Hypoglycemia Management; Teaching: Prescribed Activity/ Exercise; Referral; Medication Management *NOC:* Knowledge: Diabetes Management

ADDITIONAL NURSING DIAGNOSES/ PROBLEMS:

"Psychosocial Support"	p. 73

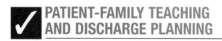

PATIENT-FAMILY TEACHING AND DISCHARGE PLANNING

See **Deficient Knowledge:** Cause, prevention, and treatment of DKA, p. 392.

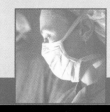

Hyperosmolar Hyperglycemic Nonketotic Syndrome   47

OVERVIEW/PATHOPHYSIOLOGY

Hyperosmolar hyperglycemic nonketotic syndrome (HHNK) syndrome, also known as *hyperosmolar coma, nonketotic hyperosmolar coma, hyperosmolar nonketotic syndrome, hyperosmolar hyperglycemic nonketotic coma,* and *nonketotic hyperglycemic hyperosmolar coma,* is a life-threatening emergency resulting from a lack of effective insulin, or severe insulin resistance, causing extreme hyperglycemia. These patients often are older adults with undiagnosed or inadequately treated type 2 diabetes mellitus (DM). Often HHNK is precipitated by a stressor, such as trauma, injury, or infection, that increases insulin demand. It is believed that enough insulin to prevent acidosis resulting from lipolysis and formation of ketone bodies is effective at the cellular level. Without adequate insulin to facilitate transport into cells, or with severe insulin resistance, glucose molecules accumulate in the bloodstream, causing serum hyperosmolality with resultant osmotic diuresis and simultaneous loss of electrolytes, most notably potassium, sodium, and phosphate. Patients may lose up to 25% of their total body water. Fluids are pulled from individual body cells by increasing serum hyperosmolality and extracellular fluid loss, causing intracellular dehydration and body cell shrinkage. Neurologic deficits (i.e., slowed mentation, confusion, seizures, strokelike symptoms, coma) can occur as a result. Loss of extracellular fluid stimulates aldosterone release, which facilitates sodium retention and prevents further loss of potassium. However, aldosterone cannot halt severe dehydration. As extracellular volume decreases, blood viscosity increases, causing slowing of blood flow. Thromboemboli are common because of increased blood viscosity, enhanced platelet aggregation and adhesiveness, and possibly patient immobility. Cardiac workload is increased and may lead to myocardial infarction. Renal blood flow is decreased, potentially resulting in renal impairment or failure. Stroke may result from thromboemboli or decreased cerebral perfusion. These severe complications, in addition to the initial precipitating disorder, contribute to a mortality of 10%-25%.

Unlike diabetic ketoacidosis, in which acidosis produces severe symptoms requiring fairly prompt hospitalization, symptoms of HHNK develop more slowly and often are non-specific. The cardinal symptoms of polyuria and polydipsia are noted first but may be ignored by older persons or their families. Neurologic deficits may be mistaken for senility. The similarity of these symptoms to those of other disease processes common to this age group may delay differential diagnosis and treatment, allowing progression of pathophysiologic processes with resultant hypovolemic shock and multiple organ failure.

HEALTH CARE SETTING

Acute care (usually intensive care) unless the condition is not severe

ASSESSMENT

See Table in "Diabetic Ketoacidosis," p. 387. **Note:** Patients with HHNK may be older than 50 yr of age and have preexisting cardiac or pulmonary disorders. The incidence of type 2 diabetes is increasing in children, teenagers, and young adults, so younger people are now presenting with HHNK syndrome. Assessment results often cannot be evaluated based on accepted normal values. Evaluate results based on what is normal or optimal for the individual patient. Central venous pressure (CVP), heart rate (HR), and blood pressure (BP) should be evaluated in terms of deviations from patient's baseline and concurrent clinical status.

DIAGNOSTIC TESTS

Serum glucose: From 400 to 1800 mg/dl is diagnostic of HHNK syndrome.

Serum chemistry: Serum values change as osmotic diuresis progresses. At late stages, patient may reflect the following electrolyte values/losses:
- *Na^+:* 125-160 mEq/L. Although patient has lost large quantities of Na^+, osmotic diuresis causes abnormally high blood concentration. The Na^+ value may appear high despite probable Na^+ deficits.
- *K^+:* less than 3.5 mEq/L.
- *Cl^-:* less than 95 mEq/L.
- *Phosphorus:* less than 1.7 mEq/L.
- *Magnesium:* less than 1.5 mEq/L.

Serum osmolality: Will be greater than 350 mOsm/L. A quick bedside calculation of serum osmolality can be obtained by using the following formula:

$$2(Na^+ + K^+) + BUN\ (mg/dl)/2.8 + Glucose\ (mg/dl)/18 = mOsm/L$$

For example: $Na^+ = 140$; $K^+ = 4.5$; $BUN = 20$; Glucose $= 120$

$$2(140 + 4.5) + 20/2.8 + 120/18 = 2\ (144.5) + 7 + 6.7$$

$$289 + 7 + 6.7 = 302.7\ mOsm/L$$

COMPLICATIONS

Complications of HHNK syndrome include arterial thrombosis, stroke, renal failure, heart failure, multiple organ failure, cerebral edema, malignant dysrhythmias, and gram-negative sepsis (from infection that may have caused the problem to ensue).

Nursing Diagnosis:

Deficient Knowledge:

Causes, prevention, and treatment of HHNK

Desired Outcome: Within the 24-hr period before hospital discharge, patient and significant other verbalize understanding of causes, prevention, and treatment of HHNK.

INTERVENTIONS	RATIONALES
Assess patient's health care literacy (language, reading, comprehension). Assess culture and culturally specific information needs.	This assessment helps ensure that information is presented in a manner that is culturally and educationally appropriate.
Determine patient's understanding of HHNK and its treatment. Enable patient to verbalize fears and feelings about the diagnosis; correct any misconceptions.	This enables the nurse to reinforce, as needed, information about the disease process of DM and HHNK syndrome and common early symptoms of worsening diabetes, including polyuria, polydipsia, polyphagia, dry and flushed skin, and increased irritability.
Teach importance of testing blood glucose levels as prescribed before meals and at bedtime. As indicated, review testing procedure with patient.	Blood glucose monitoring is essential for calculating appropriate basal, mealtime, and supplemental insulin dosages.
Explain that fasting morning blood glucose greater than 140 mg/dl should be reported to health care provider.	Reporting this value enables prompt adjustment in insulin dose based on blood glucose levels.
Stress importance of dietary changes as prescribed by health care provider. Provide referral to a dietitian as needed.	Typically, the person with type 2 DM is obese and will be on a reduced-calorie diet with fixed amounts of carbohydrate, fat, and protein. Fats should be polyunsaturated and proteins chosen from low-fat sources.
Teach importance of eating three meals per day at regularly scheduled times and a bedtime snack.	Mealtime insulin should be administered within the 30 min before a meal (regular insulin) or 15 min before or after a meal (analogue short-acting insulins such as Humalog, Novolog, or Apidra). If meals are not spaced appropriately, patients may experience hyperglycemia or hypoglycemia between meals.
Explain that increased or decreased food intake will necessitate adjustment in insulin dosage.	Mealtime insulin dose is calculated based on the average amount of carbohydrates in the patient's diet. If meal consumption changes, the insulin dose must change accordingly to ensure adequate control of blood glucose.
Caution about importance of taking oral hypoglycemic agents as prescribed.	Oral hypoglycemic agents must be taken as prescribed or patient may become hypoglycemic or hyperglycemic.
In addition, explain that exogenous insulin or insulin analogues may be required during periods of physical and emotional stress and that blood glucose levels should be monitored closely during these times.	Increased stress creates insulin resistance, which may prompt hyperglycemia even though the patient's food intake remains constant.
For patients with type 2 DM, explain benefits of regular exercise for maintaining blood glucose levels.	Exercise increases insulin effectiveness and reduces serum triglyceride and cholesterol levels, thus also decreasing risk of atherosclerosis. Aerobic exercises, such as walking or swimming, are most effective in lowering blood glucose levels.

Continued

INTERVENTIONS	RATIONALES
Caution patient to always monitor blood glucose level before exercise.	A level greater than 250 mg/dl is indicative of abnormal metabolism. In this case, exercise would be a stressor, resulting in further elevation of blood glucose.
Explain need for measures to prevent infection, such as good hygiene and meticulous daily foot care. Stress importance of avoiding exposure to communicable diseases. Explain that the following indicators of infection necessitate prompt medical treatment: fever, chills, tachycardia, diaphoresis, and nausea and vomiting. In addition, teach patient and significant other to be alert to wounds or cuts that do not heal, burning or pain with urination, and cough that is productive of sputum.	Hyperglycemia indicates glucose is not entering cells. Without glucose, all body system functions are impaired, because cells are unable to do 100% of work required. Immune system dysfunction results from the lack of energy production at the cellular level of all components of the immune system.
Provide the following address of the ADA: American Diabetes Association at *www.diabetes.org*.	Patient may acquire pamphlets and magazines related to diabetes, its complications, and treatment.

••• **Related NIC and NOC labels:** *NIC:* Teaching: Disease Process; Teaching: Prescribed Diet; Teaching: Prescribed Medication; Hyperglycemia Management; Hypoglycemia Management; Medication Administration; Subcutaneous; Teaching: Prescribed Activity/Exercise; Behavior Modification; Health Education; Nutrition Management; Referral *NOC:* Diabetes Management

ADDITIONAL NURSING DIAGNOSES/ PROBLEMS:

"Psychosocial Support"	p. 73
"Seizure Disorders" for **Risk for Trauma** related to musculoskeletal, oral, and airway vulnerability secondary to seizure activity	p. 325
"Diabetic Ketoacidosis" for **Deficient Fluid Volume**	p. 389
Risk for Infection	p. 390
Ineffective Tissue Perfusion: Peripheral	p. 392

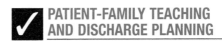 **PATIENT-FAMILY TEACHING AND DISCHARGE PLANNING**

See **Deficient Knowledge:** Causes, Prevention, and Treatment of HHNK syndrome, p. 396.

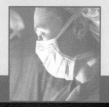

Hyperthyroidism 48

OVERVIEW/PATHOPHYSIOLOGY

Hyperthyroidism is a clinical syndrome caused by excessive circulating thyroid hormone. Because thyroid activity affects all body systems, excessive thyroid hormone exaggerates normal body functions and produces a hypermetabolic state. *Lymphocytic* ("painless") and *postpartum thyroiditis* are autoimmune disorders that result in thyroid inflammation with release of stored thyroid hormone into systemic circulation. Postpartum thyroiditis may ensue several months after delivery and remain active for several months, sometimes followed by hypothyroidism lasting several months. *Subacute (granulomatous) thyroiditis* is considered a viral syndrome, which results in a painful, enlarged thyroid with overactive thyroid until the virus is controlled. Hyperthyroid symptoms also result from ingestion of too much thyroid replacement medication.

Graves' disease (diffuse toxic goiter) accounts for approximately 85% of reported cases of hyperthyroidism. It is characterized by spontaneous exacerbations and remissions that appear to be unaffected by therapy. The cause of Graves' disease is unknown, but recent advances in diagnostic techniques have isolated an immunoglobulin known as long-acting thyroid stimulator in a majority of patients with this disorder, suggesting that Graves' disease is an autoimmune response.

The most severe form of hyperthyroidism is *thyrotoxic crisis*, or *thyroid storm*, which results from a sudden surge of large amounts of thyroid hormones into the bloodstream, causing an even greater increase in body metabolism. This is a *medical emergency*. Precipitating factors include infection, trauma, and emotional stress, all of which increase demands on body metabolism. Thyrotoxic crisis also can occur following thyroidectomy because of manipulation of the gland during surgery.

HEALTH CARE SETTING

Primary care with possible hospitalization resulting from complications

ASSESSMENT

Signs and symptoms: Nervousness, irritability, alteration in appetite, weight loss or gain, rapid pulse (usually noted by patient), irregular heartbeats, menstrual irregularities, fatigue, heat intolerance, increased perspiration, frequent defecation or diarrhea, anxiety, restlessness, tremor, and insomnia.

Physical assessment: Tachycardia, palpitations, widened pulse pressure, exophthalmos, diplopia, hyperpyrexia, enlargement of the thyroid gland, dependent lower extremity edema, muscle weakness, hyperreflexia, fine tremor, fine hair, thin skin, hypercholesterolemia, impaired glucose tolerance, and stare and/or lid lag. Occasionally males may present with gynecomastia.

Thyrotoxic crisis (thyroid storm): Acute exacerbation of some or all the above signs, marked tachycardia, hyperpyrexia, central nervous system (CNS) irritability, and sometimes coma or heart failure.

History/risk factors: Family history of hyperthyroidism is a significant factor for development of this disorder. Another important factor is presence of thyroid nodules or nodular toxic goiters in which one or more thyroid adenomas hyperfunction autonomously. Amiodarone use has caused thyroid dysfunction in 14%-18% of individuals taking this commonly used antidysrhythmic drug. Patients should have thyroid studies done before the drug is initiated and be monitored subsequently afterward.

DIAGNOSTIC TESTS

Serum thyroid-stimulating hormone (thyrotropin): Most commonly used test to detect thyroid dysfunction. It is decreased in the presence of disease.

Serum T_4 (thyroxine) or free T_4: Elevated in the presence of disease. It may be more accurate than thyroid-stimulating hormone (TSH) if patients have been recently treated for hyperthyroidism or if receiving high doses of thyroid replacement therapy. Thyroxine should be monitored along with TSH for the first year of therapy, especially in older adults.

Serum T_3 (thyroxine triiodothyronine) radioimmunoassay or free T_3: Elevated in the presence of disease.

Serum thyroid autoantibodies: Can detect TSH receptor antibodies and thyroid-stimulating immunoglobulins, which may be present if autoimmune disease is present.

Doppler ultrasonography: To diagnose size of the gland and abnormal densities, which can indicate presence of nodules.

Radioiodine (^{131}I) uptake and thyroid scan: Clarifies gland size and detects presence of hot or cold nodules.

^{123}I scintiscan/thyroid scintigraphy: Defines functional characteristics of the gland to help determine cause of hyperthyroidism.

Nursing Diagnosis:

Ineffective Protection

related to potential for thyrotoxic crisis (thyroid storm) secondary to emotional stress, trauma, infection, or surgical manipulation of the gland

Desired Outcomes: Patient is free of symptoms of thyroid storm as evidenced by normothermia; BP 90/60 mm Hg or more (or within patient's baseline range); HR 100 bpm or less; and orientation to person, place, and time. If thyroid storm occurs, it is noted promptly and reported immediately.

INTERVENTIONS	RATIONALES
Measure and report rectal or core temperature greater than 38.3° C (101° F).	An increased temperature often is the first sign of impending thyroid storm.
Monitor vital signs hourly in patients in whom thyroid storm is suspected.	These assessments may reveal evidence of hypotension and increasing tachycardia and fever, which occur with thyroid storm.
Monitor patient for signs of heart failure. Immediately report significant findings to health care provider, and prepare to transfer patient to intensive care unit if they are noted.	Signs of heart failure (jugular vein distention, crackles, decreased amplitude of peripheral pulses, peripheral edema, and hypotension) can occur as an effect of thyroid storm. If not aggressively monitored and managed, thyroid storm can lead to lethal cardiac and hemodynamic compromise.
Provide a cool, calm, protected environment. Reassure patient and explain all procedures before performing them. Limit the number of visitors.	These measures minimize emotional and physical stress, which can precipitate thyroid storm.
Ensure good handwashing and meticulous aseptic technique for dressing changes and invasive procedures. Advise visitors who have contracted or been exposed to a communicable disease either not to enter patient's room or to wear a surgical mask, if appropriate.	These measures reduce risk of infection, which is a precipitating factor in development of thyroid storm.
In the Presence of Thyroid Storm	
Assess for hyperthermia, and as prescribed, administer acetaminophen.	Acetaminophen will decrease temperature secondary to the fever associated with thyroid storm.
Caution: Avoid giving aspirin.	Aspirin is contraindicated because it releases thyroxine from protein-binding sites and increases free thyroxine levels, which would exacerbate symptoms of thyroid storm.
Provide cool sponge baths, or apply ice packs to patient's axilla and groin area. If high temperature continues, obtain prescription for a hypothermia blanket.	These actions will decrease the fever caused by thyroid storm.
Administer propylthiouracil (PTU) as prescribed.	PTU will prevent further synthesis and release of thyroid hormones. The most severe side effect of this drug is leukopenia, which increases the possibility that patient may acquire an infection. Patients should discontinue the drug at the first sign of infection and obtain a complete blood count. If the blood count is normal, medication is promptly resumed. Rash, another side effect, can be treated easily with antihistamines.
Administer propranolol as prescribed.	Propranolol will block sympathetic nervous system (SNS) effects. It reduces heart rate (HR) and blood pressure (BP), which are elevated as a result of hyperthyroidism.
Administer IV fluids as prescribed.	Fluid volume deficit may occur because of increased fluid excretion by the kidneys or excessive diaphoresis. IV fluids will provide adequate hydration and prevent vascular collapse.
Carefully monitor intake and output (I&O) hourly.	Hourly assessment of I&O will reveal fluid overload or inadequate fluid replacement, either of which necessitates prompt intervention. Decreasing output with normal specific gravity may indicate decreased cardiac output, whereas decreasing output with increased specific gravity can signal dehydration.

Continued

INTERVENTIONS	RATIONALES
Administer sodium iodide as prescribed, 1 hr after administering PTU.	Iodine is necessary for subsequent production of thyroid hormones following resolution of the crisis. **Caution:** If given before PTU, sodium iodide can exacerbate symptoms in susceptible persons.
Administer small doses of insulin as prescribed.	This will help control hyperglycemia.
	Hyperglycemia can occur as an effect of thyroid storm because of the release of stress hormones as part of the body's response to the hypermetabolic state. Stress hormones create insulin resistance.
Administer prescribed supplemental O_2 as necessary.	O_2 demands are increased as metabolism increases.

••• Related NIC and NOC labels: *NIC:* Emergency Care; Environmental Management; Risk Identification *NOC:* Safety Status: Physical Injury

Nursing Diagnosis:

Imbalanced Nutrition: Less Than Body Requirements

related to hypermetabolic state and/or inadequate nutrient absorption

Desired Outcomes: By a minimum of 24 hr before hospital discharge, patient has adequate nutrition as evidenced by stable weight and a positive nitrogen balance. Within 24 hr of the instruction, patient lists types of foods that are necessary to restore a normal nutritional state.

INTERVENTIONS	RATIONALES
Provide foods high in calories, protein, carbohydrates, and vitamins. Teach patient about foods that will provide optimal nutrients.	This will help restore a normal nutritional state for patients with hyperthyroidism.
Provide between-meal snacks.	Snacks will help maximize patient's consumption and provide needed calories.
Administer vitamin supplements as prescribed, and explain their importance to patient.	Vitamins provide essential nutrients to facilitate appropriate digestion/absorption of foods that contribute to energy production.
Administer prescribed antidiarrheal medications.	These medications increase absorption of nutrients from the gastrointestinal tract.
Weigh patient daily, and report significant losses to health care provider.	Weight assessment is a useful indicator of nutritional status.

••• Related NIC and NOC labels: *NIC:* Nutrition Management; Weight Gain Assistance; Teaching: Prescribed Diet; Medication Management *NOC:* Nutritional Status: Nutrient Intake

Nursing Diagnosis:

Disturbed Sleep Pattern

related to accelerated metabolism

Desired Outcome: Within 48 hr of hospital admission, patient relates attainment of sufficient rest and sleep.

INTERVENTIONS	RATIONALES
Adjust care activities to patient's tolerance.	It may be necessary to alter care regimen to comply with patient's rest/sleep disturbance.
Provide frequent rest periods of at least 90-min duration. If possible, arrange for patient to have bedrest in a quiet, cool room with nonexertional activities such as reading, watching television, working crossword puzzles, or listening to soothing music.	Patients will have difficulty relaxing. Therefore all efforts must be made to provide a calm, quiet environment to promote rest/sleep.

Continued

INTERVENTIONS	RATIONALES
Assist with walking up stairs or other exertional activities if needed.	If patient is tired, more assistance is needed until rest/sleep pattern normalizes.
Administer short-acting sedatives (e.g., lorazepam) as prescribed.	These medications promote rest.
After administering these agents, raise side rails and caution patient not to smoke in bed.	These actions protect patient, who will be drowsy after taking these sedatives.

••• **Related NIC and NOC labels:** *NIC:* Energy Management; Sleep Enhancement; Self-Care Assistance; Environmental Management; Medication Management *NOC:* Rest; Sleep

Nursing Diagnosis:

Anxiety

related to SNS stimulation

Desired Outcomes: Within 24 hr of hospital admission, patient is free of harmful anxiety as evidenced by an HR of 100 bpm or less, RR 12-20 breaths/min with normal depth and pattern (eupnea), and absence of or decrease in irritability and restlessness. Patient and significant others verbalize knowledge about the causes of the patient's behavior.

INTERVENTIONS	RATIONALES
Assess for signs of anxiety; administer short-acting sedatives as prescribed.	Short-acting sedatives (e.g., alprazolam or lorazepam) reduce anxiety.
Provide a quiet environment away from loud noises or excessive activity.	This will help reduce stress and anxiety.
Limit number of visitors and the amount of time they spend with patient. Advise significant others to avoid discussing stressful topics and refrain from arguing with the patient.	These measures will help reduce stress and anxiety.
Administer propranolol as prescribed.	Propranolol reduces symptoms of anxiety, tachycardia, and heat intolerance.
Reassure patient that anxiety symptoms are related to the disease process and that treatment decreases their severity.	Reassurance helps patient regain emotional control/reduce emotional stress through better understanding of the cause and treatment.
Inform significant others that patient's behavior is physiologic and should not be taken personally.	Reassuring family members helps them regain emotional control/reduce their stress regarding patient's unusual behaviors.

••• **Related NIC and NOC labels:** *NIC:* Anxiety Reduction; Counseling; Medication Administration; Environmental Management *NOC:* Anxiety Control

Nursing Diagnosis:

Impaired Tissue Integrity: Corneal

related to dryness that can occur with exophthalmos in persons with Graves' disease

Desired Outcome: Within 24 hr of admission, patient's corneas are moist and intact.

INTERVENTIONS	RATIONALES
Teach patient to wear dark glasses.	This will help protect the corneas. Dark glasses also protect those individuals who are photosensitive.
Administer lubricating eyedrops as prescribed.	Eyedrops will supplement lubrication and decrease SNS stimulation, which can cause lid retraction.
If appropriate, apply eye shields or tape eyes shut at bedtime.	Hyperthyroidism can result in severe exophthalmos that prevents eyelids from closing fully, making the corneas vulnerable to injury.
Administer thioamides as prescribed.	Thioamides maintain normal metabolic state and halt progression of exophthalmos.

••• **Related NIC and NOC labels:** *NIC:* Eye Care; Medication Administration: Eye *NOC:* Tissue Integrity: Skin and Mucous Membranes

Nursing Diagnosis:

Disturbed Body Image

related to exophthalmos or surgical scar on the neck

Desired Outcome: Within the 24-hr period before hospital discharge, patient verbalizes measures for disguising exophthalmos or surgical scar and exhibits self-acceptance.

INTERVENTIONS	RATIONALES
Encourage patient to communicate feelings of frustration.	Such communication may help patients relieve stress that would otherwise further stimulate the hypophyseal/thyroid/adrenal axis.
Advise patient to wear dark glasses.	Dark glasses will disguise exophthalmos while also protecting corneas from photosensitivity.
Suggest measures that can disguise the scar.	Customized jewelry, high-necked clothing such as turtlenecks, or loose-fitting scarves are examples of measures that will help disguise the scar.
Suggest that after incision has healed, patient can use makeup colored in his or her skin tone.	This will decrease visibility of the scar.
Caution patient that creams are contraindicated until incision has healed completely, and even then may not minimize scarring.	This is standard postoperative teaching for most surgical procedures.
	Patients are advised by some health care providers to increase vitamin C intake up to 1 g/day to promote healing. Some surgeons also advise against direct sunlight to the operative site for 6-12 mo to avoid hyperpigmentation of the incision. Instruct patient accordingly.
For additional information, see this nursing diagnosis in "Psychosocial Support," p. 80.	

••• **Related NIC and NOC labels:** *NIC:* Body Image Enhancement; Active Listening; Coping Enhancement; Counseling; Emotional Support *NOC:* Body Image

Nursing Diagnosis:

Deficient Knowledge:

Potential for side effects from iodides and thioamides or stopping thioamides abruptly

Desired Outcome: Within the 24-hr period before hospital discharge, patient verbalizes knowledge about potential side effects of prescribed medications, signs and symptoms of hypothyroidism and hyperthyroidism, and importance of following the prescribed medical regimen.

INTERVENTIONS	RATIONALES
Assess patient's health care literacy (language, reading, comprehension). Assess culture and culturally specific information needs.	This assessment helps ensure that materials are presented in a manner that is culturally and educationally appropriate.
Explain importance of taking antithyroid medications daily, in divided doses, and at regular intervals as prescribed.	A knowledgeable patient is more likely to adhere to the treatment regimen.
Teach indicators of hypothyroidism.	Indicators of hypothyroidism (e.g., early fatigue, weight gain, anorexia, constipation, menstrual irregularities, muscle cramps, lethargy, inability to concentrate, hair loss, cold intolerance, and hoarseness) may occur from excessive medication. Signs and symptoms that necessitate medical attention because the medications that cause them may require dose adjustment include cold intolerance, fatigue, lethargy, and peripheral or periorbital edema.
Teach side effects of thioamides and symptoms that necessitate medical attention.	Appearance of a rash, fever, or pharyngitis can occur in the presence of agranulocytosis, a recognized side effect of thioamides. This necessitates medical attention to adjust the dose or change the medication.
Alert patients taking iodides to signs of worsening hyperthyroidism.	Signs of worsening hyperthyroidism (high body temperature, palpitations, rapid HR, irritability, anxiety, and feelings of restlessness or panic) may signal need for medication dosage adjustment to manage the problem and should be reported promptly for timely intervention.

••• **Related NIC and NOC labels:** *NIC:* Teaching: Prescribed Medication *NOC:* Knowledge: Medication; Knowledge: Treatment Regimen

Nursing Diagnosis:

Acute Pain

related to surgical procedure

Desired Outcomes: Within 2 hr of surgery, patient's subjective perception of pain decreases, as documented by a pain scale. Objective indicators, such as hesitation before turning or moving the head, are absent or diminished.

INTERVENTIONS	RATIONALES
Document degree and character of patient's pain, including precipitating events. Devise a pain scale with patient, rating pain on a scale of 0 (no pain) to 10 (worst pain).	This assessment will enable nurse to determine trend of the pain and degree of pain relief obtained.
Inform patient to clasp hands behind neck when moving.	This measure will minimize stress on the incision.
After health care provider has removed surgical clips and drain, teach patient to perform gentle range-of-motion (ROM) exercises for the neck.	While the surgical clips and drain are in place, mobility of the neck is limited, leading to tight neck muscles. Following removal of these devices, gentle ROM is done to help relax the neck muscles and decrease pain.
For other interventions, see "Pain," p. 39.	

••• **Related NIC and NOC labels:** *NIC:* Pain Management; Positioning *NOC:* Comfort Level; Pain Control

Nursing Diagnosis:

Impaired Swallowing (or risk for same)

related to edema or laryngeal nerve damage resulting from surgical procedure

Desired Outcomes: Patient reports swallowing with minimal difficulty, has minimal or absent hoarseness, and is free of symptoms of respiratory dysfunction as evidenced by RR 12-20 breaths/min with normal depth and pattern (eupnea) and absence of inspiratory stridor. Laryngeal nerve damage, if it occurs, is detected promptly and reported immediately.

INTERVENTIONS	RATIONALES
Monitor respiratory status for dyspnea, choking, inspiratory stridor, inability to swallow.	These are signs of postsurgical edema. Edema in the neck may impinge on the pharynx or esophagus, making swallowing more difficult.
Also assess patient's voice.	Although slight hoarseness is normal after surgery, hoarseness that persists is indicative of laryngeal nerve damage and should be reported to health care provider promptly. If bilateral nerve damage is present, upper airway obstruction and dysphagia can occur.
Elevate head of bed (HOB) 30-45 degrees.	Elevating HOB enables gravity to facilitate swallowing and promotes edema reduction.
Support patient's head with flat or cervical pillows so that it is in a neutral position with the neck (does not flex or hyperextend).	This position minimizes incisional stress and reduces chance of choking and dysphagia.
Keep tracheostomy set and O$_2$ equipment at the bedside at all times.	This equipment will be used for emergency treatment in the event upper airway obstruction occurs.
Gently suction upper airway as needed.	Patients can aspirate retained secretions if edema and/or laryngeal nerve problems are present. Using gentle, rather than aggressive, suctioning avoids stimulating laryngospasm.
Administer analgesics promptly and as prescribed.	This will minimize pain and anxiety and enhance patient's ability to swallow.

••• **Related NIC and NOC labels:** *NIC:* Airway Suctioning; Positioning; Surveillance *NOC:* Aspiration Control; Swallowing Status; Swallowing Status: Esophageal Phase; Swallowing Status: Pharyngeal

---

ADDITIONAL NURSING DIAGNOSES/ PROBLEMS:

"Perioperative Care"	p. 45

 PATIENT-FAMILY TEACHING AND DISCHARGE PLANNING

When providing patient-family teaching, focus on sensory information, avoid giving excessive information, and initiate a visiting nurse referral for necessary follow-up teaching. Part of the initial assessment should include asking about existing knowledge of the disease, ability for self-management, and psychologic acceptance. Include verbal and written information about the following:

✓ Diet high in calories, protein, carbohydrates, and vitamins. Inform patient that as a normal metabolic state is attained, the diet may change.

✓ Medications, including drug name, purpose, dosage, schedule, precautions, and potential side effects. Also discuss drug-drug, food-drug, and herb-drug interactions.

✓ Changes that can occur as a result of therapy, including weight gain, normalized bowel function, increased strength of skeletal muscles, and a return to normal activity levels.

✓ Importance of continued and frequent medical follow-up; confirm date and time of next appointment.

✓ Indicators that necessitate medical attention, including fever, rash, or sore throat (side effects of thioamides), and symptoms of hypothyroidism (see p. 407) or worsening hyperthyroidism.

✓ For patients receiving radioactive iodine, importance of not holding children to the chest for 72 hr following therapy because children are more susceptible to the effects of radiation. Explain that there is negligible risk for adults.

✓ Importance of avoiding physical and emotional stress early in the recuperative stage and maximizing coping mechanisms for dealing with stress. See **Health-Seeking Behaviors:** Relaxation technique effective for stress reduction, p. 172.

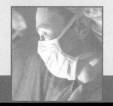

Hypothyroidism 49

OVERVIEW/PATHOPHYSIOLOGY

Hypothyroidism is a condition in which there is an inadequate amount of circulating thyroid hormone, causing a decrease in metabolic rate that affects all body systems.

Primary hypothyroidism accounts for 90% of cases of hypothyroidism and is caused by pathologic changes in the thyroid itself. The most common cause of the disease in the United States is chronic autoimmune thyroiditis (Hashimoto's disease). *Secondary hypothyroidism* is caused by dysfunction of the anterior pituitary gland, which results in decreased release of thyroid-stimulating hormone (TSH). *Tertiary hypothyroidism* is caused by a hypothalamic deficiency in the release of thyrotropin-releasing hormone (TRH).

When hypothyroidism is untreated, or when a stressor such as infection affects an individual with hypothyroidism, a life-threatening condition known as *myxedema coma* can occur. The clinical picture of myxedema coma is that of exaggerated hypothyroidism, with dangerous hypoventilation, hypothermia, hypotension, and shock. Coma and seizures can occur as well. Myxedema coma usually develops slowly, has a greater than 50% mortality rate, and requires prompt and aggressive treatment.

HEALTH CARE SETTING

Primary care with possible hospitalization resulting from complications

ASSESSMENT

Signs and symptoms can progress from mild early in onset to life threatening.

Signs and symptoms: Early fatigue, weight gain from fluid retention, anorexia, lethargy, cold intolerance, hoarseness, ataxia, memory and mental impairment, decreased concentration, menstrual irregularities or heavy menses, infertility, constipation, depression, and muscle cramps.

Physical assessment: Possible presence of goiter, bradycardia, hypothermia, deepened voice, hyperlipidemia, and obesity. Skin may appear yellow and dry, cool, and coarse, and hair may be thin, coarse, and brittle. The tongue may be enlarged (macroglossia), and reflexes may be slowed.

Myxedema coma: Hypoventilation, hypoglycemia, hypothermia, hypotension, bradycardia, and shock.

History/risk factors:

Primary hypothyroidism: Dietary iodine deficiency, thyroid gland radioablation for hyperthyroidism management, thyroid atrophy or fibrosis of unknown cause, radiation therapy to the neck, surgical removal of all or part of the gland, drugs that suppress thyroid activity including propylthiouracil and iodides, invasion of the thyroid gland by tumor (e.g., lymphoma), drugs including lithium and interferon, or a genetic dysfunction resulting in inability to produce and secrete thyroid hormone.

Secondary hypothyroidism: Pituitary tumors, postpartum necrosis of the pituitary gland, hypophysectomy.

DIAGNOSTIC TESTS

TSH: Most commonly used test to detect thyroid dysfunction. It will be elevated unless the disease is longstanding or severe.

Free thyroxine index and T$_4$ (thyroxine) levels: Decreased with hypothyroidism.

^{131}I scan and uptake: Will be less than 10% in a 24-hr period. In secondary hypothyroidism, uptake increases with administration of exogenous TSH.

Doppler ultrasonography: To diagnose gland size and abnormal densities, which may be present if nodules are present.

Thyroid autoantibodies: Presence of thyroperoxidase autoantibodies or antithyroglobulin autoantibodies signals chronic autoimmune thyroiditis.

<u>Nursing Diagnosis:</u>

Ineffective Breathing Pattern (or risk for same)

related to upper airway obstruction occurring with enlarged thyroid gland and/or decreased ventilatory drive caused by greatly decreased metabolism

Desired Outcomes: Patient has an effective breathing pattern as evidenced by RR 12-20 breaths/min with normal depth and pattern (eupnea), normal skin color, O_2 saturation 95% or more, and absence of adventitious breath sounds. Alternatively, if ineffective breathing pattern occurs, it is detected, reported, and treated promptly.

INTERVENTIONS	RATIONALES
Assess rate, depth, and quality of breath sounds, and be alert to presence of adventitious sounds or decreasing or crowing sounds.	This enables nurse to be alert to presence of adventitious sounds (e.g., from developing pleural effusion) or decreasing or crowing sounds (e.g., from swollen tongue or glottis).
Be alert to signs of inadequate ventilation. Immediately report significant findings to health care provider.	Decreased respiratory rate, shallow breathing, and circumoral or peripheral cyanosis are signs of inadequate ventilation. Ventilatory insufficiency in a patient with hypothyroid condition can indicate onset of heart failure secondary to impending myxedema coma/hypothyroid crisis.
Measure Sao_2 intermittently or continuously in patients with decreased ventilatory drive.	Decreasing O_2 saturation may signal need for oxygen supplementation in symptomatic patients.
Teach patient coughing, deep breathing, and use of incentive spirometer. Suction upper airway prn.	These measures help clear secretions that may increase with hypoventilation.
For patient experiencing respiratory distress, be prepared to assist health care provider with intubation or tracheostomy and maintenance of mechanical ventilatory assistance or transfer patient to intensive care unit (ICU).	Patient likely will need emergency treatment and intensive care.

••• **Related NIC and NOC labels** *NIC:* Airway Management; Airway Insertion and Stabilization; Cough Enhancement; Respiratory Monitoring; Emergency Care; Mechanical Ventilation; Oxygen Therapy; Ventilation Assistance *NOC:* Respiratory Status: Airway Patency; Respiratory Status: Ventilation

<u>Nursing Diagnosis:</u>

Excess Fluid Volume

related to compromised regulatory mechanisms occurring with adrenal insufficiency

Desired Outcome: By a minimum of 24 hr before hospital discharge, patient is normovolemic as evidenced by urinary output 30 ml/hr or more, stable weight, nondistended jugular veins, presence of eupnea, and peripheral pulse amplitude 2+ or more on a 0-4+ scale.

INTERVENTIONS	RATIONALES
Monitor intake and output hourly for evidence of decreasing output.	Decreasing output signals fluid retention leading to hypervolemia.
Weigh patient at same time every day, with same clothing, and using same scale. Report increasing weight gain to health care provider.	Increasing weight gain signals fluid retention, leading to hypervolemia/volume overload.
	Weighing patient at the same time and under the same conditions avoids discrepancies that could reflect inaccurate losses or gains.
Monitor for indicators of heart failure. Report significant findings to health care provider.	Indicators of heart failure include jugular vein distention, crackles, shortness of breath, dependent edema of extremities, and decreased amplitude of peripheral pulses. Lack of thyroid hormones can decrease the heart rate and force of contractions, leading to heart failure. Associated fluid retention worsens the problem.

Continued

INTERVENTIONS / RATIONALES

INTERVENTIONS	RATIONALES
Restrict fluid and sodium intake as prescribed.	This helps prevent fluid retention that could lead to volume overload.
Use a rate control device to administer IV fluids.	This will prevent accidental fluid overload.

••• **Related NIC and NOC labels:** *NIC:* Fluid Monitoring; Fluid/Electrolyte Management; Hypervolemia Management; Vital Signs Monitoring; Cardiac Care: Acute *NOC:* Fluid Balance

Nursing Diagnosis:

Activity Intolerance

related to weakness and fatigue secondary to slowed metabolism and decreased cardiac output caused by pericardial effusions, atherosclerosis, and decreased adrenergic stimulation

Desired Outcome: During activity patient rates perceived exertion at 3 or less on a 0-10 scale and exhibits cardiac tolerance to activity as evidenced by HR 20 bpm or less over resting HR, SBP 20 mm Hg or less over or under resting SBP, warm and dry skin, and absence of crackles (rales), murmurs, chest pain, and new dysrhythmias.

INTERVENTIONS	RATIONALES
Monitor vital signs and apical pulse at frequent intervals.	This enables nurse to be alert to hypotension, slow pulse, dysrhythmias, decreasing urine output, and changes in mentation, which along with complaints of chest pain or discomfort may signal heart failure/impending pulmonary edema.
Ask patient to rate perceived exertion (RPE). See **Risk for Activity Intolerance** in "Prolonged Bedrest," p. 61, for details.	An RPE more than 3 on a 0-10 scale is a signal of cardiac intolerance during exertion and also a sign that patient should stop or modify the activity causing the exertion.
Promptly report significant changes to health care provider.	This will help prevent progression of heart failure to cardiac arrest.
Balance activity with adequate rest.	Rest decreases workload of the heart.
As prescribed, administer IV isotonic solutions such as normal saline.	Isotonic solutions help prevent or ameliorate hypotension. Hypotension ensues as a result of reduced sympathetic nervous system stimulation, which causes decreased cardiac output and hypotension.
Assist patient with range of motion and other in-bed exercises and consult with health care provider about implementation of exercises that require greater cardiac tolerance. For details, see **Risk for Activity Intolerance**, p. 61, and **Risk for Disuse Syndrome**, p. 63.	Exercise prevents problems caused by immobility.

••• **Related NIC and NOC labels:** *NIC:* Energy Management; Exercise Promotion *NOC:* Energy Conservation

Nursing Diagnosis:

Risk for Infection

related to compromised immunologic status secondary to alterations in adrenal function

Desired Outcome: Patient is free of infection as evidenced by normothermia, absence of adventitious breath sounds, normal urinary pattern and characteristics, and well-healing wounds.

INTERVENTIONS	RATIONALES
Be alert to early indicators of infection. Notify health care provider of significant findings.	Fever; erythema, swelling, or discharge from wounds or IV sites; urinary frequency, urgency, or dysuria; cloudy or malodorous urine; presence of adventitious sounds on auscultation of lung fields; and changes in color, consistency, and amount of sputum are early indicators of infection. Prompt assessment and treatment can halt their progression to prevent complications such as myxedema coma, a life-threatening condition.
Provide meticulous care of indwelling catheters.	This minimizes risk of urinary tract infection.
Use sterile technique when performing dressing changes and invasive procedures.	Nonintact skin and invasive procedures can lead to bacterial ingress.
Provide good skin care.	Open sores are sites of ingress for bacteria.
Advise visitors who have contracted or been exposed to a communicable disease not to enter patient's room or to wear a surgical mask, if appropriate.	This will minimize risk of systemic infection in patients who are immunocompromised.

••• **Related NIC and NOC labels:** *NIC:* Infection Protection; Risk Identification; Surveillance; Infection Control; Environmental Management; Incision Site Care; Wound Care *NOC:* Immune Status; Infection Status

Nursing Diagnosis:

Risk for Imbalanced Nutrition: More Than Body Requirements

related to slowed metabolism

Desired Outcomes: Patient does not experience weight gain. Within the 24-hr period before hospital discharge, patient verbalizes understanding of rationale and measures for dietary regimen.

INTERVENTIONS	RATIONALES
Provide a diet that is high in protein and low in calories.	This diet will promote weight loss.
As prescribed, restrict or limit sodium intake and foods high in sodium content.	This measure decreases edema caused by fluid retention.
Teach patient about foods to augment and foods to limit or avoid.	Foods high in protein and low in calories and sodium will help with weight control while patient is in a hypometabolic/fluid-retaining state.
Provide small, frequent meals of appropriate foods patient particularly enjoys.	This promotes weight control and decreases chance of patient overeating if allowed to get too hungry.
Encourage foods that are high in fiber content (e.g., fruits with skins, vegetables, whole grain breads and cereals, nuts).	Adding bulk to the diet improves gastric motility, which will help elimination that may be decreased as a result of slowed metabolism.
Administer vitamin supplements as prescribed.	This measure will help patients who are unable to consume appropriate recommended daily allowance minimum requirements on their restricted diets.

••• **Related NIC and NOC labels:** *NIC:* Nutrition Management; Teaching: Prescribed Diet; Weight Management *NOC:* Nutritional Status: Food and Fluid Intake; Weight Control

Nursing Diagnosis:

Constipation

related to inadequate dietary intake of roughage and fluids, prolonged bed rest, and/or decreased peristalsis secondary to slowed metabolism

Desired Outcome: Within 48-72 hr of admission, patient relates attainment of his or her normal pattern of bowel elimination.

INTERVENTIONS	RATIONALES
Be alert to decreasing bowel sounds and presence of distention and increases in abdominal girth.	These indicators can occur with ileus or fecal impaction and lead to an obstructive process, which is fairly common in hypothyroidism, especially in older adults.
Encourage patient to maintain a diet with adequate roughage and fluids. Ensure that fluid intake in persons without underlying cardiac or renal disease is at least 2-3 L/day.	Such foods as fruits with skins, fruit juices, cooked fruits, vegetables, whole grain breads and cereals, and nuts provide bulk, which will promote bowel elimination by increasing peristalsis and, coupled with increased fluid intake, add moisture to keep stool moving through the intestines/colon.
Administer stool softeners and laxatives as prescribed.	These agents minimize constipation by moistening stool and increasing peristalsis. **Caution:** Suppositories are contraindicated because of risk of stimulating the vagus nerve, which would further decrease heart rate (HR) and blood pressure (BP).
Advise patient to increase amount of exercise.	Exercise promotes regularity by increasing peristalsis. Exercise also tones gastrointestinal muscles to hold intestines/colon in place, which seems to facilitate bowel elimination.

••• **Related NIC and NOC labels:** *NIC:* Bowel Management; Exercise Promotion; Fluid Management; Nutrition Management; Medication Administration *NOC:* Bowel Elimination; Hydration

Nursing Diagnosis:
Disturbed Sensory Perception

related to altered sensory reception, transmission, or integration secondary to cerebral retention of water

Desired Outcomes: Patient verbalizes orientation to person, place, and time. Alternately, if signs of myxedema coma appear, they are detected, reported, and treated promptly.

INTERVENTIONS	RATIONALES
Monitor patient's mental status at frequent intervals by assessing orientation to person, place, and time.	Increasing lethargy or confusion can signal onset of myxedema coma, which necessitates immediate medical attention.
Reorient patient frequently. Have a clock and calendar visible, and use radio or television for orientation.	This ensures that the patient has information necessary to answer neurologic assessment questions appropriately.
Clearly explain all procedures to patient before performing them. Provide adequate time for patient to ask questions.	This promotes better understanding of procedures for a patient who may have memory impairment.
If necessary, remind patient to complete activities of daily living such as bathing and brushing hair.	Same as above.
Encourage visitors to discuss topics of special interest to patient.	This will enhance patient's alertness.
Administer thyroid replacement hormones as prescribed.	These hormones will increase metabolic rate, which in turn will promote cerebral blood flow. Patients are started on low doses that are increased gradually, based on serial laboratory tests (TSH and T_4), and adjusted until the TSH is in a normal range. This dose titration prevents hyperthyroidism caused by too much exogenous hormone. Therapy is continued for the patient's lifetime. **Note:** For patients with secondary hypothyroidism, thyroid supplements can promote acute symptoms and therefore are contraindicated.

••• **Related NIC and NOC labels:** *NIC:* Cognitive Stimulation; Reality Orientation; Medication Management *NOC:* Cognitive Orientation

Nursing Diagnosis:

Ineffective Protection: Myxedema Coma

related to inadequate response to treatment of hypothyroidism or stressors such as infection

Desired Outcomes: Patient is free of symptoms of myxedema coma as evidenced by HR 60 bpm or greater, BP 90/60 mm Hg or greater (or within patient's normal range), RR 12 breaths/min or more with normal depth and pattern (eupnea), and orientation to person, place, and time. Alternatively, if myxedema coma occurs, it is detected, reported, and treated promptly.

INTERVENTIONS	RATIONALES
Monitor patient for circumoral or peripheral cyanosis and decrease in level of consciousness (LOC). Immediately report significant findings to health care providers.	These are signs of hypoxia, which is a signal that patient may be about to experience cardiac arrest.
Double-check medication doses carefully before administration, especially barbiturates and sedatives.	Because of alterations in metabolism (decreased metabolism prolongs drug action times), patients with hypothyroidism do not tolerate barbiturates and sedatives, and therefore central nervous system depressants are contraindicated unless absolutely necessary to manage the patient during a crisis.
Monitor patient for signs of toxicity if sedatives or barbiturates are administered.	Signs of toxicity include decreased LOC and decreases in BP or ventilatory effort.
Monitor serum electrolytes and glucose levels.	In myxedema coma, patient may have decreasing Na$^+$ (less than 137 mEq/L) and glucose (less than 80 mg/dl).
In the presence of myxedema coma, implement the following:	
- Restrict fluids or administer hypertonic saline as prescribed.	This will correct hyponatremia.
- Use infusion control device.	This device maintains accurate infusion rate of IV fluids.
- As prescribed, administer IV thyroid replacement hormones with IV hydrocortisone and IV glucose.	In the treatment of hypoglycemia, rapid IV administration of thyroid hormone can precipitate hyperadrenalism. This can be avoided by concomitant administration of IV hydrocortisone.
- Monitor for signs of heart failure. Notify health care provider of any significant findings.	Jugular vein distention, crackles (rales), shortness of breath, peripheral edema, weakening peripheral pulses, and hypotension are signs of heart failure, which can occur secondary to hypothyroidism and lead to myxedema coma. Hypotension is treated with administration of IV isotonic fluids, such as normal saline and lactated Ringer's solution. Hypotonic solutions, such as 5% dextrose in water, are contraindicated because they can decrease serum Na$^+$ levels further. Because of altered metabolism, these patients respond poorly to vasopressors.
- Prepare to transfer patient to ICU. Keep oral airway and manual resuscitator at the bedside in the event of seizure, coma, or the need for ventilatory assistance.	This enables emergency treatment for a decreased ventilatory drive.

••• **Related NIC and NOC labels:** *NIC:* Risk Identification; Emergency Care *NOC:* Safety Status: Physical Injury

✓ PATIENT-FAMILY TEACHING AND DISCHARGE PLANNING

When providing patient-family teaching, focus on sensory information, avoid giving excessive information, and initiate a visiting nurse referral for necessary follow-up teaching. Part of the initial assessment should include asking about existing knowledge of the disease, ability for self-management, and psychologic acceptance. Include verbal and written information about the following:

✓ Medications, including drug name, purpose, dosage, schedule, precautions, and potential side effects. Also discuss drug-drug, food-drug, and herb-drug interactions. Remind patient that thioamides, iodides, and lithium are contraindicated because they decrease thyroid activity. Be sure patient is aware that thyroid replacement medications are to be taken for life.

✓ Dietary requirements and restrictions, which may change as hormone replacement therapy takes effect.

✓ Expected changes that can occur with hormone replacement therapy: increased energy level, weight loss, and decreased peripheral edema. Neuromuscular problems should improve as well.

✓ Importance of continued, frequent medical follow-up; confirm date and time of next medical appointment.

✓ Importance of avoiding physical and emotional stress, and ways for patient to maximize coping mechanisms for dealing with stress. See **Health-Seeking Behaviors:** Relaxation technique effective for stress reduction, p. 172.

✓ Signs and symptoms that necessitate medical attention, including fever or other symptoms of upper respiratory, urinary, or oral infections and signs and symptoms of hyperthyroidism, which may result from excessive hormone replacement.

✓ Available resources:
- The American Thyroid Association at *www.thyroid.org*
- Thyroid Foundation of America at *www.tsh.org*
- The Hormone Foundation at *www.hormone.org*

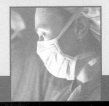

Syndrome of Inappropriate Antidiuretic Hormone 50

OVERVIEW/PATHOPHYSIOLOGY

Syndrome of inappropriate antidiuretic hormone (SIADH) is caused by release of ADH from the pituitary gland without regard to serum osmolality, plasma volume, or blood pressure (BP), resulting in excessive water retention and hyponatremia. The action of ADH increases reabsorption of water in the last segment of the distal tubules and collecting ducts of the kidney. ADH secretion usually is stimulated by one of three mechanisms: (1) increased serum osmolality, (2) decreased plasma volume, or (3) decreased BP. SIADH requires differential diagnosis from other problems that promote elevation of vasopressin and resultant hyponatremia because of an appropriate response to hypovolemic or hypotensive stimuli. SIADH is seen in postoperative and oncology patients and in individuals with multiorgan dysfunction syndrome. Sometimes it is present but not diagnosed because of mild or transient symptoms.

In the presence of excessive ADH, water that normally would be excreted is reabsorbed into the circulation, resulting in water retention and eventually water intoxication. The retained water expands extracellular fluid volume, causing serum osmolality and Na^+ to decrease because of dilutional effects. Decreased serum osmolality causes movement of water into the cells, which can result in cerebral edema. Further water retention results in increased glomerular filtration rate and decreased aldosterone secretion, and more Na^+ is filtered out into the urine.

Water intoxication, cerebral edema, and severe hyponatremia cause altered neurologic/mental status, which if untreated may lead to death.

HEALTH CARE SETTING

Acute care

ASSESSMENT

Signs and symptoms: Decreased urine output with concentrated urine. Signs of water intoxication may appear, including altered level of consciousness (LOC), fatigue, headache, diarrhea, anorexia, nausea, vomiting, and seizures. **Note:** Because of loss of Na^+, edema will not accompany the fluid volume excess.

Physical assessment: Weight gain without edema, elevated BP, altered mental status.

History of: Cancers of the lung, pancreas, duodenum, and prostate, which can secrete a biologically active form of ADH. Other common causes include pulmonary disease (e.g., tuberculosis, pneumonia, chronic obstructive pulmonary disease, empyema), acquired immunodeficiency syndrome, head trauma, brain tumor, intracerebral hemorrhage, meningitis, and encephalitis. Positive-pressure ventilation, physiologic stress, chronic metabolic illness, and a wide variety of medications (chlorpropamide, acetaminophen, oxytocin, narcotics, general anesthetic, carbamazepine, thiazide diuretics, tricyclic antidepressants, neuroleptics, angiotensin-converting enzyme inhibitors, cancer chemotherapy agents) all have been linked to SIADH.

DIAGNOSTIC TESTS

Serum Na^+ level: Decreased to less than 137 mEq/L.

Plasma osmolality: Decreased to less than 275 mOsm/kg.

Urine osmolality: Elevated disproportionately relative to plasma osmolality.

Urine Na^+ level: Increased to more than 200 mEq/L. Urine Na^+ level (e.g., increased) is best evaluated in comparison with serum Na^+ level (e.g., decreased).

Urine specific gravity: More than 1.030.

Plasma ADH level: Elevated.

Nursing Diagnosis:

Excess Fluid Volume

related to compromised regulatory mechanisms resulting in increased serum ADH level, renal water reabsorption, and renal Na^+ excretion

415

Desired Outcome: Patient becomes normovolemic (and normonatremic) within 7 days of onset of symptoms, as evidenced by orientation to person, place, and time; intake that approximates output plus insensible losses; stable weight; CVP 2-6 mm Hg; BP 90-140/60-85 mm Hg or within patient's normal range; and HR 60-100 bpm.

INTERVENTIONS	RATIONALES
Monitor for clinical signs of hypervolemia and hyponatremia. Promptly report significant findings or changes to health care provider.	Decreasing LOC, elevated BP and central venous pressure (CVP), urine output less than 30 ml/hr, and weight gain are signs of excess fluid volume that occur with SIADH and should be reported promptly for medical intervention.
Monitor laboratory results for hyponatremia and indicators of water intoxication. Report significant findings to health care provider.	Normal values are as follows: urine specific gravity, 1.010-1.020; serum Na$^+$, 137-147 mEq/L; urine osmolality, 300-1090 mOsm/kg; serum osmolality, 280-300 mOsm/kg. Decreased serum Na$^+$ and plasma osmolality, urine osmolality elevated disproportionately in relation to plasma osmolality, and increased urine Na$^+$ are values that are seen with SIADH. Water retention secondary to increased ADH secretion dilutes blood and results in reduced amounts of more concentrated urine.
Maintain fluid restriction as prescribed to prevent hypervolemia and water intoxication. Explain necessity of this treatment to patient and significant other. Do not keep water or ice chips at the bedside. Ensure precise delivery of fluid administered IV by using a monitoring device.	Restricting fluids to the amount manageable by the kidneys will allow restoration of normal serum Na$^+$ levels and osmolality without complications from drug therapy.
Elevate head of bed (HOB) 10-20 degrees.	A slightly elevated HOB promotes venous return and thus reduces ADH release. Excess fluid volume can sometimes result in cerebral edema that may add to problems with neural regulation of ADH secretion.
Administer demeclocycline, lithium, furosemide, or bumetanide as prescribed; carefully observe and document patient's response.	These drugs promote water excretion.
Administer hypertonic NaCl as prescribed.	This may be given if the patient has severe hyponatremia. Rate of administration usually is based on serial serum Na$^+$ levels. Supplemental Na$^+$ solutions may be administered with IV furosemide (Lasix) or bumetanide (Bumex) or osmotic diuretics, such as mannitol, to promote water excretion.
Make sure that specimens for laboratory tests are drawn on time and results are reported to health care provider promptly.	Serum blood levels of sodium are assessed to determine if patient has hypernatremia as a result of aggressive treatment.
Institute seizure precautions as indicated.	Seizures can occur in the presence of hyponatremia, which results from the excess fluid volume present in SIADH. Padded side rails, supplemental oxygen, and oral airway at the bedside, as well as side rails up at all times when staff member is not present, prevent patient injury in the event of seizure.

••• **Related NIC and NOC labels**: *NIC:* Fluid/Electrolyte Management; Electrolyte Management: Hyponatremia; Fluid Monitoring; Laboratory Data Interpretation; Neurologic Monitoring; Vital Signs Monitoring; Cerebral Edema Management; Medication Administration *NOC:* Electrolyte and Acid-Base Balance; Fluid Balance

Nursing Diagnosis:

Ineffective Protection

related to potential for increased intracranial pressure (IICP), diabetes insipidus (DI), cerebrospinal fluid (CSF) leak, hemorrhage, and infection secondary to transsphenoidal hypophysectomy

Desired Outcomes: Optimally, patient demonstrates normal level of mental acuity; verbalizes orientation to person, place, and time; and is free of indicators of injury caused by complications of transsphenoidal hypophysectomy. Immediately after instruction, patient and significant other verbalize understanding of importance of avoiding Valsalva-type maneuvers; describe signs and symptoms of IICP, DI, and infection; and verbalize importance of notifying staff of postnasal drip or excessive swallowing.

INTERVENTIONS	RATIONALES
Assess for changes in mental status or LOC, sluggish or unequal pupils, and changes in respiratory rate or pattern.	These are indicators of IICP. Neurologic deterioration may necessitate computerized axial tomography (CT) scan.
Monitor patient for decreased vision, eye muscle weakness, abnormal extraocular eye movements, double vision, and airway obstruction. Report significant findings to health care provider.	The surgery may interfere with cranial nerves governing eye movements and visual acuity—II, III, IV, and VI.
Measure intake and output hourly for 24 hr, and monitor urine specific gravity q1-2h. Monitor weight daily for evidence of loss.	Output greater than 200 ml/hr for 2 consecutive hr or a total of 500 ml/hr and specific gravity less than 1.007 are found with DI, as is weight loss resulting from increased fluid loss.
Teach signs of DI to patient, including polydipsia, polyuria, and decreased urine specific gravity.	DI can occur as a result of the edema caused by manipulating the pituitary stalk and usually is transitory
Report significant findings to health care provider.	The presence of DI necessitates fluid replacement to correct for excessive fluid loss.
Inspect nasal packing at frequent intervals. Note the number of times mustache dressing is changed.	These assessments will determine if frank bleeding or CSF leakage is present on the packing or dressing. Expect nasal packing removal in about 3-4 days.
Test serous drainage for the presence of CSF using a glucose reagent strip.	CSF contains glucose. However, because blood also contains glucose, testing should be done only on drainage that appears to be clear.
Monitor patient for complaints of postnasal drip or excessive swallowing.	These are signs that CSF may be draining down the back of patient's throat.
Caution: In the presence of suspected CSF, elevate HOB, and immediately report any suspicious drainage.	Raising HOB decreases the potential for bacteria entering the brain. Presence of CSF represents a serious breach in cranial integrity.
Elevate HOB 30 degrees.	This elevation will help decrease ICP and swelling. Dexamethasone may be prescribed to reduce cerebral swelling.
Explain that coughing, sneezing, and other Valsalva-type maneuvers must be avoided.	These actions can stress the operative site and increase ICP, causing CSF leakage.
Teach patient to cough or sneeze with an open mouth if either is unavoidable. Remind patient that nose blowing should be avoided until the nasal mucosa is healed (about 1 mo).	Pressure is high in the nasopharynx and sinuses if the mouth is closed when the patient coughs or sneezes. Opening the mouth will reduce this pressure and hence stress on the incisional area.
Advise patient about importance of mouth breathing and possibility of having a soft nasal airway.	Nasal passages may not be patent. Patient likely would be more comfortable breathing through the mouth.
As indicated, obtain prescription for a mild cathartic or stool softener.	This will help prevent straining with bowel movements.
Do not allow patient to brush teeth. Provide mouthwash (e.g., hydrogen peroxide diluted with water to half strength) and sponge-tipped applicator for oral hygiene. Advise that initially diet will be liquid but will progress quickly to soft food.	These actions prevent disturbance in operative site integrity. Front teeth should not be brushed until incision has healed (about 10 days).
Monitor for extreme erythema or swelling at the suture line.	These are signs of infection, which can lead to meningitis and must be reported promptly.
Advise patient that sense of smell usually returns in about 2-3 wk and taste of foods may improve at that time.	Swollen nasal passages alter sense of smell and ability to taste foods. As swelling resolves and healing ensues, senses of smell and taste normalize.
Be alert to and teach the following signs and symptoms of infection, which necessitate medical attention: fever, nuchal rigidity, moderate to severe headache, and photophobia.	These signs of infection also may signal impending meningitis. However, periorbital edema, milder headache, and tenderness over the sinuses for 2-3 days are common and can be relieved by cold compresses.

••• **Related NIC and NOC labels**: *NIC:* Neurologic Monitoring; Postanesthesia Care; Respiratory Monitoring; Vital Signs Monitoring; Airway Management; Positioning *NOC:* Neurological Status: Consciousness

ADDITIONAL NURSING DIAGNOSES/ PROBLEMS:

"Diabetic Ketoacidosis" for **Risk for Injury** related   p. 391
  to altered cerebral function

PATIENT-FAMILY TEACHING AND DISCHARGE PLANNING

When providing patient-family teaching, speak slowly and simply, avoid giving excessive information, and initiate a visiting nurse referral for necessary follow-up teaching. Include verbal and written information about the following:

✓ Importance of fluid restriction for the prescribed period. Assist patient with planning permitted fluid intake (e.g., by saving liquids for social and recreational situations as indicated).

✓ How to safely enrich diet with Na⁺ and K⁺ salts, particularly if ongoing diuretic use is prescribed.

✓ How to use daily weight measurements to assess hydration status.

✓ Signs of water intoxication and hyponatremia: altered LOC, fatigue, headache, nausea, vomiting, and anorexia, any of which should be reported promptly to health care provider.

✓ Medications, including drug name, dosage, route, purpose, precautions, and potential side effects. Also discuss drug-drug, food-drug, and herb-drug interactions. Encourage patient to report to health care provider all alternative and complementary health strategies being used.

✓ Importance of continued medical follow-up; confirm date and time of next medical appointment.

✓ How to obtain a medical alert bracelet and identification card outlining diagnosis and emergency treatment by contacting MedicAlert Foundation at *www.medicalert.org*.

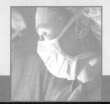

Abdominal Trauma 51

OVERVIEW/PATHOPHYSIOLOGY

Abdominal trauma accounts for nearly 7 million emergency department visits in the United States annually. Abdominal trauma may cause serious injury to major organs. It is essential to understand the mechanism of the injury (blunt, penetrating, or combination) and abdominal organs affected to avoid complications in the recovery period. Astute serial assessments in the posttraumatic period may prevent serious consequences and avoid life-threatening situations. Abdominal injuries often are associated with multisystem trauma. See also discussions under "Pneumothorax/Hemothorax," p. 131; "Spinal Cord Injury," p. 333; and "Traumatic Brain Injury," p. 361.

Common injuries to abdominal organs may be predicted with knowledge of the injury mechanism and location. Thoracic and musculoskeletal trauma, especially below the fourth rib, may be associated with abdominal trauma. Solid organs (liver, kidneys, spleen) tend to fracture and bleed with trauma; hollow organs (stomach, intestines) may collapse or rupture, releasing caustic substances into the peritoneum. Injury also may result from movement of organs within the body, particularly at the transition between rigidly fixed and mobile organs. Injury to the urinary bladder is not common but may be associated with pelvic fractures. Rectal and vaginal examinations are necessary to assess for bleeding.

Blunt trauma may be caused by falls, assaults, motor vehicle collisions, or sports injuries and involve direct transmission of energy to solid or hollow organs, most commonly affecting the spleen and liver. Splenic injury should be suspected in the presence of left lower rib fractures. Rupture may not be immediately obvious, reinforcing the need for ongoing assessments. Pain radiating to the left shoulder (Kehr's sign) may indicate blood beneath the diaphragm from splenic bleeding. Pain radiating to the right shoulder may indicate injury to the liver. Other organs that may be affected by blunt trauma include the kidneys and, occasionally, the pancreas and small and large intestines. Bleeding is the most common complication, resulting in increased morbidity and mortality. Abdominal vessels are injured in about 10% of blunt abdominal trauma patients and can quickly lead to shock and death if not recognized. Signs of blood loss may be nonspecific. Young healthy patients can lose 50% of their blood volume and appear stable.

Penetrating trauma may be caused by gunshot, stabbing, or impalement. If the lower esophagus and stomach are injured by penetration, complications from release of irritating gastric fluids into the peritoneum and free air below the diaphragm may be present. Penetrating injuries may occur to the liver, small intestine, and mesentery. External appearance of the wound may not accurately represent internal damage.

HEALTH CARE SETTING

Emergency care, trauma center, acute care surgical unit, rehabilitation center

ASSESSMENT

As with all trauma patients, immediate life-threatening problems are identified and treatment begun before the more detailed secondary and focused assessments.

Caution: Recently injured patients should be evaluated for peritoneal signs (generalized abdominal pain or tenderness, guarding of abdomen, abdominal wall rigidity, rebound tenderness, abdominal pain with movement or coughing, abdominal distention, and decreased or absent bowel sounds) by the same professional at hourly intervals. Notify health care provider immediately if patient develops peritoneal signs, evidence of shock, gastric or rectal bleeding, or gross hematuria.

Vital signs and hemodynamic measurements: Vital signs (VS) should be assessed frequently to detect changes early. Gradual or sudden changes may be the heralding signs of hemorrhage following trauma, with tachycardia, impaired capillary refill, and hypotension key indicators of bleeding or shock. Ventilatory excursion may be diminished because of pain, thoracic injury, or limited diaphragmatic movement caused by abdominal distention.

Pain: Mild tenderness to severe abdominal pain may be present, with pain either localized to the site of injury or diffuse. Blood or fluid collection within the peritoneum causes irritation and may cause involuntary guarding, distention, rigidity, and rebound tenderness.

Gastrointestinal symptoms: Nausea and vomiting are gastrointestinal (GI) symptoms that may be present following blunt or penetrating trauma secondary to bleeding or obstruction. **Note:** Absence of signs and symptoms, especially in patients who have sustained head or spinal cord injury, does not exclude presence of major abdominal injury.

Inspection: Abrasions and ecchymoses are suggestive of underlying injury. For example, ecchymosis over the left upper quadrant (LUQ) suggests possible splenic injury. Ecchymotic areas around the umbilicus or flanks are suggestive of retroperitoneal bleeding. Erythema and ecchymosis across the lower abdomen suggest intestinal or bladder injury caused by lap belts. Ecchymoses may take hours to days to develop, depending on rate of blood loss. Abdominal distention may signal bleeding, free air, or inflammation.

Auscultation: Auscultate before percussion and palpation to avoid stimulating the bowel and confounding assessment findings. Bowel sounds may be decreased or absent with abdominal organ injury, intraperitoneal bleeding, or recent surgery. However, the presence of bowel sounds does not exclude significant abdominal injury. Bowel sounds in the chest could indicate a ruptured diaphragm with small bowel herniation into the thorax. Bowel sounds should be auscultated frequently, especially in the first 24-48 hr after injury. Absence of bowel sounds is suggestive of ileus or other complications, such as bleeding, peritonitis, or bowel infarction. Presence of an abdominal bruit (turbulent blood flow through vessels) could indicate arterial injury.

Note: Percuss and palpate painful areas last. If patient's pain is severe, do not percuss or palpate, inasmuch as more advanced studies are indicated for evaluation.

Percussion: Tympany suggests the presence of gas. Percussion may reveal unusually large areas of dullness over ruptured blood-filled organs (e.g., a fixed area of dullness in the LUQ suggests a ruptured spleen).

Palpation: Tenderness or pain to palpation suggests abdominal injury. Blood or fluid in the abdomen can result in signs and symptoms of peritoneal irritation.

DIAGNOSTIC TESTS

WBC count: Leukocytosis is expected immediately after injury. Splenic injuries in particular result in rapid development of a moderate to high white blood cell (WBC) count. A later increase in WBCs or a shift to the left reflects an increase in the number of neutrophils, which signals inflammatory response and possible intraabdominal infection. In patients with abdominal trauma, ruptured abdominal viscera must be considered as a potential source of infection.

Platelet count: Mild thrombocytosis is seen immediately after traumatic injury. After massive hemorrhage, thrombocytopenia may be noted. Platelet transfusion usually is not required unless spontaneous bleeding is present.

Glucose: Glucose is initially elevated because of catecholamine release and insulin resistance associated with major trauma. Glucose metabolism is abnormal after major hepatic resection, and patients should be monitored to prevent hypoglycemic episodes.

Amylase: Elevated serum levels are associated with pancreatic or upper small bowel injury, but values may be normal even with severe injury to these organs.

Liver function tests: Elevations reflect hepatic injury.

Arterial blood gases: May reveal respiratory compromise or metabolic acidosis.

Type and cross match: If blood replacement is anticipated.

Note: A flow sheet for serial laboratory values will help pinpoint changes that might otherwise go unnoticed.

X-ray examination: Initially, flat and upright chest x-ray examinations exclude chest injuries (commonly associated with abdominal trauma) and establish a baseline. Subsequent chest x-ray examinations aid in detecting complications, such as atelectasis and pneumonia. In addition, chest and pelvic x-ray examinations may reveal fractures, missiles, foreign bodies, free intraperitoneal air, hematoma, or hemorrhage. Plain abdominal films are not useful in blunt trauma because they cannot define blood in the peritoneum.

Ultrasound: Ultrasound is a rapid, noninvasive assessment tool for detecting intraabdominal hemorrhage. The Focused Assessment Sonogram for Trauma (FAST) has a sensitivity, specificity, and accuracy rate of more than 90% in detecting 100 ml or more of intraabdominal blood or fluid. It can neither image the retroperitoneum nor determine etiology of the bleeding. A single negative FAST cannot absolutely exclude intraabdominal bleeding.

CT scan: Can reveal organ-specific blunt abdominal injury and quantify the amount of blood in the abdomen. Computerized axial tomography (CT) images the ureters and can detect extravasation of urine. Disadvantages are the expense and time required to perform the examination. Patients with positive CT scan require diagnostic laparotomy. **Caution:** A patient in unstable condition should be accompanied by a nurse during the CT scan.

Diagnostic peritoneal lavage: Involves insertion of a peritoneal dialysis catheter into the peritoneum to check for intraabdominal bleeding. This procedure is much less common since FAST and CT scan have become available. It may be indicated for confirmed or suspected blunt abdominal trauma for the following patients: (1) those in whom signs and symptoms of abdominal injury are obscured by intoxication, head or spinal cord trauma, opioids, or unconsciousness; (2) any patient with equivocal assessment findings. Diagnostic peritoneal lavage is unnecessary for patients who have obvious intraabdominal bleeding or other indications for immediate laparotomy.

Laparotomy: The "gold standard" for intraabdominal injuries, it enables complete evaluation of the abdomen and retroperitoneum. It is mandatory in all patients with hypotension, penetration of the abdominal wall, peritonitis, air in the abdomen, and in most cases of organ-specific injury noted on CT scan.

Occult blood: Gastric contents, urine, and stool are tested for occult blood because bleeding can occur as a result of direct injury and later complications.

Angiography: Angiography is performed rarely, but may be needed with blunt trauma to evaluate injury to spleen, liver, pancreas, duodenum, and retroperitoneal vessels when other diagnostic findings are equivocal. **Caution:** Because of the large amount of contrast material used during this procedure, ensure adequate hydration and monitor urine output closely for 24-48 hr, especially in older patients or patients with preexisting cardiovascular or renal disease. Decreased urinary output and increased BUN and creatinine may indicate contrast-associated acute tubal necrosis.

Nursing Diagnosis:

Ineffective Breathing Pattern

related to pain from injury or surgical incision, chemical irritation of blood or bile on pleural tissue, and diaphragmatic elevation caused by abdominal distention

Desired Outcome: Within 24 hr of admission or surgery, patient is eupneic with RR 12-20 breaths/min and clear breath sounds.

INTERVENTIONS	RATIONALES
Note quality of breath sounds, RR, presence/absence of cough, and sputum characteristics.	Individuals sustaining abdominal trauma are likely to be tachypneic, with the potential for poor ventilatory effort. If not reversed, this could result in atelectasis and pneumonia.
Monitor oximetry readings q2-4h; report significant findings.	O$_2$ saturation less than 92% usually signals need for supplemental oxygen.
Administer supplemental oxygen as prescribed. Monitor and document effectiveness.	Supplemental O$_2$ is delivered until patient's arterial blood gas or oximetry values while breathing room air are acceptable.
Encourage and assist patient with coughing, deep breathing, incentive spirometry, and turning q2-4h.	These measures help prevent pneumonia and atelectasis.
Administer analgesics at dose and frequency that relieves pain and associated impaired chest excursion.	Reducing pain will enable full chest excursion for better oxygenation.
Instruct patient in methods to splint abdomen.	This information will help the patient reduce pain on movement, coughing, and deep breathing, which in turn will aid the respiratory effort.
For additional interventions, see "Perioperative Care" **Ineffective Breathing Pattern,** p. 50.	

••• **Related NIC and NOC labels:** *NIC:* Respiratory Monitoring; Oxygen Therapy; Cough Enhancement; Pain Management; Teaching: Procedure/Treatment *NOC:* Respiratory Status: Ventilation; Vital Signs Status

Nursing Diagnosis:

Deficient Fluid Volume

related to active loss secondary to bleeding/hemorrhage

Desired Outcomes: Within 4 hr of admission or on definitive repair (e.g., surgery), patient is normovolemic as evidenced by SBP 90 mm Hg or higher (or within patient's baseline range), HR 60-100 bpm, CVP 2-6 mm Hg (5-12 cm H$_2$O), urinary output at least 30 ml/hr, warm extremities, brisk capillary refill (2 sec or less), distal pulses at least 2+ on a 0-4+ scale, and absence of orthostasis.

INTERVENTIONS	RATIONALES
In *recently injured* patients, monitor blood pressure (BP) hourly or more frequently in the presence of obvious bleeding or unstable VS. Be alert to increasing diastolic blood pressure (DBP) and decreasing systolic blood pressure (SBP). In *stable postoperative* patients, perform routine VS assessment.	Even a small but sudden decrease in SBP signals need to notify health care provider, especially with a trauma patient in whom extent of injury is unknown. Most trauma patients are young, and excellent neurovascular compensation results in a near normal BP until there is large intravascular volume depletion.
Monitor for cool and pale extremities, delayed capillary refill (2 sec or more), and absent or decreased strength of distal pulses.	These are physical indicators of fluid volume deficit.
Be alert to decreasing BP; tachycardia (heart rate [HR] more than 100 bpm); tachypnea (respiratory rate [RR] more than 20 breaths/min); anxiety (early); and confusion, lethargy, and coma (later).	These are clinical indicators of fluid volume deficit. If signs are present, they need to be reported immediately for prompt intervention.

Continued

INTERVENTIONS	RATIONALES
Monitor HR and cardiovascular status hourly until patient's condition is stable. Note and report sudden increases or decreases in HR or BP, especially if associated with indicators of fluid volume deficit, as noted previously.	Tachycardia and hypotension occur with fluid volume deficit/bleeding. VS should be assessed frequently to detect changes early.
In patient with evidence of volume depletion or active blood loss, administer prescribed fluids rapidly through large-caliber (18-gauge or larger) IV catheters.	Massive blood loss is frequently associated with abdominal injuries. Restoration and maintenance of adequate volume are essential. Initially, Ringer's lactate or similar balanced salt solution is given. Packed red blood cells are given to replace blood loss, especially with hemoglobin less than 9.0. Patients with abdominal trauma must have two large-bore IV lines inserted peripherally or centrally. Anticipate aggressive fluid replacement.
Evaluate IV flow rate frequently during rapid volume resuscitation, and monitor patient closely.	These assessments will help prevent fluid volume overload and complications such as heart failure (see p. 181).
Caution: Large volumes of fluid require warming.	Warming is necessary to prevent hypothermia.
Measure central venous pressure (CVP) q1-4h if indicated.	Low or decreasing values are likely. Sudden decreases in CVP, especially if associated with other indicators of fluid volume deficit, as just noted, are signs of significant volume depletion and should be reported promptly.
Measure urinary output hourly (or when patient voids). Be alert to decreasing urinary output and to infrequent voidings. Before administering diuretics, evaluate patient for evidence of fluid volume deficit, as just noted.	Low urine output usually reflects inadequate intravascular volume in the patient with abdominal trauma.
Measure all bloody drainage from drainage tubes or catheters, noting drainage color (e.g., coffee ground, burgundy, bright red). Monitor for, and measure when possible, bloody stools.	These measurements provide an estimate of ongoing blood loss.
Note frequency of dressing changes because of saturation with blood.	This assessment enables an estimate of the amount of blood lost via wound site.
Note and report significant increases in amount of drainage, especially if it is bloody.	An increase in bloody drainage signifies bleeding, and immediate intervention may be required to maintain hemodynamic stability.

••• **Related NIC and NOC labels:** *NIC:* Fluid Management; Fluid Monitoring; Hypovolemia Management; Fluid Resuscitation; Intravenous Insertion; Intravenous Therapy; Vital Signs Management; Blood Products Administration; Invasive Hemodynamic Monitoring; Shock Prevention *NOC:* Fluid Balance

Nursing Diagnosis:

Acute Pain

related to irritation caused by intraperitoneal blood or secretions, actual trauma or surgical incision, and manipulation of organs during surgery

Desired Outcomes: Within 4 hr of admission, patient's subjective perception of pain decreases, as documented by pain scale. Nonverbal indicators, such as grimacing, are absent or diminished. Patient's pain is controlled without sedation.

INTERVENTIONS	RATIONALES
Evaluate for presence of preoperative and postoperative pain. Devise a pain scale with patient, rating discomfort from 0 (no pain) to 10 (worst pain).	Preoperative pain is anticipated and is a vital diagnostic aid. Location and character of postoperative pain also can be important. For example, incisional and some visceral pain can be anticipated, but intense or prolonged pain, especially when accompanied by other peritoneal signs, can signal bleeding, bowel infarction, infection, or other complications. Autonomic nervous system response to pain can complicate assessment of abdominal injury and hypovolemia. A pain scale helps quantify pain and determine subsequent relief obtained.

Continued

INTERVENTIONS	RATIONALES
Administer analgesics as prescribed and indicated.	An alert patient should not suffer severe pain while awaiting surgical evaluation. Administer postoperatively prescribed analgesics on a continual or regular schedule promptly with additional analgesia as needed, or provide patient-controlled analgesia (PCA). Analgesics are helpful in relieving pain and in aiding the recovery process by promoting greater ventilatory excursion. As the severity of pain lessens, alternative analgesics such as nonsteroidal antiinflammatory drugs (e.g., ketorolac, ibuprofen) may be prescribed if not contraindicated by patient history or gastric bleeding.
Encourage patient to request analgesic before pain becomes severe.	Prolonged stimulation of pain receptors results in increased sensitivity to painful stimuli and will increase amount of drug required to relieve pain.
Be aware that intoxication often is involved in traumatic events.	Patients may be drug or alcohol users, with a higher-than-average tolerance for opioids, requiring adjusted dosage for adequate pain relief. These individuals may suffer symptoms of alcohol withdrawal (tremors, weakness, tachycardia, elevated BP, delusions, agitation, hallucinations) or narcotic withdrawal (lacrimation, rhinorrhea, anxiety, tremors, muscle twitching, mydriasis, nausea, abdominal cramps, vomiting), and this will necessitate prompt recognition and treatment.
	In addition, opioids can decrease GI motility and may delay return to normal bowel function.
Monitor PCA, if prescribed, and document effectiveness, using pain scale.	For this and other interventions/rationales, see discussions in "Pain," p. 39.
Incorporate such measures as positioning, back rubs, and distraction to aid in pain reduction. Provide these instructions to patient and family members.	Nonpharmacologic maneuvers support analgesia therapy in reducing pain.

••• **Related NIC and NOC labels:** *NIC:* Pain Management; Medication Management: Patient-Controlled Analgesia (PCA) Assistance; Teaching: Procedure/Treatment; Distraction; Simple Massage; Positioning *NOC:* Comfort Level; Pain Control; Pain: Disruptive Effects; Pain Level

Nursing Diagnosis:

Risk for Infection

related to inadequate primary defenses secondary to disruption of the GI tract (particularly of the terminal ileum and colon) and traumatically inflicted open wound; multiple indwelling catheters and drainage tubes; and compromised immune state caused by blood loss and metabolic response to trauma

Desired Outcome: Patient is free of infection as evidenced by temperature less than 37.7° C (100° F); HR 100 bpm or less; no significant changes in mental status; orientation to person, place, and time; and absence of unusual erythema, edema, tenderness, warmth, or drainage at surgical incisions or wound sites.

INTERVENTIONS	RATIONALES
Monitor VS for temperature increases and associated increases in heart and respiratory rates. Notify health care provider of sudden temperature elevations.	These signs are indicators of infection.
Evaluate mental status, orientation, and level of consciousness (LOC) q8h.	Mental status changes, confusion, or deterioration from baseline LOC can signal infection.
Ensure patency of all surgically placed tubes or drains. Irrigate or attach to low-pressure suction as prescribed. Maintain continuity of closed drainage systems; use sterile technique when emptying drainage and recharging suction containers. Promptly report loss of tube patency.	Blocked drainage systems may promote infection and abscess formation. Maintaining a closed drainage system and using sterile technique decrease risk of infection.

Continued

INTERVENTIONS	RATIONALES
Evaluate incisions and wound sites for unusual erythema, warmth, tenderness, edema, delayed healing, and purulent or unusual drainage.	These signs are evidence of localized infection.
Note amount, color, character, and odor of all drainage.	Foul-smelling or abnormal drainage can occur with infection and should be reported for prompt intervention.
Administer antibiotics in a timely fashion. Reschedule parenteral antibiotics if a dose is delayed more than 1 hr. Check blood levels as indicated (e.g., with vancomycin and gentamicin).	Failure to administer antibiotics on schedule may result in inadequate blood levels and treatment failure.
As prescribed, administer pneumococcal vaccine to patients with total splenectomy.	This measure minimizes risk of postsplenectomy sepsis.
Administer tetanus immune globulin and tetanus toxoid as prescribed.	Risk for tetanus following trauma increases if patient has not been immunized within the past 10 years.
Change dressings as prescribed, using sterile technique; change one dressing at a time.	These interventions prevent infection and cross-contamination from various wounds.
Use drains, closed drainage systems, or drainage bags to remove and collect GI secretions.	These measures prevent contamination of surgical incision site.
If patient has or develops evisceration, do not reinsert tissue or organs. Place a sterile, saline-soaked gauze over evisceration, and cover with a sterile towel until the evisceration can be evaluated by the surgeon.	Evisceration is an emergent, life-threatening situation. Preventing infection and maintaining homeostasis is essential until surgical intervention can be made.
Keep patient on bedrest in semi-Fowler's position with knees bent.	Semi-Fowler's position with knees bent reduces strain on eviscerated organs. Bedrest will minimize disruption to the abdominal organs, preventing further tissue damage and risk of infection.
Maintain NPO (nothing by mouth) status for patient.	Patient may need emergency surgery.

••• **Related NIC and NOC labels:** *NIC:* Environmental Management; Incision Site Care; Infection Control: Intraoperative; Vital Signs Monitoring; Wound Care; Tube Care: Gastrointestinal; Immunization/Vaccination Management; Infection Protection; Laboratory Data Interpretation; Medication Administration *NOC:* Infection Status; Immune Status

Nursing Diagnosis:

Ineffective Tissue Perfusion: Gastrointestinal (or risk for same)

related to interrupted blood flow to abdominal viscera secondary to vascular disruption or occlusion or related to moderate to severe hypovolemia caused by hemorrhage

Desired Outcomes: Patient has adequate GI tissue perfusion as evidenced by normoactive bowel sounds; soft, nondistended abdomen; and return of bowel elimination. Gastric secretions, drainage, and excretions are negative for occult blood.

INTERVENTIONS	RATIONALES
Auscultate for bowel sounds hourly in recently injured patients and q8h during recovery phase.	Absent or diminished bowel sounds may be anticipated for up to 72 hr after trauma or surgery. Prolonged or sudden absence of bowel sounds may signal bowel ischemia or infarction and must be reported promptly for intervention.
Evaluate patient for peritoneal signs.	Signs of peritoneal irritation (generalized abdominal pain or tenderness, guarding of abdomen, abdominal wall rigidity, rebound tenderness, abdominal pain with movement or coughing, abdominal distention, and decreased or absent bowel sounds) may occur acutely secondary to injury or may not develop until days or weeks later if complications caused by slow bleeding or other mechanisms occur.
Ensure adequate intravascular volume (see discussion in **Deficient Fluid Volume,** earlier).	Adequate intravascular volume optimizes organ perfusion.

Continued

INTERVENTIONS	RATIONALES
Evaluate laboratory data for evidence of bleeding (e.g., serial hematocrit [Hct]) or organ ischemia (e.g., elevated liver function tests).	Optimal values are Hct more than 30%; aspartate aminotransferase (AST) 5-40 IU/L; alanine aminotransferase (ALT) 5-35 IU/L. Decreases in Hct occur with bleeding. Increases in AST or ALT are especially reflective of hepatic injury.
Document amount and character of GI secretions, drainage, and excretions.	Changes suggestive of bleeding (presence of frank or occult blood), infection (e.g., increased or purulent drainage), or obstruction (e.g., failure to eliminate flatus or stool within 72 hr after surgery) may signal presence of a complication that necessitates timely intervention.

••• **Related NIC and NOC labels:** *NIC:* Hypovolemia Management; Intravenous Therapy; Laboratory Data Interpretation; Vital Signs Monitoring; Bleeding Reduction: Gastrointestinal; Bowel Management *NOC:* Tissue Perfusion: Abdominal Organs

Nursing Diagnoses:

Risk for Impaired Skin Integrity

related to risk of exposure to irritating GI drainage

Impaired Tissue Integrity (or risk for same)

related to direct trauma and surgery, catabolic posttraumatic state, and altered circulation

Desired Outcome: Patient exhibits wound healing, and skin remains nonerythremic and intact.

INTERVENTIONS	RATIONALES
Promptly change all dressings that become soiled with drainage or blood. Protect skin surrounding tubes, drains, or fistulas, keeping the areas clean and free from drainage.	Gastric and intestinal secretions and drainage are irritating and can lead to skin excoriation.
If necessary, apply ointments, skin barriers, or drainage bags. Apply reusable dressing supports such as Montgomery straps or tubular mesh gauze. Consult wound, ostomy, continence (WOC) enterostomal therapy (ET) nurse for complex or involved cases.	These measures prevent excessive injury to surrounding skin.
Inspect wounds, fistulas, and drain sites at routine intervals.	These measures identify signs of irritation, infection, and ischemia (i.e., erythema, edema, purulent drainage) for prompt intervention.
Identify infected and devitalized tissue. Aid in their removal by irrigation, wound packing, or preparing patient for surgical débridement.	Removal of devitalized tissue is essential for wound healing to progress.
Ensure adequate protein and calorie intake (see **Imbalanced Nutrition,** following).	Adequate nutrition is necessary in order for tissue healing to occur.
For more information, see "Managing Wound Care," p. 559.	

••• **Related NIC and NOC labels:** *NIC:* Skin Surveillance; Infection Protection; Skin Care: Topical Treatments; Wound Care; Nutrition Management; Incision Site Care; Wound Irrigation *NOC:* Tissue Integrity: Skin and Mucous Membranes

Nursing Diagnosis:

Imbalanced Nutrition: Less Than Body Requirements

related to decreased intake secondary to disruption of GI tract integrity (traumatic or surgical) and increased need secondary to hypermetabolic posttrauma state

Desired Outcome: By at least 24 hr before hospital discharge, patient has adequate nutrition as evidenced by maintenance of baseline body weight and positive or balanced nitrogen (N) state.

INTERVENTIONS	RATIONALES
Collaborate with health care provider, dietitian, and pharmacist to estimate patient's metabolic needs based on type of injury, activity level, and nutritional status before injury.	For example, patients with hepatic or pancreatic injury may have difficulty with blood sugar regulation; patients with trauma to upper GI tract may be fed enterally, but feeding tube must be placed distal to the injury; patients with disruption of GI tract may require feeding gastrostomy or jejunostomy tube; patients with major hepatic trauma may have difficulty with protein tolerance.
	In addition, patients with abdominal trauma have complex nutritional needs because of the hypermetabolic state associated with major trauma and traumatic or surgical disruption of normal GI function. Often, infection and sepsis contribute to negative nitrogen (N) state and increased metabolic needs. Prompt initiation of enteric feedings and administration of supplemental calories, proteins, vitamins, and minerals is essential for healing. Parenteral feedings are given if oral feedings cannot be used.
Ensure patency of gastric or intestinal tubes.	Gastric decompression prevents accumulation of gas or fluid in the stomach and reduces the chance of aspiration while promoting healing and return of bowel function. The tube usually remains in place until bowel function returns, as detected by positive bowel sounds, passage of flatus, and decreased gastric output via the tube.
Use caution and consult surgeon before irrigating nasogastric (NG) or other tubes that have been placed in or near recently sutured organs.	Some NG tubes are sutured in place; irrigation or movement of the tube could disrupt sutures and cause bleeding.
Confirm placement of feeding tube before each tube feeding. After initial insertion, check x-ray film for position of feeding tube. Mark to determine tube migration, secure tubing in place, and reassess q4h and before each feeding.	Insufflation with air and aspiration of stomach contents do not always confirm placement of small-bore feeding tubes.
Assess pH of gastric aspirate.	A pH less than 5 signals gastric placement. However, acid blockade drugs may alter pH.
Do not start enteral feeding until bowel function returns (i.e., bowel sounds are present, patient experiences hunger).	Peristalsis is often decreased following trauma/surgery.
Avoid opioid analgesics; administer prescribed nonnarcotic analgesics (e.g., ketorolac) instead.	Opioid analgesics decrease GI motility and may contribute to nausea, vomiting, abdominal distention, and ileus.
For more information, see "Providing Nutritional Support," p. 565.	

••• **Related NIC and NOC labels:** *NIC:* Enteral Tube Feeding; Gastrointestinal Intubation *NOC:* Nutritional Status

Nursing Diagnosis:

Post-trauma Syndrome

related to life-threatening accident or event resulting in trauma

Desired Outcomes: By at least 24 hr before hospital discharge, patient verbalizes aspects of the psychosocial impact of the event and does not exhibit signs of severe stress reaction, such as display of inconsistent affect, suicidal or homicidal behavior, or extreme agitation or depression. Patient cooperates with the treatment plan.

INTERVENTIONS	RATIONALES
Evaluate mental status at regular intervals. Be alert to indicators of severe stress reaction, such as display of affect inconsistent with statements or behavior, suicidal or homicidal statements or actions, extreme agitation or depression, and failure to cooperate with instructions related to care.	Many victims of major abdominal trauma sustain life-threatening injury. The patient is often aware of the situation and fears death. Even after the physical condition stabilizes, the patient may have a prolonged or severe reaction triggered by recollection of the trauma.
Consult specialists such as psychiatrist, psychologist, psychiatric nurse practitioner, or pastoral counselor if patient displays signs of severe stress reaction described previously.	The patient likely needs specialized intervention.
Consider organic causes that may contribute to posttraumatic response.	Severe pain, alcohol intoxication or withdrawal, electrolyte imbalance, metabolic encephalopathy, and impaired cerebral perfusion are potential contributors to the posttraumatic response and should be treated accordingly.

For other interventions, see "Psychosocial Support," p. 73.

••• **Related NIC and NOC labels:** *NIC:* Coping Enhancement; Spiritual Support; Counseling *NOC:* Coping

ADDITIONAL NURSING DIAGNOSES/ PROBLEMS:

"Perioperative Care"	p. 45
"Prolonged Bedrest"	p. 61
"Psychosocial Support" (particularly **Disturbed Body Image**)	p. 80
"Fecal Diversions"	p. 455

PATIENT-FAMILY TEACHING AND DISCHARGE PLANNING

Anticipate extended physical and emotional rehabilitation for patient and significant other. When providing patient-family teaching, focus on sensory information, avoid giving excessive information, and initiate a visiting nurse referral for necessary follow-up teaching. Include verbal and written information about the following:

✓ Self-management: Assessment of patient's ability to manage own care should be completed before hospital discharge. Identification of support persons to assist with care should be initiated early.

✓ Probable need for emotional care, even for patients who have not required extensive physical rehabilitation. Provide referrals to support groups for trauma patients and family members.

✓ Availability of rehabilitation programs, extended care facilities, and home health agencies for patients unable to accomplish self-care on hospital discharge.

✓ Availability of rehabilitation programs for substance abuse, as indicated. Immediately after the traumatic event,

patient and family members are very impressionable, making this period an ideal time for the substance abuser to begin to resolve the problem.

✓ Medications, including drug name, purpose, dosage, schedule, precautions, and potential side effects. Also discuss drug-drug, herb-drug, and food-drug interactions. Encourage patients taking antibiotics to take medications for prescribed length of time, even though they may be asymptomatic. If patient received tetanus immunization, ensure that he or she receives a wallet-size card documenting the immunization.

✓ Wound and catheter care. Have patient or caregiver describe and demonstrate proper technique before hospital discharge.

✓ Activity: Restrictions and recommendations should be reviewed thoroughly with patient and caregivers. An at-home assessment may be necessary if activity is severely limited or adaptations are necessary. Consider referral to occupational therapist (OT) or physical therapist (PT).

✓ Diet/nutrition: Review diet recommendations with patient/family. If enteral or parenteral feeding is necessary, have patient or caregiver describe and demonstrate correct technique before hospital discharge. Home health care services may be warranted for support and evaluation.

✓ Importance of seeking medical attention if indicators of infection or bowel obstruction occur (e.g., fever, severe or unusual abdominal pain, nausea and vomiting, unusual drainage from wounds or incisions, a change in bowel habits).

✓ Injury prevention: Following traumatic injury, patient and family members are especially likely to respond to injury prevention education. Provide instructions on proper seatbelt applications (across pelvic girdle rather than across soft tissue of lower abdomen), safety for infants and children, and other factors suitable for individuals involved.

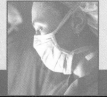

Appendicitis 52

OVERVIEW/PATHOPHYSIOLOGY

Appendicitis is the most commonly occurring inflammatory lesion of the bowel and one of the most common reasons for abdominal surgery. Appendicitis occurs most often in adolescents and young adults, especially males. The appendix is a blind, narrow tube that extends from the inferior portion of the cecum and does not serve any known useful function. Appendicitis is usually caused by obstruction of the appendiceal lumen by a fecalith (hardened bit of fecal material), inflammation, a foreign body, or a neoplasm. Obstruction prevents drainage of secretions that are produced by epithelial cells in the lumen, thereby increasing intraluminal pressure and compressing mucosal blood vessels. This tension eventually impairs local blood flow, which can lead to necrosis and perforation. Inflammation and infection result from normal bacteria invading the devitalized wall. Mild cases of appendicitis can heal spontaneously, but severe inflammation can lead to a ruptured appendix, which can cause local or generalized peritonitis.

HEALTH CARE SETTING

Acute care surgical unit. Inpatient status for ruptured appendix with peritonitis; 1-day length of stay for suspected acute appendicitis without complications.

ASSESSMENT

Signs and symptoms vary because of differences in anatomy, size, and age. The sequence of symptoms can be significant in the differential diagnosis. Abdominal discomfort, indigestion, and bowel irregularity occur first.

Early stage: Pain usually occurs in either the epigastric or umbilical area and may be vague and diffuse or associated with mild cramping. Nausea and vomiting are not always present, but if they occur, they follow the onset of pain. Fever and leukocytosis occur later.

Intermediate (acute) stage: Over a period of a few hours, pain shifts from the midabdomen or epigastrium to the right lower quadrant (RLQ) at McBurney's point (approximately 2 inches from the anterior superior iliac spine on a line drawn from the umbilicus) and is aggravated by walking, coughing, and movement. Pain may be accompanied by a sensation of constipation (gas-stoppage sensation). Anorexia, malaise, occasionally diarrhea, and diminished peristalsis also can occur.

On physical assessment, patient experiences pain in the RLQ elicited by light palpation of the abdomen; presence of rebound tenderness; RLQ guarding, rigidity, and muscle spasms; tachycardia; low-grade fever; absent or diminished bowel sounds; and pain elicited with rectal examination. A palpable, tender mass may be felt in the peritoneal pouch if the appendix lies within the pelvis. **Note:** Physical assessment is performed in four steps—inspection, auscultation, percussion, and palpation—in that order, to avoid stimulating the abdomen by palpation and percussion, which can affect bowel sounds.

Acute appendicitis with perforation: Increasing, generalized pain; recurrence of vomiting. On physical assessment patient usually exhibits temperature increases to more than 38.5° C (101.4° F) and generalized abdominal rigidity. Typically, patient remains rigid with flexed knees. Presence of abscess can result in a tender, palpable mass. The abdomen may be distended.

DIAGNOSTIC TESTS

Abdominal CT scan: Has accuracy rate of 95% overall and should be performed before a laparotomy.

White blood cell count with differential: Reveals presence of leukocytosis and an increase in neutrophils. A shift to the left with more than 75% neutrophils is a consistent finding in later stages of appendicitis.

Abdominal ultrasound: May be done to rule out appendicitis or conditions that mimic it, such as Crohn's disease, diverticulitis, or gastroenteritis. Higher success rate for diagnosis is found in children.

Abdominal x-ray examination: May reveal presence of a fecalith. About half of these patients may have x-ray findings of localized air-fluid levels, increased soft tissue density in the RLQ, and indications of localized ileus. If perforation has occurred, the presence of free air is noted.

Urinalysis: To rule out genitourinary conditions mimicking appendicitis; may reveal microscopic hematuria and pyuria. This test result usually is normal.

IV pyelogram: May be performed to rule out ureteral stone or pyelitis.

Nursing Diagnosis:

Risk for Infection

related to inadequate primary defenses (danger of rupture, peritonitis, abscess formation) secondary to inflammatory process

Desired Outcomes: Patient is free of infection as evidenced by normothermia, HR 100 bpm or less, BP at least 90/60 mm Hg, RR 12-20 breaths/min with normal depth and pattern (eupnea), absence of chills, soft and nondistended abdomen, and bowel sounds 5-34/min in each abdominal quadrant. Following instruction, patient verbalizes rationale for not administering enemas or laxatives preoperatively and enemas postoperatively, and demonstrates compliance with the therapeutic regimen.

INTERVENTIONS	RATIONALES
Assess and document quality, location, and duration of pain, presence of nausea, and patient's positioning.	Signs of worsening appendicitis that can lead to rupture include pain that becomes accentuated; generalized, recurrent vomiting; and patient assuming a side-lying or supine position with flexed knees. Pain that worsens and then disappears is a signal that rupture may have occurred.
Monitor vital signs for elevated temperature, increased pulse rate, hypotension, and shallow/rapid respirations; assess abdomen for presence of rigidity, distention, and decreased or absent bowel sounds. Report significant findings to health care provider.	Any of these indicators can occur with rupture.
Monitor for ambulation with a limp or pain with hip extension.	Retrocecal abscess may irritate the psoas muscle as it traverses the area of posterior RLQ of the abdomen and results in pain with hip extension.
Caution patient about the danger of preoperative self-treatment with enemas and laxatives.	Enemas and laxatives increase peristalsis, which increases risk of perforation and hence peritonitis and sepsis. Enemas should be avoided until approved by health care provider (usually several weeks after surgery). If constipation occurs postoperatively, health care provider may prescribe laxatives/stool softeners at bedtime after the third day.
Teach postoperative incisional care, as well as care of drains if patient is to be discharged with them.	Maintaining a clean incision and avoiding contamination of drains help prevent infection in areas in which the skin is no longer intact.
	An incisional drain may be inserted in the presence of abscess, rupture, or peritonitis to facilitate drainage of exudate and peritoneal fluid and avoid complications of infection.
Provide instructions for prescribed antibiotics if patient is to be discharged with them. See "Peritonitis," p. 474, for more information.	Antibiotics prevent or treat systemic infection from a ruptured appendix.

●●● **Related NIC and NOC labels:** *NIC:* Infection Protection; Incision Site Care; Vital Signs Monitoring; Health Education; Teaching: Procedure/Treatment *NOC:* Infection Status; Wound Healing: Primary Intention

Nursing Diagnoses:

Acute Pain/Nausea

related to inflammatory process

Desired Outcomes: Within 1-2 hr of pain-relieving interventions, patient's subjective perception of pain and nausea decreases, as documented by pain scale. Objective indicators, such as grimacing, are absent or diminished.

INTERVENTIONS	RATIONALES
Assess and document quality, location, and duration of pain. Devise a pain scale with patient, rating discomfort from 0 (no pain) to 10 (worst pain). Assess and document nausea in the same way.	These characteristics of discomfort may be seen during the following stages of appendicitis: *Early stage:* Abdominal pain (either epigastric or umbilical) that may be vague and diffuse, nausea and vomiting, fever, and sensitivity over appendix area. *Intermediate (acute) stage:* Pain that shifts from epigastrium to RLQ at McBurney's point (approximately 2 inches from anterior superior iliac spine on a line drawn from umbilicus) and is aggravated by walking or coughing. The pain may be accompanied by a sensation of constipation (gas-stoppage sensation). Anorexia, malaise, occasional diarrhea, and diminished peristalsis also can occur. *Acute appendicitis with perforation:* Increasing, generalized pain; recurrence of vomiting; increasing abdominal rigidity.
Medicate with antiemetics, sedatives, and analgesics as prescribed; evaluate and document patient's response, using the pain scale.	These agents reduce nausea and pain. Opioids are avoided until diagnosis is certain because they mask clinical signs and symptoms.
Encourage patient to request medication *before* symptoms become severe.	Prolonged stimulation of pain receptors results in increased sensitivity to painful stimuli and will increase the amount of drug required to relieve the discomfort.
Keep patient NPO (given nothing by mouth) before surgery.	Being NPO helps prevent aspiration during anesthesia when gag reflex is compromised. After surgery, nausea and vomiting usually disappear.
If prescribed, insert gastric tube.	A gastric tube enables decompression in preoperative patients with severe nausea and vomiting.
Teach technique for slow, diaphragmatic breathing.	This technique reduces stress and helps promote comfort by relaxing tense muscles.
Help position patient for optimal comfort.	Many patients find comfort from a side-lying position with knees bent, whereas others find relief when supine with pillows under knees (avoiding pressure on popliteal area).

••• **Related NIC and NOC labels:** *NIC:* Medication Management; Pain Management; Nausea Management; Positioning; Progressive Muscle Relaxation *NOC:* Comfort Level; Pain Control; Pain Level

ADDITIONAL NURSING DIAGNOSES/ PROBLEMS:

"Perioperative Care"	p. 45

 PATIENT-FAMILY TEACHING AND DISCHARGE PLANNING

When providing patient-family teaching, focus on sensory and avoid giving excessive information. Include verbal and written information about the following:

✓ Medications, including drug name, dosage, purpose, schedule, precautions, and potential side effects. Also discuss drug-drug, food-drug, and herb-drug interactions.

✓ Care of incision, including dressing changes and bathing restrictions if appropriate.

✓ Indicators of infection: fever, chills, incisional pain, redness, swelling, and purulent drainage.

✓ Postsurgical activity precautions: avoid lifting heavy objects (more than 10 lb) for the first 6 wk or as directed, be alert to and rest after symptoms of fatigue, get maximum rest, gradually increase activities to tolerance.

✓ Importance of avoiding enemas for the first few postoperative weeks. Caution patient about need to check with health care provider before having an enema.

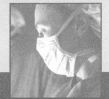

Cholelithiasis, Cholecystitis, and Cholangitis   53

OVERVIEW/PATHOPHYSIOLOGY

Gallstones may be found anywhere in the biliary system. They may cause pain and other symptoms or remain asymptomatic for years. *Cholelithiasis* is characterized by the presence of stones in the gallbladder. *Choledocholithiasis* is the term used to describe gallstones that have migrated to the common bile duct. Gallstones are classified as cholesterol or pigment stones. Cholesterol stones are more common in the United States and represent approximately 80% of cases. Black-pigment stones result from an increase of calcium and unconjugated bilirubin and are associated with cirrhosis and chronic hemolysis. Brown-pigment stones are the predominant type found in native Asians and may be associated with bacterial infection of the bile. Precipitating factors for stone formation include disturbances in metabolism, biliary stasis, obstruction, hypertriglyceridemia, and infection. Gallstones are especially prevalent in women who are multiparous, are taking estrogen therapy, or use oral contraceptives. Other risk factors include obesity, dietary intake of fats, sedentary lifestyle, and familial tendencies. The incidence increases with age, and it is estimated that one of every three persons who reach 75 years of age has gallstones. Cholelithiasis is commonly seen in disease states such as diabetes mellitus, regional enteritis, and certain blood dyscrasias. Usually cholelithiasis is asymptomatic until a stone becomes lodged in the cystic tract. If the obstruction is unrelieved, biliary colic (intermittent painful episodes) and cholecystitis can ensue.

Cholecystitis is most commonly associated with cystic duct obstructions caused by impacted gallstones; however, it may also result from stasis, bacterial infection, or ischemia of the gallbladder. Cholecystitis involves acute inflammation of the gallbladder and is associated with pain, tenderness, and fever. With obstruction, structural changes such as swelling and thickening of the gallbladder walls can occur. If the edema is prolonged, the walls become scarred and fibrosed and the constant pressure of bile can lead to mucosal irritation. As a complication of the impaired circulation and edema, pressure ischemia and necrosis can develop, resulting in gangrene or perforation. With chronic cholecystitis, stones almost always are present and the gallbladder walls are thickened and fibrosed.

Cholangitis is the most serious complication of gallstones and is more difficult to diagnose than either cholelithiasis or cholecystitis. It is caused by an impacted stone in the common bile duct, resulting in bile stasis, bacteremia, and septicemia if left untreated. Cholangitis is most likely to occur when an already infected bile duct becomes obstructed. Mortality rate is high if not recognized and treated early.

HEALTH CARE SETTING

Primary care; acute care

ASSESSMENT

Cholelithiasis: History of intolerance to fats and occasional discomfort after eating. As the stone moves through the duct or becomes lodged, a sudden onset of mild, aching pain occurs in the mid-epigastrium after eating (especially after a high-fat meal) and increases in intensity during a colic attack, potentially radiating to the right upper quadrant (RUQ) and right subscapular region. Nausea, vomiting, tachycardia, mild fever, and diaphoresis also can occur. Many individuals with gallstones are entirely asymptomatic.

Cholecystitis: History of intolerance to fats and discomfort after eating, including regurgitation, flatulence, belching, epigastric heaviness, indigestion, heartburn, chronic upper abdominal pain, and nausea. Amber-colored urine, clay-colored stools, pruritus, jaundice, steatorrhea, fever, and bleeding tendencies can be present if there is bile obstruction. Symptoms may be vague. An acute attack may last 7-10 days, but it usually resolves in several hours.

Cholangitis: Fever is present in nearly all patients with bacterial cholangitis. Jaundice, chills, mild and transient pain, mental confusion, and lethargy are part of the presenting symptoms. Leukocytosis and elevated bilirubin are present in 80% of cases.

PHYSICAL ASSESSMENT

Cholelithiasis: Palpation of the RUQ reveals a tender abdomen during colic attack. Otherwise, between attacks, the examination is usually normal.

Cholecystitis: Palpation elicits tenderness localized behind the inferior margin of the liver. With progressive symptoms, a tender, globular mass may be palpated behind the lower border of the liver. Rebound tenderness and guarding also may be present. With the patient taking a deep breath, palpation over the RUQ elicits Murphy's sign (pain and inability to inspire when the examiner's hand comes in contact with the gallbladder).

Cholangitis: RUQ tenderness is present in 90% of cases. Peritoneal signs (abdominal pain, tenderness, guarding, decreased or absent bowel sounds, nausea) are not common and only occur in 15% of patients. Hypotension and mental confusion are present in severe cases.

DIAGNOSTIC TEST

Ultrasonography: With its 95% accuracy, ultrasonography is the preferred test for confirming the presence of gallstones, as well as their number, color, and size. Ultrasonography of the gallbladder and biliary tract may be used to determine gallstone location and detect tumors.

Hydroxyliminodiacetic acid scan: Radioisotopic scan that is highly sensitive for diagnosis of acute cholecystitis. Hydroxyliminodiacetic acid (HIDA) is injected IV, absorbed in the liver, and then excreted in the biliary system. An obstructing stone in the cystic duct prevents HIDA from filling the gallbladder.

Endoscopic retrograde cholangiopancreatography: Visualization and evaluation of the biliary tree or pancreatic duct. Endoscopic retrograde cholangiopancreatography (ERCP) is the gold standard for diagnosing choledocholithiasis.

Radiologic studies: For example, oral cholangiogram, IV cholangiogram, nuclear scans, and percutaneous transhepatic cholangiogram may be performed to determine patency of biliary or cystic ducts and help rule out other conditions that mimic gallstone disease. Chest, abdominal, upper gastrointestinal (GI), and barium enema x-ray examinations often are used to rule out pulmonary or other GI disorders.

CT scan: Computerized axial tomography (CT) scan used to detect dilated bile ducts and presence of gallbladder cysts, tumors, abscesses, perforated gallbladder, and other complications of gallbladder disease.

Oral cholecystogram: Measures gallbladder function and demonstrates number and size of gallstones. This test requires ingestion of iodine-based tablets (i.e., Telepaque) at night, with x-ray films obtained the following morning. In 25% of cases, a second dose the next night may be needed for adequate visualization. As an alternative, the patient may be given a double dose of contrast on the initial night. Failure to visualize the gallbladder indicates a nonfunctioning gallbladder, usually because of complete obstruction of the cystic duct or chronic irritation of the gallbladder wall. Diarrhea may be caused by the iodine tablets and sometimes results in nonvisualization of the gallbladder. Ultrasound often takes the place of this test.

Complete blood count with differential: To assess for presence of infection or blood loss.

Bilirubin tests (serum and urine) and urobilinogen tests (urine and fecal): To differentiate among hemolytic disorders, hepatocellular disease, and obstructive disease. Usually there is an increase of bilirubin in the plasma and urine with biliary disease.

Serum liver enzyme test: Usually normal in cholecystitis but often becomes abnormal in the presence of prolonged cholecystitis or common duct stones.

Prothrombin time: To assess for prolonged clotting time secondary to faulty vitamin K absorption.

Electrocardiogram: To rule out cardiac disease.

Nursing Diagnoses:

Acute Pain/Nausea

related to obstructive or inflammatory process

Desired Outcomes: Patient's subjective perception of discomfort decreases within 1 hr of intervention, as documented by pain scale. Nonverbal indicators, such as grimacing, are absent or diminished.

INTERVENTIONS	RATIONALES
Monitor patient for pain or other discomfort. Devise a pain scale with patient, rating discomfort on a scale of 0 (no pain) to 10 (worst pain).	This assessment enables a more objective measurement of discomfort and subsequent relief obtained.
Explain that a low Fowler's position will minimize discomfort.	This position decreases tension on abdominal contents to promote comfort.
Teach patient about the prescribed diet that will promote comfort.	The prescribed diet will prevent nausea and spasms. Diet varies according to the patient's condition. During an acute attack, NPO (nothing by mouth) status with IV fluids may be instituted. With severe nausea and vomiting, a gastric tube is inserted and attached to low, intermittent suction. Diet advances to patient's tolerance, and small, frequent feedings of a low-fat diet are recommended for both the acute and chronic conditions. This diet minimizes the secretion of bile salts and subsequent gallbladder spasms. After cholecystectomy, a low-fat diet is used initially, and fatty foods may be introduced gradually to the patient's level of tolerance.

Continued

INTERVENTIONS	RATIONALES
Administer bile salt–binding agent (e.g., cholestyramine) as prescribed.	Cholestyramine and colestipol bind with bile salts in the intestine to facilitate their excretion and may be given to provide relief from pruritus caused by prolonged obstructive jaundice.
Provide cool Alpha Keri baths and cold water or ice for topical application; use soft linens on the bed.	These measures help control itching.
Administer analgesics as prescribed.	Nonsteroidal antiinflammatory drugs or opioid analgesics may be indicated, depending on pain severity. For postoperative patients, epidural, continuous IV, and patient-controlled infusions of opioid analgesics are used with increasing frequency and superior efficacy (see "Pain," p. 39 for more information). Recently, IV ketorolac q6h for 4-8 doses has shown benefit in controlling postoperative pain with these patients, reducing need for opioid analgesics. It should not be used for more than 3-5 days because of its toxic effects. While meperidine has long been used as the opioid of choice to prevent sphincter of Oddi spasms, there is risk of severe respiratory depression associated with cumulative effects of this drug.
Administer acid suppression therapy if prescribed.	This therapy neutralizes gastric hyperacidity and reduces associated pain.
Administer antiemetics as prescribed.	Antiemetics (e.g., hydroxyzine, ondansetron, prochlorperazine, promethazine) are given to control nausea and vomiting.

••• **Related NIC and NOC labels:** *NIC:* Pain Management; Nausea Management; Analgesic Administration; Positioning; Cold Application; Environmental Management: Comfort *NOC:* Comfort Level; Pain Control; Pain Level

Nursing Diagnosis:

Risk for Injury

related to potential for postsurgical perforation or recurrence of biliary obstruction

Desired Outcomes: Patient is free of symptoms of postsurgical perforation as evidenced by diminishing dark brown drainage of less than 1000 ml/day and presence of a soft and nondistended abdomen. Patient is free of symptoms of recurring biliary obstruction as evidenced by normal skin color, brown-colored stools, and straw-colored urine.

INTERVENTIONS	RATIONALES
Monitor color of the skin, sclera, urine, and stool.	If obstruction recurs and bile is forced back into the bloodstream, jaundice will be present, urine will be amber, and stools will be clay colored (clay color is normal if bile is drained via a T-tube). Brown color should return to stools once bile begins to drain normally into the duodenum.
Note and record color, amount, odor, and consistency of drainage from T-tube or wound drain q2h on day of surgery and at least every shift thereafter.	Initially drainage will be dark brown with small amounts of blood and can amount to 500-1000 ml/day. Greater amounts of blood or drainage should be reported to health care provider. Amount should subside gradually as swelling diminishes in the common duct and drainage into duodenum normalizes.
Ensure that drainage collection devices are positioned lower than the level of the common bile duct.	This will prevent reflux of drainage when patient is ambulating.

Continued

INTERVENTIONS

Be alert to abdominal distention, rigidity, and complaints of diaphragmatic irritation (caused by inflammation or bleeding and in this case is pain referred to the right shoulder) along with cessation or significant decrease in amount of drainage. If these signs occur, notify health care provider immediately and anticipate tube replacement with a 14-French catheter.

RATIONALES

These are indicators of a dislodged or clogged drainage tube causing bile leakage into the abdomen or backup of bile, necessitating timely intervention.

●●● **Related NIC and NOC labels:** *NIC:* Surveillance: Safety; Risk Identification *NOC:* Safety Status: Physical Injury

---

ADDITIONAL NURSING DIAGNOSES/ PROBLEMS:

"Perioperative Care"	p. 45
"Hepatitis" for **Risk for Impaired Skin Integrity** related to pruritus	p. 465

 PATIENT-FAMILY TEACHING AND DISCHARGE PLANNING

When providing patient-family teaching, focus on sensory information, avoid giving excessive information, and initiate a visiting nurse referral for necessary follow-up monitoring of postoperative patients. Include verbal and written information about the following:

✓ Notifying health care provider if the following indicators of recurrent biliary obstruction occur: dark urine, pruritus, jaundice, clay-colored stools. Inform patient that loose stools may occur for several months as the body adjusts to the continuous flow of bile.

✓ Medications, including drug name, dosage, schedule, purpose, precautions, and potential side effects. Also discuss drug-drug, food-drug, and herb-drug interactions.

✓ Care of dressings and tubes if patient is discharged with them, and monitoring of incision and drain sites for signs of infection (e.g., fever, persistent redness, pain, purulent discharge, swelling, increased local warmth).

✓ Importance of maintaining a diet low in fat and eating frequent, small meals for medically managed patients.

✓ Importance of follow-up appointments with health care provider; reconfirm time and date of next appointment.

✓ Avoiding alcoholic beverages during first 2 postoperative months to minimize risk of pancreatic involvement.

✓ Necessity of postsurgical activity precautions: avoid lifting heavy objects (more than 10 lb) for first 4-6 wk or as directed, rest after periods of fatigue, get maximum amounts of rest, and gradually increase activities to tolerance. Postsurgical patients may experience fatty food intolerance (e.g., flatulence, cramps, diarrhea) for several months postoperatively until the body acclimates to loss of the gallbladder.

✓ For more information contact the following organizations:

- National Institute of Diabetes & Digestive & Kidney Diseases at *www.niddk.nih.gov*
- American Gastroenterological Association at *www.gastro.org*

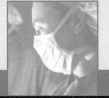

Cirrhosis 54

OVERVIEW/PATHOPHYSIOLOGY

Cirrhosis is a chronic, serious disease in which normal configuration of the liver is changed, resulting in cell death. When new cells are formed, the resulting scarring causes disruption of blood and lymph flow. Although pathologic changes do not occur for many years, structural changes gradually lead to total liver dysfunction. Manifestations of cirrhosis are related to hepatocellular necrosis and portal hypertension. Complications caused by cellular failure are similar to those of acute hepatitis and include inability to metabolize bilirubin and resultant jaundice; difficulty producing serum proteins, including albumin and certain clotting factors; hyperdynamic circulation and decreased vasomotor tone; pulmonary changes (ventilation-perfusion mismatch) and sometimes cyanosis; changes in nitrogen (N) metabolism (e.g., inability to convert ammonia to urea); and difficulty metabolizing some hormones (especially the sex hormones). Complications related to portal hypertension include development of ascites, bleeding esophageal and gastric varices, portal-systemic collaterals, encephalopathy, and splenomegaly.

Alcoholic (Laënnec's) cirrhosis: Associated with long-term alcohol abuse; accounts for 50% of all cirrhosis cases. Changes in liver structure caused by cirrhosis are irreversible, but compensation of liver function can be achieved if the liver is protected from further damage by cessation of alcohol consumption and proper nutrition. The histologic definition of this form of cirrhosis is micronodular cirrhosis.

Postnecrotic cirrhosis: Associated with history of viral hepatitis (hepatitis B virus or hepatitis C virus) or hepatic damage from drugs or toxins and is the leading type of cirrhosis in the Western world, Asia, and Africa. This type appears to predispose the patient to the development of a hepatoma. The histologic definition of this form of cirrhosis is macronodular cirrhosis.

Biliary cirrhosis: Associated with chronic retention of bile and inflammation of bile ducts; accounts for 15% of all cirrhosis cases. The histologic definition of this form of cirrhosis is mixed nodular cirrhosis; it may be further classified as follows.

Primary biliary cirrhosis (nonsuppurative destructive cholangitis): An inflammatory disease of intrahepatic bile ducts. This slowly progressive disease has other findings, including steatorrhea, xanthomatous (yellow tumors) neuropathy, osteo-porosis, and portal hypertension. Hypercholesterolemia, hyperlipidemia, and hepatomegaly are found in approximately 85% of patients with primary biliary cirrhosis (PBC).

Secondary biliary cirrhosis: Results from chronic obstruction to bile flow, usually from an obstruction outside the liver, such as calculi, neoplasms, or biliary atresia.

HEALTH CARE SETTING

Primary care with possible hospitalization for complications

ASSESSMENT

Signs and symptoms: Up to 40% of patients with cirrhosis have no symptoms. Others exhibit symptoms in varying degrees, depending on the degree of impaired hepatocellular function. Symptoms may include weakness, fatigability, weight loss, pruritus, fever, anorexia, nausea, occasional vomiting, abdominal pain, diarrhea, menstrual abnormalities, sterility, impotence, loss of libido, hematemesis. Urine may be dark (brownish) because of the presence of urobilinogen, and stools may be pale and clay colored because of the absence of bilirubin.

Physical assessment: Jaundice, hepatomegaly, ascites, peripheral edema, pleural effusion, and fetor hepaticus (a musty, sweetish odor on the breath). There may be slight changes in personality and behavior, which can progress to coma (a result of hepatic encephalopathy); spider angiomas, testicular atrophy, gynecomastia, pectoral and axillary alopecia (a result of hormonal changes); splenomegaly; hemorrhoids (a result of portal hypertension complications); spider nevi; purpuric lesions; and palmar erythema. Asterixis (i.e., jerking movements of the hands and wrists when the wrists are dorsiflexed with the fingers extended) may be present in advanced cirrhosis.

History of: Excessive alcohol ingestion; hepatitis B, C, or D infection; exposure to hepatotoxic drugs or chemicals; biliary or metabolic disease; poor nutrition.

DIAGNOSTIC TESTS

Hematologic: Red blood cells are decreased in hypersplenism and decreased with hemorrhage. White blood cells are decreased with hypersplenism and increased with infection. Platelet counts are less than normal.

Serum biochemical tests:

Bilirubin levels: Elevated because of failure in hepatocyte metabolism and obstruction in some instances. Very high or persistently elevated levels are considered a poor prognostic sign.

Alkaline phosphatase levels: Normal to mildly elevated in most cases; in PBC it is elevated 2-3 times normal.

Aspartate aminotransferase (AST) and alanine aminotransferase (ALT) levels: Usually elevated to more than 300 U with acute failure and normal or mildly elevated with chronic failure. ALT is more specific for hepatocellular damage.

Albumin levels: Reduced, especially with ascites. Persistently low levels suggest a poor prognosis. This test is not a perfect indicator of liver function because it is affected by poor nutrition and fluid status.

International normalized ratio: Elevated with severe hepatocellular dysfunction because the liver synthesizes clotting factors, particularly vitamin K–dependent factors.

Na$^+$ levels: Normal to low. Na$^+$ is retained but is associated with water retention, which results in normal serum Na$^+$ levels or even a dilutional hyponatremia. Often severe hyponatremia is present in the terminal stage and is associated with tense ascites and hepatorenal syndrome.

K$^+$ levels: Slightly reduced unless patient has renal insufficiency, which would result in hyperkalemia. Chronic hypokalemic acidosis is common in patients with chronic alcoholic liver disease.

Glucose levels: Hypoglycemia possible because of impaired gluconeogenesis and glycogen depletion in patients with severe or terminal liver disease.

Blood urea nitrogen levels: May be slightly decreased because of failure of Krebs cycle enzymes in the liver or elevated because of bleeding or renal insufficiency.

Ammonia levels: Elevation expected because of inability of the failing liver to convert ammonia to urea and shunting of intestinal blood via collateral vessels. Gastrointestinal (GI) hemorrhage or an increase in intestinal protein from dietary intake increases ammonia levels. **Note:** Keep patient NPO (nothing by mouth) except for water for 8 hr before drawing the ammonia level. Notify laboratory of all antibiotics taken by patient because antibiotics may lower the ammonia level.

Coagulation: Prothrombin time (PT) is prolonged and, in severe liver disease, unresponsive to vitamin K therapy. Coagulation abnormalities usually include factor V, but also factors II, VII, IX, and X.

Urine tests: Urine bilirubin is increased; urobilinogen is normal or increased; and proteinuria may be present.

Liver biopsy: Obtains a specimen of liver for microscopic analysis and diagnosis of cirrhosis, hepatitis, or other liver disease. After local anesthetic is administered and patient's skin is prepared, a large needle is inserted into the eighth or ninth intercostal space in the midaxillary line. It is critical that patient hold his or her breath at the end of expiration to elevate the liver maximally. Patient movement or failure to sustain expiration can result in puncture through the lung rather than the liver. Type and crossmatching sometimes are performed before the procedure in anticipation of hemorrhagic complications. Percutaneous liver biopsy is contraindicated in patients with markedly prolonged PT or very low platelet counts because of the risk of hemorrhage. In these patients, a transvenous biopsy via the jugular and hepatic vein may be attempted instead. Open liver biopsy, or minilaparotomy, also may be done for liver biopsy.

Barium swallow: Used in nonemergency situations (i.e., for patients without active bleeding) to verify presence of gastroesophageal varices. **Note:** Patient should be NPO from midnight until completion of test. Because of the constipating effects of barium, enemas should be given on patient's return from the procedure.

Radiologic studies: Ultrasound differentiates hemolytic and hepatocellular jaundice from obstructive jaundice and shows hepatomegaly and intrahepatic tumors. Computerized axial tomography (CT) scan of the liver/spleen is performed to evaluate size and location of tumors and nodules and to rule out gallbladder disease. Percutaneous transhepatic cholangiography reveals extent of obstruction via contrast dye. Endoscopic retrograde cholangiopancreatography (ERCP) is a fiberoptic technique used to show obstructions of the common bile and pancreatic ducts as potential causes of jaundice. Liver scans enable visualization of the spleen and liver via injection of radioisotopes. **Note:** After injection of the dye, patient may experience nausea, vomiting, and transient elevated temperature.

Angiographic studies: Establish portal vein patency and visualize portosystemic collateral vessels to determine cause of and effective treatment for variceal bleeding. Portal venous anatomy must be established before such operations as portal systemic shunt or hepatic transplantation. In patients with previously constructed surgical shunts, loss of patency may be confirmed as a factor leading to the present bleeding episode. The most common procedure is portal venography by indirect angiography. The femoral artery is catheterized, and contrast material is injected into the splenic artery. Contrast material flows through the spleen into the splenic and portal veins.

- Hepatic vein wedge pressure is measured by introducing a balloon catheter into the femoral vein and threading it into a hepatic vein branch.
- Direct access to the portal vein may be achieved through transhepatic portography. During this procedure, varices may be obliterated by injection of thrombin or gel foam into veins that supply the varices. **Note:** Transhepatic portography involves a direct puncture through the liver and has many of the same risks as liver biopsy. Patients returning from this procedure should be positioned on their right side and monitored closely.

Esophagoscopy: Visualizes the esophagus and stomach directly via a fiberoptic esophagoscope. Varices in the esophagus and upper portion of the stomach are identified, and attempts are made to identify the exact source of bleeding. Variceal bleeding may be treated by sclerotherapy, electrocautery, laser, vasoconstrictive agents, or other methods during the endoscopic procedure.

Peritoneoscopy or laparoscopy: Visualizes the liver (to identify characteristic "hobnailed" appearance in cirrhosis) and allows for biopsy.

Electroencephalogram: Traces the electrical impulses of the brain to detect or confirm encephalopathy. Electroencephalographic changes occur very early, usually before behavioral or biochemical alterations.

Psychometric testing: Evaluates for hepatic encephalopathy. A common test is the Reitan number connection (trail-making) test. Patient's speed and accuracy at connecting a series of numbered circles are evaluated at intervals. A daily handwriting test is an easy check of intellectual deterioration or improvement.

Nursing Diagnosis:

Imbalanced Nutrition: Less Than Body Requirements

related to anorexia, nausea, or malabsorption

Desired Outcome: By at least 24 hr before hospital discharge, patient demonstrates progress toward adequate nutritional status as evidenced by stable weight and balanced or positive N state.

INTERVENTIONS	RATIONALES
Monitor intake and output (I&O); weigh patient daily.	These measures will help assess adequacy of diet/nutritional intake.
Explain dietary restrictions. Encourage patient to eat foods that are permitted within dietary restrictions.	With fluid retention and ascites, sodium and fluids are restricted. Usually half the calories are supplied as carbohydrates to provide adequate energy when liver damage may prevent efficient liver metabolism and storage of carbohydrates.
Monitor ammonia level if it is available.	If the ammonia level rises (normal levels are whole blood 70-200 mcg/dl and plasma 56-150 mcg/dl), protein and foods high in ammonia also will be restricted. The action of intestinal bacteria on protein increases blood ammonia levels, which causes or worsens the coma state. Protein is restricted in hepatic coma or precoma states. Lactulose may be given to neutralize intraluminal ammonia.
Encourage small, frequent meals.	This helps ensure adequate nutrition without causing bloating from large meals.
Or, administer parenteral or enteral nutrition if prescribed (see "Providing Nutritional Support," p. 565).	Parenteral nutrition is administered in the presence of GI dysfunction. Enteral nutrition may be used in patients with a functional gut who are not eating adequately or at all.
Encourage significant other to bring desirable foods as permitted.	Patients are more likely to consume foods they like.
Administer vitamin and mineral supplements as prescribed.	For example, folic acid may be given for macrocytic anemia and vitamin K for a prolonged PT.
Administer the following prescribed medications: acid suppression agents, antiemetics, and cathartics.	These agents decrease gastric distress, which may facilitate intake.
Manage prescribed therapies such as diuresis, colloid replacement, and paracentesis.	These therapies relieve/mobilize ascites and decrease pressure on intraabdominal structures, which may facilitate intake.
Promote bedrest.	Rest reduces metabolic demands on the liver.
Provide soft diet if patient has esophageal varices that are not bleeding.	A soft diet will minimize risk of bleeding/hemorrhage. Patients with bleeding esophageal varices are NPO.
Encourage abstinence of alcohol in patients with alcoholic cirrhosis.	This remains the primary intervention in patients with alcohol-induced cirrhosis. Abstinence can result in healing of reversible factors of alcoholic liver disease over a period of months. Continued use of alcohol will further damage the liver to the point of irreversibility.

••• **Related NIC and NOC labels:** *NIC:* Nutrition Management; Nutrition Therapy; Teaching: Prescribed Diet; Enteral Tube Feeding; Gastrointestinal Intubation; Sustenance Support; Total Parenteral (TPN) Administration *NOC:* Nutritional Status; Nutritional Status: Nutrient Intake; Nutritional Status: Food & Fluid Intake

Nursing Diagnosis:

Impaired Gas Exchange

related to alveolar hypoventilation secondary to shallow breathing occurring with ascites or pleural effusion, altered oxygen-carrying capacity of the blood secondary to erythrocytopenia, and possible ventilation/perfusion mismatching.

Desired Outcome: Within 24 hr of admission, patient has adequate gas exchange as evidenced by $Paco_2$ 45 mm Hg or less, Pao_2 80 mm Hg or more, O_2 saturation greater than 92%, and RR 12-20 breaths/min with normal depth and pattern (eupnea).

INTERVENTIONS	RATIONALES
Monitor arterial blood gas values and pulse oximetry; notify health care provider of Pao_2 less than 80 mm Hg or O_2 saturation 92% or less. Administer oxygen as prescribed.	These values usually signal need for supplemental oxygen.
Obtain baseline abdominal girth measurement, and measure girth either daily or every shift. Measure around same circumferential area each time; mark site with indelible ink. Report significant findings to health care provider.	An increase in abdominal girth indicates increased ascitic fluid accumulation, which can cause pressure on the diaphragm with subsequent dyspnea.
During complaints of dyspnea or orthopnea, assist patient into semi-Fowler's or high Fowler's position.	These positions promote gas exchange, which is likely to be altered by pressure of ascitic fluid on the diaphragm.
Encourage patient to change positions and deep-breathe at frequent intervals.	Deep breathing expands the alveoli and aids in mobilizing secretions to the airway.
If secretions are present, ensure that patient coughs frequently.	Coughing further promotes mobilization of secretions and clears them.
Notify health care provider of spiking temperatures, chills, diaphoresis, and adventitious breath sounds.	These are indicators of respiratory infection, which can lead to complications such as pneumonia and respiratory distress. Patients with severe cirrhosis are weak, and, with poor maintenance of secretions, are more susceptible to infections.
Position patient in a side-lying position during episodes of vomiting.	This position decreases risk of aspiration, which could result in respiratory complications such as pneumonia.

••• **Related NIC and NOC labels:** *NIC:* Oxygen Therapy; Airway Management; Chest Physiotherapy; Positioning; Respiratory Monitoring; Aspiration Precautions; Cough Enhancement; Laboratory Data Interpretation *NOC:* Respiratory Status: Gas Exchange

Nursing Diagnosis:

Ineffective Protection

related to increased risk of esophageal bleeding secondary to portal hypertension and altered clotting factors

Desired Outcome: Patient is free of esophageal bleeding as evidenced by BP at least 90/60 mm Hg; HR 100 bpm or less; warm extremities; distal pulses greater than 2 on a 0-4 scale; brisk capillary refill (less than 2 sec); and orientation to person, place, and time.

INTERVENTIONS	RATIONALES
Monitor vital signs (VS) q4h (or more frequently if VS are outside of patient's baseline values).	Upper GI hemorrhage is common in patients with chronic liver disease and can result from esophageal varices, portal hypertensive gastropathy, duodenal or gastric ulcers, or Mallory-Weiss tear (mucosal laceration at the juncture of the distal esophagus and proximal stomach). Early diagnosis is essential to enable appropriate intervention. Hypotension and increased heart rate (HR), as well as cool extremities, delayed capillary refill, decreased amplitude of distal pulses, mental status changes, and decreasing level of consciousness (LOC), are indicators of hypovolemia and hemorrhage.

Continued

INTERVENTIONS	RATIONALES
Teach patient to avoid swallowing foods that are chemically or mechanically irritating.	Rough or spicy foods, hot foods, hot liquids, and alcohol may be injurious to the esophagus and result in bleeding.
Teach patient the importance of avoiding actions such as coughing, sneezing, lifting, or vomiting.	These actions increase intraabdominothoracic pressure, which can result in bleeding.
Administer stool softeners as prescribed.	Stool softeners help prevent straining with defecation, which puts patient at risk for bleeding.
Inspect stools for presence of blood; perform stool occult blood test as indicated.	This is an assessment for bleeding within the GI tract.
Monitor PT for abnormality.	Normal range is 10.5-13.5 sec; a PT that is prolonged signals that patient is at risk for bleeding.
Assess patient for signs of bleeding and notify health care provider of significant findings.	Melena and hematemesis are signs of bleeding. Altered VS, irritability, air hunger, pallor, and weakness are signs of significant bleeding and necessitate prompt intervention.
As appropriate, encourage intake of foods rich in vitamin K (e.g., spinach, cabbage, cauliflower, liver).	These foods help decrease PT.
As often as possible, avoid invasive procedures such as giving injections and taking rectal temperatures.	If patient's clotting is altered, invasive procedures could result in prolonged bleeding.
Monitor patient undergoing injection sclerotherapy for increased HR, decreased blood pressure (BP), pallor, weakness, and air hunger.	These are signs of esophageal perforation caused by sclerotherapy, whether by injection, cautery, or the scope itself.
If signs of perforation occur, notify health care provider immediately, keep patient NPO, and prepare for gastric suction. Administer antibiotics as prescribed to prevent infection.	NPO status and gastric suction prevent leakage of fluid, secretions, or food through the perforation into the mediastinum. This emergency situation necessities immediate intervention.

••• **Related NIC and NOC labels:** *NIC:* Bleeding Precautions; Emergency Care; Hemorrhage Control *NOC:* Coagulation Status

Nursing Diagnosis:

Disturbed Sensory Perception

related to increased risk of neurosensory changes secondary to hepatic coma occurring with cerebral accumulation of ammonia or GI bleeding

Desired Outcome: Patient verbalizes orientation to person, place, and time; exhibits intact signature; and is free of symptoms of injury caused by neurosensory changes.

INTERVENTIONS	RATIONALES
Perform a baseline assessment of patient's personality characteristics, LOC, and orientation. Enlist aid of significant other to help determine slight changes in personality or behavior.	Having a baseline assessment will help determine subsequent changes in patient's personality or behavior, which could progress to hepatic coma if left unchecked.
Have patient demonstrate signature daily.	If writing deteriorates, ammonia levels may be increasing.
Be alert to generalized muscle twitching and asterixis (flapping tremor induced by dorsiflexion of wrist and extension of fingers). Report significant findings to health care provider.	Asterixis may be present in advanced cirrhosis.
Remind patient to avoid protein and foods high in ammonia, such as gelatin, onions, and strong cheeses.	The diseased liver cannot convert ammonia to urea, and buildup of ammonia adds to progression of hepatic encephalopathy.
Monitor for indicators of GI bleeding, including melena or hematemesis. Report bleeding promptly to health care provider.	GI bleeding can precipitate hepatic coma.
Keep side rails up and bed in its lowest position, and assist patient with ambulation when need is determined.	These measures protect the patient from injury that could be precipitated by a confused state. Because of patient's encephalopathy and resulting neurosensory changes, reminders and reorientation are necessary to help ensure patient's safety.

Continued

INTERVENTIONS	RATIONALES
Avoid opioid analgesics and phenothiazines. Use caution when administering sedatives, antihistamines, and other agents affecting central nervous system.	Opioids and sedatives are metabolized by the liver and therefore are contraindicated. Small doses of benzodiazepines with a short half-life, such as oxazepam (Serax), may be administered if absolutely necessary.

••• **Related NIC and NOC labels:** *NIC:* Reality Orientation; Environmental Management; Neurologic Monitoring: Surveillance: Safety; Nutrition Management *NOC:* Cognitive Orientation; Muscle Function

Nursing Diagnosis:

Excess Fluid Volume

related to compromised regulatory mechanism with sequestration of fluids secondary to portal hypertension and hepatocellular failure

Desired Outcome: By at least 24 hr before hospital discharge, patient is normovolemic as evidenced by stable or decreasing abdominal girth, RR 12-20 breaths/min with normal depth and pattern (eupnea), HR 100 bpm or less, edema 1 or less on a 0-4 scale, and absence of crackles (rales).

INTERVENTIONS	RATIONALES
Obtain baseline abdominal girth measurement.	A baseline assessment enables comparison for subsequent assessments. Girth measurements indicate amount of ascitic fluid in the abdomen and provide information regarding effectiveness of medical treatment.
Place patient in supine position and mark abdomen with indelible ink. Measure girth daily or every shift as appropriate.	These measures ensure accurate serial measurements from same circumferential site.
Monitor weight and I&O.	Output should be equal to or exceed intake. Weight loss should not exceed 0.23 kg/day (½ lb/day) except in the presence of massive edema, which would permit a greater loss. Rapid diuresis from diuretics can lead to loss or shifts in electrolytes, particularly sodium, leading to encephalopathy and elevated creatinine.
Assess degree of edema from 1 (barely detectable) to 4 (deep, persistent pitting), and document accordingly.	The presence of edema signals excess sodium intake or low serum albumin. Low albumin levels are associated with ascites; persistently low levels suggest a poor prognosis.
Monitor serum Na$^+$ and K$^+$ values and report abnormalities to health care provider.	Optimal values are serum Na$^+$ 137-147 mEq/L and serum K$^+$ 3.5-5 mEq/L. Na$^+$ is retained but is associated with water retention, which results in normal serum Na$^+$ levels or even a dilutional hyponatremia. Severe hyponatremia is present in the terminal stage and is associated with tense ascites and hepatorenal syndrome. K$^+$ may be slightly reduced unless patient has renal insufficiency, which would result in hyperkalemia. Chronic hypokalemic acidosis is common in patients with chronic alcoholic liver disease.
Be alert to dyspnea, basilar crackles that do not clear with coughing, orthopnea, and tachypnea.	These are clinical indicators of pulmonary edema, which occurs from excess fluid volume in the circulatory system. Symptoms also may be present with pleural effusion caused by a small defect in the right hemidiaphragm, which develops with acute, rapid shortness of breath as the abdomen decompresses.
Give frequent mouth care, and provide ice chips to help minimize thirst.	These measures help minimize thirst while not compounding problems with fluid volume excess.

Continued

INTERVENTIONS

INTERVENTIONS	RATIONALES
As indicated, remind patient to avoid food and nonfood items that contain sodium, such as antacids, baking soda, and some mouthwashes.	Sodium may be restricted because of retention by the kidneys.
Elevate lower extremities.	This will decrease peripheral edema.
Apply antiembolism hose or support stockings, sequential compression devices, or pneumatic foot compression devices as prescribed.	These garments/devices decrease peripheral edema by external compression of the extremities.
Monitor for signs of variceal hemorrhage (see **Ineffective Protection,** earlier).	Rapid increases in intravascular volume can precipitate variceal hemorrhage in susceptible patients.
Teach patient to inhale against resistance, using a blow bottle if a LeVeen peritoneovenous or Denver shunt is in place.	Inhaling against resistance raises intraperitoneal pressure sufficiently to enable ascitic fluid to flow through the shunt.

●●● **Related NIC and NOC labels:** *NIC:* Fluid/Electrolyte Management; Laboratory Data Interpretation; Nutrition Management; Respiratory Monitoring *NOC:* Fluid Balance

ADDITIONAL NURSING DIAGNOSES/ PROBLEMS:

"Hepatitis" for **Deficient Knowledge:** Causes of   p. 464
hepatitis and modes of transmission

PATIENT-FAMILY TEACHING AND DISCHARGE PLANNING

When providing patient-family teaching, focus on sensory information, avoid giving excessive information, and initiate a visiting nurse referral for necessary follow-up teaching of any skilled care needed after discharge. Include verbal and written information about the following:

✓ Medications, including drug name, purpose, dosage, schedule, precautions, and potential side effects. Also discuss drug-drug, food-drug, and herb-drug interactions.

✓ Dietary restrictions, in particular that of sodium, protein, and ammonia.

✓ Potential need for lifestyle changes, including avoiding alcoholic beverages. Stress that alcohol cessation is a major factor in survival of this disease. Include appropriate referrals (e.g., to Alcoholics Anonymous, Al-Anon, and Alateen). As appropriate, provide referrals to community nursing support agencies.

✓ Awareness of hepatotoxic agents, especially over-the counter drugs, including acetaminophen and aspirin.

✓ Importance of breathing exercises (see p. 440) when ascites is present.

✓ Indicators of variceal bleeding/hemorrhage (i.e., vomiting blood, change in LOC) and need to inform health care provider if they occur.

✓ Telephone numbers to call in case questions or concerns arise about therapy or disease after discharge. Additional general information can be obtained by contacting National Institute of Diabetes & Digestive & Kidney Diseases at *www. niddk.nih.gov.*

✓ For patients awaiting transplantation, provide the following information: The United Network for Organ Sharing at *www.unos.org.*

✓ As an additional information source, refer patients to American Liver Foundation at *www.liverfoundation.org.*

Crohn's Disease 55

OVERVIEW/PATHOPHYSIOLOGY

Crohn's disease (CD), also known as *regional enteritis, granulomatous colitis,* or *transmural colitis,* is a chronic inflammatory disease that can involve any part of the gastrointestinal (GI) tract from the mouth to the anus. Usually the disease occurs segmentally, demonstrating discontinuous areas of disease with segments of healthy bowel in between. In 45%-50% of cases, the end of the ileum and cecum/ascending colon are involved (ileocolitis); in 35% of cases, the terminal ileum is affected (ileitis); and in 20% of cases, the colon alone is affected (Crohn's colitis). A small number of patients have involvement of the jejunum, duodenum, stomach, esophagus, and mouth; in these cases, the ileum, colon, or both are also involved. Approximately 30%-35% of patients have perianal fistulas, fissures, or abscesses. The disease affects all layers of the bowel: the mucosa, submucosa, circular and longitudinal muscles, and serosa, predisposing to intestinal strictures and fistulas. A family history of this disease or ulcerative colitis occurs in 15%-20% of affected patients.

The cause of CD is unknown, but theories include infection, immunologic factors, environmental factors, and genetic predisposition. In a genetically susceptible subject, an outside agent or substance, such as a bacterium, virus, or other antigen, interacts with the body's immune system to trigger the disease or may cause damage to the intestinal wall, initiating or accelerating the disease process. The resulting inflammatory response continues unregulated by the immune system. As a result, inflammation continues to damage the intestinal wall, causing the symptoms of CD. Initial treatment is nonoperative, individualized, and based on symptomatic relief. Because surgery is not a cure for CD, it is reserved for complications rather than used as a primary form of therapy.

Since the end of World War II, the incidence of CD has increased steadily, whereas that of ulcerative colitis (UC) has stabilized. This rise may reflect increased diagnostic awareness rather than increased incidence of CD. There is a 20-fold increase in risk of inflammatory bowel disease (IBD) in first-degree relatives of individuals with CD. CD is generally diagnosed between the ages of 15 and 35, but it also can occur in young children and in people 70 years of age or older. Prevalence is slightly higher in women than in men. CD, like UC, is seen more frequently in the Caucasian population and in Ashkenazi Jews than in nonwhite populations and in people of non-Jewish descent. It is more prevalent in urban, developed countries with temperate climates than in rural, more southern countries. However, increasing incidence is being observed in Japan and South America. Cigarette smoking has been shown to increase the risk of developing CD and is associated with resistance to medical therapy and recurrence of disease after surgery. There have been studies in the United Kingdom and the United States promoting the idea that CD is caused by a bacterium, raising important questions for further research.

HEALTH CARE SETTING

Primary care, with possible hospitalization resulting from complications

ASSESSMENT

Signs and symptoms: Clinical presentation varies as a direct reflection of the location of the inflammatory process and its extent, severity, and relationship to contiguous structures. Sometimes onset is abrupt, and the patient can appear to have appendicitis, UC, intestinal obstruction, or a fever of obscure origin. Acute symptoms include right lower quadrant (RLQ) pain, tenderness, spasm, flatulence, nausea, fever, and diarrhea. A more typical picture is insidious onset with more persistent but less severe symptoms, such as vague abdominal pain, unexplained anemia, and fever. Diarrhea—liquid, soft, or mushy stools—is the most common symptom. The presence of gross blood is rare. Abdominal pain is a common symptom, and it may be colicky or crampy, initiated by meals, centered in the lower abdomen, and relieved by defecation because of chronic partial obstruction of the small intestine, colon, or both. As the disease progresses, anorexia, malnutrition, weight loss, anemia, lassitude, malaise, and fever can occur in addition to fluid, electrolyte, and metabolic disturbances.

Physical assessment: In early stages, examination is often normal but may demonstrate mild tenderness in the abdomen over the affected bowel. In more advanced disease, a palpable mass may be present, especially in the RLQ with terminal ileum involvement. Persistent rectal fissure, large ulcers, perirectal abscess, or rectal fistula is the first indication of disease in 15%-25% of patients with small bowel involvement and in 50%-75% of patients with colonic involvement. Rectovaginal, abdominal, and enterovesical fistulas also can occur. Extraintestinal manifestations characteristic of UC do occur, but less commonly (10%-20%).

DIAGNOSTIC TESTS

Stool examination: Usually reveals occult blood; frank blood may be noted in stools of patients with colonic involvement or with ulcerations and fistulas of the rectum. A few patients have presenting symptom of bloody diarrhea. Stool cultures and smears rule out bacterial and parasitic disorders. Specimens are also examined for fecal fat.

Sigmoidoscopy: Evaluates possible colonic involvement and obtains rectal biopsy. The finding of granulomas on mucosal biopsy argues strongly for the diagnosis of CD. However, because granulomas are more numerous in the submucosa, suction biopsy of the rectum provides deeper, larger, and less traumatized specimens for a better diagnostic yield than mucosal biopsy obtained through an endoscope.

Colonoscopy: May help differentiate CD from UC. Characteristic patchy inflammation (skip lesions) rules out UC. However, colonoscopy usually does not add useful diagnostic information in the presence of positive findings from sigmoidoscopy or radiologic examination. When diagnosis is unclear and there is a question of malignancy, colonoscopy provides the means of directly visualizing mucosal changes and obtaining biopsies, brushings, and washings for cytologic examination. Colonoscopy also may assist in planning for surgery by documenting the extent of colonic disease. **Note:** Because of risk of perforation, this procedure may be contraindicated in patients with acute phases of Crohn's colitis or when deep ulcerations or fistulas are known to be present.

Endoscopic ultrasonography: Aids in diagnosis of perirectal fistula and abscesses and in detecting transmural depth of inflammation in the bowel or esophagus, using an endoscopically placed ultrasound probe.

Small bowel enteroscopy: Permits visualization of the upper GI tract to identify areas of inflammation and bleeding to the level of the midjejunum.

Wireless capsule: Permits visualization of the small intestine to identify abnormalities. The patient swallows a large capsule that contains a small disposable camera; images are transmitted to a receiver on the patient's waist. **Note:** Use is contraindicated if strictures exist, because strictures can prevent the capsule from progressing through the intestine; surgical removal of the capsule may be required.

Barium enema and upper GI series with small bowel follow-through: Contribute to diagnosis of CD. Involvement of only the terminal ileum or segmental involvement of the colon or small intestine almost always indicates CD. Thickened bowel wall with stricture (string sign) separated by segments of normal bowel, cobblestone appearance, and presence of fistulas and skip lesions are common findings. A double-contrast barium enema technique may increase sensitivity in detecting early or subtle changes. **Note:** Barium enema may be contraindicated in patients with acute phases of Crohn's colitis because of risk of perforation. Upper GI barium series is contraindicated in patients in whom intestinal obstruction is suspected.

CT scan: Complements information gathered via endoscopy and conventional radiography. In advanced disease, computerized axial tomography (CT) scanning clearly delineates extraluminal complications (e.g., abscess, phlegmon, bowel wall thickening, mesenteric inflammation). CT scan has been used also to percutaneously drain fistulas (colovesicular, enterovesicular, colovaginal, enterocolonic) and to evaluate perirectal disease, enterocutaneous fistula, and sinus tracts.

Serum antibody testing: In difficult to diagnose cases, may be helpful in differentiating CD from UC.

Radionuclide imaging: IV indium-111– or technetium-99–labeled leukocytes migrate to areas of active inflammation and are then identified by scans performed after 4 and 24 hr. This procedure aids in differentiating CD from UC and evaluating abscess and fistula formation.

Blood tests: Are nonspecific for diagnosis of CD but help determine whether the inflammatory process is active and evaluate patient's overall condition. Anemia may be present and may be microcytic because of iron deficiency from chronic blood loss and bone marrow depression secondary to chronic inflammatory process or megaloblastic because of folic acid or vitamin B_{12} deficiency (usually seen only in patients with extensive ileitis causing malabsorption). Increased white blood cell (WBC) count and sedimentation rate reflect disease activity and inflammation. Hypoalbuminemia corresponds with disease activity and results from decreased protein intake, extensive malabsorption, and significant enteric loss of protein. Hypokalemia is seen in patients with chronic diarrhea; hypophosphatemia and hypocalcemia are seen in patients with significant malabsorption. Liver function studies may be abnormal secondary to pericholangitis.

Urinalysis and urine culture: May reveal urinary tract infection secondary to enterovesicular fistula.

Tests for malabsorption: Because patients with active, extensive disease (especially when it involves the small intestine) may develop malabsorption and malnutrition, the following tests are clinically significant: D-xylose tolerance test (for upper jejunal involvement); Schilling test (for ileal involvement); serum albumin, carotene, calcium, and phosphorus levels; and fecal fat (steatorrhea).

Nursing Diagnosis:

Deficient Fluid Volume

related to active loss secondary to diarrhea or presence of GI fistula

Desired Outcomes: Patient is normovolemic within 24 hr of admission as evidenced by balanced I&O, urinary output 30 ml/hr or more, specific gravity 1.010-1.030, BP 90/60 mm Hg or higher (or within patient's normal range), RR 12-20 breaths/min, stable weight, good skin turgor, and moist mucous membranes. Patient reports that diarrhea is controlled.

INTERVENTIONS	RATIONALES
Monitor intake and output (I&O) and urinary specific gravity, weigh patient daily, and monitor laboratory values to evaluate fluid and electrolyte status.	These assessments monitor for fluid loss and electrolyte imbalance. GI fluid losses (nasogastric [NG] suction, vomiting, diarrhea, fistula) can lead to hyponatremia, hypokalemia, and hypochloremia. Optimal values are serum K^+ 3.5-5.0 mEq/L, serum Na^+ 137-147 mEq/L, and serum Cl^- 95-108 mEq/L. Critical values: K^+ less than 2.5 or more than 6.5 mEq/L, Na^+ less than 120 or more than 160 mEq/L, Cl^- less than 80 or more than 115 mEq/L.
Monitor frequency and consistency of stools. Keep a stool count, and measure volume of liquid stools.	These assessments monitor for presence and amount of blood, mucus, fat, and undigested food, which occur secondary to the underlying inflammatory process.
Monitor patient for the presence of thirst, poor skin turgor, dryness of mucous membranes, fever, and concentrated (specific gravity greater than 1.030) and decreased urinary output.	These are indicators of dehydration.
Maintain patient on parenteral replacement of fluids, electrolytes, and vitamins as prescribed.	Patients with involvement of the small intestine often require supplementation of vitamins and minerals, especially calcium, iron, folate, and magnesium secondary to malabsorption or to compensate for foods excluded from the diet. Patients with extensive ileal disease or resection often require vitamin B_{12} replacement, and if bile salt deficiency exists, cholestyramine and medium-chain triglycerides may be needed to control diarrhea and reduce fat malabsorption and steatorrhea. Vitamin D deficiency is common in these patients and may require replacement with cholecalciferol.
When patient is taking food PO, provide diet as prescribed. Assess tolerance to diet by determining incidence of cramping, diarrhea, and flatulence. Modify diet plan accordingly.	Bland diets low in residue, roughage, and fat but high in protein, calories, carbohydrates, and vitamins provide good nutrition and reduce excessive stimulation of the bowel. A diet free of milk, milk products, gas-forming foods, alcohol, and iced beverages reduces cramping and diarrhea.
	Elemental diets (e.g., Vivonex, Ensure) that are free of bulk and residue, low in fat, and digested in the upper jejunum provide good nutrition with low fecal volume to enable bowel rest in selected patients. Use of elemental diets is being investigated for effectiveness as primary therapy as an alternative to steroids and bowel rest in treating patients with acute Crohn's disease.

••• **Related NIC and NOC labels:** *NIC:* Fluid Management; Electrolyte Monitoring; Intravenous Therapy; Laboratory Data Interpretation; Diarrhea Management; Blood Products Administration *NOC:* Fluid Balance; Bowel Elimination; Electrolyte & Acid-Base Balance

Nursing Diagnoses:

Risk for Infection/Ineffective Protection

related to potential complications caused by intestinal inflammatory disorder

Desired Outcomes: Patient is free from indicators of infection and intraabdominal injury as evidenced by normothermia; HR 60-100 bpm; RR 12-20 breaths/min; normal bowel sounds; absence of abdominal distention, rigidity, or localized pain and tenderness; absence of nausea and vomiting; negative culture results; no significant change in mental status; and orientation to person, place, and time.

INTERVENTIONS	RATIONALES
Monitor for abdominal distention, abdominal rigidity, and increased episodes of nausea and vomiting.	These are indicators of intestinal obstruction. Contributing factors to development of intestinal obstruction include use of opioids and prolonged use of antidiarrheal medication.
Monitor for fever, increased respiratory rate (RR) and heart rate (HR), chills, diaphoresis, and increased abdominal discomfort.	These indicators can occur with intestinal perforation, abscess or fistula formation, or generalized fecal peritonitis and septicemia. **Note:** Systemic therapy with corticosteroids and antibiotics can mask development of these complications.
Evaluate mental status, orientation, and level of consciousness q2-4h.	Mental cloudiness, lethargy, and increased restlessness can occur with peritonitis and septicemia.
Obtain cultures of blood, urine, fistulas, or other possible sources of infection, as prescribed, if patient has a sudden temperature elevation. Monitor culture reports, and notify health care provider promptly of any positive results.	Abscesses or fistulas to the abdominal wall, bladder, or vagina are common in Crohn's disease and are potential sources of infection, as are abscesses or fistulas to other loops of small bowel and colon.
If draining fistulas or abscesses are present, change dressings and pouching system or irrigate tubes or drains as prescribed. Note color, character, and odor of all drainage. Refer to a wound, ostomy, continence (WOC) nurse for fistula management as needed.	Foul-smelling or abnormal drainage, which can signal infection, or loss of tube/drain patency should be reported to health care provider promptly for intervention.
Administer antibiotics as prescribed and on prescribed schedule.	Maintaining the therapeutic serum level of antibiotics will help control suppurative complications (e.g., bacterial overgrowth) and perianal fistulas in patients with mild to moderate colonic or ileocolonic CD. In patients who are allergic, intolerant, or unresponsive to sulfasalazine, metronidazole appears to be effective in colonic disease and in promoting healing of perianal disease. Long-term use of metronidazole is limited because of potential for peripheral neuropathy and other side effects. Patients with bacterial overgrowth in the small intestine may be treated with broad-spectrum antibiotics. Ciprofloxacin may be useful in treating patients who are intolerant or unresponsive to metronidazole therapy.
Administer immunosuppressive immunomodulatory agents and biologic agents as prescribed.	These agents aid in healing, especially with refractory disease or active disease unresponsive to conventional therapy; reduce drainage of perianal and cutaneous fistulas; reduce steroid dosage; and maintain remission. Oral immunosuppressive agents include azathioprine and 6-mercaptopurine (6-MP). IV cyclosporine has been used to treat refractory CD and treatment-resistant fistulas. Because of toxicity and side effects, only short-term use is recommended and its role has been diminished with the advent of infliximab. IM and subcutaneous methotrexate provide both immunosuppressive and antiinflammatory effects. The biologic agent infliximab is used IV for treatment and maintenance of remission in moderate to severe, active disease that is unresponsive to conventional treatment and for treatment and maintenance of remission of fistulizing disease.

Continued

INTERVENTIONS	RATIONALES
Use good handwashing technique before and after caring for patient, and dispose of dressings and drainage using proper infection control techniques (see p. 781).	These measures prevent transmission of potentially infectious organisms.

••• **Related NIC and NOC labels:** *NIC:* Infection Control; Infection Protection; Medication Administration; Specimen Management; Wound Care *NOC:* Infection Status

Nursing Diagnoses:

Acute Pain/Nausea

and abdominal cramping *related to* intestinal inflammatory process

Desired Outcomes: Patient's subjective perception of discomfort decreases within 4 hr of intervention, as documented by pain scale. Objective indicators, such as grimacing, are absent or diminished.

INTERVENTIONS	RATIONALES
Monitor and document characteristics of discomfort, and assess whether it is associated with ingestion of certain foods or with emotional stress. Devise a pain scale with patient, rating discomfort from 0 (no discomfort) to 10 (worst discomfort). Eliminate foods that cause cramping and discomfort.	The discomfort of pain, nausea, and abdominal cramping may be associated with certain foods or emotional stress. A pain scale will help determine degree of relief obtained after interventions have been implemented.
As prescribed, keep patient NPO (nothing by mouth) and provide parenteral nutrition.	These measures allow bowel rest, which will help alleviate discomfort.
Administer antidiarrheal medications and analgesics as prescribed.	These medications are given to reduce abdominal discomfort. Codeine or loperamide often reduces diarrhea with a concomitant decrease in abdominal cramping. Anticholinergics are not recommended because they may mask obstructive symptoms and precipitate toxic megacolon. For these reasons, antidiarrheal medications should be administered with caution.
Assess patient's response to these medications. Report significant findings to health care provider.	If patient does not respond appropriately to standard antidiarrheal medications and mild sedation, the presence of obstruction, bowel perforation, or abscess formation is suspected.
Instruct patient to request analgesic before pain becomes severe.	Prolonged stimulation of pain receptors results in increased sensitivity to painful stimuli and increases the amount of drug required to relieve discomfort.
Provide nasal and oral care at frequent intervals.	These measures lessen discomfort from NPO status and presence of NG tube.
Administer antiemetic medications before meals.	These agents enhance appetite when nausea is a problem.
For additional information, see "Pain," p. 39.	

••• **Related NIC and NOC labels:** *NIC:* Medication Management; Pain Management; Nausea Management; Anxiety Reduction; Bowel Management *NOC:* Comfort Level

Nursing Diagnosis:

Diarrhea

related to intestinal inflammatory process

Desired Outcome: Patient reports a reduction in frequency of stools and a return to more normal stool consistency within 3 days of hospital admission.

INTERVENTIONS	RATIONALES
If patient is experiencing frequent and urgent passage of loose stools, provide covered bedpan or commode or be sure bathroom is easily accessible and ready to use at all times.	Providing easy access to bedpan, commode, or bathroom reduces stress and enables patient to cope with diarrhea more effectively.
Empty bedpan or commode promptly.	This intervention will control odor and decrease patient's anxiety and self-consciousness.
Administer antidiarrheal medication as prescribed.	These agents decrease fluidity and number of stools. Codeine and loperamide often reduce diarrhea. Anticholinergics are not recommended because they may mask obstructive symptoms and precipitate toxic megacolon. Therefore, antidiarrheal medications should be administered with caution.
Administer cholestyramine as prescribed.	This agent controls diarrhea if bile salt deficiency (because of ileal disease or resection) is contributing to this problem.
Eliminate or decrease fat content in the diet.	Fat can increase diarrhea in individuals with malabsorption syndromes.
Restrict raw vegetables and fruits; whole-grain cereals; condiments; gas-forming foods; alcohol; iced and carbonated beverages; and, in lactose-intolerant patients, milk and milk products.	These foods and beverages also can precipitate diarrhea and cramping. When remission occurs, a less restricted diet can be tailored to the individual patient, excluding foods known to precipitate symptoms.

••• **Related NIC and NOC labels:** *NIC:* Diarrhea Management; Anxiety Reduction; Bowel Management; Medication Administration *NOC:* Symptom Severity

Nursing Diagnosis:

Activity Intolerance

related to generalized weakness secondary to intestinal inflammatory process

Desired Outcome: Patient adheres to prescribed rest regimen and sets appropriate goals for self-care as the condition improves (optimally within 3-7 days of admission).

INTERVENTIONS	RATIONALES
Keep patient's environment quiet.	This will facilitate needed rest.
Assist patient with activities of daily living (ADL) and plan nursing care to provide maximum rest periods.	Adequate rest is necessary to sustain remission.
Facilitate coordination of health care providers. Provide 90 min for undisturbed rest.	This enables rest periods between care activities.
As prescribed, administer sedatives and tranquilizers.	These agents promote rest and reduce anxiety.
As patient's physical condition improves, encourage self-care to greatest extent possible and assist patient with setting realistic, attainable goals.	These measures enable patient to increase endurance incrementally to his or her tolerance and prevent problems associated with prolonged bedrest.
For additional information, see **Risk for Activity Intolerance,** p. 61, in "Prolonged Bedrest."	

••• **Related NIC and NOC labels:** *NIC:* Energy Management; Self-Care Assistance; Environmental Management; Mutual Goal Setting *NOC:* Energy Conservation; Self-Care: Activities of Daily Living; Endurance

Nursing Diagnosis:

Deficient Knowledge:

Drugs used during exacerbations of Crohn's disease

Desired Outcome: Immediately following teaching, patient verbalizes accurate information about drugs used during exacerbations of Crohn's disease.

INTERVENTIONS	RATIONALES
Teach patient about the following:	
Sulfasalazine	This medication is given to treat acute exacerbations of colonic and ileocolonic disease. Although sulfasalazine does not prevent recurrence of Crohn's disease, patients who respond tend to benefit from long-term therapy and relapse when the agent is discontinued. It appears to be more effective in patients with mild-to-moderate disease limited to the colon than in those with disease limited to the small bowel.
- Folic acid supplements are necessary during treatment.	Sulfasalazine impairs folate absorption.
- Have blood count done within first 4 mo of treatment.	WBCs may be lowered with this drug, and anemia can occur (uncommon).
- Have liver enzymes checked within first year of treatment.	Hepatitis, though uncommon, has occurred.
- Notify physician immediately if discoloration of skin or urine occurs.	Sulfasalazine may produce orange-yellow discoloration of skin and urine and could cause contact lenses to turn yellow.
- Males may want to check for infertility by sperm analysis.	Infertility has occurred in some men, though it reverses when patient stops taking the drug.
- Be alert to the following side effects: fever, skin rash, joint pain, nausea, headache, or fatigue when dose exceeds 4 tablets/day.	Most side effects are sulfa related and caused by the sulfa component of the drug.
5-Aminosalicylic acid (5-ASA) preparations	5-ASA is used in patients unable to tolerate sulfasalazine. Slow-release mesalamine (Pentasa) and enteric-coated mesalamine (Asacol) are used for mildly to moderately active ileocolonic and ileal disease and for maintenance therapy in selected patients. They may delay or prevent postoperative recurrence when initiated soon after ileal and colonic resection.
- Patients on prolonged treatment must have annual kidney profile and urine examination, including blood urea nitrogen (BUN) and creatinine.	There is risk of kidney damage with high doses (above 4000 mg/day).
Corticosteroids	These agents reduce the active inflammatory response, decrease edema in moderate-to-severe forms, and control exacerbations in chronic disease. Oral route is most effective for disease limited to the small intestine.
- Check blood pressure (BP) during each clinic/office visit.	Hypertension is a side effect.
- Test blood glucose after 1 mo of therapy, then q3mo.	Increased blood glucose level can occur.
- Schedule eye examination q6mo and bone density evaluation every few years for patients taking steroids longer than 12 mo.	There is potential for cataract formation and osteoporosis with long-term treatment.
- Be alert to rounding of face (moon face), acne, increased appetite and weight gain, red marks/blotches on skin, facial hair, severe mood swings, weakness, and leg cramps.	These are typical side effects with steroids.
- As active disease subsides, prednisone is tapered.	The goal is eventual elimination of the drug.
- In some cases of chronic disease, continuous corticosteroid therapy may be necessary.	Many patients with Crohn's disease become steroid dependent, meaning they are symptomatic with low-dose therapy (5-15 mg/day) or with total discontinuation of the drug.

Continued

INTERVENTIONS	RATIONALES
- A new nonsystemic steroidal agent, budesonide, is approved for treatment of mild to moderate active disease involving the ileum and cecum/ascending colon.	It provides benefits of traditional therapy with reduced side effects. It is used for flare-ups but not commonly for maintenance therapy.
- Avoid grapefruit and grapefruit juice when taking budesonide.	They may increase drug effects.
- Topical therapy is an effective route.	Topical therapy with hydrocortisone has controlled inflammation via retention enemas for patients with proctosigmoiditis (involvement to 40 cm); suppositories have been used for patients with Crohn's proctitis.
Immunosuppressive immunomodulatory agents	These agents allow dosage reduction or withdrawal of corticosteroids in steroid-dependent patients, are used for maintenance therapy with a lower relapse rate, and aid in healing and reducing drainage of perianal fistulas.
- If taking 6-mercaptopurine (6-MP), check blood cell counts every other week until dose has been stable for 6 mo. Then monitor every month for 3 mo, then once every 3 mo.	Lowered WBC count can occur, as can anemia (rare).
- Be alert to the following when taking 6-MP: allergic reaction (fever, skin rash, joint aches) and inflammation of the pancreas.	These are possible side effects.
- IV cyclosporine has been used to treat refractory Crohn's disease and treatment-resistant fistulas. (Its role has been diminished with advent of biologic agent infliximab.)	Oral cyclosporine has not proved to be effective for maintenance therapy because relapse occurs when dosage is reduced or stopped. Because of the frequency and severity of toxicity and side effects, short-term IV administration is the best method for cyclosporine.
- If taking cyclosporine, check BP at 2-wk intervals.	Elevated BP can occur.
- Monitor kidney function, including BUN and creatinine.	Decreased kidney function can occur.
- Parenteral (IM, subcutaneous) methotrexate provides both immunosuppressive and antiinflammatory effects and allows for reduction or cessation of steroid therapy in some patients with chronically active Crohn's disease.	However, incidence of side effects and toxicity limit its use in many patients.
- Methotrexate is used with extreme caution in people who consume significant quantities of alcohol. Blood cell counts and liver enzymes are checked monthly for first 3 mo, then at 3-mo intervals.	This drug can affect the liver.
- Methotrexate is contraindicated in pregnancy or in women anticipating pregnancy.	It may cause fetal death and congenital abnormalities; can be transferred via breast milk.
Biologic agent: infliximab (Remicade)	This agent blocks tumor necrosis factor (TNF)-alpha, a protein that escalates inflammation. Infliximab is used intravenously to treat and maintain remission of moderate to severe active disease unresponsive to conventional therapy. It is used to treat and maintain remission in fistulizing disease and may be effective for use in tapering steroids.
- Patient should be alert to and report sore throat, upper respiratory infection, abscesses, sinusitis, and bronchitis.	These are signs of infection. There is risk of altered immune response with this drug.
- There is risk of malignancy.	Lymphoma has occurred in some patients.
- Infusion related reactions that occur during or shortly after the drug is given include fever, chills, headache, low BP, rash, muscle and joint pain, chest pain, itching, and shortness of breath. Teach patient to watch for reactions during and up to 2 hours after infusion.	These reactions usually are of short duration and almost always respond to treatment with acetaminophen, antihistamines, corticosteroids, or epinephrine as prescribed.
- Tuberculosis skin test should be performed before therapy is initiated.	Treatment of latent tuberculosis infection is needed before starting infliximab therapy.
- Patient needs to inform health care provider of infliximab use before receiving vaccines.	Live-virus vaccines should not be administered until infliximab therapy stops, since infliximab may affect normal immune response.
- Ensure that patient verbalizes accurate knowledge about purpose, precautions, and potential side effects of any prescribed drug he or she will be taking.	A knowledgeable individual is more likely to adhere to the therapeutic regimen and promptly report untoward side effects to health care provider.

••• **Related NIC and NOC labels:** *NIC:* Teaching: Prescribed Medication *NOC:* Knowledge: Medication

ADDITIONAL NURSING DIAGNOSES/PROBLEMS:

Perioperative Care	p. 45
Psychosocial Support	p. 73
"Fecal Diversions: Colostomy, Ileostomy, and Ileal Pouch Anal Anastomosis" for **Risk for Impaired Skin Integrity/Impaired Tissue Integrity**	p. 456
Bowel Incontinence	p. 458
Disturbed Body Image	p. 459

✓ PATIENT-FAMILY TEACHING AND DISCHARGE PLANNING

When providing patient-family teaching, focus on sensory information, avoid giving excessive information, and initiate a visiting nurse referral for necessary follow-up teaching. Include verbal and written information about the following:

✓ Medications, including drug name, rationale, dosage, schedule, route of administration, precautions, and potential side effects. Also discuss drug-drug, herb-drug, and food-drug interactions.

✓ Signs and symptoms that necessitate medical attention, including fever, nausea and vomiting, abdominal discomfort, any significant change in appearance and frequency of stools, or passage of stool through the vagina or stool mixed with urine, any of which can signal recurrence or complications of CD.

✓ Importance of dietary management to promote nutritional and fluid maintenance and prevent abdominal cramping, discomfort, and diarrhea.

✓ Importance of perineal/perianal skin care after bowel movements.

✓ Importance of balancing activities with rest periods, even during remission, because adequate rest is necessary to sustain remission.

✓ Referral to community resources, including the following organization: Crohn's & Colitis Foundation of America, Inc., at *www.ccfa.org*.

✓ Importance of follow-up medical care, including supportive psychotherapy, because of the chronic and progressive nature of CD.

In addition, if patient has a fecal diversion (colostomy or ileostomy):

✓ Care of incision, dressing changes, and bathing.

✓ Care of stoma and peristomal skin, use of ostomy equipment, and method for obtaining supplies.

✓ Gradual resumption of ADL, excluding heavy lifting (more than 10 lb), pushing, or pulling for 6-8 wk to prevent incisional herniation.

✓ Referral to community resources, including home health care agency, WOC/ET nurse, local ostomy association, and the United Ostomy Association of America at *uoaa.org*.

✓ Importance of reporting signs and symptoms that require medical attention, such as change in stoma color from the normal bright and shiny red; lesions of stomal mucosa that may indicate recurrence of disease; peristomal skin irritation; diarrhea or constipation, fever, chills, abdominal pain, distention, nausea, and vomiting; and incisional pain, local increased temperature, drainage, swelling, or redness.

Fecal Diversions: Colostomy, Ileostomy, and Ileal Pouch Anal Anastomoses

56

OVERVIEW/PATHOPHYSIOLOGY

For a discussion of ulcerative colitis, see p. 487; for a discussion of Crohn's disease, see p. 445.

HEALTH CARE SETTING

Acute care on surgical unit, primary care, home care after hospital discharge

SURGICAL INTERVENTIONS

It is sometimes necessary to interrupt continuity of the bowel because of intestinal disease or its complications. A fecal diversion may be necessary to divert stool around a diseased portion of the bowel or, more commonly, out of the body. A fecal diversion can be located anywhere along the bowel, depending on location of the diseased or injured portion, and it can be permanent or temporary. The most common sites for fecal diversion are the colon and ileum.

Colostomy: Created when the surgeon brings a portion of the colon to the surface of the abdomen. An opening in the exteriorized colon permits elimination of flatus and stool through the stoma. Any part of the colon may be diverted into a colostomy.

Transverse colostomy: Most commonly created stoma to divert feces on a temporary basis. Surgical indications include relief of bowel obstruction before definitive surgery for tumors, inflammation, or diverticulitis and colon perforation secondary to trauma. Stool can be liquid to pastelike or soft and unformed, and bowel elimination is unpredictable. A temporary colostomy may be double barreled, with a proximal stoma through which stool is eliminated and a distal stoma, called a mucus fistula, adjacent to the proximal stoma. More commonly, a loop colostomy is created with a supporting rod placed beneath it until the exteriorized loop of colon heals to the skin.

Descending or sigmoid colostomy: Usually a permanent fecal diversion. Rectal cancer is the most common cause for surgical intervention. Stool is usually formed, and some individuals may have stool elimination at predictable times.

In a permanent colostomy, the surgeon brings the severed end of the colon to the abdominal skin surface. The diseased or injured portion of the colon and/or rectum is resected and removed. To create the stoma, the colon above the skin surface is rolled back on itself to expose the mucosal surface of the intestine. The end of the cuff is sutured to the subcutaneous tissues with absorbable sutures to hold it in place as it heals.

Temporary colostomy: Typically created when there is significant inflammation in the diseased portion of the bowel (e.g., perforated diverticulum or ulcerative colitis) or when rectum-sparing surgery is performed for colorectal cancer. When a temporary colostomy is created, the severed end of the colon is brought through the abdominal wall as for a permanent colostomy. The diseased or injured portion of the colon is resected and removed. The remaining rectum or rectosigmoid is oversewn and left in the peritoneal cavity; it is referred to as Hartmann's pouch. After the inflammatory process has resolved (e.g., 3-6 mo), the colostomy is taken down and reattached to the bowel of Hartmann's pouch, thus reconstructing continuity of the bowel and normal bowel elimination.

Cecostomy or ascending colostomy: Not a common procedure. A temporary diverting colostomy is used to bypass an unresectable tumor. The stool from an ascending colostomy is soft, unformed, pastelike, semiliquid, or liquid, and bowel elimination is unpredictable. Surgical procedure is similar to that with transverse colostomies.

Ileostomy

Conventional (Brooke) ileostomy: Created by bringing a distal portion of the resected ileum through the abdominal wall. A permanent ileostomy is created by the same procedure discussed with a permanent colostomy. Surgical indications include UC, CD, and familial adenomatous polyposis (FAP) requiring excision of the entire colon and rectum. For any ileostomy, the output is usually liquid (or, more rarely, pastelike) and is eliminated continually. The more proximal the ileostomy, the more active are digestive enzymes within

455

the effluent (stool) and the greater their potential for irritation to exposed skin around the stoma. A collection pouch is worn over the stoma on the abdomen to collect gas and fecal discharge.

Temporary ileostomy: Usually a loop stoma with or without a supporting rod in place beneath the loop of the ileum until the exteriorized loop of ileum heals to the skin. The purpose is to divert the fecal stream away from a more distal anastomotic site or fistula repair until healing has occurred.

Continent (Kock pouch) ileostomy: An intraabdominal pouch constructed from approximately 30 cm of distal ileum. Intussusception of a 10-cm portion of ileum is performed to form an outlet nipple valve from the pouch to the skin of the abdomen, where a stoma is constructed flush with the skin. The intraabdominal pouch is continent for gas and fecal discharge and is emptied approximately four times daily by inserting a catheter through the stoma. No external pouch is needed, and a Band-Aid or small dressing is worn over the stoma to collect mucus. Surgical indications include UC and FAP requiring removal of the colon and rectum. CD is generally a contraindication for this procedure because the disease can recur in the pouch, necessitating its removal. A long-term complication of Kock pouch is pouchitis. See under Ileal pouch anal anastomosis (IPAA) next, with the exception that tenesmus is not a symptom for a patient with a Kock pouch.

Ileal pouch anal anastomosis (IPAA) or restorative proctocolectomy: A two-stage surgical procedure developed to preserve fecal continence and prevent the need for a permanent ileostomy. During the first stage after total colectomy and removal of the rectal mucosa, an ileal reservoir or pouch is constructed and lowered into position in the pelvis just above the rectal cuff. Then the ileal outlet from the pouch is brought down through the cuff of the rectal muscle and anastomosed to the anal canal. The anal sphincter is preserved, and the resulting ileal pouch provides a storage place for feces. A temporary diverting ileostomy is required for 2-3 mo to allow healing of the anastomosis. The second stage occurs when the diverting ileostomy is taken down and fecal continuity is restored. Initially, the patient experiences fecal incontinence and 10 or more bowel movements per day. After 3-6 mo, the patient experiences decreased urgency and frequency with 4-8 bowel movements per day. This procedure is an option for patients requiring colectomy for UC or FAP. Its use is controversial in patients with CD. It is contraindicated with incontinence problems. *Pouchitis* is a long-term complication of IPAA. Its cause is unknown but may be due to stasis of bacteria in the ileal pouch. Symptoms include increased stool frequency, cramping, tenesmus, and bleeding. Pouchitis is effectively treated with metronidazole or ciprofloxacin. Probiotics also may be effective in preventing and maintaining remission in patients with recurrent pouchitis.

Nursing Diagnoses:

Risk for Impaired Skin Integrity: Peristomal

related to exposure to effluent or sensitivity to appliance material

Impaired Tissue Integrity: Stomal (or risk for same)

related to improperly fitted appliance resulting in impaired circulation

Desired Outcomes: Patient's stomal and peristomal skin and tissue remain nonerythremic and intact.

INTERVENTIONS	RATIONALES
After colostomy or conventional ileostomy (permanent or temporary)	
Apply a pectin, gelatin, methylcellulose-based, or synthetic solid-form skin barrier around stoma.	This barrier will protect peristomal skin from irritation caused by contact with stool or small bowel effluent.
Cut an opening in the skin barrier the exact circumference of the stoma or as recommended by manufacturer. Remove release paper and apply sticky surface directly to peristomal skin.	For some pouching systems, the skin barrier may be a separate barrier to be used with an adhesive-backed pouch, part of a two-piece system, or an integral part of a one-piece pouch system. Pectin-based paste also may be used to "caulk" around the barrier and compensate for irregular surfaces on peristomal skin. A pectin-based paste may prevent undermining of the barrier with effluent and protect skin immediately adjacent to the stoma.
Remove the skin barrier and inspect skin q3-4d. Monitor peristomal skin for erythema, erosion, serous drainage, bleeding, and induration. Carefully document abnormal findings, and report them to health care provider.	These indicators may signal presence of infection, irritation, or sensitivity to materials placed on the skin.

Continued

INTERVENTIONS	RATIONALES
Discontinue use of irritating materials, and substitute other materials.	This will help heal and protect irritated and/or denuded skin.
Patch-test patient's abdominal skin.	This will determine sensitivity to suspected materials.
Recalibrate skin barrier opening to size of stoma with each change.	Stomas become less edematous over a period of weeks after surgery, necessitating changes in the size of the skin barrier opening. The skin barrier opening should be the exact circumference of the stoma, or as recommended by the manufacturer, to prevent contact of stool with skin. Commercial templates are available to aid in estimating size of the opening needed for the skin barrier. Burning, itching, and odor are signs that stool or effluent may have contacted the skin. In order to prevent skin irritation or breakdown, the skin barrier should be changed immediately.
Empty pouch when it is one-third to one-half full of stool and/or gas.	This helps ensure maintenance of a secure pouch seal. A pouch with a larger amount of stool and/or gas could break the seal.

After continent ileostomy (Kock pouch)

INTERVENTIONS	RATIONALES
Avoid stress on ileostomy catheter and its securing suture.	This will prevent tissue destruction and catheter dislodgement.
As prescribed, maintain catheter on low, continuous suction or gravity drainage.	The catheter was inserted through the stoma into the continent ileostomy pouch during surgery to prevent stress on the nipple valve and maintain pouch decompression so that suture lines are allowed to heal without stress or tension.
Monitor site for erythema, induration, drainage, or erosion around the stoma. Report significant findings to health care provider.	These are signs of infection, irritation, or sensitivity to materials placed on the skin.
Check catheter q2h for patency, and irrigate with sterile saline (30 ml). Notify health care provider if solution cannot be instilled, if there are no returns from the catheter, or if leakage of irrigating solution or pouch contents appears around catheter.	These measures check for and help prevent catheter obstruction. Instilling 30 ml of saline will clear the catheter and liquefy the secretions/effluent without adding unnecessary pressure on the pouch walls and areas of anastomosis.
Change 4 × 4 dressing around stoma q2h or as often as it becomes wet.	This will help prevent peristomal skin irritation.
Report presence of frank bleeding to health care provider.	Normally, drainage will be serosanguineous at first and mixed with mucus.
Assess stoma for viability with each dressing change.	The stoma should be red in color and moist and shiny with mucus. A stoma that is pale, dark purple to black, or dull in appearance may indicate circulatory impairment and should be documented and reported to health care provider immediately.

After ileal pouch anal anastomosis (IPAA)

INTERVENTIONS	RATIONALES
After first stage of the operation, perform routine care for temporary diverting ileostomy.	See earlier discussion for "After colostomy or conventional ileostomy (permanent or temporary)."
Maintain perineal/perianal skin integrity by gently cleansing the area with water and cotton balls or soft tissues.	After first stage of the operation, patient may have incontinence of mucus.
Avoid soap.	Soap can cause itching and irritation.
Use absorbent pad at night.	This will absorb oozing mucus from the anus.
After second stage of the operation (when temporary diverting ileostomy is taken down), monitor patient's defecation pattern.	Expect patient to experience frequency and urgency of defecation.
Wash perineal/perianal area with warm water or commercial perineal/perianal cleansing solution, using squeeze bottle, cotton balls, or soft tissues.	This will promote comfort and cleanse the perineal/perianal area to ensure skin integrity.
Do not use toilet paper. If desired, dry the area with hair dryer on a cool setting.	Toilet paper can cause skin irritation. A hair dryer, on a cool setting, will prevent skin irritation potentially caused by other materials.
Provide sitz baths.	These will promote comfort and help clean the perineal/perianal area.
Apply protective skin sealants or ointments.	This will help maintain skin integrity.
	Note: Skin sealants containing alcohol should not be used on irritated or denuded skin because the high alcohol content would cause a painful burning sensation; apply only to intact skin.

••• **Related NIC and NOC labels:** *NIC:* Skin Surveillance; Circulatory Precautions; Incision Site Care; Ostomy Care; Skin Care: Topical Treatments; Self-Care Assistance: Bathing/Hygiene *NOC:* Tissue Integrity: Skin and Mucous Membranes

Nursing Diagnosis:

Bowel Incontinence

related to disruption of normal function with fecal diversion

Desired Outcomes: Within 2-4 days after surgery, patient has bowel sounds and eliminates gas and stool via the fecal diversion. Within 3 days after teaching has been initiated, patient verbalizes understanding of measures that will maintain normal elimination pattern and demonstrates care techniques specific to the fecal diversion.

INTERVENTIONS	RATIONALES
After colostomy and conventional ileostomy (permanent and temporary)	
Monitor intake and output (I&O). Empty stool from bottom opening of pouch and assess quality and quantity of stool. Record volume of liquid stool and its color and consistency.	This assessment documents return of normal bowel function and its quality and quantity. Expect serosanguinous to serous liquid drainage and flatus initially. Colostomy output of clear brown, liquid stool usually begins within 3-4 days. Ileostomy output of liquid, bilious effluent usually begins within 24-48 hours. Output consistency thickens as solid food is ingested and varies with type of ostomy.
If colostomy is not eliminating stool after 3-4 days and bowel sounds have returned, gently insert a gloved, lubricated finger into the stoma.	This may reveal presence of a stricture at skin or fascial levels and presence of any stool within reach of examining finger.
	To stimulate elimination of gas and stool, health care provider may prescribe colostomy irrigation. (For procedure, see **Deficient Knowledge:** Colostomy irrigation procedure, p. 460.)
After continent ileostomy (Kock pouch)	
Monitor I&O, and record amount, color, and consistency of output.	Expect bright red blood or serosanguinous liquid drainage from Kock pouch during early postoperative period.
As gastrointestinal (GI) function returns after 3-4 days, monitor and document color and character of output.	Expect drainage to change from blood-tinged to greenish brown liquid. When ileal output appears, suction (if used) is discontinued and pouch catheter is connected to or maintained on gravity drainage.
Check and irrigate catheter q2h and as needed.	This will maintain catheter patency. As patient's diet progresses from clear liquids to solid food, ileal output thickens. If patient reports abdominal fullness in area of pouch along with decreased fecal output, catheter placement and patency should be assessed.
When patient is alert and taking food by mouth, teach catheter irrigation procedure, which should be performed q2h; demonstrate how to empty pouch contents through the catheter into the toilet. Before hospital discharge, teach patient how to remove and reinsert catheter.	Irrigation liquefies effluent for easier flow through the catheter. Frequent irrigations prevent overdistention of the pouch.
	Teaching, followed by return demonstration, helps ensure that learning has occurred and facilitates retention of that information.
After ileal pouch anal anastomosis (IPAA)	
Monitor output from IPAA.	This assessment monitors quantity, quality, and consistency of output. Also see earlier discussion "After colostomy or conventional ileostomy (permanent or temporary)" for the monitoring of output from temporary diverting ileostomy.
Monitor patient for temperature elevation accompanied by perianal pain and discharge of purulent, bloody mucus from drains and anal orifice. Report significant findings to health care provider.	These are signs of infection or anastomotic leak, which should be reported for prompt intervention.
If drains are present, irrigate them as prescribed.	Irrigation helps maintain patency, decrease stress on suture lines, and decrease incidence of infection.
After first stage of the operation, advise patient to wear small pad in perianal area to absorb mucus drainage.	This will prevent soiling of outer garments. After first stage of the operation, patient may experience oozing of mucus from the anus.
After second stage of the operation (when temporary diverting ileostomy is taken down), monitor patient's output.	Expect incontinence and 15-20 bowel movements per day with urgency when patient is on a clear-liquid diet. Expect number of bowel movements to decrease to 6-12/day and consistency to thicken when patient is eating solid foods.

Continued

INTERVENTIONS	RATIONALES
Assist with perianal care, and apply protective skin care products.	This helps maintain perineal/perianal skin integrity. If nocturnal incontinence is especially troublesome, the catheter can be placed in the reservoir and connected to gravity drainage bag overnight.
Administer hydrophilic colloids and antidiarrheal medications as prescribed.	These agents decrease frequency and fluidity of stools.
Provide diet consultation.	Patient can learn about foods that cause liquid stools (spinach, raw fruits, highly seasoned foods, green beans, broccoli, prune and grape juices, alcohol) and increase intake of foods that cause thick stools (cheese, ripe bananas, applesauce, creamy peanut butter, gelatin, pasta).
Reassure patient that frequency and urgency are temporary and that as the reservoir expands and absorbs fluid, bowel movements should become thicker and less frequent.	This reassurance may decrease anxiety about the disruption of usual bowel pattern.

••• **Related NIC and NOC labels:** *NIC:* Bowel Management; Ostomy Care; Nutrition Management *NOC:* Bowel Elimination; Tissue Integrity: Skin and Mucous Membranes

Nursing Diagnosis:

Disturbed Body Image

related to presence of fecal diversion

Desired Outcome: Within 5-7 days after surgery, patient demonstrates actions that reflect beginning acceptance of the fecal diversion and incorporates changes into self-concept as evidenced by acknowledging body changes, viewing the stoma, and participating in the care of the fecal diversion.

INTERVENTIONS	RATIONALES
Monitor patient for expressed fears about the fecal diversion.	Many fears may be expressed by patients experiencing a fecal diversion. Some patients view incontinence as a return to infancy. The following fears may be expected: physical, social, and work activities will be curtailed significantly; rejection, isolation, and feelings of uncleanliness will occur; everyone will know about the altered pattern of fecal elimination; and loss of voluntary control may occur.
Encourage patient to discuss feelings and fears; clarify any misconceptions. Involve family members in discussions because they too may have anxieties and misconceptions.	Fears and anxieties about body image may be reduced by talking about them. Such discussions also enable clarification about misconceptions.
Provide a calm and quiet environment for patient and significant other to discuss the surgery. Initiate an open, honest discussion.	An open discussion enables understanding of patient's perspective of the impact the diversion will have and assists in development of an individualized plan of care that will help patient.
Monitor carefully for and listen closely to expressed or nonverbalized needs.	Each patient will react differently to the surgical procedure.
Encourage patient to participate in care.	Optimally, this will promote patient's acceptance of the fecal diversion and enhance a sense of control.
Assure patient that physical, social, and work activities will not be affected by presence of a fecal diversion.	Resuming previous lifestyle with minimal disruption is an essential component of the patient's rehabilitation. It helps rebuild a sense of independence and self-esteem.
Expect patient to have fears about sexual acceptance. If you are uncomfortable talking about sexuality with patients, be aware of these potential concerns and arrange for a consultation with someone who can speak openly and honestly about these problems.	Although these fears usually are not expressed overtly, concerns center on change in body image; fears about odor and the ostomy appliance interfering with intercourse; conception, pregnancy, and discomfort from perianal wound and scar in women; and impotence and failure to ejaculate in men, especially after more radical dissection of the pelvis in patients with cancer.

Continued

INTERVENTIONS	RATIONALES
Consult patient's health care provider about a visit by another person with an ostomy.	Patients gain reassurance and build positive attitudes and body image by seeing a healthy, active person who has undergone the same type of surgery, and it expands patient's support system as well.

••• **Related NIC and NOC labels:** *NIC:* Active Listening; Anxiety Reduction; Coping Enhancement; Emotional Support; Ostomy Care; Support Group; Body Image Enhancement *NOC:* Body Image

Nursing Diagnosis:

Deficient Knowledge:

Colostomy irrigation procedure

Desired Outcome: Within 3 days after initiation of teaching, patient demonstrates proficiency with the procedure for colostomy irrigation.

INTERVENTIONS	RATIONALES
Instruct patient about the following steps and have patient return demonstration:	The prescribed colostomy irrigation is taught to patient with permanent descending or sigmoid colostomy. Colostomy irrigation is performed daily or every other day so that wearing a pouch becomes unnecessary. An appropriate candidate is a patient who has one or two formed stools each day at predictable times (same as normal stool elimination pattern before illness). In addition, the patient must be able to manipulate the equipment, remember the technique, and be willing to spend approximately 1 hr/day performing the procedure. It may take 4-6 wk for the patient to have stool elimination regulated with irrigation.
	A return demonstration with explanation for each step will enable nurse to determine patient's knowledge level and facilitate learning retention for the patient.
Position irrigating sleeve over colostomy, centering stoma in opening. Secure sleeve in place with adhesive disk on the sleeve or with a sleeve belt.	The irrigation sleeve provides controlled diversion of stool and irrigation solution into the toilet.
Fill enema/irrigation container with 500-1000 ml (1-2 pints) warm water. With patient in a sitting position on toilet or on a chair facing toilet, position sleeve so that it empties into toilet. Hang enema/irrigation container so that the bottom surface is at patient's shoulder level.	Volume of water must be titrated for each patient to affect colon distention without causing cramping or excessive stretching of colon wall.
Open slide or roller clamp and flush tubing; reclamp tubing.	This removes air from the tubing.
Gently dilate stoma with a gloved finger lubricated with water-soluble lubricant.	This enables patient to identify direction of intestinal lumen and presence or absence of obstructing stool or stomal stenosis.
Lubricate cone, with or without attached catheter, and slowly insert into stoma.	This prevents bowel perforation. If cone has attached catheter, catheter should be inserted no more than 3 inches.
Hold the cone gently, but firmly, in place against stoma.	This prevents backflow of irrigant.
Let water slowly enter stoma from the container through the tubing; allow 15 min for fluid to enter the colon.	This prevents cramping caused by too-rapid infusion.
Note: If cramping occurs while water is flowing, stop the flow and leave cone in place until cramping passes, then flow of water may be resumed.	This likely will stop the cramping. If cramping does not resolve, the colon is probably ready to evacuate and should be allowed to do so.
After water has entered colon, advise patient to hold cone in place for a few seconds and then gently remove it.	This ensures complete infusion of water.
Leave sleeve in place for 30-40 min.	This enables water and stool to be eliminated.

Continued

INTERVENTIONS	RATIONALES
When elimination is complete, remove irrigation sleeve and cleanse and dry peristomal area.	Cleaning and drying the skin helps prevent skin irritation.
Apply a small dressing or security pouch over colostomy between irrigations.	This collects mucus drainage from the stoma. **Note:** During initial adaptation period, a drainable pouch is worn between irrigations to collect expected spillage of stool.

••• **Related NIC and NOC labels:** *NIC:* Teaching: Procedure *NOC:* Knowledge: Treatment Regimen

---

ADDITIONAL NURSING DIAGNOSES/ PROBLEMS:

"Perioperative Care"	p. 45
"Psychosocial Support"	p. 73

✓ PATIENT-FAMILY TEACHING AND DISCHARGE PLANNING

When providing patient-family teaching, focus on sensory information, avoid giving excessive information, and initiate a visiting nurse referral for necessary follow-up teaching. Include verbal and written information about the following:

✓ Medications, including drug name, rationale, dosage, schedule, route of administration, precautions, and potential side effects. Also discuss drug-drug, herb-drug, and food-drug interactions.

✓ Importance of dietary management to promote nutritional and fluid maintenance.

✓ Care of incision, dressing changes, and permission to take baths or showers once sutures and drains are removed.

✓ Care of stoma, care of peristomal and perianal skin, use of ostomy equipment, and method for obtaining supplies.

✓ Gradual resumption of ADL, excluding heavy lifting (more than 10 lb), pushing, or pulling for 6-8 wk to prevent development of incisional herniation.

✓ Referral to community resources including home health care agency; wound, ostomy, continence (WOC) nurse; local ostomy association; and the United Ostomy Association of America at *www.uoaa.org.*

✓ Importance of follow-up care with health care provider and WOC/ET nurse; confirm date and time of next appointment.

✓ Importance of reporting signs and symptoms that require medical attention, such as change in stoma color from normal bright and shiny red; peristomal or perianal skin irritation; any significant changes in appearance, frequency, and consistency of stools; fever, chills, abdominal pain, or distention; and incisional pain, increased local warmth, drainage, swelling, or redness; and signs and symptoms of pouchitis, including diarrhea, cramping, tenesmus, and bleeding.

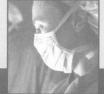
Hepatitis 57

OVERVIEW/PATHOPHYSIOLOGY

Viral hepatitis may be caused by one of five viruses that are capable of infecting the liver: hepatitis A (HAV), B (HBV), C (HCV), D or delta (HDV), or E (HEV). A sixth virus, hepatitis G (HGV), has been isolated in a few cases of hepatitis caused by other viruses of the five common strains. It is not known what the role of HGV is in liver disease, nor are clinical manifestations, natural history, or pathogenesis known. However, it has been found in 1.5% of blood donors, sometimes along with other hepatotropic viruses and sometimes alone. It also has been found in IV drug users, hemodialysis patients, and hemophiliacs. Although symptomatology is similar among all the hepatitis viruses, immunologic and epidemiologic characteristics are different. When hepatocytes are damaged, necrosis and autolysis can occur, which in turn lead to abnormal liver functioning. Generally these changes are completely reversible after the acute phase. In some cases, however, massive necrosis can lead to acute liver failure and death.

Chronic hepatitis is inflammation of the liver for more than 6 mo. The term is used to describe a spectrum of inflammatory liver diseases ranging from mild chronic persistent hepatitis to severe chronic active hepatitis. Forms of chronic hepatitis are associated with infection from HBV, HCV, and HDV; viral infections such as cytomegalovirus (CMV); excessive alcohol consumption; inflammatory bowel disease; and autoimmunity (chronic active lupoid hepatitis).

Alcoholic hepatitis occurs as a result of tissue necrosis caused by alcohol abuse; it is nonviral and noninfectious. Generally it is a precursor to cirrhosis (see p. 437), but it may occur simultaneous with cirrhosis.

Jaundice is discoloration of body tissues from increased serum levels of bilirubin (total serum bilirubin more than 2.5 mg/dl). Jaundice may be seen in any patient with impaired hepatic function and occurs as bilirubin begins to be excreted through the skin. There is also an increased excretion of urobilinogen and bilirubin by the kidneys, resulting in darker, almost brownish, urine. Jaundice is classified as follows.

Prehepatic (hemolytic): Caused by increased production of bilirubin following erythrocyte destruction. Prehepatic jaundice is implicated when the indirect (unconjugated) serum bilirubin is more than 0.8 mg/dl.

Hepatic (hepatocellular): Caused by the dysfunction of the liver cells (hepatocytes), which reduces their ability to re-move bilirubin from the blood and form it into bile. Hepatic jaundice is also implicated with indirect serum bilirubin and is associated with hepatitis.

Posthepatic (obstructive): Caused by an obstruction of the flow of bile out of the liver and resulting in backed-up bile through the hepatocytes to the blood. Posthepatic jaundice is implicated when direct serum bilirubin is more than 0.3 mg/dl.

HEALTH CARE SETTING

Primary care, with possible brief hospitalization resulting from complications

ASSESSMENT

Signs and symptoms: Nausea, vomiting, malaise, anorexia, muscle or joint aches, fatigue, irritability, slight to moderate temperature increases, epigastric discomfort, dark urine, clay-colored stools, pruritus, aversion to smoking.

Acute hepatic failure: Nausea, vomiting, and abdominal pain tend to be more severe. Jaundice is likely to appear earlier and deepen more rapidly. Mental status changes (possibly progressing to encephalopathy), coma, seizures, ascites, sharp rise in temperature, significant leukocytosis, coffee-ground emesis, gastrointestinal (GI) hemorrhage, purpura, shock, oliguria, and azotemia all may be present.

Physical assessment: Presence of jaundice; palpation of lymph nodes and abdomen may reveal lymphadenopathy, hepatomegaly, and splenomegaly. Liver size usually is small with acute hepatic failure.

History of: Clotting disorders, multiple blood transfusions, excessive alcohol ingestion, parenteral drug use, exposure to hepatotoxic chemicals or medications, travel to developing countries.

DIAGNOSTIC TESTS

Immunoglobulins: Chronic infection markers are present for HBV, HCV, and HDV. They are HBsAG, anti-HBc IgG for hepatitis B; anti-HCV (enzyme-linked immunosorbent assay) recombinant immunoblot assay (RIBA) for hepatitis C; and anti-HDV IgG for hepatitis D.

Serum enzymes: Aspartate aminotransferase (AST) and alanine aminotransferase (ALT) are initially elevated and then drop. Gamma-glutamyl transpeptidase (GGT) is elevated early in liver disease and persists as long as cellular damage continues.

Other hematologic tests: Total bilirubin is elevated, and prothrombin time (PT) is prolonged. Differential white blood cell (WBC) count reveals leukocytosis, monocytosis, and atypical lymphocytes.

Urine tests: Reveal elevation of urobilinogen, mild proteinuria, and mild bilirubinuria.

Liver biopsy: Performed percutaneously or via laparoscopy to collect a specimen for histologic examination to confirm differential diagnosis.

Nursing Diagnosis:

Fatigue

related to decreased metabolic energy production secondary to liver dysfunction, which causes faulty absorption, metabolism, and storage of nutrients

Desired Outcome: By at least 24 hr before hospital discharge, patient relates decreasing fatigue and increasing energy.

INTERVENTIONS	RATIONALES
Take a diet history to determine food preferences. Consult dietitian regarding increased intake of carbohydrates or other high-energy food sources within prescribed dietary limitations. Encourage significant other to bring in desirable foods if permitted. Monitor and record intake.	In general, dietary management consists of giving palatable meals as tolerated without overfeeding. If oral intake is substantially decreased, parenteral or enteral nutrition may be initiated. Sodium restrictions may be indicated in the presence of fluid retention. Protein is moderately restricted, or eliminated, depending on the degree of mental status changes (i.e., encephalopathy). If no mental status changes are noted, normal amounts of high biologic value protein are indicated to facilitate tissue healing, promote energy, and decrease fatigue. All alcoholic beverages are strictly forbidden. When appetite and food selection are poor, vitamins may be given to supplement dietary intake.
Encourage small, frequent feedings, and provide emotional support during meals.	Smaller and more frequent meals are usually better tolerated in patients who are fatigued, nauseated, and anorexic.
Provide rest periods of at least 90 min before and after activities and treatments.	Rest facilitates recovery after the body has experienced stress and may be indicated when symptoms are severe, with a gradual return to normal activity as symptoms subside.
Avoid activity immediately after meals.	Exercise after meals increases potential for nausea and vomiting, which could cause loss of nutrients and exacerbate fatigue.
Keep frequently used objects within easy reach.	This will help conserve patient's energy.
Decrease environmental stimuli; provide back massage and relaxation tapes; and speak with patient in short, simple terms.	These measures promote rest and sleep.
Administer acid suppression therapy, antiemetics, antidiarrheal medications, and cathartics as prescribed.	These agents minimize gastric distress and promote absorption of nutrients, which will help provide energy and reverse feelings of fatigue.

••• **Related NIC and NOC labels:** *NIC:* Energy Management; Nutrition Management; Sleep Enhancement; Simple Relaxation Therapy; Nutrition Therapy: Environmental Management *NOC:* Energy Conservation; Nutritional Status: Energy

Nursing Diagnosis:

Deficient Knowledge:

Causes of hepatitis and modes of transmission

Desired Outcome: Within the 24-hr period before hospital discharge, patient verbalizes knowledge about the causes of hepatitis and measures that help prevent transmission.

INTERVENTIONS

INTERVENTIONS	RATIONALES
Assess patient's health care literacy (language, reading, comprehension). Assess culture and culturally specific information needs.	This assessment helps ensure that information is presented in a manner that is culturally and educationally appropriate.
Assess patient's knowledge about the disease process, and educate as necessary.	Determining patient's level of knowledge will facilitate development of an individualized teaching plan.
Make sure patient knows you are not making moral judgments about alcohol/drug use or sexual behavior.	This will promote patient's confidence in you.
Teach patient and significant other importance of wearing gloves and using good handwashing technique if contact with body fluids such as urine, blood, wound exudate, or feces is possible.	These measures help prevent spread of infection.
If appropriate, advise patients with HAV that crowded living conditions with poor sanitation should be avoided.	This information may prevent recurrence.
Remind patients with HBV and HCV that they should modify sexual behavior as directed by health care provider. Explain that blood donation is no longer possible.	For patients with HBV and HCV, contact with blood is a likely mode of transmission, and blood contact can occur with some types of sexual activity. For patients with HBV, sexual contact is a likely mode.
Advise patients with HBV that their sexual partners should receive HBV vaccine.	For patients with HBV, sexual contact is a likely mode of transmission.
Refer patient to drug treatment programs as necessary.	Drug use can further damage the liver.

••• **Related NIC and NOC labels:** *NIC:* Teaching: Disease Process; Risk Identification; Health Education; Teaching: Safe Sex; Behavior Modification; Infection Protection; Substance Use Prevention; Infection Control; Immunization/Vaccination Management *NOC:* Knowledge: Disease Process; Knowledge: Health Behaviors; Knowledge: Infection Control

Nursing Diagnosis:

Risk for Impaired Skin Integrity

related to pruritus secondary to hepatic dysfunction

Desired Outcome: Patient's skin remains intact.

INTERVENTIONS	RATIONALES
Keep patient's skin moist by using tepid water or emollient baths, avoiding alkaline soap, and applying emollient lotions at frequent intervals.	Hot water and alkaline soaps can dry the skin and may cause irritation in patients with sensitive skin. Emollients and lipid creams (i.e., Eucerin) are used to keep patient's skin moist and supple.
Encourage patient not to scratch skin and to keep nails short and smooth. Suggest use of knuckles if patient must scratch. Wrap or place gloves on patient's hands (especially comatose patients).	These measures help prevent skin breakdown and infection. Knuckles and gloved hands are less traumatic to the skin and tissue than fingernails.
Treat any skin lesion promptly.	This will help prevent infection. Pathogens can enter the body through nonintact skin.
Administer antihistamines as prescribed; observe closely for excessive sedation.	Antihistamines may be used for symptomatic relief of pruritus. However, if used, they are administered with caution and in low doses because they are metabolized by the liver.
Encourage patient to wear loose, soft clothing; provide soft linens (cotton is best).	These measures help prevent abrasions caused by tight clothing or rough material on skin that is already compromised.
Keep environment cool.	Cool temperatures help prevent further skin irritation caused by perspiration.
Change soiled linen as soon as possible.	This measure helps prevent further irritation caused by waste products or fluids having constant skin contact.

••• **Related NIC and NOC labels:** *NIC:* Skin Surveillance; Bathing; Skin Care: Topical Treatments; Nail Care *NOC:* Tissue Integrity: Skin & Mucous Membranes

Nursing Diagnosis:

Ineffective Protection

related to increased risk of bleeding secondary to decreased vitamin K absorption, thrombocytopenia

Desired Outcome: Patient is free of bleeding as evidenced by negative tests for occult blood in the feces and urine, absence of ecchymotic areas, and absence of bleeding at the gums and injection sites.

INTERVENTIONS	RATIONALES
Monitor PT levels daily.	These assessments detect prolonged PT. Optimal range for PT is 10.5-13.5 sec. In hepatitis, PT is prolonged because of inability of the liver to produce coagulation factors.
Monitor platelet count daily.	These assessments detect thrombocytopenia. Optimal range is 150,000-400,000/mm^3. In hepatitis, platelet count is decreased because of decrease in production of thrombopoietin or platelet pooling caused by splenomegaly and portal hypertension.
Monitor hematocrit (Hct) and hemoglobin (Hgb) daily.	These assessments detect decreases that may indicate occult bleeding. Optimal ranges are Hct 40%-54% (male) and 37%-47% (female) and Hgb 14-18 g/dl (male) and 12-16 g/dl (female).
Handle patient gently (e.g., when turning or transferring).	This measure helps minimize risk of bleeding within the tissues.
Minimize IM injections. Rotate sites, and use small-gauge needles. Administer medications orally or IV when possible.	Bleeding may result from use of large-bore needles. Rotating sites helps prevent tissue damage caused by frequent injections in same tissue.
Apply moderate pressure after an injection, but do not massage site.	These measures minimize bleeding at injection site while preventing excessive pressure on tissue.
Observe for ecchymotic areas. Inspect gums, and test urine and feces for bleeding. Report significant findings to health care provider.	These assessments detect early signs of bleeding potential and abnormal bleeding sources.
Teach patient to use electric razor and soft-bristle toothbrush.	These measures minimize risk of bleeding from cuts or abrasions caused by razor or hard bristles.
Administer vitamin K as prescribed.	For patients with prolonged PT, vitamin K is a cofactor that modifies clotting factors to provide a site for calcium binding—an essential part of the clotting function. Patients with severe hepatic failure may not respond to vitamin K and may require transfusions of fresh frozen plasma.

••• **Related NIC and NOC labels:** *NIC:* Bleeding Precautions; Bleeding Reduction; Blood Products Administration *NOC:* Coagulation Status

ADDITIONAL NURSING DIAGNOSES/ PROBLEMS:

"Cirrhosis" for **Ineffective Protection,** if the patient develops encephalopathy   p. 440

✓ PATIENT-FAMILY TEACHING AND DISCHARGE PLANNING

When providing patient-family teaching, focus on sensory information, avoid giving excessive information, and initiate a visiting nurse referral for necessary follow-up teaching. Include verbal and written information about the following:

✓ Importance of rest and getting adequate nutrition. When appropriate, provide a list of high biologic value protein food sources or protein foods to avoid and sample menus to demonstrate how these foods may be incorporated into or excluded from the diet. Instruct patient to eat frequent, small meals; to eat slowly; and to chew all food thoroughly. Teach patient to rest for 30-60 min after meals. Initiate dietitian consult as needed for diet instruction.

✓ Importance of avoiding hepatotoxic agents, including over-the-counter (OTC) drugs. Examples of OTC drugs include aspirin and other salicylates, nonsteroidal antiinflammatory drugs, acetaminophen, alcohol, and vitamin A.

✓ Prescribed medications (e.g., multivitamins), including drug name, purpose, dosage, schedule, potential side effects, and precautions. Also discuss drug-drug, food-drug, and herb-drug interactions.

✓ Importance of informing health care providers, dentists, and other health care workers of hepatitis diagnosis.

✓ Potential complications, including delayed healing, skin injury, and bleeding tendencies.

✓ Importance of avoiding alcohol during recovery.

✓ Referral to alcohol/drug treatment programs as appropriate.

✓ Provide information about organizations available for education:

- Hepatitis Foundation International at *www.hepfi.org*
- Centers for Disease Control and Prevention at *www.cdc.gov/ncidod/diseases/hepatitis/index.htm*
- National Digestive Diseases Information Clearinghouse (NDDIC) at *http://digestive.niddk.nih.gov/resources/patient.htm*

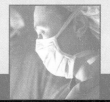

Pancreatitis 58

OVERVIEW/PATHOPHYSIOLOGY

The pancreas serves both endocrine (hormonal) and exocrine (nonhormonal) functions. (Pancreatic endocrine function is discussed in Diabetes Mellitus, p. 377). The exocrine portion comprises 98% of its tissue mass. Exocrine secretions, which are produced by the acini cells, empty through a series of lobular ducts into the main pancreatic duct, where they are released into the duodenum. Exocrine function is the secretion of potent enzymes, proteases, lipases, and amylases that act to reduce proteins, fats, and carbohydrates respectively into simpler chemical substances. Pancreatic proteases (trypsin, chymotrypsin, carboxypeptidases A and B, elastase, and phospholipase A) aid in protein digestion. Pancreatic lipase acts on fats to produce glycerides, fatty acids, and glycerol; pancreatic amylase acts on starch to produce disaccharides. The pancreas also secretes sodium bicarbonate to neutralize the strongly acidic gastric contents as it enters the duodenum. The resultant mixture of acids and bases provides an optimal pH of 8.3 for activation of pancreatic enzymes.

Pancreatitis, which can be acute or chronic, is an inflammation of the pancreas with varying degrees of edema, hemorrhage, and necrosis. The damage can lead to fibrosis, stricture, and calcifications. Acute pancreatitis occurs when pancreatic ductal flow becomes obstructed and digestive enzymes escape from the pancreatic duct into surrounding tissue. Self-destruction of the pancreas produces edema, hemorrhage, and necrosis of pancreatic and surrounding tissue. Biochemical abnormalities and disruption of cardiopulmonary, renal, metabolic, and gastrointestinal (GI) function are likely. Pancreatitis has been associated with gallstones, alcoholism, surgical manipulation, abdominal trauma, abdominal vascular disease, heavy metal poisoning, infectious agents (viral, bacterial, mycoplasma, parasitic), and some allergic reactions. Pancreatitis also is associated with familial hyperlipidemia and can be induced by endoscopic retrograde cholangiopancreatography (ERCP). The majority of acute pancreatitis cases are mild, require a short hospitalization, and leave no long-term adverse effects. Severe acute pancreatitis (SAP) involving multiple organ failure occurs in approximately 25% of cases but accounts for 98% of deaths associated with acute pancreatitis. Complications of acute pancreatitis include pancreatic abscess, hemorrhage, pancreatic pseudocyst, fistula formation, and transient hypoglycemia. Acute, life-threatening complications include renal failure, hemorrhagic pancreatitis, septicemia, adult respiratory distress syndrome (ARDS), shock, and disseminated intravascular coagulation (DIC).

Chronic pancreatitis is characterized by varying degrees of pancreatic insufficiency, which results in decreased production of enzymes and bicarbonate and malabsorption of fats and proteins. The digestion of fat is affected most severely. As a result, a high-fat content in the bowel stimulates water and electrolyte secretion, which produces diarrhea. The action of bacteria on fecal fat produces flatus, fatty stools (steatorrhea), and abdominal cramps. Often diabetes mellitus (DM) occurs as a result of chronic pancreatitis because of damage to the insulin-producing beta cells and resultant deficient insulin production. Chronic pancreatitis is also associated with complications of DM, chronic pain, maldigestion, pseudocysts, and bleeding.

HEALTH CARE SETTING

Primary care with hospitalization for acute pancreatitis and complications of chronic pancreatitis

ASSESSMENT

Acute pancreatitis: Symptoms vary according to severity of the attack. Sudden onset of constant, severe epigastric pain often occurs after a large meal or alcohol intake. Pain frequently radiates to the back or left shoulder and is somewhat relieved by a sitting position with the spine flexed. It is caused by biliary tree obstruction, enzymes irritating pancreatic and surrounding tissue, and the resulting edema. Nausea and vomiting, sometimes with persistent retching, usually occur and are caused by bowel hypermotility or ileus. Pain may be increased after vomiting because of increased pressure on the ducts, leading to further obstructions of secretions and tissue damage. Fever is usually present as well as hypotension and tachycardia. Jaundice suggests biliary tree obstruction. Extreme malaise, restlessness, respiratory distress, and diminished urinary output may be present. Hypovolemic shock may be present with hemorrhagic events, or distributive shock may occur secondary to systemic inflammatory response syndrome.

Physical assessment: Diminished or absent bowel sounds, suggesting presence of ileus; mild to moderate ascites; generalized abdominal tenderness; tachypnea, crackles (rales) at lung bases related to atelectasis, and interstitial fluid accumulation; diminished ventilatory excursion related to splinting and guarding with pain; low-grade fever (37.7°-38.8° C [100°-102° F]) or pronounced fever with abscess or sepsis; and agitation, confusion, and altered mental status may occur because of electrolyte/metabolic abnormalities or acute alcohol withdrawal. Gray-blue discoloration of the flank (Grey Turner's sign) or blue-red discoloration around the umbilicus (Cullen's sign) sometimes is present with pancreatic hemorrhage.

Chronic pancreatitis: Constant, dull epigastric pain; steatorrhea resulting from malabsorption of fats and protein; severe weight loss; and onset of symptoms of DM (polydipsia, polyuria, polyphagia). In addition, chemical addiction is often seen because of the chronic pain.

History of: Biliary tract disease; chronic excessive alcohol consumption; physical trauma to the abdomen (especially in young people); peptic ulcer disease; viral infection; ERCP; cystic fibrosis; neoplasms; shock; and use of certain medications, such as estrogen-containing oral contraceptives, glucocorticoids, sulfonamides, chlorothiazides, and azathioprine.

DIAGNOSTIC TESTS:

Serum amylase: When significantly elevated (more than 500 units/dl), rules out acute abdomen conditions, such as cholecystitis, appendicitis, bowel infarction/obstruction, and perforated peptic ulcer, and confirms presence of pancreatitis. These levels return to normal 48-72 hr after onset of acute symptoms, even though clinical indicators may continue. Sensitivity is limited in patients with alcoholic pancreatitis and hypertriglyceridemia.

Serum lipase: Has higher specificity and sensitivity than serum amylase. It rises more slowly than serum amylase and persists longer. Both lipase and amylase levels reflect the degree of necrotic pancreatic tissue. Higher cost and the few additional benefits of this test limit its use.

Blood glucose: Hyperglycemia occurs because of interference with beta cell function. It is transient with acute pancre-

atitis but common with chronic pancreatitis, during which DM is likely to develop.

Ultrasound, MRI, CT scan: May reveal an enlarged and edematous pancreatic head or abscess, pseudocyst, or calcification.

MR cholangiopancreatography: Used to visualize pancreatic and common bile ducts and may be used if an ERCP is not feasible.

ERCP: A combined endoscopic-radiographic tool that is used to study the degree of pancreatic disease via assessment of biliary-pancreatic ductal systems. It allows direct visualization of the ampulla of Vater, diagnoses biliary stones and duct stenosis, and distinguishes cancer of the pancreas from pancreatic calculi. ERCP is not performed until the acute episode has subsided.

Potassium: Hyperkalemia will occur in the presence of tissue damage, metabolic acidosis, and renal failure in severe cases.

Serum calcium and magnesium: May be lower than normal. On electrocardiogram, hypocalcemia is evidenced by prolonged QT segment with a normal T wave.

Complete blood count: Elevated white blood cells (WBCs) caused by inflammatory process. Polymorphonuclear bodies may increase if bacterial peritonitis is present secondary to duodenal rupture. Hematocrit (Hct) may be elevated or decreased.

BUN and serum creatinine: To evaluate renal function.

Urinalysis: May show presence of glycosuria, which can signal the onset of DM. Elevated urine amylase levels are useful diagnostically when serum levels have dropped off. An elevated specific gravity reflects the presence of dehydration.

Abdominal x-ray examination: May show dilation of the small or large bowel and presence of pancreatic calcification in chronic pancreatitis.

Secretin stimulation test: To diagnosis chronic pancreatitis.

Nursing Diagnosis:

Deficient Fluid Volume

related to active loss secondary to nasogastric (NG) suctioning, vomiting, diaphoresis, or pooling of fluids in the abdomen and retroperitoneum

Desired Outcome: Patient is normovolemic within 8 hr of admission as evidenced by HR 60-100 bpm, CVP 2-6 mm Hg (5-12 cm H_2O), brisk capillary refill (less than 2 sec), peripheral pulse amplitude greater than 2+ on a 0-4+ scale, urinary output at least 30 ml/hr, and stable weight and abdominal girth measurements.

INTERVENTIONS	RATIONALES
Monitor vital signs (VS) q2-4h.	This assessment enables detection of a falling blood pressure (BP) and increasing heart rate (HR) (100-140 bpm), which can occur with moderate to severe fluid loss.

Continued

INTERVENTIONS	RATIONALES
Measure intake and output (I&O) and central venous pressure (CVP), if available, q2-4h. Weigh patient daily, and note trends. Correlate weights with I&O ratios.	CVP less than 2 mm Hg can occur with volume-related hypotension, and output greater than intake signals fluid loss. Weight decreases when fluid is lost or intake is insufficient. Fluid loss requires immediate replacement to prevent shock and acute renal failure. Approximately 1 kg weight = 1 L fluid.
Measure orthostatic VS initially and q8h.	This enables detection of decreasing BP and increasing HR on standing, which suggests need for crystalloid and/or colloid volume expansion.
Administer parenteral solutions and plasma volume expanders as prescribed.	These measures help maintain adequate circulating blood volume. Examples of blood volume expanders include albumin and plasma protein fraction.
Monitor closely for adventitious breath sounds, increased weight, and drop in Hct without concomitant blood loss.	These are signs of fluid overload and potentially of pulmonary edema as a result of overly aggressive fluid resuscitation. In cases of severe, acute pancreatitis, patients develop a profound loss of circulating blood volume and need adequate fluid resuscitation quickly, sometimes as much as 5-6 L/day. This increases risk for fluid overload, especially if patient has been hypotensive and the kidneys are not functioning well enough to handle the large amounts of fluid. The fluid overload can lead to pulmonary edema and respiratory failure. In fact, respiratory dysfunction is the most frequent complication of severe, acute pancreatitis and one of the main causes of early death.
Be alert to positive Chvostek's sign (facial muscle spasm) and Trousseau's sign (carpopedal spasm), muscle twitching, tetany, or irritability.	These signs are indicators of hypocalcemia, which can occur with electrolyte loss.
Administer electrolytes (K^+, Ca^{2+}) as prescribed.	These electrolytes help prevent cardiac dysrhythmias, tetany, and other problems caused by their specific decreases.
Monitor values of the following for irregularities: Hct, Hgb, WBCs, Ca^{2+}, glucose, blood urea nitrogen (BUN), creatinine, and K^+.	Irregularities can occur in patients with infection, inflammatory response, and bleeding caused by necrotic pancreas and would be outside the following normal values: Hct 40%-54% (male) and 37%-47% (female); Hgb 14-18 g/dl (male) and 12-16 g/dl (female); Ca^{2+} 8.5-10.5 mg/dl (4.3-5.3 mEq/L); glucose 145 mg/dl (2-hr postprandial) and 65-110 mg/dl (fasting); BUN 6-20 mg/dl; K^+ 3.5-5 mEq/L; and WBCs 4500-11,000 mm^3.

••• **Related NIC and NOC labels:** *NIC:* Fluid/Electrolyte Management; Electrolyte Monitoring; Laboratory Data Interpretation; Vital Signs Monitoring; Blood Products Administration *NOC:* Electrolyte and Acid-Base Balance; Fluid Balance

Nursing Diagnosis:

Acute Pain

related to inflammatory process of the pancreas

Desired Outcomes: Within 6 hr of intervention, patient's subjective perception of discomfort decreases, and it is controlled within 24 hr, as documented by pain scale. Nonverbal indicators, such as splinting of abdominal muscles, are absent or diminished.

INTERVENTIONS	RATIONALES
Assess for and document degree and character of patient's discomfort. Devise a pain scale with patient, rating discomfort on a scale of 0 (no pain) to 10 (worst pain).	Pain characteristics may signal varying problems (see Assessment section). Baseline and subsequent use of pain scale helps determine effectiveness of pain relief.
Assess patient's previous responses to pain and previously effective pain relief measures. Consider possible cultural and spiritual influences.	Patient's previous history of pain and how well it was managed influence perceptions and trust in present pain relief measures. Some cultures allow less outward show of pain, whereas others do not prohibit expressions of pain.

Continued

INTERVENTIONS	RATIONALES
Ensure that patient maintains limited activity or bedrest.	Rest helps minimize pancreatic secretions and pain.
Maintain NPO (nothing by mouth) status, and monitor NG tube function.	NPO status and NG suction are initiated early in the course of illness to decrease stimulus for pancreatic secretions and reduce stress in the GI tract. After acute pain and ileus have resolved, the patient is given clear liquids and diet is advanced as tolerated.
Administer analgesics, steroids, histamine H$_2$-receptor blockers, anti-emetics, and other medications as prescribed. Be alert to patient's response to medications, using pain scale.	Analgesics reduce discomfort associated with pancreatitis. Steroids may be given to reduce inflammation in certain types of pancreatitis when infection is not a problem.
	Histamine H$_2$-receptor blockers are given to reduce gastric acid secretion, which stimulates pancreatic enzymes. Antiemetics (e.g., hydroxyzine, ondansetron, prochlorperazine, promethazine) are given for nausea and vomiting. Antacids are given to neutralize gastric acid and reduce associated pain. **Note:** Both morphine and meperidine may cause spasms at the sphincter of Oddi, although meperidine may be less likely to do so. However, large doses and prolonged use of meperidine can lead to seizures. Response varies with the individual. Pentazocine may be used as an alternative analgesic.
Instruct patient to request analgesic before pain becomes severe.	Pain is more easily managed when it is treated before it becomes severe. If analgesic is ineffective, health care provider should be notified because patient may require another intervention. Optimally, analgesics are administered via patient-controlled pumps.
Avoid IM injections in individuals with clotting or bleeding complications.	Transdermal analgesic or small, frequent doses of IV opioids usually are more effective than IM injections, which also increase the risk of bleeding in individuals with bleeding/clotting complications.
Assist patient in attaining a position of comfort.	A sitting or supine position with knees flexed often helps relax abdominal muscles.
Emphasize nonpharmacologic pain interventions (e.g., relaxation techniques, distraction, guided imagery, massage). See **Health-Seeking Behaviors:** Relaxation technique effective for stress reduction, p. 172.	These interventions are especially important for patients in whom chronic pancreatitis develops and who are prone to chemical dependence.
Prepare significant other for personality changes and behavioral alterations associated with extreme pain and opioid analgesic. Reassure them that these are normal responses.	Pancreatitis can be very painful. Family members sometimes misinterpret patient's lethargic or unpleasant disposition and may even blame themselves.
Monitor patient's respiratory pattern and level of consciousness (LOC) closely.	Both may be depressed by the large amount of opioids usually required to control pain.
	Note: Opioid analgesics also decrease intestinal motility and delay return to normal bowel function.
Report O$_2$ saturation less than 92%.	Continuous pulse oximetry identifies decreasing oxygen saturation associated with hypoventilation. Values less than 92% often signal need for supplemental oxygen.
Consider referral to a pain management team.	A pain management team can help with conventional pain control measures during acute pain situations in patients with chronic or frequent bouts of pancreatitis or with low pain tolerance. Less conventional measures such as nerve blocks that interfere with transmission of pain sensations along visceral nerve fibers are effective in the relief of pancreatic pain. Bilateral splanchnic nerve or left celiac ganglion blocks may be performed as well.

For additional pain interventions, see "Pain," p. 39.

●●● **Related NIC and NOC labels:** *NIC:* Pain Management; Medication Management; Analgesic Administration; Positioning; Patient-Controlled Analgesia Assistance; Simple Massage; Simple Relaxation Therapy; Distraction; Family Support *NOC:* Comfort Level; Pain Control; Pain: Disruptive Effects

Nursing Diagnosis:

Impaired Gas Exchange (or risk for same)

related to ventilation-perfusion mismatching secondary to atelectasis or accumulating pulmonary fluid

Desired Outcome: Patient has adequate gas exchange as evidenced by RR 12-20 breaths/ min with normal depth and pattern (eupnea); oxygen saturation greater than 92%; no significant changes in mental status; orientation to person, place, and time; and breath sounds that are clear and audible throughout the lung fields.

INTERVENTIONS	RATIONALES
Monitor and document respiratory rate (RR) q2-4h as indicated by patient's condition. Note pattern, degree of excursion, and whether patient uses accessory muscles of respiration. Report significant deviations from baseline to health care provider.	Irregular pattern, decreased chest excursion, and use of accessory muscles of respiration occur with impending respiratory compromise (can occur with ARDS and respiratory failure) and may be a sign of inadequate pain control or worsening pancreatitis.
Auscultate both lung fields q4-8h.	Presence of abnormal (crackles, rhonchi, wheezes) or diminished breath sounds can occur with fluid overload (see discussion in **Deficient Fluid Volume,** earlier) or atelectasis.
Monitor sputum production, and promptly report to health care provider an increase or color change (from clear to white to yellow to green) in respiratory secretions.	Copious secretions that change color can indicate respiratory tract infection; copious secretions without color changes can occur with pulmonary edema.
Be alert to changes in mental status, restlessness, agitation, and alterations in mentation.	These are early signs of hypoxia.
Monitor pulse oximetry q8h or as indicated (report oxygen saturation 92% or less). Monitor arterial blood gas results as available (report Pao_2 less than 80 mm Hg).	These decreased values usually signal need for supplementary oxygen.
Administer oxygen as prescribed. Monitor oxygen delivery system at regular intervals.	Hypoxia is an early sign of impending respiratory failure and necessitates oxygen delivery.
Elevate head of bed 30 degrees or higher, depending on patient comfort.	This position optimizes ventilation and oxygenation.
If pleural effusion or other defect is present on one side, position patient with unaffected lung dependent.	This position maximizes ventilation-perfusion relationship, which optimizes oxygenation.
Avoid overaggressive fluid resuscitation.	This could lead to hypoxia, heart failure, pleural effusions, and respiratory failure. See discussion on **Deficient Fluid Volume,** earlier.
Explain to patient and significant other that patient is at risk for hypostatic pneumonia.	Pancreatitis results in decreased production of surfactant, and pain limits adequate respiratory excursion, increasing potential for hypostatic pneumonia.
Teach use of hyperinflation device (e.g., incentive spirometer) followed by coughing exercises. Explain that emphasis of this therapy is on inhalation to expand the lungs maximally. Ensure that patient inhales slowly and deeply 2× normal tidal volume and holds the breath at least 5 sec at end of inspiration. Monitor patient's progress and document in nurses' notes.	Deep breathing expands alveoli and aids in mobilizing secretions to the airways, while coughing further mobilizes and clears secretions. Ten breaths/hr is recommended to maintain adequate alveolar inflation.
When appropriate, teach methods of splinting wounds or upper abdomen.	Splinting helps reduce pain and enable effective cough.
Teach cascade cough (i.e., a succession of more short and forceful exhalations) to patients who cannot cough effectively.	A cascade cough helps keep lung expanded when abdominal pain would not otherwise enable deep cough.
Encourage activity as prescribed.	Activity helps mobilize secretions and promote effective airway clearance.

••• **Related NIC and NOC labels:** *NIC:* Oxygen Therapy; Chest Physiotherapy; Positioning; Respiratory Monitoring; Cough Enhancement; Pain Management *NOC:* Respiratory Status: Gas Exchange; Tissue Perfusion: Pulmonary

Nursing Diagnosis:

Risk for Infection

related to potential for tissue destruction with resulting necrosis secondary to release of pancreatic enzymes

Desired Outcome: Patient remains free of infection as evidenced by body temperature less than 37.7° C (less than 100° F); negative culture results; HR 60-100 bpm; RR 12-20 breaths/min; BP within patient's normal range; and orientation to person, place, and time.

INTERVENTIONS	RATIONALES
Check patient's temperature q4h.	An increase may signal infection. **Note:** Hypothermia may precede hyperthermia in some individuals, particularly older adults.
Monitor BP, HR, and RR q4h.	Increases in HR (up to 100-140 bpm) and RR are associated with infection of the necrotic pancreatic tissue. BP may be either transiently high or low with significant orthostatic hypotension.
If there is a sudden elevation in temperature, obtain specimens for culture of blood, sputum, urine, wound, drains, and other sites as indicated. Monitor culture reports, and report findings promptly to health care provider.	Cultures enable detection of developing necrotic pancreas or presence of abscess.
Evaluate patient's mental status, orientation, and LOC q4-8h. Document and report significant deviations from baseline.	Impairments may occur with alcohol withdrawal, hypotension, electrolyte imbalance, hypoxia, and from the sepsis associated with the necrotic, infected pancreas.
Administer parenteral antibiotics in a timely fashion. Reschedule antibiotics if a dose is delayed for more than 1 hr.	These measures help maintain bacteriocidal serum levels. Failure to administer antibiotics on schedule can result in inadequate blood levels and treatment failure.
Observe all secretions and drainage for changes in appearance or odor that may signal infection.	Sputum, for example, can become more copious and change in color from clear to white to yellow to green.
Use good handwashing technique before and after caring for patient and dispose of dressings and drainage carefully.	This measure helps prevent transmission of potentially infectious agents.

••• Related NIC and NOC labels: *NIC:* Infection Control; Infection Protection; Laboratory Data Interpretation; Medication Administration; Respiratory Monitoring; Vital Signs Monitoring *NOC:* Infection Status

Nursing Diagnosis:

Imbalanced Nutrition: Less Than Body Requirements

related to anorexia, dietary restrictions, and digestive dysfunction

Desired Outcome: Patient maintains baseline body weight and exhibits a positive or balanced nitrogen (N) state on N studies by 24 hr before hospital discharge.

INTERVENTIONS	RATIONALES
Be alert to dysphagia, polydipsia, and polyuria.	These indicators of a hyperglycemic state reflect need for health care provider evaluation and intervention to ensure proper metabolism of carbohydrates if endocrine function is impaired. Hyperglycemia occurs because of interference with beta cell function. It is transient with acute pancreatitis but common with chronic pancreatitis, during which DM is likely to develop.
Monitor capillary blood sugar levels for presence of hyperglycemia. Adjust insulin amounts according to capillary blood glucose levels, as prescribed.	Laboratory values of fasting blood sugar and bedside monitoring of blood glucose may reveal abnormalities in blood glucose levels and direct the appropriate insulin therapy (see "Diabetes Mellitus," p. 377, for more information).

Continued

INTERVENTIONS	RATIONALES
Deliver enteral or parenteral nutrition as prescribed.	Enteral feedings are being used with increasing frequency but should be infused past the ligament of Treitz to avoid pancreatic stimulation. Parenteral nutrition likely is instituted if distal enteral feedings are unobtainable or unsuccessful within 5-7 days.
Provide oral hygiene at frequent intervals.	This measure enhances appetite and minimizes nausea.
When the gastric tube is removed, provide diet as prescribed.	Small, high-carbohydrate, low-fat meals at frequent intervals (six per day) with protein added according to patient's tolerance is the usual diet for patients with pancreatitis.
Instruct patient to avoid coffee, tea, alcohol, and nicotine or other gastric irritants.	These are stimulants that increase pancreatic enzyme secretion.
Weigh patient daily to assess gain or loss.	Progressive weight loss may signal need to change diet or provide enzyme replacement therapy.
Note amount and degree of steatorrhea (foamy, foul-smelling stools high in fat content).	This is an indicator of fat intolerance, which is common with chronic pancreatitis. Steatorrhea can indicate recurrence of disease process or ineffectiveness of drug therapy and should be reported to health care provider.
As prescribed, administer pancreatic enzyme supplements.	Pancreatic enzyme supplements are given before introducing fat into the diet to enable its digestion.
If prescribed, administer other dietary supplements that support nutrition and caloric intake.	These supplements, which may include products that consist of medium-chain triglycerides (MCTs) such as MCT oil, do not require pancreatic enzymes for absorption.
Avoid administering pancreatin with hot foods or drinks.	Heat deactivates its enzyme activity.
Provide meals in small feedings throughout the day.	Smaller, more frequent meals may help alleviate bloating, nausea, and cramps experienced by some patients.

••• **Related NIC and NOC labels:** *NIC:* Nutrition Management; Nutrition Therapy; Teaching: Prescribed Diet; Sustenance Support
NOC: Nutritional Status; Nutritional Status: Food & Fluid Intake

ADDITIONAL NURSING DIAGNOSES/ PROBLEMS:

"Pain"	p. 39
"Perioperative Care"	p. 45
"Providing Nutritional Support"	p. 565

 PATIENT-FAMILY TEACHING AND DISCHARGE PLANNING

When providing patient-family teaching, focus on sensory information, avoid giving excessive information, and initiate a visiting nurse referral for necessary follow-up teaching. Include verbal and written information about the following:

✓ Cause for current episode of pancreatitis, if known, so that recurrence may be avoided.

✓ Alcohol consumption, which can cause or exacerbate chronic pancreatitis.

✓ Availability of chemical dependency programs to prevent/treat drug dependence, which is a common occurrence with chronic pancreatitis; or to treat alcoholism. Discuss availability of community support groups, such as the following:

- Alcoholics Anonymous at *www.alcoholics-anonymous.org*
- Narcotics Anonymous at *www.na.org*

✓ Diet: frequent, small meals that are high in carbohydrates and protein. Food should be bland until gradual return to normal diet is prescribed. Remind patient to avoid enzyme stimulants, such as coffee, tea, nicotine, and alcohol.

✓ Medications, including drug name, purpose, dosage, schedule, precautions, and potential side effects. Also discuss drug-drug, food-drug, and herb-drug interactions.

✓ Signs and symptoms of DM, including fatigue, weight loss, polydipsia, polyuria, and polyphagia.

✓ Necessity of medical follow-up; confirm time and date of next medical appointment.

✓ Potential for recurrence of steatorrhea as evidenced by foamy, foul-smelling stools that are high in fat content.

✓ Weighing daily at home; importance of reporting weight loss to health care provider.

✓ If surgery was performed, the indicators of wound infection: redness, swelling, discharge, fever, pain, or increased local warmth.

✓ For more information, contact National Institute of Diabetes & Digestive & Kidney Diseases at *www.niddk.nih.gov.*

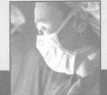

Peptic Ulcers 59

OVERVIEW/PATHOPHYSIOLOGY

Peptic ulcers are erosions of the upper gastrointestinal (GI) tract mucosa, potentially extending through the muscularis mucosa and into the muscularis propria. They may occur anywhere the mucosa is exposed to the erosive action of gastric acid and pepsin. Commonly, ulcers are gastric or duodenal, but the esophagus, surgically created stomas, and other areas of the upper GI tract may be affected. Autodigestion of mucosal tissue and ulceration are associated with increased acidity of the stomach juices or increased sensitivity of the mucosal surfaces to erosion. Erosions can penetrate deeply into the mucosal layers and become a chronic problem, or they can be more superficial and manifest as an acute problem resulting from severe physiologic or psychologic trauma, infection, or shock (stress ulceration of the stomach or duodenum). Both duodenal and gastric ulcers can occur in association with high-stress lifestyle, smoking, use of irritating drugs, as well as secondary to other diseases. Ulceration may occur as a part of Zollinger-Ellison syndrome, in which gastrinomas (gastrin-secreting tumors) of the pancreas or other organs develop. Gastric acid hypersecretion and ulceration subsequently occur. However, the most common causes of peptic ulcer disease are use of nonsteroidal antiinflammatory drugs (NSAIDs) and infection with *Helicobacter pylori (H. pylori)*.

H. pylori, a gram-negative, spiral-shaped bacterium with four to six flagella on one pole, was first isolated from gastric biopsies in 1983. *H. pylori* can reside below the mucosa of the stomach because it produces the enzyme *urease*, which hydrolyses urea to ammonia and carbon dioxide, providing a buffering alkaline halo. Infection can go undetected for years because there may be no symptoms until gastric or duodenal ulceration or gastritis occurs. Transmission of *H. pylori* has been determined to be by fecal-oral and oral-oral routes of transmission. A high duodenal acid load is one of the characteristics of duodenal ulcer disease inasmuch as it reduces concentration of bile acids that normally inhibit growth of *H. pylori*. Gastric ulcers tend to occur on the lesser curvature of the stomach. Ulcers in both locations are characterized by slow healing leading to metaplasia. In turn, a greater colonization with *H. pylori* causes slow healing and results in a vicious cycle.

Serious and disabling complications, such as hemorrhage, GI obstruction, perforation, peritonitis, or intractable ulcer pain, are common. With treatment, ulcer healing usually occurs within 4-6 wk (gastric ulcers can take as long as 12-16 wk to heal), but there is potential for recurrence in the same or another site.

HEALTH CARE SETTING

Primary care; acute care for complications

ASSESSMENT

Signs and symptoms: Burning, gnawing, dull pain typically 1-3 hr after eating. Discomfort occurs more often between meals and at night. With duodenal ulcer, eating usually alleviates discomfort; with gastric ulcer, pain often worsens after meals. Older adults have less sensory perception in the stomach and may not experience pain as a symptom. In addition, 40% of patients with active ulcers deny abdominal pain. However, on examination there may be findings of ulcers, gastritis, and other conditions. Even so, pain symptoms warrant further investigation.

Hematemesis, melena, dizziness, and syncope are associated with an actively bleeding ulcer. Sudden, severe epigastric pain, often radiating to the right shoulder, suggests perforation of an ulcer. Pain described as piercing through to the back suggests penetration of the ulcer into adjacent posterior structures in the abdomen.

Physical assessment: Tenderness over the involved area of the abdomen. With perforation, there is severe pain (see "Peritonitis" for more information) and rebound tenderness. With penetration, the pain is usually altered by changes in back position (extension or flexion).

History of: NSAID use; chronic or acute stress; smoking; use of irritating agents such as caffeine, alcohol, corticosteroids, salicylates, reserpine, indomethacin, or phenylbutazone; disorders of the endocrine glands, pancreas, or liver; and hypersecretory conditions, such as Zollinger-Ellison syndrome.

DIAGNOSTIC TESTS

Endoscopy: Allows visualization of the stomach (gastroscopy), duodenum (duodenoscopy), both stomach and duodenum (gastroduodenoscopy), or the esophagus, stomach, and duodenum (esophagogastroduodenoscopy) via passage of a lighted, fiberoptic, flexible tube. Patient is NPO (given nothing by mouth) for 8-12 hr before the procedure, and written consent is required. Before the test, a sedative is administered

477

to relax the patient, and an opioid analgesic may be given to prevent pain. Local anesthetic may be sprayed into the posterior pharynx to ease passage of the tube. A biopsy may be performed as part of the endoscopy procedure. Biopsied tissue may be sent for histologic examination and for culture and sensitivity to identify *H. pylori* infection. Postprocedure care involves maintaining NPO status for ½-1 hr; ensuring return of the gag reflex before allowing the patient to eat (if local anesthetic was used); administering throat lozenges or analgesics as prescribed; and monitoring for complications, such as bleeding or perforation (e.g., hematemesis, pain, dyspnea, tachycardia, hypotension).

H. pylori testing: Serum antigen testing identifies exposure to *H. pylori* bacteria; this is the least expensive means of identifying *H. pylori* infection. However antibody tests remain positive many months after successful therapy and are not reliable for assessing therapy effectiveness. A breath test is available to identify *H. pylori* infection by detecting carbon dioxide and ammonia as by-products of the action of the bacterium's urease in the patient's expired air. Histologic identification of the microorganism and culture are other direct tests for *H. pylori*. Direct tests and stool antigen testing require discontinuation of all drugs that suppress *H. pylori* for 2 wk before testing.

Barium swallow: Uses contrast agent (e.g., barium) to detect abnormalities. Patient should maintain NPO status and not smoke for at least 8 hr before the test. Postprocedure care involves administration of prescribed laxatives and enemas to facilitate passage of the barium and prevent constipation and fecal impaction.

CBC: Reveals a decrease in hemoglobin (Hgb), hematocrit (Hct), and red blood cells when acute or chronic blood loss accompanies ulceration.

Stool for occult blood: Positive if bleeding is present.

Gastric secretion analysis: Performed rarely due to general unavailability of pentagastrin. Its lack of clinical utility makes it a useful diagnostic tool only in patients who have hypergastrinemia or when evaluating for gastric cancer. A nasogastric (NG) tube is passed, and the stomach contents are aspirated and analyzed for the presence of blood and free hydrochloric acid. Achlorhydria (absence of free hydrochloric acid) suggests gastric cancer, whereas mildly elevated levels suggest gastric ulcer. Excessive elevation of free hydrochloric acid occurs with Zollinger-Ellison syndrome. A tubeless gastric analysis involves administration of a gastric stimulant followed by a resin dye. A urine specimen is obtained 2 hr later and analyzed for the presence of dye. Absence of dye indicates achlorhydria. The patient is NPO for at least 8 hr before either test.

Nursing Diagnosis:

Ineffective Protection

related to potential for bleeding, obstruction, and perforation secondary to ulcerative process

Desired Outcome: Patient is free of signs and symptoms of bleeding, obstruction, perforation, and peritonitis as evidenced by negative results for occult blood testing, passage of stool and flatus, soft and nondistended abdomen, good appetite, and normothermia.

INTERVENTIONS	RATIONALES
Assess for hematemesis and melena. Check all NG aspirate, emesis, and stools for occult blood. Report positive findings.	Bleeding can occur with an ulcerative process.
Monitor results of complete blood count (CBC) and coagulation studies.	Hct less than 40% (male) or less than 37% (female) and Hgb less than 14 g/dl (male) or less than 12 g/dl (female) are indicators of bleeding and should be reported promptly.
	The incidence of peptic ulcers is increased in cirrhosis patients, in whom clotting factors are altered. Partial thromboplastin time (PTT) greater than 70 sec or prothrombin time (PT) greater than 12.5 sec are longer than normal clotting times.
If indicated, insert a gastric tube.	A gastric tube will enable evacuation of blood from the stomach, monitoring of bleeding, and gastric lavage as prescribed.
Do not use gastric tubes in patients who have or are suspected of having esophageal varices.	Trauma from tube insertion could result in hemorrhage.
Monitor O_2 saturation via oximetry and report O_2 saturation less than 92%.	Usually patients with O_2 saturation less than 92% require oxygen supplementation.
If patient is actively bleeding or if Hct is low, administer prescribed O_2.	A low Hct or Hgb indicates an anemic state, which means there is less available Hgb for oxygen transport.

Continued

INTERVENTIONS

INTERVENTIONS	RATIONALES
Monitor and note abdominal pain, abnormal (increased peristalsis, "rushes," or "tinkles") or absent bowel sounds, distention, anorexia, nausea, vomiting, and inability to pass stool or flatus.	These are indicators of obstruction, a serious complication of peptic ulcers, which necessitates prompt notification of health care provider for rapid intervention.
Be alert to sudden or severe abdominal pain, distention, and rigidity; fever; nausea; and vomiting. Notify health care provider immediately of significant findings. See "Peritonitis," p. 481, for more information.	These are indicators of perforation and peritonitis, serious complications of peptic ulcers, which necessitate prompt notification of health care provider for rapid intervention.
Teach signs and symptoms of GI complications and importance of reporting them promptly to staff or health care provider if they occur.	A knowledgeable patient likely will report these signs promptly, which will enable rapid treatment.

••• **Related NIC and NOC labels:** *NIC:* Bleeding Precautions *NOC:* Coagulation Status

Nursing Diagnosis:

Impaired Tissue Integrity

related to exposure to chemical irritants (gastric acid, pepsin)

Desired Outcomes: Patient verbalizes knowledge of necessary lifestyle alterations within the 24-hr period before hospital discharge and demonstrates compliance with medical recommendations for peptic ulcer throughout the hospital stay. Gastric and duodenal mucosal tissues heal and remain intact as evidenced by reduced or absent pain and absence of bleeding.

INTERVENTIONS	RATIONALES
Encourage patient to avoid foods that seem to cause pain or increase acid secretion.	Although this response is highly individualized, foods that cause pain or increase acid secretion worsen mucosal erosion.
Advise patient to avoid coffee, caffeine, alcohol, aspirin, and NSAIDs.	These foods and drugs are associated with increased acidity and GI erosions.
If applicable, recommend strategies for smoking cessation.	Smoking impairs ulcer healing and has been associated with a higher incidence of complications and the need for surgical repair of the ulcer.
Administer *H. pylori* eradication therapy for *H. pylori*–associated ulceration.	Highest eradication rates are obtained with either of the following regimens: (1) proton pump inhibitor (PPI), clarithromycin 500 mg twice daily, and either amoxicillin or metronidazole for 2 wk; (2) ranitidine bismuth citrate, clarithromycin 500 mg twice daily, and either amoxicillin, metronidazole, or tetracycline for 2 wk; or (3) PPI, bismuth, metronidazole, and tetracycline for 1-2 wk.
	PPIs deactivate the enzyme system that pumps hydrogen ions (H^+) from the parietal cells, thus inhibiting gastric acid secretion. They are used for short-term treatment of active duodenal and gastric ulcers and for long-term treatment of hypersecretory conditions.
	Giving PPIs with antimicrobials increases the intragastric pH needed for antimicrobials to be effective.
Administer acid suppression therapy as prescribed.	This therapy is given for acute episodes of ulceration.
- Histamine H_2-receptor blockers (e.g., cimetidine, ranitidine, nizatidine, famotidine)	These agents are administered PO or IV to suppress secretion of gastric acid and facilitate ulcer healing. They also can be used prophylactically for limited periods of time, especially in patients susceptible to stress ulceration. They are administered with meals at least 1 hr apart from antacids because antacids can reduce their absorption. They are available both as prescription and over-the-counter (OTC), and while time to relief obtained is longer than with antacids, their effects last longer.

Continued

INTERVENTIONS

INTERVENTIONS	RATIONALES
- Sucralfate	This is an antiulcer agent that coats the ulcer with a protective barrier so that healing can occur. This drug must be taken before meals and at bedtime. It should not be taken within 30 min of antacids because acid facilitates adherence of sucralfate to the ulcer.
- Antacids	Antacids are administered orally or through an NG tube to provide quick, symptomatic relief, facilitate ulcer healing, and prevent further ulceration. They can be administered prophylactically in patients who are especially susceptible to ulceration. Antacids are administered after meals and at bedtime or give periodically via NG tube for patients who are intubated.
- PPIs (e.g., omeprazole, esomeprazole, lansoprazole, pantoprazol, rabeprozole)	PPIs deactivate the enzyme system that pumps hydrogen ions (H^+) from the parietal cells, thus inhibiting gastric acid secretion. They are used for short-term treatment of active duodenal and gastric ulcers and for long-term treatment of gastroesophageal reflux disease and hypersecretory conditions. Omeprazole is now available OTC for heartburn.
- Misoprostol	This is a synthetic prostaglandin E_1 analogue that enhances the body's normal mucosal protective mechanisms and decreases acid secretion. The drug may be used in the healing and prevention of NSAID-induced ulcers for people requiring high doses of NSAIDs for treatment of arthritis and other chronic pain conditions. This drug is used with caution in women of childbearing years who could be pregnant because it can cause abortion.
Stress importance of taking medications at prescribed intervals, not just for symptomatic relief of pain.	Initial pain relief does not mean the ulcer is completely healed.
Refer patient to community resources and support groups for assistance in smoking cessation or abstinence from drinking.	Smoking increases acid secretions and decreases mucosal blood flow, thereby inhibiting ulcer healing. Alcohol also slows the healing process.

••• **Related NIC and NOC labels:** *NIC:* Bleeding Reduction: Gastrointestinal; Nutrition Management; Medication Management *NOC:* Tissue Integrity: Skin and Mucous Membranes

ADDITIONAL NURSING DIAGNOSES/ PROBLEMS:

"Perioperative Care"	p. 45
"Crohn's Disease" for **Acute Pain**, **Nausea**	p. 449

PATIENT-FAMILY TEACHING AND DISCHARGE PLANNING

When providing patient-family teaching, focus on sensory information, avoid giving excessive information, and initiate a visiting nurse referral for necessary follow-up teaching of skilled needs. Include verbal and written information about the following:

✓ Importance of following prescribed diet to facilitate ulcer healing, prevent exacerbation or recurrence, or control postsurgical dumping syndrome. If appropriate, arrange consultation with dietitian.

✓ Medications, including drug name, rationale, dosage, schedule, precautions, and potential side effects. Also discuss drug-drug, food-drug, and herb-drug interactions.

✓ Signs and symptoms of exacerbation and recurrence, as well as potential complications.

✓ Care of incision line and dressing change technique, as necessary.

✓ Signs of wound infection, including persistent redness, swelling, purulent drainage, local warmth, fever, and foul odor.

✓ Role of lifestyle alterations in preventing exacerbation or recurrence of ulcer, including smoking cessation, stress reduction (see **Health-Seeking Behavior:** Relaxation technique effective for stress reduction, p. 172), decreasing or eliminating consumption of alcohol, and avoidance of irritating foods and drugs. Note that histamine H_2-receptor blockers are more effective in individuals who are nonsmokers.

✓ Referral to health care specialist for assistance with stress reduction as necessary.

✓ Referrals to community support groups, such as Alcoholics Anonymous at *www.alcoholics-anonymous.org*.

✓ Referrals to other reliable websites:
• National Digestive Diseases Information Clearinghouse at *www.digestive.niddk.nih.gov*
• American Gastroenterologic Association at *www.gastro.org* (use Patient Center link)

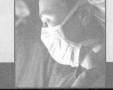

Peritonitis 60

OVERVIEW/PATHOPHYSIOLOGY

Peritonitis is the inflammatory response of the peritoneum to offending chemical and bacterial agents invading the peritoneal cavity. The inflammatory process can be local or generalized and may be classified as primary, secondary, or tertiary, depending on pathogenesis of the inflammation. Primary peritonitis, such as spontaneous bacterial peritonitis, occurs without a recognizable cause. Secondary peritonitis is caused by abdominal injury or rupture of abdominal organs. Common events include abdominal trauma, postoperative leakage of gastrointestinal (GI) content or blood into the peritoneal cavity, intestinal ischemia, ruptured or inflamed abdominal organs, poor sterile techniques (e.g., with peritoneal dialysis), and direct contamination of the bloodstream. Tertiary peritonitis is a persistent abdominal sepsis without a focus of infection, and it may follow treatment of a previous episode of peritonitis. The peritoneum responds to invasive agents by attempting to localize the infection with a shift of the omentum (the "guardian of the abdominal cavity") to wall off the inflamed area. Inflammation of the peritoneum results in tissue edema, development of fibrinous exudate, and hypermotility of the intestinal tract. As the disease progresses, paralytic ileus occurs, and intestinal fluid, which then cannot be reabsorbed, leaks into the peritoneal cavity. As a result of the fluid shift, cardiac output and tissue perfusion are reduced, leading to impaired cardiac and renal function. If infection or inflammation continues, respiratory failure and shock can ensue. Peritonitis often is progressive and can be fatal. It is the most common cause of death following abdominal surgery, and mortality is dictated by the patient's overall health, including nutritional and immune status and organ function.

HEALTH CARE SETTING

Acute care surgical unit, critical care unit

ASSESSMENT

Signs and symptoms:

Early findings: Acute abdominal pain with movement, anorexia, nausea, vomiting, chills, fever, rigor, malaise, weakness, hiccoughs, diaphoresis, absence of bowel sounds, and abdominal distention and rigidity (often described as boardlike).

Later findings: Dehydration (e.g., thirst, dry mucous membranes, oliguria, concentrated urine, poor skin turgor).

Physical assessment: Presence of tachycardia, hypotension, and shallow and rapid respirations caused by abdominal distention and discomfort. Often the patient assumes a supine position with knees flexed or side-lying with knees drawn up toward the chest. Palpation usually reveals peritoneal irritation as shown by distention, abdominal rigidity with general or localized tenderness, guarding, and rebound or cough tenderness. However, as many as one fourth of these patients will have minimal or no indications of peritoneal irritation. Auscultation findings include hyperactive bowel sounds during the gradual development of peritonitis and absence of bowel sounds or infrequent high-pitched sounds ("tinkling" or "squeaky") during later stages if paralytic ileus occurs. Mild ascites may be present as demonstrated by shifting areas of dullness on percussion.

History of: Abdominal surgery, peptic ulcer disease, cholecystitis, acute necrotizing pancreatitis, GI disorders, acute salpingitis, ruptured appendix or diverticulum, trauma, peritoneal dialysis.

DIAGNOSTIC TESTS

Serum tests: May reveal presence of leukocytosis, usually with a shift to the left (may be the only sign of tertiary peritonitis); hemoconcentration; elevated blood urea nitrogen (BUN); and electrolyte imbalance, particularly hypokalemia. Hypoalbuminemia and prolonged prothrombin time (PT), in combination with leukocytosis, are especially characteristic.

ABG values: May reveal hypoxemia (Pao_2 less than 80 mm Hg) or acidosis (pH less than 7.40).

Urinalysis: Often performed to rule out genitourinary involvement (e.g., pyelonephritis).

Paracentesis for peritoneal aspiration with culture and sensitivity: May be performed to determine presence of blood, bacteria, bile, pus, and amylase content and identify causative organism. Gram stain of ascitic fluid is positive in only about 25% of these patients. Ascitic fluid with a white blood cell (WBC) count greater than 500/mm³ with more than 25% polymorphonuclear leukocytes is especially characteristic. Blood-ascitic fluid albumin gradient greater than 1.1 g/dl, reduced pH of ascitic fluid (less than 7.31), and serum lactic acid elevation more than 33 mg/dl aid in confirmation of the diagnosis.

Abdominal x-ray examination: To determine presence of distended loops of bowel and abnormal levels of fluid and gas, which usually collect in the large and small bowel in the presence of a perforation or obstruction. "Free air" under the diaphragm also may be visualized, which indicates a perforated viscus.

Chest x-ray examination: Abdominal distention may elevate the diaphragm. Pain from peritonitis may limit respiratory excursion and lead to associated infiltrates in the lower lobes. In later stages, changes in serum osmolality allow for pleural effusions to occur.

Contrast x-ray examination: May be used to identify specific intestinal pathologic conditions. Water-soluble contrast (e.g., meglumine diatrizoate) may be used to evaluate suspected upper GI perforation.

CT scan and ultrasound: May be used to evaluate abdominal pain and more clearly delineate nondistinct areas found by plain abdominal x-ray examination. Magnetic resonance imaging (MRI) has not been an effective adjunct in abdominal surveys because of motion artifacts.

Radionuclide scans: Gallium, hepatoiminodiacetic acid (HIDA) (lidofenin) and liver-spleen scans may be used to identify intraabdominal abscess.

Nursing Diagnoses:

Acute Pain/Nausea

related to inflammatory process, fever, and tissue damage

Desired Outcomes: Patient's subjective perception of pain decreases within 1 hr of intervention, as documented by a pain scale. Nonverbal indicators, such as grimacing and abdominal guarding, are absent or diminished.

INTERVENTIONS	RATIONALES
Assess and document character and severity of discomfort q1-2h. Devise a pain scale with patient, rating discomfort on a scale of 0 (no pain) to 10 (worst pain).	This assessment will not only define the type of pain but it will monitor relief of discomfort obtained to determine effectiveness of the treatment.
After diagnosis has been made, administer opioids, other analgesics, and sedatives as prescribed.	These medications relieve severe pain and discomfort once the diagnosis has been confirmed. Because potent analgesics can mask diagnostic symptoms, opioids should not be administered until surgical evaluation has been completed.
Encourage patient to request analgesic *before* pain becomes severe. Document relief obtained, using the pain scale.	Pain management is more effective when analgesia is given before pain becomes too severe. Prolonged stimulation of pain receptors results in increased sensitivity to painful stimuli and will increase the amount of drug required to relieve pain.
Keep patient on bedrest. Provide a restful and quiet environment.	Rest minimizes pain, which can be aggravated by activity and stress.
Instruct patient in methods to splint abdomen.	Splinting reduces pain on movement, coughing, and deep breathing.
Keep patient in a position of comfort, usually semi-Fowler's position with knees bent.	This position promotes fluid shift to the lower abdomen, which will reduce pressure on the diaphragm and enable deeper and easier respirations. Raising the knees will decrease stress on the abdominal wall.
Explain all procedures.	Information helps minimize anxiety, which can exacerbate discomfort.
Offer mouth care and lip moisturizers at frequent intervals.	Oral care helps relieve discomfort from continuous or intermittent suction, dehydration, and NPO (nothing by mouth) status.
Administer antiemetics (e.g., hydroxyzine, ondansetron, prochlorperazine, promethazine) as prescribed; instruct patient to request medication *before* nausea becomes severe.	These medications, when given early, combat nausea and vomiting before they become more difficult to control.
See "Pain," p. 39, for other pain interventions.	

••• Related NIC and NOC labels: *NIC:* Medication Management; Anxiety Reduction; Environmental Management: Comfort; Medication Administration; Positioning; Splinting; Nausea Management *NOC:* Comfort Level

Nursing Diagnosis:

Impaired Gas Exchange

related to alveolar hypoventilation and decreased depth of respirations secondary to guarding with abdominal pain or distention

Desired Outcomes: Patient has an effective breathing pattern as evidenced by PaO_2 at least 80 mm Hg; oxygen saturation greater than 92%; BP at least 90/60 mm Hg (or within patient's baseline range); HR 100 bpm or less; and orientation to person, place, and time. Eupnea occurs within 1 hr after pain-relieving intervention.

INTERVENTIONS	RATIONALES
Monitor vital signs (VS), arterial blood gas (ABG), and oximetry results for evidence of hypoxemia.	The following are indicators of hypoxemia and usually signal the need for supplemental oxygen: PaO_2 less than 80 mm Hg and low oxygen saturation (92% or less), and to the following clinical signs: hypotension, tachycardia, tachypnea, restlessness, confusion or altered mental status, central nervous system depression, and possibly cyanosis.
Auscultate lung fields. Note and document presence of adventitious breath sounds.	This assessment monitors ventilation and detects pulmonary complications, such as pleural effusion. Pleural effusion, an accumulation of fluid in the pleural space, can develop in later stages of peritonitis because of changes in serum osmolality. Decreased breath sounds and pleural friction rub are diagnostic of pleural effusion.
Keep patient in semi-Fowler's or high Fowler's position; encourage deep breathing and coughing.	These positions aid respiratory effort and promote deep breathing to enhance oxygenation and coughing to clear pulmonary secretions.
Instruct patient in splinting abdomen.	Splinting enables better chest excursion to facilitate respiratory hygiene.
Administer oxygen as prescribed.	Oxygen supports increased metabolic needs and treats hypoxia.

••• Related NIC and NOC labels: *NIC:* Laboratory Data Interpretation; Oxygen Therapy; Chest Physiotherapy; Positioning; Respiratory Monitoring; Cough Enhancement *NOC:* Respiratory Status: Gas Exchange

Nursing Diagnoses:

Risk for Injury/Risk for Infection

related to potential for worsening/recurring peritonitis or development of septic shock secondary to inflammatory process

Desired Outcome: Patient is free of symptoms of worsening/recurring peritonitis or septic shock as evidenced by normothermia, BP at least 90/60 mm Hg (or within patient's normal range), HR 100 bpm or less, absence of chills, presence of eupnea, urinary output at least 30 ml/hr, CVP 2-6 mm Hg (5-12 cm H_2O), decreasing abdominal girth measurements, and minimal tenderness to palpation.

INTERVENTIONS	RATIONALES
Assess abdomen q1-2h during acute phase and q4h once patient is stabilized.	Bowel sounds initially may be frequent but later are absent as peritonitis advances.
Lightly palpate abdomen for evidence of increasing rigidity or tenderness.	This would signal disease progression. If patient experiences increased pain on removal of your hand, rebound tenderness is present.
Measure abdominal girth.	Girth measurements monitor for increasing distention, which would signal development of ascites.
Use a permanent marker to identify placement of tape measure. Notify health care provider of significant findings.	This ensures consistent site of measurement by caregivers.
If prescribed, insert gastric tube and connect it to suction.	Suction prevents or decreases distention.

Continued

INTERVENTIONS	RATIONALES
Monitor skin and VS at least q2h and more frequently if patient's condition is unstable. Be alert to signs of septic shock: increased temperature, hypotension, tachycardia, shallow and rapid respirations, urine output less than 30 ml/hr, and central venous pressure (CVP) less than 2 mm Hg (less than 5 cm H$_2$O).	In the early (warm) stage of shock, skin usually is warm, pink, and dry secondary to peripheral venous pooling, and blood pressure (BP) and CVP begin to drop. In the late (cold) stage of shock, extremities become pale and cool because of decreasing tissue perfusion.
Administer antibiotics as prescribed; ensure close adherence to schedules for maintenance of bacteriocidal serum levels.	Combination broad-spectrum antibiotic therapy is rapidly begun to ensure treatment of gram-negative bacilli and anaerobic bacteria. Common agents include cephalosporins (cefotaxime, cefepime), aminoglycosides (gentamicin), ampicillin, floxacin (Floxin), and metronidazole. Antibiotics are commonly administered IV and may also be directly instilled into the peritoneal cavity via surgically placed catheters.
Collect peak and trough antibiotic determinations as prescribed.	Peak and trough levels are drawn at specific times around the antibiotic dose. Peak levels indicate if there is enough drug in the bloodstream and the dose is high enough. The trough level indicates if the kidneys/liver are clearing the drug adequately.
Monitor complete blood count for presence of leukocytosis, which signals infection, and hemoconcentration (increased hematocrit [Hct] and hemoglobin [Hgb]), which occurs with decreased plasma volume.	Normal values are as follows: WBC 4500-11,000/mm^3; Hgb 14-18 g/dl (male) or 12-16 g/dl (female); Hct 40%-54% (male) or 37%-47% (female). With peritonitis, WBC count usually is greater than 20,000/mm^3. Notify health care provider of significant findings.
Maintain sterile technique with dressing changes and all invasive procedures.	This prevents/reduces spread of infection.
Teach signs and symptoms of recurring peritonitis and importance of reporting them promptly if they occur: fever, chills, abdominal pain, vomiting, and abdominal distention.	An informed individual likely will report these signs promptly for rapid treatment.

••• **Related NIC and NOC labels:** *NIC:* Risk Identification; Infection Control; Infection Protection; Vital Signs Monitoring; Medication Administration; Tube Care: Gastrointestinal *NOC:* Infection Status

Nursing Diagnosis:

Imbalanced Nutrition: Less Than Body Requirements

related to vomiting and intestinal suctioning

Desired Outcome: By at least 24 hr before hospital discharge, patient demonstrates optimal progress toward adequate nutritional status as evidenced by stable weight and balanced or positive nitrogen (N) state.

INTERVENTIONS	RATIONALES
Keep patient NPO as prescribed during acute phase.	Oral fluids are not resumed until patient has passed flatus and the gastric/intestinal tube has been removed. If patient has an ileus, a nasogastric tube will be inserted to decompress the abdomen.
Reintroduce oral fluids gradually once motility has returned, as evidenced by presence of bowel sounds, decreased distention, and passage of flatus.	This ensures that patient will tolerate fluids through the intestines, which may have become irritated from the inflammatory process.
Support patient with peripheral parenteral nutrition or total parenteral nutrition (TPN), as prescribed, depending on duration of acute phase (usually by day 5).	If the GI tract is nonfunctioning, TPN usually is initiated in the early stages to promote nutrition and protein replacement.
Administer replacement fluids, electrolytes, and vitamins as prescribed.	This maintains hydration and restores electrolytes and nutrients lost in gastric/intestinal tube output and fluid shifts. Daily measurements of serum electrolytes and calculations of fluid volume are performed to determine necessary types of fluid and electrolyte replacement. Crystalloids, colloids (albumin, Plasmanate), blood, and blood products may be administered to correct hypovolemia, hypoproteinemia, and anemia.

Continued

INTERVENTIONS	RATIONALES
Instruct patient in rationale for tube placement and NPO status; underlying pathologic condition (as appropriate); need for close monitoring of fluid intake and output; and, eventually, diet advancement.	A knowledgeable patient likely will adhere to the treatment regimen and report symptoms that would necessitate timely intervention.

●●● **Related NIC and NOC labels:** *NIC:* Nutrition Therapy; Nutritional Monitoring; Teaching: Prescribed Diet; Enteral Tube Feeding; Fluid/Electrolyte Management; Gastrointestinal Intubation; Total Parenteral Nutrition Administration; Intravenous Therapy; Laboratory Data Interpretation *NOC:* Nutritional Status; Nutritional Status: Food and Fluid Intake; Nutritional Status: Nutrient Intake

ADDITIONAL NURSING DIAGNOSES/ PROBLEMS:

"Perioperative Care"	p. 45
"Prolonged Bedrest" for **Risk for Activity Intolerance**	p. 61
Risk for Disuse Syndrome	p. 63
"Providing Nutritional Support" for care of patients receiving enteral or parenteral feedings	p. 565

PATIENT-FAMILY TEACHING AND DISCHARGE PLANNING

When providing patient-family teaching, focus on sensory information, avoid giving excessive information, and initiate a visiting nurse referral for necessary monitoring of wound care and follow-up teaching. Include verbal and written information about the following:

✓ Medications, including drug name, dosage, schedule, purpose, precautions, and potential side effects. Also discuss drug-drug, food-drug, and herb-drug interactions.

✓ Activity alterations as prescribed by health care provider, such as avoiding heavy lifting (more than 10 lb), resting after periods of fatigue, getting maximum amounts of rest, and gradually increasing activities to tolerance.

✓ Notifying health care provider of the following indicators of recurrence: fever, chills, abdominal pain, vomiting, abdominal distention.

✓ If patient has undergone surgery, indicators of wound infection: fever, pain, chills, incisional swelling, persistent erythema, purulent drainage.

✓ Importance of follow-up medical care; confirm date and time of next medical appointment.

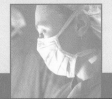

Ulcerative Colitis 61

OVERVIEW/PATHOPHYSIOLOGY

Ulcerative colitis (UC) is a nonspecific, chronic inflammatory disease of the mucosa and submucosa of the colon. Generally the disease begins in the rectum and sigmoid colon, but it can extend proximally and uninterrupted as far as the cecum. In 30%-50% of cases, the rectum (proctitis) or rectosigmoid (proctosigmoiditis) is affected; in 30%-40% of cases, the disease extends to the splenic flexure (left-sided or distal colitis); and in 20%-30% of cases, the disease extends proximally to involve the entire colon (pancolitis). In some instances, a few centimeters of distal ileum are affected. This is sometimes referred to as *backwash ileitis*, and it occurs in only about 10% of patients with UC involving the entire colon. In the majority of patients, extent of colonic involvement is maintained from onset through the disease course, with the patient experiencing flare-ups and remissions. UC initially affects the mucosal layer. Eventually small mucosal layer abscesses form that ultimately penetrate the submucosa, spread horizontally, and allow sloughing of the mucosa, creating ulcerative lesions. The muscular layer (muscularis) generally is not affected, but the serosal layer may have congested and dilated blood vessels.

The cause of UC is unknown, but theories posit an interaction of external agents, host responses, and genetic immunologic factors creating the pathogenic responses. In a genetically susceptible subject, an outside agent or substance, such as a bacterium, virus, or other antigen, interacts with the body's immune system to trigger the disease or may cause damage to the intestinal wall, initiating or accelerating the disease process. The resulting inflammatory response continues unregulated by the immune system. As a result, inflammation continues damaging the intestinal wall, causing symptoms of UC. Medical therapy is based upon symptomatic relief. The goals are to terminate the acute attack, induce and maintain remission, maintain quality of life, and prevent complications, both disease-related and therapy-related. Surgical intervention is indicated only when the disease is intractable to medical management or when the patient develops a disabling complication. Total proctocolectomy cures UC and results in construction of a permanent fecal diversion.

The most firmly established risk factor for developing inflammatory bowel disease (IBD) is a positive family history. There is a 10-fold increase in risk of IBD in first-degree relatives of patients with UC. Individuals with UC develop colonic adenocarcinomas at 10 times the rate of the general population. UC can occur at any age, but is generally diagnosed in the third decade of life with a second peak in the fifth and sixth decades. There is no difference in gender distribution; however, men are more likely than women to be diagnosed in the fifth and sixth decades of life. Incidence is higher in the Caucasian population and in Ashkenazi Jews than in nonwhite populations and in people of non-Jewish descent. UC is more prevalent in urban, developed countries with temperate climates than in rural, more southern countries. It is more common in nonsmokers and former smokers, suggesting that smoking has a protective effect and may decrease severity of symptoms. Appendectomy before age 20 may reduce risk.

HEALTH CARE SETTING

Primary care; acute care for complications

ASSESSMENT

Signs and symptoms: Bloody diarrhea (the cardinal symptom). The clinical picture can vary from acute episodes with frequent discharge of watery stools mixed with blood, pus, and mucus, accompanied by fever, abdominal pain, rectal urgency, and tenesmus, to loose or frequent stools, to formed stools coated with a little blood. However, nearly two thirds of patients have crampy abdominal pain and varying degrees of fever, vomiting, anorexia, weight loss, and dehydration. Remissions and exacerbations are common. Extracolonic manifestations also can occur, including polyarthritis, skin lesions (erythema nodosum, pyoderma gangrenosum), liver impairment, and ophthalmic complications (iritis, uveitis). Extracolonic manifestations may precede overt bowel disease, and their clinical activity may be related or unrelated to the clinical activity of the bowel disease.

Physical assessment: With mild disease, there is no significant abdominal tenderness; left lower quadrant (LLQ) cramps are commonly relieved by defecation. With moderate disease, abdominal pain and tenderness may be present; mild fever (temperature 99°-100° F), anemia (hematocrit [Hct] 30%-40%), and hypoalbuminemia (3.0-3.5 g/dl) may be present. With severe disease, abdominal pain and tenderness are present, especially in the LLQ; distention and a tender, spastic anus also may be present; fever (temperature greater than 100° F), severe anemia (Hct less than 30%), and impaired nutrition with hypoalbuminemia (less than 3.0 g/dl) and weight loss are present. With rectal examination, the mucosa may feel gritty and the examining gloved finger may be covered with blood, mucus, or pus.

Risk factors: Duration of active disease more than 10 yr, pancolitis, and family history of colonic cancer.

DIAGNOSTIC TESTS

Stool examination: Reveals presence of frank or occult blood. Stool cultures and smears rule out bacterial and parasitic disorders. **Note:** Collect specimens before barium enema is performed.

Sigmoidoscopy: Reveals red, granular, hyperemic, and extremely friable mucosa; strips of inflamed mucosa undermined by surrounding ulcerations, which form pseudopolyps; and thick exudate composed of blood, pus, and mucus. **Note:** Enemas should not be given before the examination because they can produce hyperemia and edema and may cause exacerbation of the disease. A limited prep may be given to facilitate visualization during examination.

Colonoscopy: Will help determine extent of the disease and differentiate UC from Crohn's disease (CD) through both endoscopic appearance and histologic examination of biopsy tissues. Serial colonoscopy is also performed to monitor patients with chronic UC at risk for colon carcinoma. **Note:** This test may be contraindicated in patients with acute disease because of risk of perforation or hemorrhage.

Rectal biopsy: Aids in differentiating UC from carcinoma and other inflammatory processes.

Barium enema: Reveals mucosal irregularity from fine serrations to ragged ulcerations, narrowing and shortening of the colon, presence of pseudopolyps, loss of haustral markings, and presence of spasms and irritability. Double-contrast technique may facilitate detection of superficial mucosal lesions. With a double-contrast technique, barium is instilled into the colon as with a conventional barium enema, but most of the barium is then withdrawn and the colon is inflated with air, which causes a thin coating of barium to line the intestinal wall. The double-contrast technique has become the "gold standard" for evaluating patients for colitis. **Note:** Because they produce hyperemia and edema and may cause exacerbation of the disease, irritant cathartics and enemas should not be given before the examination.

Abdominal plain films (flat plate): An important tool for screening severely ill patients when colonoscopy and barium enema are contraindicated. An abdominal flat plate may reveal fecal residue, appearance of mucosal margins, widening or thickening of visible haustra, and colonic wall diameter. In patients with suspected ileus, obstruction, or perforation, the flat plate film reveals abnormal gas and fluid levels or presence of free air in the peritoneal cavity.

CT scan: Used to identify suspected complications of UC (i.e., toxic megacolon, pneumatosis coli).

Serum antibody testing: Several serum antibodies are being evaluated for aiding in the development of noninvasive diagnostic techniques for UC. Some of these tests have been found to be useful in differentiating UC from CD.

Radionuclide imaging: To identify extent of disease activity, especially when colonoscopy and barium enema are contraindicated. Injections of indium-111–labeled autologous leukocytes are used to identify areas of active inflammation.

Blood tests: Anemia, with hypochromic microcytic red blood indices in severe disease, usually is present because of blood loss, iron deficiency, and bone marrow depression. White blood cell (WBC) count may be normal to markedly elevated in severe disease. Sedimentation rate usually is increased according to illness severity. Hypoalbuminemia and negative nitrogen (N) state occur in moderately severe to severe disease and result from decreased protein intake, decreased albumin synthesis in the debilitated condition, and increased metabolic needs. Electrolyte imbalance is common; hypokalemia is often present because of colonic losses (diarrhea) and renal losses in patients taking high doses of corticosteroids. Bicarbonate may be decreased because of colonic losses and may signal metabolic acidosis.

Nursing Diagnosis:

Deficient Fluid Volume

related to active loss secondary to diarrhea and gastrointestinal bleeding/hemorrhage

Desired Outcome: Patient is normovolemic within 24 hr of admission as evidenced by balanced intake and output (I&O), urine output 30 ml/hr or more, urine specific gravity less than 1.030, good skin turgor, moist mucous membranes, stable weight, BP 90/60 mm Hg or more (or within patient's normal range), and RR 12-20 breaths/min.

INTERVENTIONS	RATIONALES
Monitor I&O and urine specific gravity; weigh patient daily; and monitor laboratory values to evaluate fluid, electrolyte, and hematologic status.	These assessments evaluate fluid, electrolyte, and hematologic status. Optimal values are serum K$^+$ 3.5 mEq/L or greater, Hct 40%-54% (male) and 37%-47% (female), hemoglobin (Hgb) 14-18 g/dl (male) and 12-16 g/dl (female), and red blood cells (RBCs) 4.5-6.0 million/mm^3 (male) and 4.0-5.5 million/mm^3 (female). Critical values: K$^+$ less than 2.5 or greater than 6.5 mEq/L, Hct less than 15% or greater than 60%, Hgb less than 5.0 g/dl or greater than 20 g/dl. Hypokalemia is common because of the prolonged diarrhea. Prolonged anemia may result in decreased Hct, Hgb, and RBCs.
Monitor frequency and consistency of stool. For frequent bowel movements, keep a stool count; measure liquid stools. Assess and record presence of blood, mucus, fat, and undigested food.	Although bloody diarrhea is most commonly seen, the patient may experience acute episodes with frequent discharge of watery stools mixed with blood, pus, and mucus, accompanied by fever, abdominal pain, rectal urgency, and tenesmus; loose or frequent stools; or formed stools coated with a little blood.
Monitor for thirst, poor skin turgor (may not be a reliable indicator of hydration in the older adult), dryness of mucous membranes, fever, and concentrated (specific gravity greater than 1.030) and decreased urinary output.	These are indicators of dehydration.
Monitor for hypotension, increased heart rate (HR) and respiratory rate (RR), pallor, diaphoresis, and restlessness. Assess stool for quality (e.g., is it grossly bloody and liquid?) and quantity (e.g., is it mostly blood or mostly stool?). Report significant findings to health care provider.	These are signs of hemorrhage.
Provide parenteral replacement of fluids, electrolytes, and vitamins as prescribed.	These measures maintain the acutely ill patient, and are guided by laboratory test results.
Administer blood products and iron as prescribed.	This will help correct existing anemia and losses caused by hemorrhage.
Provide bland, high-protein, high-calorie, low-residue diet, as prescribed when patient is taking food PO.	Nutritional management varies with patient's condition. In severely ill patients, total parenteral nutrition (TPN) along with NPO (nothing by mouth) status is prescribed to replace nutritional deficits while allowing complete bowel rest and improving patient's nutritional status before surgery. For less severely ill patients, a low-residue elemental diet provides good nutrition with low fecal volume to allow bowel rest. A bland, high-protein, high-calorie, low-residue diet with vitamin and mineral supplements and excluding raw fruits and vegetables provides good nutrition and decreases diarrhea. Milk and wheat products are restricted to reduce cramping and diarrhea in patients with lactose and gluten intolerance.
Assess tolerance to diet.	Cramping, diarrhea, and flatulence are signs that patient is not tolerating the diet.

••• **Related NIC and NOC labels:** *NIC:* Fluid Management; Electrolyte Monitoring; Fluid Management; Laboratory Data Interpretation; Vital Signs Monitoring; Diarrhea Management; Blood Products Administration; Total Parenteral Nutrition; Hemorrhage Control *NOC:* Fluid Balance

Nursing Diagnoses:

Risk for Injury/Risk for Infection

related to potential for perforation secondary to deeply inflamed colonic mucosa

Desired Outcome: Patient is free of signs of perforation as evidenced by normothermia; HR 60-100 bpm; RR 12-20 breaths/min with normal depth and pattern (eupnea); normal bowel sounds; absence of abdominal distention, tympany, or rebound tenderness; negative culture results; no mental status changes; and orientation to person, place, and time.

INTERVENTIONS	RATIONALES
Monitor for fever, chills, increased respiratory and heart rates, diaphoresis, and increased abdominal discomfort.	These indicators can occur with perforation of the colon and potentially result in localized abscess or generalized fecal peritonitis and septicemia. **Note:** Systemic therapy with corticosteroids and antibiotics can mask the development of this complication.
Report any evidence of sudden abdominal distention associated with preceding symptoms.	Together these indicators can signal toxic megacolon. Factors contributing to development of this complication include hypokalemia, barium enema examinations, and use of opioids and anticholinergics. Surgery to prevent perforation is indicated in patients with fulminant disease or toxic megacolon whose condition worsens or does not improve in 48-72 hr.
Monitor WBC counts.	Patients with severe UC can have markedly elevated WBC counts—greater than $20,000/mm^3$ and occasionally as high as $50,000/mm^3$. Critical values are less than $2500/mm^3$ and greater than $30,000/mm^3$.
Evaluate mental status, orientation, and level of consciousness q2-4h.	Mental cloudiness, lethargy, and increased restlessness can signal impending or actual septic shock.
If patient has a sudden temperature elevation, culture blood and other sites as prescribed. Monitor culture reports, notifying health care provider promptly of any positive cultures.	A temperature spike can signal septicemia; a culture will identify causative organism if present.
Administer antibiotics as prescribed and in a timely fashion.	This measure ensures optimal blood levels of the effective therapeutic dose in order to kill the bacteria and control infection in the patient with acute pancolitis or toxic megacolon since secondary bacterial infection of deeply inflamed mucosa is likely.
	Antibiotics are not indicated in the management of mild to moderate disease, in that infectious agents are not believed to be responsible for UC.

••• **Related NIC and NOC labels:** *NIC:* Infection Protection; Laboratory Data Interpretation; Medication Administration; Specimen Management; Vital Signs Monitoring *NOC:* Infection Status; Safety Status: Physical Injury

Nursing Diagnoses:

Acute Pain/Nausea

related to abdominal cramping and the intestinal inflammatory process

Desired Outcomes: Within 4 hr of intervention, patient's subjective perception of discomfort decreases as documented by pain scale. Objective indicators, such as grimacing, are absent or diminished.

INTERVENTIONS	RATIONALES
Monitor and document characteristics of discomfort, and assess whether it is associated with ingestion of certain foods or medications or with emotional stress. Devise a pain scale with patient, rating discomfort from 0 (no pain) to 10 (worst pain). Eliminate foods that cause cramping and discomfort.	These assessments help determine discomfort trigger and degree to which discomfort is alleviated following intervention.
As prescribed, maintain patient on NPO or TPN to provide bowel rest.	These measures provide bowel rest, which should help alleviate symptoms.
Provide nasal and oral care at frequent intervals.	These measures lessen discomfort from NPO status, nausea, or presence of nasogastric (NG) tube.
Keep patient's environment quiet. Facilitate coordination of health care providers to provide rest periods between care activities. Allow 90 min for undisturbed rest.	Rest promotes healing.

Continued

INTERVENTIONS

INTERVENTIONS	RATIONALES
Administer sedatives and tranquilizers as prescribed.	These agents promote rest and reduce anxiety, which optimally will lessen symptoms.
Administer hydrophilic colloids, anticholinergics, and antidiarrheal medications as prescribed.	These agents relieve cramping and diarrhea. **Note:** Opioids and anticholinergics should be administered with extreme caution because they contribute to development of toxic megacolon.
Instruct the patient to request medication before discomfort becomes severe.	Cramping and diarrhea are more easily controlled if they are treated before they become severe.
Monitor for intensification of symptoms. Notify health care provider of significant findings.	This can indicate presence of complications, which should be treated promptly.

••• **Related NIC and NOC labels:** *NIC:* Medication Management; Bowel Management; Sleep Enhancement; Nausea Management *NOC:* Comfort Level

Nursing Diagnosis:

Diarrhea

related to inflammatory process of the intestines

Desired Outcome: Patient's stools become normal in consistency, and frequency is lessened within 3 days of admission.

INTERVENTIONS	RATIONALES
Monitor and record amount, frequency, and character of stools. When possible, measure liquid stools.	Although bloody diarrhea is the cardinal symptom, the clinical picture can vary from acute episodes with frequent discharge of watery stools mixed with blood, pus, and mucus, accompanied by fever, abdominal pain, rectal urgency, and tenesmus, to loose or frequent stools, to formed stools coated with a little blood.
Provide covered bedpan, commode, or bathroom that is easily accessible and ready to use at all times.	This will control odor and decrease patient's anxiety and self-consciousness.
Empty bedpan and commode promptly.	This will remove source of odor and decrease patient's anxiety about incontinence.
Administer hydrophilic colloids, anticholinergics, and antidiarrheal medications as prescribed.	These agents decrease fluidity and number of stools. Opioids and anticholinergics should be administered with extreme caution because they contribute to development of toxic megacolon.
Administer topical corticosteroid or aminosalicylate preparations and antibiotics via retention enema, as prescribed.	These agents reduce mucosal inflammation in patients with mild disease limited to the rectum and sigmoid colon. In patients with acute moderate to severe disease and with more extensive (pancolonic) disease, oral or IV corticosteroid therapy is initiated. In patients not responding to steroids or aminosalicylates, immunosuppressive immunomodulatory therapy may be initiated to reduce inflammation.
If patient has difficulty retaining the enema for the prescribed amount of time, consult health care provider about use of corticosteroid foam.	Corticosteroid foam is easier to retain and administer.
Administer probiotics or fish oil, as prescribed.	Probiotics are beneficial bacteria that restore balance to the intestinal environment, with resulting reduction in inflammation. Omega-3 fatty acids found in fish oil appear to benefit patients with active UC by decreasing inflammation; they must be taken in large quantity.
Monitor serum electrolytes, particularly K$^+$, for abnormalities. Alert health care provider to K$^+$ less than 3.5 mEq/L. (Critical value: K$^+$ less than 2.5 mEq/L.)	Hypokalemia is often present because of colonic losses (diarrhea) and renal losses in patients taking high doses of corticosteroids.

••• **Related NIC and NOC labels:** *NIC:* Fluid/Electrolyte Management; Diarrhea Management; Electrolyte Management: Hypokalemia; Laboratory Data Interpretation; Anxiety Reduction; Medication Administration *NOC:* Electrolyte and Acid-Base Balance; Symptom Severity

Nursing Diagnosis:

Risk for Impaired Skin Integrity: Perineal/Perianal

related to persistent diarrhea

Desired Outcome: Patient's perineal/perianal skin remains intact with no erythema.

INTERVENTIONS	RATIONALES
Provide materials or assist patient with cleansing and drying perineal area after each bowel movement. Use a nonirritating cleansing agent.	These measures help keep skin clean and intact.
Apply protective skin care products (skin preparations, gels, or barrier films).	These products prevent irritation caused by frequent liquid stools and maintain perianal skin integrity. Skin care products containing alcohol should not be used on broken or denuded skin because the alcohol content causes a painful burning sensation.
Administer hydrophilic colloids, anticholinergics, and antidiarrheal medications as prescribed.	These agents decrease fluidity and number of stools. **Note:** Opioids and anticholinergics should be administered with extreme caution because they contribute to development of toxic megacolon.

••• **Related NIC and NOC labels:** *NIC:* Bathing; Bowel Incontinence Care; Skin Care: Topical Treatments; Diarrhea Management; Perineal Care; Self-Care Assistance: Bathing/Hygiene *NOC:* Tissue Integrity: Skin & Mucous Membranes

Nursing Diagnosis:

Deficient Knowledge:

Purpose and precautions for medications used with ulcerative colitis

Desired Outcome: Immediately following teaching (if patient is not hospitalized) or within the 24-hr period before hospital discharge, patient verbalizes accurate information about drugs used with UC, including their purpose and necessary precautions.

INTERVENTIONS	RATIONALES
Teach Patient about the Following:	
Antiinflammatory agents	Corticosteroids reduce mucosal inflammation.
Dosage and routes of administration vary with severity and extent of the disease.	In patients with mild disease limited to the rectum and sigmoid colon, rectal instillation of steroids (enema, foam, or suppository) may induce or maintain remission. In patients with more extensive (pancolonic) and acute active disease, oral corticosteroid therapy with prednisone or prednisolone usually is initiated. In severely ill patients with fulminant disease, IV corticosteroids are given.
Once clinical remission is achieved, IV and oral corticosteroids are tapered until discontinuation.	These medications have not been shown to prolong remission or prevent future exacerbations.
Sulfasalazine	This agent helps maintain remissions and is effective in the treatment of mild to moderate attacks of ulcerative colitis and appears to decrease frequency of subsequent relapse. Sulfasalazine is considered inferior to corticosteroids in the treatment of severe attacks of disease; once remission has been attained by use of corticosteroid therapy, sulfasalazine appears to be superior to systemic corticosteroids in the maintenance of remission.
To avoid side effects of sulfapyridine, several agents have been developed using a variety of delivery mechanisms that allow release of the active agent in the colon or ileum. These agents include the 5-aminosalicylic acid (5-ASA) derivatives: mesalamine (in enteric-coated and time-release forms), olsalazine, and balsalazide. These three agents are useful alternatives for patients unable to tolerate sulfapyridine; however, these agents have their own side effects.	When administered orally, sulfasalazine is broken down by colonic bacteria into its two constituents: 5-ASA, which is considered the active therapeutic component, and sulfapyridine, which is the carrier and responsible for the side effects experienced by more than one third of the individuals treated with this therapy.

Continued

INTERVENTIONS	RATIONALES
Topical therapy is an effective route for proctitis or proctosigmoiditis.	Mesalamine suppository or foam is used for proctitis; mesalamine retention enema is used for proctosigmoiditis.
Combination therapy of mesalamine enema and oral mesalamine may be used.	Combination therapy may be more effective than using oral form alone.
Immunosuppressive/immunomodulatory therapy	This therapy reduces inflammation in patients not responding to steroids and sulfasalazine; in patients unwilling or unable to undergo colectomy; or as an alternative to steroid dependency. Azathioprine and 6-mercaptopurine have been used alone and in combination with steroids.
Immunosuppressive/immunomodulatory therapy has been used to maintain remission in patients with frequent relapses.	These agents may have steroid-sparing and steroid-enhancing effects and are used with the goal of gradually withdrawing, or substantially reducing, the dosage of corticosteroids.
Advise patient of the need to be closely monitored.	Therapy may be necessary for 3-6 mo to achieve therapeutic response, and this amount of time can result in hematologic toxicity.
IV cyclosporine has been used cautiously in severe, intractable ulcerative colitis. If there is no response within 4-7 days, cyclosporine is unlikely to be effective.	Cyclosporine is toxic and associated with many side effects and thus is used with caution.

••• **Related NIC and NOC labels:** *NIC:* Teaching: Prescribed Medication *NOC:* Knowledge: Medication

ADDITIONAL NURSING DIAGNOSES/ PROBLEMS:

"Perioperative Care" if surgery is performed	p. 45
"Psychosocial Support"	p. 73
"Fecal Diversions"	p. 455
Risk for Impaired Skin Integrity: Peristomal/ Impaired Skin Integrity: Stomal	p. 456
Bowel Incontinence	p. 458
Disturbed Body Image	p. 459

 PATIENT-FAMILY TEACHING AND DISCHARGE PLANNING

When providing patient-family teaching, focus on sensory information, avoid giving excessive information, and initiate a visiting nurse referral for necessary follow-up teaching. Include verbal and written information about the following:

✓ Medications, including drug name, rationale, dosage, schedule, route of administration, precautions, and potential side effects. Also discuss drug-drug, herb-drug, and food-drug interactions. **Note:** Caution patients receiving high-dose steroid therapy about abrupt discontinuation of steroids to prevent precipitation of adrenal crisis. Withdrawal symptoms include weakness, lethargy, restlessness, anorexia, nausea, and muscle tenderness. Instruct patient to notify health care provider if these symptoms occur.

✓ Signs and symptoms that necessitate medical attention, including fever, nausea and vomiting, diarrhea or constipation, and any significant change in appearance and frequency of stools, any of which can signal exacerbation of the disease.

✓ Dietary management to promote nutritional and fluid maintenance and prevent abdominal cramping, discomfort, and diarrhea.

✓ Importance of perineal care after bowel movements.

✓ Enteral or parenteral feeding instructions if patient is to supplement diet or is NPO.

✓ Referral to community resources, including the Crohn's & Colitis Foundation of America, Inc., at *www.ccfa.org.*

✓ Importance of follow-up medical care, particularly for patients with long-standing disease because so many of them develop colonic adenocarcinoma.

✓ Referral to a mental health specialist if recommended by health care provider.

In addition, if patient has a fecal diversion (colostomy, ileostomy, or ileal pouch anal anastomosis):

✓ Care of incision, dressing changes, and permission to take baths or showers once sutures and drains are removed.

✓ Care of stoma, peristomal/perianal skin, or perineal wound; use of ostomy equipment; and method for obtaining supplies. Sitz baths may be indicated for perineal wound.

✓ Medications that are contraindicated (e.g., laxatives) or that may not be well tolerated or absorbed (e.g., antibiotics, enteric-coated tablets, long-acting tablets).

✓ Gradual resumption of activities of daily living, excluding heavy lifting (more than 10 lb), pushing, or pulling for 6-8 wk to prevent incisional herniation.

✓ Referral to community resources, including home health care agency, wound, ostomy, continence nurse, the local ostomy association, and the United Ostomy Association of America at *www.uoaa.org*.

✓ Importance of reporting signs and symptoms that require medical attention, such as change in stoma color from the normal bright and shiny red; peristomal or perianal skin irritation; diarrhea; incisional pain, local increased temperature, drainage, swelling, or redness; signs and symptoms of fluid and electrolyte imbalance; and signs and symptoms of mechanical or functional obstruction.

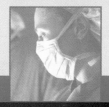

Anemias of Chronic Disease 62

OVERVIEW/PATHOPHYSIOLOGY

Erythropoietin (EPO) is a naturally occurring protein hormone produced and released by the kidneys (90%) and liver (10%). The kidneys are stimulated to release EPO in response to low blood oxygenation. EPO then stimulates stem cells in the bone marrow to develop and produce red blood cells (RBCs). Individuals with decreased renal function (e.g., chronic kidney disease [CKD]) often become anemic because their kidneys cannot produce EPO. In other chronic conditions, bone marrow fails to compensate (because of a blunted response to EPO) for decreased red cell survival adequately by increasing RBC production. In these cases, erythropoietin rarely is an important cause of underproduction of red cells except in renal failure. However, development of recombinant human erythropoietin (epoetin alpha) has provided dramatic benefits for patients with CKD, patients receiving chemotherapy for cancer, and patients undergoing treatment for infection with human immunodeficiency virus (HIV).

HEALTH CARE SETTING

Primary care; acute care for blood transfusion or treatment for sequelae of CKD

ASSESSMENT

Chronic indicators: Patient may be asymptomatic or have brittle hair and nails and pallor. In the presence of severe and chronic disease, shortness of breath, dizziness, and fatigue may be present even at rest. History of CKD, dialysis therapy, cancer within the bone marrow (e.g., leukemia), cancer chemotherapy, or therapy for HIV infection also may be factors.

Acute indicators: Fatigue, decreased ability to concentrate, cold sensitivity, menstrual irregularities, and loss of libido.

Physical assessment: Tachycardia, palpitations, tachypnea, exertional dyspnea, pale mucous membranes, pale nail beds, vertigo.

DIAGNOSTIC TESTS

Blood count: Usually RBCs and hemoglobin (Hgb) are decreased, and hematocrit (Hct) is low because the percentage of RBCs in the total blood volume is decreased.

Ferritin: Normal or increased. However, if it is less than 30 mcg/L, there is a coexisting iron deficiency.

Peripheral blood smear to examine RBC indices: Morphology reveals normocytic and normochromic erythrocytes (normal or slightly low mean corpuscular volume [MCV]).

Total iron-binding capacity: Decreased.

Reticulocyte count: Normal to slightly elevated.

Serum iron levels: Decreased.

Cobalamine, folate: Normal.

Nursing Diagnosis:

Activity Intolerance

related to anemia and decreased oxygen-carrying capacity of the blood occurring with decreased RBCs

Desired Outcome: After treatment, Hgb and Hct levels are within medical goals and patient perceives exertion at 3 or less on a 0-10 scale and tolerates activity as evidenced by RR 12-20 breaths/min, presence of eupnea, HR 100 bpm or less, and absence of dizziness and headaches.

INTERVENTIONS	RATIONALES
Assess patient for signs of activity intolerance. Ask patient to rate perceived exertion (see "Prolonged Bedrest" for **Risk for Activity Intolerance,** p. 61).	Dyspnea on exertion, dizziness, palpitations, headaches, and verbalization of increased exertion level (rate perceived exertion [RPE] more than 3) are signs of activity intolerance and decreased tissue oxygenation, and patient should stop or modify the activity until signs of increased exertion are no longer present with the activity.
Assess patient for risk of falling and implement appropriate strategies.	Because of the potentially slow, progressive nature of this anemia, patients may not be aware of weaknesses and limitations leading to reductions in strength and balance.
As indicated, monitor oximetry; report O_2 saturation 92% or less.	O_2 saturation 92% or less may signal need for supplementary oxygen.
Administer oxygen as prescribed; encourage deep breathing.	Both measures augment oxygen delivery to the tissues.
Facilitate coordination of care providers, allowing time for at least 90 min of undisturbed rest.	Fewer interruptions in rest enable patients to benefit from the undisturbed rest/sleep they need until the anemia is resolved.
Encourage gradually increasing activities to tolerance as patient's condition improves.	This promotes endurance while preventing problems caused by prolonged bedrest.
	An effective measure is setting mutually agreed on goals with patient (e.g., "Let's plan this morning's activity goals. Do you think you could walk up and down the hall once, or twice?" or appropriate amount, depending on patient's tolerance).
Administer blood components (usually packed RBCs) through an 18-gauge catheter as prescribed.	This will increase the number of circulating RBCs, which in turn will increase the blood's oxygen-carrying capacity.
Double-check type and crossmatching and patient identifiers with a colleague, and monitor for and report signs of transfusion reaction.	These measures reduce risk of delivering wrong type of blood to the patient and enable rapid treatment if transfusion reaction occurs.
Reassure patient that symptoms usually are relieved and tolerance for activity increased with therapy.	Therapy likely will include erythropoietin replacement (recombinant EPO [epoetin-α]), 150 units/kg IV 3 times each week, or 600 units/kg subcutaneously once each week, or darbepoietin alfa 200 mcg every 2 weeks. Red cell production is improved through additional EPO (red cells are not responsive to normal EPO levels in chronic conditions).
	In addition, iron and other supplements (cobalamine, folate) may be given to replenish Hgb and depleted iron and other deficiencies if needed. People with chronic disease, especially older individuals, may not have normal dietary intake of these substances. Supplements will maximize normal erythropoiesis.

••• **Related NIC and NOC labels:** *NIC:* Activity Therapy; Energy Management; Exercise Promotion; Oxygen Therapy; Mutual Goal Setting
NOC: Endurance; Energy Conservation; Activity Tolerance

PATIENT-FAMILY TEACHING AND DISCHARGE PLANNING

When providing patient-family teaching, focus on sensory information, avoid giving excessive information, and initiate a visiting nurse referral for necessary follow-up teaching. Include verbal and written information about the following:

✓ Importance of a well-balanced diet, especially iron intake, if appropriate, which is found in foods such as red meat, dark green vegetables, legumes, and certain fruits (apricots, figs, raisins). Refer to clinical dietitian as prescribed.

✓ Special instructions for taking iron, if appropriate, depending on type prescribed. Therapy may need to be continued for 4-6 mo to replace iron stores adequately.

✓ Necessity for EPO replacement therapy to be continued for duration of the underlying condition.

✓ When self-administering EPO, importance of *not* shaking medication vial before taking it. Shaking the vial may denature glycoprotein in the solution and render it biologically inactive. Any discolored solution or solution with particulate matter should not be used.

✓ Other medications, including drug name, dosage, purpose, schedule, precautions, and potential side effects. Also discuss drug-drug, herb-drug, and food-drug interactions.

✓ Risks and benefits for RBC transfusion (as explained by health care provider) and necessity for signed consent to the transfusion.

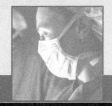

Disseminated Intravascular **63** Coagulation

OVERVIEW/PATHOPHYSIOLOGY

Disseminated intravascular coagulation (DIC) is an acute coagulation disorder characterized by paradoxical clotting and hemorrhage. The sequence usually progresses from massive clot formation, depletion of clotting factors, and activation of diffuse fibrinolysis to hemorrhage. DIC occurs secondary to widespread coagulation factors in the bloodstream caused by extensive surgery, burns, shock, sepsis, neoplastic diseases, or abruptio placentae; extensive destruction of blood vessel walls caused by eclampsia, anoxia, or heat stroke; or damage to blood cells caused by hemolysis, sickle cell disease, or transfusion reactions. While clotting and bleeding occur simultaneously, organ failure related to thromboses of vital organs (e.g., renal, pulmonary) is usually the primary life-threatening concern. Prompt assessment of the disorder can result in a good prognosis. Usually, affected patients are transferred to the intensive care unit (ICU) for careful monitoring and aggressive therapy. DIC may be classified as low-grade (compensated or chronic) or fulminant (acute).

HEALTH CARE SETTING

Acute care/critical care unit

ASSESSMENT

Clinical indicators: Bleeding of abrupt onset; oozing from venipuncture sites or mucosal surfaces; bleeding from surgical sites; and presence of hematuria, blood in stool (melena or hematochezia), spontaneous ecchymosis (bruising), petechiae, purpura fulminans, pallor, or mottled skin. The patient also may bleed from the vagina (menometrorrhagia), nose (epistaxis), and mucous membranes. Joint pain and swelling may signal bleeding into joints. Complaint of headache or mental status changes may indicate intracranial hemorrhage. Symptoms of hypoperfusion can occur, including decreased urine output and abnormal behavior.

Physical assessment: Abdominal assessment may reveal signs of gastrointestinal (GI) bleeding, such as guarding; distention (increasing abdominal girth measurements); hyperactive, hypoactive, or absent bowel sounds; and a rigid, board-like abdomen. With significant hemorrhage, patients may exhibit the following: systolic blood pressure (SBP) less than 90 mm Hg and diastolic blood pressure (DBP) less than 60 mm Hg; heart rate (HR) greater than 100 bpm; peripheral pulse amplitude 2+ or less on a 0-4+ scale; respiratory rate (RR) greater than 22 breaths/min; shortness of breath; urinary output less than 30 ml/hr; secretions and excretions positive for blood; cool, pale, clammy skin; lack of orientation to person, place, and time; or changes in mental status.

Risk factors: Infection, burns, trauma, hepatic disease, hypovolemic shock, severe hemolytic reaction, malignancy, obstetric complications, and hypoxia.

DIAGNOSTIC TESTS

Serum fibrinogen: Low because of abnormal consumption of clotting factors in the formation of fibrin clots.

Platelet count: Less than 250,000/mm^3.

Fibrin split products: Increased, indicating widespread dissolution of clots. Fibrinolysis produces fibrin split products (FSPs), also known as fibrin degradation products (FDPs), as an end product.

D-dimers: The byproducts of fibrinolysis, D-dimers are increased in DIC and, along with increased FDPs, are considered diagnostic of DIC.

Prothrombin time: Normal, low, or possibly increased because of depletion of clotting factors.

Partial thromboplastin time: Normal, low, or possibly high because of depletion of clotting factors.

Peripheral blood smear: Shows fragmented red blood cells (RBCs; schistocytes).

Nursing Diagnosis:

Ineffective Tissue Perfusion: Cardiopulmonary, Peripheral, Renal, and Cerebral

related to coagulation/fibrinolysis processes

Desired Outcome: Following treatment, patient has adequate cardiopulmonary, peripheral, renal, and cerebral perfusion as evidenced by BP 90/60 mm Hg or greater and HR 100 bpm or less (or within patient's baseline range); peripheral pulse amplitude 2+ or greater on a 0-4+ scale; urinary output 30 ml/hr or more; equal and normoreactive pupils; normal/baseline motor function; orientation to person, place, and time; and no mental status changes.

INTERVENTIONS	RATIONALES
Assess for coagulation and bleeding:	
- Monitor vital signs (VS), particularly BP, HR, and peripheral pulses.	Decreased BP, increased HR, and decreased amplitude of peripheral pulses may signal that coagulation and thrombus formation are occurring. This in turn can lead to digital ischemia and gangrene.
- Perform neurologic checks, including orientation, mental status assessments, pupillary reaction to light, level of consciousness (LOC), and motor response.	Deficits may signal that cerebral perfusion is ineffective and should be reported promptly. Signs may be general, such as increased confusion, agitation, or seizures, and become more focal, such as a unilateral widened pupil. If signs of impaired cerebral perfusion occur, it is important to protect patient from injury caused by cerebral impairment by implementing fall precautions as appropriate.
- Monitor intake and output (I&O); report significant findings.	Output less than 30 ml/hr in the presence of adequate intake may indicate renal vessel thrombosis.
- Monitor for hemorrhage from surgical wounds, GI and genitourinary (GU) tracts, and mucous membranes.	Hemorrhage is a potential risk after fibrinolysis.
- Monitor oxygen saturation via pulse oximetry q4h or as indicated; report oxygen saturation 92% or less.	Oxygen perfusion may be compromised by pulmonary emboli and/or pulmonary hemorrhage. Oxygen saturation 92% or less often signals need for supplement oxygen.
Monitor laboratory work for values suggestive of DIC.	Increased D-dimer values, low serum fibrinogen (less than 200 mg/dl), low platelet count (less than 250,000/mm^3), increased FSPs (9 mcg/ml or greater), possible increased prothrombin time (PT) (greater than 11-15 sec), and possible increased partial thromboplastin time (PTT) (greater than 40-100 sec) are common with DIC.
Report significant findings to patient's health care provider; prepare for emergent blood product transfusion, medical support, and transfer to ICU if condition worsens.	Patient may require careful monitoring and aggressive therapy.
Administer antithrombin agents as prescribed.	Antithrombin III and drotrecogin alfa are used for their anticoagulant and antiinflammatory effects.

••• Related NIC and NOC labels: *NIC:* Bleeding Precautions; Embolus Precautions; Laboratory Data Interpretation; Oxygen Therapy; Vital Signs Monitoring; Emergency Care; Neurologic Monitoring *NOC:* Circulation Status; Tissue Perfusion: Cardiac; Tissue Perfusion: Pulmonary; Vital Signs Status; Tissue Perfusion: Cerebral; Tissue Perfusion: Abdominal Organs; Tissue Perfusion: Peripheral

Nursing Diagnosis:

Ineffective Protection

related to increased risk of bleeding secondary to hemorrhagic component of DIC

Desired Outcome: Patient is free of signs of bleeding as evidenced by SBP 90 mm Hg or greater; HR 100 bpm or less (or within patient's normal range); RR 12-20 breaths/min with normal depth and pattern (eupnea); urinary output equal to 30 ml/hr or more; secretions and excretions negative for blood; stable abdominal girth measurements; orientation to person, place, and time; and no changes in mental status.

INTERVENTIONS	RATIONALES
Monitor VS and LOC at frequent intervals; report significant changes.	Hypotension, tachycardia, dyspnea, disorientation, and changes in mental status can signal hemorrhage.
Caution: Be careful of pressure used with BP cuffs. Inflate cuff only as high as needed to obtain reading. Alternate arms with each BP check.	Frequent BP readings may cause bleeding under the cuff. Alternating arms reduces repeated tissue trauma.
Assess for abdominal pain, abdominal distention, changes in bowel sounds, and a boardlike abdomen.	These are signs of GI bleeding.
Assess puncture sites regularly.	This assessment will detect external bleeding or oozing.
When possible, treat bleeding sites with ice, pressure, rest, and elevation.	In addition, some health care providers promote use of thrombin-soaked gauze, such as Gelfoam, or topical thrombin powder.
Be alert to visual changes, headache, and joint pain.	Visual changes may signal retinal hemorrhage. Joint pain and headache are other signs that bleeding may be occurring.
Monitor coagulation and other hematologic laboratory values.	Increased PT (more than 11-15 sec) is a sign that clotting factors are depleted and patient is at risk for hemorrhage.
Prevent or promptly control retching, vomiting, coughing, and straining with bowel movements. Avoid giving IM injections, and minimize venipunctures as appropriate.	These measures minimize the potential for bleeding.
Post "Bleeding Precautions" signs.	This will notify all healthcare providers that venipuncture sites may require additional manual pressure to stop bleeding.
Use a reagent-screening agent to check stool, urine, emesis, and nasogastric drainage for blood.	A positive test signals presence of blood in the GI/GU tracts and should be reported to health care provider promptly for rapid intervention.
Administer blood products (packed RBCs, platelets, fresh frozen plasma [FFP]), and IV fluids as prescribed.	These products help counteract deficiencies causing the bleeding and support blood volume. Cryoprecipitate or FFP may be used if fibrinogen is low; platelets may be given if they are less than 10,000/mm^3 or if there is bleeding.
Teach patient to use electric shaver and soft-bristle toothbrush and avoid forceful nose blowing (dab instead), bending down (head lower than the heart), and potentially traumatic procedures (e.g., enemas, rectal temperatures).	These precautions reduce the risk of bleeding. Razors, hard bristles, thermometers, and enema nozzles, for example, could break the skin and mucous membranes, causing bleeding.
Report significant findings to patient's health care provider. Prepare for emergent blood product transfusion, medical support, and transfer to ICU if condition worsens.	Patient may require aggressive therapy and careful monitoring.

••• **Related NIC and NOC labels:** *NIC:* Bleeding Precautions; Blood Products Administration; Bleeding Reduction *NOC:* Coagulation Status

Nursing Diagnoses:

Risk for Impaired Skin Integrity or Impaired Tissue Integrity

related to altered circulation secondary to hemorrhage and thrombosis

Desired Outcome: Patient's skin and tissue remain nonerythremic and intact.

INTERVENTIONS	RATIONALES
Assess patient's skin, noting changes in color, temperature, and sensation.	Erythema that does not clear after removal of pressure or changes in color, sensation, and temperature may signal decreased perfusion that can lead to tissue damage.
Ensure that patient turns q2h, and consider use of sheepskin on elbows and heels and enhanced pressure-distribution mattress padding. Do not pull on extremities when turning patient.	These measures eliminate or minimize pressure points that could damage the skin/tissue.
As prescribed, encourage active range of motion (ROM) of all extremities q2h.	ROM exercise reduces tissue pressure and promotes circulation.
Keep patient's extremities warm.	Warmth helps prevent tissue hypoxia, which would increase risk of tissue damage/necrosis.
Use alternatives to tape to hold dressings in place, such as gauze wraps or net gauze.	Tape removal could damage fragile skin and tissue.
If patient has areas of breakdown, see "Managing Wound Care," p. 559.	

••• **Related NIC and NOC labels:** *NIC:* Pressure Management; Skin Surveillance; Circulatory Precautions *NOC:* Tissue Integrity: Skin and Mucous Membranes

ADDITIONAL NURSING DIAGNOSES/ PROBLEMS:

"Pulmonary Embolus" for **Ineffective Protection**   p. 139
related to increased risk of bleeding or hemorrhage secondary to anticoagulation therapy

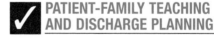 **PATIENT-FAMILY TEACHING AND DISCHARGE PLANNING**

See patient's primary diagnosis.

Polycythemia 64

OVERVIEW/PATHOPHYSIOLOGY

Polycythemia is a chronic disorder characterized by excessive production of red blood cells (RBCs), platelets, and myelocytes. As these increase, blood volume, blood viscosity, and hemoglobin (Hgb) concentration increase, causing excessive workload for the heart and congestion of some organs (e.g., liver, kidney).

Secondary polycythemia results from an abnormal increase in erythropoietin production (e.g., because of hypoxia that occurs with chronic lung disease or prolonged living in altitudes greater than 10,000 ft) or with renal tumors. *Polycythemia vera* is a primary disorder of unknown cause most often affecting men of Jewish descent, with onset in late midlife. *Polycythemia vera* results in increased RBC mass, leukocytosis, and slight thrombocytosis. Because of increased viscosity and decreased microcirculation, mortality is high if the condition is left untreated. In addition, there is potential for this disorder to evolve into other hematopoietic disorders, such as acute leukemia.

HEALTH CARE SETTING

Primary care; acute care for complications

ASSESSMENT

Signs and symptoms: Fatigue, muscle pain, headache, dizziness, paresthesias, visual disturbances, dyspnea, thrombophlebitis, joint pain, painful pruritus, night sweats, chest pain, and a feeling of "fullness," especially in the head.

Physical assessment: Hypertension, engorgement of retinal blood veins, crackles (rales), weight loss, cyanosis, changes in mentation or mood (delirium, psychotic depression, mania), ruddy complexion (especially palmar aspects of hands and plantar surfaces of feet), splenomegaly, hepatomegaly, gastrointestinal (GI) disturbances (ulcers, GI bleed).

DIAGNOSTIC TESTS

Complete blood count: Increased RBC mass (8-12 million/mm^3), Hgb (18-25 g/dl), hematocrit (Hct) (more than 54% in men and 49% in women), and leukocytes; and overproduction of thrombocytes are diagnostic of polycythemia.

Platelet count: Elevated as a result of increased production.

Bone marrow aspiration: Reveals RBC proliferation.

Uric acid levels: May be increased because of increased nucleoprotein, an end product of RBC breakdown.

Erythropoietin levels: Elevated in secondary polycythemia and decreased in polycythemia vera.

O_2 saturation: Normal (greater than 92%).

Nursing Diagnosis:

Acute Pain

related to headache, angina, pruritus, and abdominal and joint discomfort *secondary to* altered circulation occurring with blood hyperviscosity

Desired Outcomes: Within 1 hr of intervention, patient's subjective perception of discomfort decreases, as documented by pain scale. Objective indicators, such as grimacing, are absent or diminished. Lifestyle behaviors are not compromised because of discomfort.

501

INTERVENTIONS	RATIONALES
Assess for presence of headache, angina, abdominal pain, and joint pain. Devise a pain scale with patient, rating discomfort from 0 (no pain) to 10 (worst pain).	The patient provides a personal baseline report, enabling nurse to more effectively monitor subsequent increases and decreases in pain. Use of a pain intensity scale allows more accurate documentation of discomfort and subsequent relief obtained after analgesia has been administered.
Be alert to patient complaints of calf pain and tenderness.	These are indicators of peripheral thrombosis, which should be reported promptly for immediate intervention.
In the presence of joint or skin discomfort, rest the joint and elevate the extremity. Use gentle range-of-motion (ROM) exercises as tolerated. Caution patient to avoid crossing legs and wearing restrictive clothing. Apply cool compresses or ice.	Elevation may help increase circulation and prevent pooling of hyperviscous blood in the joints. ROM helps improve circulation. Ice is used (short term) to decrease severe joint pain. **Note:** In the presence of pruritus, skin may become painful and swollen, exacerbated by heat or exposure to water. Topical antihistamines or lotions generally are not helpful.
Administer analgesics as prescribed.	Analgesics reduce pain.
Note: Avoid analgesics containing aspirin or nonsteroidal antiinflammatory drugs unless prescribed by health care provider.	These drugs may exacerbate bleeding associated with thrombocytosis (high number of ineffective platelets) but may be helpful in alleviating microvascular symptoms.
Instruct patient to request analgesic before pain becomes too intense.	Pain is easier to control before it becomes severe. Prolonged stimulation of pain receptors results in increased sensitivity to painful stimuli and will increase the amount of drug required to relieve pain.
Encourage use of nonpharmacologic pain control, such as relaxation and distraction.	These are pain measures that potentiate analgesics and do not have side effects.
For more information, see "Pain," p. 39.	

••• **Related NIC and NOC labels:** *NIC:* Pain Management; Analgesic Administration; Positioning; Simple Relaxation Therapy; Distraction; Heat/Cold Application *NOC:* Comfort Level

Nursing Diagnosis:

Ineffective Tissue Perfusion: Renal, Peripheral, and Cerebral

related to blood hyperviscosity

Desired Outcome: Following treatment, patient has adequate renal, peripheral, and cerebral perfusion as evidenced by urinary output 30 ml/hr or more; peripheral pulses 2+ or more on a scale of 0-4+; distal extremity warmth; adequate (baseline) muscle strength; no mental status changes; and orientation to person, place, and time.

INTERVENTIONS	RATIONALES
Monitor intake and output; report significant findings.	Urine output less than 30 ml/hr in the presence of adequate intake can signal renal congestion and decreased perfusion.
Palpate peripheral pulses and assess distal extremities.	Pulse amplitude 2+ or less on a scale of 0-4+ and coolness in distal extremities can signal disruption of peripheral tissue perfusion secondary to hyperviscosity of the blood.
Monitor for muscle weakness and decreases in sensation and LOC.	These are indicators of thrombosis.
If these indicators are present, assist with ambulation or initiate fall prevention measures, depending on degree of deficit.	These measures reduce risk of further thrombosis as well as protect patient from injury caused by declining neurologic status.
In the absence of signs of cardiac and renal failure, provide prescribed IV hydration and encourage fluid intake to decrease viscosity.	Inadequate hydration can increase blood viscosity and contribute adversely to polycythemia.
Encourage patient to change position qh when in bed or to exercise and ambulate to tolerance.	These measures promote circulation and reduce the risk of thrombosis.

Continued

INTERVENTIONS	RATIONALES
Instruct patient to avoid tight or restrictive clothing.	Tight clothing could impede blood flow/circulation, increasing the risk of thromboses.
Administer myelosuppressive agents, as prescribed.	Chemotherapy agents are given to inhibit bone marrow function and reduce overproduction of blood cells. For example, hydroxyurea (preferred), busulfan, and/or radioactive phosphorus may be given, especially for older adults and those refractive to other agents. Myeloablative chemotherapy followed by hematopoietic stem cell transplant from an HLA-matched donor to reconstitute patient's bone marrow may be used in younger patients who do not respond to other therapies.
If patient smokes, encourage enrollment in a smoking cessation program.	Smoking significantly increases the potential of a thromboembolic event.

••• **Related NIC and NOC labels:** *NIC:* Embolus Precautions; Circulatory Precautions; Hypovolemia Management; Neurologic Monitoring; Medication Administration *NOC:* Circulation Status; Neurological Status; Tissue Perfusion: Cerebral; Tissue Perfusion: Abdominal Organs; Tissue Perfusion: Peripheral; Tissue Perfusion: Renal

Nursing Diagnosis:

Imbalanced Nutrition: Less Than Body Requirements

related to anorexia secondary to feelings of fullness occurring with organ system congestion

Desired Outcome: By at least 24 hr before hospital discharge, patient exhibits adequate nutrition as evidenced by maintenance of or return to baseline body weight or a 1- to 2-lb weight gain.

INTERVENTIONS	RATIONALES
Weigh patient daily.	This will help identify trend of patient's nutritional status.
Monitor fluid volume intake; encourage intake if necessary.	These measures will maximize hydration and vascular blood flow.
Encourage patient to eat small, frequent meals. Document intake.	Smaller, more frequent meals usually are better tolerated than larger, less frequent meals.
Request that significant other bring in patient's favorite foods if they are unavailable in the hospital.	This promotes the likelihood that patient will eat.
Advise patient to avoid spicy foods and to eat mild foods.	Mild foods are better tolerated.
Teach patient to avoid intake of iron and citrus with meals.	These restrictions help minimize abnormal RBC proliferation and iron overload. Citrus increases absorption of iron.
As indicated, obtain dietary consultation.	Such a referral will enable more detailed instruction/discussion about foods to eat and those to avoid.
Teach patient or significant other how to record and maintain fluid and food intake diary.	This will help them monitor trends in food intake and ensure monitoring of hydration status.

••• **Related NIC and NOC labels**: *NIC:* Nutritional Monitoring; Fluid Monitoring; Weight Gain Assistance; Teaching: Prescribed Diet *NOC:* Nutritional Status; Nutritional Status: Food & Fluid Intake

Nursing Diagnosis:

Ineffective Tissue Perfusion: Cerebral and Cardiopulmonary (or risk for same)

related to hypovolemia secondary to phlebotomy

Desired Outcome: Patient has adequate cerebral and cardiopulmonary perfusion as evidenced by no mental status changes; orientation to person, place, and time; HR 100 bpm or less; BP 90/60 mm Hg or greater (or within patient's baseline range); absence of chest pain; and RR 20 breaths/min or less.

INTERVENTIONS	RATIONALES
Assess for tachycardia, hypotension, chest pain, or dizziness during procedure; notify patient's health care provider of significant findings.	These are signs of deficient fluid volume as a result of phlebotomy. Blood is withdrawn from the vein to decrease blood volume (and decrease Hct to 45%). Usually 500 ml is removed every 2-4 days until Hct is 42%-47%. For the older adult, 250-300 ml is removed.
During phlebotomy procedure, keep patient recumbent.	This position helps prevent dizziness or hypotension as a result of phlebotomy.
After the procedure, assist patient into a sitting position for 5-10 min before ambulation.	This will help prevent orthostatic hypotension. For more information about orthostatic hypotension, see "Prolonged Bedrest" for **Ineffective Tissue Perfusion: Cerebral,** p. 66.
Teach patients, especially those who are older and chronically ill, about potential for orthostatic hypotension and need for caution when standing for at least 2-3 days after phlebotomy.	This information will help protect against injury caused by falling as a result of orthostatic hypotension.

••• **Related NIC and NOC labels:** *NIC:* Fluid Monitoring; Hypovolemia Management; Vital Signs Monitoring; Positioning *NOC:* Circulation Status; Vital Signs Status; Tissue Perfusion: Cerebral

 PATIENT-FAMILY TEACHING AND DISCHARGE PLANNING

When providing patient-family teaching, focus on sensory information, avoid giving excessive information, and initiate a visiting nurse referral for necessary follow-up teaching. Include verbal and written information about the following:

✓ Need for continued medical follow-up, including potential for phlebotomy.

✓ Medications, including drug name, purpose, dosage, schedule, precautions, and potential side effects. Also discuss drug-drug, herb-drug, and food-drug interactions.

✓ Importance of augmenting fluid intake (e.g., greater than 2.5 L/day) to decrease blood viscosity and avoiding smoking; provide smoking cessation information as appropriate.

✓ Signs and symptoms that necessitate medical attention: angina, muscle weakness, numbness and tingling of extremities, decreased tolerance to activity, mental status changes, joint pain, and bleeding.

✓ Nutrition: Importance of maintaining balanced diet to increase resistance to infection, and limiting dietary or supplemental intake of iron to help minimize abnormal RBC proliferation and iron overload.

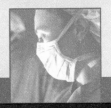

Thrombocytopenia 65

OVERVIEW/PATHOPHYSIOLOGY

Thrombocytopenia is a relatively common coagulation disorder that results from a decreased number of platelets. It can be congenital or acquired, and it is classified according to cause. Causes include deficient production of thrombocytes, as occurs with bone marrow disease (e.g., leukemia, aplastic anemia) or accelerated platelet destruction occurring from loss or increased use, as in hemolytic anemia, disseminated intravascular coagulation (DIC), or damage by prosthetic heart valves, as well as hypersplenism and hypothermia. Potential triggers include an autoimmune disorder, severe vascular injury, and spleen malfunction. In addition, thrombocytopenia can occur as a side effect of certain medications, such as heparin. Regardless of cause or trigger, the disorder affects coagulation and hemostasis. With chemical-induced thrombocytopenia, prognosis is good after withdrawal of the offending drug. Prognosis for other types depends on the form of thrombocytopenia and the individual's baseline health status and response to treatment. **Note:** Thrombocytopenia may be the first sign of systemic lupus erythematosus (SLE) or infection.

Thrombotic thrombocytopenic purpura (TTP) is an acute, often fatal disorder caused by deficiency of a plasma enzyme that normally inactivates the von Willebrand clotting factor (vWF) when it is not needed. vWF is the most important protein that mediates platelet adhesion to damaged endothelial surfaces. *Idiopathic thrombocytopenic purpura (ITP)* is believed to be an immune disorder specifically involving antiplatelet immunoglobulin G (IgG), which destroys platelets. The acute form is most often seen in children (2-6 yr of age) and may be related to a previous viral infection. The chronic form is seen more often in adults (18-50 yr of age) and is of unknown origin.

Heparin-induced thrombocytopenia (HIT) is a disorder in which heparin triggers an antibody response; the heparin-antibody complexes bind to platelet surfaces, causing activated platelets to aggregate, leading to further thrombosis and, because of increased utilization, thrombocytopenia. Because the platelets are activated (although low in number), HIT is uniquely associated with both arterial and venous thrombosis rather than bleeding.

HEALTH CARE SETTING

Primary care; hospitalization for complications

ASSESSMENT

Chronic indicators: Long history of mild bleeding or hemorrhagic episodes from the mouth, nose, gastrointestinal (GI) tract, or genitourinary (GU) tract. Increased bruising (ecchymosis) and petechiae also have been noted.

Acute indicators: Fever, splenomegaly, acute and severe bleeding episodes, weakness, lethargy, malaise, hemorrhage into mucous membranes, gum bleeding, and GU or GI bleeding. Prolonged bleeding can lead to a shock state with tachycardia, shortness of breath, and decreased level of consciousness (LOC). Optic fundal hemorrhage decreases vision and may preclude potentially fatal intracranial hemorrhage. **Note:** With TTP and HIT, the individual may exhibit signs associated with platelet thrombus formation, such as skin necrosis, and ischemic organ failure (decreased renal function or neurologic changes).

History of: Recent infection, myeloproliferative disease, or aplastic anemia; recent vaccination; binge alcohol consumption; positive family history of thrombocytopenia; or use of chlorothiazide, digitalis, quinidine, rifampin, sulfisoxazole, chloramphenicol, phenytoin, or heparin.

DIAGNOSTIC TESTS

Platelet count: Can vary from only slightly decreased to nearly absent. Less than 100,000/mm^3 is significantly decreased; less than 20,000/mm^3 results in a serious risk of hemorrhage.

Peripheral blood smear: May reveal megathrombocytes (large platelets), which are present during premature destruction of platelets, as well as reticulocytosis and fragmented red cells.

Lactate dehydrogenase: May be elevated.

Bilirubin: Increased.

Complete blood count: Low hemoglobin (Hgb) and hematocrit (Hct) levels because of blood loss; white blood cell (WBC) count usually within normal range.

Coagulation studies

Bleeding time: Increased because of decreased platelets.

Partial thromboplastin time: May be increased or normal.
Prothrombin time: May be increased or normal.
International normalized ratio: Increased.
International sensitivity index: Increased.
Bone marrow aspiration: Reveals increased number of megakaryocytes (platelet precursors) in the presence of ITP

and HIT but may be decreased in other causes of thrombocytopenia.

Antibody screen: May be positive because of the presence of IgG platelet antibodies or positive HIT antibody tests.

Nursing Diagnosis:

Ineffective Protection

related to increased risk of bleeding secondary to decreased platelet count

Desired Outcome: Patient is free of the signs of bleeding as evidenced by secretions and excretions negative for blood, BP 90/60 mm Hg or greater or within patient's baseline range, HR 100 bpm or less, RR 12-20 breaths/min with normal depth and pattern (eupnea), and absence of bruising or active bleeding.

INTERVENTIONS	RATIONALES
Assess patient for hematuria, melena, epistaxis, hematemesis, hemoptysis, menometrorrhagia, bleeding gums, petechiae, or severe ecchymosis. Teach patient to be alert to and report these indicators promptly as well as any headache or changes in vision.	These are signs of bleeding that could occur as a result of thrombocytopenia. These signs should be reported promptly for timely intervention.
Monitor platelet count daily and coagulation studies at least weekly or as prescribed.	Optimal range is 150,000-400,000/mm³. Less than 100,000/mm³ is significantly decreased; less than 20,000/mm³ results in a serious risk of hemorrhage.
Ensure that there is a current type and crossmatch in the blood bank for RBCs.	RBC transfusions would be necessary to help maintain intravascular volume in the event acute bleeding occurs.
Prevent or promptly control symptoms that can trigger bleeding, such as retching, vomiting, coughing, and straining with bowel movements.	Straining and similar actions increase intracranial pressure and can result in intracranial hemorrhage.
When possible, avoid venipuncture. If performed, apply pressure on site for 5-10 min or until bleeding stops. Do not give IM injections. If injections are necessary, use subcutaneous route with a small-gauge needle.	Patient is at risk for prolonged bleeding because of the decreased platelet count.
Advise patient to avoid straining at stool.	Straining increases intracranial pressure and can result in intracranial hemorrhage.
Obtain prescription for stool softeners, if indicated. Teach patient anticonstipation routine as described in "Prolonged Bedrest" for **Constipation**, p. 67.	These measures help prevent constipation, thereby minimizing need to strain at stool.
Administer corticosteroids as prescribed.	Corticosteroids enhance vascular integrity and diminish platelet destruction.
Teach patient to use electric razor and soft-bristle toothbrush.	These items minimize risk of injury and hence bleeding.
Instruct patient about the association of alcohol consumption, smoking, and use of aspirin or nonsteroidal antiinflammatory drugs (NSAIDs) with increased risk of bleeding.	Alcohol may suppress bone marrow production of blood cells, smoking affects circulation, and aspirin and NSAIDs reduce platelet adhesion.
Administer platelet-increasing agents as prescribed.	*Intravenous immunoglobulin (IV IgG)* increases platelet count by impeding the antibody production that destroys platelets.
	Recombinant interleukin 11 stimulates megakaryocyte differentiation and platelet production in cancer patients who have thrombocytopenia, but clinical benefit over use of platelets is controversial.
	IV anti-D immune globulin increases platelet count by impeding production of antibodies that destroy platelets.

Continued

INTERVENTIONS	RATIONALES
Administer platelets as prescribed.	Platelet transfusion is used if platelet destruction or deficient formation is the primary cause of the disorder, or risk of increased microthrombi and organ ischemia is not of primary concern. It provides only temporary relief because the half-life of platelets is only 3-4 days and may be even shorter with ITP (i.e., minutes to hours). Platelet transfusions should be avoided in patients with TTP or active HIT except in life-threatening or organ-threatening hemorrhage. If used, HLA-matched or cross-matched platelets may improve clinical response.
Double-check blood product and type with a colleague, and monitor for and report signs of transfusion reaction, including chills, back pain, dyspnea, hives, and wheezing.	These precautions help ensure that patient receives correct blood product and type, which otherwise could result in transfusion reaction.
Make sure patient has been informed of risks and benefits of all blood product transfusions by health care provider and that patient signs consent to the transfusion.	Although risk of life-threatening reactions and infections is low, patients must be informed as to the risks and benefits by the health care provider according to the Paul Gann Act.

••• **Related NIC and NOC labels:** *NIC:* Bleeding Precautions; Blood Products Administration *NOC:* Coagulation Status

Nursing Diagnosis:

Ineffective Tissue Perfusion: Cerebral, Peripheral, and **Renal** (or risk for same)

related to interrupted blood flow secondary to presence of thrombotic component, which results in sensitization and clumping of platelets in the blood vessels

Desired Outcome: Patient's cerebral, peripheral, and renal perfusions are adequate as evidenced by no mental status changes; orientation to person, place, and time; normoreactive pupillary responses; absence of headaches, dizziness, and visual disturbances; peripheral pulses greater than 2+ on a 0-4+ scale; and urine output 30 ml/hr or more.

INTERVENTIONS	RATIONALES
Assess for changes in mental status, LOC, and pupillary response. Monitor for headaches, dizziness, or visual disturbances.	These changes and findings are indicators of ineffective cerebral tissue perfusion.
Palpate peripheral pulses on all extremities. Compare distal extremities for color, warmth, and character of pulses.	Pulse amplitude 2+ or less on a 0-4+ scale is a signal of ineffective peripheral tissue perfusion (thrombosis), as are differences in color, warmth, and pulse character when comparing one extremity to the other.
Assess urine output.	Adequate renal perfusion is reflected by urine output 30 ml/hr or more for 2 consecutive hr. Amounts less than that may signal decreased renal perfusion as a result of thrombosis.
Monitor patient's fluid intake.	Patient should be well hydrated (2-3 L/day) to increase perfusion to the small vessels.

••• **Related NIC and NOC labels:** *NIC:* Neurologic Monitoring; Embolus Care: Peripheral; Fluid Management *NOC:* Tissue Perfusion: Cerebral; Tissue Perfusion: Peripheral; Tissue Perfusion: Abdominal Organs

Nursing Diagnosis:

Acute Pain

related to joint discomfort secondary to hemorrhagic episodes or blood extravasation into the tissues

Desired Outcomes: Within 1 hr of intervention, patient's subjective perception of discomfort decreases, as documented by pain scale. Objective indicators, such as grimacing, are absent or diminished.

INTERVENTIONS	RATIONALES
Monitor patient for presence of fatigue, malaise, and joint pain. Devise a pain scale with patient, rating discomfort on a scale of 0 (no pain) to 10 (worst pain).	This assessment will help determine the degree and type of discomfort. The pain scale also will help assess degree of relief obtained after treatment/intervention.
Maintain a calm, quiet environment. Facilitate coordination of care providers, allowing time for periods of undisturbed rest.	These measures promote rest, which will help decrease discomfort and fatigue.
Elevate legs. Support legs with pillows.	These measures help minimize joint discomfort in the lower extremities.
Avoid gatching bed at the knee. Choose chairs with or provide padding on seats.	These measures help prevent occlusion of popliteal vessels.
Use a bed cradle; provide socks, as needed, for warmth.	A bed cradle will decrease pressure on tissues of the lower extremities. Decreased circulation results in extremity coolness.
Administer analgesics as prescribed. Reassess pain and document relief obtained, using the pain scale.	Analgesics reduce pain. The pain scale will help assess degree of relief obtained after treatment/intervention.
Caution: Avoid use of aspirin and NSAIDs.	These agents are contraindicated because of their antiplatelet action, which would increase risk of bleeding.
Instruct patient to request analgesic before pain becomes severe.	Pain is more readily controlled when it is treated before it gets severe. Prolonged stimulation of pain receptors results in increased sensitivity to painful stimuli and will increase the amount of drug required to relieve pain.

See "Pain," p. 39, for more information.

●●● **Related NIC and NOC labels:** *NIC:* Management; Analgesic Administration; Environmental Management: Comfort; Positioning *NOC:* Comfort Level; Pain Control; Pain: Disruptive Effects; Pain Level

ADDITIONAL NURSING DIAGNOSES/ PROBLEMS:

"Perioperative Care" for **Risk for Deficient Fluid Volume** *related to* postoperative bleeding/hemorrhage   p. 51

 PATIENT-FAMILY TEACHING AND DISCHARGE PLANNING

When providing patient-family teaching, focus on sensory information, avoid giving excessive information, and initiate a visiting nurse referral for necessary follow-up teaching. Include verbal and written information about the following:

✓ Importance of preventing trauma, which can cause bleeding.

✓ Seeking medical attention for any signs of bleeding, infection, or clotting. Review signs and symptoms of common infections, such as upper respiratory, urinary tract, and wound infections. Signs and symptoms of common infections are described in "Care of the Renal Transplant Recipient," **Risk for Infection,** p. 239. Also teach patient to assess for hematuria, melena, hematemesis, hemoptysis, menometrorrhagia, oozing from mucous membranes, and petechiae.

✓ Importance of regular medical follow-up for laboratory studies.

✓ If patient is discharged taking corticosteroids, an explanation of side effects of steroids, including weight gain, headache, capillary fragility, hypertension, moon facies, thinning of arms and legs, mood changes, acne, buffalo hump, edema formation, risk of GI hemorrhage, delayed wound healing, and increased appetite. Review need to take medication with food, immediately take missed doses, and not precipitously discontinue medication.

✓ Other medications, including drug name, dosage, purpose, schedule, precautions, and potential side effects. Also discuss drug-drug, herb-drug, and food-drug interactions.

✓ Importance of obtaining a medical alert bracelet and identification card outlining diagnosis and emergency treatment. Contact MedicAlert Foundation at *www.medicalert.org.*

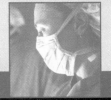

Amputation 66

OVERVIEW/PATHOPHYSIOLOGY

Amputation, the removal of part or all of a limb through bone, is now less commonly performed as an orthopedic surgical intervention than it was before advances in antibiotic therapy, treatment for musculoskeletal neoplasms, and microsurgery/limb salvage techniques. Lower extremity amputation may still be the treatment of choice for complications of diabetes mellitus (DM) such as peripheral vascular disease (PVD) and for osteomyelitis or severe trauma. Persons with PVD account for approximately 80% of lower extremity amputations in the Western world. On rare occasions, amputation may be necessary because of congenital limb deficiencies in infants and children.

While the majority of lower extremity amputations are performed due to disease, most upper extremity amputations are the result of trauma. Amputation and prosthesis use may offer the patient improved functional ability.

HEALTH CARE SETTING

Critical care unit, acute care surgical unit, orthopedic rehabilitation unit

ASSESSMENT

Chronic disease: Patients with advanced PVD often complain of extremity pain in a definable muscle group (usually calf muscles) precipitated by exercise and promptly relieved by rest. This pain is distinguished from that of diabetic neuropathy, which is distributed along dermatomes rather than confined to a specific muscle group; neuropathy is also constant and unrelated to exercise. The affected limb is often a dark red color (rubor) when it is dependent; atrophy of skin and subcutaneous tissue may be apparent. Amputation also may be needed because of metabolic disorders (e.g., osteosarcoma of Paget's disease), or massive muscle necrosis that results from an acute thromboembolic event or untreated compartment syndrome. The patient also may have a tumor of bone or soft tissue, but amputation in this case is much less common than in the past because of the advent of sophisticated limb salvage procedures.

Trauma: A mangled extremity is common with high-energy injuries. The patient may have multiple injuries, and surgical priority must be given to those injuries that may be life threatening. Trauma may result in a complete amputation, a near or partial amputation, or a segmental amputation of an extremity.

DIAGNOSTIC TESTS

Ankle-arm (ankle-brachial) index: The most widely used noninvasive test for evaluating PVD. Blood pressure is measured at the ankle and in the arm while patient is at rest. Measurements are then repeated at both sites after patient has walked 5 min on a treadmill. Ankle-brachial index (ABI) is calculated by dividing the highest blood pressure at the ankle by the highest recorded pressure in either arm. A decrease in the ABI result with exercise can aid in predicting severity of the vascular disease and is a sensitive indicator that significant PVD is present.

Doppler ultrasound: Evaluates blood flow to the extremities. It can reliably distinguish exercise-related effects from severe ischemia.

Transcutaneous O_2 pressure: Measured after oxygen sensors are applied to the skin. By determining oxygen tension (desired value is 30-50 mm Hg), the surgeon can map out areas of lesser perfusion in the affected extremity. This test offers the most accurate assessment of blood supply and the best prediction of residual limb healing potential.

Angiography: Confirms circulatory impairment to determine appropriate level for amputation. This invasive study involves radiographic imaging after injection of a radiopaque substance into a blood vessel. It is most useful if patient is a candidate for angioplasty or arterial reconstruction.

Xenon-133: A radioactive isotope injected intradermally at the midpoint of the intended incision for amputation. Skin clearance of this agent reflects skin blood flow as a measure of the appropriate level of amputation.

Nursing Diagnoses:

Acute Pain/Chronic Pain

related to phantom limb sensation

Desired Outcome: Within 24 hr of intervention, patient's subjective perception of pain decreases as documented by pain intensity rating scale.

INTERVENTIONS	RATIONALES
Ensure adequate pain management before elective amputation surgery.	This measure decreases the likelihood that phantom limb sensation will develop. Patients with unrelieved preoperative pain are more likely to experience phantom limb sensation.
Explain that continued sensations often arise postoperatively from the amputated part and may be painful, irritating, or simply disconcerting.	This information prepares patient for the potential experience of phantom limb sensation.
Assist in use of a pain intensity rating scale.	This scale enables more accurate documentation of patient's pain experience and the effects of analgesia.
Administer simple analgesics, nonsteroidal antiinflammatory drugs, opioid analgesics, and adjuncts as prescribed and reassess their effectiveness in approximately 1 hr using pain intensity rating scale. Document preintervention and postintervention pain scores.	Although opioids provide effective treatment of incisional pain, they may be ineffective for phantom limb sensation because they do not alter response of afferent nerves to noxious stimuli. Higher opiate doses are often required to treat phantom limb sensation.
	Anticonvulsants such as gabapentin and topiramate may be effective for neuropathic pain, and baclofen may be used to control spasms and cramps in the phantom limb. Tricyclic antidepressants (e.g., amitriptyline) not only offer analgesia but also may be used to elevate mood and alleviate insomnia. A lidocaine patch also may be helpful when applied near the surgical wound. Beta-blockers such as propanolol have been used as adjuncts but their efficacy is unclear.
Teach patient to use counterirritation to manage painful sensations.	Counterirritation manages painful sensations by providing a new stimulus to compete with the patient's pain.
As indicated, use transcutaneous electrical nerve stimulation (TENS) on the contralateral limb.	TENS may provide effective short-term management of phantom limb sensation. Use on the residual limb has been associated with exacerbation of pain and should be avoided.
Also consider interventions such as distraction, guided imagery, relaxation, and biofeedback.	These nonpharmacologic methods augment pharmacologic pain relief.
Instruct patient to begin to massage residual limb 3 wk postoperatively.	Massage will desensitize the area in preparation for prosthesis. Early prosthesis may reduce incidence of phantom limb sensation.
	After surgical wound healing is complete, vigorous stimulation of the end of the residual limb may be prescribed. This can be accomplished by hitting the end of the limb with a rolled towel.
Encourage patient to consider use of sympathetic blocking agents, acupuncture, ultrasound, and injection with local anesthetics.	These are other modalities for decreasing phantom limb sensation.
Refer patient to a pain clinic.	Pain clinics enable a comprehensive interdisciplinary program to manage chronic phantom limb sensation.
Explore impact phantom limb pain may have on patient's ability to function on the job or in interpersonal relationships.	Attempts to cope with chronic pain can deplete patient's resources, leaving little energy for job and relationships.
For more information, including use of patient-controlled analgesia, see "Pain," p. 39.	

••• Related NIC and NOC labels: *NIC:* Medication Management; Pain Management; Biofeedback; Positioning; Simple Guided Imagery; Simple Massage; Simple Relaxation Therapy; Transcutaneous Electrical Nerve Stimulation; Cutaneous Stimulation; Distraction *NOC:* Comfort Level; Pain Control; Pain: Disruptive Effects; Depression Control

Nursing Diagnosis:

Risk for Disuse Syndrome

related to severe pain and immobility secondary to amputation

Desired Outcomes: Within 24 hr of instruction, patient verbalizes understanding of the prescribed exercise regimen and performs exercises independently. Patient is free of symptoms of contracture as evidenced by optimal range of motion (ROM) of joints and maintenance of muscle mass.

INTERVENTIONS	RATIONALES
Establish with the patient a goal for pain management, using both pharmacologic and nonpharmacologic measures.	Effective pain management promotes early movement and ambulation, which in turn aid in prevention of flexion contractures. An early return to activity also prevents loss of muscle strength and increases local circulation to improve wound healing.
If prescribed, elevate affected extremity for the first 24 hr postoperatively.	During the first 24 hr after surgery, elevation decreases swelling and therefore aids in pain management and mobility. Elevation is discontinued after this period to prevent hip flexion contracture.
Caution: Perform extremity elevation and ROM exercises *only* if prescribed by health care provider.	A residual limb with deficient vascular supply must not be elevated in order to avoid further compromise of circulation.
Assist in performance of ROM exercises daily for mobility of proximal joints.	Performance of ROM exercises contributes to optimal joint function and decreases the risk for development of flexion contractures.
On the second postoperative day, ensure that patient keeps the residual limb flat when at rest.	This position will decrease risk for hip flexion contracture. Other strategies to prevent contracture include assisting patient to lie prone for 1 hr qid.
Teach patient to perform prescribed exercises that increase strength of muscle extensors.	Prescribed exercises may include the following: - Above-knee amputation *(AKA):* Patient attempts to straighten hip from a flexed position against resistance or perform gluteal-setting exercises. - Below-knee amputation *(BKA):* Patient attempts to straighten knee against resistance or perform quadriceps exercises. Patient also should perform exercises for AKA.

••• Related NIC and NOC labels: *NIC:* Exercise Therapy: Joint Mobility; Exercise Therapy: Muscle Control; Positioning; Pain Management; Teaching: Prescribed Activity/Exercise *NOC:* Immobility Consequences: Physiological; Mobility Level

Nursing Diagnoses:

Disturbed Body Image/Ineffective Role Performance

related to loss of limb

Desired Outcome: Within 72 hr of surgery, patient begins to show adaptation to loss of limb and demonstrates interest in resuming role-related responsibilities.

INTERVENTIONS	RATIONALES
Encourage use of a prosthesis (if prescribed) immediately after surgery.	Whether the amputation is the result of trauma, chronic illness, or cancer, the patient is likely to experience a period of grieving. Disbelief and anger often mark the initial response. The patient may believe attainment of independence and future goals is impossible. Early use of a prosthesis offers a prompt return to mobility and patient's resumption of typical activities.

Continued

INTERVENTIONS	RATIONALES
Gently encourage patient to look at and touch residual limb and verbalize feelings about the amputation. Provide privacy for patient and significant other to express feelings regarding the amputation.	The patient may have a stereotyped image of disability and unattractiveness following amputation. Sometimes these emotions are suppressed during rehabilitation and reemerge as time passes. Addressing stereotypical thinking early in recovery and actively involving patient in education will help provide patient with a sense of participation and control. All caregivers must show an accepting attitude and encourage significant other to accept patient's new appearance.
Assist patient with adapting to loss of limb while maintaining a sense of what is perceived as the normal self.	Strategies to accomplish this include introducing patient to others who have successfully adapted to a similar amputation. Teaching aids such as books, pamphlets, audiovisuals, and videotapes can be used to demonstrate how others have adapted to amputation.
Discuss ways patient may alter task performance to continue to function in vocational and interpersonal roles.	Assistive devices may be needed for continued functioning in current vocational role. If patient's health precludes continued performance in the current vocational role, referral and counseling for retraining may be needed.
For patient who continues to have difficulty adapting to the amputation, provide a referral to an appropriate resource person such as a psychologist or psychiatric nurse.	Trained professionals can help explore the impact of amputation on patient's life and review strategies for adaptation.

●●● **Related NIC and NOC labels:** *NIC:* Body Image Enhancement; Amputation Care; Coping Enhancement; Grief Work Facilitation; Counseling; Support Group; Role Enhancement; Normalization Promotion *NOC:* Body Image; Psychosocial Adjustment: Life Change; Coping; Role Performance

Nursing Diagnosis:

Deficient Knowledge:

Care of the residual limb and prosthesis; signs and symptoms of skin irritation or pressure necrosis

Desired Outcomes: Within 24 hr of hospital discharge, patient verbalizes knowledge about care of the residual limb and prosthesis and independently returns demonstration of wrapping the residual limb. Patient verbalizes knowledge about indicators of pressure necrosis and irritation from the shrinkage device or prosthesis.

INTERVENTIONS	RATIONALES
Assess patient's health care literacy (language, reading, comprehension). Assess culture and culturally specific information needs.	This assessment helps ensure that materials are presented in a manner that is culturally and educationally appropriate.
Teach Patient about the Following:	
- For the first 24 hr after surgery, elevate residual limb as prescribed.	Elevation reduces edema and pain.
- After this period, keep the lower residual limb flat when at rest in bed.	A flat position reduces risk of hip flexion contracture after the first 24 hr after surgery.
- When in a chair, elevate the lower residual limb.	Elevating the lower residual limb reduces dependent edema when the patient is in a chair.
- Teach application of a shrinkage device such as an elastic wrap or sock.	A shrinkage device molds the residual limb in patients for whom prosthesis fitting is prescribed. Application of elastic wrap is begun with a recurrent turn over distal end of residual limb; then diagonal circumferential turns are made, overlapping to two-thirds the width of the wrap. Wrapping in a circular pattern may compromise blood supply to the residual limb. The shrinkage device should be wrapped snugly but not too tight to avoid impeding circulation and healing. It should remain smooth and free of wrinkles to avoid causing skin breakdown or uneven shrinkage of the residual limb.

Continued

INTERVENTIONS	RATIONALES
Ensure that all tissue is contained by the elastic wrap.	The goal of wrapping is to form a cone-shaped residual limb. If any tissue is allowed to bulge, proper fitting of prosthesis will be difficult.
Perform rewrapping, combined with careful inspection of residual limb, q4-6h, or more often if the elastic wrap becomes loose.	Assessment of the limb at regular intervals will detect skin impairment and allow early intervention. Rewrapping also assures that the elastic wrap remains snug enough to effectively mold the residual limb for the prosthesis.
Use extra padding with moleskin or lamb's wool.	Extra padding prevents irritation to areas that are susceptible to pressure.
Teach patient to monitor residual limb for skin abrasions, blisters, and hair follicle infection.	These are indicators of skin irritations or pressure necrosis caused by shrinkage device or prosthesis.
Explain that if erythema persists after massage, patient should notify health care provider.	Persistent erythema may be an early sign of pressure sore development.
If prescribed, instruct patient to leave any open areas on residual limb exposed to air for 1-hr periods qid.	Prolonged dressing of wounds can trap moisture that can contribute to wound maceration. Exposure to air allows the wound surface to dry naturally to facilitate healing. Verify wound care preferences with patient's surgeon.
Teach a daily routine of skin cleansing with soap and water.	Soap and water have adequate antibacterial effects. Washing also helps toughen skin on the residual limb in preparation for wearing the prosthesis. Patient should be taught to avoid applying lotions, alcohol, powder, or oils unless they are prescribed because these can cause excessive wound dryness.
Instruct patient to dry residual limb thoroughly before any shrinkage device is applied.	Retained moisture can cause skin maceration, which would contribute to fungal growth.
The shrinkage device must be changed daily, washed with mild soap and water, and dried thoroughly before reapplication.	Use of a soiled shrinkage device can contribute to wound infection.
Instruct patient to begin to massage residual limb 3 wk postoperatively.	Massage will break up adherent scar tissue and prepare skin for stress of prosthesis wear.
Ensure that patient receives complete instructions in the care of the prosthesis by a certified prosthetist-orthotist or nurse expert.	Patient needs to be encouraged to accept the residual limb and become adept at self-care in order to be independent as quickly as possible.

••• **Related NIC and NOC labels:** *NIC:* Teaching: Procedure/Treatment; Teaching: Psychomotor Skill *NOC:* Knowledge: Treatment Procedures; Knowledge: Treatment Regimen

ADDITIONAL NURSING DIAGNOSES/ PROBLEMS:

Constipation related to decreased mobility and use of opioid analgesics   p. 519

"**Fractures**" for **Self-Care Deficit: Dressing/Grooming, Bathing/Hygiene** related to physical limitations secondary to cast, immobilizer, or orthotic devices   p. 519

Impaired Physical Mobility related to musculoskeletal impairment and adjustment to new walking gait with assistive device.   p. 531

"**Osteoarthritis**" for **Sexual Dysfunction** related to pain, decreased joint function, or body image changes that interfere with sexual performance   p. 532

 PATIENT-FAMILY TEACHING AND DISCHARGE PLANNING

When providing patient-family teaching, focus on sensory information, avoid giving excessive information, and make appropriate referrals (e.g., visiting or home health nurse, community health resources) for follow-up teaching. Include verbal and written information about the following:

✓ Medications and supplements, including name, dosage, purpose, schedule, precautions, and potential side effects. Also discuss drug-drug, herb-drug, and food-drug interactions.

✓ How and where to purchase necessary supplies and equipment for self-care.

✓ Care of residual limb and prosthesis.

✓ Indicators of wound infection that require medical attention such as swelling, persistent redness, purulent discharge, local warmth, systemic fever, and pain. Suggest use of a small hand mirror if needed to examine incision and residual limb.

✓ Prescribed exercise regimen, including rationale for each exercise, number of repetitions for each, and frequency of exercise periods.

✓ Ambulation with assistive devices and prosthesis on level and uneven surfaces and on stairs. Patient should demonstrate independence before hospital discharge. For patient with upper extremity amputation, independence with performance of activities of daily living should be demonstrated before discharge.

✓ Importance of follow-up care, date of next appointment, and a telephone number to call if questions arise.

✓ Referral to visiting, public health, or home health nurses as necessary for ongoing care after hospital discharge. Also consider referral to appropriate resource person if patient has continued difficulty with grief or body image disturbance.

✓ Referral to community resources, including local amputation support activities, and to Amputee Resource Foundation of America at *www.amputeeresource.org.*

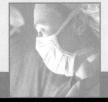

Fractures 67

OVERVIEW/PATHOPHYSIOLOGY

A fracture is a break in continuity of a bone. It occurs when stress is placed on the bone that exceeds its biologic loading capacity. Most commonly the stress is the result of trauma. Pathologic fractures can occur when the bone's decreased loading capacity cannot tolerate even normal stress, as with osteoporosis.

HEALTH CARE SETTING

Emergency care, acute care, primary care

ASSESSMENT

Physical findings: Include loss of normal bony or limb contours, edema, ecchymosis, limb shortening, decreased range of motion (ROM) of adjacent joints, and false motion (occurs outside a joint). Patient may describe crepitus, but this should not be elicited by health care provider because of risk of injury to surrounding soft tissues. Complicated or complex fractures can present with signs and symptoms of perforated internal organs, neurovascular dysfunction, joint effusion, or excessive joint laxity. Open fractures involve a break in the skin and will demonstrate a wound in the area of suspected fracture, or bone may be exposed in the wound.

Acute indicators: Fractures cause either insidious and progressive pain or sudden onset of severe pain and are usually associated with trauma or physical stress, such as jogging, strenuous exercise, or a fall. In the event of pathologic fracture, the patient typically describes signs and symptoms associated with the underlying pathology.

Complications: Chronic fracture can result from *delayed union*, which is failure of bone fragments to unite within the normally accepted time frame for that bone's healing. *Nonunion* is demonstrated by nonalignment and lost function secondary to lost bony rigidity. *Pseudoarthrosis* is a state in which the fracture fails to heal and a false joint develops at the fracture site. *Avascular necrosis* occurs when the fracture interrupts blood supply to a segment of bone, which eventually dies. *Myositis ossificans* involves heterotrophic bone formation (abnormal, out of the normal area) and occurs most commonly in the arms, thighs, and hips. *Complex regional pain syndrome* (or *reflex sympathetic dystrophy*) is an incompletely understood process that results in chronic pain out of proportion to the injury, with reduced function, joint stiffness, and trophic changes in soft tissue and skin following a traumatic event such as a fracture. Other fracture complications include altered sensation, limb length discrepancies, and chronic lymphatic or venous stasis.

Note: Any patient with a suspected fracture should be treated as though a fracture is present until it is ruled out. Interventions should include immobilization of the affected area and careful monitoring of neurovascular function distal to the injury. Any restrictions to swelling (e.g., rings, wristwatches, bracelets) should be removed before they can contribute to neurovascular dysfunction.

DIAGNOSTIC TESTS

Most fractures are identified easily with standard anteroposterior (AP) and lateral x-ray examination. Occasionally special radiographic views are needed, such as the mortise view with bimalleolar ankle fractures (showing joint spaces between the fibula, tibia, and talus) or x-ray examination through the open mouth to identify fractures of the odontoid process. Magnetic resonance imaging may be useful in evaluating complicated fractures, but its ability to identify different bone densities is limited. Intraarticular fractures may be diagnosed with arthroscopy. Bone scans, computerized axial tomography (CT) scans, tomograms, stereoscopic films, and arthrograms also can be used.

Nursing Diagnosis:

Acute Pain

related to injury, surgical repair, and/or rehabilitation therapy

Desired Outcomes: Within 1-2 hr of intervention, patient's subjective perception of pain decreases as indicated by a lower pain intensity rating. Patient demonstrates ability to perform activities of daily living (ADL) with minimal complaints of discomfort.

INTERVENTIONS	RATIONALES
Assist in use of a pain intensity rating scale to evaluate pain and analgesic relief on a scale of 0 (no pain) to 10 (worst pain imaginable).	Use of a pain intensity scale enables more accurate documentation of pain and subsequent relief obtained after analgesia has been administered. The patient provides a personal baseline report, enabling nurse to more effectively monitor subsequent increases and decreases in pain.
If intraarticular anesthetic or opioid was administered intraoperatively, advise patient that lack of pain in the immediate postoperative period should *not* be mistaken for ability to move the joint excessively.	Patients with minimal postoperative pain may be tempted to become overly active, thereby putting unnecessary stress on the fracture site. Prescribed activity must be carefully followed to avoid additional injury to the affected extremity.
If patient-controlled analgesia (PCA) or epidural analgesia is used, verify with another nurse that PCA or epidural pump contains prescribed medication and concentration with prescribed settings for patient dosing, continuous infusion, and/or clinician-activated bolus.	Verification of pump settings is critical to the safe delivery of the analgesia.
If appropriate, instruct hospitalized surgical patient in use of PCA or epidural analgesia.	Understanding principles of PCA or epidural analgesia will help patient obtain better pain management.
Instruct family/significant other that only the patient may administer a dose of analgesia from the PCA pump.	If the family administers medication via the PCA pump, patient may experience negative effects from overmedication (e.g., excessive sedation).
If PCA or epidural analgesia is used, monitor effectiveness of patient's pain management while observing for excessive sedation, respiratory depression, and decreased level of consciousness. Keep appropriate reversal agent readily available.	Excessive sedation may necessitate administration of appropriate reversal agent. Most commonly, naloxone is used for opioid-induced side effects, and ephedrine is given for hypotensive crisis associated with epidural administration of anesthetics such as bupivacaine.
Assist patient to coordinate time of peak effectiveness of analgesics with periods of exercise or ambulation.	Careful timing of analgesics enables patient to achieve optimal pain management before exercise or ambulation. Participation in the exercise regimen contributes to expediency of patient's recovery.
As prescribed, administer nonsteroidal antiinflammatory drugs (NSAIDs) and monitor effectiveness of patient's pain management, as well as adverse effects.	Because of potential for excessive bleeding following NSAID administration, it is important to monitor for hemorrhage at surgical site.
Avoid giving NSAIDs and anticoagulants if patient is receiving epidural analgesia.	NSAIDs and anticoagulants should not be prescribed during administration of epidural analgesia because of risk of bleeding into the epidural space, which may cause lower extremity impairment through pressure on spinal nerves.
Use nonpharmacologic methods of pain management, such as guided imagery, relaxation, massage, distraction, biofeedback, heat or cold therapy, and music therapy. Traditional nursing interventions such as back rubs and repositioning should also be included in pain management plan of care.	Nonpharmacologic methods can augment pharmacologic pain management strategies. These methods may be critical for a patient who is resistant to use of analgesics.

••• Related NIC and NOC labels: *NIC:* Medication Management: Pain Management; Analgesic Administration; Biofeedback; Patient-Controlled Analgesic Assistance; Simple Guided Imagery; Simple Massage; Simple Relaxation Therapy; Distraction; Heat/Cold Application; Music Therapy *NOC:* Comfort Level; Pain Control; Pain Level

Nursing Diagnosis:

Risk for Peripheral Neurovascular Dysfunction

related to interruption of capillary blood flow secondary to increased pressure within the myofascial compartment (compartment syndrome)

Desired Outcomes: Patient has adequate peripheral neurovascular function in the involved extremity as evidenced by normal muscle tone, brisk (less than 2 sec) capillary refill (or capillary refill consistent with the contralateral extremity), normal tissue pressures (15 mm Hg or less), minimal edema or tautness, and absence of paresthesia. Patient verbalizes understanding of the importance of reporting symptoms indicative of impaired neurovascular function.

INTERVENTIONS	RATIONALES
Assess patient's pain at regular intervals, immediately informing physician of increased pain not managed by analgesia.	Increased pain, or pain out of proportion to the injury, is the first sign of developing compartment syndrome (pain = first "P").
Monitor neurovascular status at regular intervals by checking temperature (circulation), movement, and sensation in affected extremity.	Paresthesia (second "P"), pallor (third "P"), and poikilothermia (coolness due to diminished blood flow to distal tissues) (fourth "P") are additional signs of developing compartment syndrome. True paralysis (fifth "P") is a late sign of compartment syndrome, which indicates significant ischemia/limb impairment. **Note:** With the exception of pain and paresthesia, the so-called 5 P's are not reliable for diagnosis, and the presence or absence of them should not affect injury management.
In response to changes in neurovascular condition, contact health care provider promptly. Adjust constricting device as prescribed (e.g., bivalving cast, loosening elastic wrap around splint); wrap a dressing around a split cast.	When swelling places patient at risk for acute compartment syndrome, the constricting device (e.g., cast, splint, circumferential dressing) must be loosened down to skin level to prevent further swelling and compromise to the affected extremity. Dressing around split cast aids in continued immobilization of fracture fragments.
Teach patient and significant other symptoms of neurovascular compromise that should be immediately reported (e.g., changes in temperature, sensation, or ability to move digits of affected extremity).	Awareness of the risk of compartment syndrome will enable patient to respond more quickly to possible symptoms and reduce delay in treatment.
Monitor tissue pressures as prescribed if an intracompartmental pressure device is available. Alert health care provider to pressures higher than 15 mm Hg.	Sustained high pressures may indicate developing compartment syndrome; if pressures exceed systolic blood pressure, perfusion to the extremity is threatened. Continued monitoring of high-risk patients (e.g., adolescents or young adults with traumatic injury; confused or developmentally disabled patients who cannot accurately report symptoms) should be done to avoid possible complications.
Apply ice and elevate affected extremity when prescribed.	A fractured limb is typically elevated for the first 24 hours to decrease swelling. Ice is applied to cause vasoconstriction in the area of injury, which decreases edema and aids in pain management. Because edema can contribute to development of compartment syndrome, these early interventions may be critical.
Caution: When acute compartment syndrome is suspected, however, avoid use of ice and elevation.	Ice and elevation may further compromise vascular supply in an extremity that is already experiencing ischemia secondary to developing compartment syndrome.

••• **Related NIC and NOC labels:** *NIC:* Peripheral Sensation Management; Positioning: Neurologic; Risk Identification; Circulatory Care: Venous Insufficiency; Circulatory Precautions; Pressure Management *NOC:* Neurological Status: Spinal Sensory/Motor Function; Tissue Perfusion: Peripheral

Nursing Diagnosis:

Impaired Physical Mobility

related to musculoskeletal pain and use of immobilization devices

Desired Outcomes: By at least 24 hr before hospital discharge, patient maintains appropriate body alignment with external fixation devices in place or demonstrates setup and use of home traction device. Patient uses mobility aids safely. Patient verbalizes understanding of use of analgesics and adjunctive methods to decrease pain.

INTERVENTIONS	RATIONALES
Teach patient proper body alignment when applying and using external fixation device, most commonly with joints in neutral position.	Maintenance of a neutral position decreases risk of contracture formation, which would affect patient's mobility.
If orthotic devices are used to maintain position, teach exercises and ROM to do when the device is removed.	Prolonged use of the orthotic can cause impaired joint mobility. Exercise at regular intervals will help maintain joint flexibility.

Continued

INTERVENTIONS	RATIONALES
Teach patient and significant other active and/or passive ROM of adjacent joints q8h as appropriate.	ROM exercises help preserve joint mobility and decrease risk of contracture formation.
When appropriate, instruct patient and significant other in care of an extremity in traction, and signs and symptoms of complications (e.g., pressure necrosis, impaired neurovascular function, pin site infection).	Knowledge in these areas will help ensure optimal healing and prompt treatment in case of problems.
Instruct patient and significant other in care of an extremity in external fixator, performance of prescribed exercises while in fixator, and signs and symptoms of complications.	Knowledge in these areas will help ensure optimal healing and prompt treatment in case of problems.
Instruct patient and significant other in care of casted extremity and in signs and symptoms of complications (e.g., skin maceration, impaired neurovascular function, disuse osteoporosis).	A knowledgeable patient should be able to demonstrate cast care, demonstrate and describe assessment of neurovascular status of the distal extremity, describe assessment of evidence of pressure necrosis beneath cast, demonstrate performance of prescribed exercises, and describe prevention of skin maceration and disuse osteoporosis to ensure optimal healing and prompt treatment in case of problems.
Instruct patient in use of crutches, walker, or other mobility aids.	Appropriate use allows patient's early mobilization and decreases risk of additional injury.
Instruct patient and significant other in use of analgesics and nonpharmacologic pain management methods.	Effective pain management will increase patient's ability to participate in appropriate exercise and activity.

••• Related NIC and NOC labels: *NIC:* Exercise Therapy: Joint Mobility; Exercise Therapy: Muscle Control; Body Mechanics Promotion; Teaching: Prescribed Activity/Exercise; Pain Management; Positioning; Traction/Immobilization Care; Cast Care: Maintenance; Circulatory Precautions; Neurologic Monitoring; Pressure Management; Skin Surveillance *NOC:* Mobility Level

Nursing Diagnoses:

Risk for Impaired Skin Integrity and/or Impaired Tissue Integrity

related to irritation and pressure secondary to presence of an immobilization device (e.g., cast, splint)

Desired Outcomes: Within 8 hr of immobilization device application, patient verbalizes knowledge about indicators of pressure necrosis. Patient relates absence of discomfort under immobilization device and exhibits intact skin when the device is removed.

INTERVENTIONS	RATIONALES
When assisting with application of cast or other immobilization device, ensure that adequate padding is put on bony prominences of affected extremity.	Bony prominences are at risk for skin breakdown. Padding decreases pressure over these areas.
While a cast is drying, handle it only with palms of the hand.	Handling a wet cast with fingers can cause indentations that create pressure points on underlying skin. Using palms of the hands ensures a smooth surface as the cast dries and decreases likelihood of underlying pressure points.
Ensure that all cast surfaces are alternately exposed to air.	Exposure to air facilitates drying of the cast.
Petal edges of plaster casts with tape or moleskin.	Petaling prevents cast crumbs from falling into cast. These crumbs can cause pressure areas or skin irritation/impairment.
Pad surfaces of other immobilization devices as well.	Padding decreases pressure on skin underneath the devices.

Continued

INTERVENTIONS	RATIONALES
Instruct patient never to insert anything between immobilization device and skin.	Use of a coat hanger or stick can cause skin irritation that leads to infection. It also may cause bunching of the cotton material placed between the cast and skin, which would result in pressure points under the cast.
In the presence of severe itching, advise patient to notify health care provider.	Health provider may prescribe a medication to relieve itching.
Teach indicators of pressure necrosis under immobilization device such as pain, burning sensation, foul odor from opening, or drainage on the device.	An informed individual is more likely to report these findings quickly, which will enable prompt treatment to avoid further impairment.

••• Related NIC and NOC labels: *NIC:* Pressure Management; Skin Surveillance; Circulatory Precautions; Cast Care Management; Traction/Immobilization Care *NOC:* Tissue Integrity: Skin and Mucous Membranes

Nursing Diagnosis:

Constipation

related to decreased mobility and use of opioid analgesics

Desired Outcomes: Within 8 hr of immobilization device application, patient verbalizes understanding of strategies to maintain normal bowel elimination. Patient maintains bowel elimination in his/her normal pattern.

INTERVENTIONS	RATIONALES
As indicated, teach current influences on impaired bowel elimination.	Decreased mobility, use of opioid analgesics, and inconsistent food intake are examples of situations that can adversely influence bowel elimination.
Encourage choice of diet items that will facilitate normal bowel elimination.	Such high-fiber foods as bran, whole grains, nuts, raw and coarse vegetables, and fruits with skins add bulk to stool to promote bowel elimination.
If not contraindicated, encourage patient to drink adequate fluids.	Fluid intake helps promote soft stool for easier elimination.
If patient desires, request prescription for stool softener and/or laxative. Reassess bowel elimination for response to medication, and initiate additional treatment as needed to return normal bowel function.	Pharmacologic intervention may be needed to maintain normal bowel elimination. If stool softener or laxative is ineffective, patient may require enema administration to assist with elimination.
Encourage mobility to the extent of prescribed activity parameters.	Mobility promotes peristalsis and hence improves bowel elimination. Because of this, the patient should not be left in bed or allowed to use a bedside commode if he or she can tolerate additional mobility.

••• Related NIC and NOC labels: *NIC:* Bowel Management; Exercise Promotion; Fluid Management; Nutrition Management *NOC:* Bowel Elimination; Hydration

Nursing Diagnoses:

Self-Care Deficit: Dressing/Grooming, Bathing/Hygiene

related to physical limitations secondary to cast, immobilizer, or orthotic devices

Desired Outcome: Within 48 hr of initiation of immobilization, patient demonstrates optimal performance of ADL.

INTERVENTIONS	RATIONALES
Ensure that patient receives appropriate treatment as prescribed for pain.	Unrelieved pain can severely limit patient's mobility in a cast or immobilizer, making performance of self-care tasks difficult or impossible.
Incorporate a structured exercise regimen that will increase strength and endurance. Direct the regimen toward development of those muscle groups needed for specific activity deficit.	Patients with insufficient strength to manipulate immobilized extremities need planned exercise to assist them in managing self-care while in a cast or immobilizer. Increased strength and endurance contribute to independence in self-care.
As indicated, refer patient to occupational therapy, and use assistive devices and dressing/grooming aids as needed based on assessment of patient's self-care limitations.	Use of appropriate assistive devices maximizes patient's self-care ability. Sock donners, long-handled reachers and brushes, raised toilet seats, and other devices may help minimize stress on joints. Clothing also can be adapted for greater ease in dressing (e.g., zipper pulls, Velcro closures); adaptive clothing also accommodates a cast or external fixator.
When needed, teach significant other how to assist patient with self-care activities.	Although independence with self-care is the goal, involvement of the significant other can minimize need for skilled home services. A knowledgeable significant other also can reinforce professional health instructions given to patient.
Refer to care management/social services department of hospital.	Patient may require assistance with funding for purchasing assistive equipment or arranging home help. Care management/social services staff are also aware of community agencies that loan equipment or have other volunteer services.

••• **Related NIC and NOC labels:** *NIC:* Self-Care Assistance: Bathing/Hygiene; Self-Responsibility Facilitation; Exercise Promotion: Muscle Control; Self-Care Assistance: Dressing/Grooming; Pain Management *NOC:* Self-Care Activities of Daily Living

Nursing Diagnosis:

Deficient Knowledge:

Function of external fixation, performance of pin care, and signs and symptoms of pin site infection

Desired Outcomes: By at least 24 hr before hospital discharge, patient verbalizes knowledge of rationale for the external fixator and indicators of pin site infection. Patient also demonstrates performance of pin care.

INTERVENTIONS	RATIONALES
Assess patient's health care literacy (language, reading, comprehension). Assess culture and culturally specific information needs.	This assessment helps ensure that information is presented in a manner that is culturally and educationally appropriate.
Teach rationale for use of fixator with type of fracture or injury, emphasizing patient benefits.	A patient who is knowledgeable about essential parts of the device and their purposes is more likely to handle the device judiciously to ensure bone fragment immobilization. External fixation consists of skeletal pins that penetrate the fracture fragments and are attached to universal joints. These joints are in turn attached to rods, which provide stabilization and form a frame around the fractured limb for immobilization.
Instruct patient and significant other to *avoid* using external fixator as a handle or support for moving extremity.	Repeated use of external fixator in this manner may lead to loosening of skeletal pins and loss of bone fragment immobilization.
Teach patient and significant other to support extremity with pillows, two hands, slings, and other devices as necessary.	Adequate support of the extremity prevents stress on skeletal pins. Stress on pins can contribute to loosening and loss of bone fragment immobilization.

Continued

INTERVENTIONS	RATIONALES
Instruct patient and significant other in pin care as prescribed by health care provider.	For external fixator pins, some health care providers require daily cleansing with dilute hydrogen peroxide or other skin preparation solution. Iodine-based mixtures may cause corrosion of some fixation devices.
If prescribed, teach patient and significant other how to apply antibacterial ointments and small dressings to pin sites. Follow health care provider's instruction for removal of buildup of crusts from serous drainage at pin sites.	
Teach patient to monitor pin sites for indicators of infection, including persistent redness, swelling, drainage, increasing pain, and local warmth and body temperature greater than 101° F (38.3° C). Instruct patient to report significant findings immediately to health care provider.	Patient and/or significant other must recognize signs of infection and report them to health care provider for prompt evaluation and treatment.
If an orthotics device is used, ensure that patient and/or significant other is aware of its purpose, knows to check for areas of excessive pressure, and is aware of schedule for adjunctive/ROM exercises.	Orthotics may be added to the external fixator to prevent wristdrop, footdrop, contracture, or other joint dysfunction. Device should be kept clean and dry to decrease risk for infection at pin sites.
Advise patient of need for maintaining adequate fracture immobilization and for follow-up care.	Failure to immobilize the fracture adequately may lead to delayed union, malunion, or nonunion. Follow-up assessment of the device will ensure that fracture immobilization is maintained.

••• **Related NIC and NOC labels:** *NIC:* Teaching: Procedure/Treatment; Teaching: Individual *NOC:* Knowledge: Illness Care

 PATIENT-FAMILY TEACHING AND DISCHARGE PLANNING

When providing patient-family teaching, focus on sensory information, avoid giving excessive information, and make appropriate referrals (e.g., visiting or home health nurse, community health resources) for follow-up teaching. Include verbal and written information about the following:

✓ Medications and supplements, including name, dosage, purpose, schedule, precautions, and potential side effects. Also discuss drug-drug, herb-drug, and food-drug interactions.

✓ Use of nonpharmacologic methods of pain management.

✓ Appropriate use of elevation and thermotherapy.

✓ Importance of performing prescribed exercises.

✓ Rationale for therapy (i.e., casting, external fixation, internal fixation).

✓ Precautions of therapy.

• *Casts:* Caring for cast, monitoring neurovascular function of distal extremity and for evidence of pressure necrosis beneath cast, preventing skin maceration, preventing disuse osteoporosis.

• *Internal fixation devices:* Caring for wound, noting signs of wound infection and monitoring for delayed infection, following appropriate weight-bearing prescription for lower extremity fracture.

• *External fixator:* Demonstrating pin care, monitoring pin sites for signs of infection, knowing when to notify health care provider of problems with fixator, using prescribed orthotics, monitoring neurovascular function of distal extremity.

✓ Use of assistive devices/ambulatory aids. Ensure that patient can perform return demonstration and is independent with devices/aids before hospital discharge.

✓ Materials necessary for wound care at home, with names of agencies that can provide additional supplies.

✓ Importance of follow-up care, date of next appointment, and telephone number to call if questions arise.

✓ For all patients who receive allograft bone for bone graft and who have questions about these grafts, resources for information include the following organizations:

• American Red Cross at *www.redcross.org*
• AlloSource at *www.allosource.org*

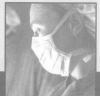

Joint Replacement Surgery 68

OVERVIEW/PATHOPHYSIOLOGY

Total Hip Arthroplasty

Total hip arthroplasty (THA) involves surgical resection of the hip joint and its replacement with an endoprosthesis. THA may be necessary for conditions such as osteoarthritis, rheumatoid arthritis, Legg-Calvé-Perthes disease, avascular necrosis (AVN), and benign or malignant bone tumors. Because conservative treatments usually fail to decrease the impact of disease on the patient's functional ability, surgery becomes the next best alternative. Arthroscopy, osteotomy, excision, or arthrodesis (joint fusion) may be considered before the patient and surgeon choose THA.

Historically, THA has been restricted to older patients because life of the implant has been unknown. However, younger patients with severe disease are now undergoing this procedure. Advanced age is not an absolute contraindication for THA because poor surgical outcomes appear to be related more to comorbidities than to aging alone. Contraindications to surgery include recent or active joint sepsis, arterial impairment or deficit to the extremity, neuropathic joint, and patient's inability to cooperate in postoperative interventions and rehabilitation.

If patient's condition indicates, replacement of only the femoral head can be accomplished with a bipolar or universal endoprosthesis. With THA, however, both femoral and acetabular components will be replaced. A typical prosthesis design includes a polyethylene-lined metal cup that fits over a metal femoral component. Metal-on-metal, ceramic-on-polyethylene, and ceramic-on-ceramic components are also used. The ceramic-on-ceramic components show very little wear and have minimal particle debris, thus extending the life of hip replacement. Components may be secured in place with cement (polymethylmethacrylate [PMMA]), or noncemented components with porous or roughened surfaces that may be chosen to enable bony ingrowth. Because cemented components typically allow early weight bearing, they may be ideal for the patient whose activities do not place great demand on the joint but who would benefit from early mobility. The noncemented arthroplasty requires early weight-bearing restriction but accepts more strenuous activity after the patient's recovery.

Early complications of infection, breakage, and loosening now occur less commonly because of improved surgical techniques. Infection risk has been substantially decreased with administration of prophylactic antibiotics. However, potential complications still include dislocation and aseptic loosening of components. The patient is also at risk for deep vein thrombosis (DVT).

Total Knee Arthroplasty

Total knee arthroplasty (TKA) involves surgical resection of the knee joint and its replacement with an endoprosthesis. TKA may be necessary for conditions such as osteoarthritis, rheumatoid arthritis, gouty arthritis, hemophilic arthritis, and severe knee trauma. Because conservative treatments have failed to decrease the impact of disease on functional ability in most patients, surgery is the next best alternative. Arthroscopy, osteotomy, hemiarthroplasty, arthrodesis (joint fusion), or use of a joint spacer may be considered before the patient and surgeon choose TKA.

Contraindications to surgery include recent or active sepsis in the joint, arterial impairment or deficit in the extremity, neuropathic joint, and inability of the patient to cooperate in postoperative interventions and rehabilitation. Infection in the operative joint is a possible complication, with the risk increased for patients with diabetes mellitus, immunosuppression, or significant peripheral vascular disease. Incidence of DVT ranges from 40% to 60% if prophylaxis is not initiated. Risk of dislocation is minimal, but component loosening is a long-term complication that may necessitate revision arthroplasty.

HEALTH CARE SETTING

Acute care surgical unit; rehabilitation unit

DIAGNOSTIC TESTS

Various tests are combined with patient history and physical findings to confirm presence of conditions that necessitate joint replacement. X-ray examination is commonly required, and arthroscopy may be useful in confirming extent of joint pathology and in identifying appropriate prosthesis.

Nursing Diagnosis:

Risk for Peripheral Neurovascular Dysfunction

related to interrupted arterial blood flow secondary to compression from abduction wedge after THA, and edema or use of bulky postoperative dressing after TKA

Desired Outcomes: Patient maintains adequate peripheral neurovascular function distal to operative site as evidenced by warmth, normal color, and ability to dorsiflex/plantar flex foot and feel sensations with testing of the area enervated by peroneal and tibial nerves. Patient verbalizes knowledge about peripheral neurovascular complications and importance of promptly reporting signs of impairment.

INTERVENTIONS	RATIONALES
Perform neurovascular assessment of the operative leg along with vital signs (VS) as prescribed by the surgeon or in accordance with hospital policy. Compare to nonoperative leg and preoperative baseline assessment. Notify health care provider of significant findings.	Pressure from the abductor wedge (THA) or a bulky knee dressing (TKA) can interrupt arterial blood flow and compress the peroneal and tibial nerves. These nerves provide movement and sensation to the calf and foot muscles. The peroneal nerve runs superficially by the fibular neck; it is assessed by testing sensation in the first web space between the great and second toes and by having patient dorsiflex the foot. The tibial nerve, a branch of the sciatic nerve, is assessed by testing sensation on the bottom of the foot and by having patient plantar flex the foot. Loss of sensation or movement signals impaired nerve function and must be promptly reported to health care provider.
Apply cold therapy as prescribed at operative site.	Swelling increases intracompartmental pressure in the lower leg, potentially interrupting arterial blood flow and compromising nerve function. Ice application is an important early intervention to decrease swelling.
Ensure that patient is aware of potential for neurovascular impairment and importance of promptly reporting alterations in sensation, strength, movement, temperature, and color of operative extremity.	These are signals of impaired nerve function. Nerve damage can lead to severe disability with footdrop and paresthesias. Patient's awareness of signs of impairment leads to prompt reporting, enabling health care providers to initiate appropriate treatment in a timely way.
Encourage patient to perform prescribed exercises (e.g., ankle pumps, heel slides) as a means of stimulating circulation to distal extremity.	Exercises stimulate circulation to distal extremity and decrease risk for neurovascular dysfunction.

••• **Related NIC and NOC labels:** *NIC:* Peripheral Sensation Management; Surveillance; Traction/Immobilization Care; Exercise Promotion; Circulatory Care: Arterial Insufficiency; Circulatory Precautions; Pressure Management *NOC:* Muscle Function; Tissue Perfusion: Peripheral

Nursing Diagnosis:

Ineffective Tissue Perfusion (or risk for same)

related to possible development of DVT

Desired Outcome: Patient exhibits adequate tissue perfusion in the lower extremities as evidenced by maintenance of normal skin temperature and absence of calf pain and/or swelling.

INTERVENTIONS	RATIONALES
Encourage patient to perform calf pumping/ankle circle exercises.	These exercises cause calf muscle contraction. As the contracted muscles tighten on the veins, blood return to the heart is increased, and risk for thrombus development is decreased.
Encourage patient to perform prescribed exercises and participate fully in physical therapy (PT) program.	Early mobilization decreases risk of thrombus formation.
Discuss use of anticoagulants and other modalities.	Because of increased risk of DVT with joint replacement surgery, the surgeon typically prescribes anticoagulant therapy.

Continued

INTERVENTIONS	RATIONALES
Encourage patient to wear antiembolic stockings, intermittent pneumatic compression devices, or venous foot pump compression devices whenever in bed or chair.	These devices compress leg muscles and promote blood return to the heart, decreasing risk for thrombus development.
Administer anticoagulants as prescribed and monitor results of any associated blood tests, ensuring that health care provider has been informed of laboratory results.	Low-molecular-weight heparin (e.g., enoxaparin), heparin derivative (e.g., fondaparinux), or unfractionated heparin is administered by subcutaneous injection. Oral warfarin also may be used for DVT prevention. The patient should be knowledgeable about risks associated with anticoagulant use in order to report adverse effects in a timely way. Review **Ineffective Protection** in "Pulmonary Embolus," p. 139.
Promptly report to health care provider patient's complaints of swelling, warmth, or pain/tenderness along vein tracts in lower extremities.	Close monitoring for these signs of thrombosis is imperative to ensure timely treatment. Patient awareness of indicators also contributes to early identification and treatment of potential thrombotic complications.

••• **Related NIC and NOC labels:** *NIC:* Circulatory Care: Venous Insufficiency; Skin Surveillance; Embolus Precautions; Circulatory Precautions *NOC:* Tissue Perfusion: Peripheral

Nursing Diagnosis:

Risk for Deficient Fluid Volume

related to postoperative hemorrhage or hematoma formation following joint replacement surgery

Desired Outcome: Within 36 hr of surgery, patient is free of symptoms of excessive bleeding or hematoma formation as evidenced by maintenance of HR, RR, and BP within patient's normal range; balanced intake and output; output from wound drain 10 ml/hr or less; brisk capillary refill (less than 2 sec or consistent with preoperative assessment); peripheral pulses 2+ or more on 0-4+ scale; and warmth and normal color in the operative extremity distal to the surgical site.

INTERVENTIONS	RATIONALES
When taking VS, monitor drainage from wound drainage system and on surgical dressing. Promptly report to health care provider output from drainage system that exceeds 50 ml/hr.	During wound closure, it is possible that a bleeding vessel may be overlooked or that bleeding will begin later during patient's recovery. Careful monitoring of wound drainage will detect excessive output.
Carefully evaluate patient's VS, subjective complaints, and neurovascular activity. Report significant findings.	Patient complaints of warmth beneath dressing, sensation of "things crawling" under dressing, increasing pressure or pain, or coolness distal to area of surgery can occur with hemorrhage or hematoma formation.
Reassess VS at regular intervals for hypotension and increasing pulse rate.	These are signs of shock or hemorrhage.
Reassess at regular intervals for pallor, decreased posterior tibial or dorsalis pedis pulses, slowed capillary refill, or coolness of distal extremity.	These signs can occur with hemorrhage or hematoma formation.
If hemorrhage or hematoma formation is suspected, notify health care provider promptly for intervention.	Interventions may include limb elevation or application of elastic wrap to provide direct pressure on site of bleeding.
If patient's VS are indicative of shock related to suspected hemorrhage or hematoma formation and health care provider is unavailable, expose the surgical area by loosening dressing.	This will enable direct inspection of and pressure to the area. Direct pressure will usually control hemorrhage; if not, a thigh-high blood pressure (BP) cuff over sheet wadding will serve as a tourniquet until health care provider arrives for definitive therapy.

••• **Related NIC and NOC labels:** *NIC:* Fluid Monitoring; Hypovolemia Management; Shock Management: Volume; Vital Signs Monitoring; Bleeding Precautions; Bleeding Reduction; Hemorrhage Control; Shock Prevention *NOC:* Fluid Balance

Nursing Diagnosis:

Deficient Knowledge:

Appropriate activity precautions to decrease risk for dislocation of the operative hip

Desired Outcome: At least 24 hr before hospital discharge, patient verbalizes knowledge about potential for dislocation of the operative hip and activity precautions that decrease risk for dislocation.

Note: The following discussion relates to the posterolateral approach for THA; other approaches require different positional restrictions.

INTERVENTIONS	RATIONALES
Assess patient's health care literacy (language, reading, comprehension). Assess culture and culturally specific information needs.	This assessment helps ensure that materials are presented in a manner that is culturally and educationally appropriate.
During preoperative instruction, advise patient of the potential for postoperative dislocation.	A knowledgeable patient is more likely to understand the rationale for and adhere to activity and positional restrictions. Risk of dislocation remains high until the periarticular tissues heal around the endoprosthesis (approximately 6 wk). If dislocation occurs once, the potential for recurrence is increased because of stretching of the periarticular tissues. A confirmed dislocation is treated with closed reduction using general anesthesia. Recurrent dislocations may require revision arthroplasty or surgery to tighten periarticular tissues.
Show patient an endoprosthesis and describe how it can be dislocated when positional restrictions are not followed (i.e., flexion of the hip past 90 degrees, internal rotation, or adduction).	Actually seeing how certain positions result in dislocation will help patient understand need for and adhere to positional restrictions.
During preoperative instruction, explain and demonstrate use of ambulatory aids and assistive devices for activities of daily living (ADL) that enable independence without violating positional restrictions.	Preoperative introduction to ambulatory aids and ADL assistive devices makes their postoperative use easier because of patient familiarity with devices and techniques for use.
After surgery, reinforce position restrictions and discuss activities that may violate restrictions, including pivoting on the operative leg, sitting on a toilet seat of regular height, bending over to tie shoelaces, or crossing legs.	Following a THA using the posterolateral approach, the patient may use an abduction wedge to prevent internal rotation and keep the hip from crossing the midline (i.e., maintain abducted position). Avoidance of flexion past 90 degrees is required to decrease risk of dislocation.
Also discuss weight bearing as indicated.	For the patient with a cemented prosthesis, the surgeon may prescribe full weight bearing or weight bearing as tolerated. The patient is able to become mobile within 1-2 days because of the immediate fixation of the components. The patient with a noncemented prosthesis will have restricted weight bearing for approximately 6 wk until bony ingrowth into the components has been shown on x-ray.
Advise patient of the need for assistive devices for use at home after discharge. Provide contact information for businesses that sell these items. Ensure that patient verbalizes and demonstrates understanding of the positional restrictions and muscle-strengthening exercises and can perform ADL independently using appropriate assistive devices.	Self-care tasks such as dressing, bathing, and toileting will necessitate use of assistive devices such as a long-handled reacher and sock donner. The patient with posterior precautions will need bathroom equipment such as an elevated toilet seat. PT generally includes a prescription for muscle-strengthening exercises and gait training with a walker or crutches to maximize patient's mobility. Exercises also target the upper extremities because their weakness can make it difficult for patient to use walker or crutches.
Instruct patient to report pain in hip, buttock, or thigh, or prolonged limp after hospital discharge.	These symptoms may indicate prosthesis loosening.

••• Related NIC and NOC labels: *NIC:* Teaching: Procedure/Treatment; Teaching: Psychomotor Skill; Teaching: Individual; Teaching: Prescribed Activity/Exercise *NOC:* Knowledge: Treatment Regimen

Deficient Knowledge:

Continuous passive movement (CPM) and other prescribed exercises for involved extremity following TKA

Desired Outcome: Within 30 min of instruction, patient verbalizes understanding of CPM machine use and returns a demonstration of prescribed exercises.

INTERVENTIONS	RATIONALES
Assess patient's health care literacy (language, reading, comprehension). Assess culture and culturally specific information needs.	This assessment helps ensure that materials are presented in a manner that is culturally and educationally appropriate.
Provide instructions for muscle-strengthening and joint ROM exercise regimen. Provide written instructions that describe the exercises, listing frequency and number of repetitions for each one.	These exercises will facilitate return of normal joint function and reinforce gains in joint mobility through use of CPM. An effective method is to teach appropriate exercise, demonstrate it, and then have patient return the demonstration.
Teach use of CPM machine. For patient with prescribed postdischarge CPM, ensure understanding of need to use CPM machine for appropriate amount of time each day.	The CPM machine supplements PT in rehabilitating the operative knee and restoring joint ROM.
Provide contact information in the event that patient has questions after hospital discharge.	Patient may need a contact with whom to discuss possible problems with CPM machine as well as achievements with CPM therapy.

••• **Related NIC and NOC labels:** *NIC:* Teaching: Prescribed Activity/Exercise; Exercise Promotion; Teaching: Individual; Activity Therapy *NOC:* Knowledge: Prescribed Activity

Impaired Physical Mobility

related to postoperative musculoskeletal pain and immobilization devices

Desired Outcomes: By at least 24 hr before hospital discharge, patient demonstrates appropriate use of ambulatory aids. Patient verbalizes understanding of use of analgesics and adjunctive methods to decrease pain when performing prescribed exercises or activity.

INTERVENTIONS	RATIONALES
Reinforce teaching by physical therapist on use and care of ambulatory aids such as walker or crutches. Include use of ambulatory aid on stairs or in other situations the patient may experience at home after discharge.	Patient needs to be aware of equipment maintenance and techniques for their safe use to avoid injury.
Reinforce teaching by physical therapist on exercises that improve muscle strength and increase joint flexibility.	Improved muscle strength and joint flexibility contribute to earlier mobilization and safe use of ambulatory aids. Both lower extremity and upper extremity exercises should be included in the prescribed regimen.
Instruct patient and significant other in use of analgesics and nonpharmacologic pain management methods.	Effective pain management will enable patient to become mobile more quickly, decreasing risk of complications associated with impaired physical mobility.

••• **Related NIC and NOC labels:** *NIC:* Exercise Therapy: Ambulation; Exercise Therapy: Joint Mobility; Exercise Therapy: Muscle Control; Body Mechanics Promotion; Fall Prevention; Pain Management; Teaching: Prescribed Activity/Exercise *NOC:* Mobility Level; Joint Movement: Active; Ambulation: Walking

---

ADDITIONAL NURSING DIAGNOSES/ PROBLEMS:

"Fractures" for **Acute Pain** related to injury, surgical   p. 515
repair, and/or rehabilitation therapy

"Osteoarthritis" for **Sexual Dysfunction** related to   p. 532
pain, decreased joint function, or body image
changes that interfere with sexual performance

✓ PATIENT-FAMILY TEACHING AND DISCHARGE PLANNING

When providing patient-family teaching, focus on sensory information, avoid giving excessive information, and make appropriate referrals (e.g., visiting or home health nurse, community health resources) for follow-up teaching. Include verbal and written information about the following:

✓ Medications and supplements, including name, dosage, purpose, schedule, precautions, and potential side effects. Also discuss drug-drug, herb-drug, and food-drug interactions.

✓ Any precautions related to wound care and signs of infection (i.e., persistent redness or pain, swelling or localized warmth, fever, purulent drainage), or other complications of surgery.

✓ Need to consult health care provider about possible prophylactic antibiotics before any minor surgical procedure (e.g., dental surgery).

✓ Activity and weight-bearing restrictions related to surgical approach and choice of prosthesis.

✓ Use of prescribed immobilization device such as abductor wedge for patients with THA.

✓ Use of CPM machine, if prescribed for home use by patients with TKA.

✓ Frequency of exercise and rationale for exercise performance. Ensure that patient independently demonstrates each exercise.

✓ For ADL and ambulation, ensure that patient demonstrates independence in use of walker/crutches and assistive devices before hospital discharge.

✓ Assessment of neurovascular status at least four times daily, including need to immediately report to physician symptoms such as numbness and tingling or coolness in extremity.

✓ Importance of follow-up care, date of next appointment, and a telephone number to call if questions arise.

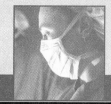

Osteoarthritis 69

OVERVIEW/PATHOPHYSIOLOGY

Osteoarthritis (OA) is the most prevalent articular disease in adults 65 yr of age and older. OA has been known by many names, including degenerative joint disease (DJD), degenerative arthritis, or hypertrophic arthritis. It is no longer regarded as a wear-and-tear condition that occurs as a normal result of aging. In fact, joint changes that result from arthritis can be distinguished readily from age-related changes in articular cartilage of an asymptomatic older adult. In OA, chondrocytes within the joint fail to synthesize good-quality matrix in terms of both resistance and elasticity; this makes the cartilage more prone to deterioration. OA is recognized as a process in which all joint structures produce new tissue in response to joint injury or cartilage destruction. This chronic, progressive disease is characterized by gradual loss of articular cartilage combined with thickening of the subchondral bone and formation of bony outgrowths (osteophytes) at the joint margins. Affected individuals experience increasing pain, deformity, and loss of function. Prevalence of OA varies among different populations, but it is a universal human problem that actually may begin by 20-30 yr of age. The majority of people are affected by 40 yr of age, but few experience symptoms until after 50 or 60 yr of age. Before 50 yr of age, men are affected more often than women. After 50 yr of age, however, incidence of OA is twice as great in women than in men.

OA may be classified as either *idiopathic* or *secondary.* Idiopathic OA occurs in individuals with no history of joint injury or disease or of systemic illness that might contribute to the development of arthritis. Aging may be one influence on the deterioration of cartilage in arthritic joints, but additional evidence suggests existence of an autosomal recessive trait for gene defects that causes premature cartilage destruction. Prevalence of OA in postmenopausal women also suggests involvement of one or more hormonal factors in initiation of the disease. In contrast, secondary OA has an identifiable cause. Any condition or event that directly damages or overloads articular cartilage or causes joint instability can result in arthritic changes. Secondary OA typically occurs in younger individuals because of congenital processes (e.g., Legg-Calvé-Perthes disease), trauma, repetitive occupational stress, joint hemorrhage, or infection.

OA is characterized by *site specificity,* with certain synovial joints showing higher disease prevalence. These include the weight-bearing joints (hips, knees); cervical and lumbar spine;

distal interphalangeal (DIP), proximal interphalangeal (PIP), and metacarpophalangeal (MCP) joints in the hands; and metatarsophalangeal (MTP) joints in the feet (bunion deformity, or hallux valgus). The hips are most often affected in men and the hands in women, especially after menopause.

HEALTH CARE SETTING

Primary care

ASSESSMENT

Signs and symptoms: Joint pain and stiffness are typically the dominant symptoms and most common reason for seeking medical evaluation. However, because onset of pain is typically insidious, the patient may not be able to recall exactly when it began, often describing an "aching" asymmetric pain that increases with joint use and is relieved by rest, especially in early stages of OA. Patients often report pain that is worse with using stairs, standing, and walking; less pain is experienced at night and when sitting. As the disease progresses, however, night pain or pain at rest is likely to occur. The patient also may confirm that pain increases with cool, damp, and rainy weather. This has been attributed to changes in intra-articular pressure associated with the fall in barometric pressure that precedes inclement weather. Joint stiffness ranges from slowness to pain with initial movement. Early morning stiffness is common but typically lasts less than 30 min. Stiffness after periods of rest or inactivity (*articular gelling* or *gel phenomenon*) is also characteristic of OA but resolves within several minutes. Patient may describe a squeaking, creaking, or grating with movement (*crepitus*) caused by loose cartilage particles in the joint capsule.

Physical assessment: Pairs of joints should be compared for symmetry, size, shape, color, appearance, temperature, and pain. Bony enlargement is common, and affected joints are likely to be tender to palpation. Reduced range of motion (ROM) is extremely common in osteoarthritic joints and contributes greatly to disability. Generally it is related to osteophyte formation, joint surface incongruity from severe loss of cartilage, or spasm and contracture of surrounding muscle. Locking during movement may be accentuated by mild effusion and soft tissue swelling; large effusions are uncommon in OA and in fact would suggest other processes such as septic arthritis or gout. Crepitation during passive movement is present in more than 90% of patients with knee OA and indicates

529

loss of cartilage integrity. Deformities may include Heberden's nodes on DIP joints and Bouchard's nodes on PIP joints of the hands. Almost 50% of patients with knee OA have a joint malalignment, typically a varus deformity due to cartilage loss in the medial compartment. Leg length discrepancy may be noted due to loss of joint space in advanced hip OA. In addition, muscular atrophy may be seen in advanced disease secondary to joint splinting for pain relief.

DIAGNOSTIC TESTS

OA almost always can be diagnosed by history and physical examination.

Laboratory tests: To rule out other arthropathic conditions (e.g., rheumatoid arthritis, septic arthritis) and to establish baselines before starting therapy.

CBC: Suggested for patients who will be taking nonsteroidal antiinflammatory drugs (NSAIDs) for arthritis symptom management, with additional complete blood count (CBC) studies prescribed periodically to screen for anemia caused by occult gastrointestinal (GI) bleeding.

Renal and liver function tests: For older adults starting aspirin or NSAID therapy, with further testing done every 6 mo to monitor for occasional side effects such as electrolyte imbalance, hepatitis, or renal insufficiency.

RF and ESR: Neither excludes a diagnosis of OA in the older patient. About 20% of healthy older adults are rheumatoid factor (RF)-positive, and erythrocyte sedimentation rate (ESR) tends to rise with age. ESR evaluation is useful to rule out chronic conditions such as polymyalgia rheumatica. Synovial fluid analysis is another reliable method for differentiating OA from other arthritic disorders.

X-ray examination: Radiographic findings do not always correlate with severity of patient's clinical symptoms. With disease progression, x-ray examination reveals joint space narrowing, osteophytes at joint margins, subchondral cysts, and altered shape of bone ends that suggests bone remodeling.

MRI scan: Much more sensitive than x-ray examination in marking progression of joint destruction.

Nursing Diagnoses:

Chronic Pain/Acute Pain

related to arthritic joint changes and associated therapy

Desired Outcomes: Within 1-2 hr of intervention, patient's subjective perception of pain decreases as documented by a pain intensity scale. Patient demonstrates ability to perform ADL with minimal discomfort.

INTERVENTIONS	RATIONALES
Assist patient in use of a pain intensity rating scale to evaluate pain and analgesic relief on a scale of 0 (no pain) to 10 (worst pain imaginable).	Use of a pain intensity scale allows more accurate documentation of pain and subsequent relief obtained after analgesia has been administered. The patient provides a personal baseline report, enabling the nurse to more effectively monitor subsequent increases and decreases in pain.
Administer simple analgesics, NSAIDs, and opioid analgesics as prescribed and reassess their effectiveness in approximately 1 hr using pain intensity rating scale. Document preintervention and postintervention pain scores. Observe for adverse effects of NSAIDs, such as GI bleeding or renal failure.	Pain management is a treatment priority because no drug is available to reverse effects of OA. Acetaminophen is now recommended by the American College of Rheumatology as the initial treatment for OA pain, with doses up to 1000 mg qid. If acetaminophen proves to be ineffective, low dose over-the-counter NSAIDs or salicylates are recommended for patients with normal renal function and no prior history of GI problems. Prescriptive NSAID doses are indicated if pain persists or worsens. Traditional NSAIDs, such as ibuprofen or naproxen sodium, may increase patient's risk of gastric ulceration or renal impairment because of their inhibition of cyclooxygenase-1 (Cox-1), which reduces prostaglandin levels in the stomach and kidneys. Traditional NSAIDs also decrease synthesis of renal prostaglandins, thus reducing renal circulation. Newer NSAIDs (e.g., celecoxib) with cyclooxygenase-2 (Cox-2) selectivity have shown less GI toxicity. However, two Cox-2 inhibitors were withdrawn from the market after several large studies showed increased cardiovascular risk after 18 mo of use; additional long-term studies are underway. Traditional NSAIDs can be taken with a proton pump inhibitor to minimize GI effects. Salicylates (e.g., aspirin) are still preferred by many patients and doctors for pain management. An opioid analgesic can be safely added to acetaminophen or NSAID therapy if pain is unremitting.

Continued

INTERVENTIONS	RATIONALES
Advise patient to coordinate time of peak effectiveness of analgesic or NSAID with periods of exercise or other use of arthritic joints.	Careful timing of analgesics enables patient to achieve optimal pain relief before exercise or ambulation. Participation in the exercise regimen expedites patient's recovery.
Apply topical analgesics as prescribed.	Topical application provides some pain relief for the OA patient. Capsaicin cream in particular has been shown to reduce knee pain significantly when used along with regular arthritis medications. Necessity for several applications daily often leads to poor adherence to treatment.
Use nonpharmacologic methods of pain management, such as guided imagery, relaxation, massage, distraction, biofeedback, heat or cold therapy, and music therapy. Include traditional nursing interventions such as back rubs and repositioning in the pain management plan of care.	Nonpharmacologic methods can augment pharmacologic pain management strategies. These methods may be critical for a patient who is resistant to the use of analgesics. Thermal therapy in particular may lessen pain and stiffness. Ice can be helpful during episodes of acute inflammation, whereas heat therapy may be beneficial for stiffness. Heat therapy is delivered via numerous modalities, including hot packs, ultrasound, whirlpool, paraffin wax, and massage.
Teach patient about use and purpose of biologic agents.	Glucosamine sulfate and chondroitin sulfate have rapidly gained popularity because of perceived effects on cartilage regeneration. Neither supplement is directly incorporated into the extracellular matrix, so their rapid action suggests an antiinflammatory effect. The dietary supplement S-adenosylmethionine (SAM-e) is believed to play a role in cell growth and repair and also may provide arthritis pain relief.
Caution patient to avoid joint immobilization for more than a week.	Additional stiffness and discomfort can result from prolonged rest.
As indicated, refer patient to occupational therapy, and advise use of assistive devices and dressing/grooming aids as needed based on assessment of patient's pain-related self-care limitations.	Use of appropriate assistive devices decreases pain during attempts at self-care. Sock donners, long-handled reachers and brushes, raised toilet seats, and other devices may help minimize stress on joints. Clothing also can be adapted for greater ease in dressing (e.g., zipper pulls, Velcro closures); adaptive clothing also accommodates a cast or external fixator.

●●● **Related NIC and NOC labels:** *NIC:* Medication Management; Analgesic Administration; Biofeedback; Emotional Support; Patient-Controlled Analgesia Assistance; Positioning; Simple Guided Imagery; Simple Massage; Distraction; Heat/Cold Application; Music Therapy; Simple Relaxation Therapy; Splinting *NOC:* Comfort Level; Pain Control; Pain: Disruptive Effects

Nursing Diagnosis:

Impaired Physical Mobility

related to musculoskeletal impairment and adjustment to a new walking gait with assistive device

Desired Outcomes: Within 1 wk of instruction, patient demonstrates adequate upper body strength for use of an assistive device. Patient demonstrates appropriate use of assistive device on flat and uneven surfaces.

INTERVENTIONS	RATIONALES
Before beginning gait training, ensure patient has necessary strength of upper extremities for using prescribed assistive device.	Many older adults in particular have impaired upper body strength. Upper extremities must be strong enough to support patient's body weight and allow safe use of prescribed assistive devices such as crutches or walker.
As indicated, teach armchair push-ups to attain and maintain triceps muscle strength.	Armchair push-ups target the triceps muscles, which are critically important for safe ambulation with crutches or walker. The patient should be encouraged to do 10 repetitions several times daily if possible to improve triceps muscle strength.

Continued

INTERVENTIONS	RATIONALES
Be sure that height of walker, crutches, or cane allows patient to have approximately 15 degrees of elbow flexion when ambulating.	The assistive device must be appropriately sized to the patient to enable safe use.
Ensure that crutch tops rest 1-1.5 inches (width of two fingers) below axillae.	This position avoids upper extremity paresthesias caused by pressure of crutch tops on the brachial plexus.
Describe and demonstrate use of prescribed assistive device, supervising return demonstration. Ensure that patient can safely get in and out of a motor vehicle.	Return demonstration and supervised practice help ensure that patient will be able to use the device safely on different surfaces and in multiple settings. Ambulation should begin in small increments on a flat surface and progress to all surfaces the patient is expected to encounter.

••• **Related NIC and NOC labels:** *NIC:* Exercise Therapy: Ambulation; Body Mechanics Promotion; Exercise Promotion: Strength Training; Teaching: Prescribed Activity/Exercise *NOC:* Ambulation: Walking; Mobility Level

Nursing Diagnosis:

Deficient Knowledge:

Potential interaction between NSAIDs and herbal products

Desired Outcome: Within 1-2 hr of instruction, patient verbalizes understanding of potential interactions between NSAIDs and herbal products that potentiate bleeding.

INTERVENTIONS	RATIONALES
Assess patient's health care literacy (language, reading, comprehension). Assess culture and culturally specific information needs.	This assessment helps ensure that materials are presented in a manner that is culturally and educationally appropriate.
Determine patient's use of NSAIDs and herbal products that potentiate bleeding (e.g., ginkgo, ginger, turmeric, chamomile, kelp, horse chestnut, garlic, dong quai).	Bleeding risk may be increased when both NSAIDs and herbal products are used for treatment of arthritis symptoms.
	Herbal supplements, particularly ginger and turmeric, have been shown to reduce the pain and inflammation of arthritis. However, patient needs to be aware that these herbs can potentiate bleeding.
Teach signs of occult bleeding such as black or tarry stools, hematuria, and coughing up or vomiting blood.	A knowledgeable patient is more likely to recognize and report signs of occult bleeding in order to get prompt treatment.
Advise patient to discuss with health care provider use of herbal products while taking NSAIDs for arthritis symptom management.	Health care provider should be aware of any products that increase patient's bleeding risk.

••• **Related NIC and NOC labels:** *NIC:* Teaching: Prescribed Medication; Health Education; Risk Identification; Medication Management *NOC:* Knowledge: Medication; Knowledge: Personal Safety; Knowledge: Treatment Regimen

Nursing Diagnosis:

Sexual Dysfunction

related to pain, decreased joint function, or body image changes that interfere with sexual performance

Desired Outcome: Within 1 wk of intervention, patient describes increased physical and psychological comfort during sexual intimacy.

INTERVENTIONS	RATIONALES
Discuss possible problems with sexual performance related to decreased joint function, pain, or body image.	This discussion encourages patients to verbalize feelings related to body image changes, pain experience, and mobility that may impact interest and ability to have sexual intercourse.
Instruct patient about disease process and alternative positions that promote comfort during sexual intercourse.	Understanding the impact of OA on mobility will allow patient to choose positions that decrease stress on joints during sexual intercourse.
Encourage patient to use relaxation strategies (e.g., warm bath) to alleviate pain and stiffness before sexual intercourse.	Relaxation strategies decrease muscle tension, which contributes to joint pain, and allow increased flexibility of connective tissues that support the joints.
Encourage use of analgesics before sexual intercourse to enable easier movement.	Careful timing of analgesics enables patient to achieve optimal pain management before sexual intercourse.
Discuss other ways to preserve intimacy (e.g., caressing and holding) in a relationship if intercourse is difficult.	Exploration of additional ways to demonstrate intimacy will reinforce patient's ability to maintain/strengthen the relationship despite effects of OA.

••• **Related NIC and NOC labels:** *NIC:* Sexual Counseling; Medication Management *NOC:* Sexual Functioning

ADDITIONAL NURSING DIAGNOSES/ PROBLEMS:

"Rheumatoid Arthritis" for **Self-Care Deficit: Dressing/Grooming** related to pain and limitations in joint range of motion	p. 543
Fatigue related to state of discomfort, effects of prolonged immobility, and psychoemotional demands of chronic illness	p. 544

PATIENT-FAMILY TEACHING AND DISCHARGE PLANNING

When providing patient-family teaching, focus on sensory information, avoid giving excessive information, and initiate a visiting nurse/home health or community services referral for necessary follow-up teaching whenever possible. Include verbal and written information about the following:

✓ Medications and supplements, including name, dosage, purpose, schedule, precautions, and potential side effects. Also discuss drug-drug, herb-drug, and food-drug interactions.

✓ Importance of laboratory follow-up (e.g., blood or urine testing) for needed monitoring while patient is taking selected medications.

✓ Proper use of heat or cold therapy, as appropriate to joint condition.

✓ Importance of joint protection, with balance of rest and activity.

✓ Use, care, and replacement of orthotics and assistive devices.

✓ Weight reduction, if appropriate.

✓ If surgery was performed, any precautions related to procedure, wound care, and signs of infection (i.e., persistent redness or pain, swelling or localized warmth, fever, purulent drainage) or other complications of surgery.

✓ Importance of follow-up care, date of next appointment, and a telephone number to call if questions arise.

✓ Referral to community resources, including local arthritis support activities, such as Arthritis Foundation at *www.arthritis.org*.

✓ Additional information on arthritis may be available through National Institute of Arthritis and Musculoskeletal and Skin Diseases (NIAMS) Information Clearinghouse, Information Specialist, at *www.nih.gov/niams/health info*.

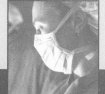

Osteoporosis 70

OVERVIEW/PATHOPHYSIOLOGY

Osteoporosis ("porous bone") is the most common metabolic bone disease. It is characterized by reduction in both bone mass and bone strength, while bone size remains constant. These changes make bone more brittle and susceptible to fractures. Osteoporosis affects 10 million people in the United States, while 18 million more have low bone mass. Osteoporosis is responsible for up to 1.5 million fractures annually. One in three women and one in six men have the disease; women are four times more likely than men to develop osteoporosis. Three types of osteoporosis have been identified: postmenopausal, senile, and secondary.

Postmenopausal osteoporosis: Affects females primarily; clinical symptoms appear 10-15 yr after menopause as a result of lack of estrogen.

Senile osteoporosis: Affects both males and females, more commonly after 70 yr of age; related to poor nutritional status and decreased physical activity.

Secondary osteoporosis: Affects both males and females; results from another disease process (e.g., chronic kidney failure/liver disease, diabetes mellitus, rheumatoid arthritis), nutritional abnormalities (e.g., malnutrition, hypercalciuria, protein deficiency), medications and therapies (e.g., glucocorticoids, anticoagulants, anticonvulsants, cyclosporines, excessive thyroid replacement therapy, radiation therapy), and disuse (e.g., spinal cord injury/loss of biomechanical function, long-term bedrest).

HEALTH CARE SETTING

Primary care; acute care for complications. Individuals with osteoporosis are seen in all health care settings for primary diagnoses other than osteoporosis.

ASSESSMENT

Signs and symptoms: Because of the insidious onset of osteoporosis, most individuals are not diagnosed until they experience an acute fracture or receive radiographic evidence from x-ray examinations obtained for other conditions (e.g., chest x-ray examination to confirm pneumonia). Vertebral compression fractures can develop gradually, resulting in back discomfort and loss of height. Severe chronic flexion of the vertebral spine (kyphosis or "dowager's hump") may inhibit function of multiple organ systems (e.g., gastrointestinal [GI], respiratory). With severe spinal deformities, patient often describes difficulty in obtaining clothes that fit well.

Risk factors

Unchangeable factors: Gender, age, family history, body size (small frame, slight build), ethnicity (Caucasian, Asian).

Changeable factors: Hormone levels (surgical or physiologic menopause, hypogonadism), diet (lifelong low-calcium intake, decreased protein intake, increased caffeine intake).

Lifestyle factors: Smoking, alcohol use, sedentary activity level.

Other influences: Medications, hyperthyroidism, hyperparathyroidism, multiple myeloma, transplantation, chronic diseases.

DIAGNOSTIC TESTS

Use of one or more tests is common.

Laboratory tests: Cannot accurately determine bone density or fracture risk, but serum and urinary markers of bone remodeling can help in determining disease cause. For example, urinary calcium may be elevated even if serum calcium is normal. Biochemical markers of bone resorption (e.g., osteocalcin) may be useful for both initial assessment and for monitoring treatment effectiveness for confirmed disease.

Standard anteroposterior and lateral x-ray examinations of the spine: Provide a diagnosis for osteoporotic fractures or kyphosis. They have limited use in diagnosing disease before a fracture, however, because changes are not evident on plain films until at least 30% of bone mineral density has been lost.

Bone mineral density tests: Can measure amount of bone in specific areas of the skeleton to predict risk of fracture. Dual energy x-ray absorptiometry (DEXA) is the "gold standard" for measuring bone density by testing bone mass in the spine, hip, and wrist. This method is precise and economical; short procedure times mean minimal radiation exposure. Quantitative computed tomography measures bone density at sites throughout the body but is most often used in the spine. It is accurate but costly and delivers a considerable amount of radiation. In the heel, quantitative ultrasound compares favorably with density measurements obtained by DEXA. It is also an easy, low-cost, radiation-free diagnostic aid.

Bone biopsy: Useful in differential diagnosis of metabolic bone diseases such as osteoporosis and osteomalacia. It also can be useful for diagnosis in individuals with early onset of osteoporosis (age less than 50 yr) or those with severe demineralization.

Nursing Diagnosis:

Health-Seeking Behaviors:

Prevention of osteoporosis, its treatment, and importance of adequate dietary calcium intake/supplementation

Desired Outcome: Within 48 hr of instruction, patient verbalizes knowledge of the disease process, possible treatments, and importance of adequate calcium intake.

INTERVENTIONS	RATIONALES
Ensure that patient understands the silent nature of osteoporosis and realizes that treatment may be less effective if not initiated until symptoms arise.	Because of the insidious onset of osteoporosis, most individuals are not diagnosed until they experience an acute fracture or receive radiographic evidence from x-rays obtained for other conditions (e.g., chest x-ray to confirm pneumonia).
Include instruction on osteoporosis prevention as a routine part of health teaching for children, adolescents, and adults.	Adults need to recognize factors that increase their risk for osteoporosis (e.g., female gender, increasing age, small frame, Caucasian or Asian race). Children and adolescents are still experiencing bone growth, and their bone quality can be improved through awareness of osteoporosis prevention strategies.
Teach patient about proper nutrition in relation to calcium intake.	A knowledgeable patient is more likely to adhere to prevention and treatment strategies. Appropriate nutrition is the foundation of osteoporosis prevention and treatment, and consistent calcium intake is especially important. See **Imbalanced Nutrition: Less Than Body Requirements,** later, for more information.
Ensure that health care provider has recommended or approves use of calcium supplements for patient.	Although calcium is important to bone health, excessive calcium intake can lead to nephrolithiasis in susceptible individuals.
Teach patient that calcium supplements come in numerous forms, but calcium carbonate is the best choice.	The most effective form is calcium carbonate (e.g., OsCal), which is best absorbed in an acidic environment such as the stomach. It delivers approximately 40% calcium. Bone meal and dolomite should be avoided because they may contain high amounts of lead or other toxic substances.
Teach patient to recognize amount of *elemental calcium* available in supplements and to verbalize the recommended calcium dosage.	*Elemental calcium* refers to the amount of calcium in a supplement that is available for the body to absorb. Total weight in grams listed on the supplement label will reflect the weight of the calcium plus its binder (carbonate, citrate, lactate, gluconate). Adults 19-50 yr of age should take 1000 mg of calcium daily, and individuals 51 yr and older should take 1200 mg of calcium daily through diet and supplements.
Teach patient not to take calcium and iron supplements at the same time.	The two elements bind with each other, and absorption of both will be impaired.
Evaluate patient's medication profile.	Because calcium may reduce absorption of other medications, the nurse should carefully time administration of all patient's medications to ensure maximal absorption.
Caution patient to avoid taking more than 500-600 mg of calcium at one time and to spread doses over entire day.	Excessive intake can lead to hypercalcemia, which may cause muscle weakness, constipation, and heart block.
Remind patient to drink a full glass of water with each supplement.	Adequate hydration minimizes risk of developing renal calculi.
Remind patient of need for sunlight to enable vitamin D activation.	Exposure to sunlight is needed for cutaneous synthesis of vitamin D, but prolonged exposure does not necessarily increase the amount of vitamin D that is synthesized. An average of 15 minutes of exposure to hands, face, arms, and legs typically meets the vitamin D requirement for most people.
Instruct patient to avoid vitamin D supplementation if dietary intake is adequate.	Supplements may be needed by institutionalized persons, those living in extreme northern or southern latitudes, and people with limited sun exposure. Excessive intake is discouraged because of risk of toxicity. Recommended amounts of vitamin D include 200 IU through age 50 yr, 400 IU for ages 51-70 yr, and 600 IU for those 71 yr or older.

Continued

INTERVENTIONS	RATIONALES
If hormone replacement therapy (HRT) has been prescribed, explain its purpose, action, and precautions.	HRT is not routinely recommended for treatment of chronic disease and is prescribed only after risks and benefits have been evaluated for each patient. Women are encouraged to talk to their health care providers about their personal risks and benefits. Benefits should be weighed against any risk of heart disease, stroke, and breast cancer, and health care providers should identify other prevention and treatment options when appropriate. The Food and Drug Administration also suggests using the lowest possible dose for the shortest period of time to manage symptoms of menopause.
Teach patient about possible medications prescribed for treatment of osteoporosis, indications for use, possible side effects, administration time and method, and need for follow-up laboratory tests.	A knowledgeable patient is likely to adhere to the drug therapy and report necessary signs and symptoms to ensure prompt treatment of untoward side effects.
- Anabolic steroids	These medications improve bone density, but masculinizing side effects are usually prohibitive.
- Calcitonin-salmon	Calcitonin exerts a powerful inhibitory effect on osteoclasts to prevent bone resorption. It has also been used prophylactically in patients with low bone mineral density but no other symptoms of osteoporosis. It should be taken in conjunction with a high-calcium diet or with calcium supplementation and adequate amounts of vitamin D.
- Alendronate (Fosamax) - Risedronate (Actonel) - Ibandronate (Boniva)	Bisphosphonates are nonhormonal oral preparations. Their highly selective inhibition of osteoclast activity is greater than that of calcitonin and accomplished without disturbing normal bone formation. Alendronate and risedronate may be taken once daily or weekly, and ibandronate requires only monthly administration. However, dosing restrictions may make adherence to the treatment regimen difficult. All bisphosphonates must be taken with plain water on first rising, and the patient must refrain from eating or drinking for at least 30 min after taking it and remain in an upright position during this time to avoid esophageal damage.
- Raloxifene (Evista)	In the class of medications known as selective estrogen receptor modulators (SERMs), raloxifene has had consistently positive effects on bone mineral density without stimulating the endometrium and contributing to cancer risk. Studies have also documented decreased fracture risk in postmenopausal women, including those with prior osteoporotic fracture. Raloxifene can be given at any time of day without regard to meals. The patient should be taught to avoid prolonged immobility during travel because of the increased risk for venous thromboembolism.
- Teriparatide (Forteo)	Teriparatide is approved for treatment of osteoporosis in men and postmenopausal women at high risk for fracture. Teriparatide is a synthetic form of parathyroid hormone, which is the primary regulator of calcium and phosphate metabolism in bones. Daily injections of teriparatide stimulate new bone formation leading to increased bone mineral density.
Teach patient about importance of weight-bearing exercise and associated precautions.	Weight-bearing exercise contributes to increased bone density and prevents bone loss. Individuals with established osteoporosis should avoid vigorous unsupervised exercise, and their exercise regimen should not include spinal flexion through activities such as toe touches and sit-ups. Rotational exercises such as golf and bowling may lead to vertebral injury by creating excessive compressive forces. Walking is generally considered a safe weight-bearing exercise.

••• **Related NIC and NOC labels:** *NIC:* Health Education; Risk Identification; Teaching: Individual; Health Screening; Nutrition Management
NOC: Health Promoting Behavior

Nursing Diagnosis:

Risk for Injury

related to decreased bone density secondary to osteoporosis

Desired Outcome: Within 24 hr of instruction, patient describes strategies to decrease risk for fall or fracture.

INTERVENTIONS	RATIONALES
Identify factors that can contribute to falls via a fall risk assessment tool. Refer to health care provider for additional evaluation of any identified deficits as necessary.	Confusion/dementia, cardiovascular disorders, decreased mobility, generalized weakness, abnormal elimination needs, impaired vision or hearing, and use of medications that affect blood pressure, balance, or level of consciousness can lead to falls and possible fracture in a patient with decreased bone density.
Instruct patient and family about need to reduce/eliminate environmental hazards that may increase risk for falls in the home.	Patient and family need to assess home for poor lighting, scatter rugs, electrical cords or oxygen tubing that cross floors or halls, and narrow stairs without adequate railing.
Encourage patient to avoid unnecessarily limiting activity because of fear of falling.	Inactivity can place individual at greater risk for fractures by further decreasing bone density and contributing to muscle atrophy.
Instruct patient to avoid lifting objects heavier than 5-10 pounds.	Lifting puts patient with osteoporosis at risk for vertebral compression fractures. The patient needs strategies to maintain routine without increasing risk for vertebral injury. Patients interested in holding young grandchildren should be encouraged to have child crawl, climb, or be placed in lap.
Teach exercise regimen that improves balance.	Aerobic walking and strength training via upper and lower body exercises have been shown to improve standing balance, which will help decrease risk of falls.
Encourage adequate calcium and vitamin D intake.	Calcium and vitamin D contribute to bone health and minimize risk of injury in case a fall occurs. Other prescribed medications such as bisphosphonates or SERMs must be consistently taken as prescribed for optimal bone health.

••• **Related NIC and NOC labels:** *NIC:* Environmental Management: Safety; Risk Identification; Fall Prevention: Surveillance: Safety *NOC:* Safety Behavior: Home Physical Environment; Safety Status: Falls Occurrence

Nursing Diagnosis:

Imbalanced Nutrition: Less Than Body Requirements

Of foods/supplements containing calcium and vitamin D

Desired Outcomes: Within 24 hr of instruction, patient demonstrates adequate intake of calcium and vitamin D. Patient plans a 3-day menu that provides sufficient intake of both.

INTERVENTIONS	RATIONALES
Teach purpose and recommended daily intake for calcium and vitamin D.	Proper nutrition is the foundation of osteoporosis prevention and treatment. Consistent calcium intake alone cannot prevent or cure osteoporosis, but it is an important part of an overall prevention or treatment program.

Continued

INTERVENTIONS	RATIONALES
	Premenopausal women (19-50 yr of age) need 1000 mg of calcium daily. After menopause, requirements rise to 1200 mg daily. Adolescents (13-18 yr of age) need 1300 mg of calcium daily to maintain bone health. Oral calcium supplements (as calcium carbonate) may help perimenopausal women who have inadequate dietary intake and may compensate for inadequate intestinal absorption of calcium in post-menopausal women. Vitamin D is needed for adequate intestinal absorption and usage of calcium. Dietary sources include dairy products and vitamin-enriched cereals.
Verify patient's ability to select foods high in calcium, including cheese and milk.	If patient is unable to tolerate dairy products, explore other food choices that can ensure adequate calcium intake (e.g., broccoli, sardines).
Provide sample menus that include adequate daily amounts of calcium and vitamin D. Guide patient in developing a 3-day menu that includes appropriate intake of foods containing calcium and vitamin D.	Sample menus demonstrate easy ways in which adequate calcium and vitamin D can be incorporated into the daily diet.
Teach necessity for appropriate exposure to sunlight to prevent vitamin D deficiency.	Even casual sun exposure can prevent vitamin D deficiency. Patient should be outside 15 minutes daily but can achieve this by walking into and out of stores during normal routine.
If patient has limited exposure to sunlight (e.g., resident of a long-term care facility), discuss Vitamin D supplementation to ensure adequate calcium absorption.	Supplementation will ensure adequate vitamin D intake. See previous discussion in **Health-Seeking Behaviors.**

••• **Related NIC and NOC labels:** *NIC:* Nutritional Counseling; Teaching: Prescribed Diet *NOC:* Nutritional Status

ADDITIONAL NURSING DIAGNOSES/ PROBLEMS:

"Fractures" for **Constipation** related to decreased mobility and use of opioid analgesics   p. 519

"Osteoarthritis" for **Chronic Pain/Acute Pain** related to arthritic joint changes and associated therapy   p. 530

Impaired Physical Mobility related to musculoskeletal impairment and adjustment to new walking gait with an assistive device   p. 531

Sexual Dysfunction related to pain, decreased joint function, or body image changes that interfere with sexual performance   p. 532

Self-Care Deficit: Dressing/Grooming related to pain and limitations in joint range of motion   p. 543

"Rheumatoid Arthritis" for **Disturbed Body Image** related to development of joint deformities   p. 545

PATIENT-FAMILY TEACHING AND DISCHARGE PLANNING

When providing patient-family teaching, focus on sensory information, avoid giving excessive information, and make appropriate referrals (e.g., visiting or home health nurse, community health resources) for follow-up teaching. Include verbal and written information about the following:

✓ Description of disease process and recommended treatment.

✓ Medications and supplements, including name, dosage, purpose, schedule, precautions, and potential side effects. Also discuss drug-drug, herb-drug, and food-drug interactions.

✓ Prescribed dietary regimen, including rationale for food choices.

✓ Prescribed exercise regimen, including need to avoid movements that twist or compress the spine (e.g., sit-ups).

✓ Importance of establishing fall prevention measures in the home (e.g., placing handrail in tub or shower, installing night-lights, avoiding use of throw rugs). Arrange for home visit from a nurse or physical therapist as necessary.

✓ Importance of reporting to health care provider any indicators of pathologic fracture (i.e., deformity, pain, edema, ecchymosis, limb shortening, false motion, decreased range of motion, or crepitus). Stress need to promptly report any indicators of vertebral fractures (e.g., paresthesias, weakness, paralysis, or loss of bowel or bladder function) due to risk for possible spinal cord or nerve compression.

✓ Importance of follow-up care, date of next appointment, and telephone number to call if questions arise.

✓ Referral to community resources, including local osteoporosis support activities:

- National Osteoporosis Foundation at *www.nof.org*.
- National Institute of Arthritis and Musculoskeletal and Skin Diseases (NIAMS) Information Clearinghouse, Information Specialist, at *www.niams.nih.gov*.

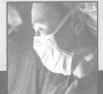

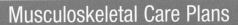

Rheumatoid Arthritis 71

OVERVIEW/PATHOPHYSIOLOGY

Rheumatoid arthritis (RA) is a chronic systemic disease associated with severe morbidity and functional decline caused by inflammation of connective tissue, primarily in the synovial joints. Mortality rates of persons with RA are double that of the general population, particularly if their disease is not well-controlled. Individuals with RA are at increased risk for heart attack and stroke. Women are affected two to three times more often than men. Although no single known cause exists for RA, theory suggests that it occurs in a susceptible host who initially experiences an immune response to an antigen. Because complex genetic factors appear to be involved, the antigen is probably not the same in all patients. Autoimmunity has been suggested as a cause because of association of RA with occurrence of rheumatoid factor (RF), the antibody against an abnormal immunoglobulin G (IgG). Support for a genetic predisposition has come from studies of disease clusters in families, and formal genetic studies have confirmed this familial aggregation. No microorganism has been cultured from blood and synovial tissue or fluid with enough reproducibility to determine an infectious etiology for RA. In addition, no environmental factors have been identified as disease precipitators.

The immune response appears to center on synovial tissue, where disease changes are first seen. Synovitis develops when immune complexes are deposited onto the synovial membrane or superficial articular cartilage. As hypertrophied synovium invades surrounding tissues, highly vascularized fibrous exudate (*pannus*) forms to cover the entire articular cartilage. Pannus also scars and shortens adjacent tendons and ligaments to create the laxity, subluxation, and contractures characteristic of RA.

HEALTH CARE SETTING

Primary care; acute care for complications

ASSESSMENT

Signs and symptoms: Nonspecific symptoms such as fatigue, anorexia, weight loss, and generalized stiffness may precede onset of joint complaints. Stiffness typically becomes more localized as time progresses. Morning joint stiffness lasting at least 1 hr is common, but it may in fact last as long as 4 hr. Patient often complains of joint pain and swelling, especially in hands and wrists. Knees, ankles, and metatarsophalangeal joints also may be affected. Patient describes increasing difficulty with mobility and performance of activities of daily living.

Physical assessment: During early disease, examination may reveal spindle-shaped fingers, with swan-neck and boutonnière deformities becoming apparent because of flexion contractures that occur with disease progression. Ulnar deviation, a "zigzag" wrist deformity, is also likely. Metatarsal-head subluxation and hallux valgus (bunion) in the feet may lead to walking disability and pain. Affected symmetric (bilateral) joints are typically swollen, red, warm, and tender with decreased range of motion (ROM). Subcutaneous nodules may be noted over bony prominences, extensor surfaces, or juxta-articular areas; hoarseness may be evident if nodules have invaded the vocal chords. Patient also may exhibit guarded movement and gait abnormalities due to joint changes.

DIAGNOSTIC TESTS

Diagnosis of RA is based primarily on physical findings and patient history. Radiographic studies are not usually needed to make a diagnosis. Laboratory results are helpful in confirming diagnosis and monitoring disease progression.

Rheumatoid factor: Positive in about 85% of patients. Higher titers appear to be correlated with severe and unremitting disease. However, the RF titer has little prognostic value, and serial titers have no usefulness in following disease process.

Antinuclear antibodies: Elevated titers seen in 5%-20% of patients.

Erythrocyte sedimentation rate and C-reactive protein: Elevation is a general indicator of active inflammation.

Synovial fluid analysis: Fluid is opaque with cloudy yellow appearance, with elevated white blood cell count and polymorphonuclear leukocytes in the presence of RA. Glucose level will be lower than serum glucose.

X-ray examination of affected joints: Radiographs may be inconclusive in early disease but baseline films, especially of the hands, aid in monitoring disease progression. Presence of erosions also helps determine prognosis. With advanced disease, loss of articular cartilage leads to narrowed joint space. Subluxation and joint malalignment can be identified on x-ray film, reflecting changes noted on physical examination. Osteopenia or osteoporosis may be evident in the RA patient who has been treated with corticosteroids.

Bone scan: Detects early synovial changes.

Arthroscopy: Reveals pale, hypertrophic synovium with destruction of cartilage and formation of fibrous scar tissue.

Nursing Diagnosis:

Deficient Knowledge:

Drugs used in RA treatment

Desired Outcome: Immediately following teaching, patient verbalizes accurate information about prescribed RA drugs.

INTERVENTIONS	RATIONALES
Teach patient about all drugs prescribed for treatment of arthritis: indications for use, possible side effects, administration time and method, and need for follow-up laboratory tests.	Drug therapy remains the cornerstone of an interdisciplinary approach to care for RA. A knowledgeable patient is likely to comply with the drug therapy and report necessary signs and symptoms to ensure prompt treatment of untoward side effects.
Disease-Modifying Antirheumatic Drugs (Dmards)	Accurate, timely diagnosis is critical to initiation of DMARDs, which have been shown to control active synovitis and prevent joint erosions and damage. Their early use is critical because they have been shown to slow the erosive course of RA and are now considered to be a first-line therapy in disease treatment. Nonsteroidal antiinflammatory drugs (NSAIDs) are often prescribed along with DMARDs to allow optimal management of pain and swelling until the slower acting disease-modifying agent begins to exert its effect.
- Methotrexate	Most frequently prescribed by rheumatologists in the United States in doses of 7.5-25 mg weekly PO or IM.
- Gold	Has been a standard therapy for more than 60 yr (25-50 mg IM every 1-4 wk or 3-6 mg PO daily).
- Other DMARDs	Include sulfasalazine (2000-3000 mg daily), hydroxychloroquine (200-400 mg daily), penicillamine (250-1000 mg daily), cyclosporin (1.5-2.5 mg/kg daily), cyclophosphamide (1-2 mg/kg daily), and leflunomide (10-20 mg daily).
Teach patient that laboratory monitoring of renal and liver function is necessary with all DMARDs.	Because the potential is great for renal and hepatic toxicity with DMARDs, patient should be instructed to complete all follow-up laboratory tests as prescribed.
Biologic Response Modifiers (BRMs)	BRMs interfere with cell surface antigens of modulating cytokines to manage RA symptoms in patients with moderate to severe disease who have not responded to DMARDs. Adalimumab, etanercept, and infliximab block a cytokine known as tumor necrosis factor alpha (TNF-α), while anakinra blocks interleukin-1 (IL-1). BRMs are frequently given with a DMARD.
Explain that because most BRMS are given subcutaneous by self-injection, they may not be appropriate for all RA patients.	Self-administration by RA patients may be problematic because of muscle weakness and joint deformity. If patient does not have a family member/significant other who can be taught the injection technique, the nurse may need to request a home health visit or determine patient's ability to return to an outpatient clinic for medication administration. Infliximab is given IV, often in the physician's office, and offers an alternative to subcutaneous administration.
Teach patient to minimize exposure to ill individuals and immediately report personal illness to the physician.	Both DMARDs and BRMs cause immunosuppression, and can increase patient's risk for illness. Illness, particularly if resistant to conventional treatment (e.g., common cold), should be reported immediately to the physician for more aggressive treatment.
NSAIDs	A number of NSAIDs provide largely equal analgesic and antiinflammatory effects in the treatment of RA. They do not affect disease progression and their use in alleviating RA symptoms may in fact delay initiation of DMARD therapy or referral to a rheumatologist.

Continued

INTERVENTIONS	RATIONALES
Teach patient that traditional NSAIDs (e.g., ibuprofen, naproxen sodium) are cyclooxygenase-1 (Cox-1) inhibitors that are linked to increased risk for gastrointestinal (GI) toxicity, and patient should recognize signs and symptoms of internal bleeding or GI ulceration.	The patient must be able to seek prompt medical attention for any suspected bleeding or ulceration.
Advise that the Cox-2 inhibitor celecoxib offers an alternative to traditional NSAIDs.	Myocardial infarction (MI), transient ischemic attack (TIA), or stroke patients who require antiplatelet therapy can safely use celecoxib because it has no effect on bleeding time or platelet aggregation.
Corticosteroids	Injection of corticosteroids directly into affected joints can temporarily relieve the pain and inflammation of RA exacerbations. Low-dose oral prednisone may be useful in selected patients to minimize disease activity until the prescribed DMARD becomes therapeutic.
Explain that caution is necessary in long-term use of oral corticosteroids.	Corticosteroids have been associated with development of avascular necrosis or osteoporosis and therefore should not be a mainstay of treatment for the patient with RA. Patients who take corticosteroids should receive additional instruction on risks associated with long-term use.
Antibiotics	Minocycline is the only antibiotic to be studied carefully for use in treatment of RA. It can improve mild-to-moderate symptoms but has no DMARD properties. Side effects such as skin discoloration, dizziness, GI upset, and autoimmune phenomenon (including hepatitis) frequently lead to discontinuation of therapy.
Future Drug Therapies	Research on underlying causes of inflammation associated with RA may lead to development of new medications or new uses for previously marketed medications. The nurse should listen carefully to patient's stated interest in any other pharmacologic therapies and inform health care provider of patient's willingness to try additional treatments. Other TNF inhibitors may be available soon, including a fully humanized and longer acting medication. Biologics that target other cytokines, such as IL-6 and IL-8, are in clinical trials. Also being studied are a number of so-called next generation biologics, which include co-stimulatory blockers that inhibit receptors such as CD 40 to block the initial signaling and chain of chemical reactions that is believed to turn on the immune system.

••• **Related NIC/NOC labels:** *NIC:* Teaching: Individual; Teaching: Prescribed Medication; Analgesic Administration; Medication Management; Pain Management *NOC:* Knowledge: Illness Care; Knowledge: Medication; Knowledge: Treatment Regimen

Nursing Diagnosis:

Self-Care Deficit: Dressing/Grooming

related to pain and limitations in joint ROM

Desired Outcome: Within 1 wk of instruction, patient verbalizes/exhibits increased independence in dressing/grooming.

INTERVENTIONS	RATIONALES
Determine impact of pain and limitations in joint ROM on dressing/grooming activities.	Recognition of extent to which the disease has affected patient's ability to perform dressing/grooming activities independently enables nurse and patient to develop an individualized care/teaching plan for dressing/grooming.

Continued

INTERVENTIONS	RATIONALES
Assess pain and ROM in joints used in dressing/grooming (e.g., small joints in hands; elbows, shoulders, knees).	Independence in dressing/grooming can be quickly lost as small joints become affected by the disease. Strategies for self-care must take into consideration any limitations in the small joints.
Teach patient to coordinate time of peak effectiveness of prescribed analgesics and antiinflammatory drugs with periods of joint use for dressing/grooming.	Careful timing of analgesics enables patient to achieve optimal pain management before initiating dressing/grooming activities that can stress small joints.
Teach patient to perform exercises that increase joint flexibility and decrease pain during joint use for dressing/grooming.	Joint flexibility is critical to patient's ability to perform dressing/grooming activities independently. Pain should be minimized to facilitate joint use for dressing/grooming.
Refer patient to occupational therapist to evaluate need for dressing/grooming aids.	The occupational therapist is able to evaluate need for dressing/grooming aids. Sock donners, buttoners, long-handled reachers and brushes, raised toilet seats, and other devices may help minimize stress on joints. Clothing also can be adapted to encourage independence in dressing (e.g., zipper pulls, elastic shoelaces, Velcro closures).

••• **Related NIC and NOC labels:** *NIC:* Self-Care Assistance: Dressing/Grooming; Exercise Therapy: Joint Mobility; Pain Management *NOC:* Self-Care: Activities of Daily Living; Self-Care: Dressing; Self-Care: Grooming

Nursing Diagnosis:

Fatigue

related to state of discomfort, effects of prolonged mobility, and psychoemotional demands of chronic illness

Desired Outcome: Within 24 hr of instruction and interventions, patient verbalizes a reduction in fatigue.

INTERVENTIONS	RATIONALES
Investigate patient's sleep pattern and suggest strategies that facilitate adequate rest (e.g., warm bath at bedtime).	Adequate rest helps patient maintain a more normal routine and decreases risk of disease exacerbation.
Assist patient to evaluate food preparation methods that may contribute to fatigue.	For example, patient might set table for next day's breakfast before going to bed at night, use convenience foods whenever possible, or prepare food while seated on a stool at the kitchen counter.
Assess patient's ability to manage pain and encourage use of interventions to maximize quality of rest periods.	Effective use of pain management interventions will allow improved quality to rest periods.
Encourage patient to pace activities and allow adequate rest periods during the day.	Balance of rest and activity keeps patient from becoming fatigued. Fatigue contributes to stress and possible disease exacerbations.
Assess patient's stress or psychoemotional distress. Suggest coping strategies or refer patient to appropriate clinical specialist in psychiatric nursing.	Stress and psychoemotional distress may increase fatigue and exacerbate disease symptoms. By understanding patient's response to chronic illness, family/significant other are more likely to support efforts to maintain routine activities. If patient is unable to develop and use effective coping strategies independently, referral may be warranted.
Discuss rationale for a stepped approach to exercise that increases endurance and strength without fatiguing patient. Encourage patient to set realistic exercise goals and share them with associated health care providers.	Endurance and strength should be increased gradually. An aggressive exercise program may cause fatigue and exacerbation of disease symptoms.

Continued

INTERVENTIONS	RATIONALES
Instruct patient in use of assistive devices.	A variety of devices are available to support small joints during routine activities and to assist with ambulation, thus minimizing stress and fatigue. The patient who uses appropriate assistive devices is also generally able to continue with routine activities and avoid social isolation.
Assist patient to evaluate time that fatigue occurs, its relationship to necessary activities, and activities that relieve or aggravate symptoms.	With planning, patient should be able to optimize ability to participate in routine and recreational activities. Patient also can anticipate fatigue-producing activities and plan rest periods accordingly.

••• **Related NIC and NOC labels:** *NIC:* Activity Therapy; Exercise Promotion; Energy Management; Sleep Enhancement; Coping Enhancement; Mood Management; Pain Management *NOC:* Endurance; Energy Conservation; Psychomotor Energy

Nursing Diagnosis:

Disturbed Body Image

related to development of joint deformities

Desired Outcome: Within 1 mo of intervention, patient verbalizes positive adjustment to body image changes.

INTERVENTIONS	RATIONALES
Provide anticipatory counseling about possible joint deformities/body image changes following initial diagnosis, including ways for patient to prepare for reaction of others.	Awareness of the likelihood of deformity will enable patient to develop strategies that make routine encounters and regular activities easier. Patient also can anticipate times when RA deformities may be especially apparent and respond in ways that will minimize potential embarrassment or inconvenience. For example, the nurse may tell the patient, "As the disease progresses, you will notice deformities in your hands that affect your ability to write a check. To make this process easier and to minimize negative reactions of cashiers and other customers, you can write your check before you enter the store and fill in the purchase amount at the cash register."
Routinely assess patient for negative body image.	Manifestations of negative body image may be different in each patient. Examples may include refusal to discuss or participate in care, withdrawal from social contacts, and avoidance of intimate relationships. Early identification of changing body image provides opportunity for overcoming isolating effects of the disease.
Assess patient for negative feelings about body image linked specifically to use of assistive devices/mobility aids.	The nurse can assist in selection of the least obtrusive aids that will help patient maintain a more normal body image.
Encourage participation in support groups for patients with RA.	Support group members can be good role models for successful coping.
Ask patient to complete the Baird Body Image Assessment Tool or other self-assessment survey to determine subjective response to physical changes.	This tool encourages patient to consider meaning and impact of any physical changes and helps the nurse advise on strategies to cope with those changes.
Demonstrate positive regard for patient and acceptance of any physical changes associated with chronic illness.	The nurse's consistent positive regard will help the patient avoid equating self with the disease process. It is critical that the patient recognize the disease as a separate entity rather than the defining element of his/her life.

••• **Related NIC and NOC labels:** *NIC:* Body Image Enhancement; Active Listening; Coping Enhancement; Counseling; Emotional Support; Anticipatory Guidance; Behavior Modification *NOC:* Body Image; Psychosocial Adjustment: Life Change

ADDITIONAL NURSING DIAGNOSES/ PROBLEMS:

"Osteoarthritis" for **Chronic Pain/Acute Pain** related   p. 530
    to arthritic joint changes and associated therapy

Impaired Physical Mobility related to   p. 531
    musculoskeletal impairment and adjustment to
    new walking gait with an assistive device

Deficient Knowledge: Potential interaction between   p. 532
    NSAIDs and herbal products

Sexual Dysfunction related to pain, decreased joint   p. 532
    function, or body image changes that interfere
    with sexual performance

✓ PATIENT-FAMILY TEACHING AND DISCHARGE PLANNING

When providing patient-family teaching, focus on sensory information, avoid giving excessive information, and make appropriate referrals (e.g., visiting or home health nurse, community health resources) for follow-up teaching. Include verbal and written information about the following:

✓ Treatment regimen, including physical therapy and exercises, systemic rest/principles of joint protection, and thermotherapy.

✓ Importance of laboratory follow-up (e.g., blood or urine testing) for needed monitoring while patient is taking selected medications.

✓ Medications and supplements, including name, dosage, schedule, precautions, and potential side effects. Also discuss drug-drug, herb-drug, and food-drug interactions.

✓ Nutrition: Research has shown several positive connections between food or nutritional supplements (e.g., omega-3 fatty acids) and some types of arthritis, including RA. However, there are also many claims that special diets, foods, or supplements can cause harm in arthritis. Some specific diets that are known to have harmful side effects include those that rely on large doses of alfalfa, copper salts, or zinc or the so-called immune power diet or the low-calorie/low-fat/low-protein diet. Patients who are taking methotrexate may experience folic acid deficiency that requires supplementation.

✓ Potential complications of disease and therapy, as well as need to recognize and seek medical attention promptly if they occur.

✓ Potential concurrent pathologic conditions, such as pericarditis and ocular lesions, and need to report them promptly to health care provider.

✓ Use, care, and replacement of splints, orthotics, and assistive devices.

✓ Use of adjunctive aids as appropriate, including long-handled reacher, long-handled shoehorn, elastic shoelaces, Velcro fasteners, crutches, walker, and cane.

✓ Referral to visiting/public health or home health nurses as necessary for ongoing care after discharge.

✓ Importance of follow-up care, date of next appointment, and telephone number to call if questions arise.

✓ Referral to community resources, including local arthritis support activities, and to the following:

- Arthritis Foundation at *www.arthritis.org*
- American Academy of Pediatrics at *www.aap.org*
- National Institute of Arthritis and Musculoskeletal and Skin Diseases (NIAMS) Information Clearinghouse, Information Specialist, at *www.niams.nih.gov*

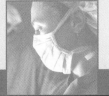

Caring for Individuals with Human Immunodeficiency Virus 72

OVERVIEW/PATHOPHYSIOLOGY

Acquired immunodeficiency syndrome (AIDS) is a life-threatening illness caused by the human immunodeficiency virus (HIV). AIDS is characterized by disruption of cell-mediated immunity. This breakdown of the immune system is manifested by opportunistic infections such as *Pneumocystis jiroveci* pneumonia (PCP) (previously *Pneumocystis carinii* pneumonia) or tumors such as Kaposi's sarcoma (KS). According to the Centers for Disease Control and Prevention (CDC), the HIV epidemic in the United States continues to grow with an estimated 40,000 new HIV infection cases per year (CDC, 2005).

Confirmed routes of transmission of HIV infection include the following:

- *Blood*: Exposure to HIV-infected blood by sharing of unsterile needles or other drug paraphernalia, unsterile invasive instruments, exposure to needlesticks or sharps, transfusion with contaminated blood, mucocutaneous exposure to blood or other infected body fluids.
- *Semen*: Exposure to HIV-infected semen during male to male or male to female sexual activity. Anal receptive sex with an HIV-infected person is the greatest sexual risk for exposure to HIV.
- *Vaginal fluid*: Exposure to HIV-infected vaginal fluids.
- *Breast milk*: Infant exposure to HIV-infected breast milk from HIV-infected woman.
- *Perinatal*: Fetal exposure to HIV during all stages of pregnancy with the highest rates of transmission during labor and delivery.

HIV infection has transcended all racial, social, sexual, and economic barriers, and all persons who engage in high-risk behaviors are at risk of transmission.

It is estimated that the average time span between infection with HIV and seroconversion (development of a positive HIV antibody test) is 3-12 wk, although antibody response may be absent for 6-12 mo. Therefore a negative test does not guarantee absence of infection. Individuals with a recent history of high-risk behavior and a negative HIV antibody test should be retested at 3-mo intervals for 6-12 mo and follow the guidelines for safer sex practices. Anyone with a positive HIV antibody test must be considered infectious and capable of transmitting the virus.

To a minimal extent, health care workers who come into contact with body substances of patients are also at risk. Understanding and practicing stringent infection control is essential for all health care workers. Review Appendix A, p. 783, for a discussion of the handling of blood and body fluids for all patients. Postexposure prophylaxis is available for prevention of HIV transmission in case an occupational or high-risk nonoccupational exposure occurs, but is most effective when initiated soon after exposure.

HIV targets CD4+ T cells, weakening the immune system. When the immune system has been significantly depleted of CD4+ T cells, the body becomes increasingly vulnerable to various infections. This phase of HIV infection is called AIDS. Thus, HIV is a chronic viral disease that covers a wide spectrum of illnesses and symptoms for a variable course of time. Although not all individuals will follow the classic disease progression, the stages of illness, when therapy is not initiated, are described under "Assessment."

Since the introduction of ART (antiretroviral therapy) there has been a dramatic reduction in HIV-related morbidity and mortality. Strict adherence to a combination of antiretroviral agents slows viral replication at different points in the life cycle of HIV within the CD4+ T cell. Use of combinations of these antiretroviral agents reduces the amount of circulating virus (viral load). This viral load reduction has been shown to enable immune system recovery and slow progression of the disease, resulting in reduction in symptoms and opportunistic diseases, prolonging survival time, and improving quality of life.

Maintenance of a positive attitude by the patient and caregivers is an essential element in the therapeutic plan, but an honest approach to this life-threatening illness is also important. This plan must include discussion of adherence to medication, ongoing follow-up, and prevention of HIV transmission to others through safe sex and risk reduction.

HEALTH CARE SETTING

Primary care, hospice, and home care with possible hospitalization resulting from complications or occurrence of opportunistic infections

ASSESSMENT

HIV risk assessment: Because of continued transmission of HIV infection and incidence of new infections regardless of race, gender, sexual preference, or age, continuous HIV risk assessment and prevention education within all clinical settings is essential. Health care providers have a responsibility to assess each patient's risk for HIV infection and be sensitive to issues of sexual orientation and practices, as well as cultural values, norms, and traditions. A risk assessment should be used not only for the purpose of recommending testing, but also for development of a "patient-centered" risk reduction plan.

Key components of conducting a sexual history:

- Focus on sexual "behaviors" rather than on categories or labels.
- Avoid making assumptions about individuals.
- Ask about specific sexual behavior rather than ask general questions.
  - For example, "How many sexual partners have you had?" "In the last 5 years?" "In the last month?"
  - "Do you have sex with men, women, or both?"
  - "When is the last time you had sex while under the influence of drugs or alcohol?"
- Ask nonjudgmentally about traditional and nontraditional sexual practices.
  - "What type of sexual intercourse (vaginal, anal, oral) do you have with your partner(s)?"
  - "When you have anal or oral intercourse, are you the insertive or receptive partner?"
- It is essential that clinicians provide patients with risk reduction information in a consistent and continuous process within the clinical care relationship. This intervention should include development of specific skills and ongoing monitoring of patient successes and continued challenges.

Key components of conducting a drug history:

- Focus on specific drug-using behaviors. For example:
  - "Do you use alcohol or tobacco?" If so, ask how much and how often.
  - "Have you ever injected any kind of drug?"
  - "What drugs do you use?" "What drugs do you inject?"
  - "When did you last inject drugs?" "When did you last share needles?"
  - "Do you clean your works?" "How do you do this?"
- Avoid making assumptions about individuals because drug use occurs in all socioeconomic groups.
- Convey a nonjudgmental attitude.

Stages of HIV disease (for untreated individuals): The four stages of HIV infection can be categorized as acute infection, asymptomatic, symptomatic, and AIDS.

Acute or primary infection: Period of rapid viral replication during which the person may experience flulike symptoms at the time of seroconversion.

Asymptomatic stage: Immune system continues to mount a massive response to HIV, causing a drop in viral load but viral replication continues. It may last 10 yr or more and the person may remain free of symptoms or opportunistic infections.

Early symptomatic stage: Rate of viral replication remains relatively constant; however, gradual failure of the immune system results in inability to control the virus, causing increased viral load.

Advanced stage, AIDS: The immune mechanism for virus control fails, resulting in large amounts of circulating virus and significant destruction of CD4+ T cells. Clinical manifestations include wasting and opportunistic diseases such as neoplasms and viral, bacterial, and fungal infections. Dementia also can occur, characterized by cognitive impairment and mood changes.

Physical assessment: The following indicators are commonly seen with HIV infection.

General: Fever, night sweats, weight loss.

Cutaneous: Herpes zoster or simplex lesions, seborrheic or other dermatitis, fungal infections of the skin (moniliasis, candidiasis) or nail beds (onychomycosis), KS lesions, petechiae, warts.

Head/neck: "Cotton-wool" spots visualized on funduscopic examination; oral KS; candidiasis (thrush); hairy leukoplakia; aphthous ulcers; enlarged, hard, and occasionally tender lymph nodes.

Respiratory: Tachypnea, dyspnea, diminished or adventitious breath sounds (crackles [rales], rhonchi, wheezing).

Cardiac: Tachycardia, friction rub, gallops, murmurs.

Gastrointestinal: Enlargement of liver or spleen, nausea, vomiting, diarrhea, constipation, hyperactive bowel sounds, abdominal distention.

Genital/rectal: KS lesions, herpetic lesions, candidiasis, balanitis, warts, syphilitic chancres, warts, rectal or cervical dysplasia, fistulas.

Neuromuscular: Flattened affect, apathy, withdrawal, memory deficits, headache, muscle atrophy, speech deficits, gait disorders, generalized weakness, incontinence, neuropathy.

DIAGNOSTIC TESTS

A variety of diagnostic tests are used for specific reasons in the course of HIV disease. The following tests are used to determine HIV infection. Because it can take up to 6-12 mo to develop enough antibodies to test positive, the person may be infected but test negative. This is often referred to as the "window period" for HIV infection. Individuals who test negative should be retested in 3-6 mo to confirm seronegativity.

ELISA: The "gold standard" test for HIV. Enzyme-linked immunosorbent assay (ELISA) tests for presence of HIV antibody. An initially reactive ELISA should be repeated on the same specimen. If reactive, a confirmatory Western blot (WB) is performed. A positive ELISA with a confirmatory WB signals infection with HIV.

Western blot: A confirmatory test used to detect immune response to the specific viral proteins of HIV. A reactive WB is defined by a specific pattern of protein bands separated by electrophoresis on a strip of nitrocellulose paper; three of the following bands must be present for reactivity: p24 (see the following), gp41, and gp210 or gp160.

p24 antigen test: Detects HIV p24 antigen in serum, plasma, and cerebrospinal fluid (CSF) of infected individuals.

Its advantage is that it may detect viral antigen (HIV p24) early in the course of infection before seroconversion.

Immunofluorescence assay: Tests for HIV antibody and is equivalent to the WB.

OraSure test system: Food and Drug Administration (FDA)-approved noninvasive HIV test on saliva. The test detects IgG for determining antibody presence. Sensitivity and specificity are comparable to serologic testing.

Rapid tests: Several relatively new FDA-approved rapid antibody tests indicate presence of HIV antibodies in oral fluid, serum, and/or whole blood within approximately 20-40 min. Confirmation of positive results with a WB is imperative. This method of testing is ideal when a rapid result is critical and assists in increasing the number of persons obtaining results.

Monitoring Tests

With use of ART in the clinical management of HIV disease, monitoring tests have become increasingly essential in making appropriate clinical treatment decisions. These clinical decisions are based not only on clinical symptoms but also on the person's CD4+ T-cell count and viral load. Based on the current Department of Health and Human Services (DHHS) HIV treatment guidelines, asymptomatic persons, depending on these measurements, are appropriate candidates for initiation of ART.

CD4+ T-cell count: A measure of the amount of CD4+ T cells per milliliter in the blood. It is a marker for the impact of HIV infection on the immune system and the individual's susceptibility to infections. With increased viral load there is a reduction in CD4+ T-cell counts because of destruction of these lymphocytes by HIV. A CD4+ T-cell count of less than 200 is diagnostic of AIDS.

Viral load testing: Only 3%-4% of the virus is located in the plasma. The remaining 90+% is located in lymphoid tissues and other blood cells. The viral load test measures the free virus in the plasma but not in these other areas. It is used to determine response of antiretroviral treatment, monitor development of drug resistance, and determine need to change antiretroviral treatment. When a patient is on ART, the viral load should be undetectable.

Viral resistance testing: Testing for viral resistance to specific antiretroviral drugs. It is used to determine, before initiating treatment, if the virus is already resistant to a specific agent. It is also used to assess treatment failure and assist in determining appropriate changes in the introduction of new or alternative antiretroviral agents. There are two different types of resistance testing: (1) genotypic tests, which look for genetic mutations that have been linked to drug resistance, and (2) phenotypic tests, which assess which drugs best stop HIV growth in a laboratory setting.

Nursing Diagnosis:

Impaired Gas Exchange

related to altered oxygen supply secondary to presence of pulmonary infiltrates, hyperventilation, and sepsis

Desired Outcomes: After treatment/intervention, patient has adequate gas exchange as evidenced by RR 12-20 breaths/min with normal depth and pattern (eupnea) and absence of adventitious sounds, nasal flaring, and other clinical indicators of respiratory dysfunction. By hospital discharge, patient's oximetry demonstrates O_2 saturation greater than 92% or ABG results as follows: Pao_2 80 mm Hg or higher; $Paco_2$ 35-45 mm Hg; pH 7.35-7.45.

INTERVENTIONS	RATIONALES
Assess respiratory status q2h noting rate, rhythm, depth, and regularity of respirations.	Use of accessory muscles, flaring of nares, presence of adventitious sounds, cough, changes in color or character of sputum, or cyanosis occur with respiratory dysfunction. See discussion in next nursing diagnosis about adventitious sounds that can occur with opportunistic infections that have pulmonary signs and symptoms.
As indicated, assess O_2 saturation via oximetry. Report significant findings.	O_2 saturation 92% or less may signal need for supplementary oxygen and should be reported to health care provider.
Monitor arterial blood gas (ABG) results closely for decreased $Paco_2$ and increased pH.	Decreased $Paco_2$ (less than 35 mm Hg) and increased pH (greater than 7.40) can occur with hyperventilation.
As prescribed, initiate or adjust oxygen therapy.	This measure helps ensure optimal oxygenation as determined by ABG values.
Administer oxygen with humidity.	Humidity alleviates convective losses of moisture and relieves mucous membrane irritation, which can predispose patient to coughing spells.

Continued

INTERVENTIONS	RATIONALES
Instruct patient to report changes in cough, as well as dyspnea that increases with exertion.	These indicators may be seen with opportunistic respiratory disease.
Provide chest physiotherapy as prescribed. Encourage use of incentive spirometry at frequent intervals.	These measures help maintain adequate tidal volume.
Reposition patient q2h.	Repositioning helps prevent stasis of lung fluids.
Monitor for changes in color or character of sputum; obtain sputum for culture and sensitivity as indicated.	Changes in color and character of patient's sputum may signal infection; a culture confirms infection type.
Group nursing activities to provide patient with uninterrupted periods of rest, optimally 90-120 min at a time.	Rest promotes optimal chest excursion.
When administering TMP-SMX for PCP, monitor closely for rash, fever, or bone marrow suppression (leukopenia, neutropenia).	These are side effects of TMP-SMX.
If administering pentamidine for PCP, be alert to hypotension, hypoglycemia, hyperglycemia, or nephrotoxicity.	These side effects necessitate frequent blood pressure (BP) checks and fingersticks for blood sugar levels.
If administering corticosteroids, be alert for additional infections/other potential side effects.	Side effects of corticosteroids include masking of and increased susceptibility to infection. Corticosteroids may be given for PCP when Pa_{O_2} is less than 70 mm/Hg or arterial alveolar O_2 gradient is more than 35 mm/Hg.
Administer sedatives and analgesics judiciously.	This measure will help prevent or minimize the respiratory depression that can occur with these drugs.

••• Related NIC and NOC labels: *NIC:* Acid-Base Monitoring; Oxygen Therapy; Chest Physiotherapy; Energy Management; Respiratory Monitoring; Laboratory Data Interpretation; Vital Signs Monitoring; Medication Management; Positioning *NOC:* Respiratory Status: Gas Exchange; Vital Signs Status; Tissue Perfusion: Pulmonary; Ventilation

Nursing Diagnosis:

Risk for Infection

related to inadequate immune system function, malnutrition, or side effects of chemotherapy

Desired Outcome: Patient is free of additional infections, as evidenced by appropriate cultures or biopsies.

INTERVENTIONS	RATIONALES
Assess for persistent fevers, night sweats, fatigue, involuntary weight loss, persistent and dry cough, persistent diarrhea, and headache.	These are indicators of opportunistic infections that can occur as a result of breakdown of the patient's immune system.
Monitor laboratory data, especially complete blood count, differential, erythrocyte sedimentation rate, and cultures, to evaluate course of infection. Be alert to abnormal results and notify health care provider of significant findings.	Increased/positive values may signal presence/type of infection.
Monitor temperature and vital signs at frequent intervals. Perform a complete physical assessment at least q8h.	These assessments identify changes from baseline assessment that signal fever or sepsis. In addition to increased temperature, other signs include diaphoresis, confusion or mental status changes, decrease in level of consciousness, increased heart rate (HR), and decreased BP secondary to the vasodilator effect of the increased body temperature.
Assess for changes in breath sounds.	Diminished or adventitious sounds may indicate opportunistic disease and/or an increasing level of pulmonary infiltrates. PCP is commonly seen in HIV disease when the immune system is extremely compromised (CD4+ T-cell counts below 200). Other opportunistic infections that can manifest with pulmonary signs and symptoms include *Mycobacterium tuberculosis* (MTB) and bacterial pneumonia.
Maintain strict sterile technique for all invasive procedures.	This helps prevent introduction of new pathogens.

Continued

INTERVENTIONS

RATIONALES

INTERVENTIONS	RATIONALES
Assist patient in maintaining meticulous body hygiene.	This measure helps prevent spread of organisms from body secretions into skin breaks, especially if patient has diarrhea.
Encourage patient to engage in frequent breathing or incentive spirometry exercises.	These exercises promote pulmonary health, which will help prevent respiratory infections.
Use caution when performing postural drainage and chest physiotherapy, if prescribed.	Patient may be too ill to tolerate these activities.
Monitor sites of invasive procedures for erythema, swelling, local warmth, tenderness, and purulent exudate.	These are signs of localized infection.
Enforce good handwashing techniques before and after contact with patient.	Handwashing minimizes risk of transmitting infectious organisms from staff and other patients.
Teach patient home care considerations for infection prevention after hospital discharge (see "Patient-Family Teaching and Discharge Planning").	This reinforces importance of infection protection and promotes adherence after hospital discharge.
Caution: When providing care to patients with active tuberculosis (TB) or unknown TB status, wear respiratory protection consistent with current recommendations from CDC and Occupational Safety and Health Administration.	This helps prevent spread of disease. See "Pulmonary Tuberculosis," p. 143, and "Infection Prevention and Control," p. 783, for more information.

••• **Related NIC and NOC labels:** *NIC:* Infection Protection; Laboratory Data Interpretation; Risk Identification; Surveillance; Communicable Disease Management; Environmental Management; Incision Site Care; Vital Signs Monitoring; Bathing; Chest Physiotherapy; Perineal Care *NOC:* Immune Status; Infection Status

Nursing Diagnosis:

Diarrhea

related to opportunistic infections; medication side effects, including chemotherapy; HIV-related gastrointestinal (GI) changes; or tube feeding/food intolerance

Desired Outcome: By the time of hospital discharge, patient has formed stools and a bowel elimination pattern that is normal for him or her.

INTERVENTIONS	RATIONALES
Be alert to cool and clammy skin, increased HR (greater than 100 bpm), increased respiratory rate (RR) (greater than 20 breaths/min), and decreased urinary output (less than 30 ml/hr).	These are signs of hypovolemia that could result from prolonged diarrhea.
Monitor for anxiety, confusion, muscle weakness, cramps, dysrhythmias, weak pulse, and decreased BP.	These are indicators of electrolyte imbalance that could occur because of fluid loss.
Maintain accurate intake and output.	This measure monitors for changes in fluid volume status.
Assess stool for blood, fat, and undigested materials.	This may reveal presence of infection or feeding tube intolerance.
Monitor stool cultures.	Cultures identify infectious organisms that could be causing the diarrhea.
If patient is being given tube feedings, dilute strength or decrease rate of infusion to prevent "solute drag."	Solute drag (concentrated solutions that pull water into the bowel lumen) may be the cause of the diarrhea.
Encourage patient to increase fluid intake as long as there are no fluid restrictions.	Increased hydration helps prevent dehydration.
Encourage foods high in potassium and sodium.	These foods help replace electrolyte loss.
Protect anorectal area by keeping it cleansed and using compounds such as zinc oxide or sitz baths.	This measure prevents or slows skin excoriation caused by diarrhea.
Teach patient to avoid large amounts (greater than 300 mg/day) of caffeine.	Caffeine increases peristalsis and can promote diarrhea.

••• **Related NIC and NOC labels:** *NIC:* Diarrhea Management; Medication Management; Electrolyte Management: Hypokalemia; Electrolyte Management: Hyponatremia; Specimen Management; Skin Care: Topical Treatments; Perineal Care *NOC:* Electrolyte and Acid-Base Balance; Bowel Elimination; Symptom Severity

Nursing Diagnosis:

Imbalanced Nutrition: Less Than Body Requirements

related to diarrhea and nausea associated with side effects of medications, malabsorption, anorexia, dysphagia, and fatigue

Desired Outcomes: By hospital discharge, patient has adequate nutrition as evidenced by stable weight, retinol-binding protein 4-5 mg/dl, serum albumin 3.5-5.5 g/dl, and a state of nitrogen (N) balance or a positive N state. Patient states that nausea and other GI side effects associated with ART are controlled.

INTERVENTIONS	RATIONALES
Assess nutritional status daily, noting weight, caloric intake, and protein values.	Progressive weight loss, wasting of muscle tissue, loss of skin tone, and decreases in total protein can adversely affect wound healing and impair patient's ability to withstand infection.
Provide small, frequent, high-calorie, high-protein meals, allowing sufficient time for patient to eat. Offer supplements between feedings.	Smaller, more frequent meals may be more easily tolerated. Higher calorie/protein meals will provide the adequate nutrition necessary to promote healing.
Provide supplemental vitamins and minerals as prescribed.	These supplements replace deficiencies.
Provide oral hygiene before and after meals.	Oral hygiene minimizes anorexia and helps treat stomatitis, which can occur as a side effect of chemotherapy.
If patient feels isolated socially, encourage significant other to visit at mealtimes and bring patient's favorite high-calorie, high-protein foods from home.	Patient likely will benefit from socialization at mealtime, which also may promote intake of these high-calorie, high-protein foods.
If patient is nauseated, provide instructions for deep breathing and voluntary swallowing.	These measures help decrease stimulation of the vomiting center.
Administer antiemetics as prescribed.	Antiemetics help prevent or minimize nausea.
Encourage patients to request medication as early as possible.	Nausea/vomiting is easier to control when it is treated before it gets too severe or is prolonged.
If patient is dysphagic, encourage intake of fluids that are high in calories and protein; provide different flavors and textures for variation.	Fluids may be better tolerated than foods when the patient has dysphagia because they are less irritating; fluids that contain supplemental nutrients will help ensure optimal intake.
As prescribed, deliver isotonic tube feeding for patients who are unable to eat.	Isotonic fluids will help prevent diarrhea associated with hypertonic or hypotonic fluids.
Check placement of gastric tube before each feeding.	This precaution helps prevent instillation of fluids into the respiratory tract.
Evaluate residual feeding q4h.	This measure assesses the amount of feeding that has not been absorbed. Usually feedings are not delivered if residual is 50-100 ml.
Keep head of bed elevated 30 degrees while feeding, and position patient in a right side-lying position.	This position facilitates gastric emptying and helps prevent aspiration.
Discuss potential need for total parenteral nutrition (TPN) with health care provider.	TPN promotes caloric intake in patients whose caloric intake is insufficient.

••• **Related NIC and NOC labels:** *NIC:* Nutrition Management; Nutritional Monitoring; Enteral Tube Feeding; Total Parenteral Nutrition Administration; Sustenance Support; Electrolyte Management *NOC:* Nutrition Status; Nutritional Status: Food and Fluid Intake; Nutritional Status: Nutrient Intake

Nursing Diagnosis:

Impaired Tissue Integrity (or risk for same)

related to cachexia and malnourishment, diarrhea, side effects of chemotherapy, skin infections, altered nutritional status, and decreased mobility

Desired Outcome: At hospital discharge, patient's tissue is intact.

INTERVENTIONS	RATIONALES
Assess and document skin integrity, noting temperature, moisture, color, vascularity, texture, lesions, and areas of excoriation or poor wound healing. Evaluate lesions for location, dissemination, weeping, or significant changes. Report any changes or symptoms of infection to the clinician.	A thorough baseline assessment of patient's skin integrity should be performed to which subsequent assessments are compared in order to determine improving or worsening condition.
Note and record presence of herpes lesions, especially those that are perirectal.	This assessment enables appropriate systemic treatment.
As needed, turn and reposition patient q2h; or encourage patient to change position frequently.	These measures prevent prolonged pressure on dependent body parts, which could cause breakdown in skin that is already at risk.
Provide pressure relief mattress, as indicated.	These mattresses reduce pressure on body tissues.
Teach patient to use mild, hypoallergenic, nondrying soaps or lanolin-based products for bathing and to pat rather than rub skin to dry it. When appropriate, use lotions and emollients.	These measures soften and prevent/relieve itching of dry, flaky skin.
Use soft sheets on the bed, avoiding wrinkles. If patient is incontinent, use rectal device (e.g., fecal incontinence bags, rectal tube).	These measures protect the skin and help prevent perirectal excoriation and skin breakdown.
Assist patient toward a state of N balance by promoting adequate amounts of protein and carbohydrates (see discussion under **Imbalanced Nutrition**, earlier).	This measure promotes skin and tissue healing.
Ensure that patient receives minimum daily requirements of vitamins and minerals; supplement them as necessary.	These supplements promote skin and tissue healing.
Encourage range-of-motion (ROM) and weight-bearing mobility, when possible.	These measures increase circulation to skin and tissue, which will help improve skin/tissue integrity.

••• **Related NIC and NOC labels:** *NIC:* Wound Care; Nutrition Management; Pressure Management; Skin Surveillance; Bathing; Diarrhea Management; Perineal Care *NOC:* Tissue Integrity: Skin and Mucous Membranes

Nursing Diagnosis:

Acute Pain/Chronic Pain

related to physical and chemical factors associated with prolonged immobility, side effects of chemotherapy, neoplasms, infections, and peripheral neuropathy

Desired Outcomes: Within 1-2 hr of intervention, patient's subjective perception of pain decreases, as documented by pain scale. Nonverbal indicators of discomfort, such as grimacing, are absent or diminished.

INTERVENTIONS	RATIONALES
Assess and record the following: location, onset, duration, and factors that precipitate and alleviate patient's pain. With patient, establish a pain scale, rating pain from 0 (no pain) to 10 (worst pain).	Competent pain management requires frequent and thorough assessment of these factors. Using a pain scale provides an objective measurement that enables assessment of pain management strategies.
Administer analgesics as prescribed. Encourage patient to request medication before the pain becomes severe.	Pain that is allowed to become severe is more difficult to control. Prolonged stimulation of pain receptors results in increased sensitivity to painful stimuli and will increase the amount of drug required to relieve pain.

Continued

INTERVENTIONS	RATIONALES
Provide heat or cold applications to affected areas (e.g., apply heat to painful joints and cold packs to reduce swelling associated with infections or multiple venipunctures).	Heat and cold applications are effective nonpharmacologic measures that reduce pain, as well as augment effects of analgesics.
Encourage patient to engage in diversional activities (e.g., soothing music; quiet conversation; reading; slow, rhythmic breathing).	Diversion is a means of increasing pain tolerance and decreasing its intensity.
Teach techniques such as deep breathing, biofeedback, and relaxation exercises (see **Health-Seeking Behaviors:** Relaxation technique effective for stress reduction, p. 172).	These techniques reduce pain intensity by decreasing skeletal muscle tension.
Discuss with health care provider the desirability of a capped venous catheter for long-term blood withdrawal.	This measure will help reduce pain in patients in whom frequent venipunctures cause discomfort.
Administer back rubs and massage.	These measures promote relaxation and comfort.
For other interventions, see "Pain," p. 39.	

••• **Related NIC and NOC labels:** *NIC:* Pain Management; Medication Management; Analgesic Administration; Biofeedback; Simple Massage; Simple Relaxation Therapy; Distraction; Heat/Cold Application; Music Therapy *NOC:* Comfort Level; Pain Control; Pain: Disruptive Effects; Pain Level

Nursing Diagnosis:

Activity Intolerance

related to generalized weakness secondary to fluid and electrolyte imbalance, arthralgia, myalgia, dyspnea, fever, pain, hypoxia, and effects of chemotherapy

Desired Outcome: Before hospital discharge, patient rates perceived exertion at 3 or less on a 0-10 scale and exhibits tolerance to activity as evidenced by HR 20 bpm or less over resting HR, RR 20 breaths/min or less, and SBP 20 mm Hg or less over or under resting SBP.

INTERVENTIONS	RATIONALES
Assess HR, RR, and BP before and immediately after activity, and ask patient to rate his or her perceived exertion. See "Prolonged Bedrest" for **Activity Intolerance**, p. 61, for details about perceived exertion.	This assessment monitors patient's tolerance to activity.
	If patient's rate of perceived exertion (RPE) is more than 3 or he or she exhibits signs of activity intolerance, the activity should be stopped or modified.
Monitor oximetry or ABG values to ensure that patient is oxygenated adequately; adjust oxygen delivery accordingly.	Oxygen saturation 92% or less may signal need for supplemental oxygen or an increase in oxygen delivery.
Monitor electrolyte levels.	This helps determine if muscle weakness is caused by hypokalemia.
Plan adequate (90- to 120-min) rest periods between scheduled activities. Adjust activities as appropriate.	This will help reduce patient's energy expenditure.
As much as possible, encourage regular periods of exercise.	Exercise helps prevent cardiac intolerance to activities, which can occur quickly after periods of prolonged inactivity.
Advise patient to keep anecdotal notes (perhaps in journal format) on exacerbation and remission of signs and symptoms.	Anecdotal notes are useful tools for self-examination as well as for reporting to health care provider, who may use this information to alter or modify treatment or develop new strategies.

••• **Related NIC and NOC labels:** *NIC:* Energy Management; Exercise Promotion; Oxygen Therapy; Vital Signs Monitoring *NOC:* Activity Tolerance; Endurance: Energy Conservation

Nursing Diagnosis:

Impaired Environmental Interpretation Syndrome

related to physiologic changes and impaired judgment secondary to infection, space-occupying lesion in the central nervous system (CNS), or HIV dementia

Desired Outcomes: Following intervention, patient verbalizes orientation to person, place, and time. Optimally, by hospital discharge, patient correctly completes exercises in logical reasoning, memory, perception, concentration, attention, and sequencing of activities.

INTERVENTIONS	RATIONALES
Assess for minor alterations in personality traits that cannot be attributed to other causes, such as stress or medication.	This assessment may help rule out medication side effects or opportunistic diseases.
Assess for slowing of all cognitive functioning, with problems in the areas of attention, concentration, memory, perception, logical reasoning, and sequencing of activities.	These are signs of dementia.
Encourage patient to report persistent headaches, dizziness, or seizures.	These indicators may signal CNS involvement.
Note any cranial nerve involvement that differs from patient's past medical history.	Most commonly the fifth (trigeminal), seventh (facial), and eighth (acoustic) nerves are involved in infectious processes of the CNS.
Assess for signs of mental aberration, blindness, aphasia, hemiparesis, or ataxia.	These indicators may signal presence of a demyelinating disease. Blindness, for example, can occur with an opportunistic infection.
Divide activities into small, easily accomplished tasks.	Pacing activities decreases frustration and increases likelihood of completion.
Maintain a stable environment (e.g., do not change location of furniture in room).	A stable environment helps patient remain familiarized with immediate surroundings.
Write notes as reminders; maintain calendar of appointments. Provide some mechanism (e.g., pillbox) to ensure medication adherence.	Patient will require these reminders to complete tasks, take medications, and make appointments as independently as possible.
Teach importance of reporting increasing severity of headaches, blurred vision, gait disturbances, or blackouts. Notify health care provider of all significant findings.	These indicators identify neurologic changes that necessitate treatment intervention.

••• Related NIC and NOC labels: *NIC:* Dementia Management; Reality Orientation; Environmental Management; Learning Facilitation; Medication Management *NOC:* Cognitive Orientation; Information Processing; Memory; Safety Behavior: Home Physical Environment

Nursing Diagnosis:

Deficient Knowledge:

Disease process, prognosis, lifestyle changes, and treatment plan

Desired Outcome: Before hospital discharge, patient verbalizes accurate information about the disease process, prognosis, behaviors that increase risk of transmitting the virus to others, and treatment plan.

INTERVENTIONS	RATIONALES
Assess patient's health care literacy (language, reading, comprehension). Assess culture and culturally specific information needs.	This assessment helps ensure that information is presented in a manner that is culturally and educationally appropriate.
Assess patient's knowledge about HIV disease, including pathophysiologic changes that will occur, ways the disease is transmitted, and how to prevent other infections. Correct misinformation and misconceptions as necessary.	This assessment enables formulation of an individualized teaching plan to improve patient's health and quality of life.

Continued

INTERVENTIONS	RATIONALES
Assess patient's knowledge about ART and viral resistance. Correct mis-information and misconceptions as necessary.	This information enables nurse to formulate individualized teaching plans to improve adherence and help prevent viral resistance to ART.
Inform patient of private and community agencies that are available to help with tasks such as handling legal affairs, cooking, housecleaning, and nursing care. Provide telephone numbers and addresses for HIV support groups and self-help groups.	Lack of knowledge about these services and groups may add unnecessary stress to patient's illness.
Provide literature that explores myths and realities of HIV disease process.	This information assists patients with engaging in activities that will improve, rather than harm their health.
Teach importance of how to inform sexual partners of HIV condition and reduce high-risk behaviors known to transmit the virus.	These measures reduce risk of transmitting virus to others.
Involve significant other in the teaching and learning process.	Involving the significant other in the teaching process not only provides information to him or her but enables the significant other to reinforce teaching for the patient as well.
Provide patient and significant other with names and addresses or phone numbers of HIV resources (see "Patient-Family Teaching and Discharge Planning").	These resources provide information about current therapies, support services, and funding for medications.

●●● **Related NIC and NOC labels:** *NIC:* Teaching: Disease Process; Behavior Modification; Teaching: Safe Sex; Discharge Planning; Health Care Information Exchange *NOC:* Knowledge: Health Behaviors; Knowledge: Health Resources; Knowledge: Illness Care; Knowledge: Infection Control; Knowledge: Disease Process: Knowledge: Treatment Regimen

Nursing Diagnosis:

Anxiety

related to threat of death, significant life changes, and social isolation

Desired Outcome: Following intervention, patient expresses feelings and is free of harmful anxiety as evidenced by HR 100 bpm or less, RR 20 breaths/min or less with normal depth and pattern (eupnea), and BP within patient's normal range.

INTERVENTIONS	RATIONALES
Monitor for verbal or nonverbal expressions of anxiety, fear, or depression.	Inability to cope, apprehension, guilt for past actions, uncertainty, concerns about rejection and isolation, and suicidal ideation are likely signs of anxiety/fear or depression.
Spend time with patient and encourage expression of feelings and concerns. Support effective coping patterns (e.g., by allowing patient to cry or talk rather than denying his or her legitimate fears and concerns).	Before patients can learn effective coping strategies, they must first clarify their feelings. Verbalizing feelings in a nonthreatening, nonjudgmental environment can help patients deal with unresolved/unrecognized issues that may be contributing to the current stressor.
Provide accurate information about HIV disease, related diagnostic procedures, and emerging treatments.	Some fears and anxieties may be realistic, whereas others may necessitate clarification based on current treatment information.
If patient hyperventilates, teach him or her to mimic your normal respiratory pattern (eupnea).	This is an effective calming technique.

●●● **Related NIC and NOC labels:** *NIC:* Anxiety Reduction; Active Listening; Calming Technique; Coping Enhancement; Presence *NOC:* Anxiety Control; Coping; Fear Control

Nursing Diagnosis:

Disturbed Body Image

related to biophysical changes secondary to KS lesions, chemotherapy, wasting, lipodystrophy, and lipoatrophy

Desired Outcome: Before hospital discharge, patient expresses positive feelings about himself or herself to family, significant other, and primary nurse.

INTERVENTIONS	RATIONALES
Encourage patient to express feelings, especially the way he or she views or feels about self. Provide patient with positive feedback; help patient focus on facts rather than myths or exaggerations.	These measures provide an environment conducive to free expression and promote patient's understanding of health status, which may clarify misconceptions that may be contributing to the disturbed body image.
Provide a referral to a nutritionist if appropriate.	A nutrition expert will assist in establishing a healthy diet that will minimize body changes.
Provide patient with access to clergy, psychiatric nurse, social worker, psychologist, or HIV counselor as appropriate.	The patient may require specialized counseling, especially if he or she is at risk for self-harm.
Encourage patient to join and share feelings with HIV support group.	Many people benefit from support groups and sharing experiences with others who are having similar experiences.
For additional information, see "Psychosocial Support" for **Disturbed Body Image,** p. 80.	

●●● **Related NIC and NOC labels:** *NIC:* Body Image Enhancement; Active Listening; Coping Enhancement; Emotional Support; Counseling; Support Group *NOC:* Body Image; Psychosocial Adjustment: Life Change

Nursing Diagnosis:

Social Isolation

related to altered state of wellness, societal rejection, loss of support system, feelings of guilt and punishment, fatigue, and changed patterns of sexual expression

Desired Outcome: Before hospital discharge, patient communicates and interacts with others.

INTERVENTIONS	RATIONALES
Keep patient and significant other well informed about patient's status and treatment plan. Provide private periods of time for patient to communicate and interact with significant other.	Information and communication help reduce sense of isolation.
Encourage significant other to share in care of patient. Encourage physical closeness between patient and significant other. Provide privacy as much as possible.	These actions increase the amount of time for interaction and communication with significant other.
Involve patient in unit or group activities as appropriate.	Such activities reduce sense of isolation and promote socialization.
Explain significance of transmission precautions to patient.	Understanding rationale for these precautions may help patient cope with and adhere to them better and develop new approaches to life with HIV infection.
Provide link with community support services.	This provides contact with others, psychosocial support, resources, and care.

●●● **Related NIC and NOC labels:** *NIC:* Socialization Enhancement; Support System Enhancement; Active Listening; Presence; Therapy Group; Touch; Visitation Facilitation; Support Group *NOC:* Loneliness; Social Involvement; Social Support

ADDITIONAL NURSING DIAGNOSES/ PROBLEMS:

"Prolonged Bedrest"	p. 61
"Psychosocial Support"	p. 73
"Psychosocial Support for the Patient's Family and Significant Other"	p. 87
"Managing Wound Care"	p. 559
"Providing Nutritional Support"	p. 565

✔ PATIENT-FAMILY TEACHING AND DISCHARGE PLANNING

When providing patient-family teaching, focus on sensory information, avoid giving excessive information, and initiate a visiting nurse referral for necessary follow-up teaching. Include verbal and written information about the following:

✓ Importance of reporting any new symptoms of infection or changes in neurologic status (e.g., increasing severity of headaches, blurred vision, gait disturbances, blackouts) immediately to health care provider.

✓ Necessity of modifying high-risk sexual behaviors.

✓ Prescribed medications, including drug name, dosage, purpose, and potential side effects. Also discuss drug-drug, herb-drug, and food-drug interactions. Instruct patient and significant other in the necessity of taking antiretroviral medications as prescribed to avoid viral resistance.

✓ Importance of patient adherence to ART regimens, which is critical to patients and the clinicians providing and monitoring their care. Interruptions in drug treatment can lead to development of viruses resistant to specific antiretroviral drugs, which can result in treatment failure and limiting of future treatment options. Health care provider and patient partnerships characterized by shared decision making has been identified as a key component in successful HIV treatment.

✓ Strategies for promoting HIV treatment adherence. These must be customized to meet needs of each patient. The approach must be patient centered and include ongoing education, psychosocial and community support, and resources that involve both patient-directed and provider-directed strategies.

✓ Because of decreased resistance to infection, importance of limiting contact with individuals known to have active infections. In addition, pets may harbor various fungal, protozoal, and bacterial organisms in their excrement. Therefore contact with birdcages, cat litter, and tropical fish tanks should be avoided.

✓ Necessity for meticulous hygiene to prevent spread of any extant or new infectious organisms. To avoid exposure to fungi, damp areas in bathrooms (e.g., shower) should be cleaned with solutions of bleach, refrigerators should be cleaned thoroughly with soap and water, and leftover foodstuffs should be disposed of within 2-3 days.

✓ Techniques for self-assessment of early signs of infection (e.g., erythema, tenderness, local warmth, swelling, purulent exudate) in all cuts, abrasions, lesions, or open wounds.

✓ Importance of avoiding use of recreational drugs, which are believed to potentiate immunosuppressive process and lower resistance to infection.

✓ Significance and importance of refraining from donating blood.

✓ Principles and importance of maintaining a balanced diet; ways to supplement diet with multivitamins and other food sources, such as high-calorie substances (e.g., Isocal, Ensure). Because of increased susceptibility to foodborne opportunistic organisms, fruits and vegetables should be washed thoroughly; meats should be cooked thoroughly at appropriate temperatures; and raw eggs, raw fish (sushi), and unpasteurized milk should be avoided.

✓ Care of venous access device, including technique for self-administration of TPN or medications (see "Providing Nutritional Support," p. 565); care of gastric tube and administration of enteral tube feedings if appropriate.

✓ Importance of avoiding fatigue by limiting participation in social activities, getting maximum amounts of rest, and minimizing physical exertion.

✓ Importance of maintaining medical follow-up appointments.

✓ Advisability of sharing feelings with significant other or within a support group.

✓ Referral to hospice or agency that provides home help. This should occur before discharge planning begins to ensure continuity of care between hospital and home or hospice.

✓ Phone numbers to call if questions or concerns arise about hospice after discharge. Information for these patients can be obtained by contacting National Hospice Palliative Care Organization at *www.nhpco.org.*

✓ In addition, provide the following information regarding HIV resources:

- Public Health Service AIDS Hotline at (800) 342-AIDS or (800) 342-2437
- National Sexually Transmitted Diseases Hotline/ American Social Health Association at (800) 227-8922
- Local Red Cross Chapter or American Red Cross AIDS Education Office at (202) 737-8300
- CDC National Center for HIV, STD, and TB Prevention at *www.cdc.gov/hiv/resources/guidelines/index.htm*
- Association of Nurses in AIDS Care (ANAC) at *www. anacnet.org*
- NIH, National Institutes of Allergy and Infectious Diseases at *www.niaid.nih.gov*
- DHHS HIV/AIDS Treatment Information and Clinical Trials Information at *http://aidsinfo.nih.gov*
- HRSA, Bureau of HIV/AIDS at *www.hab.hrsa.gov*
- AIDS Education and Training Centers National Resource Center at *http://aids-etc.org*
- National HIV/AIDS Clinician's Post-Exposure Prophylaxis Hotline (PEPline) at (800) 448-4911, *www.ucsf.edu/hivcntr*
- National HIV/AIDS Clinician's Consultation Center at (800) 933-3413, *www.ucsf.edu/hivcntr*

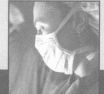

Managing Wound Care 73

A wound is a disruption of tissue integrity caused by trauma, surgery, or an underlying medical disorder. Wound management is directed at preventing infection and deterioration in wound status and promoting healing.

WOUNDS CLOSED BY PRIMARY INTENTION
OVERVIEW/PATHOPHYSIOLOGY

Clean, surgical, or traumatic wounds whose edges are closed with sutures, clips, tissue glue, or sterile tape strips are referred to as *wounds closed by primary intention*. Impairment of healing most commonly manifests as dehiscence, evisceration, or infection. Individuals at high risk for disruption of wound healing include those who are very young or very old, have diabetes mellitus with poor glucose control, smoke cigarettes, are obese, are malnourished, or are immunosuppressed (e.g., receiving steroids or other immunosuppressive drugs, undergoing chemotherapy or radiation therapy, or have immunosuppressive disease).

HEALTH CARE SETTING

Primary care, acute care, critical care

ASSESSMENT

Normal healing: Warm, reddened, indurated, tender incision line immediately after injury. After 1 or 2 days, epithelial cells migrate across the incision line and seal the wound. Over time, a pink scar is visible. After 7-9 days, a healing ridge—a palpable accumulation of scar tissue—forms. In patients who undergo cosmetic surgery, the healing ridge is purposefully avoided to minimize scar formation. Healing is complete when structural and functional integrity is reestablished.

Impaired healing: Lack of an adequate inflammatory response manifested by absence of initial redness, warmth, and induration or inflammation that persists or occurs after the fifth postinjury day; continued drainage from the incision line 2 days after injury (when no drain is present); absence of a healing ridge by the ninth day after injury; presence of purulent exudate. Older persons may not exhibit classic signs of impaired healing but only changes in cognition or functional status that lead to search for the site of infection.

DIAGNOSTIC TESTS

Culture and sensitivity of tissue by biopsy or swab: To determine optimal antibiotic. Sample is obtained from clean tissue, not from exudate, pus, or necrotic tissue. Infection is present when there are 10^5 organisms/g or more from tissue or when there is fever and drainage.

Gram stain of drainage: Done as part of the culture procedure to identify offending organism and aid in selection of preliminary antibiotics.

WBC with differential: To assess for infection.

Nursing Diagnosis:

Impaired Tissue Integrity: Wound

related to altered blood flow, metabolic disorders (e.g., diabetes mellitus [DM]), alterations in fluid volume and nutrition, and medical therapy (chemotherapy, radiation therapy, steroid or immunosuppressive drug administration)

Desired Outcome: Patient exhibits the following signs of wound healing: well-approximated wound edges; good initial postinjury inflammatory response (erythema, warmth, induration, pain); no inflammatory response past the fifth day after injury; no drainage (without drain present) 48 hr after closure; healing ridge present by postoperative day 7-9.

INTERVENTIONS	RATIONALES
Assess wound for absence of a healing ridge, presence of drainage or purulent exudate, and delayed or prolonged inflammatory response.	These signs are indications of impaired healing.
Monitor vital signs for elevated temperature and heart rate (HR). Document findings.	These are signs of infection, a manifestation of impaired wound healing.
In the hospital setting, follow sterile technique when changing dressings. If a drain is present, keep it sterile, maintain patency (e.g., empty drainage reservoir and recharge suction on closed drainage systems as needed), and handle it gently to prevent it from becoming dislodged.	Sterile technique eliminates introduction of nosocomial organisms to prevent infection. Most outpatient wound care is done with clean technique.
If wound care will be necessary after hospital discharge, teach dressing change procedure to patient and significant other.	Clean technique is used at home because most people have antibodies to familiar organisms. For immunosuppressed patients, however, sterile technique often is used at home.
In patients with DM, perform serial monitoring of capillary glucose and administer insulin as indicated to keep glucose level 110 mg/dl or less.	These measures monitor for hyperglycemia and help maintain blood glucose within normal range for persons with DM. Hyperglycemia increases risk for infection, thereby adversely affecting wound healing.
Encourage deep breathing q2h while patient is awake. Splint incision as needed. If indicated, provide incentive spirometry.	Deep breathing promotes oxygenation, which enhances wound healing.
As indicated, monitor oximetry. Report O_2 saturation 92% or less, and consult health care provider about administration of O_2.	Oxygen saturation 92% or less often signals need for supplemental oxygen to support healing.
Stress importance of position changes and activity as tolerated.	Movement, exercise, and activity promote ventilation and circulation, and hence oxygenation to the tissues.
Monitor perfusion status by checking blood pressure (BP), HR, and capillary refill time in the tissue adjacent to the incision.	These measures determine if blood flow to the area is adequate for healing. BP and HR optimally should be within patient's normal range; capillary refill should be less than 2 sec, which signals adequate tissue perfusion to the area.
Assess hydration status by monitoring peripheral pulses, moisture of mucous membranes, skin turgor, volume and specific gravity of urine, and intake and output.	Hypovolemia adversely affects wound healing.
For nonrestricted patients, ensure a fluid intake of at least 30 ml/kg body weight/day.	This ensures that patient has adequate hydration to assist with wound healing.
Provide a diet with adequate protein, vitamin C, and calories. If patient complains of feeling full with three meals per day, give more frequent small feedings. Encourage between-meal high-protein supplements (e.g., yogurt, milkshakes).	This diet promotes positive nitrogen balance and nutrients needed for wound healing. Smaller, more frequent meals are often more easily tolerated.
Monitor serum albumin and total lymphocytes for decreased values. Consult health care provider about significant findings.	Serum albumin less than 3.5 g/dl and total lymphocyte count less than 1800/mm³ may be indicators of the need for supplemental protein.
Assess wound pain using a numeric rating scale. Treat pain with pharmacologic and nonpharmacologic interventions. Anticipate pain associated with dressing change and premedicate.	Pain causes vasoconstriction and impairs healing. See "Pain," p. 39, for detail.

••• **Related NIC and NOC labels:** *NIC:* Incision Site Care; Wound Care; Fluid Management; Nutrition Management; Infection Protection; Vital Sign Status *NOC:* Skin Care: Topical Treatments, Respiratory Status: Gas Exchange; Wound Healing: Primary Intention

---

✓ **PATIENT-FAMILY TEACHING AND DISCHARGE PLANNING**

When providing patient-family teaching, focus on sensory information, avoid giving excessive information, and initiate a home health referral for necessary follow-up teaching. Include verbal and written information about the following:

✓ Local wound care, including type of equipment necessary, wound care procedure, and therapeutic and potential side effects of topical agents used. Have patient or significant other demonstrate dressing change procedure before hospital discharge.

✓ Signs and symptoms of improvement or deterioration in wound status, including those that necessitate notification of health care provider or clinic.

✓ Diet that promotes wound healing. Discuss importance of adequate protein and calorie intake. See "Providing Nutritional Support," p. 565. Involve dietitian, patient, and significant other as necessary.

✓ Activities that maximize ventilatory status: a planned regimen for ambulatory patients and deep breathing and turning (at least q2h) for those on bedrest.

✓ Importance of taking pain medication, antibiotics, multivitamins, and supplements of iron and zinc as prescribed. For all medications to be taken at home, provide the following: drug name, purpose, dosage, schedule, precautions, and potential side effects. Also discuss drug-drug, herb-drug, and food-drug interactions.

✓ Importance of follow-up care with health care provider; confirm time and date of next appointment, if known.

✓ If needed, arrange for a visit by a home health nurse before hospital discharge.

✓ How/where to obtain wound care supplies.

SURGICAL OR TRAUMATIC WOUNDS HEALING BY SECONDARY INTENTION

OVERVIEW/PATHOPHYSIOLOGY

Wounds healing by secondary intention are those with tissue loss or heavy contamination that form granulation tissue and contract in order to heal. Most often, impairment of healing is caused by contamination and inadequate blood flow, oxygenation, and nutrition. Individuals at risk for impaired healing include those who are very young or very old, have DM with poor control, smoke cigarettes, are obese, are malnourished, or are immunosuppressed (e.g., receiving steroids or other immunosuppressive drugs, undergoing chemotherapy or radiation therapy, have immunosuppressive disease).

HEALTH CARE SETTING

Acute care, critical care, primary care, long-term care, home care

ASSESSMENT

Normal healing: Initially the wound edges are inflamed, indurated, and tender. At first, granulation tissue is pink, progressing to a deeper pink and then to a beefy red; wound tissues should be moist. Epithelial cells from the tissue surrounding the wound gradually migrate across the granulation tissue. As healing occurs, the wound edges become pink, the angle between surrounding tissue and the wound becomes less acute, wound contraction occurs, and the wound gets smaller. Occasionally a wound has a tract or sinus that gradually decreases in size as healing occurs. When a drain is in place, volume, color, and odor of the drainage should be evaluated. Time frame for healing depends on wound size and location and on patient's physical and psychologic status. Healing is complete when structure and function have been reestablished.

Impaired healing: Exudate/slough/necrotic tissue on the floor and walls of the wound. Note distribution, color, odor, volume, and adherence of the exudates/slough/dead tissue and damage to skin surrounding the wound, including disruption, discoloration, swelling, local increased warmth, and increasing pain. Older persons may not exhibit classic signs of impaired healing but only changes in cognition or functional status that lead to search for the site of infection.

DIAGNOSTIC TESTS

Culture with tissue biopsy or swab: To determine presence of infection and optimal antibiotic, if appropriate.

Gram stain: Performed as part of the culture to determine characteristics of the offending organism, if present, and aid in selection of preliminary antibiotic.

CBC with WBC differential: Complete blood count (CBC) to assess hematocrit level and for presence of severe anemia (less than 25 g/dl). Increased white blood cell (WBC) count signals infection, whereas a decrease occurs with immunosuppression. Watch the differential for a shift to the left, which indicates infection. Monitor lymphocyte count ($1800/mm^3$ or less) as a sign of malnutrition.

X-ray examination/bone scan: To determine presence of osteomyelitis.

Nursing Diagnosis:

Impaired Tissue Integrity: Wound

related to presence of contaminants, metabolic disorders (e.g., DM), medical therapy (e.g., chemotherapy, radiation therapy), altered perfusion, or malnutrition

Desired Outcomes: Patient's wound exhibits the following signs of healing: initially after injury, wound edges are inflamed, indurated, and tender; with epithelialization, edges become pink; granulation tissue develops over time (identified by pink tissue that becomes beefy red); and there is no odor, exudate, or necrotic tissue. Patient or significant other successfully demonstrates wound care procedure before hospital discharge, if appropriate.

INTERVENTIONS	RATIONALES
Monitor for the following: decreased inflammatory response in first 5 days or inflammatory response that lasts more than 5 days; epithelialization slowed or mechanically disrupted or noncontiguous around the wound; granulation tissue remaining pale or excessively dry or moist; presence of odor, exudate, slough, and/or necrotic tissue.	These are signs of impaired healing.

Continued

INTERVENTIONS	RATIONALES
Cleanse drainage or secretions from skin surrounding wound with a mild disinfectant (e.g., soap and water). Do not use friction with cleansing if tissue is friable.	These measures help prevent wound contamination.
Cleanse wound with each dressing change using 100-150 ml normal saline via 35-ml syringe with an 18-gauge angiocatheter, following meticulous infection control procedures (see p. 783).	Use of an angiocatheter facilitates dislodging and removal of bacteria and loosens necrotic tissue, foreign bodies, and exudate.
When topical enzymes are prescribed, use them on necrotic tissue only and follow package directions carefully.	This measure removes necrotic tissue and spares healthy tissue. **Note:** Some agents, such as silver, deactivate the enzymes.
Apply prescribed dressings following meticulous infection control procedures (see p. 783).	Depending on patient's individual needs, these dressings keep healthy wound tissue moist. Silver dressings decrease surface bacterial counts.
Insert dressing into all tracts.	This promotes gradual closure of those areas.
Ensure good handwashing before and after dressing changes, and dispose of contaminated dressings appropriately.	These measures prevent spread of infection to patient and others.
When a drain is used, maintain its patency, prevent kinking of the tubing, and secure tubing to prevent the drain from becoming dislodged.	Drains remove excess tissue fluid or purulent drainage.
Use sterile technique when caring for drains.	Organisms may move into tissue by way of the drain. Sterile technique reduces risk of contamination and ingress of organisms.
With closed drainage systems, empty drainage reservoir and maintain suction as needed.	Suction aids in removal of excess fluid.
With negative pressure therapy, maintain pressure and change dressing as prescribed.	This therapy reduces bacterial load and enhances blood flow to support healing.
Teach patient or significant other the prescribed wound care procedure, if indicated.	Wound care may be required after patient is discharged.
See discussion of diet, supplemental oxygen, insulin, hydration, and supplemental vitamins in **Impaired Tissue Integrity**, p. 559, in Wounds Closed by Primary Intention.	

••• **Related NIC and NOC labels:** *NIC:* Wound Care; Fluid Management; Infection Control; Infection Protection; Nutrition Management; Wound Care: Closed Drainage; Wound Irrigation *NOC:* Wound Healing: Secondary Intention

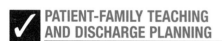

PATIENT-FAMILY TEACHING AND DISCHARGE PLANNING

See teaching and discharge planning interventions in Wounds Closed by Primary Intention, p. 560.

PRESSURE ULCERS
OVERVIEW/PATHOPHYSIOLOGY

Pressure ulcers result from a disruption in tissue integrity and are caused most often by excessive tissue pressure. High-risk patients include older persons and those who have decreased mobility, decreased level of consciousness (LOC), impaired sensation, debilitation, incontinence, sepsis/elevated temperature, or malnutrition.

HEALTH CARE SETTING

Primary care, acute care, critical care, long-term care, assisted care, home care

ASSESSMENT

High-risk individuals should be identified on admission assessment or with daily assessments during hospitalization using a standard assessment schema. Pressure ulcer severity is staged on a scale of I to IV or classified as unstageable or having suspected deep tissue injury.

Stage I: Intact skin with nonblanchable redness of a localized area over a bony prominence. Darkly pigmented skin may not exhibit blanching and may have color that differs from the surrounding area.

Stage II: Partial-thickness skin loss of dermis that presents as a shallow open ulcer with a pink bed without slough. It also may present as an intact or ruptured serum-filled blister. This assessment should not be used to describe skin tears, tape burns, perineal dermatitis, maceration, or excoriation.

Stage III: Full-thickness tissue loss. Subcutaneous fat tissue may be visible but bone, tendon, and muscle are not exposed. Slough may occur but will not obscure the depth of tissue loss. Undermining or tunneling may be present.

Stage IV: Full-thickness tissue loss with exposed bone, tendon, or muscle. Slough or eschar may be present on some parts of the wound bed. Undermining and tunneling often are present.

Unstageable: Full thickness tissue loss in which the base is covered with slough (yellow, tan, gray, green, or brown) and/or eschar (tan, brown, or black) in the wound bed.

Suspected Deep Tissue Injury: Localized area of discolored (maroon or purple) intact skin or a blood-filled blister due to damage of underlying soft tissue from pressure and/or shear. These signs may be preceded by painful, firm, mushy, boggy, warmer, or cooler tissue when it is compared to adjacent tissue.

Note: Do *not* downstage during pressure ulcer assessment. The ulcer is always described at its greatest depth (e.g., healing stage IV ulcer) because tissue lost in a pressure ulcer is not replaced; rather the hole is filled with scar tissue.

See also Surgical or Traumatic Wounds Healing by Secondary Intention, p. 561, for other assessment data.

DIAGNOSTIC TESTS

See Diagnostic Tests, p. 561, in Surgical or Traumatic Wounds Healing by Secondary Intention.

Nursing Diagnosis:

Impaired Tissue Integrity (or risk for same)

related to excessive tissue pressure

Desired Outcomes: Patient's tissue remains intact. Patient or significant other participates in preventive measures and verbalizes understanding of the rationale for these interventions.

INTERVENTIONS	RATIONALES
Identify individuals at risk, and systematically assess skin over bony prominences daily; document. Use a standard risk assessment scale such as the Braden scale (see reference section for Web site information).	High-risk patients include older persons and those who have decreased mobility, decreased LOC, impaired sensation, debilitation, incontinence, sepsis/elevated temperature, malnutrition, or previous pressure ulcer.
Establish and post a position-changing schedule.	This communicates established turning and position-changing schedule for staff and patient/family and reinforces its importance.
Assist patient with position changes.	There is an inverse relationship between pressure and time in ulcer formation; therefore heavier patients need to change position more frequently.
Ensure the following position changes:	
- Turn the bed-bound patient q1-2h and have the wheelchair-bound patient (who is able) perform push-ups in the chair q15min (and not less than q1h).	Position changes will ensure periodic relief from pressure.
- Use pillows, foam wedges, or gel pads to pad and position.	This maintains alternative positions and pads bony prominences.
- In addition, for high risk patients and those with history of previous pressure ulcers, provide pressure-relief measures more frequently.	Healed pressure ulcers have a lower pressure tolerance than uninjured skin.
- Use low Fowler's position and alternate supine position with prone and 30-degree or less elevated side-lying positions.	High Fowler's position results in increased shearing caused by sliding down in bed. A side-lying position at 30 degrees or less prevents high pressure on the trochanter.
For immobile patients, raise heels off the bed surface.	This totally relieves pressure on heels.
Lift rather than drag patient during position changes and transferring; use a draw sheet to facilitate patient movement.	Lifting minimizes friction and shear on tissue during activity.
Do not massage over bony prominences.	Massage can result in skin/tissue damage.
Cleanse at the time of soiling and at routine intervals. Use moisture barriers and disposable briefs as needed.	These measures minimize skin exposure to moisture and chemical irritants.
Use a mattress such as foam, low air loss, alternating air, gel, or water.	These mattresses reduce pressure on body tissues.

Continued

INTERVENTIONS	RATIONALES
Encourage patient to maintain or increase current level of activity.	Activity promotes blood flow, which helps prevent impaired skin/tissue integrity.

••• **Related NIC and NOC labels:** *NIC:* Bed Rest Care; Pressure Management; Circulatory Precautions; Positioning; Positioning: Wheelchair; Pressure Ulcer Prevention; Skin Surveillance; Bathing *NOC:* Immobility Consequences: Physiological; Tissue Integrity: Skin and Mucous Membranes

Nursing Diagnosis:

Impaired Tissue Integrity: Pressure Ulcer

With increased risk for further breakdown *related to* altered circulation and presence of contaminants or irritants (chemical, thermal, or mechanical)

Desired Outcomes: Stages I and II show progressive healing over days to weeks; stages III and IV may require months to heal. Following intervention and instruction, patient or significant other verbalizes causes and preventive measures for pressure ulcers and successfully participates in the plan of care to promote healing and prevent further breakdown.

INTERVENTIONS	RATIONALES
Assess ulcer and stage (see Assessment, earlier).	This assessment provides data on healing status.
Maintain a moist physiologic environment. Change dressings as needed, using meticulous infection control procedure (see p. 783).	These measures promote tissue repair and minimize contaminants.
Be sure patient's skin is kept clean with regular bathing, and be especially conscientious about washing urine and feces from the skin.	Incontinence causes chemical irritation to the skin and reduces tissue tolerance to external pressure. Soap should be used and then thoroughly rinsed from the skin.
Apply heel and elbow protection as needed.	These protectors absorb moisture and prevent shearing when patient moves.
If patient has excessive perspiration, ensure frequent bathing and change bedding as needed.	Perspiration reduces tissue tolerance.
Teach patient and significant other the importance of and measures for preventing excess pressure as a means of preventing pressure ulcers.	Knowledgeable individuals are more likely to adhere to prevention measures.
Provide wound care as needed (described under Surgical or Traumatic Wounds Healing by Secondary Intention, p. 561).	

••• **Related NIC and NOC labels:** *NIC:* Wound Care; Pressure Ulcer Prevention; Infection Protection; Pressure Management; Bathing; Diarrhea Management; Pressure Ulcer Care; Urinary Incontinence Care *NOC:* Tissue Integrity: Skin and Mucous Membranes; Wound Healing: Secondary Intention

ADDITIONAL NURSING DIAGNOSES/PROBLEMS:

Surgical or Traumatic Wounds Healing by Secondary Intention for **Impaired Tissue Integrity**   p. 561

PATIENT-FAMILY TEACHING AND DISCHARGE PLANNING

When providing patient-family teaching, focus on sensory information, avoid giving excessive information, and initiate a home health referral for necessary follow-up teaching. Consider including verbal and written information about the following:

✓ Location of local medical supply stores that have pressure-reducing mattresses and wound care supplies.

✓ Planning a schedule for changing patient positions.

See Wounds Closed by Primary Intention, p. 560, for other teaching and discharge planning interventions.

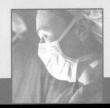

Providing Nutritional Support 74

Hospitalized patients are at high risk for developing protein-energy malnutrition. Studies have shown that 40%-50% of hospitalized surgical patients have insufficient nutrient intake. This situation may be seen in surgical patients who are given IV dextrose/electrolyte solutions alone for extended periods and in patients kept fasting for diagnostic procedures. If this state persists for more than 10-14 consecutive days in an individual with moderately or severely reduced nutritional stores, that individual should be considered and evaluated for nutritional support. When individuals are well-nourished, there are no defined time frames during which they can be without water or food before addressing artificial replacement. The best markers to use for initiation of water and food in well-nourished people are magnitude of the injury/insult to the body and amount of time the individual will be unable to resume normal oral intake.

HEALTH CARE SETTING

Acute care

ASSESSMENT

Dietary History

A dietary history is compiled to reveal adequacy of usual and recent food intake. Based on the information obtained, the nurse may identify the need to consult with a registered dietitian for additional interventions. Be alert to excesses or deficiencies of nutrients and any special eating patterns (e.g., various types of vegetarian or prescribed diets), use of fad diets, and excessive supplementation. Include in the care plan anything that impairs adequate selection, preparation, ingestion, digestion, absorption, or excretion of nutrients as follows:

- Food allergies, food aversions, and use of nutritional supplements (prescribed or over-the-counter).
- Any alternative therapies such as use of herbs.
- Any over-the-counter medications.
- Recent unplanned weight loss or gain.
- Chewing or swallowing difficulties. Include questions related to dental care, such as dentures (note presence of dentures; ask about fit of dentures or other problems), missing teeth, no teeth, and/or loose teeth.
- Nausea, vomiting, or pain with eating.
- Altered pattern of elimination (e.g., constipation, diarrhea).

- Chronic disease affecting utilization of nutrients (e.g., malabsorption, pancreatitis, diabetes mellitus).
- Surgical resection; disease of the gut or accessory organs of digestion (i.e., pancreas, liver, gallbladder).
- Currently pregnant or lactating.
- Use of medications (e.g., laxatives, antacids, antibiotics, antineoplastic drugs) or alcohol. Long-term use of drugs may affect appetite, digestion, or utilization or excretion of nutrients.

PHYSICAL ASSESSMENT

Most physical findings are not specific to a particular nutritional deficiency. Compare current assessment findings with past assessments, especially related to the following.

- Loss of muscle and adipose tissue.
  - Assess fit of clothing, rings, and watches.
  - Be aware that assessment of obese patients or individuals who have an excess of fluid accumulation due to body edema may be difficult.
  - Look for temporal wasting in individuals who have ascites or other forms of body edema.
- Work and muscle endurance.
  - Assess ability to maintain activities of daily living.
  - Query patient regarding recent changes in mobility and/or activities.
  - Muscle weakness may reflect several different deficiencies that may require additional evaluation and tests:
    Selenium
    Vitamin D
    Potassium
    Magnesium
- Changes in hair, skin, or neuromuscular function.
  - Excessive bruising or bleeding may reflect vitamin K deficiency.
  - Biotin deficiency may appear as alopecia or seborrheic dermatitis.
  - Scaly dermatitis may reflect essential fatty acid deficiency.
  - Zinc deficiency may present as sores at edges of mouth, palms of hands, and soles of feet with peeling of skin along with brittle nails.
  - Hypocalcemia may be accompanied by dry, scaling skin; brittle nails; and/or dry hair.

Anthropometric Data

Height: Used to determine ideal weight and body mass index (BMI). If patient's height is unavailable or impossible to measure, obtain an estimate from family or significant other.

Weight: Used by many to determine nutritional status, but fluctuations may be a result of amputation, dehydration, diuresis, fluid retention (renal failure, edema, third spacing), fluid resuscitation, wound dressings, or clothing. (It is helpful to remember that 1 L of fluid equals approximately 2 lb or 1 kg.) More reliable information may be obtained by asking patient to recall usual weight, weight changes (gains and losses), and time frame in which these occurred. Unintentional loss in weight of greater than 10% over a 6-mo period is considered significant and may be associated with severe malnutrition. The greater the unintentional weight loss, the more predictive this weight loss may be of mortality.

Most dietitians use the Hamwi "rule of thumb" calculation to determine ideal body weight:

Men: 106 lb for the first 5 ft, then add 6 lb for each inch over 5 ft, **or**

48 kg for the first 1.5 cm, then add 2.7 kg for each 2.54 cm over 1.5 cm

Women: 100 lb for the first 5 ft, then add 5 lb for each inch over 5 ft, **or**

45 kg for the first 1.5 cm, then add 2.3 kg for each 2.54 cm over 1.5 cm

BMI: Used to evaluate the weight of adults. One calculation and one set of standards are applicable to both men and women:

$$\text{BMI (kg m/m}^2) = \text{Weight/Height (m}^2)$$

BMI values of 19-25 are appropriate for 19-34 year olds; whereas, BMI values of 21-27 are appropriate for individuals older than 35 yr of age. Obesity is defined as BMI greater than 27.5, with severe or morbid obesity greater than 40. A BMI of 16-18.5 is considered mild to moderate malnutrition; whereas BMI less than 16 indicates severe malnutrition.

Biochemical Data

Historically, hepatic proteins (albumin, prealbumin, and transferrin) have been used by health care practitioners as a tool to evaluate nutritional status. This dates back to the diagnosis of Kwashiorkor malnutrition, a condition occurring when protein is relatively absent from the diet for a prolonged period of time. Stress-induced hypoalbuminemia occurs following a traumatic injury or acute illness and is not a reflection of malnutrition. Instead it reflects the body's physiologic response to injury and infection and will increase with recovery. However, hepatic proteins help the clinician identify the "sickest" patients who are likely to develop malnutrition in the health care setting even if well-nourished before trauma or the onset of illness.

Iron status: Measurement of red blood cell (RBC) size (i.e., mean corpuscular volume [MCV] [normal: 80-95 μm^3]) aids in determining the type of nutrient anemia. In iron-deficiency anemia, RBCs are smaller than normal, whereas in folate or vitamin B_{12} deficiencies, RBCs are larger than normal.

Estimating Nutritional Requirements

The primary goal of nutritional support is to meet the needs for body temperature, metabolic processes, and tissue repair. Having collected all the data, energy needs may be estimated using the following options.

Harris-Benedict equations: Used to determine basal energy expenditure (BEE). The following equations can be used to calculate BEE. **Note:** Weight = weight in kg; height = height in cm; age = age in yr.

BEE (Male):

$$66.5 + (13.8 \times \text{weight}) - (5.0 \times \text{height}) - (6.8 \times \text{age})$$

BEE (Female):

$$655.1 + (9.6 \times \text{weight}) - (1.9 \times \text{height}) - (4.7 \times \text{age})$$

Calorie estimation: To prevent overfeeding, calculate the total calorie intake as follows:

Average nourished patient: 25 total calories per kg of body weight

Mildly stressed patient: 30 total calories per kg of body weight

Severely stressed patient: 35 total calories per kg of body weight

Morbidly obese patient: 18 total calories per kg of body weight

Permissive hypocaloric feeding (approximately 20% less than estimated needs): Often used for patients in a septic or inflammatory state.

Distribution of calories: A relatively normal distribution of calories is adequate. Percentages of total calories from carbohydrates (CHOs), protein, and fat should equal approximately 60%, 15%-20%, and 15%-25%, respectively.

Protein requirements: Usually 0.8-1.5 g/kg/24 hr. (Protein will be restricted if patient has hepatic or renal failure that is not being treated with dialysis.)

$$1 \text{ g protein} = 4.0 \text{ kcal}$$

$$1 \text{ g nitrogen} = 6.25 \text{ g protein}$$

CHO requirements: Daily glucose administration of 9-15 g/kg/24 hr is an adequate range. Excess amounts of CHO are not utilized or tolerated. Overfeeding of CHO may lead to hyperglycemia, increased CO_2 production, hypophosphatemia, and fluid overload in short-term use or fatty liver syndrome in long-term use.

$$1 \text{ g dextrose IV} = 3.4 \text{ kcal}$$

$$1 \text{ g CHO in food} = 4.0 \text{ kcal}$$

Fat requirements: Fat can be administered in minimal quantities to satisfy needs for essential fatty acids but should not exceed 1 g fat/kg/24 hr because of the potential for suppression of the immune system.

$$1 \text{ g fat} = 9.0 \text{ calories}$$

Special diets for organ-specific pathologic conditions: Commercially available oral supplements and enteral formulas are available for patients with respiratory disease, diabetes, renal failure, hepatic failure, inflammatory bowel disease, and immune compromise. Well-designed clinical trials may not be available to support the suggested indication.

Vitamin and essential trace mineral requirements: In general, follow the recommended daily allowances (RDAs) to provide minimum quantities of vitamins, minerals, and essential fatty acids. For specific patients, supplement specific vitamins or minerals needed in increased amounts for existing disease states (e.g., burns: zinc, vitamins A and C; chronic alcohol ingestion: thiamine, folate, vitamin B_{12}).

Fluid requirements: Many factors affect fluid balance. Under usual circumstances an estimate of fluid needs can be made by providing 1 ml of free water for each calorie provided, or 30-50 ml/kg body weight. Daily loss of water includes approximately 1400 ml in urine (60 ml/hr), 350 ml via respiration, 600 ml as evaporation through skin, and about 200 ml in feces. Fluid losses are 100-150 ml/day for each degree of temperature increase above 37° C. If loss by any of these routes is increased, fluid needs increase; if loss by any of these routes is impaired, fluid restriction may be necessary. Areas to include in the nursing assessment for fluid requirements are:

- Intake and output (I&O). Evaluate that neither one is in excess of the other and for decreases in urine output.
- Daily weights. **Note:** Rapid changes may represent problems with technique or equipment rather than actual changes in body weight. If sudden increases in weight occur, look for imbalances in I&O, occurrence of edema, and dilution of serum electrolytes.
- Presence or absence of edema.
- Large wounds, burns, or open abdomen.
- Skin turgor. This assessment may be helpful in younger patients, but is less useful in older adults due to normal changes in skin elasticity that occurs with aging.

Nutritional Support Modalities

Specialized nutritional support refers to provision of an artificial formulation of nutrients via oral, enteral, or parenteral route for the treatment or prevention of malnutrition. Oral supplements are the preferred route because they are less invasive, more natural, and less costly, whereas enteral nutrition is preferred over parenteral.

Types of feeding tubes

Small-bore nasal tubes: Defined as 12 French or smaller. Require abdominal x-ray examination for confirmation of placement. Composition may be polyurethane, silicone, or polyvinyl chloride. Location cannot be verified in the gastrointestinal (GI) tract when using auscultation after injecting an air bolus, asking patient to speak, or submerging the tube's proximal tip into a glass of water. Usual length of tube is 36-55 inches and it may or may not require a stylet for insertion. The physician should determine whether the distal tip ends in the stomach or small intestine. Insertion by a nurse is determined by hospital policy. It also may be inserted by a physician using endoscopy or fluoroscopy-guided placement. Be-

cause of their diameter and composition, these tubes are easily dislocated proximally in the GI tract without any resultant external signs.

Large-bore nasal tubes: Defined as larger than 12 French. Composition is either polyurethane or polyvinyl chloride. Usual length of tube is 36 inches. Stylet is not required for insertion. Insertion may be by a nurse. Placement is confirmed by withdrawal of gastric fluid or x-ray examination.

Gastrostomy tubes: Exit stomach directly through abdominal wall and usually anchored with either a balloon or disc on the inside of the stomach. Usually they are 12 French or larger. Composition may be polyurethane, silicone, or rubber and may contain multiple ports, in addition to the main lumen, for insertion of air into the balloon and delivery of medications. Initially a physician in radiology, endoscopy, or surgery performs the insertion. If not placed during surgery (i.e., open laparotomy), the common term used to describe the tube is percutaneous endoscopically inserted gastrostomy (PEG). Reinsertion by a nurse is determined by hospital policy. Inadvertent removal of a tube in position for less than 6 wk should be considered a medical emergency and the health care provider should be contacted immediately.

Gastrostomy button: Placed into a mature gastrostomy stoma. It fits into the stoma tract flush with the outer abdominal wall. The button contains an antireflux valve to prevent leakage, but gastric samples or residuals usually cannot be obtained via the button.

Jejunostomy tubes: Placed by a physician either surgically or percutaneously (PEJ). Diameter is usually about 12-18 French. Anchoring the tube inside the jejunum presents a problem because a balloon larger than 5 ml might cause bowel obstruction. Confirmation of position requires x-ray examination with contrast. No residuals should be obtained from this tube. If the tube becomes displaced, the entry site into the jejunum will close down rapidly (approximately 20-30 min). Reinsertion by a nurse is determined by hospital policy, but it is not recommended without special training.

Gastrostomy-jejunostomy tubes: Exit stomach directly through the abdominal wall with a small-bore jejunostomy tube placed through the main lumen of the gastrostomy and the distal tip positioned in the jejunum.

Feeding sites

Stomach: Simulates normal GI functions; may be used for bolus, intermittent, or continuous feedings; indicated for patients who have intact gag or cough reflexes.

Duodenum, jejunum: Must be used for continuous feedings only to prevent dumping syndrome and diarrhea. Small-bore diameter tube is recommended.

Total Parenteral Nutrition

Total parenteral nutrition (TPN) provides some or all nutrients by the IV route. TPN is used to provide complete nutrition for patients who cannot receive enteral nutrition or to supplement nutritional needs of patients who are unable to absorb sufficient calories via the GI tract. TPN is more expensive than enteral nutrition and has the potential for developing severe complications more rapidly.

Parenteral solutions: IV solutions are customized combinations of dextrose (CHO), amino acids (protein), IV fat emulsions (fat), electrolytes, vitamins, and trace metals.

CHOs: Dextrose provides the bulk of calories and energy needs, with concentrations ranging from 5%-70%. The percentage of dextrose selected is based on the available administration site and patient's volume status. All final mixed solutions that are more than 12.5% dextrose must be administered via a central venous catheter. (If unsure or information is unavailable on the infusion container related to infusion route, consult with pharmacist or refer to hospital policy.) The average amount of CHO calories delivered is approximately 60% of the total. The more CHO delivered, the greater the potential for complications, which include fatty liver syndrome, increased CO_2 production, and hyperglycemia.

Protein: Synthetic crystalline essential and nonessential amino acid formulations are available in concentrations of 3.5%-15%. Special amino acid formulations are available that have varied the ratio of essential to nonessential amino acids for specific disorders (e.g., liver, renal disease). The amount of protein delivered depends on patient's renal and hepatic function.

Fat: IV fat emulsion (IVFE) of 10%, 20%, or 30% is an isotonic solution providing essential fatty acids and a source of concentrated calories.

$$10\% \text{ IVFE} = 1.1 \text{ calorie/ml}$$

$$20\% \text{ IVFE} = 2 \text{ calories/ml}$$

$$30\% \text{ IVFE} = 3 \text{ calories/ml}$$

When fats are mixed in the same infusion bag with the CHO and amino acids, the solution is referred to as a total nutrient admixture (TNA) or 3:1 solution (all three nutrient components in one bag). The IVFE may be given piggyback into the amino acid/dextrose infusion to infuse over 8-12 hr. The amount of IVFE administered may be reduced or removed for patients who have hypertriglyceridemia (e.g., patients receiving antirejection medication following organ transplant, or for coronary artery disease, pancreatitis, or acquired immunodeficiency syndrome [AIDS]). Determine whether patient has an egg allergy because long-chain triglycerides in IVFEs may originate from phospholipids in egg yolks. If a patient develops a rash during IVFE infusion, consider an allergy immediately. If ratio of the protein, CHO, and IVFE in the ad-

mixture is not stable, separation of the IV fats from the emulsion may occur, which is called "cracking" of the solution. The IV fats may float on top of the mixture much like an egg yolk floating in the solution or appear as an uneven yellow consistency. In addition, "oiling out" may occur, which looks like an oil slick or oil droplets on top of the solution. Return any solution that appears "different" to the pharmacy and do not use it.

Selection of administration site

Central venous catheter: Used for all IV solutions whose final concentration is greater than 12.5% dextrose or a solution with an osmolarity 800 mOsm/L or greater. (If unsure or information is unavailable on the infusion container related to infusion route, consult with a pharmacist or refer to hospital policy.) Central venous catheter (CVC) use requires a large central vein with the distal tip of the catheter in the superior vena cava. The flow of blood through the large vessels rapidly dilutes hypertonic solutions and decreases the potential for thrombophlebitis.

Peripheral venous catheter: Reserved for individuals with a need for nutritional support for short-term periods, with small nutritional requirements, and for whom CVC access is unavailable. Only a low-osmolarity solution (less than 800 mOsm/L) can be used. To reduce osmolarity of the base solution, dilution of the components is usually required. The required large volume limits the type of patients in whom this admixture can be administered. (If unsure or information is unavailable on the infusion container related to infusion route, consult with a pharmacist or refer to hospital policy.)

Transitional Feeding

A transition is necessary before discontinuing nutritional support. Reduce the percent of total calories supplied from enteral nutrition as oral intake increases to 60%-70% of estimated needs. Similarly, patients who have received TPN for more than 2-3 wk may have some mucosal atrophy of the bowel and will need a period of adjustment before the bowel can fully resume its usual functions of digestion and absorption. The best diet advancement includes starting with clear liquids, then advancing to a soft diet. Because these individuals have been ill, the lactase in their stomach has decreased, placing them at higher risk for lactose deficiency; therefore they should limit or avoid a full liquid diet because of increased incidence of bloating, nausea, and diarrhea associated with lactose deficiency.

Nursing Diagnosis:

Imbalanced Nutrition: Less Than Body Requirements

related to inability to ingest, digest, or absorb nutrients

Desired Outcome: Patient has adequate nutrition as evidenced by stabilization of weight at desired level or steady weight gain of ½-1 lb/wk; presence of wound granulation (i.e., pinkish white tissue around wound edges; wound edges approximating together), and absence of infection (see **Risk for Infection,** p. 574).

INTERVENTIONS	RATIONALES
For Oral Nutrition:	
Ensure nutritional screening and assessment of patient within 24 hr of admission; document and reassess weekly.	Hospitalized patients are at risk for developing protein-energy malnutrition. Baseline assessment enables comparison with subsequent assessments, which may reveal problems that may require interventions.
	Because no single sensitive and comprehensive nutritional assessment factor exists, multiple sources of information are used, including any of the following: historical data, nutritional history, anthropometric data, biochemical analysis of blood and urine, and duration of the disease process.
Position patient in high Fowler's position for eating.	This promotes normal position for eating and decreases risk of aspiration.
Assist with preparation of food tray for eating prn.	This ensures that all packages are opened and patient can access all food.
Involve significant other in meal rituals for companionship.	Patients who eat alone tend to eat less.
Assess for food allergies/intolerances and avoid these foods.	Individuals with celiac disease, for example, will have severe reactions that may result in malabsorption when exposed to even minute quantities of wheat and other glutens.
Provide small, frequent feedings of diet compatible with disease state and patient's ability to ingest foods.	After an illness, early satiety may be a problem. Small, frequent meals are likely to increase intake.
Respect food aversions, religious guidelines, and food preferences.	Individuals will eat more readily and frequently when consuming preferred foods that are within dietary allowances.
If appropriate, allow family and friends to bring food from home.	Patients may prefer home-cooked meals to those prepared at the hospital.
Provide liquid nutritional supplements as prescribed.	Supplements increase calories consumed and help meet RDAs for vitamins and minerals needed for recovery.
Serve supplements cold or over ice.	This will help enhance palatability.
Obtain weight weekly.	Stabilizing weight or weight gain of $\frac{1}{2}$-1 lb/wk is the usual goal if weight gain is desired. This assessment also tracks maintenance of weight.
Provide psychological support.	Emotional health influences appetite.
For Enteral or Parenteral Nutrition in the Acute Care Setting:	
Ensure nutritional screening and assessment within 24 hr of health care provider's directive; document and reassess weekly.	Hospitalized patients are at risk for developing protein-calorie malnutrition. Baseline assessment enables comparison with subsequent assessments, which may reveal problems that may require intervention. Because no single sensitive and comprehensive nutritional assessment factor exists, multiple sources of information are used, including any of the following: historical data, nutritional history, anthropometric data, biochemical analysis of blood and urine, and duration of the disease process.
Administer continuous enteral feedings using a pump at prescribed rate.	Using a continuous rate provides food and CHO at a steady infusion rate, which decreases feelings of fullness and avoids peaks in patient's blood glucose levels. Postoperative patients may experience gastric ileus and benefit from feeds delivered into the small bowel.
Check infused volume and rate q4h.	This helps ensure accuracy of delivery.
Administer intermittent feeding over 30-40 min via gravity drip.	Intermittent feeding is similar to the natural pattern of eating.
Administer TPN using a volumetric pump at prescribed rate.	There is potential for complications such as hyperglycemia, and a continuous rate for volume is better tolerated by the patient.
Check infused volume and rate q4h.	Checking volume and rate prevents volume overload and other complications that could occur when using the pump.

Continued

INTERVENTIONS	RATIONALES
Monitor laboratory data every day until stable for TPN and enteral feedings, then at least weekly: electrolytes, blood glucose, blood urea nitrogen (BUN), creatinine, phosphorus, magnesium, and calcium. Advance calories to goal over 2-3 days in patients reporting a decreased caloric intake for several days before admission.	Values outside the normal range may signal refeeding syndrome, changing metabolic status, or poor glycemic control. Refeeding syndrome is the consequence realized after a large CHO (often dextrose) infusion in a patient with previous inadequate food intake and may result in fluid retention, hypophosphatemia, hypokalemia, increased diarrhea, and cardiac dysrhythmias.
Monitor other laboratory data initially and then at least weekly: liver function tests including albumin, triglycerides (if patient at risk, i.e., pancreatitis, transplant antirejection medications, AIDS).	These laboratory values provide data about tolerance, clearance, and metabolism by organs and stabilization of the disease process.
Record I&O carefully.	This data tracks fluid balance trends.
Weigh patient initially and daily during an acute illness, then advance to weekly.	Stabilized weight or weight gain of ½-1 lb/wk is the usual goal if weight gain is an intended goal. Weight trend also assesses fluid status and disease process.
Ensure that patient receives prescribed caloric intake.	As a general rule, percentages of total calories from CHO, protein, and fat should equal approximately 60%, 15%-20%, and 15%-25%, respectively. Protein is burned for calories during the recovery phase if enough CHOs and fats are not eaten, enabling protein to be used for healing and rebuilding.
Assess for fluid imbalance, especially fluid volume excess.	Patient may be especially susceptible to fluid excess because low protein levels in the blood cause a decrease in oncotic pressure in the vessels, resulting in fluid retention.
	Fluid excess may be manifested by peripheral edema, adventitious breath sounds (especially crackles), and weight gain (1 kg = 1000 ml).

••• **Related NIC and NOC labels:** *NIC:* Nutrition Management; Weight Gain Assistance; Nutrition Therapy; Nutritional Monitoring; Enteral Tube Feeding; Total Parenteral Nutrition Administration; Intravenous Therapy; Laboratory Data Interpretation *NOC:* Nutritional Status; Nutritional Status: Food and Fluid Intake; Nutritional Status: Nutrient Intake; Weight Control

Nursing Diagnosis:

Risk for Aspiration

related to GI feeding or delayed gastric emptying

Desired Outcome: Patient is free of aspiration problems as evidenced by auscultation of clear lung sounds, VS within normal limits for the patient, and no signs of respiratory distress.

INTERVENTIONS	RATIONALES
Mark nasogastric (NG) tube to determine length exiting from the body. Check this mark to determine tube migration. Secure tubing in place per agency policy.	The NG tube can easily slide out of the nose because of nasal discharge, sweat, and loosening of the tape or tube holder.
Reassess tube position q4h and before each feeding.	If tube migration is suspected or the tube is reinserted, obtain x-ray to confirm placement.
Assess respiratory status q4h, including respiratory rate, effort, and adventitious breath sounds.	Patient's lung sounds should be clear, and there should be no signs of respiratory distress before infusing a feeding.
Monitor temperature q4h; report any parameters as defined by health care provider.	Temperature outside of parameters as defined by health care provider should be reported. An increased temperature occurs with aspiration pneumonia.
Auscultate bowel sounds q8h.	High-pitched or absent bowel sounds, abdominal distention, or nausea can occur with ileus, decreased tolerance to the feeding, and small bowel obstruction. These problems can lead to vomiting and aspiration and therefore should be reported promptly.

Continued

INTERVENTIONS	RATIONALES
Depending on patient's medical condition, raise head of bed 30 degrees or higher or place patient in a right side-lying position during and for 1 hr after administration of a bolus or intermittent feeding.	These positions promote gravity flow from the greater stomach curvature through the pylorus into the duodenum and decrease risk for aspiration.
Stop the tube feeding ½-1 hr before chest physical therapy or placing patient supine.	This measure enables complete emptying of the stomach and decreases potential for aspiration.
Check residuals per agency policy.	The best practice is to hold the feeding if residuals are 200 ml from an NG or orogastric tube or 100 ml from a gastrostomy. High-volume residuals may be a sign of intolerance because of ileus or small bowel obstruction, either of which can lead to vomiting and aspiration.
Recognize that no residuals or minimal volume should be obtained from a tube placed into the small intestine.	Unlike the stomach, the small intestine does not function as a reservoir and therefore normally will not hold volume because of forward peristalsis.
Caution: Avoid use of formulas that have been tinted with coloring to assess for aspiration.	Published case reports describe fatal metabolic acidosis secondary to the excessive use of food coloring in enteral feedings. This practice has received a warning from the Food and Drug Administration and should not be used under any circumstance
Assess for the following two syndromes associated with aspiration to assist health care provider in making the correct differential diagnosis:	
- Regurgitation or vomiting of gastric contents.	Aspiration of gastric contents is a risk factor for ventilator-associated pneumonia, which is the leading cause of hospital-associated death.
- Aspiration from the oropharynx of saliva and upper airway secretions.	Aspiration of bacteria from the oral and pharyngeal areas may cause bacterial pneumonia.

••• **Related NIC and NOC labels:** *NIC:* Aspiration Precautions; Gastrointestinal Intubation; Positioning; Respiratory Monitoring; Enteral Tube Feeding *NOC:* Aspiration Control

Nursing Diagnosis:

Diarrhea (or risk for same)

related to medications, dumping syndrome, bacterial contamination, or formula intolerance

Desired Outcome: Patient has formed stools within 2-3 days of intervention.

INTERVENTIONS	RATIONALES
Assess abdomen and GI status: bowel sounds, distention, cramping, nausea, and frequency of bowel movements.	These assessments establish a baseline and reference point from which current trend can be compared. Hyperactive bowel sounds may occur with increased stooling, along with signs and symptoms of distention, cramping, and nausea.
Ask patient to define diarrhea. Determine patient's normal stool pattern.	One loose stool does not mean patient has diarrhea. Liquid intake normally produces a pasty stool, and patient may misinterpret this as diarrhea. Enteral feedings may produce several soft formed stools per day.
Consult with health care provider regarding stopping prokinetic medication (e.g., metoclopramide).	These drugs stimulate the bowels.
Suggest a review of medications by pharmacy.	Pharmacists are knowledgeable about drugs that cause diarrhea.
Suggest stopping any stool softeners being administered.	Stool softeners may stimulate the bowels.
Consider giving yogurt or the medication equivalent.	This will replace normal flora removed by antibiotics and diarrhea.
Evaluate route of yogurt delivery.	Yogurt will clog a small-bore feeding tube.

Continued

INTERVENTIONS	RATIONALES
Consult pharmacy if patient has a history of multiple bowel surgeries, GI hypersecretion, or intestinal failure.	The pharmacist has knowledge of drugs used to treat the symptoms and complications associated with GI hypersecretion and diarrhea related to intestinal failure. Loperamide is generally used as the first-line agent.
Contact pharmacy about elixirs being administered. Discuss with health care provider and pharmacist changing form of medication or switching to another medication within the same class.	The majority of elixirs contain sorbitol, which will increase transit time in the intestines and cause diarrhea.
Collect a stool sample for bacterial culture and sensitivity.	Diarrhea may be caused by bacteria.
Collect a stool sample for ova and parasites.	Parasites can cause diarrhea.
Collect a stool sample for *Clostridium difficile* toxin.	If *C. difficile* is present, the volume of the daily stool output may exceed 500 ml and will occur whether or not the individual consumes food or enteral products. This type of diarrhea is considered secretory because the fluid is secreted from the intestinal wall and can lead to imbalances in fluid status.
Do not administer an antidiarrheal medication until stool culture is confirmed as negative.	Giving this medication when stool culture is positive increases risk for toxic megacolon and bowel perforation.
Maintain optimal hydration.	This will replace losses caused by diarrhea.
Record I&O status every shift. Obtain parameters from health care provider for notification of output.	An example of a parameter established by health care provider for a dehydrated patient would be urinary output 30 ml/hr $\times$ 4 or hourly stools of specific volume amount.
Check weight daily.	This assesses fluid status. With diarrhea, the concern is weight loss. For example, 1 kg/day could signal a loss of 1000 ml.
If patient is receiving a bolus feeding, switch to intermittent or continuous feeding.	Bolus feedings may contribute to dumping syndrome, which would result in increased diarrhea.
Follow hazard analysis and critical control point (HACCP) guidelines for handling of enteral products, feeding tube, and feeding sets.	Bacteria can grow in feeding sets and on hands of caregiver and could cause diarrhea if allowed to be transported to patient.
Change all equipment per agency policy.	Same as above.
Refrigerate all opened products, but discard after 24 hr. Date and time all products.	These products are a potential growth media for bacteria and could cause diarrhea if the product is given to the patient. All manufacturers state on their products to discard after opened for 24 hr and store in refrigerator.
Store all unopened products at room temperature (about 70° F).	This prevents clumping of proteins in the container.
Use enteral solutions at room temperature for a maximum of 12 hr when using an open delivery system vs 24-48 hr when using a closed system. Check with manufacturer guidelines for specific duration of hang time.	This reduces risk of bacterial contamination. Closed systems reduce the risk of touch contamination.
Identify tube as enteral access before attaching closed system.	This measure reduces risk of inadvertent infusion of enteral feeding into an IV port. **Note:** Spike set is IV compatible.

●●● **Related NIC and NOC labels:** *NIC:* Diarrhea Management; Medication Management; Fluid Management; Fluid Monitoring *NOC:* Bowel Elimination; Hydration

Nursing Diagnosis:

Nausea (or risk of same)

related to underlying medical condition, too rapid infusion of enteral product, food intolerance, or medication administration

Desired Outcome: Patient has no nausea with food intake.

INTERVENTIONS	RATIONALES
Give antiemetic as prescribed.	An antiemetic decreases/eliminates nausea.
Administer medication on an empty stomach only when indicated.	Medications such as analgesics may cause nausea if given without food.
Offer food in small portions, 6 times per day.	Smaller meals are better tolerated than larger meals.
Give chewing gum or hard candies prn, if permitted.	Providing some sugar to the system may stimulate the GI tract and decrease nausea.
Suggest patient brush teeth and tongue q8h and prn.	A bad taste in the mouth may increase nausea in some individuals.
If odor of food induces nausea, remove the food immediately.	This will help eliminate nausea caused by odor.
Reduce rate/min of enteral formula infusion.	Nausea may be caused by increased infusion rate, which may result in delayed gastric emptying, overdistention, or constipation.
If patient is receiving bolus infusion, change to intermittent or continuous.	Overdistention with a bolus infusion may cause or increase nausea, whereas a slower infusion rate with an intermittent or continuous infusion may be better tolerated.
Inspect abdomen for distention and auscultate bowel sounds.	Absence of bowel sounds may signal ileus. Decreased bowel sounds may indicate need to decrease feeding and check stool output. Distention may appear either with ileus or with decreased motility. These signs would necessitate notifying health care provider for intervention.
Monitor for and record flatus and bowel movements.	Decreased bowel movements and flatus may indicate ileus or partial obstruction.
If medically indicated, consider bowel suppository.	This will stimulate the intestinal tract. Nausea may occur secondary to constipation or decreased motility.
Monitor electrolytes, especially potassium.	Hypokalemia is associated with ileus and nausea.

••• **Related NIC and NOC labels:** *NIC:* Nausea Management; Medication Management; Environmental Management: Comfort; Medication Administration *NOC:* Comfort Level; Nutritional Status: Food and Fluid Intake

Nursing Diagnosis:

Constipation

related to inadequate fluid and fiber in the diet

Desired Outcome: Patient states that he or she has had a soft bowel movement within 3-4 days of this diagnosis (or within patient's usual pattern).

INTERVENTIONS	RATIONALES
If patient is receiving a formula that contains fiber and is on fluid restriction or receiving large amounts of diuretics, consider changing formula to an isotonic formula without fiber.	Fiber pulls more fluid into the intestines. When a patient is "dry" from medical therapy, there is no extra water to pull, and if no extra water is available, constipation will occur.
If patient is receiving a formula that contains fiber, assess intake of free water.	Optimally water intake should be 1 ml/calorie of intake or 30-50 ml/kg body weight in order to compensate for losses that occur normally via respirations, urination, fever, and so on.
Give free water q4h or as prescribed and after each medication.	Free water helps maintain fluid balance and patency of feeding tube, as well as promote soft stools and prevent constipation.
If medically indicated, consider a reduction in the amount of narcotics being administered.	Opioid medications are constipating. Patient may need a stool softener or motility enhancer.
Consider a stool softener, especially if patient regularly uses a laxative at home.	If patient is unable to increase water needs effectively, a stool softener will prevent straining and decrease risk of constipation.

••• **Related NIC and NOC labels:** *NIC:* Bowel Management; Constipation/Impaction Management; Fluid Management; Medication Management; Nutritional Monitoring; Enteral Tube Feeding *NOC:* Bowel Elimination; Hydration

Nursing Diagnosis:

Risk for Impaired Swallowing

related to decreased or absent gag reflex, facial paralysis, mechanical obstruction, fatigue, weight loss, or deceased strength or excursion of muscles involved in mastication

Desired Outcome: Before food or fluids are initiated, patient demonstrates adequate cough and gag reflexes and the ability to ingest foods via the phases of swallowing as instructed.

INTERVENTIONS	RATIONALES
Assess oral motor function within 24 hr of admission or on patient's progression to oral diet.	If patient has adequate oral motor functioning, oral intake can be increased. Otherwise, tube feedings should be considered to prevent aspiration.
Assess cough and gag reflexes before the first feeding.	Patients who develop gastric reflux or vomit can aspirate if their cough and gag reflexes are not intact.
Offer semisolid foods and progress to thicker textures as tolerated.	If patient is likely to have difficulty with swallowing, liquids will be the most difficult and most likely to be aspirated.
Coach patient through phases of ingesting food: opening mouth, inserting food, closing lips, chewing, transferring food from side to side in the mouth and then to the back of the oral cavity, elevating tongue to roof of mouth (hard palate), and swallowing between breaths.	With illness, muscles may become weaker and this may result in bad habits of rushing swallowing and moving food into the trachea rather than into the esophagus, where they are less likely to be aspirated.
Order extra sauces, gravies, or liquids if dryness of the oral cavity impairs patient's swallowing ability.	This moistens each bite of food for patients in whom dryness of the oral cavity impairs swallowing ability.
If tolerated, keep patient in high Fowler's position for ½ hr after eating.	This position minimizes risk of aspiration by promoting gravity flow through the stomach and into the duodenum.
Provide mouth care before and after meals and dietary supplements.	This measure ensures that all traces of food are removed, preventing subsequent aspiration.
Provide small, frequent meals.	Six smaller feedings per day may increase muscle strength needed for swallowing and be less likely to result in rushing, which could cause aspiration.
Provide foods at temperatures acceptable to patient.	Foods that are too hot or too cold could rush swallowing and lead to aspiration.
As indicated, obtain services of speech, physical, or occupational therapist.	These specialists assist in retraining or facilitating patient's swallowing.

••• **Related NIC and NOC labels:** *NIC:* Aspiration Precautions; Positioning; Risk Identification; Swallowing Therapy; Feeding; Referral
NOC: Aspiration Control; Swallowing Status

Nursing Diagnosis:

Risk for Infection

related to invasive procedures, malnutrition, and suppression of the immune system

Desired Outcome: Patient is free of infection as evidenced by temperature, pulse, and respirations within patient's normal range and absence of clinical signs of sepsis: erythema, swelling at catheter insertion site, chills, fever, and glucose intolerance.

INTERVENTIONS	RATIONALES
Weekly and prn, monitor white blood cell (WBC) count with differential for values outside normal range.	A higher value signals infection. Infection requires extra calories.
Monitor bedside glucose for values outside normal range. If the individual is glucose intolerant, begin q4h bedside assessment and administer sliding scale insulin as prescribed by health care provider.	Glucose intolerance is a sign of sepsis. An increase in glucose also promotes bacterial growth and increases risk of infection. Insulin will maintain blood glucose within normal limits.
Examine catheter insertion site (if using a transparent dressing) q12h for erythema, swelling, or purulent discharge. If using a gauze dressing, examine site at time of dressing change.	These are signs of local infection.
Use meticulous sterile technique when changing central line dressing, containers, or administration lines. Follow agency policy for central line dressing changes.	These measures reduce possibility of infection.
Consult health care provider to obtain prescription for blood cultures at two sites as outlined by the Centers for Disease Control and Prevention (CDC) in patients with a central line who are febrile with a rising WBC count.	Two positive cultures may indicate a bloodstream infection requiring antibiotic treatment.
Restrict use of lumen used for administration of TPN, if possible. Avoid drawing blood specimens or other fluids, pressure monitoring, or medication administration, if possible.	When TPN is being administered, most infections of catheters and blood are related to insertion site or tubing sets.
Change all administration sets, as established by CDC.	This is a standard infection control protocol.

••• **Related NIC and NOC labels:** *NIC:* Infection Protection; Laboratory Data Interpretation; Risk Identification; Infection Control; Incision Site Care; Nutrition Management; Tube Care: Gastrointestinal; Venous Access Devices Maintenance *NOC:* Immune Status; Infection Status

Nursing Diagnosis:

Risk for Imbalanced Fluid Volume

related to failure of regulatory mechanisms, hyperglycemia, medications, fever, infection, fluid administration, or immobility

Desired Outcome: Patient's hydration status is adequate, as evidenced by baseline VS, serum glucose less than 200 mg/dl, balanced I&O, 1-2 lb weight gain/wk, and serum electrolytes and WBC count within normal limits.

INTERVENTIONS	RATIONALES
Assess rate and volume of nutritional support q4h.	This assessment helps ensure prescribed rate and volume and prevent volume overload or deficiency.
Weigh patient daily initially, and advance to weekly.	Baseline will determine weight goals; subsequent assessments will determine efficacy of those goals.
Monitor I&O q8h or more frequently if medically indicated.	This measure assesses for imbalances and trends toward overhydration or dehydration.
Monitor electrolytes daily, and advance to a minimum of weekly, depending on patient's medical condition.	This assesses for hypovolemia or hypervolemia. Changes in sodium, chloride, and BUN levels may indicate changes in fluid status.
Monitor for signs of circulatory overload during fluid replacement.	Signs of circulatory overload may occur during fluid replacement, including peripheral edema, bounding pulse, jugular distention, and adventitious lung sounds (especially crackles). Circulatory overload is more likely to occur in older adults or individuals with heart failure or other chronic medical conditions such as renal insufficiency in which output is decreased, even if fluids are delivered properly.
If medically indicated, provide 1 ml of free water for each calorie of enteral formula provided (or 30-50 ml/kg of body weight).	This is the amount of water needed for normal metabolism and organ functioning per day.

Continued

INTERVENTIONS	RATIONALES
Monitor for hyperglycemia as follows:	Hyperglycemia may occur because of increased CHO intake or response to the stress of illness or in the presence of type 1 diabetes. Along with hyperglycemia, volume deficits may occur because of the osmotic diuresis that accompanies increased glucose.
- In patient who is not diabetic: q6h for 24-48 hr, then discontinue when patient is within normal limits per hospital laboratory standards.	
- In patient who is glucose intolerant: q4h, with sliding scale short-acting insulin prescribed and administered.	
- In patient who is diabetic: q4h, with sliding scale short-acting insulin prescribed and administered; consult with a health care provider who specializes in care of patients with diabetes.	
- Decrease frequency of fingersticks when blood glucose control is obtained.	Frequent use of a lancet for monitoring may cause patient discomfort.

●●● **Related NIC and NOC labels:** *NIC:* Fluid/Electrolyte Management; Electrolyte Monitoring; Intravenous Therapy; Laboratory Data Interpretation *NOC:* Electrolyte and Acid-Base Balance; Fluid Balance

ADDITIONAL NURSING DIAGNOSES/ PROBLEMS:

"Managing Wound Care" for **Impaired Tissue Integrity**   p. 559

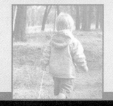

Asthma 75

OVERVIEW/PATHOPHYSIOLOGY

The prevalence of asthma and associated morbidity rates have risen over the past decade in children. Asthma is the leading cause of chronic illness in children and the third leading cause of hospitalization in children younger than age 15. An estimated 6.2 million children younger than 18 years old (1.2 million younger than 5 years old) have asthma, with 4 million having had an asthma attack in 2003. Before puberty, there is increased incidence in boys. It occurs more often in African Americans and Puerto Ricans. Asthma is the leading cause of school absences and accounts for an estimated loss of 12.8 million school days and is responsible for more hospitalizations, restricted activity, and significant health care costs than any other pediatric chronic illness. The incidence of death due to asthma has decreased over the past 5 years, yet in 2002 more than 4000 Americans died of asthma (American Lung Association, 2006). The classification of asthma is based on severity and frequency of symptoms. Daily or maintenance treatment is based on the following:

- Step 1: Mild intermittent asthma
- Step 2: Mild persistent asthma
- Step 3: Moderate persistent asthma
- Step 4: Severe persistent asthma

Asthma is a chronic, reversible (in most cases) obstructive airway disease characterized by inflammation and mucosal edema, increased sensitivity of the airways, and airway obstruction (bronchospasm and in some children, excessive, thick mucus). Increased inflammation causes increased sensitivity of the airways and is the most common feature of asthma.

HEALTH CARE SETTING

Primary care, with possible hospitalization resulting from severe acute attacks

ASSESSMENT

It is important to obtain a history of current problems as well as past episodes.

Common early warning signs: Breathing changes, sneezing, moodiness, headache, itchy/watery eyes, dark circles under eyes, easy fatigue, sore throat, trouble sleeping, chest or throat itchiness, downward trend in peak flow values, cough especially at night (hallmark symptom of asthma), slight tightness in chest.

Symptoms of acute episode: Coughing, shortness of breath, dyspnea, anxiety, apprehension, tightness in chest, and wheezing (primarily on expiration).

Severe asthma symptoms: Severe coughing, shortness of breath, tightness in chest and/or wheezing, and difficulty talking, eating, or concentrating. The mucosal edema causes shortness of breath, tachypnea or bradypnea, hunched shoulders (posturing), suprasternal and intercostal retractions, cyanosis, increasing dyspnea, nasal flaring and use of accessory muscles, extreme anxiety, and apprehension.

Symptoms of severe respiratory distress and impending respiratory failure: Profuse diaphoresis, sitting upright and refusing to lie down, suddenly becoming agitated or becoming quiet when previously agitated, decrease in or absence of wheezing.

Physical assessment: Chest has hyperresonance on percussion. Breath sounds are loud and coarse, with sonorous crackles throughout the lung fields. Prolonged expiration is noted. Coarse rhonchi may be heard, as well as generalized inspiratory and expiratory wheezing that becomes more high pitched as obstruction increases. With minimal obstruction, wheezing may be minimal or heard only on end expiration with auscultation. Breath sounds and crackles may become inaudible with severe obstruction or bronchospasm. Posturing occurs to facilitate breathing. Pulsus paradoxus (an abnormally large decrease in systolic blood pressure and pulse wave amplitude during inspiration) also may be noted because of lung hyperinflation.

Children with chronic asthma may develop a barrel chest with depressed diaphragm, elevated shoulders, and increased use of accessory muscles of respiration.

Caution: If symptoms are untreated or treated unsuccessfully, an acute asthma attack may progress to *status asthmaticus*, a severe unrelenting attack. Status asthmaticus is an acute, severe, and prolonged asthma attack in which respiratory distress continues despite vigorous therapeutic measures and may result in death.

DIAGNOSTIC TESTS

ABG values: Reveal status of oxygenation and acid-base balance. In severe asthma exacerbation with Pao_2 less than 60 mm Hg (on room air) and $Paco_2$ 42 mm Hg or greater, child may have cyanosis and may progress to respiratory failure. Arterial blood gas (ABG) values are not obtained often in children except in intensive care unit and with initial assessment in order to provide atraumatic care. If possible, topical anesthetics are used to decrease pain and anxiety with blood draws.

Pulse oximetry: Noninvasive method that reveals decreased O_2 saturation (less than 93%-95%, depending on protocol of facility) and helps provide atraumatic care.

Chest x-ray examination: To rule out pneumonia and assess for air trapping. It is also used to evaluate possible cardiomegaly secondary to pulmonary hypertension resulting from chronic obstruction. Typical findings in a child with significant asthma symptoms are hyperinflation, atelectasis, and flattened diaphragm.

Complete blood count: May show slight elevation during acute asthma, but white blood cell elevations greater than $12,000/mm^3$ or an increased percentage of band cells may indicate a respiratory infection. Eosinophils greater than $500/mm^3$ tend to suggest an allergic or inflammatory disorder.

Sputum: Gross examination may reveal increased viscosity or actual mucus plugs. Culture and sensitivity may reveal microorganisms if infection was the precipitating event. Cytologic examination will reveal elevated eosinophils, which is commonly associated with asthma.

Serum theophylline level: Important baseline indicator for patients who are receiving this therapy, although it is now considered a third-line agent and used infrequently. Current guidelines call for a serum concentration of 5-15 mcg/ml.

Theophylline toxicity can occur with serum levels greater than 20 mcg/ml. Side effects include nausea, vomiting, headache, irritability, and insomnia. Early signs of toxicity are nausea, tachycardia, irritability, and seizures. Dysrhythmias occur at serum levels greater than 30 mcg/ml.

Peak expiratory flow rate: Assesses severity of asthma by measuring maximum flow of air that can be forcefully exhaled in 1 sec using peak flow meter (PFM). Each child's peak expiratory flow rate (PEFR) varies according to age, height, sex, and race. Once personal best value is established, it is recommended that it be done 1-2 times/day in children with moderate-to-severe persistent asthma. The child should measure the PEFR three times with at least 30 sec between each measurement; then record the highest reading. Maintaining a diary or log book is beneficial and helps direct plan of care.

Pulmonary function tests: Provide an objective method of evaluating presence and degree of lung disease, as well as response to treatment, and usually can be performed reliably on children by 5 or 6 years of age. They typically show diminished maximal breathing capacity, tidal volume, and timed vital capacity.

Skin testing: The 1997 revised guidelines and 2002 update issued by the National Asthma Education and Prevention Program Expert Panel through the National Heart, Lung and Blood Institute of the National Institutes of Health recommend that all patients with persistent asthma be tested to determine sensitization to perennial allergens.

Nursing Diagnosis:

Ineffective Airway Clearance

related to bronchospasm, mucosal edema, and increased mucus production

Desired Outcomes: *Child with a significant asthma attack:* Within 48 hr of interventions/treatment, adventitious breath sounds, cough, and increased work of breathing (WOB) are decreased. Within 72 hr, RR returns to child's normal range, and retractions and nasal flaring disappear. *Child with a mild asthma attack:* Within 3 hr after interventions/treatment, adventitious breath sounds and cough are decreased, and retractions and nasal flaring are absent.

Note: WOB means ease or effort of breathing. Signs of increased WOB include nasal flaring, retractions, and use of accessory muscles.

INTERVENTIONS	RATIONALES
Assess respiratory status with initial assessment, with each vital sign check, and prn.	After establishing the baseline, changes can be detected quickly with subsequent assessments, enabling rapid intervention.
Administer nebulizer treatment/metered dose inhaler (MDI; usually albuterol) as prescribed.	These therapies decrease bronchospasm/mucosal edema, thereby opening the airway and enabling more effective airway clearance.
Assess respiratory rate (RR), heart rate (HR), O_2 saturation, and breath sounds before and several minutes after each nebulizer treatment/MDI administration.	These assessments determine child's status and effectiveness of medication in decreasing bronchospasm/mucosal edema and enabling more effective airway clearance.

Continued

INTERVENTIONS	RATIONALES
Hold albuterol treatment if HR is: - Greater than 180 bpm (children 2 to 3 yr) - Greater than 160 bpm (children 3 to 6 yr) - Greater than 140 bpm (children 6 to 12 yr) - Greater than 120 bpm (children older than 12 yr) Notify health care provider as directed.	Tachycardia is a major side effect of albuterol. When it is present, the health care provider needs to assess the patient to ensure that side effects of medication do not outweigh the benefit of decreasing bronchospasm.
Position child in high Fowler's position and encourage deep breathing.	This will ensure the child has maximum lung expansion and that medication will be dispersed more effectively, thereby improving airway clearance.
Check PEFR in children 5 yr of age and older before and after each albuterol treatment using PFM.	These assessments monitor effectiveness of medication in decreasing bronchospasm and increasing effective airway clearance. For more information about PEFR, see Diagnostic Tests section.
Use a spacer or AeroChamber with administration of MDI.	These are the most effective methods of getting maximum amount of medication delivered to a child. A mask may be required with a spacer in children less than 5 yr of age or anyone who is unable to seal lips effectively around the mouthpiece.
Encourage deep breathing and effective cough q2h while awake.	This loosens and expectorates secretions (many young children cough up secretions and swallow them) and will lead to more effective airway clearance.
Teach children 7 yr old and older breathing exercises and controlled breathing.	Children younger than 7 are diaphragmatic breathers normally. Proper diaphragmatic breathing decreases WOB and improves chest wall mobility and airway clearance.
Administer other medications (IV or PO) as prescribed (usually corticosteroids).	Corticosteroids decrease inflammation, thereby improving airway clearance. Antibiotics are only given if a bacterial infection is present.
Encourage maintenance fluids, preferably orally, that are appropriate for child's weight.	Fluids thin mucus and improve ability to expectorate it, which improves airway clearance. Some children may need IV fluids because of increased WOB.
Give child/family specific guidelines for hydration (maintenance fluids).	For example, a 2-yr-old child who needs 1200 ml/day and drinks from a 4-oz "sippy" cup, needs to drink 10 "sippy" cupfuls/day. Understanding appropriate care improves adherence to the treatment regimen and decreases symptoms.
Monitor and document intake and output (I&O) q4h. Ensure that a minimum urine output (UO) of 1 ml/kg/hr is met.	Assessing I&O on a regular basis alerts one to inadequate intake or output before the child shows signs of dehydration. Dehydration thickens secretions and decreases airway clearance.
Assess hydration status q4h, including level of consciousness (LOC), anterior fontanel (if child is younger than 2 yr old), abdominal skin turgor, and urine output.	Because of increased insensible water loss (owing to increased RR, metabolic rate, and secretions), child may still become dehydrated *even if* receiving maintenance fluids and having appropriate I&O. Ongoing assessments detect early changes and provide more prompt resolution of the problem. Dehydration thickens secretions and decreases airway clearance. Signs of dehydration include decreasing LOC, sunken fontanel, tented abdominal skin, and decreasing urine output.
Avoid iced fluids and caffeinated fluids.	These fluids may trigger bronchospasm.

••• **Related NIC and NOC labels:** *NIC:* Asthma Management; Respiratory Monitoring; Positioning; Vital Signs Monitoring; Cough Enhancement; Medication Administration: Inhalation; Fluid Monitoring *NOC:* Respiratory Status: Airway Patency; Respiratory Status: Ventilation

Nursing Diagnosis:

Fatigue

related to hypoxia and increased WOB

Desired Outcome: Within 24 hr following treatment/interventions, child exhibits decreased fatigue as evidenced by less irritability and restlessness, improved sleeping pattern, and ability to perform usual activities.

INTERVENTIONS	RATIONALES
Assess HR, RR, and WOB q4h or more frequently for increases from child's normal. Report significant findings.	Recognizing and reporting changes promptly facilitates appropriate actions that resolve the problem and decrease likelihood of fatigue.
Monitor for signs of hypoxia (restlessness, fatigue, irritability, tachycardia, dyspnea, change of LOC).	Recognizing symptoms of hypoxia promptly enables timely treatment and decreases fatigue.
Provide a calm and restful environment.	These measures promote rest and decrease stress, oxygen demand, and fatigue.
Ensure child's physical comfort. Consolidate care; organize nursing care to provide periods of uninterrupted rest and sleep.	
Encourage parents' presence, especially with younger children.	Parents' presence decreases fear and anxiety, thereby decreasing O_2 consumption and fatigue.
Encourage quiet, age-appropriate play activities as child's condition improves.	Emotional and physical comfort increase sense of well-being, promote rest, and decrease oxygen expenditure and fatigue.

••• **Related NIC and NOC labels:** *NIC:* Energy Management; Environmental Management *NOC:* Energy Conservation

Nursing Diagnosis:

Anxiety

related to illness, loss of control, and medical/nursing interventions

Desired Outcome: Following interventions/treatments, child/parents verbalize and demonstrate decreased anxiety.

INTERVENTIONS	RATIONALES
Explain all procedures/interventions performed on child (e.g., blood drawing, starting IV) to child (depending on age) and/or parents.	Knowledge often helps decrease anxiety and promotes family-centered care.
Explain purpose of equipment used on child (HR monitor, O_2 and pulse oximeter, blood pressure [BP] monitor). Use therapeutic play with equipment in children older than 3 yr.	Increased understanding of equipment decreases fear of pain, which in turn will decrease anxiety. For example, put BP cuff on a doll or teddy bear or let child put cuff on you.
Provide a quiet room where child can be closely observed.	Increased stimuli increase anxiety.
Encourage parents to stay with child if possible.	This promotes sense of security, which will decrease child's anxiety.
Avoid making parents feel guilty if they are unable to stay.	Parents are already anxious about child being ill and in a hospital.
Keep parents informed of child's progress, including what is being done and why.	This decreases their anxiety. The child easily perceives parental anxiety.
Talk quietly and calmly to child in age-appropriate language. Reassure child that you are available and will be there to help.	Establishing rapport increases trust and decreases anxiety.
Encourage transitional objects (items from child's home).	Such items increase feeling of security and decrease anxiety.
Facilitate coordination of care.	This avoids disturbing child any more than necessary, which would otherwise increase anxiety level.

••• **Related NIC and NOC labels:** *NIC:* Anxiety Level; Anxiety Reduction; Calming Technique; Presence; Therapeutic Play *NOC:* Anxiety Self-Control

Nursing Diagnosis:

Interrupted Family Processes

related to child having a chronic illness and/or emergent hospitalization

Desired Outcome: Within 1 mo of diagnosis, family provides a normal environment for the child and copes effectively with the symptoms, management, and effects of asthma.

INTERVENTIONS	RATIONALES
Teach parents to have realistic expectations about child's asthma.	Knowing what to expect enables family to cope more effectively. Expectations will vary, depending on child's developmental age and severity of asthma.
Encourage parents and siblings to focus on child as a normal child who needs some lifestyle modifications.	Child needs to be the focus, not the disease. Normalizing the environment as much as possible promotes child as the focus.
Reinforce importance of helping siblings cope with/adapt to having a sibling with a chronic illness.	This supports family-centered care and increases the likelihood of more normal family processes.
Reinforce to parents the importance of setting consistent behavior limits and not enabling secondary gain for asthma attack.	Discipline and guidelines are essential for all children to develop appropriate behavior.
Use every chance to reinforce understanding of asthma and its therapies.	Accurate knowledge enables family to cope more effectively with child's chronic illness.
Reinforce need to use PFM at least 1-2 times/day and implement child's asthma action plan.	Understanding importance of monitoring child's status enables family to cope more effectively and incorporate monitoring into daily routine, thereby promoting normalization and child's optimal health status.
Teach child/parents how to give respiratory treatments (nebulizer, MDI) correctly, using prescribed medication and administering it with proper technique.	This information eliminates confusion about correct administration of medications and method of delivery, thereby improving ability to cope with managing a chronic illness.
Encourage family to contact school (nurse, teachers, coaches) to develop a 504 plan for child.	This promotes family's coping while facilitating child's improvement. A 504 plan makes accommodations in the school environment so that the child can function better and thereby learn more effectively. For example, a child who is allergic to grass will not be assigned to a classroom with windows that open near a field of grass when the grass is being mowed.
Refer family to appropriate support groups and community agencies.	These groups/agencies help child and family function and deal with chronic illness more effectively.

●●● **Related NIC and NOC labels:** *NIC:* Family Involvement Promotion; Coping Enhancement; Family Support; Support Group *NOC:* Family Coping; Family Support During Treatment

Nursing Diagnosis:

Deficient Knowledge:

Purpose, precautions, and potential side effects of prescribed medications

Desired Outcome: Following interventions/instructions, child/parents verbalize accurate information about prescribed medication.

INTERVENTIONS	RATIONALES
Teach Parents and Patients the Following:	
Long-Term Control Medications	These are taken daily to achieve and maintain control of persistent asthma.
Cromolyn sodium/nedocromil sodium	*Antiallergic agent,* which prevents release of mast cells (e.g., histamine) after exposure to an allergen.
- Observe for and report rash, cough, bronchospasm, and nasal congestion. If used orally, be alert for headache or diarrhea. If Spinhaler is used, monitor for bronchospasm and pharyngeal irritation occurring with cromolyn.	These are potential side effects.
- Decrease in asthma symptoms should occur after medication has been taken for 4-6 wk.	Therapeutic response may occur within 2-4 wk, but maximum response occurs in 4-6 wk.
- Protect cromolyn from direct light and heat. Store oral capsules in foil pouch until ready for use.	This drug is light- and heat-sensitive.
- Store nedocromil at room temperature; do not freeze.	This drug is temperature-sensitive.
Inhaled corticosteroids, such as fluticasone (Flovent), beclomethasone (Vanceril), and flunisolide (AeroBid)	*Antiinflammation agents*
- Rinse mouth and gargle with water after oral inhalation.	This prevents thrush (oral candidiasis).
- Administer using a spacer or AeroChamber.	These devices may enhance drug delivery and efficiency of inhaled form and help decrease incidence of thrush.
- Monitor for and report ongoing cough, thrush, voice impairment, or difficulty in speaking.	If no improvement occurs, health care provider may need to adjust medication dosage.
- Do not decrease dose or discontinue without consent of health care provider.	This is a maintenance medication, and child may have exacerbation of symptoms if it is decreased or discontinued inappropriately.
Oral corticosteroids, such as prednisolone and prednisone	*Antiinflammation agents*
- Monitor for and report mood changes, seizures, increased blood sugar, diarrhea, nausea, gastrointestinal (GI) bleeding (seen in emesis, stools), weight gain, and tissue swelling.	These are side effects; dosage may need to be changed.
- Take cautiously with barbiturates, carbamazepine, phenytoin, rifampin, or isoniazid.	These medications may reduce effect of prednisone and increase risk for GI ulcer.
- Observe carefully if taking salicylates, toxoids, nonsteroidal antiinflammatory drugs (NSAIDs), or diuretics that are potassium depleting.	These drugs may increase risk for GI ulcer when taken with corticosteroids.
- Limit use of caffeine and alcohol.	They may increase risk for GI ulcer.
Caution: Inform all health care providers about steroid use.	It may be necessary to avoid vaccinations while taking prednisone. Live virus vaccines may increase risk of viral infection. Vaccines in general may have decreased effect.
- Do not change or discontinue dose without consent of health care provider.	Long-term steroid dosage needs to be decreased carefully in order to allow for gradual return of pituitary-adrenal axis functioning. Failure to do so can result in adrenal insufficiency.
Leukotriene modifiers such as montelukast (Singulair)	*Antiasthmatics; decrease inflammation and bronchoconstriction.*
- Be alert for and report headache, abdominal pain, stomachache, fatigue, dizziness, cough, diarrhea, laryngitis, pharyngitis, nausea, earache, sinus discomfort, and viral infections.	These are side effects.
- Use cautiously with phenobarbital.	Phenobarbital reduces action duration of Singulair.
Long acting beta$_2$-agonists such as salmeterol (Serevent)	*Relax bronchial smooth muscles to relieve bronchospasm*
- Be alert for and report increased HR, tremors, palpitations, dizziness, headache, and nausea.	These are side effects.
- Store canister at room temperature.	Therapeutic effect may decrease when canister is cold or hot.
- Use Serevent Diskus powder up to 6 wk after removing protective foil.	Serevent powder for inhalation is stable for 6 wk after removal from foil packet.

Continued

INTERVENTIONS	RATIONALES
Methylxanthines such as aminophylline and theophylline (rarely used now)	*Bronchodilators*
- Be alert for and report GI upset, GI reflux, diarrhea, vomiting, nausea, abdominal pain, nervousness, insomnia, agitation, dizziness, tremors, and increased pulse rate.	These are the most common side effects.
- Limit caffeine (e.g., caffeinated beverages and chocolate).	Excessive intake may increase risk of cardiovascular and central nervous system side effects.
- Limit intake of charcoal broiled foods.	Excessive intake may increase elimination/decrease effectiveness of medication.
- Check with health care provider or pharmacist before taking any other medications.	Numerous medications increase or decrease theophylline level.
Quick-Relief Medications	These drugs treat acute signs and symptoms and pretreat exercise-induced asthma.
Short-acting inhaled beta₂-agonists such as albuterol (Proventil or Ventolin) and metaproterenol (Alupent)	*Bronchodilators*
- Be alert for and report increased HR, palpitations, tremor, insomnia, nervousness, nausea, and headache.	These are side effects.
- If using an MDI, use with a tube spacer or chamber.	These devices increase drug efficiency.
- Limit caffeinated beverages if taking albuterol or metaproterenol.	Caffeine may increase side effects of albuterol or metaproterenol.
Oral and intravenous corticosteroids (also see under long-term control medication) such as methylprednisolone or prednisolone.	*Antiinflammation agents*
- Be alert for and report dizziness, headache, anxiety, GI discomfort, and cough.	These are side effects.
- Give oral medication with food or milk.	Food/milk decrease GI upset.

••• **Related NIC and NOC labels:** *NIC:* Teaching: Prescribed Medication *NOC:* Knowledge: Medication

ADDITIONAL NURSING DIAGNOSES/PROBLEMS:

"Bronchiolitis" for **Deficient Fluid Volume** p. 595

"Cystic Fibrosis" for **Impaired Gas Exchange**. However, p. 623
with asthma, be aware that oxygen saturation needs to be greater than 93%-95%, depending on agency protocol.

 PATIENT-FAMILY TEACHING AND DISCHARGE PLANNING

When providing patient/family teaching, focus on sensory information, avoid giving excessive information, and initiate a visiting nurse referral for necessary follow-up teaching and assessment. Stress importance of family-centered care (looking at the family as a unit that is the "constant" in the child's life and maintaining or improving the health of the family and its members in a holistic manner). Include verbal and written information about the following, ensuring that it is written at a level understandable to child/family:

✓ What is asthma? Discuss definition, signs and symptoms, and pathophysiology.

✓ Identification of specific triggers for child that can precipitate an attack and removal of as many as possible from environment. Asthma triggers vary for each child. Most common triggers of asthma are upper respiratory infection (URI), cigarette smoke, exercise, and weather changes. Other triggers unique to the environment are important (e.g., humid weather, frequent rainy days, local industry). Additional common triggers include pollens, dust mites, mold, cockroaches, rodents, and pet dander.

✓ Importance of personal asthma action plan with green, yellow, and red zone values specific for child. This plan is set up by health care provider based on child's best score (PEFR). Zones are established similar to a stoplight. The green zone is a score 80%-100% of child's best score and with no symptoms present. The yellow zone is a score 50%-80% of the child's best score and signals caution: the child may need extra asthma medicine. Follow guidelines in the child's personal asthma action plan. The red zone is a score that is below 50% of the child's best score and signals an emergency situation. Follow asthma action plan and call health care provider. A sample asthma action plan is available at *http://asthma.nationaljewish.org*.

✓ Correct PFM technique. Most children by 5 yr old can use PFM. Document return demonstration before discharge.

Child should check this rate at least daily and more often if rate is decreased. Child should keep a log to document PEFR.

✓ Maintaining asthma symptom diary, especially for a child with frequent symptoms.

✓ Medications, including drug name, route, purpose, type (controller: long-term management or short-acting immediate relief), dosage, precautions, and potential side effects. Also discuss drug-drug, food-drug, and herb-drug interactions.

✓ Proper technique for using MDIs with spacer (chamber) or spacer with a mask (usually for child younger than 5 yr old). Document adequate return demonstration. Remind family that over-the-counter (OTC) inhalers contain medications that can interfere with prescribed therapy. Instruct child/parent to contact health care provider before trying any OTC medications. Instruct child/parent in sequencing of inhalers; bronchodilator inhalers are used 15 min before administration of steroid inhaler.

✓ Cleaning and care of equipment—nebulizer, MDI, or other medication delivery systems, including assessment of when canister is low or empty.

✓ If child is taking oral corticosteroids while at home, instructions to ensure that he or she receives correct amount each day, especially if medication is going to be tapered.

✓ Importance of taking medication at home and at school as directed. Medication in the original bottle/canister (with prescribing label) and written prescription from health care provider are needed for child to be able to take any medication at school.

✓ Importance of knowing early warning signs before acute attack (e.g., fatigue, sneezing, sore throat, itchy/watery eyes, headache, slight tightness in chest, drop in PFM values). These differ for each child.

✓ Signs and symptoms of increased respiratory distress in children relating to age (e.g., an infant may have increased RR when sleeping, decreased interest in eating/drinking, nasal flaring, grunting, retractions). Other signs and symptoms include difficulty speaking in sentences, inability to walk short distances, hunched posture, and PFM values in red zone.

✓ Importance of avoiding contact with infectious individuals, especially those with respiratory infection.

✓ Recommendation that the child receive annual influenza and possibly pneumococcal (depends on health care provider) vaccinations.

✓ Importance of follow-up care on a regular basis (not just emergency room). Confirm date and time of next appointment.

✓ Phone numbers to call should questions or concerns arise about therapy or disease.

✓ When to call health care provider:
- To refill medications
- PEFR in yellow zone 24 hr or child has event such as coughing, wheezing, chest tightness, or shortness of breath
- PEFR in red zone or child is in increased respiratory distress
- Immediate reliever (albuterol) needed more often than q4h
- Reliever medication not helping

✓ When to call emergency medical services:
- Child is in severe respiratory distress.
- Child is gray/blue.
- Child is unable to answer questions or seems confused.

✓ Importance of communication with child's school or day care regarding child's condition, need for medication, and activity level.

✓ Legal rights of the child—Section 504 of Rehabilitation Act of 1973: Each student with a disability is entitled to accommodation needed to attend school and participate as fully as possible in school activities. This accommodation may be related to a medical condition or an education issue.

✓ Guidelines for attendance, activity level, and exercise at school/day care.

✓ Referral to community resources, such as the local and national American Lung Associations and camps for educational programs for children with asthma. Additional general information can be obtained by contacting:
- American Lung Association at *www.lungusa.org*
- Allergy & Asthma Network Mothers of Asthmatics (AANMA) at *www.aanma.org*
- Asthma and Allergy Foundation of America (AAFA) at *www.aafa.org* (Student Asthma Action Card and Child Care Asthma/Allergy Action Card are available as free downloads; look under "Education—Materials and Tools.")
- STARBRIGHT Foundation at *www.starbright.org*
- Quest for the Code Asthma CD-ROM: education and adventure for children 7-15 yr old, available free at National Library of Medicine's Virtual Asthma Exhibit at *www.nlm.nih.gov/news/breathoflifedvd.html*

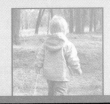

Attention Deficit 76
Hyperactivity Disorder

OVERVIEW/PATHOPHYSIOLOGY

Attention deficit hyperactivity disorder (ADHD) is a neuro-developmental disorder involving developmentally inappropriate behavior. ADHD is the second most common chronic illness in children (asthma is first) and the most commonly diagnosed mental health condition among children in the United States. The statistics per the number of school-age children affected varies from 5% (NICHY, 2004) to nearly 13% (Betz, 2006). Although the exact etiology is unknown, it probably involves a combination of biologic, genetic, and psychologic factors. It is seen more often in children who have a family member with ADHD, particularly the father, brother, or uncle. Chromosomal or genetic abnormalities such as fragile X syndrome have been seen in some children with ADHD. ADHD commonly occurs in association with oppositional disorder, conduct disorder, depression, anxiety disorder, and many developmental disorders, such as speech and language delays and learning disabilities. ADHD is more common in males than females and many children affected continue to demonstrate symptoms into adolescence and adulthood. There is some belief that ADHD is not "outgrown" but that people learn to compensate.

HEALTH CARE SETTING

Primary care

ASSESSMENT

Includes standard history and physical examination, neurologic examination, family assessment, and school assessment.

Signs and symptoms: The behaviors exhibited are not unusual aspects of any child's behavior. The difference lies in the quality of motor activity and developmentally inappropriate inattention, impulsivity, and hyperactivity displayed. The symptoms vary with developmental age and may range from a few to numerous different symptoms. The core symptoms include inattention, hyperactivity, and impulsivity. Children may experience significant functional problems such as school difficulties, academic underachievement,

troublesome interpersonal relationships with family members and peers, and low self-esteem.

Physical assessment: Physical examination includes vision and hearing screening and a detailed neurologic examination that will help rule out any severe neurologic disorders.

Guidelines for the Diagnosis of ADHD *(published by the American Academy of Pediatrics in May 2000)*:
1. Use of specific criteria for the diagnosis using the *Diagnostic and Statistical Manual of Mental Health Disorders*, 4th edition (DSM-IV) criteria.
2. Importance of obtaining information concerning the child's symptoms/behavior in more than one setting (especially from school).
3. Evaluation for coexisting conditions that may make the diagnosis more difficult or complicate treatment planning.

Multidisciplinary evaluation: Includes the primary pediatrician (and possibly a developmental pediatrician, pediatric neurologist, or pediatric psychiatrist), psychologist, pediatric/school nurse, classroom teacher, specialty teachers as appropriate, and the child's parents in order to obtain all perspectives of the child's behavior.

Detailed history: Both medical and developmental history and descriptions of the child's behavior should be obtained from as many observers as possible. Traumatic experiences and psychiatric and other disorders are ruled out, including lead poisoning, seizures, partial hearing loss, psychosis, and witnessing sexual activity and/or violence.

Psychologic testing: Valuable in determining a variety of deficits and helpful in identifying the child's intelligence and achievement level.

Behavioral checklists and adaptive scales: Helpful in measuring social adaptive functioning in children with ADHD.

DIAGNOSTIC TESTS

ADHD is a diagnosis of exclusion. There is no definitive test for ADHD.

Nursing Diagnosis:

Disturbed Thought Processes

related to inability to concentrate, control impulses, and organize thoughts in a manner appropriate for age and development

Desired Outcomes: Within 1 mo of this diagnosis, child completes activities of daily living (ADL) and shows behavioral improvement in the school setting. Within one semester, child shows improvement in academic activities.

INTERVENTIONS	RATIONALES
Encourage parents/teachers to provide a structured environment and consistency.	Structure and consistency offer opportunity for children to focus on areas that need improvement.
Promote ongoing communication between parents and teachers.	Consistency among family and teachers in reinforcing same guidelines improves the child's ability to concentrate.
Encourage parents/teachers to decrease stimuli when concentration is important.	Children with ADHD are easily distracted by extraneous stimuli. Removing those stimuli should improve concentration. For example, parents/teachers should have child do homework in a quiet area without TV or radio on or sit in a quiet section of the classroom, not near an open door.
Advise parents to work with school in determining if child is eligible for care under Individuals with Disabilities Education Act (IDEA) and therefore an Individualized Education Plan (IEP) or for Section 504 eligibility.	Many parents are unaware of the rights of disabled children. Environmental accommodation and appropriate classroom placement help children with ADHD reach their maximum potential by concentrating better, controlling impulses, and improving organizational ability. For example, for a child with ADHD, the desk may be placed in the front and on the quieter side of the classroom, and the child may be given extra time to complete tests.

••• **Related NIC and NOC labels:** *NIC:* Environmental Management *NOC:* Concentration

Nursing Diagnosis:

Chronic Low Self-Esteem

related to negative responses from others regarding behavior

Desired Outcome: Within 1 mo of this diagnosis, the child achieves at least one goal, lists strengths, and elicits fewer negative responses from others.

INTERVENTIONS	RATIONALES
Monitor the child's interactions with others.	This assessment helps determine existence/degree of negative responses from other people.
Reward positive behavior and provide limit setting as needed. Avoid negative comments and giving attention for negative behavior.	Positive reinforcement is an effective way to improve behavior and self-esteem.
Help the child set goals that are age appropriate, realistic, and achievable. Set timetable to achieve step-by-step progress until he or she accomplishes overall goal.	Achieving goals increases self-esteem. If the child has difficulty completing assignments, divide the assignment into manageable tasks. For example, for an essay assignment: day 1, make outline; day 2, begin literature search; day 3, begin writing paper; day 4, finish paper and have someone review it; day 5, finalize paper.
Encourage the child to make a list of his or her strengths. Teach self-questioning techniques (e.g., What am I doing? How is that going to affect others?). Encourage positive self-talk (e.g., I did a good job with that!). Provide feedback accordingly.	These activities encourage positive self-thought and build self-esteem.

••• **Related NIC and NOC labels:** *NIC:* Self-Esteem Enhancement; Counseling; Self-Awareness Enhancement; Emotional Support
NOC: Self-Esteem

Nursing Diagnosis:

Risk for Injury

related to increased activity level, limited judgment skills, and impulsivity

Desired Outcome: Child remains free from signs of injury.

INTERVENTIONS	RATIONALES
Reinforce to parents the importance of the child using appropriate safety equipment/protective device (e.g., seat belt, bicycle helmet).	Using this equipment/device decreases likelihood of injury.
Encourage parents to model the use of appropriate safety equipment/ protective devices.	Children are more likely to wear a seat belt or bicycle helmet if parents wear them also.
Encourage parents to set clear limits on where the child may ride a bike or play and to offer choices from several safe areas child can go.	Clear, simple guidelines are easier for a child with ADHD to focus on and follow. Allowing the child some choice improves compliance, which decreases likelihood of injury.
Encourage child's participation in active play rather than in passive activities (e.g., playing softball rather than playing video games).	Active play helps children grow physically and cognitively. It also helps the child with ADHD to redirect energy in a safe and effective manner, thus decreasing risk of injury.
Reinforce importance of parents monitoring child's activities frequently.	Adequate supervision decreases likelihood of injury.
Teach parents to reinforce positive behavior with feedback and intermittent rewards.	This encourages appropriate behavior and activity, thereby decreasing risk of injury.

••• **Related NIC and NOC labels:** *NIC:* Environmental Management; Safety; Surveillance: Safety; Area Restriction; Parent Education: Childrearing Family *NOC:* Safe Home Environment

Nursing Diagnosis:

Deficient Knowledge:

Chronicity of ADHD and its treatment

Desired Outcome: Within 1 mo of this diagnosis, child/parents verbalize accurate understanding of the chronic condition of ADHD and possible treatments.

INTERVENTIONS	RATIONALES
Determine parents' and child's understanding of ADHD. As indicated, teach them about the disorder, including the fact that it is chronic.	This assessment enables development of an individualized teaching plan. Accurate knowledge about the condition facilitates understanding of the need for treatment and ways to manage it realistically.
Discuss different treatment strategies.	This information promotes understanding that no single treatment strategy is *the* answer and that there are multiple strategies that may help the child, such as medication, behavioral/psychosocial interventions (parent training and education, behavior modification, teacher training/proper classroom placement and management, counseling, psychotherapy), combined or multimodal treatment, and biofeedback.

••• **Related NIC and NOC labels:** *NIC:* Teaching: Disease Process; Teaching: Procedure/Treatment; Parent Education: Childrearing Family *NOC:* Knowledge: Disease Process; Knowledge: Treatment Regimen

Nursing Diagnosis:

Deficient Knowledge:

Purpose, precautions, and potential side effects of prescribed medications

Desired Outcome: Within 1 wk of starting medication, child/parents verbalize accurate
information about prescribed medications.

INTERVENTIONS	RATIONALES
Teach the Following to Parents/Patients:	
Stimulant Medications	
Short, intermediate, and long-acting methylphenidate (e.g., Ritalin); short, intermediate, and long-acting dextroamphetamine (e.g., Dexedrine); mixed dextroamphetamine/amphetamine salts; and dexmethylphenidate.	Stimulants are given to promote attentiveness and decrease restlessness by increasing dopamine and norepinephrine levels, which leads to stimulation of the inhibitory system of the central nervous system (CNS).
First-line treatment:	
- Be alert for and report decreased appetite, weight loss, stomachache or headache, delayed sleep onset, jitteriness, increased crying or irritability, and social withdrawal.	These common side effects may require either dosage adjustment or change in schedule.
- Report tics (involuntary movements of a small group of muscles such as of the face).	Tics occur in 15%-30% of children and are usually transient.
- Report child becoming overfocused while on medication or appearing dull or overly restricted.	These changes are seen in children receiving too high a dose or who are overly sensitive. Decreasing dose usually resolves these problems.
- Take the medication on an empty stomach 30-45 min before meals, if possible.	Absorption of methylphenidate is increased when taken with meals, with the exception of Concerta, a long-acting form. Taking the medication at a consistent time is most important. Dosage can be adjusted to counteract effects of any decreased absorption as long as the medication is taken consistently with or without food.
- Do not crush, chew, or break sustained-release forms.	Action of medication will change and probably not be as effective.
- Take last daily dose 4-6 hr before bedtime.	This reduces potential for insomnia.
- Get all prescriptions filled at the same pharmacy or give a list of all current medications to every pharmacy used.	There are many drug interactions with these medications. An informed pharmacist can identify all potential interactions among medications. For example, methylphenidate may increase serum levels of tricyclic antidepressants, phenytoin, phenobarbital, and warfarin. Monoamine oxidase (MAO) inhibitors or general anesthetics potentiate methylphenidate.
- Limit caffeine and decongestants.	They are stimulants and can potentiate medications the child is receiving.
- Monitor height, weight, and blood pressure (BP).	Suppression of growth may occur with long-term use, and it can increase BP as well.
- Avoid amphetamine-dextroamphetamine combinations in children with structural or symptomatic heart disease.	Food and Drug Administration alert in Feb 2005 stated these combined products should not be used due to preliminary reports of sudden unexplained death. This combination could precipitate a hypertensive crisis.
- Avoid amphetamine-dextroamphetamine combinations in children who have taken an MAOI or agents with MAOI activity within the past 14 days.	
- Caution is necessary when taken by children with seizures.	These medications may lower the seizure threshold.
- Child may need periodic drug holiday (e.g., no medication during the summer) or periodic discontinuation.	This assesses patient's requirement for medication, decreases tolerance, and limits suppression of linear growth and weight.
- Be alert to and report decreased impulsiveness, improved social interaction, and increased academic productivity and accuracy.	This will indicate effectiveness of medication.

Continued

INTERVENTIONS	RATIONALES
Norepinephrine Reuptake Inhibitor	
Atomoxetine (e.g., Straterra)	This medication is given to improve attentiveness, ability to follow through on tasks with less distraction and forgetfulness, and diminish hyperactivity. Exact mechanism of action is unknown but is thought to be related to selective inhibitor of prosynaptic norepinephrine transporter, resulting in norepinephrine reuptake inhibition.
- Report headache, dizziness, insomnia, upper abdominal pain, vomiting, decreased appetite, or cough.	These are the most common side effects and may require either dosage adjustment or change in schedule.
- Report chest pain or palpitations, urinary retention or difficulty voiding, appetite loss and weight loss, or insomnia.	These are significant side effects and will require some change in either dosage or medication.
- Monitor weight on a regular basis and ensure dose prescribed is appropriate for weight before administering.	Dose is based on weight. An accurate weight is needed to get optimal effects of medication and minimal side effects.
- Monitor baseline heart rate (HR) and BP with dose increases and periodically while on therapy.	This medication may cause increased HR, increased BP, and palpitations; if so, dose needs to be adjusted. This is especially important for a child with preexisting hypertension.
- Use cautiously with Albuterol or other beta 2 agonists, vasopressor drugs, or CYP2D6 inhibitors (e.g., paroxetine, fluoxetine, quinidine).	Beta 2 agonists potentiate cardiovascular effects of this medication; CYP2D6 inhibitors may increase blood levels and toxicity.
- Do not use within 2 wk of taking MAOIs.	This may precipitate a hypertensive crisis.
- Observe closely for and report clinically worsening suicide ideation or behavioral changes, including increased aggression and hostility.	Short-term studies show increased risk of suicide ideation in children and adolescents with this medication for the first few months and after dose changes.
- Get all prescriptions filled at the same pharmacy or give a list of all current medications to every pharmacy used.	This drug interacts with many medications. An informed pharmacist can identify all potential interactions among medications.
Antidepressants	
Tricyclics imipramine (e.g., Tofranil) and desipramine (e.g., Norpramin)	These medications block norepinephrine and serotonin at nerve endings and increase action of both substances in nerve cells.
Second-line treatment:	
- Child should have a baseline evaluation of blood pressure (standing and supine), electrocardiogram (ECG), and complete blood count (CBC) with reevaluation whenever dosages change.	Dysrhythmias, ECG changes, and hypotension (especially orthostatic) are possible. Blood dyscrasias also may occur. Baseline evaluation shows status when medication is initiated and enables comparison as therapy continues.
- Be alert for and report palpitations, blurred vision, constipation, dry mouth, dental caries, sedation, urinary retention, dizziness, and drowsiness.	These common side effects may require dose adjustment. Bedtime dosing (i.e., hour of sleep [HS] dosing) during first few weeks of therapy reduces sedation.
- Do not take/give with clonidine.	This may result in hypertensive crisis.
- Get all prescriptions filled at the same pharmacy or give a list of all current medications to every pharmacy used.	These drugs interact with many medications. An informed pharmacist can identify all potential interactions among medications.
- Slowly decrease dosage per health care provider's guidelines; do not stop abruptly.	Abrupt discontinuation may cause nausea, vomiting, diarrhea, headache, trouble sleeping, vivid dreams, and irritability.
Bupropion (e.g., Wellbutrin)	This is an antidepressant, a dopamine-reuptake inhibitor whose mechanism of activity is not well understood.
- Be alert to and report CNS side effects such as seizures, agitation, headache, or tremors; weight change; dry mouth; nausea; or vomiting.	These are major side effects. Dose adjustment may be required.
- Avoid administering to a child with a history of seizures or a current or previous history of anorexia nervosa or bulimia nervosa.	This medication increases the risk of seizures in all of these patients, with the highest risk in patients with a history of seizures.
- Get all prescriptions filled at the same pharmacy or give a list of all current medications to every pharmacy used.	There are many drug interactions with this medication. An informed pharmacist can identify all potential interactions among medications. For example, many seizure medications decrease the clinical effect of bupropion, MAO inhibitors increase its toxicity, and many herbs such as kava kava and St. John's wort interact with it.

Continued

INTERVENTIONS

INTERVENTIONS	RATIONALES
- Administer doses in equally spaced time intervals.	This minimizes risk of seizures.
- Implement frequent mouth rinses and good oral hygiene.	These actions may minimize dry mouth, if this problem occurs.
- Be alert for mood changes.	This indicates effectiveness of medication.

Other Drug

INTERVENTIONS	RATIONALES
Clonidine (not listed with recommended medications by American Academy of Pediatrics but frequently used)	This medication inhibits presynaptic release of norepinephrine to act as a mood stabilizer.
- Be alert for and report dry mouth, dizziness, drowsiness, fatigue, constipation, anorexia, palpitations, and local skin reactions with patch.	These are side effects that may necessitate change in dosage.
- Do not stop medication abruptly.	Patient will go through withdrawal symptoms.
- Watch child closely if clonidine is given with CNS depressants.	Additive sedation would occur if given with CNS depressants, including alcohol, antihistamines, opioid analgesics, and sedative/hypnotics.

●●● **Related NIC and NOC labels:** *NIC:* Teaching: Prescribed Medication *NOC:* Knowledge: Medication

Nursing Diagnosis:

Compromised Family Coping

related to need for constant and close supervision of the child, hyperactivity of the child, or the stigma associated with a child with impulsive or aggressive behavior

Desired Outcome: Within 1 wk of diagnosis, family members (including siblings depending on their developmental age) discuss child's needs and develop a plan to provide the necessary support.

INTERVENTIONS	RATIONALES
Assist family with problem-solving ways of managing child's behavior and needs.	Positive reinforcement, time-out, response cost, or token rewards are examples of effective behavioral techniques for children with ADHD.
Provide handouts for caregivers explaining behavioral management techniques.	Verbal and written guidelines promote understanding. Handouts increase consistency among caregivers and improve ability to meet child's needs.
Enable family (including siblings) to vent concerns and problems.	Discussing concerns increases ability to cope with the situation.
Assist in identifying community resources for support (e.g., many school systems have ADHD support groups, local Children and Adults with ADHD [CHADD] chapter).	Support groups often help families function and cope more effectively.
Encourage family to advocate for their child within the school system (Individualized Education Plan [IEP] or 504 accommodation plan as appropriate).	This involvement/support by the family increases potential for the child to function well/succeed.

●●● **Related NIC and NOC labels:** *NIC:* Active Listening; Coping Enhancement; Family Involvement Promotion; Family Support *NOC:* Caregiver Stressors; Family Coping

ADDITIONAL NURSING DIAGNOSES/ PROBLEMS:

"Psychosocial Support for the Patient's Family and Significant Other," for relevant psychosocial care plans that would help family members cope with ADHD   p. 87

✓ PATIENT-FAMILY TEACHING AND DISCHARGE PLANNING

The child with ADHD may have a wide variety of symptoms and treatment modalities. Providing support and information about the disease is essential because of the stigma associated with ADHD. When providing child/family teaching, focus on sensory information and avoid giving excessive information. Stress family-centered care (viewing the family as a unit that is the "constant" in the child's life and maintaining or improving the health of the family and its members). Include verbal and written information about the following (ensure that written information is at a level the reader can understand):

✓ Clarification of myths and realities concerning ADHD: Child is not "bad," "lazy," or "stupid."

✓ Safety measures relative to developmental age, impulsivity, inattentiveness, and hyperactivity.

✓ Medications, including drug name; purpose; dosage; frequency; precautions; drug-drug, food-drug, and herb-drug interactions; and potential side effects.

✓ Importance of taking medication as directed at home and school. Medication in the original pharmacy bottle and written prescription from health care provider are needed for child to be able to take medication at school.

✓ Importance of consistency, structure, and routine for the child with ADHD.

✓ Importance of collaboration of family, health care provider, and school for optimal outcome.

✓ Importance of supporting siblings and including them in the "plan." Help them cope with/adapt to having a brother/sister with a chronic illness.

✓ Environmental manipulation and appropriate classroom placement, which increase child's ability to function optimally.

✓ Suggestions regarding house rules:
- Give clear, specific directions.
- Use positive rewards; don't punish.
- Implement contingency plan.

✓ Suggestions to help children with ADHD:
- Daily picture with schedule of activities and events
- Index cards with written steps or pictures
- Organized backpack and notebook
- Physical relaxation techniques
- Standing when needing to work at desk
- Two chairs (can move back and forth between them)
- Boundaries in classroom
- Provide *only* needed materials
- Include short, fast-paced tasks
- Soothing music, carpet, earplugs
- One step—student verbalizes step, student performs step, next step
- Positive self-talk and reinforcement practices

✓ Suggestions to facilitate communication between family and school, including daily written communication with teacher per behavior (gives better overall evaluation of effectiveness of medication/behavioral modification).

✓ Legal rights of the child
- Individuals with Disabilities Education Act (IDEA): Requires states to identify, diagnose, educate, and provide related services for children 3-21 yr old.
- Individualized Education Plan (IEP): Multidisciplinary team designs this plan to facilitate special education and therapeutic strategies and goals for each eligible child. Parents need to be involved in this process.
- Section 504 of Rehabilitation Act of 1973: Each student with a disability is entitled to the accommodation needed to attend school and participate as fully as possible in school activities.

✓ Signs that indicate when to contact health care provider:
- Child appears very drowsy.
- Child is unable to concentrate after being on medication several weeks.
- Child physically harms self or others.
- No improvement is seen in school performance over 1-2 mo.

✓ Importance of follow-up care, including primary pediatrician and multidisciplinary team.

✓ Referral to community resources such as support groups, pediatricians who are comfortable dealing with ADHD, child psychologists, and local community services boards, including:
- Children and Adults with Attention-Deficit/Hyperactivity Disorder (CHADD) at *www.chadd.org*
- National Information Center for Children and Youth with Disabilities (NICHCY) at *www.nichcy.org*

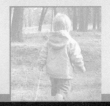

Bronchiolitis 77

OVERVIEW/PATHOPHYSIOLOGY

Bronchiolitis is an acute infection that causes inflammation and obstruction of the bronchioles, the smallest, most distal sections of the lower respiratory tract. It rarely occurs in children older than 2 years of age and has a peak incidence between 2 and 6 mo of age. Bronchiolitis is one of the major causes of hospitalization in children younger than 1 yr of age. Incidence is greatest in the winter and early spring.

Acute bronchiolitis is most often a viral infection and is usually caused by the respiratory syncytial virus (RSV). RSV is highly contagious; about two thirds of infants are infected with RSV by 1 yr of age, and almost 100% are infected by the age of 2 yr. RSV is the leading cause of lower respiratory tract disease in infants and young children, causing approximately 125,000 hospitalizations annually. Most of these infants and young children can be cared for at home, but approximately 1%-2% of those hospitalized with RSV bronchiolitis die of the disease (Lauts, 2005).

HEALTH CARE SETTING

Primary care with possible hospitalization for respiratory distress

ASSESSMENT

Initially upper respiratory infection (URI) symptoms for 2-3 days: fever, rhinorrhea, and cough.

Acute respiratory distress: Expiratory wheezing, tachypnea with respiratory rate (RR) 60-80 breaths/min or more, nasal flaring, paroxysmal nonproductive cough, increased respiratory effort or work of breathing (WOB), cyanosis, retractions, difficulty feeding because of increased RR, irritability, lethargy.

Physical assessment: Auscultation of expiratory wheezing and crackles or rhonchi. Symptoms of dehydration may be present: decreased level of consciousness (LOC), sunken anterior fontanel (if younger than 2 yr old), dry or sticky oral mucosa, decreased abdominal skin turgor, decreased urine output.

Risk factors for severe RSV bronchiolitis:
- Premature infants born at less than 35 wk gestation
- Chronic lung disease or bronchopulmonary dysplasia
- Congenital heart disease; mortality was once 50% but is now 5%
- Low socioeconomic status
- Weight less than 5 kg or birth weight less than 1500 g
- T-cell immunodeficiency

DIAGNOSTIC TESTS

Diagnosis may be made on the basis of history, physical examination, and chest radiography.

Arterial blood gases: May be done initially to determine presence/degree of hypoxemia and acid-base imbalance. Topical anesthetics are used if possible to decrease pain and anxiety (atraumatic care).

Pulse oximetry: Noninvasive method of monitoring oxygen saturation. It facilitates atraumatic care of the infant.

Chest x-ray examination: Usually shows hyperinflation with mild interstitial infiltrates, but segmental atelectasis occurs infrequently.

Complete blood count: May be normal or show mild lymphocytosis.

RSV washing on nasal or nasopharyngeal secretions: To identify cause of respiratory distress; detects RSV antigen.

Nursing Diagnosis:

Ineffective Airway Clearance

related to increased mucosal edema and secretions secondary to respiratory infection

Desired Outcomes: Within 24 hr of treatment/intervention, child exhibits decreased RR and decreased WOB. By discharge, child is able to manage respiratory secretions as evidenced by more normal RR and minimal WOB.

INTERVENTIONS	RATIONALES
Assess respiratory status q2h: LOC, RR, breath sounds, signs of increased WOB (nasal flaring, retractions, use of accessory muscles), cough, and skin and mucous membrane color.	Early identification of changes that might indicate increasing respiratory distress (decreased LOC, increased RR, adventitious or decreasing breath sounds, increased WOB, and pallor or bluish tint) ensures prompt intervention, which results in decreased severity of respiratory symptoms.
Administer racemic epinephrine or albuterol with handheld nebulizer (HHN), if prescribed.	These agents decrease mucosal edema, which will open the airway and decrease WOB. Racemic epinephrine is a specific type of epinephrine that is administered via nebulizer, generally for croup or bronchiolitis. Examples include Vaponefrin, microNefrin, and AsthmaNefrin.
Assess HR, RR, O_2 saturation, and breath sounds before and after nebulizer treatment.	These assessments monitor effectiveness of treatment and for its side effects (see next rationale).
Hold nebulizer treatment if HR is greater than 230 bpm for a child 1 yr of age or younger or greater than 180 bpm for a child older than 1 yr of age. Notify health care provider accordingly.	Tachycardia is one of the main side effects of both medications. Side effects should not outweigh the benefit of improving airway clearance.
Instill saline nose drops, wait 1-2 min, and suction nares before feedings and prn.	Instilling saline drops before suctioning is helpful if the secretions are not loose or the child sounds congested. Suctioning before feedings to clear nares will improve intake inasmuch as infants are obligate nose breathers. Suctioning too often causes nasal edema if using a bulb syringe.

••• **Related NIC and NOC labels:** *NIC:* Airway Suctioning; Vital Signs Monitoring; Respiratory Monitoring *NOC:* Respiratory Status: Airway Patency; Respiratory Status: Gas Exchange

Nursing Diagnosis:

Impaired Gas Exchange

related to edema of the bronchiole mucosa and presence of increased mucus

Desired Outcomes: Immediately following treatment/intervention, child attains O_2 saturation greater than 92%. By discharge, child maintains O_2 saturation greater than 92% on room air (unless child was O_2 dependent before the illness).

INTERVENTIONS	RATIONALES
Observe for signs and symptoms of hypoxia (restlessness, change in LOC, dyspnea). Remember that cyanosis is a late sign of hypoxia in children.	Ongoing observation results in early detection of problems and early intervention, thereby decreasing severity of the hypoxia if it occurs.
Assess respiratory status q2h: LOC, RR, breath sounds, signs of increased WOB (nasal flaring, retractions, use of accessory muscles), cough, and skin and mucous membrane color.	This ensures early identification of changes that might indicate increasing respiratory distress. See details in previous nursing diagnosis.
Monitor vital signs q2-4h and prn.	Hypoxia causes an increase in HR, RR, and blood pressure (BP). A drop in BP and decreasing RR may be signs of impending respiratory arrest.
Maintain continuous oximetry while child is on O_2 and document at least q2h.	Oximetry provides continuous monitoring of O_2 saturation and alerts nurse to changes.
Provide humidified O_2 via nasal cannula to maintain O_2 saturation greater than 92%.	Delivering oxygen increases oxygen to the tissues. Oxygen is drying to the nasal mucosa, and humidity liquefies mucus.
Report to health care provider if O_2 saturation is 92% or less.	O_2 saturation 92% or less may indicate deteriorating condition.
Position child for maximum ventilation (e.g., head elevated but without compression on diaphragm).	Children are diaphragmatic breathers until 7 yr of age. Preventing compression of the diaphragm enables optimal breathing effort.
Use cardiorespiratory monitor for infant or young child at high risk for or with history of apnea.	This monitor ensures quick detection of deterioration in status or apneic episode.

Continued

INTERVENTIONS

INTERVENTIONS	RATIONALES
Consolidate care to provide maximum rest.	Oxygen needs decrease with decreased energy expenditure.
Provide a neutral thermal environment.	An environment in which the child does not need to use any energy to cool or warm self reduces O_2 demand.

●●● **Related NIC and NOC labels:** *NIC:* Oxygen Therapy; Energy Management; Positioning; Respiratory Monitoring; Vital Signs Monitoring
NOC: Respiratory Status: Gas Exchange; Vital Signs Status

Nursing Diagnosis:

Deficient Fluid Volume

related to increased insensible loss (secondary to increased RR, fever, increased metabolic rate) and decreased intake

Desired Outcome: Within 4 hr following treatment, child has adequate fluid volume as evidenced by alertness and responsiveness, soft anterior fontanel (in child younger than 2 yr of age), moist oral mucous membrane, good skin turgor, and normal urine output (UO; e.g., infant UO more than 2-3 ml/kg/hr, toddler and preschooler UO 2 ml/kg/hr, school-age UO 1-2 ml/kg/hr, and adolescent UO 0.5-1 ml/kg/hr).

INTERVENTIONS

INTERVENTIONS	RATIONALES
Ensure that child is receiving daily maintenance fluids based on his or her weight.	Daily maintenance fluid requirements need to be met in order for child to have adequate hydration. The smaller the child, the greater the percentage of body weight is water. To meet minimal fluid requirements, calculate volume needed based on child's weight: **Up to 10 kg: 100 ml/kg/24 hr = _____** **10-20 kg: 50 ml/kg/24 hr = _____** **More than 20 kg: 20 ml/kg/24 hr = _____** **= maintenance fluid requirement** *For example, child weighs 23 kg:* 10 kg × 100 ml/kg/24 hr = 1000 ml/24 hr 10 kg × 50 ml/kg/24 hr = 500 ml/24 hr 3 kg × 20 ml/kg/24 hr = 60 ml/24 hr 23 kg ————————— 1560 ml/24 hr Maintenance fluid requirement for child weighing 23 kg is 1560 ml/24 hr.
Assess hydration status: LOC, anterior fontanel (in child younger than 2 yr old), oral mucous membranes, abdominal skin turgor, UO q4h.	Child may be receiving maintenance fluids but still be dehydrated because of increased insensible losses. Frequent assessment leads to early recognition of problems and quicker treatment. Deficient fluid volume may be evidenced by decreased LOC, sunken anterior fontanel, dry or sticky oral mucous membrane, tented abdominal skin, and decreased UO.
Monitor intake and output q2h. Weigh all diapers. Ensure minimum UO of 1 ml/kg/hr is met.	These assessments enable earlier intervention if a deficit is noted.
Monitor daily weights, using same scale at same time of day and without any clothing (including diaper).	Short-term weight changes are the most reliable measurement of fluid loss or gain.
Monitor temperature q4h and treat per health care provider's directive.	Increased body temperature increases insensible fluid loss.
Offer a variety of liquids frequently that child likes (e.g., frozen juices, Popsicles, Pedialyte, Rice-Lyte, breast milk, formula).	This replaces measurable and insensible fluid losses and helps liquefy secretions. Child is more likely to cooperate if offered preferred fluids.

Continued

INTERVENTIONS

INTERVENTIONS	RATIONALES
Do not offer PO fluids if child's RR is more than 80 breaths/min while awake.	There is increased chance of aspiration when child is tachypneic.
Administer IV fluids as prescribed.	Child may not be able to take adequate oral fluid because of respiratory distress. Administering IV fluids ensures that the child receives maintenance fluids.

••• **Related NIC and NOC labels:** *NIC:* Fluid Management: Hypovolemia Management; Intravenous Therapy; Fluid Monitoring; Fever Treatment *NOC:* Hydration; Fluid Balance

---

ADDITIONAL NURSING DIAGNOSES/ PROBLEMS:

"Asthma" for **Fatigue** related to hypoxia and increased   p. 579
    WOB

Anxiety related to illness, loss of control, and medical/   p. 580
    nursing interventions

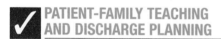

PATIENT-FAMILY TEACHING AND DISCHARGE PLANNING

When providing child/family teaching, focus on sensory information, avoid giving excessive information, and initiate a visiting nurse referral for necessary follow-up teaching and assessment as needed. Stress importance of family-centered care (viewing the family as a unit that is the "constant" in the child's life and maintaining or improving the health of the family and its members in a holistic manner). Include verbal and written information about the following (ensure that written information is at a level the reader can understand):

✓ RSV bronchiolitis: definition, signs and symptoms, basic pathophysiology, and length/progression of illness.

✓ If child is on medications, drug name, route, purpose, type, dosage, precautions, and potential side effects. Also discuss drug-drug, food-drug, and herb-drug interactions.

✓ Despite having RSV bronchiolitis, the child can develop another RSV infection.

✓ Risk factors for developing RSV bronchiolitis:
- Exposure to tobacco smoke
- Day care attendance
- School-age siblings
- Crowded living conditions (two or more children in the same bedroom)
- Multiple births and/or premature infant born at 35 wk gestation
- Born within 6 mo of RSV season (November-April)
- Formula-fed rather than breastfed

✓ Guidelines for preventing RSV infection:
- Good handwashing
- Keeping anyone with a fever or cold away from the child
- Avoiding secondhand smoke
- Avoiding crowds/day care

✓ Importance of checking hydration status at least several times a day when child is ill (i.e., the less the child weighs and the younger, the greater the percentage of body weight is water. Therefore, dehydration occurs much more quickly than it would in an older child or adult).
- Is the child alert and interactive? Child would not be as alert and interactive as normal if dehydrated.
- Check soft spot on top of the head (in children younger than 2 yr old). If it is sunken, the child may be dehydrated.
- Check inside the mouth, not the lips. If dry or sticky and the child is not a mouth breather, the child is dehydrated.
- Pinch skin on the abdomen. If it sits up like a tent instead of falling down right away, the child is dehydrated.
- How many wet diapers does the child normally have a day? If the number of diapers is decreased or they are not as wet as usual, the child may be dehydrated.

✓ How much should the child drink per day? Give parents information they can understand, such as an infant that weighs 9 kg needs 900 ml/day for maintenance fluids, which is 30 ounces. If the infant drinks from 4-oz bottles, he or she needs to take eight 4-oz bottles of fluid/day to get maintenance fluids.

✓ Use of normal saline nose drops and bulb syringe to clear nares before feedings. An infant breathes primarily through the nose until 5-6 mo old, so if the nose is congested, he or she cannot breathe and therefore cannot drink or eat.

✓ Continued prophylaxis against RSV with Synagis or RespiGam if already receiving prophylaxis or per prescription (e.g., monthly IM or IV medication that gives passive immunity against RSV during RSV season, usually November through April).

✓ Child may still have some signs and symptoms of RSV but may return to babysitter/day care if he or she doesn't have a fever and looks well after the follow-up visit to the health care provider.

✓ Importance of follow-up care; typically follow-up appointment is made within 24-48 hr after discharge.

✓ Phone number to call in case questions or concerns arise about treatment or disease after discharge.

✓ When to call health care provider:
- Fever increases.
- Rate of breathing increases (more than 60 breaths/ min).

- Nostrils flare out with each breath when child is resting (crying will cause this to happen when child is not having breathing problems).
- Chest sinks in with each breath.
- Child looks like he or she is working harder to breathe.
- Lips turn gray or blue (cold can make lips look very pale and almost blue).
- Child exhibits signs of dehydration.

✓ Importance of infant/child receiving all routine childhood immunizations and rationale for giving immunizations.

✓ Importance of cardiopulmonary resuscitation (CPR) and safety training.

✓ Refer to community resources such as local and national American Lung Associations. Additional information can be obtained by contacting:

- The American Lung Association at *www.lungusa.org* (Go to Diseases A to Z and look under R fact sheet on RSV)
- March of Dimes at *www.Marchofdimes.com* under Pregnancy and Newborn Health Education Center
- *www.rsvprotection.com* (information per disease, treatment, and prevention)

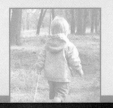

Burns 78

OVERVIEW/PATHOPHYSIOLOGY

Burn injuries represent one of the most painful and devastating traumas a person can experience. Fire and burn-related injuries are a leading cause of death from injury in children ages 1-14. Most burns in children are relatively minor and do not require hospitalization, but in 2003 an estimated 83,300 children 14 yr old and younger were treated in hospital emergency departments for burn-related injuries, 63% of which were thermal burns (hair curlers and curling irons, radiators, ovens and ranges, irons, gasoline, and fireworks being the most common causes) (SAFE KIDS, 2006).

The causative agent for burns varies depending on the child's developmental age. For instance, in children 4 yr old and younger hospitalized with burn-related injuries, about 65% are treated for scald burns caused by hot liquid or steam (e.g., coffee or soup), with the highest incidence in children younger than 2 yr of age. Chemical burns, the third most commonly seen burns in children, occur from touching or ingesting a caustic agent such as a cleaning solution and are also seen more often in younger children. The most common type of burn-related injury in older children is flame burn, which is caused by direct contact with fire (SAFE KIDS, 2006). Fires caused by children playing are the leading cause of residential fire-related death and injury in children 5 yr old and younger.

Another source of burn injury is child abuse. About 10% of all burns in children are caused by child abuse. In the presence of unusual burns such as immersion (glove and stocking) burns, burns that spare flexor surfaces, contact burns from cigarettes or irons, and zebra burn lines from contact with a hot grate, child abuse should be suspected (London, 2007). The majority of child abuse burn victims are younger than 2 yr old and are almost always younger than 10 yr old.

Factors affecting severity of the burn and seriousness of the injury:

1. Percentage of total body surface area (TBSA) burned: Use modified rule of nine for children (i.e., percentage of TBSA of head varies with age of child; at 1 yr old, it is 19%; at 5-9 yr old, it is 13%).
2. Burn depth:
   a. Superficial (first-degree) burn involves epidermis and heals in 5-10 days without scarring.
   b. Partial-thickness (second-degree) injury involves epidermis and varying degrees of the dermis. It may be superficial (usually healing in 14-21 days with variable scarring) or deep dermal (usually heals in 30 days to several months if no infection occurs and with extensive scarring).
   c. Full-thickness (third-degree) burn involves the epidermis and dermis and extends into the subcutaneous tissue. Nerve endings, sweat glands, and hair follicles are destroyed. It cannot reepithelialize and requires surgical excision and wound grafting.
   d. Fourth-degree is a full-thickness burn that involves underlying structures—muscles, fascia, and bones.
3. Wound location: Certain body areas carry a higher risk of complications and require specialized care (e.g., burns of the hand and feet and across joints can interfere with growth and development because of scar formation).
4. Age of the child: For example, the very thin skin of a premature infant would take longer to heal and be damaged more easily than that of a healthy 3-yr-old.
5. Causative agent.
6. Presence of respiratory involvement.
7. General health of the child.
8. Presence of concomitant injuries.

Children most at risk:
- Children 4 yr old and younger because of their natural curiosity and lack of awareness of danger are especially at risk for scald and contact burns and for sparkler injury.
- Children with disabilities related to developmental level or physical inability to get out of harm's way are especially at risk for scald and contact burns.
- Boys are at greater risk than girls.
- Children in homes without smoke detectors are at greatest risk for fires and fire-related death and injury.
- Males 10-14 yr old are at highest risk for fireworks-related injuries.

Differences in effects of burn injury in children:
- There is a higher mortality rate in very young children who have been severely burned compared to older children and adults with comparable burns.
- Lower temperatures and shorter exposure time can cause more severe burns in children than in adults because of the child's thinner skin.
- Larger body surface area as compared with adults puts severely burned children at increased risk for fluid and heat loss.

- The greater proportion of body fluid to mass in children increases risk of dehydration and cardiovascular problems because of less effective cardiovascular response to changing intravascular volume. The younger the child, the greater the percentage of total body weight is water and the greater his or her percentage of extracellular fluid (i.e., interstitial fluid surrounds the cell; intravascular fluid is within the blood vessels or plasma; and transcellular fluid such as spinal fluid and sweat).
- Because of smaller muscle mass and less body fat than adults, children are at increased risk for protein and calorie deficiency.
- The younger the child, the less mature the immune system and the greater the risk for infection.
- Extensive burns may result in delayed growth.
- Hypertrophic scarring is increased, and scar maturation is prolonged.

HEALTH CARE SETTING

Emergency department, with possible hospitalization for significant burns; some burns are treated in primary care and others at home

ASSESSMENT

Varies significantly depending on burn severity and seriousness of the injury.

Superficial burn (e.g., mild sunburn): Erythremic, moderate discomfort/pain, blanches with pressure, good capillary refill.

Partial-thickness burn:

- *Superficial:* Fluid-filled blisters, skin red to ivory with moist surfaces, considerable pain, blanches with pressure and refills.
- *Deep:* May or may not have fluid-filled blisters; blisters are often flat and dehydrated, making skin tissue-paper like; color is mottled, waxy white, and with dry surface. Nerve endings are intact, so pain is severe on exposure to air or water.

Full-thickness burn: Varies in color from red to tan, waxy white, brown, or black. It does not blanch with pressure. Edema is present. It has a dry, leathery appearance and lacks sensation because of destruction of nerve endings. However, because it is usually surrounded by superficial and partial-thickness burns that have intact nerve endings, adjacent areas likely will be painful.

Respiratory compromise: Upper airway edema related to injury starts within a few minutes, and the airway may occlude in minutes to a few hours, although it may be delayed up to 24-48 hr.

Respiratory distress: Abdominal breathing in a child older than 7 yr old (children are primarily abdominal breathers until that age), head bobbing with respiratory effort, nasal flaring, coughing, stridor, wheezing.

Burn shock: With severe burns (greater than 15%-20% TBSA), a type of hypovolemic shock may occur with increased heart rate (HR), increased respiratory rate (RR), low blood pressure (BP), hypothermia, pallor, cyanosis, decreased level of consciousness (LOC), and poor muscle tone.

Physical assessment: In addition to signs mentioned above, the examiner may notice singed nasal hairs and nasopharynx edema. It is also important to assess for other injuries such as fractures and internal injuries.

Complications:

- Pulmonary complications are the leading cause of death in thermal trauma: Inhalation injury, aspiration of gastric contents, bacterial pneumonia, pulmonary edema/insufficiency, and emboli.
- Wound sepsis: Disorientation is one of the first signs of overwhelming sepsis.
- Gastrointestinal complications: Impaired gastric and large bowel motility is common with burns greater than 20% TBSA.
- Encephalopathy: Hallucinations, personality changes, delirium, seizures, and coma. Although encephalopathy is relatively common, full neurologic recovery usually occurs (Hockenberry, 2003).

DIAGNOSTIC TESTS

Note: Topical anesthetics are used with blood draws, if possible, to decrease pain and anxiety and to provide atraumatic care.

Arterial blood gas level: To determine respiratory status; variations from normal may signal respiratory compromise.

Chemistries:

- **Fluid and electrolytes:** Deficits of fluid and sodium occur with burn shock.
- **Blood urea nitrogen and creatinine:** Elevations may indicate renal failure.
- **Glucose:** May be elevated in young infants. Stress may cause either hypoglycemia or pseudodiabetes, resulting in elevated glucose levels.

Nursing Diagnosis:

Deficient Fluid Volume

related to fluid shift from intravascular to interstitial compartment, increased metabolic demands, and decreased intake

Desired Outcomes: Within 4 hr following intervention/treatment, child has adequate fluid volume as evidenced by normal LOC for child, soft anterior fontanel (in child younger than 2 yr), moist oral mucous membranes, good/elastic abdominal skin turgor (on unaffected areas), and normal urine output (UO). For example, infant UO more than 2-3 ml/kg/hr, toddler and preschooler UO 2 ml/kg/hr, school-age child UO 1-2 ml/kg/hr, and adolescent UO 0.5-1 ml/kg/hr.

INTERVENTIONS	RATIONALES
Administer IV fluids as prescribed.	Fluid resuscitation is required in children with burns greater than 10% TBSA. Fluids help maintain general circulation to vital organs and capillary circulation to viable skin.
Once stabilized, ensure that child receives *at least minimum* maintenance fluids based on his or her weight.	The smaller the child, the greater the percentage of body weight is water and the larger the percentage of extracellular fluid. Because of excess fluid loss from the burn injury and increased metabolic demands related to child's age and increased catecholamine release caused by burn stress, child probably will need more than maintenance fluids. First, use this formula to determine maintenance fluids: **Up to 10 kg: 100 ml/kg/24 hr =** _____ **10-20 kg: 50 ml/kg/24hr =** _____ **More than 20 kg: 20 ml/kg/24hr =** _____ **= maintenance fluid requirement** *For example, child weighs 33 kg:* $$\frac{\begin{array}{ll} 10\ kg \times 100\ ml/kg/24\ hr & = \quad 1000\ ml/24\ hr \\ 10\ kg \times 50\ ml/kg/24\ hr & = \quad 500\ ml/24\ hr \\ 13\ kg \times 20\ ml/kg/24\ hr & = \quad 260\ ml/24\ hr \end{array}}{33\ kg \qquad\qquad\qquad\qquad 1760\ ml/24\ hr}$$ Maintenance fluid requirement for child weighing 33 kg is 1760 ml/24 hr. Remember that child probably will need *more* than maintenance fluids.
Assess intake and ouptut (I&O) q2h. Weigh all diapers, 1 ml = 1 g. Ensure minimum urine output of 1 ml/kg/hr is met. Assess hydration status q4h: LOC, anterior fontanel (in child younger than 2 yr old), oral mucous membrane, abdominal skin turgor, and urine output. **Note:** Edema may occur around the burn or from fluid shifts.	Child may be receiving maintenance fluids but still be dehydrated because of increased insensible water losses, especially in a child with burns. Frequent assessment leads to early detection of problems and quicker treatment. Signs of impaired hydration include decreasing LOC, sunken fontanel, dry and sticky oral mucous membranes, tenting of abdominal skin, and decreased UO.
Monitor vital signs (VS), capillary refill, and LOC q4h for changes related to hypovolemia.	Hypovolemia may be present because of reduced circulating blood volume that occurs with plasma loss in burns. Tachycardia, changes in tissue perfusion (e.g., capillary refill more than 2 sec), and alteration in LOC are early signs of hypovolemic shock. BP will be normal initially because increased systemic vascular resistance helps to maintain it. However, perfusion with a normal BP may be inadequate to meet the body's demands. Therefore decreased BP can be a late sign of hypovolemia in children.
Monitor daily weights, using same scale at same time of day and with same amount of clothing (no clothes, including diaper in infants).	Short-term weight changes are the most reliable measurement of fluid loss or gain. Excessive weight gain indicates fluid retention, which could interfere with wound healing; weight loss could signal dehydration or excessive fluid loss, which also would interfere with wound healing.
Alert health care provider promptly to significant findings or changes.	This helps ensure timely treatment.

●●● **Related NIC/NOC labels:** *NIC:* Fluid Management; Fluid Monitoring; Hypovolemia Management; Intravenous (IV) Therapy; Vital Signs Monitoring; Shock Prevention *NOC:* Fluid Balance; Hydration

Nursing Diagnosis:

Acute Pain

related to thermal injuries and medical-surgical interventions

Desired Outcome: Within 30 min to 1 hr after treatment/intervention, child's pain level is decreased (2 or less on FACES 0-5 scale or 4 or less on FLACC [face, legs, activity, cry, consolability] or numeric 0-10 scale) or at a level acceptable to child.

INTERVENTIONS	RATIONALES
Establish pain scale appropriate for child's developmental level (e.g., FLACC, Wong-Baker FACES, or numeric scales).	A pain scale increases ability to accurately assess pain and degree of relief obtained.
Assess level of pain q2-4h, as well as before and after pain medication administration (e.g., 1 hr after PO medications, 10-20 min after IV medications).	These assessments detect early changes in pain level and assess effectiveness of pain medications.
Provide pain medications/nonpharmacologic pain relief measures around the clock on a regular basis, not prn.	Scheduled rather than prn pain relief provides better and more reliable pain control. Prolonged stimulation of pain receptors results in increased sensitivity to painful stimuli and will increase the amount of drug needed to relieve pain. Pain relief measures such as distraction; relaxation; repositioning; guided imagery; cutaneous stimulation such as massage, heat, or cold; and positive self-talk increase effectiveness of medication.
Explain how patient-controlled analgesia (PCA) works and that child cannot give self too much medication. Encourage child/parent to use PCA when needed if it is available.	Most experts believe that when a child is capable of pushing the button on the pump, usually by 5-6 yr of age, he or she can self-administer pain medication. Some facilities allow PCA by proxy—the parent or nurse can administer the medication if the child is too ill or cannot understand the concept of pushing the button to relieve the pain.
Reassure parent that addiction rarely occurs when medication is used to relieve pain.	Fear of addiction may decrease use of pain medication.
Premedicate child before painful procedures. Use topical anesthetic to decrease trauma of blood draws/IV insertion, if possible (atraumatic care).	Pain medications given before painful procedures will help control pain. Time frame before procedure depends on route (e.g., 10-20 min IV and 1 hr PO).
Explain all procedures at developmental level appropriate for child.	Anxiety increases pain; knowing what to expect may decrease anxiety.

••• **Related NIC and NOC labels:** *NIC:* Pain Management; Medication Management; Patient-Controlled Analgesia Assistance; Positioning; Distraction; Simple Relaxation Therapy; Simple Guided Imagery; Cutaneous Stimulation; Anxiety Reduction *NOC:* Comfort Level

Nursing Diagnoses:

Impaired Skin Integrity/Impaired Tissue Integrity

related to burn injury

Desired Outcomes: The skin/graft site heals without signs of infection (e.g., drainage, erythema, edema, or pain). Superficial burns heal within 5-10 days without scarring; deep partial-thickness burns heal within 30 days with varying degrees of scarring.

INTERVENTIONS	RATIONALES
Carefully clean wound and tissue immediately surrounding wound as prescribed.	Cautious cleansing is necessary to avoid damaging the epithelialization of granulating skin and decrease risk of infection. Infection would further damage the already traumatized tissue, disrupt epithelialization, and delay healing.
Débride wound as prescribed.	Débridement promotes healing by removing dead or injured tissue so that the wound has an environment conducive to healing.

Continued

INTERVENTIONS	RATIONALES
Apply ointment and/or dressings as prescribed using clean/sterile technique.	These measures protect the wound, decrease risk of infection, and promote healing.
Monitor child and wound/graft site/donor site q4h for signs and symptoms of infection.	These assessments ensure prompt recognition of problems, more rapid treatment, and maximum healing. Infection indicators include change in LOC, hypothermia or hyperthermia, odor, drainage, increased edema, increased erythema, and increased pain.
Monitor graft q4h for evidence of hematoma, edema, or sloughing of graft; notify health care provider promptly if noted.	Early recognition of the problem and prompt treatment increase chance of saving the graft.
Minimize child scratching and picking at wound using methods appropriate for developmental age.	This promotes better wound healing and decreases scarring.
	Methods for developmental age include:
	- Young child: distraction and supervision
	- Older child: explanations of importance of not scratching, picking, or hitting wound
Offer high-calorie, high-protein meals and snacks, providing foods that the child likes.	Child has increased metabolism and catabolism because of burn injury and therefore needs increased calories and protein to promote positive nitrogen balance, which facilitates healing. Offering foods that the child likes increases likelihood of increased intake.
Administer vitamins and minerals (e.g., vitamins A, B, C, zinc, and iron) as prescribed.	These supplements facilitate wound healing and epithelialization.
Perform active (or ensure passive) range-of-motion (ROM) exercises to affected joints as prescribed.	These exercises promote reabsorption of edema, prevent contracture formation, and improve healing.
Position for minimal stress/pressure on wound/graft.	Proper positioning promotes healing and protects wound/graft. For example, do not allow child to lie on wound; use a cradle to keep sheets/blankets off the graft site.

For more detailed information, see "Managing Wound Care," p. 559.

••• **Related NIC and NOC labels:** *NIC:* Wound Care; Infection Protection; Positioning; Medication Administration; Nutrition Management; Wound Irrigation; Skin Care: Topical Treatments *NOC:* Tissue Integrity: Skin & Mucous Membranes; Wound Healing: Secondary Intention

Nursing Diagnosis:

Risk for Infection

related to loss of skin barrier/denuded skin, increased metabolic demands, altered nutritional status, invasive procedures/lines, and the hospital environment

Desired Outcome: Child exhibits wound healing without signs of burn wound infection (e.g., odor, drainage, increased erythema or edema, increased pain) or systemic infection (e.g., pneumonia or septicemia).

Note: See interventions and rationales for **Impaired Skin Integrity/Impaired Tissue Integrity** plus the following:

INTERVENTIONS	RATIONALES
Wash hands before and after working with child.	Handwashing is the best method of preventing nosocomial infection.
Use gloves as indicated, following standard precautions.	Gloves provide additional level of protection for patient by reducing risk of contamination of open wounds by bare hands of caregivers. (Wearing gloves also protects caregiver from contact with patient's open wounds.)

Continued

INTERVENTIONS	RATIONALES
Screen visitors for colds or other infectious illnesses before they enter child's room.	Child has altered immune response and is at greater risk for infection because of the following: - Open wounds or denuded skin have lost the protective skin barrier and are potential entry sites for infection. - Decreased circulation to the burned area compromises the body's ability to fight infection at the tissue level because fewer leukocytes (white blood cells, which act as scavengers and fight infection) are able to reach damaged tissue. - Mature neutrophils, the body's first line of defense against bacterial infection and severe stress, are decreased as immature neutrophils increase to digest products of burn injury.
Monitor VS q4h and notify health care provider of findings indicative of infection (e.g., temperature 36° C or less or 38.5° C or greater, HR 100 bpm or greater, or RR 30 breaths/min or more, but will vary depending on age of child).	Early signs of infection/sepsis include tachycardia, tachypnea, and fever or hypothermia. Early recognition of abnormality enables prompt treatment and less serious infection.
Monitor LOC q4h.	Disorientation is one of the first signs of overwhelming sepsis/septic shock in burn patients.
Monitor for signs of pneumonia q4h (varies depending on age of child).	Early recognition facilitates prompt treatment and a less severe infection. - Infant: fever, restlessness, anxiety, grunting, nasal flaring, retractions, tachypnea, head bobbing - Child and adolescent: fever, chills, cough, chest pain, restlessness, anxiety, tachypnea
Position child with head elevated 15-30 degrees for 1-2 hr after meals.	This position decreases incidence of aspiration of gastric contents, which could lead to aspiration pneumonia.
Depending on developmental age, ensure that child turns, coughs, and deep breathes or uses incentive spirometer q2h while awake. Younger children can blow bubbles or blow on a pinwheel.	Deep breathing expands alveoli and aids in mobilizing secretions to the airways, and coughing further mobilizes and clears the secretions to help prevent pneumonia.
Assess IV sites (peripheral or central access) q4h for signs of infection (e.g., erythema, warmth, edema).	There is potential for increased rate of infection because of child's altered immune response and because IV site is another entry site for bacteria.
For more information, see Appendix A for "Infection Prevention and Control," p. 783.	

●●● **Related NIC and NOC labels:** *NIC:* Infection Protection; Respiratory Monitoring; Aspiration Precautions; Wound Care *NOC:* Immune Status; Infection Status; Wound Healing: Secondary Intention

Nursing Diagnosis:

Imbalanced Nutrition: Less Than Body Requirements

related to hypermetabolic state and decreased appetite

Desired Outcome: Within 1 wk of intervention/treatment, child exhibits adequate nutrition as evidenced by maintenance of or gaining weight.

INTERVENTIONS	RATIONALES
Provide high-calorie, high-protein meals and snacks, as well as foods high in vitamin C content.	Because of smaller muscle mass and less body fat than adults, children are at increased risk for protein and calorie deficiency. This diet provides positive nitrogen balance and nutrients needed for wound healing. Energy requirements increase according to size of the burn; caloric requirements may be 2 to 3 times normal because of increased metabolic rate. High-protein meals replace protein lost by exudation.

Continued

INTERVENTIONS	RATIONALES
Ensure that child is receiving adequate nutrients. Discuss child's needs with health care provider.	If this cannot be accomplished orally, enteral or parenteral feedings may be necessary. Burns will not heal well without adequate nutrients.
Provide foods that the child likes and encourage child to feed self as much as possible.	These measures stimulate appetite and promote cooperation.
Try to minimize anorexia in the following ways:	Anorexia occurs in many children with burn injury.
- Offer small, frequent meals.	- Child may eat better with 4-5 small meals/day rather than 3 large meals.
- Make meal times pleasant with attractive meals, companionship, and no treatments or unpleasant interruptions.	- Eating is more likely to occur in a more "homelike" environment.
Maintain neutral thermal environment.	Caloric expenditure is minimized when child does not need to use energy to cool or heat body.
Monitor I&O q4h.	This assessment determines whether the child is receiving appropriate intake and has adequate output.
Monitor for hypoglycemia.	Hypoglycemia can result from the stress of injury as glycogen stores in the liver are rapidly depleted.
Monitor for hyperglycemia.	Hyperglycemia can occur because of mobilization of glucagon and decreased insulin production.
Ensure that child is having a normal stooling pattern. Monitor for constipation or diarrhea and notify health care provider if either occurs.	Constipation caused by decreased activity and intake could further affect intake because of discomfort and thus interfere with weight gain.
	Diarrhea would decrease weight as well.
Weigh weekly on the same scale at the same time of day with the same amount of clothing.	Consistency with weight measurements helps ensure more accurate results. Weight is a reliable indicator of nutritional status.

••• **Related NIC and NOC labels:** *NIC:* Nutrition Monitoring; Enteral Tube Feeding; Nutrition Management; Weight Gain Assistance; Total Parenteral Nutrition Administration *NOC:* Nutritional Status; Nutritional Status: Nutrient Intake

Nursing Diagnosis:

Disturbed Body Image

related to child's perception of altered appearance and mobility/skills

Desired Outcomes: Child receives emotional support from the onset of injury and discusses feelings related to change in appearance and mobility/skills after wound healing begins. Within 48-72 hr of this diagnosis, child relates at least one positive example of his or her appearance/abilities and expresses realistic expectations for the future.

INTERVENTIONS	RATIONALES
Ensure a positive attitude when caring for the child.	This shows acceptance and encourages expectation the child will get better.
Point out positive aspects of child's appearance/abilities. Ask child during subsequent care to give examples of positive aspects.	Positive reinforcement encourages child to focus on positive aspects rather than on deficits.
Encourage child to provide for developmentally appropriate self-care as much as his or her condition allows.	Encouragement enables child to focus on tasks that he or she can do and promotes positive self-image in the process.
Give honest answers to child and family regarding care and appearance.	Honesty facilitates building of a trusting nurse-patient/family relationship and assists in developing realistic expectations.
Assess support systems and coping mechanisms used in previous stressful situations.	Optimally, this assessment will mobilize previous effective strategies to assist child in dealing with current altered appearance and mobility/skills.
Arrange for continued schooling, depending on age of child.	This decreases isolation and provides normalization, which may help self-image.

Continued

INTERVENTIONS	RATIONALES
Promote peer contact if possible and prepare peers for child's appearance.	These measures facilitate acceptance and support.
Support appropriate adaptive behaviors.	This measure builds on strengths.
Encourage verbalization about feelings regarding appearance and changes in lifestyle.	This will help identify child's concerns and anxieties, enabling nurse to provide more realistic feedback about appearance if appropriate and aid in working on coping strategies.
Point out evidence of healing.	This promotes sense of hope.
Discuss ways child can "cover up" disfigurement, dressings, and pressure garments.	This facilitates coping. Examples include clothing (e.g., turtleneck sweaters, larger shirt than normal), wigs, makeup.
Assist child in devising a plan to address and cope with reactions of others.	This will increase sense of control. Role playing may help child perfect this plan.
Facilitate transition back to day care, school, and home environment. Encourage communication of family and medical staff with other care providers, including school nurse and teachers.	These measures prepare other children and caregivers for change in child's appearance and encourage them to make transition a positive experience.

••• **Related NIC and NOC labels:** *NIC:* Body Image Enhancement; Active Listening; Anxiety Reduction; Coping Enhancement; Emotional Support; Self-Awareness Enhancement; Support System Enhancement; Self-Modification Assistance *NOC:* Body Image

ADDITIONAL NURSING DIAGNOSES/ PROBLEMS:

"Psychosocial Support"	p. 73
"Psychosocial Support for the Patient's Family and Significant Other"	p. 87
"Managing Wound Care" for more details regarding wound treatment	p. 559
"Asthma" for **Anxiety**	p. 580
"Cystic Fibrosis" for **Impaired Gas Exchange** (for children with inhalation injury)	p. 623

✔ PATIENT-FAMILY TEACHING AND DISCHARGE PLANNING

When providing patient/family teaching, focus on sensory information, avoid giving excessive information, and initiate visiting nurse referral for necessary follow-up teaching and assessment as needed. Stress importance of family-centered care (viewing the family as a unit that is the "constant" in the child's life and maintaining or improving the health of the family and its members in a holistic manner). Include verbal and written information about the following (ensure that written information is at a level the reader can understand):

✓ Type of burn and normal healing time.
✓ Wound care as appropriate:
- Administering oral pain medication about 1 hr before wound care if needed
- Cleaning wound
- Applying ointment
- Applying dressing

✓ Treatment of pain (e.g., administering medication on a regular basis, which gives better control and assists healing process; use of nonmedication adjuncts such as distraction).
✓ Signs and symptoms of burn wound, graft site, or donor site infection:
- Purulent drainage or odor
- Increased redness or swelling
- Temperature 101.5° F or greater
✓ Ways to prevent infection:
- Good handwashing before and after caring for wound
- Dressing changes performed in a clean area with good light
- Making sure that dressing stays clean and dry
✓ Methods of preventing scars and contractures:
- Wearing pressure garments as prescribed (usually 23 hr/day)
- Wearing splints as prescribed (over top of pressure garment)
- ROM exercises as prescribed and demonstrated by physical therapist (PT)
- Child performing as many activities of daily living as possible (e.g., feeding self, combing hair, dressing self)
✓ Care of healing skin:
- May be dry: Apply lotion (cocoa butter is most often recommended) but avoid those containing alcohol or lanolin.
- May be itchy: Use lotion, prescribed medication (e.g., Benadryl), distraction.
- Bathing: Use lukewarm water and be gentle!
- Protect new skin over burned area.
✓ Wear comfortable clothing, not constrictive.
✓ Try to avoid hitting or bumping area.
✓ Protect from sun with clothing and sunscreen (SPF 15 or higher).

✓ Do not stay out in cold weather; burned area is sensitive to cold.

✓ If child is on any medications: drug name; route; purpose; type; dosage; precautions; drug-drug, food-drug, and herb-drug interactions; and potential side effects.

✓ Demonstrate drawing up and administering medication and having family member perform return demonstration.

✓ Nutritional needs (child needs increased calories and protein to heal well):

- Make pudding with Ensure instead of milk (increases calories).
- Eat small, frequent meals or three meals with nutritious snacks between meals.
- Make mealtime a social, shared time. Turn off TV.
- Feed child when he or she is well rested.
- If receiving tube feeding: procedure for checking placement and administering feeding, checking residual, and recognizing and reporting problems.
- Vitamins that help skin heal: A and C (oranges, grapefruit, tomatoes, broccoli, and carrots).
- Protein promotes skin healing: meat, fish, eggs, peanut butter, chicken, and milk.

✓ Importance of adequate fluid intake to promote healing (child should receive at least maintenance fluids or more per health care provider). How much should the child drink per day? Give parents information they can understand, such as an infant that weighs 9 kg needs 900 ml/day for maintenance fluids, which is 30 oz. If the infant drinks from 4-oz bottles, he or she needs to take eight 4-oz bottles of fluid/day to get maintenance fluids. An older child weighing 40 kg would need 1900 ml/day for maintenance fluids. If this child drinks from 12-oz glasses, he or she would need at least five and a half 12-oz glasses/day. These examples are only for maintenance fluids; child may need 1½-2 times maintenance fluids to stay well hydrated, depending on size and stage of healing of the burn injury.

✓ Importance of checking hydration status at least several times a day while the child is still healing from the burn. The less the child weighs and the younger he or she is, the greater the percentage of body weight is water. Therefore dehydration occurs much more quickly than it would in an older child or adult. The child may still be losing fluid from the burn and using more energy to heal, therefore using more fluid.

- Is the child alert and interactive? Child would not be as alert and interactive as normal if dehydrated.
- Check soft spot on top of the head (in children younger than 2 yr old). If it is sunken in, the child may be dehydrated.
- Check inside the mouth, not the lips. If dry or sticky and the child is not a mouth breather, the child is dehydrated.
- Pinch skin on the abdomen. If skin sits up like a tent instead of falling down right away, the child is dehydrated.
- How many wet diapers does the child normally have a day or how many times does he or she normally void? If the number of diapers is decreased, they are not as wet

as usual, or the child is voiding less often, he or she may be dehydrated.

✓ Adjustment after burn injury, which is often prolonged and painful. Family and individual psychosocial support is important. Reinforce importance of helping siblings cope/adjust to having a sibling with a potentially long-term injury.

✓ Growth and development (realistic expectations of what child should be doing at different ages and encouragement of activities that promote normal growth and development).

✓ Feelings that child may experience with reentry to school/society, which vary depending on developmental age and severity of burn: fear, anger, guilt, depression, withdrawal, altered body image, anticipating peer response.

✓ Potential for regression. This is normal after a stressful event.

✓ Developmentally related risks for burn injuries (see introductory data).

✓ Tips for childproofing the home:

- Set water heater thermostat at 120° F or less or install antiscald devices in faucets and showerheads in buildings where one does not have access to the water tank (e.g., apartment buildings).
  - Water temperature of 120° takes 2.5 min for partial-thickness burn.
  - Water temperature of 130° takes 15 sec for partial-thickness burn.
  - Water temperature of 140° takes 2.5 sec for partial-thickness burn.
- The younger the child, the thinner the skin, and the quicker and more deeply the burn that occurs.
- Never leave a young child alone, especially in the kitchen or bathroom, even to answer the telephone for a minute. Take the child with you.
- Turn pot handles toward back of the stove and use back burners when cooking.
- Cover stovetop knobs.
- Keep appliance cords out of child's vision and reach (e.g., coffee pot), especially if appliance contains hot food or liquid.
- Cover unused electrical outlets with appropriate outlet covers (not the ones that just plug in).
- Keep hot foods and liquids away from table and counter edges.
- Do not leave hot foods or liquids on a table with a tablecloth that child can reach.
- Never carry or hold child and hot food and/or beverage at the same time.
- Stress dangers of open flames; explain what "hot" means.
- Place protective cover in front of radiator, fireplace, or other heating element.
- Keep matches, gasoline, lighters, and all other flammable materials locked away and out of child's reach.
- Teach children how to "stop, drop, and roll" if their clothes catch on fire and how to crawl to safety if a fire occurs in the building they are in.

- Over 6 mo old, apply sunscreen with SPF 15 or higher when child is exposed to sunlight.
✓ Additional tips for preventing fire-related injuries:
- Install smoke detectors in home in every bedroom and on each level. Test them monthly and change batteries at least yearly. Having smoke detectors cuts the risk of dying in a fire by 50%.
- Have at least two multipurpose dry chemical fire extinguishers: one in the kitchen and one in workshop or area where potential sources of fire exist (e.g., water heater or furnace). Check monthly for signs of damage, corrosion, tampering, and leaks. Always call the fire department before using the fire extinguisher. Use the PASS method (*p*oint, *a*im at the base of the fire, *s*queeze the handle, and *s*weep from side to side).
- Set up a home emergency fire escape plan and have practice drills using escape plan at least quarterly. Include a meeting place outside the home in your plan.

✓ First-aid emergency care for burn injury: Put burned area under cool running water immediately, remove clothing, cover burned area loosely with bandage or clean cloth, seek medical assistance.

✓ Importance of follow-up care with health care provider, PT, and any other specialists involved.

✓ Telephone numbers to call for health care provider, home health nurse, and PT in case any questions or concerns about treatment or injury arise after discharge.

✓ When to call health care provider:
- If child is not eating well or showing signs of dehydration
- If there is unmanageable behavior at home or school
- If there are any signs of infection (e.g., healing burn area or donor site looks, feels, or smells different—red, warm,

swollen, very tender to touch or there is foul smelling drainage)
- If there is itching that is not controlled with lotion or medication
- If the healing/healed area cracks open or splits
- If contracture occurs
- If child's temperature is higher than 101.5° F
- If dressing change is painful despite giving pain medication as prescribed

✓ Referral to community resources, such as National SAFE KIDS Campaign, public health nurse, home health agencies, community support groups, camps for children with burns, psychologists, and financial counseling as appropriate. Additional general information can be obtained by contacting the following organizations:
- National SAFE KIDS Campaign at *www.safekids.org*
- Shriners Hospitals "Burn Prevention Tips" from *www.shrinershq.org/files/hospitals/Cincinnati/pdf/Guide_to_Ch_Burn_Inj.pdf*
- Alisa Ann Ruch Burn Foundation at *www.aarbf.org*
- Burn survivor assistance; prevention materials from Phoenix Society for Burn Survivors, Inc., at *www.phoenix-society.org*
- Assistance locating local resources on Phoenix Society Web site: Look under resources, click on USA, and then click on desired state, where listings of burn centers, burn camps, and support groups can be found. "You Can Do It" video for teens is available for a nominal charge.
- USFA (United States Fire Association) for Kids: For fire safety instructions at *www.usfa.fema.gov/kids/flash.shtm*

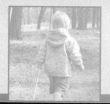

Cerebral Palsy 79

OVERVIEW/PATHOPHYSIOLOGY

Cerebral palsy is a term used to describe a group of chronic conditions affecting body movement and muscle coordination. It is caused by damage to one or more specific areas of the brain, which typically occurs before birth during fetal development but can occur during or shortly after birth—usually before age 5 yr. Cerebral palsy is the most common physical disability of childhood with about 8000 neonates and infants as well as an additional 1200 to 1500 preschool age children being diagnosed each year (UCP, 2001). There is an increased incidence in premature or very low-birth-weight babies. It is nonprogressive, although secondary conditions (e.g., muscle spasticity) can develop and may remain the same, improve, or deteriorate. A child with cerebral palsy may have intellectual, perceptual, and language deficits. A large number of factors may contribute to cerebral palsy, either singly or multifactorially. Events occurring before birth that can disrupt normal development of the brain cause cerebral palsy in about 70% of cases, whereas lack of oxygen during labor and delivery contributes to only a small minority of cases (March of Dimes, 2004). No identifiable cause is found in many cases. There are three main types of cerebral palsy, and there may be a mixture of types.

- **Spastic:** May involve one or both sides. Hypertonicity is present with poor control of posture, balance, and coordinated movements. The patient has difficulty with fine and gross motor skills. The majority of children have this type.
- **Dyskinetic/athetoid:** Involuntary and uncontrolled body movement.
- **Ataxic:** Disturbed sense of balance and depth perception.
- **Mixed:** Combination of spasticity and athetosis.

HEALTH CARE SETTING

Primary care, with possible hospitalization for surgery or pneumonia

ASSESSMENT

Involves physical assessment along with a detailed health history. Ongoing developmental surveillance is important. Cerebral palsy is not usually diagnosed until 6-12 mo of age.

Signs and symptoms: Clinical manifestations vary tremendously from child to child. Some children may have a mild problem with ataxia, whereas some may be severely affected. The universal clinical manifestation is delayed gross motor development. Other common problems are abnormal motor performance, alterations of muscle tone (hypertonicity or hypotonicity), abnormal postures, reflex abnormalities, and numerous associated disabilities and problems, including intellectual impairment, attention deficit hyperactivity disorder (ADHD), seizures, drooling, feeding and speech problems, orthopedic complications, increased incidence of dental problems, and visual and hearing problems.

Physical assessment: Involves evaluation of range of motion (ROM), muscle strength and tone, abnormal movements, and contractures.

DIAGNOSTIC TESTS

Primary method of diagnosis is neurologic examination with developmental screening and history. Other diagnostic testing might include the following:

Electroencephalogram: Can rule out seizure disorders or slowly growing brain tumor.

Neuroimaging tests: To determine site of brain injury and provide clues to potential causes, as well as rule out slow growing brain tumors.

Cytologic studies: Genetic evaluation is done to determine if a progressive degenerative disease is present or symptoms are part of a syndrome.

Metabolic studies: To rule out metabolic defects (e.g., Guthrie blood test for phenylketonuria or serum galactose levels for galactosemia).

Electrolyte levels: To assess for and rule out electrolyte imbalance that may be causing symptoms.

Nursing Diagnosis

Imbalanced Nutrition: Less Than Body Requirements

related to chewing and/or swallowing difficulty and motor problems/activity

Desired Outcome: Within 1 wk of intervention/treatment, child exhibits improved intake and maintains or gains weight.

INTERVENTIONS	RATIONALES
Provide high-calorie meals and snacks.	Child likely will need increased calories because of increased muscle activity (i.e., spasticity or dyskinetic movements).
Provide foods that child likes.	This measure will stimulate appetite and promote cooperation in eating.
Encourage child to feed self as much as possible.	Allowing child to try to feed self may increase intake by decreasing frustration of having no control over other matters.
Make meal times pleasant with no interruptions, a relaxed environment, attractive meals, eye contact, and conversation appropriate for child.	This encourages focusing on eating, thereby increasing intake.
Approach child with a greeting that alerts him or her that movement or a change in activity is going to occur.	This prevents a startle reflex, which interferes with ability to chew and swallow successfully.
Use the following aids and techniques to facilitate feeding; seek input from occupational/speech therapists:	These measures improve likelihood of adequate oral intake.
- Let child know that food is coming.	This prepares child for meal and increases likelihood of successful feeding.
- Put a bib on child.	This signals for child that it is mealtime.
- Ensure proper positioning.	Proper positioning decreases incidence of aspiration and gastroesophageal reflux (GER) and improves intake. Firmly supporting child through the hips and trunk provides a stable base for sitting up. Keeping head and neck in a midline, neutral position, prevents aspiration and enables better oral muscular control.
- Place spoon in middle of child's mouth, placing pressure on the tongue.	This measure prevents tonic bite reflex and tongue thrust.
- Sit in front of child.	This facilitates eye contact, conversation, and use of prescribed therapy techniques.
- Hold jaw with hand.	This promotes jaw control.
- If child has GER, position sitting up for 30 min to 1 hr after meal.	This position decreases incidence of GER and ultimately improves intake.
- Make sure that food and liquid are the proper texture (e.g., pureed or bite size) and temperature for the child.	Some children aspirate when taking regular liquids (they need them to be thickened), and some children cannot chew.
Monitor intake and output.	This assessment reveals if child is receiving adequate nutrients and has adequate output.
Weigh weekly on same scale, at same time of day, and with child wearing same clothing.	Consistency with weight measurements helps ensure more accurate results. Child is receiving adequate nutrients if maintaining or gaining weight (as long as weight gain is not excessive). If weight is decreasing, diet may need to be supplemented.
Ensure that child is receiving adequate nutrients. If child is unable to take sufficient nutrients orally, discuss child's needs with health care provider.	Because of difficulty swallowing and increased motor activity, some children are unable to take sufficient nutrients orally, necessitating enteral feedings, which do not require adequate swallowing.

●●● **Related NIC and NOC labels:** *NIC:* Nutrition Management; Nutritional Monitoring; Enteral Tube Feeding; Self-Care Assistance: Feeding; Feeding *NOC:* Nutritional Status; Nutritional Status: Food & Fluid Intake

Risk for Injury

related to physical disability, perceptual or cognitive impairment, seizures, and/or lack of knowledge regarding injury/accident prevention

Desired Outcomes: Child remains free from signs and symptoms of injury. Parents verbalize accurate knowledge about how to provide a safe environment for the child.

INTERVENTIONS	RATIONALES
Educate family about ways of childproofing the home based on child's developmental age.	This information reduces child's risk for injury in the home. Examples include: - No furniture or tables with sharp edges. - No scatter rugs or polished floors. - Remove small or sharp objects from reach. - Use a protective helmet for the child prone to falls.
Teach family ways in which to institute seizure precautions as appropriate. General suggestions include:	This information helps prevent injury caused by seizures. **Note:** Not all children with cerebral palsy have seizures.
- Keep side rails raised when child is napping or sleeping (there are toddler side rails that can be used on beds at home).	This will protect child from falling out of bed with a seizure or from spastic movements or posturing.
- Keep side rails and hard objects padded (e.g., bumper guards on side rails that can be secured well).	This will prevent child from being injured during a seizure.
- Do not pad bedside rails with pillows.	Pillows can cause suffocation or slide out from under the side rail.
- Ensure that the child wears or carries medical identification describing his/her condition.	Seizures can be confused with other medical conditions and may be misdiagnosed in an emergency.
Teach family how to secure child properly in wheelchair, positioning devices, and motor vehicle. General suggestions include: - Secure all straps and belts, ensuring that they fit snugly. - Put brakes on wheelchair when transferring child or while child is sitting in it. - Use appropriate child safety restraint system (based on developmental age, not just chronologic age) whenever child is in a motor vehicle.	This information decreases chance of injury by falling as a result of spasticity, posturing, or lack of muscular control. There are many different systems used to secure children.
Review with family safe, appropriate toys for developmental age and physical limitations.	No sharp, small, or easily shattered toys should be allowed for a child who may fall during a seizure or is prone to falling. Aspiration/choking on small toys occurs frequently in children who are developmentally 3 yr of age or younger.

••• **Related NIC and NOC labels:** *NIC:* Fall Prevention; Surveillance: Safety; Environmental Management; Seizure Precautions; Parent Education: Childrearing Family; Health Education *NOC:* Safety Behavior: Home Physical Environment; Safety Status: Physical Injury; Safety Status: Falls Occurrence

Impaired Physical Mobility

related to neuromuscular impairment

Desired Outcome: Within 1 mo after intervention/treatment, child demonstrates improved mobility, and parents demonstrate correct use of splints/braces and physical therapy techniques.

INTERVENTIONS	RATIONALES
Encourage performance of developmental tasks such as sitting, crawling, and walking, as appropriate.	These tasks help to stretch and strengthen muscles.
Reinforce use of physical therapy exercises.	These exercises facilitate optimum muscular development by strengthening and promoting muscle coordination.
Provide incentives to move.	Developmentally appropriate incentives (e.g., a mobile for an infant functioning at a 4-mo-old level) increase likelihood of child trying to move.
Encourage rest before locomotion activities.	Spasticity and abnormal posturing increase when child is tired. Being rested before attempting locomotion improves chance of accomplishing goal.
Incorporate play into mobility exercises.	This is the normal activity of a child and encourages cooperation.
Instruct parents in correct use of orthoses.	Orthoses help prevent contractures, protect skin, and maintain or improve function.
Encourage parents to be active in child's daily physical and occupational therapy.	Parental involvement facilitates integration of therapy skills into child's activities of daily living (ADL) and promotes continuity of care.
Evaluate child's response to therapy on a regular basis.	Ongoing evaluation of effectiveness of current plan increases chance of success because modifications or changes can be made in a timely manner, as necessary.

••• **Related NIC and NOC labels:** *NIC:* Body Mechanics Promotion; Energy Management; Exercise Promotion; Teaching: Prescribed Activity/Exercise *NOC:* Mobility Level

Nursing Diagnoses:

Self-Care Deficit: Bathing/Hygiene, Dressing/Grooming, Toileting

related to neuromuscular impairment

Desired Outcome: Within 1 mo following intervention/treatment, child begins to assist with or perform ADL.

INTERVENTIONS	RATIONALES
Assess child's developmental and intellectual level.	This assessment enables development of an individualized care plan for assisting child with ADL.
Encourage child to assist with care as much as possible, depending on developmental age and capabilities.	This facilitates child in performing optimum level of self-care.
Encourage parents to have realistic expectations of what the child can do.	Likelihood of success is increased if child is given tasks that he or she can accomplish. For example, an 18-mo-old functioning at the level of a 6-mo-old would not be able to feed self with a spoon.
Use toys and activities that encourage maximum participation by child and improve motor and sensory function.	Improved fine motor control will enable child to accomplish more self-care tasks. For example, in a 5-yr-old with poor fine motor control, putting together large "pop beads" may be an appropriate activity.
Set a series of small goals for child to accomplish. Avoid undue pressure.	Child may be unable or not ready to accomplish final goal but may be able to complete one small task at a time (e.g., picking up brush, holding brush correctly, and then brushing hair).
Encourage use of adaptive clothing and utensils and consumption of finger foods.	These measures facilitate success in self-care. Examples include clothing that opens up in front with self-adhering closures rather than buttons, shoes with self-adhering straps rather than shoe strings, large spoons with padded handles, finger foods and foods that will not slide off the eating utensil.

Continued

INTERVENTIONS	RATIONALES
Provide guidance for toilet training based on developmental age and physical/cognitive abilities.	This is a significant developmental milestone for families and one that causes the most problems in healthy children. Realistic expectations improve chances of child being successful. Methods of toilet training may need to be changed based on child's abilities. For example, a 4-yr-old functioning at the level of a 1-yr-old would not be physically or cognitively ready to be toilet trained.
Stress importance of good oral hygiene and regular dental care. Provide suggestions for how to accomplish this.	There is an increased incidence of dental caries in children with cerebral palsy because of improper dental hygiene (may result from spastic or clonic movements that cause gagging or biting down on toothbrush or from oral hypersensitivity), congenital enamel defects, high carbohydrate intake without proper brushing, dietary imbalance with poor nutritional intake, inadequate fluoride, and difficulty with mouth closure and drooling. Up to 90% of children with cerebral palsy have malocclusion, as well. A child with gum overgrowth from seizure medications, for example, will have gums that bleed easily. Teeth should be brushed after every meal with a soft toothbrush, and child should see dentist q3-6mo for checkup and cleaning beginning at 2-3 yr old.

••• **Related NIC and NOC labels:** *NIC:* Self-Care Assistance: Bathing/Hygiene; Self-Care Assistance: Dressing/Grooming; Self-Care Assistance: Feeding; Self-Care Assistance: Toileting *NOC:* Self-Care: Activities of Daily Living

Nursing Diagnosis:

Impaired Verbal Communication

related to hearing loss, neuromuscular impairment, and difficulty with articulation

Desired Outcome: Within 1 mo of intervention/treatment, child's ability to communicate needs to caregivers improves.

INTERVENTIONS	RATIONALES
Coordinate with speech therapist if child has difficulty with articulation and/or feeding.	Early interventions maximize speech and feeding potential in children with poor control of oral musculature.
Reinforce importance of using speech therapy techniques, including nonverbal methods of communicating, jaw control, and appropriate feeding techniques.	This facilitates goals of speech therapy, which include improving communication and feeding ability, thereby decreasing child's frustration with inability to communicate or eat orally. Increased control of oral musculature improves ability to chew, swallow, and speak.
Speak slowly and clearly when talking with child.	This gives child time to understand speech.
Listen closely to what child says and ask him or her to repeat it if you cannot understand.	Ignoring or not listening to child increases frustrations with failure to communicate.
Use assistive devices such as pictures or flash cards.	These devices promote child's communication ability and mutual understanding of what is being said.
Help family obtain assistive equipment for child.	Such equipment facilitates child's nonverbal communication. Examples include typewriter, communication board, and computer with voice synthesizer. These may be acquired through the school system or funded by Medicaid.

••• **Related NIC and NOC labels:** *NIC:* Active Listening; Communication Enhancement: Hearing Deficit; Communication Enhancement: Speech Deficit; Communication Enhancement: Visual Deficit *NOC:* Communication Ability; Communication: Expressive Ability; Communication: Receptive Ability

ADDITIONAL NURSING DIAGNOSES/ PROBLEMS:

"Psychosocial Support"   p. 73

"Psychosocial Support for the Patient's Family   p. 87
    and Significant Other" for **Interrupted Family
    Processes**

"Seizures and Epilepsy" for care of the patient   p. 323
    undergoing seizures

Fatigue related to increased energy   p. 579
    expenditure

"Asthma" for **Interrupted Family Processes**   p. 581
    related to child having a chronic illness

✓ **PATIENT-FAMILY TEACHING AND DISCHARGE PLANNING**

When providing patient-family teaching, focus on sensory information and avoid giving excessive information. Stress family-centered care (viewing the family as a unit that is the "constant" in child's life and maintaining or improving the health of the family and its members). The child with cerebral palsy may have a wide range of symptoms with varying degrees of severity. Providing support, as well as information about cerebral palsy, is essential in dealing with a lifelong disabled child. Include verbal and written information (ensure that written information is at a level the reader can understand) about the following:

✓ Importance of the multidisciplinary team to evaluate and monitor child on a regular basis and involvement of early intervention programs/school for optimum outcome.

✓ Early intervention program with Individualized Family Service Plan (IFSP) for children from birth to 3 yr old or Individualized Education Plan (IEP) for children 3-21 yr old.

✓ Safety measures appropriate for physical disability and developmental level, including childproofing home.

✓ Medications, including drug name; purpose; dosage; frequency; precautions; drug-drug, food-drug, and herb-drug interactions; and potential side effects.

✓ Carrying a list of medications, dosage, and frequency. Both parents and child should carry this list.

✓ Nutrition, including special formulas, foods, and devices/techniques to help child feed self.

✓ Importance of meticulous oral hygiene, especially if receiving seizure medication that causes gum overgrowth and gums to bleed easily (i.e., brush after each meal with a soft toothbrush and see dentist q3-6mo for cleaning and checkups beginning at 2-3 yr old).

✓ Methods to facilitate communication.

✓ Correct use and care of orthoses and adaptive equipment.

✓ Seizure precautions and care during and after a seizure, if child has seizures.

✓ Routine immunizations, including yearly influenza vaccine and possibly pneumococcal vaccine.

✓ List of telephone numbers to call in case questions or concerns arise about therapy or treatment plan.

✓ Importance of helping siblings cope with/adapt to having a brother/sister with a lifelong disability.

✓ Importance of finding respite care, such as family, friends, support group.

✓ Referral to community resources, such as national and local Cerebral Palsy Association, local community services board, and any available respite care resources.

✓ Additional information can be obtained from:
- United Cerebral Palsy Association at *www.ucpa.org*
- Exceptional Parent Magazine, "Parenting Your Child or Young Adult with a Disability or Special Healthcare Needs" at *www.eparent.com*
- Easter Seals Disability Services at *www.easterseals.com*
- March of Dimes at *www.marchofdimes.com*

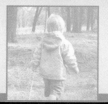

Child Abuse and Neglect 80

OVERVIEW/PATHOPHYSIOLOGY

The problem of child abuse and neglect, formerly called "battered child syndrome," is now recognized as a serious threat to children in the United States. Approximately 3 million cases of suspected abuse/neglect are reported each year, and experts estimate the actual number of incidents of abuse/neglect is 3 times greater than those reported. In 2003, 32% of reported cases were substantiated with about 1500 fatalities (Child Help, 2006). Many more children are left permanently disabled, and thousands of victims are overwhelmed by this trauma for the rest of their lives.

Child abuse and neglect occur in all cultural, ethnic, occupational, and socioeconomic groups. It is not usually a single event but rather a pattern of behavior that occurs over time. The following factors increase the likelihood of abuse or neglect occurring in families:

- **Parental characteristics:** Predisposition to maltreatment (perhaps having been victims themselves), substance abuse, lack of parenting skills, poor impulse control, and emotional immaturity.
- **Child characteristics:** Temperament, physical or cognitive disability that predisposes child to injury, chronic illness or disability, being born to unmarried parents, or hyperactivity.
- **Environmental characteristics:** Divorce, marital problems, financial strain, poor housing, isolation from support of families or friends.
- **Societal factors:** Increased violence, children viewed as property and not valued, physical methods of punishment, lack of willingness in community to become involved in family violence issues.

The highest incidence of child abuse and neglect occurs in children younger than 3 yr old, with the rate declining as children get older (except for sexual abuse). In 2003, more than 60% of victims suffered neglect, 18.9% suffered physical abuse, 9.9% were sexually abused, 4.9% suffered emotional or psychological maltreatment, and 2.3% were medically neglected. In addition, about 17% of the children experienced "other" types of maltreatment such as abandonment, threats of harm to the child, and congenital drug addiction (ACF, HHS, 2003). About one third of the victims experience more than one type of maltreatment. The perpetrators most often are the parents. Terms include:

- **Child maltreatment:** A broad term that includes intentional physical abuse or neglect, emotional abuse or neglect, and sexual abuse (younger than 18 yr old) usually by an adult caregiver, most often the parent.
- **Physical abuse:** The deliberate infliction of physical injury or pain. It may result from punching, beating, kicking, biting, bruising, shaking, burning, or otherwise harming a child and can occur from overdiscipline or physical punishment.
- **Physical neglect:** Failure to provide basic necessities such as food, clothing, shelter, and a safe environment in which the child can grow and develop normally.
- **Emotional abuse:** Deliberate attempt to destroy or significantly impair self-esteem or competence by rejecting, ignoring, criticizing, isolating, or terrorizing the child. The most common form is verbal abuse or "belittling."
- **Emotional neglect:** Failure to meet the child's needs for affection, attention, and emotional support. The most common feature is absence of normal parent-child attachment and interaction.
- **Sexual abuse:** Contacts or interactions between a child and an adult for the adult's sexual gratification, with or without physical contact. It includes pedophilia and all forms of incest and rape. It also includes fondling, oral-genital contact, all forms of intercourse, exhibitionism, voyeurism, and involvement of children in the production of pornography. It is believed to be one of the most common but underreported crimes against children.
- **Medical care neglect:** Failure to provide needed treatment to infants or children who generally have life-threatening or serious medical conditions.
- **Munchausen syndrome by proxy:** Abuse inflicted on a child in which a parent (usually the mother) fabricates symptoms and falsifies medical history or actually causes an illness that results in evaluation and treatment.
- **Shaken baby syndrome (SBS):** Caused by violent shaking of an infant or young child (usually younger than 2 yr old), resulting in severe injury. There are high mortality rates in infant victims, averaging 20% to 25% (AAP,

2001). About 25% of "shaken babies" die of their injuries (Torpy, 2003), and most of the remaining victims suffer permanent physical damage (brain damage, blindness, paralysis, mental retardation, seizures) of varying degrees.

HEALTH CARE SETTING

Primary care or emergency department with possible hospitalization resulting from complications. Abuse/neglect also may be found during hospitalization for other reasons.

ASSESSMENT

Note: History is critical in making a diagnosis. Frequently in child abuse/neglect cases, the history is inconsistent with injury severity, or it changes during evaluation. It is essential that the nurse taking the history be nonjudgmental and report factual information. This is difficult to do at times, and collegial support is beneficial. History and physical examination will determine needed diagnostic tests.

Physical abuse: Acts out violently against others; frightened of parents or caregivers; avoids changing clothes (e.g., in gym class); old, new, and multiple injuries; burn or restraint injuries; questionable bruises and welts; questionable burns (e.g., imprint or immersion); questionable fractures (e.g., spiral fracture); questionable lacerations or abrasions (e.g., human bite marks); skull fractures; or internal abdominal injuries.

Physical neglect: Consistently hungry; poor hygiene (e.g., diaper rash or lice) or inappropriate dress for weather; consistently left without supervision; abandoned; begging or stealing for food; constant fatigue and listlessness; frequently absent or tardy for school; failure to gain weight or failure to thrive (FTT); developmentally delayed; assumes adult responsibility; given inappropriate food, drink, or medication; reportedly ingests harmful substances.

Emotional abuse or neglect: Antisocial or destructive behavior; sleep disorders; habit disorders such as biting, head banging, rocking, or thumb sucking (in an older child); demanding behaviors; self-destructive, suicide attempt; overly adaptive behavior; emotional or intellectual developmental delays; speech disorders.

Sexual abuse: Recurrent abdominal pain; genital, urethral, or anal trauma; sexually transmitted diseases; recurrent urinary tract infections; enuresis (involuntary discharge of urine) or encopresis (incontinence of stool not caused by organic defect or illness); pregnancy; sleep disturbances (e.g., nightmares and night terrors); appetite disturbances (e.g., anorexia or bulimia); neurotic or conductive disorders; withdrawal, guilt, or depression; temper tantrums (in older children); aggressive behaviors; suicidal or runaway threats or behaviors;

hysterical or conversion reactions; excessive masturbation; sexualized play in developmentally immature children; school problems; promiscuity; reluctance to change clothes. Many children have normal genital examinations.

Munchausen syndrome by proxy: Signs and symptoms only occur when the perpetrator (usually the mother) is present. Common presenting indicators include poisoning, seizures, apnea, bleeding, vomiting, diarrhea, fever, and even cardiopulmonary arrest.

SBS: Often there are no external signs of injury other than change in level of consciousness. The child may have history of poor feeding, vomiting, lethargy, and irritability occurring for several days or weeks. More severe shaking may cause brain damage, seizures, blindness, paralysis, and death. On ophthalmologic examination, retinal hemorrhages are seen. Anterior fontanel may be tense or full when infant is quiet.

DIAGNOSTIC TESTS

Radiographs of injured area or skeletal survey: Certain findings on x-ray examination are strong indicators of physical abuse. These include metaphyseal "corner" or "bucket handle" fractures of long bones in infants, spiral fractures of long bones in nonambulatory infants, and multiple fractures of ribs or long bones in varying stages of healing. These findings may help distinguish abuse from osteogenesis imperfecta (an inherited condition marked by abnormally brittle bones that are subject to fracture).

CT scan or MRI scan: May reveal subdural hematoma and subarachnoid hemorrhage, hallmark signs of SBS. Computerized axial tomography (CT) scans and magnetic resonance imaging (MRI) scans may also diagnose abdominal injuries from abuse.

Ophthalmology examinations: May reveal retinal hemorrhages (usually bilateral), hallmark signs of SBS.

Bone scans: Detect soft tissue and bone trauma, especially in locating unseen fractures or bone injuries. For example, they can define rib fractures, which are difficult to assess because of overlying structures such as the heart, lungs, and liver.

Coagulation studies: Used in children with many bruises in different stages to differentiate abuse from a medical condition such as leukemia or bleeding or clotting disorders.

Complete blood count: Helps rule out medical condition in child with FTT.

Forensic evaluation: In sexually abused children, it may be done to identify evidence such as semen or detect sexually transmitted disease.

Nursing Diagnosis:

Risk for Injury

related to family history of neglect or physical, emotional, or sexual abuse

Desired Outcome: Following intervention/treatment, child exhibits no further evidence of abuse or neglect.

INTERVENTIONS	RATIONALES
Assess child's physical and mental status as follows: - Note bruises, scars, or other signs of abuse. - Note unusual interactions or responses of child.	A thorough evaluation should be done on all children in all health care settings. Abuse occurs in all cultural and socioeconomic groups and may not be the admitting diagnosis.
Observe interactions between child and family.	Signs of abuse or neglect may be detected in the way the child interacts with parents and other adults. For example, a child who is emotionally neglected may not want to be held or have eye contact with the parent or other adult.
Obtain detailed history.	This may detect a pattern of injury or neglect or lack of correlation between history and severity of injury; or history may change as examination progresses.
Keep factual, detailed, objective records for documentation.	Medical records may be subpoenaed as evidence in court proceedings and therefore need to be as detailed and objective as possible. Being factual (i.e., no opinions, impressions, or interpretations) is imperative. Records should include the following: - Physical condition (e.g., "Three small, well-delineated, circular lesions, approximately 3-5 mm in diameter and 1 mm in depth, dark purple-red, noted on sole of left foot"). - Pictures, which are most beneficial in documenting injuries, need to be dated and kept in patient's chart. - Child's behavioral response to parents, others, and environment (e.g., child with FTT often does not verbally or physically interact with anyone). - Specific comments of child, parents, or other family members and developmental age of child.
Use nonjudgmental, nonthreatening manner when interacting with child's parents.	Frequently it is unclear who actually abused the child. Child is more likely to be helped if parents trust staff. If parents feel alienated by staff, they may deny child access to care. Parents will be more receptive to teaching in a trusting environment.
Report all cases of suspected child abuse or neglect.	All 50 states consider health care workers mandatory reporters of child abuse/neglect.
Keep child in a safe environment in the hospital (e.g., near the nurses' station).	Suspected abuser may be restricted from visiting, or only certain individuals may be approved to visit.
Assist in removing child from unsafe situation (whether verbal or physical neglect or abuse is suspected). Report any suspicious behavior to Social Services in the hospital and Child Protective Services in the community.	Nurses are mandated reporters of suspected neglect or abuse in all 50 states.
Refer families to social agencies for assistance with finances, food, clothing, and health care.	These measures help ameliorate causes of neglect.
Collaborate with multidisciplinary health care team involved with case.	This provides continual evaluation of progress/status of child in hospital, foster care, or on return to home.
Help parents identify events that precipitate an abusive act (i.e., crying is a major trigger) and alternative ways to deal with release of anger (e.g., role playing).	This may prevent further abuse for this child or siblings.

●●● **Related NIC and NOC labels:** *NIC:* Risk Identification; Abuse Protection Support: Child; Health Screening; Surveillance: Safety
NOC: Parenting: Social Safety

Nursing Diagnosis:

Risk for Impaired Parenting

related to child's, caregiver's, or situational characteristics that precipitate child abuse or neglect

Desired Outcome: Within 1 wk following interventions, parents demonstrate more positive interactions with the child and more appropriate parenting activities, and verbalize accurate understanding of normal expectations for the child.

INTERVENTIONS	RATIONALES
Identify families at risk for abuse/neglect.	Identifying at-risk families is the first step in helping prevent abuse or neglect. Such families tend to have immature, single parents; parents who were abused as children; premature infant; child younger than 3 yr old or with a chronic illness or disability; parental substance abuse; limited social network/support.
Observe parents' interactions with child.	This is the best way to get a realistic view of the relationship. For example, when feeding the child, the parent may avoid making eye contact or touching the child unless absolutely necessary.
Assess parents' strengths and weaknesses, normal coping behaviors, and presence or absence of support systems.	This assessment provides the basis for developing an appropriate plan of care and making necessary referrals.
Demonstrate age-appropriate child-rearing practices, especially communication and discipline.	Parents may care for their child in the way their parents cared for them and may not know age-appropriate child-rearing practices.
Teach alternative methods of discipline, such as rewards, time-out, consequences, and verbal disapproval.	Parents may not know any nonviolent methods of discipline.
Provide care for child until parent is ready to provide care.	This allows parents time to "relax" and observe age-appropriate care.
Encourage parents to participate in care of child. Reinforce positive behaviors.	This helps build self-esteem and confidence in parents to improve interactions.
Focus on positive aspects of child (e.g., "What beautiful eyes your child has" or "Tell me something your child is good at").	Parents may have negative view of child, and this gives them another perspective.
Teach family what to expect in terms of growth and development for their child—physical, psychosocial, and cognitive—through role modeling and having parents return demonstration.	Parents will incorporate information better if not "instructed" and feeling as though they are being criticized. This increases their knowledge and reinforces accurate expectations of what is normal for the child.
Also provide education about nutrition, care related to activities of daily living, routine well-child care, manifestations of illness, and importance of caring/loving attitude in dealing with children.	This information increases realistic expectations and chance of positive parenting.
Convey nonjudgmental attitude of genuine concern.	Such an attitude facilitates developing trust and respect and enables parents to observe and develop better methods of caring for the child.
Refer family to appropriate social agencies to assist with financial support, adequate housing, employment, and so on.	This ameliorates risk factors of abuse/neglect.
Help identify support systems for parents such as extended family, neighbors, or support groups.	Support systems decrease family stress and hence decrease risk of abuse/neglect.

••• **Related NIC and NOC labels:** *NIC:* Abuse Protection Support: Child; Developmental Enhancement: Child; Risk Identification; Surveillance: Safety; Family Support; Self-Esteem Enhancement; Self-Modification Assistance; Support Group *NOC:* Parenting: Social Safety

Nursing Diagnoses:

Fear/Anxiety

related to maltreatment, powerlessness, and potential loss of parents

Desired Outcome: Within 72 hr following interventions, child verbalizes source of fear/anxiety and exhibits more interactivity and sociability and less withdrawal.

INTERVENTIONS	RATIONALES
Provide consistent caregivers and an age-appropriate safe environment.	These measures help relieve child's anxiety and provide a positive role model for family.
Reassure child about his or her personal safety.	Verbal reassurance increases sense of security.
Demonstrate acceptance of child but do not reinforce inappropriate behaviors.	Children need acceptance, as well as guidance regarding appropriate behaviors.
Support child in talking about family or stressful events.	Verbalization of fears/anxieties decreases their impact on children.
Do not ask too many questions.	This may upset child and interfere with other professionals' interrogations.
Encourage play, especially with family or dollhouse activity.	Play is the "work of the child" and may help reveal types of relationships perceived by child. This could include, for example, playing with dolls that represent father, mother, and siblings or drawing pictures of events. The child may tell the story of events with dolls. Drawings often depict fears and reactions to experiences.
Incorporate therapeutic play into care activities if possible.	This helps children cope with new, frightening experiences in a non-threatening way. For example, have child check blood pressure on doll before checking it on him or her.
Treat child as you would other children, not as an "abused" victim.	This encourages child to interact with others rather than promoting isolation.
Offer choices whenever possible regarding clothing, diet, and other activities of daily living (ADL); recreation time; and socialization time.	Being allowed to make choices provides a sense of control and decreases sense of powerlessness, and hence anxiety.

••• **Related NIC and NOC labels:** *NIC:* Anxiety Reduction; Active Listening; Coping Enhancement; Security Enhancement; Therapeutic Play; Abuse Protection Support *NOC:* Anxiety Control; Fear Control

PATIENT-FAMILY TEACHING AND DISCHARGE PLANNING

When providing patient-family teaching, focus on sensory information, avoid giving excessive information, and initiate a visiting nurse referral for necessary follow-up teaching and assessment. Stress family-centered care (viewing the family as a unit that is the "constant" in the child's life and maintaining or improving the health of the family and its members in a holistic manner). Include verbal and written information about the following, ensuring that it is written at a level understandable to the child/family:

✓ Care related to any specific injury.

✓ Realistic expectations for individual child related to:

• Growth and development (e.g., regression is normal after a child has been hospitalized or severely stressed)

• Nutrition (e.g., toddler's food jags—may only want one food for every meal for several days)

✓ Guidelines based on developmental level:

• Safety (e.g., preschooler does not understand danger of chasing a ball across the street)

• Need for love and attention

✓ Methods of handling normal developmental problems that increase parent's stress level (e.g., toddler's negativism, temper tantrums, toilet training, and need for rituals and routines).

✓ Demonstration of care related to ADL; observe return demonstration by parents.

✓ Importance of regular well-child visits and provision of routine well-child care.

✓ Suggestions for nonviolent, age-appropriate methods of disciplining child (e.g., reward, time-out, consequences, and verbal disapproval).

✓ Identification of stressful situations for parents and ways to deal with them. For example, if an infant cries for prolonged periods, make sure that infant is clean and dry and is not uncomfortable, hungry, or ill; put infant in crib on his or her back and go out of the room. DO NOT SHAKE THE BABY. This can cause severe damage.

✓ Review of situations/circumstances that precipitate abuse/violence and of methods to deal with anger constructively.

✓ Importance of providing child with positive reinforcement of appropriate behavior to build self-esteem.

✓ Teaching child the difference between "good touch" and "bad touch."

✓ Name or place a child can go if being abused (e.g., neighborhood "safe house").

✓ Suggestions for local support systems (e.g., extended family members, church members, neighbors).

✓ Referrals to community resources, such as parenting classes, support groups, public health nurse, social worker, and financial counseling if appropriate. Additional general information can be obtained by contacting the following organizations:

- Parents Anonymous, Inc., at *www.parentsanonymous.org*. This group provides support and resources for overwhelmed families.
- National Child Abuse Hotline at (800) 4-A-CHILD (1-800-422-4453) or *www.childhelpusa.org*
- Prevent Child Abuse America at *www.preventchildabuse.org*
- Shaken Baby Alliance at *www.shakenbaby.com*
- National Center on Shaken Baby Syndrome at *www.dontshake.com*

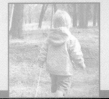

Cystic Fibrosis 81

OVERVIEW/PATHOPHYSIOLOGY

Cystic fibrosis (CF) is a chronic, progressive multisystem disease in which there is a dysfunction of the exocrine (mucus-producing) glands and abnormal transport of sodium and chloride across the epithelium. This results in abnormally thick secretions, causing obstruction of the small passageways of many organs. CF is an autosomal recessive hereditary disease with more than 1000 gene mutations. This is why there is such a wide variation in clinical manifestations.

In the recent past, CF was described as the most common lethal genetic illness in white children. The median life expectancy has improved dramatically from 7.5 years in 1966 (Hockenberry, 2003) to 36.8 years in 2006 (CFF, 2006). The median life expectancy has increased 5 years over the past 4 years because of earlier diagnosis, antibiotic therapy, improved nutritional management, and recent breakthroughs in treatment.

About 30,000 people in the United States have CF, and more than 40% are 18 yr old or older. CF occurs in approximately 1 in every 3200 live Caucasian births (1 in every 3500 live births of all Americans). More than 10 million Americans are genetic carriers (CFF, 2006).

HEALTH CARE SETTING

Primary care, with possible hospitalization for CF exacerbation or other complications

ASSESSMENT

Initially involves overall appraisal, including monitoring general activity, physical findings, nutritional status, and chest x-ray examination.

Signs and symptoms: Vary widely, as does the severity of involvement of specific organ systems. Patients tend to have periods without acute symptoms and then periods with acute exacerbation of symptoms. The first clinical manifestation may be meconium ileus in a newborn, or the patient may not have symptoms for months or years.

Most of the usual symptoms are caused by the following:

- **Progressive chronic obstructive lung disease:** Initially wheezing and dry cough, progressing to paroxysmal cough that frequently causes posttussive emesis. Other signs include increased dyspnea, barrel chest, mild to severe clubbing of nail beds, cyanosis, and repeated pulmonary infec-

tions that cause scarring and bronchiectasis. Numerous complications such as pneumothorax and hemoptysis often occur.

- **Pancreatic enzyme deficiency** resulting from duct blockage (present in 80%-85% of children with CF): Stools that are frothy (bulky and large), foul smelling, fat containing (steatorrhea), and float (four *F*'s of CF); voracious appetite initially, progressing to loss of appetite late in the disease; weight loss, marked tissue wasting, protuberant abdomen with thin extremities, failure to thrive (FTT), anemia; and evidence of deficiency of fat-soluble vitamins (A, D, E, K). Complications include pancreatic fibrosis leading to glucose intolerance, diabetes mellitus (DM), and pancreatitis. Incidence of DM is greater in children with CF than in the general population. CF-related DM is found in 35% of adults 20-29 yr old and in 43% of those older than 30 yr (CFF, 2005).

- **Sweat gland dysfunction** resulting in increased sodium and chloride concentrations. Infant "tastes" salty and is more susceptible to dehydration.

Other GI complications: Include intestinal obstruction in infants, distal intestinal obstruction syndrome in adolescents and adults, and rectal prolapse, which occurs in 20% of children with CF (keepkidshealthy, 2006) usually younger than 5 yr old.

Liver complications: Biliary cirrhosis and gallbladder dysfunction.

DIAGNOSTIC TESTS

CF has been called the "great imitator" because signs of chronic respiratory infection and FTT are symptoms of many other childhood conditions.

Chest x-ray examination: Shows characteristic patchy atelectasis and chronic obstructive emphysema.

Pulse oximetry: Reveals decreased oxygen saturation.

Complete blood count: Increased white blood cells with increased neutrophils on differential count will be present with infection.

Pilocarpine iontophoresis (quantitative sweat chloride test): Production of sweat is stimulated with a special device, and the sweat is collected and measured. Diagnosis is made with sodium and chloride levels greater than 60 mEq/L (levels of 40-60 are considered suggestive and should be repeated) and the presence of clinical symptoms or a family history of CF. Sweat test is not usually done before 4-6 wk of age because the infant has decreased sweat production until then.

Pulmonary function tests (after 5-6 yr old): Assess degree of pulmonary disease and response to therapy and help distinguish between restrictive and obstructive pulmonary disease. In the presence of CF the test will show decreased vital capacity (VC) and tidal volume, increased airway resistance, increased residual volume, and decreased FEV_1 (forced expiratory volume in 1 sec) and FEV_1/VC ratio.

Stool fat and/or enzyme analysis to determine pancreatic involvement: For digestive enzymes, stool must be fresh or frozen immediately. Trypsin (breaks down dietary proteins) is either absent or severely diminished in children with CF. For fat content (steatorrhea), stool is collected over 72 hr with

documented and measured intake. The test will show significant increase in fat content because of malabsorption.

Sputum culture: For identification of infective organisms and sensitivity of these organisms. Many resistant organisms develop because of the frequency of respiratory infections.

Immunoreactive trypsinogen test: Newborn screening test that can be done at the same time as phenylketonuria and other screening tests. This test enables early detection and treatment of CF and is done several days after birth. If positive, it is confirmed by a mutation analysis (i.e., genetic testing). The combination of these two tests is sensitive 90%-100% of the time.

DNA analysis of chorionic villi or amniotic fluid: Can establish prenatal diagnosis.

Nursing Diagnosis:

Ineffective Airway Clearance

related to thick, tenacious mucus in airways

Desired Outcome: Immediately following treatment/interventions, child expectorates mucus and exhibits improved airway clearance as evidenced by improved breath sounds and HR and RR within child's normal limits.

INTERVENTIONS	RATIONALES
Assess heart rate (HR), respiratory rate (RR), and breath sounds.	This assessment establishes baseline data from which to compare later findings. With ineffective airway clearance, the child will have increased HR and RR. Breath sounds may be decreased with little air movement because of the blocked airway, or adventitious sounds may be increased because of mucus in the airway.
Assist child with sputum expectoration (may be done by respiratory therapist):	
- Assess HR, RR, breath sounds, and O_2 saturation before nebulization and after chest physiotherapy.	Assessment before and after treatment monitors effectiveness of treatment.
- Position child in an upright sitting position, ensuring that he or she does not slouch.	This position facilitates maximum inhalation of medication and improves effectiveness of cough to clear secretions out of airways.
- Administer nebulization (albuterol) as prescribed 1 hr before or 2 hr after meals.	This treatment opens bronchi and loosens secretions. It usually causes considerable coughing followed by expectoration of mucus and sometimes vomiting from excessive coughing. Scheduling in relation to meals is essential to provide maximum benefit of treatment and prevent interference with nutrient ingestion. Treatment before breakfast helps loosen secretions that built up overnight. Treatment before bedtime helps clear secretions that would otherwise provide a medium for bacterial growth.
- Perform chest physiotherapy after nebulizer treatment. Examples follow.	This helps to loosen secretions, which will facilitate their expectoration. This treatment is performed at least 2-4 times/day for maintenance/routine daily care. Method used depends on age of child, effectiveness of technique, child/parent's ability to perform/tolerate technique, and preference of child/parent.
- *Chest percussion and postural drainage for 20-30 min*	Chest percussion loosens secretions, and postural drainage facilitates drainage of secretions so that they can be expectorated.

Continued

INTERVENTIONS

- *Mucus clearance device (e.g., flutter valve) used for 5-15 min*

- *Airway clearance system (e.g., The Vest).*

- Suction as necessary.

Ensure that child is receiving at least maintenance fluids.

Administer dornase alfa (Pulmozyme) as prescribed.

RATIONALES

This handheld pipelike device has a plastic mouthpiece on one end that child breathes into. On the other end of the pipe a stainless steel ball rests inside a plastic circular cone. Exhaling into the device vibrates the airways, thereby loosening mucus from the airway walls and accelerating airflow, which facilitates upward movement of mucus so that it can be more readily cleared. This device is very effective and gives child control because it can be used without assistance of others.

This inflatable vest fits like a life jacket and is connected by tubes to a generator. The vest inflates and deflates rapidly, applying gentle pressure to the chest. It provides high frequency chest wall oscillation to help loosen secretions and increase mucus expectoration.

For infants/young children or if there is a large volume of mucus, assistance may be needed to clear secretions from the airway. However, children usually cough sufficiently after nebulizer treatment and chest physiotherapy to clear secretions independently.

Hydration thins and loosens secretions for easier expectoration.

This medication thins mucus, which will facilitate expectoration.

●●● **Related NIC and NOC labels:** *NIC:* Airway Suctioning; Chest Physiotherapy; Positioning; Vital Signs Monitoring; Cough Enhancement; Medication Administration: Inhalation *NOC:* Respiratory Status: Gas Exchange; Respiratory Status: Airway Patency

Nursing Diagnosis:

Impaired Gas Exchange

related to airway obstruction secondary to air trapping in alveoli and airways narrowed by tenacious mucus

Desired Outcome: Within 2 hr following treatment/intervention, child has adequate gas exchange as evidenced by O_2 saturation greater than 92% (or consistent with child's baseline).

INTERVENTIONS

Along with vital signs, assess respiratory status q2-4h, or more frequently as indicated by child's condition.

Ensure continuous monitoring of pulse oximetry readings; report low value (usually 92% or lower).

Monitor for behavioral indicators of hypoxia.

Be alert to changes in child's skin color.

Position child in high Fowler's position and/or leaning forward.

Deliver O_2 along with humidity via most appropriate delivery system and at rate prescribed.

Monitor child on O_2 delivery closely.

RATIONALES

Increased HR and RR would occur with impaired gas exchange, as would chest retractions, increased work of breathing (WOB), nasal flaring, and use of accessory muscles of respiration. These are signs of respiratory distress necessitating prompt intervention/treatment.

Decreased O_2 saturation can indicate need for initiation of/increased O_2.

Restlessness, mood changes, and/or change in level of consciousness are early signs of O_2 deficiency.

Cyanosis of the lips and nail beds is a late indicator of hypoxia and a signal of the need for prompt treatment/intervention.

These positions promote comfort and optimal gas exchange by enabling maximal chest expansion.

The child's developmental age helps determine the most effective delivery system and flow rate (e.g., nasal cannula for infants with liter flow rate less than 4). Humidity use replaces convective losses of moisture.

O_2-induced CO_2 narcosis is a hazard of O_2 therapy in the child with chronic pulmonary disease. If O_2 saturation is consistently greater than 96%, for example, it is likely that the flow rate can be decreased slowly by small increments.

Continued

INTERVENTIONS	RATIONALES
Encourage games or physical exercise appropriate to child's condition (e.g., blowing bubbles or walking) but avoid overexertion.	Breathing more deeply facilitates clearing of mucus and improves oxygenation.
Provide neutral thermal environment for child.	This is a room temperature in which the body does not have to use as much energy to stay warm or cool off, thereby enabling child to use energy to grow or heal. With decreased energy demands, more O_2 is available to ensure these needs are met.

••• **Related NIC and NOC labels:** *NIC:* Oxygen Therapy; Energy Management; Positioning; Respiratory Monitoring; Vital Signs Monitoring *NOC:* Respiratory Status: Gas Exchange; Vital Signs Status

Nursing Diagnosis:

Imbalanced Nutrition: Less Than Body Requirements

related to decreased appetite (advanced disease) or increased metabolic requirements because of increased WOB, infection, and/or malabsorption

Desired Outcome: By discharge or within 7 days after treatment/intervention, patient maintains or gains weight and does not have more than 2 or 3 stools per day.

INTERVENTIONS	RATIONALES
Administer pancreatic enzymes with meals and snacks per health care provider's prescription if child has pancreatic insufficiency (80%-85% of children with CF).	Replacement of enzymes is necessary for proper digestion and absorption of nutrients. Failure to replace pancreatic enzymes would affect child's growth and ability to fight infection.
For young children unable to swallow a capsule, mix powder, granules, or contents of the capsule with a small amount of carbohydrate food.	Protein foods break down this enzyme and can burn mouths of infants and young children. Using smallest amount of food possible (e.g., 1-2 tsp of applesauce) helps ensure that the child receives all the medication.
Do not administer with formula/milk in a bottle or cup.	Pancreatic enzymes curdle milk and formula. In addition, the child may not receive all the medication and may not take milk/formula in the future if he or she associates it with medication.
Monitor and document frequency and appearance of stools.	Pancreatic enzymes are adjusted to provide normal stooling (i.e., decreased enzymes given with constipation; increased enzymes given with frequent, bulky, foul-smelling stools that float). Normal stooling indicates increased absorption of nutrients.
Provide well-balanced, high-calorie, high-protein diet (usually 1.5-2 times recommended daily allowance).	Only 80%-85% of nutrients are absorbed in children with CF who have gastrointestinal (GI) involvement.
Provide adequate salt, especially with fever, hot weather, or exercise.	Patient is at risk for electrolyte imbalance (hyponatremia) because sodium concentration in sweat of a child with CF is 2-5 times greater than that of a child without CF.
Administer fat-soluble vitamins in water-miscible form (i.e., mixed in a suspension that will not separate) as prescribed.	This counteracts malabsorption of fat-soluble vitamins (A, D, E, and K). Examples of water-miscible forms of vitamins include Aquasol A and ADEK.
Administer iron preparations as prescribed.	Malabsorption can cause iron deficiency.
Administer supplemental tube feedings (nasogastric tube [NGT] or gastric tube [GT]) or total parenteral nutrition (TPN) as prescribed.	Measures described in previous interventions alone are not always effective in child exhibiting FTT. Supplemental feedings via NGT, GT, or TPN provide increased calories to treat malnutrition.
Ensure daily weight measurements in the hospital and teach importance of weekly weight measurements at home.	This assesses effectiveness of nutritional interventions. If the child is losing weight, he or she may not be receiving adequate nutrients or may not be absorbing nutrients properly.

••• **Related NIC and NOC labels:** *NIC:* Nutrition Management; Medication Management; Nutrition Therapy; Sustenance Therapy; Enteral Tube Feeding; Total Parenteral Nutrition *NOC:* Nutritional Status: Nutrient Intake

Nursing Diagnosis:

Deficient Knowledge:

Purpose, precautions, and potential side effects of prescribed medications

Desired Outcome: Within 1 wk of diagnosis or change in medication, patient/parent
verbalizes accurate information about prescribed medications.

INTERVENTIONS	RATIONALES
Teach the Following to Patient/Parent for the Prescribed Drugs	
Aerosolized Bronchodilators: Albuterol	This medication helps open the bronchi for easier expectoration of mucus. Route is via nebulizer or metered-dose inhalers (MDIs).
- Be alert for and report palpitations, increased HR, chest pain, muscle tremors, dizziness, headache.	These are side effects that may indicate the need for dosage adjustment.
- Be alert for and report nervousness, central nervous system (CNS) stimulation, hyperactivity, and insomnia.	These are side effects that occur more often in younger children than in adults.
- All above symptoms, as well as dry mouth, may occur with MDI. Notify prescriber if they persist.	These are additional side effects.
- Limit caffeinated beverages.	Caffeine may increase side effects such as CNS stimulation and insomnia.
- Do not take with beta-adrenergic blocking agents (e.g., propranolol), monoamine oxidase inhibitors (MAOIs), tricyclic antidepressants.	Propranolol antagonizes action of albuterol. MAOIs potentiate sympathomimetic effects. Tricyclic antidepressants increase cardiovascular effects.
- Do not take with other sympathomimetics.	Albuterol increases cardiovascular effects.
- Rinse mouth with water following each inhalation of MDI.	Rinsing helps moisten dry mouth and throat.
Aerosolized Mucolytic Enzymes: Dornase Alfa (Pulmozyme)	This medication thins secretions and optimally decreases number of pulmonary infections.
- Use with appropriate nebulizer system.	A nebulizer unit is available that is made specifically to administer this medication.
- Be alert to and report hoarseness, pharyngitis, laryngitis, rash, chest pain, and conjunctivitis.	Typically side effects are mild and subside within a few weeks.
- Do not dilute or mix with other drugs in nebulizer.	These actions may deactivate the drug.
- Store in refrigerator and discard if unopened vials are subjected to room temperature for more than 24 hr.	Room temperature may deactivate medication.
- Protect from strong light. Discard if solution is cloudy or discolored.	These are signs that the medication may be deactivated.
Aerosolized Antibiotics: Tobramycin (Tobi)	This medication helps fight infection, which would cause increased symptoms.
- Be alert to and report hoarseness, shortness of breath, increased cough, pharyngitis, and hoarseness.	These are side effects.
- Store in refrigerator. Date and time the drug when removing it from refrigerator.	Tobi can only be used for 28 days when stored at room temperature.
- Do not use if cloudy or contains particles.	These are signs that the medication is compromised.
- Protect from intense light.	Light adversely affects Tobi.
- Do not take with dornase alfa (Pulmozyme).	When tobramycin and Pulmozyme are mixed, a precipitate may form.
- Take bronchodilator first, then chest physiotherapy, then other inhaled medications, and tobramycin last.	This is the most effective method of administration because when airways are clear, absorption of Tobi is enhanced.
- Ensure that serum aminoglycoside level is monitored for patients on high-dose aerosolized tobramycin.	This identifies patients who are significant absorbers and may be at risk for ototoxicity and nephrotoxicity.
Pancreatic Enzymes	These enzymes increase food and nutrient absorption.
- As prescribed, take with meals and snacks within 30 min of eating.	Taking enzymes in this manner promotes degradation and absorption of nutrients just consumed.

Continued

INTERVENTIONS

- If patient is an infant or young child, may open capsule and give in small amount of nonfat, nonprotein food (e.g., 1-2 tsp applesauce).

- Do not mix with milk or formula.

- Do not chew microspheres or microtabs; swallow capsules or tablets whole.

- Monitor stools for frequency and appearance.

- Do not take if allergic to pork or patient has acute or chronic pancreatitis.

- Be alert for and report nausea, abdominal cramps, mouth irritation, sneezing, constipation, or diarrhea.

- Notify prescriber if patient is taking H2 antagonists or gastric acid pump inhibitors (e.g., ranitidine, cimetidine, omeprazole).

Vitamins/Minerals

- Take vitamins A, D, E, and K in water-miscible form as prescribed.

Antibiotics—Usually IV (e.g., Ticarcillin, Tobramycin)

- Take as prescribed, usually for at least 10 days and often for several weeks.

- Monitor for side effects specific to each individual antibiotic.

RATIONALES

Protein foods break down this enzyme and can burn mouth in infant/young child.

Pancreatic enzymes curdle milk or formula.

Chewing or mouth retention before swallowing may cause mucosal irritation and stomatitis.

Constipation or increased stooling (more than 3 stools/day) indicates need to adjust dosage.

These are contraindications for use.

These are side effects that may indicate the need for dosage adjustment.

These agents increase effectiveness of pancreatic enzymes; dosage adjustment may be needed.

They supplement overall diet.

The water-miscible form enables absorption of fat-soluble vitamins.

These medications are used to treat infections.

Children with CF have frequent respiratory infections and often develop drug resistance. Antibiotics may need to be given for an extended time.

Side effects vary, depending on specific antibiotic.

••• **Related NIC and NOC labels:** *NIC:* Teaching: Prescribed Medication *NOC:* Knowledge: Medication

ADDITIONAL NURSING DIAGNOSES/PROBLEMS:

"Psychosocial Support" for relevant nursing diagnoses that pertain to patient's psychologic status in dealing with a chronic and potentially fatal illness — p. 73

"Psychosocial Support for the Patient's Family and Significant Other" for relevant nursing diagnoses for family members dealing with a chronic and potentially fatal illness in their loved one — p. 87

"Diabetes Mellitus" for **Risk for Infection** related to chronic disease process — p. 381

"Asthma" for **Anxiety** related to illness, loss of control, and medical/nursing interventions — p. 580

Interrupted Family Processes — p. 581

"Burns" for **Disturbed Body Image** related to delayed puberty, copious sputum and chronic cough, inability to maintain weight, and/or possible presence of GT — p. 605

 PATIENT-FAMILY TEACHING AND DISCHARGE PLANNING

When providing child-family teaching, focus on sensory data, avoid excessive information, and initiate a visiting nurse referral for necessary follow-up assessment or teaching. Stress family-centered care (viewing the family as a unit that is the "constant" in the child's life and maintaining or improving the health of the family and its members in a holistic manner). Include verbal and written information about the following and ensure that written information is at a level the reader can understand:

✓ Basic information about disease process with emphasis on respiratory and GI components.

✓ Remission/maintenance and exacerbation aspects of this chronic disease process.

✓ Diet, including rationale for increased calories and protein (usually two to three snacks/day).

✓ Administration of pancreatic enzymes with meals and snacks (usually a fractional dose given with snacks).

- If patient is an infant or young child, may mix contents of capsule, granules, or powder with a small amount of applesauce or other carbohydrate food.

- Do not chew or bite capsule or enteric-coated microspheres.

- Do not administer in bottle or cup with fluid.

✓ Need for salt replacement and free access for child to salt, especially during hot weather, fever, diarrhea, or vomiting.

✓ GI symptoms that signal malabsorption and inadequate enzyme replacement (e.g., bloating, abdominal cramping and distention, and diarrhea).

✓ Need to monitor stools (constipation indicates too much enzyme; frequent fatty loose stools indicate insufficient enzyme).

✓ Administration of nebulizer treatment and chest physiotherapy (i.e., chest percussion and postural drainage, mucus clearance device [e.g., FLUTTER] or a vest airway clearance system [e.g., The Vest]). Nebulizer treatment is done first (1 hr before or 2 hr after meals), followed by chest physiotherapy. Stress the importance of routine pulmonary toilet because thickened mucus is an ideal medium for bacterial growth, which causes pulmonary infections.

✓ Cleaning and care of equipment (e.g., nebulizer attachments for albuterol and Pulmozyme).

✓ Medications, including drug name; route; purpose; dosage; precautions; drug-drug, food-drug, and herb-drug interactions; and potential adverse effects.

✓ Importance of taking medication at home and at school as directed. Medication in the original container (with prescribing label) and written prescription from health care provider are needed for child to be able take medication at school.

✓ Importance of regular medical follow-up care:
- Routine immunizations plus pneumococcal vaccinations and yearly influenza vaccination
- Prompt attention to infection (fever, increased coughing, green sputum)
- Regular visits with health care provider

✓ Team care approach, including pediatrician, school nurse and teachers, pulmonologist, or infectious disease physician. Ensure that a genetic referral is made.

✓ Realistic expectations for the child, especially concerning growth and development, participation in school activities and sports, and child's participation/responsibility for self-care.

✓ Child's legal rights: Section 504 of Rehabilitation Act of 1973. Each student with a disability (physical or mental impairment) is entitled to accommodation in order to attend school and participate as fully as possible in school activities. A child with significant pulmonary involvement may need to be excused from class for 15-30 min after receiving a nebulizer treatment and chest physiotherapy because of excessive coughing and expectoration of mucus, or the class schedule might need to be rearranged to accommodate required treatment.

✓ Telephone numbers to call in case questions or concerns arise about therapy or disease after discharge.

✓ When to call health care provider:
- Increased respiratory effort (e.g., increased RR, nasal flaring, retractions)
- Excessive coughing and/or coughing up blood
- Color change: pallor or cyanosis (blue around mouth or eyes)
- Temperature increase to greater than 101.5° F lasting more than a few days or a low-grade fever lasting for a week or more
- Weight loss
- Abdominal pain or distention, with or without constipation

✓ Referral to community resources such as support groups, specialists working with children affected by CF, CF care center if available, and genetic counselors.

✓ Additional information can be obtained by contacting:
- Cystic Fibrosis Foundation at *www.cff.org*
- STARBRIGHT Foundation at *www.starbright.org*
- Information for FLUTTER mucus clearance device, high-calorie shakes, and pancreatic enzymes at *www. axcanscandipharm.com*
- Information for The Vest at *www.thevest.com*
- CareFirst for CF at *www.axcan.com/pub/carefirst. php?lang=*. This program helps ease financial burden of infants (includes children up to 2 years of age). It must be prescribed by health care provider.
- Comprehensive Care Program for CF at *www.axcan. com//pub/comprehensive.php?lang=1*. This program provides additional support for CF patients by helping reduce cost of therapy (includes a certificate for a FLUTTER mucus clearance device).

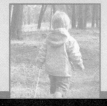

Diabetes Mellitus in Children 82

OVERVIEW/PATHOPHYSIOLOGY

Diabetes mellitus (DM) is the most common childhood endocrine disorder and one of the most costly chronic diseases of childhood. It is a disorder of carbohydrate metabolism marked by hyperglycemia and glycosuria, and it results from inadequate production or use of insulin. The major classifications seen in children are as follows:

- **Type 1 DM:** There is an absolute deficiency of insulin secretion resulting from destruction of beta cells, causing hyperglycemia and ketosis. This destruction is often an immune-mediated or related response. Previously it was called insulin-dependent DM (IDDM) or juvenile onset diabetes. Historically, this was the primary type of diabetes seen in children. Currently, approximately 176,500 people younger than 20 have diabetes in the United States. Type 1 DM is found in 1 in every 400-600 children and more than 13,000 children are diagnosed with type 1 DM each year. Incidence peaks during puberty (10-12 yr in girls and 12-14 yr in boys), although children have been diagnosed in infancy. About 75% of all newly diagnosed cases of type 1 DM occur in individuals younger than 18 years old (National Diabetes Education Program or NDEP, 2006). These children are dependent on insulin for survival and to prevent diabetic ketoacidosis (DKA). Even with insulin, type 1 diabetes shortens the life span by 15 yr.

- **Type 2 DM:** There is an insulin resistance with this type, so there is a relative, not absolute, insulin deficiency. Previously this was called non–insulin-dependent DM (NIDDM) or adult-onset DM. In the 1990s, there was an alarming epidemic of children developing type 2 DM. Children as young as 8 yr old with an average age of 13-14 yr old were being diagnosed. Currently, 8%-45% [depending on geographic location (Diabetes Care, 2004)] with some studies showing 30%-50% of children newly diagnosed with diabetes have type 2 DM. Previously, less than 5% of children were diagnosed with type 2 DM. Being overweight is a strong risk factor for type 2 DM, and recent data from the Centers for Disease Control and Prevention noted that about 10%-15% of children and adolescents in the United States are overweight—double the number 2 decades ago—and the incidence is increasing. Sedentary lifestyle is another significant risk factor. There is also an increased risk of developing type 2 diabetes in African-American, Hispanics/Latino-American, Asian and Pacific Islander-American, and Native-American populations (NDEP, 2006).

- **Mature-onset diabetes of youth (MODY):** This type involves impaired insulin secretion with minimal or no defects in insulin action, usually in individuals younger than 25 yr old and symptomatic only with stress or infection.

- For information on other types, see the adult Diabetes Mellitus care plan, p. 377.

HEALTH CARE SETTING

Primary care, with possible hospital admission because of complications

ASSESSMENT

Signs and symptoms: These are the same as in the adult DM care plan except children with type 2 DM usually have hypertension, dyslipidemia, and acanthosis nigricans (hypertrophy or thickening of skin with gray, brown, or black pigmentation chiefly in axilla, other body folds, and sometimes on hands, elbows, and knees). Females may have vaginitis because of long-standing glycosuria. DKA also may occur in children and adolescents.

COMPLICATIONS

Potential for acute crisis: This is the same as in the adult DM care plan with the addition of *idiopathic cerebral edema* in resolving DKA, which occurs more often in children than in adults. The patient may have headache and lethargy or be asymptomatic. Symptoms can start with abrupt change in level of consciousness (LOC); pupils dilated, fixed, or unequal; papilledema; decorticate or decerebrate posturing; rapid progression to deep coma, respiratory arrest, or brain death (herniation of brain stem).

Long-term complications: Micro and macro complications are very aggressive in children with type 2 DM. They occur over a much shorter time frame than is usually seen in adults.

DIAGNOSTIC TESTS

In 2006, the American Diabetes Association (ADA) published the position statement *Diagnosis and Classification of Diabetes Mellitus*. This and the 2005 ADA Statement *Care of Children and Adolescents with Type 1 Diabetes* define the following terms:

Fasting plasma glucose: Will reveal a value 126 mg/dl or higher. Fasting is defined as no caloric intake for at least 8 hr. This is the recommended test for children, and it should be confirmed by a second positive test on another day in an asymptomatic child.

- *Normal plasma glucose:* A value less than 100 mg/dl.
- *Impaired fasting glucose:* 100-125 mg/dl or impaired glucose tolerance if 2 hr postprandial plasma glucose is 140-199 mg/dl. Impaired fasting plasma glucose or impaired glucose tolerance should be monitored on a regular basis but losing weight and increased activity can prevent or delay onset of DM.
- *Screening recommendations* (ADA, Consensus Statement Type 2 Diabetes in the Young: The Evolving Epidemic, 2004) for type 2 DM:
  - Overweight or at risk for overweight (body mass index greater than 85th percentile for age and sex, weight for height greater than 85th percentile, or weight greater than 120% of ideal for height)
  PLUS
  - Two or more of the following risk factors:
    Family history of type 2 DM in first- and second-degree relatives
    Belonging to certain race/ethnic groups (Native-American, African-American, Hispanic/Latino-American, Asian/South Pacific Islanders)
    Signs of insulin resistance or conditions associated with insulin resistance (acanthosis nigricans, hypertension, dyslipidemia, polycystic ovarian syndrome)
    If listed factors present, testing should be done (1) every 2 years starting at age 10 or (2) at onset of puberty, if it occurs at a younger age. Preferred test is fasting plasma glucose.

Two-hour postprandial plasma glucose: Will reveal a value 200 mg/dl or greater during oral glucose tolerance test. It is not usually done in children.

Random/casual plasma glucose: Symptoms of diabetes (polyuria, polydipsia, polyphagia, unexplained weight loss)

and a random/casual plasma glucose 200 mg/dl or greater are diagnostic of diabetes and no further testing is required.

Glycosylated hemoglobin or hemoglobin A1C: Assesses control of blood glucose over preceding 2 to 3 mo. Normal range for glycosylated hemoglobin A1C (HbA$_1$C) is 4%-7%. Range in children varies depending on age, with higher glucose levels allowed in younger children. Values differ depending on test done (NDEP, 2006):

- Younger than 6 yr old: HbA$_1$C 7.5%-8.5%
- 6-12 yr old: HbA$_1$C less than 8%
- Adolescent: HbA$_1$C less than 7.5%

Fasting lipid panel, if type 2 diabetes suspected: Dyslipidemia is frequently seen in children in type 2 DM and also needs to be treated. Values vary depending on age of child and if reference range is in conventional units or international units.

Basic metabolic panel (electrolytes, glucose, blood urea nitrogen, creatinine): Serum glucose will be elevated, usually greater than 250 mg/dl. Sodium and potassium may be lost because of osmotic diuresis. The higher the glucose level, the greater the dehydration and loss of electrolytes. Serum potassium may be normal on admission, but after fluid and insulin administration, rapid return of potassium to the cells decreases serum potassium, which necessitates monitoring for cardiac dysrhythmias. Blood urea nitrogen and creatinine likely will be elevated because of dehydration. Also, renal dysfunction occurs when serum glucose level rises to greater than 600 mg/dl.

Thyroid-stimulating hormone and thyroxine: Thyroid hormone increases gluconeogenesis (synthesis of glucose from noncarbohydrate sources such as amino acids and glycerol) and peripheral use of glucose. Elevated or decreased value would impact carbohydrate metabolism and therefore plasma glucose. Normal range varies for children depending on their age and type of reference units reported.

Ketones: Elevated when insulin is not available and the body starts to break down stored fats for energy. Ketone bodies are by-products of this fat breakdown, and they accumulate in the blood and urine. Normal range for children is 0 with the qualitative test and 0.5-3 mg/dl (conventional units) or 5-30 mg/L (international units) with the quantitative test.

Nursing Diagnosis:

Deficient Knowledge:

Blood glucose monitoring

Desired Outcome: Within 48 hr of this diagnosis, child/family demonstrates and verbalizes accurate understanding of proper blood glucose monitoring and when to monitor for ketones.

INTERVENTIONS	RATIONALES
Discuss reasons for blood glucose testing.	Understanding purpose of performing tests facilitates adherence. Reasons for blood glucose testing include: - Allows child to relate "how I feel at this time" with actual blood glucose level. - Gives child/family some control. - Enables understanding of effects of food, exercise, insulin, and/or stress. - Enables adjustments in insulin or diet.
Demonstrate correct use of glucometer the child will use at home and proper technique for fingerstick.	There are many different models and strips available commercially. Each system functions a little differently, and it could be overwhelming having to learn a new system at home without assistance or guidance. General guidelines include: - Use side of finger, not tip for fingersticks. Sides of the fingers have fewer nerve endings and hurt less. In addition, using sides decreases loss of sense of touch in fingertips. - Clean hands with soap and warm water. Cleansing helps reduce risk of infection. Warm water facilitates circulation and hence blood flow. - Avoid regular use of alcohol to cleanse skin. Any trace of alcohol left on the skin will interfere with the chemical reaction involved in checking blood glucose. It is okay to use occasionally (e.g., at a picnic), but the finger must be dried carefully and the first drop of blood discarded. Repeated use of alcohol also can lead to thickening of the skin, making fingerstick more difficult and painful. - Hold hand down, not up, to facilitate blood flow.
Discuss when blood glucose testing should be done.	Knowledge and understanding facilitate adherence. - Testing normally should be done before each meal and bedtime snack. Checking blood glucose on a regular basis and documenting findings help determine if adjustments need to be made in insulin/diet/exercise/medication by assessing pattern of blood glucose levels. - If child is sick, blood sugar is checked q4h. Risk of hyperglycemia is increased when child is ill (e.g., with headache, fever, sore throat) or has an infection owing to stress on the body and increased energy demands. Stress causes the adrenal gland to produce more epinephrine, norepinephrine, and cortisol. These stress hormones are "antiinsulin" in their actions, so blood glucose increases and ketones are formed by the liver, breaking down fat stores for energy. As blood glucose increases, the three *P's* occur, causing dehydration as well as nausea and vomiting owing to ketosis. Blood glucose testing will determine if changes need to be made in insulin and if health care provider should be contacted. - Blood sugar is checked with hypoglycemic or hyperglycemic symptoms to identify which event is occurring and therefore facilitate proper treatment.
If blood glucose is greater than 250 mg/dl or if child is ill, check urine for ketones with every void.	The body starts breaking down stored fats for energy because it cannot use blood glucose for energy. Ketone bodies are by-products of this fat breakdown and can lead to DKA if not controlled/treated.
Demonstrate use of diary or log to record blood glucose levels, ketones, insulin dose, diet, exercise, and any comments.	Information in this log provides good overview of how the child is doing and assists health care provider in making adjustments based on pattern seen in log/diary.
Instruct child/family when to call health care provider per blood glucose levels or ketones.	Understanding when to call improves adherence and decreases complications such as DKA: - Blood glucose greater than 250 mg/dl 3 times in a row - Blood glucose less than 70 mg/dl twice in 1 wk - Ketones moderate or large

••• **Related NIC and NOC labels:** *NIC:* Hyperglycemia Management; Hypoglycemia Management *NOC:* Knowledge: Diabetes Management

<u>Nursing Diagnosis:</u>

Deficient Knowledge:

Causes, signs and symptoms, and treatment of hypoglycemia and hyperglycemia

Desired Outcome: Immediately following teaching, child/family verbalizes accurate understanding of possible causes, signs and symptoms, and treatment of hypoglycemia and hyperglycemia.

INTERVENTIONS	RATIONALES
Define hypoglycemia for child and family.	Knowledge facilitates early recognition of problem, enabling prompt treatment. Hypoglycemia is defined as a low blood glucose level (less than 60-70 mg/dl) that occurs rapidly with signs and symptoms noted within minutes to an hour. Hypoglycemia is a potential emergency and needs to be treated promptly.
Teach child and family causes of hypoglycemia.	Understanding causes of hypoglycemia optimally will help child/parent decrease occurrences. Causes include: - Too little food or not eating on time - Increased exercise/activity with no increased intake - Too much insulin
Teach child and family to recognize early and late signs and symptoms of hypoglycemia.	Signs and symptoms of hypoglycemia should prompt child or family to check blood glucose level. - Early signs occurring secondary to adrenaline release are trembling, tachycardia, sweating, headache, anxiety, and hunger. - Later signs and symptoms occurring secondary to cerebral glucose deficit are dizziness, personality/mood changes, slurred speech, loss of coordination, and decreased LOC. Some children may not show early symptoms of adrenaline release or if younger than 6 yr old may not recognize early symptoms.
Teach child and family best method of assessing and treating hypoglycemia.	Some signs and symptoms of hypoglycemia and hyperglycemia are difficult to distinguish from one another, but the treatments are different. It is essential to know which reaction a child is experiencing to treat it effectively. Measures include: - Checking blood sugar to determine if child is hypoglycemic. - In the presence of hypoglycemia, giving 15 g of readily absorbed carbohydrates such as 4 oz orange juice, 6 oz regular soda, 4 glucose tablets, or 6 LifeSavers. If blood glucose is not increased or the child is still having signs and symptoms of hypoglycemia in 15 min, treatment is repeated. This will elevate plasma glucose level and relieve symptoms of hypoglycemia. Understanding of appropriate initial treatment improves ability to treat hypoglycemia successfully. - In addition, if it is not time for a meal or snack within 1 hr, giving complex carbohydrates and protein such as bread or crackers with peanut butter or cheese sustains glucose level inasmuch as readily absorbed carbohydrates (fast-acting or simple sugars) will be out of the system in 45-60 min. Complex carbohydrates (e.g., crackers) take 2-3 hr and proteins (e.g., cheese or peanut butter) 3-4 hr to be metabolized. Knowledge of appropriate follow-up treatment and understanding necessity of this treatment improve ability to resolve situation successfully.
Teach strategies to prevent hypoglycemia by identifying pattern of activity or time of day that precedes reactions.	Knowledge of these patterns enables child/family to prevent or decrease incidence of hypoglycemia. For example, patient/parent should record in log/diary all unusual events or change in activity or diet to help identify patterns.

Continued

INTERVENTIONS	RATIONALES
Teach care if child is unable to eat, drink, or swallow or is unconscious.	Knowing appropriate treatment improves outcome. - Glucagon (subcutaneous or IM) is administered if available to raise blood glucose level when child is unable to drink or eat fast-acting carbohydrate. - If glucagon is not available, child should be positioned on side and honey, corn syrup, or Cake Mate gel rubbed inside the cheek. This position prevents aspiration, especially if giving glucagon, because vomiting may occur. Fast-acting/simple sugars are absorbed through the oral mucosa without danger of aspiration.
Define hyperglycemia.	This helps differentiate between hyperglycemia and hypoglycemia. Knowledge enables recognition and discernment of which reaction child is experiencing. Hyperglycemia is defined as blood glucose levels higher than target range. Signs and symptoms appear within hours to several days (see signs and symptoms, below).
Teach child and family causes of hyperglycemia.	Understanding situations that can result in hyperglycemia (e.g., increased food intake, too little insulin, decreased exercise, infection or illness, and emotional stress) can help child/family avoid such events.
Teach signs and symptoms of hyperglycemia.	Recognition of hyperglycemia enables earlier and more effective treatment and prevents development of DKA. Signs and symptoms include the three *P's* (polydipsia, polyuria, polyphagia), fatigue, fruity-smelling breath, weight loss.
Teach treatment for hyperglycemia.	Interventions prevent DKA through early treatment. These include: - If blood glucose level is greater than 250 mg/dl, urine should be checked for ketones. - If ketone results are trace to small, child should drink extra water and be rechecked for ketones in 2 hr. - If ketone results are medium to large, health care provider should be contacted.
Teach patient to call health care provider if blood glucose is greater than 250 mg/dl 3 times in a row.	Provider may need to adjust insulin.

••• **Related NIC and NOC labels:** *NIC:* Hyperglycemia Management; Hypoglycemia Management *NOC:* Knowledge: Diabetes Management

Nursing Diagnosis:

Deficient Knowledge:

Meal planning and its relationship to blood glucose

Desired Outcome: Within 48 hr after teaching, child/family demonstrates ability to perform meal planning based on blood glucose levels.

INTERVENTIONS	RATIONALES
Teach the action that different foods (carbohydrates, fats, proteins) have on blood glucose level.	This information facilitates understanding of need for adhering to prescribed diet. For example, carbohydrates raise blood sugar, and simple sugars raise blood sugar more rapidly. Fats and proteins have less immediate effect on blood sugar level.
Involve dietitian in developing and instructing child/family about prescribed meal plan.	Dietitians have expertise in designing a plan appropriate for children based on age, cultural background, preferences, and caloric needs. Including these variables in the meal plan increases knowledge, understanding, and hence likelihood of compliance.

Continued

INTERVENTIONS	RATIONALES
Use handouts from dietitian and guidelines in diabetes book used by facility for diabetes education (see resources at end of care plan) to review prescribed diet.	Written and verbal explanations increase understanding and promote adherence.
As indicated, teach carbohydrate counting.	Understanding the diet plan increases ability to continue this regimen at home and improves compliance as well. Counting grams of carbohydrate and matching them with amount of insulin is the diet used most often in children. A no-concentrated-sweets diet is another plan used in some facilities.
Review child's normal schedule and set up a schedule that includes time for blood glucose tests, medication, meals, and snacks.	Having a written schedule facilitates child's/family's adjustment to new routines. Meal plan is tailored to child and his or her activity level. Ongoing assessment enables change as necessary and/or a follow-up dietary consultation.
Assess weight on admission and daily thereafter (same time of day, same scales, same amount of clothing).	Whether child is maintaining or gaining weight may be an indicator of effectiveness of diet and treatment and/or compliance.
Identify ideal blood glucose levels for child based on age.	Diet and activity levels vary more in the younger child. Generally at 6 yr old, a child is more likely to have hypoglycemia and less likely to recognize early signs and symptoms, so ideal blood glucose values are kept in a higher range. Range (mg/dl) varies slightly before meals and at bedtime/overnight:
	- Younger than age 6 yr: 100-180 ante cebum (ac), 110-200 hour of sleep (HS)
	- School age (6-12 yr): 90-180 ac, 100-180 HS
	- Older child or adolescent (13-19 yr): 90-130 ac, 90-150 HS (NDEP, 2006)
Instruct family to write meal plans for several days implementing use of prescribed foods.	This is one method of assessing and promoting family's understanding of diet instruction.
Provide scenarios for family when blood glucose is outside normal range and have them identify ways of adjusting diet, insulin, and/or exercise to get closer to blood glucose goal. Include how to adjust insulin and meal plan if ill and cannot eat.	This information facilitates development of problem-solving skills within family and assesses family's understanding of interaction among blood glucose, insulin, diet, and exercise.

••• **Related NIC and NOC labels:** *NIC:* Teaching: Prescribed Diet; Nutrition Management *NOC:* Knowledge: Diabetes Management

ADDITIONAL NURSING DIAGNOSES/ PROBLEMS:

"Psychosocial Support"   p. 73

"Psychosocial Support for the Patient's Family and   p. 73
    Significant Other"

Interrupted Family Processes   p. 88

Compromised Family Coping   p. 89

"Diabetes Mellitus" in the adult care plans for   p. 379
    Risk for Unstable Glucose Level

Risk for Infection   p. 381

Impaired Skin Integrity   p. 382

Deficient Knowledge: Proper insulin administration   p. 382
    and dietary precautions for promoting
    normoglycemia

"Asthma" for **Anxiety** related to illness, loss of   p. 580
    control, and medical/nursing interventions

"Asthma" for **Interrupted Family Processes**   p. 581

PATIENT-FAMILY TEACHING AND DISCHARGE PLANNING

Children with DM may have different classifications of DM with varying symptoms and complications. When providing patient-family teaching, focus on sensory information, avoid giving excessive information, and initiate a visiting nurse referral for necessary follow-up teaching and assessment. A part of initial assessment should include asking about existing knowledge of the disease, ability for self-care by child and/or family, and psychologic acceptance. Stress family-centered care (viewing the family as a unit that is the "constant" in the child's life and maintaining or improving the health of the family and its members). Include verbal and written information (ensuring that written material is at a level the reader can understand) about the following:

✓ DM: definition, type child has, brief pathophysiology, characteristics of specific type.

✓ Major influences on blood sugar control: diet, exercise, insulin/oral medication, stress/infection.

✓ Diet prescribed for child (most often carbohydrate-counting or no-concentrated-sweets diet). The diet is also low in fat and high in fiber to prevent or decrease problems with blood fats, especially cholesterol and triglycerides. Provide rationale for three meals and two to three snacks on a consistent schedule.

✓ Exercise/activity: lowers blood glucose, helps maintain normal cholesterol levels, increases circulation, and is an essential part of a child's life. If exercise is increased or has a different time frame than usual, it may be necessary to adjust diet (add 15-30 g carbohydrates for each 45-60 min of exercise), insulin, or oral medications.

✓ Stress or illness/infection: increases blood glucose level; therefore adjustments may be necessary in diet and/or insulin dosage.

✓ Insulin: type of insulin; characteristics of particular insulin, including onset, peak, and duration; dose prescribed; and dosing schedule.
- Have child/parent demonstrate drawing up each prescribed dose (e.g., lispro and NPH before breakfast, lispro before supper, and NPH at bedtime).
- Rotation of injection sites:
  - Insulin absorption varies by site (most rapidly in abdomen, then in the arms, in the hips, and slowest in the thighs).
  - Insulin absorption is affected by injection site. Massage after injection, exercise of injected limb, and body temperature increase the rate of absorption.
  - Use all spots in one site before you move on to another site or use the same site for every morning injection and the same site for every evening injection until all spots have been used (gives same absorption of insulin).
- Have child/parent administer insulin using proper technique.
- At least two people (one could be the child) need to know how to draw up and administer insulin.

✓ Other medications, including drug name; purpose; dosage; frequency; precautions; drug-drug, food-drug, and herb-drug interactions; and potential side effects.

✓ Honeymoon phase or period: may occur a short time after diagnosis, usually within 2 to 8 wk, and usually lasts 1-3 mo, but may last up to a year. Insulin requirement decreases. The child is *not* cured. The insulin requirement will increase again.

✓ Acute complications of DM: hypoglycemia and hyperglycemia
- Possible causes
- Signs and symptoms
- Treatment

✓ Long-term complications (avoid addressing for now if child has just been diagnosed): microvascular, macrovascular, joint contractures.

✓ Blood glucose monitoring: See details in **Deficient Knowledge:** Blood glucose monitoring.

✓ Sick-day plan of care
- Always give insulin.
- Check blood sugar at least q4h and urine ketones with each void. Document in log/diary.

- If small amount of ketones, increase fluid intake.
- If child does not feel like eating, then give fluids with sugar such as fruit juice, regular soda, and regular Jell-O, and broth-type soups (provides some electrolytes and extra fluid) unless blood sugar is greater than 200 mg/dl. Then give diet fluids.
- Call health care provider or nurse educator for the following:
  - Nausea and vomiting
  - Fruity odor to breath
  - Deep, rapid respirations
  - Decreasing LOC
  - Moderate or high ketones in urine
  - Persistent hyperglycemia greater than 250 mg/dl (3 times in a row)

✓ Prevention of infection:
- Have good body hygiene with special attention to feet.
- Report any breaks in skin and treat promptly.
- Wear only properly fitting shoes and do not go barefooted.
- Get regular dental checkups.
- Need for pneumococcal and yearly influenza vaccines.

✓ Importance of child wearing medical alert necklace or bracelet (depending on age) and carrying a card that states child has diabetes, the type of diabetes, child's name, address, phone number, and health care provider's name and number.

✓ Psychosocial adjustment:
- Reactions of child: shock, denial, and sadness
- Reaction of parents: grief reaction

✓ Delegation of tasks to child, based on age (with supervision):
- Toddler/preschooler: Chooses and cleans finger for puncture; tries to identify word or phrase to describe feeling of hypoglycemia. Help choose food; give child a choice of appropriate options.
- School-age child: Performs finger puncture and blood glucose test. Pushes plunger down on insulin syringe after needle is inserted by parent or gives own injection. Performs ketone test on urine. Recognizes need to eat on time to avoid hypoglycemia. Verbalizes the treatment for hypoglycemia.
- Older school-age child: Records blood glucose values in log/diary. May draw up and inject insulin. Knows meal plan. Can choose correct foods for snacks.
- Adolescent: Looks for patterns in blood glucose values. Recognizes when to test for ketones. Initiates treatment for ketones (increased fluids). Can plan meals and snacks based on dietary plan. Can choose appropriate food at a party.

✓ Coordination of care. Need to talk with school nurse and/or other adults who are in close contact with child (e.g., teachers, scout leaders, day care provider).

✓ Legal rights of the child:
- Individuals with Disabilities Education Act (IDEA): Mandates federal government to provide funding to education agencies, state and local, to facilitate free and appropriate education to qualifying students with dis-

abilities. This includes children with diabetes because diabetes can, at times, adversely affect school performance in some students. If this can be proved, school is then required to develop an Individualized Education Plan (IEP).

- IEP: Designed by multidisciplinary team to facilitate special education and therapeutic strategies and goals for each child. Child does not have to be in special education classes. Parents need to be involved in this process.

- Section 504 of Rehabilitation Act of 1973: Each student with a disability is entitled to accommodation in order to attend school and participate as fully as possible in school activities. This accommodation may be related to a medical condition or an education issue. For example, child may leave the classroom to use bathroom facilities without raising hand and will not be penalized for excessive absences from school that are caused by the diabetes. The 504 plan may include as many accommodations as necessary for child to function well at school. Composition of the 504 team may include teachers, school nurse, therapists (physical, occupational, or speech therapist), psychologist, and parents and child as appropriate for child's needs. Input from health care provider is vital.

✓ Necessity of having health care provider's prescription form at school detailing guidelines for when to check blood sugar and administer medication or treatment for diabetes-related problems, as well as medications in the original container with prescribing label intact.

✓ Goals of care for child with diabetes:

- Focus is on child with diabetes, *not* on the diabetic child.
- Child will have appropriate growth (height and weight).
- Child will have age-appropriate lifestyle (development).
- Child will have near normal HbA$_1$C (varies with age).
- Child will not have acute complications (hypoglycemia or hyperglycemia).
- Child will have minimal serious complications associated with long-term diabetes.
- Child will be able to perform age-appropriate self-care tasks.

✓ Importance of follow-up care and regular visits to health care provider and any other specialists working with child, such as dietitian, physical therapist, or endocrinologist.

✓ Telephone numbers for family to call if any questions arise about therapy or disease after discharge.

✓ When to call health care provider:

- Increased blood sugar greater than 250 mg/dl 3 times in a row
- More than two episodes of hypoglycemia per week
- Moderate-to-large amount of ketones in urine

✓ Diabetes camps, which are a fun way for children to learn more about their diabetes and feel less isolated. Listing is available at *www.childrenwithdiabetes.com*. (Under keyword search, type in "camp.")

✓ Referrals to community resources, such as local and national chapters of the American Diabetes Association and Juvenile Diabetes Foundation, public health nurses or home health nurse, diabetes nurse educator or endocrinologist, community teaching programs or support groups for children, diabetes camps, or other resources as necessary.

✓ See "Diabetes Mellitus," p. 385, for additional family teaching and discharge planning suggestions and resources.

✓ Additional resources include the following:

- Children with Diabetes at *www.childrenwithdiabetes. com/index_cwd.htm*. This is an online community for kids, families, and adults with diabetes. Sample 504 and IEP available. Rufus, the teddy bear with diabetes, is available here.
- Juvenile Diabetes Research Foundation International (JDRF) at *www.jdrf.org*
- American Association of Diabetes Educators at *www. aadenet.org*
- Chase HP. *Understanding Insulin-Dependent Diabetes*, ed 11, 2006. Available at *www.childrensdiabetesfdn.org*. To order, call (800) 695-2873 ($25.00)
- Travis LB. *An Instructional Aid on Insulin-Dependent Diabetes Mellitus*, ed 12, 2004. Available at *www.Designersink. com*. To order, call (512) 832-0611 ($21.50)
- Blood glucose diary, carbohydrate and calorie counter, videos from Novo Nordisk Pharmaceuticals, Inc., at *www.novonordisk-us.com*

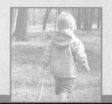

Fractures in Children 83

OVERVIEW/PATHOPHYSIOLOGY

Fractures are common childhood injuries and usually the result of trauma (falls, motor vehicle accidents, sports injuries, child abuse) or bone disease with abnormally fragile bones (osteogenesis imperfecta). Fractures usually result from increased mobility and immature understanding of potentially dangerous situations. Fractures in infancy are most often caused by trauma or child abuse.

Important variables that affect care of fractures in children as compared with adults:
- Children's bones heal faster than adults'; the younger the child, the faster the bone heals.
- Children's bones are softer than adults'; rather than breaking, they bend or buckle.
- Children's bones have a thicker periosteum and increased amount of immature bone.
- Children's bones have an open growth plate or epiphysis. Damage to the growth plate can interrupt and alter growth.
- Children usually only complain when something is wrong. Restlessness, extended periods of crying, and calling for the parent more than usual, as well as disuse of affected extremity, or increased use of unaffected extremity after a fall or injury are signals that more investigation of the event is needed.

Most frequent types of fractures in children:
- **Bends or plastic deformation:** A child's flexible bone can be bent 45 degrees or more before breaking and remains bent when the force is removed. The ossification of bones begins at birth and continues until the child is 18-21 yr old. The less ossified the bone, the more easily it bends. Thus, this type of injury occurs only in children, most often in the ulna and fibula.
- **Buckle or torus fracture:** Compression of the porous bone as a result of minimal angular trauma. It causes a bulge at the fracture site and occurs most often in young children, usually in the distal radius or ulna.
- **Greenstick:** Break occurs through the periosteum on one side of the bone but only bows or buckles the other side. It occurs most often in the forearm.
- **Complete fracture:** Break divides the bony fragments. The four types include spiral fracture (from rotational force, often associated with child abuse, especially in infants), oblique, transverse, and epiphyseal.

Most common fracture sites in children: Ulna, clavicle, tibia, and femur.

Most fractures are treated with closed reduction and immobilization of affected area. Developmental age is key to the cause of injury (falls, motor vehicle accidents, sports) and type of fracture.

HEALTH CARE SETTING

Emergency department, with possible hospitalization

ASSESSMENT

Child's symptoms, trauma history (should match physical examination), and physical examination are all part of the assessment profile.

Signs and symptoms: Vary with location, severity, and type of injury. Pain or tenderness at site, decreased range of motion (ROM) or immobility, deformity at fracture site, crepitus, gross motion at injured site, edema, erythema, ecchymosis, muscle spasm, and inability to bear weight may be present.

Physical assessment: Assess for location of deformity, swelling, ecchymosis, and pain. Check vital signs and perform neurovascular assessment.

DIAGNOSTIC TESTS

X-ray examination: Most effective tool for determining type and location of a fracture. Much of the skeleton of infants and young children is composed of radiolucent growth cartilage that does not appear on radiographs. Observation of gross deformity and point tenderness may be more reliable in diagnosing extremity fractures than would an x-ray. X-rays of unaffected limb may be obtained for comparison. Radiography of the suspected limb fractures should include joint above and below with a minimum of two views. X-rays are also taken after fracture reduction and often during healing process to assess progress.

CT scan, MRI scan, bone scan: May be needed to evaluate fracture in certain circumstances.

Nursing Diagnosis:

Acute Pain

related to fracture and other injury

Desired Outcome: Following treatment/intervention, child's report of pain/pain level is less than 2 on a 5-point scale (e.g., FACES scale), less than 4 on a 10-point scale (e.g., numeric scale), or child exhibits behavior consistent with pain less than 4 on a 10-point scale (e.g., FLACC [face, legs, activity, cry, consolability] scale).

INTERVENTIONS	RATIONALES
Establish a pain scale appropriate for child (FLACC, Wong-Baker FACES, Oucher, Poker Chip, numeric) and use it to assess pain before and after analgesia administration and at least q4h.	This helps determine degree of pain and effectiveness of pain medication.
Administer pain medication around the clock for first 24-48 hr or depending on severity of injury.	This decreases or prevents pain more effectively than when given prn. Prolonged stimulation of pain receptors results in increased sensitivity to painful stimuli and will increase the amount of drug required to relieve pain.
Administer analgesia via IV or PO route. If using the IM route, use topical anesthetic.	These measures facilitate atraumatic care and encourage child to give accurate pain rating. Child may fear a "shot" and deny pain or refuse pain medication.
Position, align, and support affected body part.	Appropriate positioning decreases tension on affected area, thereby decreasing pain.
Use nonpharmacologic pain control measures as appropriate for child depending on developmental age.	These are adjuncts to pain medication and include rocking, play, toys, music, distraction, relaxation techniques, humor, and massage.
Ice and elevate extremity, especially for the first 48 hr.	These measures decrease edema, thereby decreasing pain.
Notify health care provider if relief from pain is not obtained 1 hr after PO pain medication was given and after using all above measures.	Medication may need to be adjusted for optimal pain control. It also may signify a fracture complication.

●●● **Related NIC and NOC labels:** *NIC:* Pain Management; Analgesic Administration; Humor; Positioning; Cold Application; Distraction; Simple Massage; Music Therapy *NOC:* Comfort Level; Pain Level

Nursing Diagnosis:

Ineffective Tissue Perfusion: Peripheral

related to edema or immobilization following fracture

Desired Outcome: Child's neurovascular checks are within normal limits within 24 hr of fracture as evidenced by digits that are warm and sensitive to touch, brisk capillary refill (2 sec or less), peripheral pulse amplitude greater than 2+ on a 0-4+ scale, and minimal or decreased swelling in affected limb.

INTERVENTIONS	RATIONALES
Perform neurovascular checks (color, sensation, pulses, warmth, swelling) qh for first 24 hr and then q2-4h. Use a measuring tape in millimeter increments to compare circumference of area distal to the injury to that of noninjured limb. Or, depending on size of child, you should be able to insert one or two fingers into the cast opening.	These checks help determine presence of decreased peripheral tissue perfusion in the injured limb, which would be evidenced by darker or lighter color than opposite extremity, decreased sensation, decreased or absent pulse, skin cool to touch, and increased swelling distal to the injury.

Continued

INTERVENTIONS	RATIONALES
Be alert to subjective and behavioral indicators of decreasing perfusion.	Complaints of constant or increasing pain (especially on passive movement of the digits) and numbness or tingling in the digits of the injured extremity are subjective indicators of decreasing perfusion. Constant crying or increasing irritability may be seen in young children.
Elevate extremity.	This helps prevent/decrease edema, thereby promoting tissue perfusion.
Apply ice during the first 48 hr.	Most swelling occurs during the first 48 hr. Ice helps decrease edema, thereby promoting tissue perfusion.
Notify health care provider immediately if tissue perfusion deteriorates quickly from baseline.	Child may be developing or experiencing compartment syndrome, **an emergency situation**. For details, see "Fractures" in the adult care plans for **Risk for Peripheral Neurovascular Dysfunction** related to interruption of capillary blood flow secondary to increased pressure within the myofascial compartment, p. 516.
Encourage child to move digits.	Moving toes or fingers in the affected limb improves circulation, thereby decreasing edema and increasing tissue perfusion. **Note:** Inability to move digits is another sign of compartment syndrome.

••• **Related NIC and NOC labels:** *NIC:* Neurologic Monitoring; Positioning; Circulatory Precautions *NOC:* Tissue Perfusion: Peripheral

Nursing Diagnosis:

Risk for Impaired Skin Integrity

related to presence of immobilization device (bandages, splint, cast)

Desired Outcome: Child's skin remains intact while wearing immobilization device.

INTERVENTIONS	RATIONALES
Assess for erythema or irritation caused by the immobilization device q4h. - Check edges of immobilization device above and below fracture site. - If edges are rough, petal moleskin to smooth edges.	Ongoing assessment results in early detection and treatment, thereby decreasing risk of break in skin integrity.
Run hand over immobilization device to feel for indentations or "hot" spots q4h.	Indentations can cause skin breakdown/pressure. Hot spots (after cast has dried) may indicate an infection that might occur as a result of a break in skin integrity.
Feel around edges of immobilization device for tightness q4h.	This determines if cast/immobilization device fits appropriately and is not too tight or loose. Examiner should be able to insert fingers between cast and child's skin after it dries. If cast is too tight, it will cause pressure, which can result in decreased tissue perfusion and skin breakdown. If cast is too loose, it can rub on the skin and cause skin breakdown.
Instruct child/family not to put powder or corn starch under cast.	These products may cake and cause skin irritation and breakdown.
Suggest that family use cool air blown from fan or hair dryer to relieve itching or rub unaffected extremity.	These distraction techniques may keep child from itching or putting things inside cast to scratch and cause skin breakdown.
Caution child/family not to put anything inside cast to scratch skin.	This can cause skin breakdown or become lodged inside cast.
Encourage position changes q2-4h as appropriate.	This improves circulation by preventing prolonged pressure at same area.

••• **Related NIC and NOC labels:** *NIC:* Pressure Management; Skin Surveillance; Cast Care: Maintenance; Positioning; Traction/Immobilization Care *NOC:* Tissue Integrity: Skin and Mucous Membranes

ADDITIONAL NURSING DIAGNOSES/ PROBLEMS:

"Prolonged Bedrest" for such nursing diagnoses as **Risk for Activity Intolerance,**   p. 61

Risk for Disuse Syndrome,   p. 63

and **Constipation,** which occur with prolonged immobilization   p. 67

"Psychosocial Support" for such care plans as **Fear,** which child may experience as a result of injury and treatment   p. 76

"Psychosocial Support for Patient's Family and Significant Other" for such care plans as **Interrupted Family Processes,** which may occur with child's injury   p. 87

"Fractures" for care plans that discuss self-care deficits   p. 519

"Asthma" for **Anxiety** related to illness, loss of control, and medical/nursing interventions   p. 580

"Child Abuse and Neglect" for all diagnoses   p. 615

✓ PATIENT-FAMILY TEACHING AND DISCHARGE PLANNING

When providing child-family teaching, focus on sensory data, avoid giving excessive information, and initiate a visiting nurse referral for necessary follow-up teaching as needed. All information should emphasize that which is developmentally appropriate for the child. Stress family-centered care (viewing the family as a unit that is the "constant" in the child's life and maintaining or improving the health of the family and its members in a holistic manner). Include written and verbal information about the following (ensuring that information is at a level the reader can understand):

✓ Proper care of immobilization device. See **Risk for Impaired Skin Integrity,** earlier.

✓ Medications, including drug name; purpose; dosage; frequency; precautions; drug-drug, food-drug; and herb-drug interactions; and potential adverse effects.

✓ Importance of taking medications at home and at school as directed. Medication in the original bottle (with prescribing label) and written prescription from health care provider are needed for the child to be able to take medication at school.

✓ Legal rights of the child—Section 504 of Rehabilitation Act of 1973: Each student with a disability (whether temporary or permanent) is entitled to accommodation needed to attend school and participate as fully as possible in school activities. This accommodation may be related to a medical or an education issue. The 504 team for this child includes teachers, school nurse, possibly therapists, and parents and child, with input from health care provider. For example, a child with a long leg cast who has to go up and down steps to change classes would need accommodation—either staying in the same room all day, leaving one class early enough to be able to get to the next class, having someone else carry his or her books, or possibly having a teacher provide lessons at home. As many accommodations can be made as necessary for the child to be able to be successful in school.

✓ Adjustments needed for activities of daily living.

✓ Age-appropriate (developmental age, not just chronologic age) safety measures to help prevent further injuries:
- Childproof home and play area (include what is appropriate for *all* children in home).
- Avoid use of baby walkers, which are responsible for many injuries in infants.
- Proper use of protective equipment (e.g., car safety seats, bicycle helmets).
- Adaptation of child safety restraint system to accommodate cast/immobilization device.
- Importance of supervising young children while playing.
- Realistic expectations for child.

✓ When to call health care provider:
- Child complains of pain consistently in the same spot or pain seems to be getting worse.
- Child has tingling or numbness of toes or fingers.
- Child cannot feel something touching fingers or toes.
- Red or sore areas appear around cast edges.
- Child's fingers or toes are cold when in a warm environment.
- Child's nails stay pale when pressing on them and releasing pressure.
- Child's nails look blue even after elevating limb.
- Child's fingers or toes become very swollen several days after injury. Most swelling should occur in the first 48 hr.
- A foul smell comes from the cast.
- A "hot" spot is felt on the cast.
- Staining appears on the cast that was not there when child first came home. This could be an infected area or pressure sore.
- Child complains of constant itching that nothing helps.
- Cast is too tight or too loose.
- The cast starts to break down or fall apart or has indented areas. The cast may need to be reinforced or replaced to provide appropriate support for the injured area.
- Swelling after the first few days, pain, numbness, tingling, red marks or sores, and foul smell are serious signs of a problem. Talk with child's health care provider immediately. If health care provider is unavailable, go to nearest emergency care facility.

✓ Importance of follow-up care.

✓ Referral to community resources for assistance as needed (e.g., in providing safe home environment and transport to accommodate cast/immobilization device). Additional information can be obtained by contacting the local children's hospital, Social Services, and the following organizations:
- National SAFE KIDS Campaign at *www.safekids.org*
- Easter Seals at *www.easterseals.com*

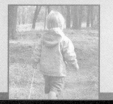

Gastroenteritis 84

OVERVIEW/PATHOPHYSIOLOGY

Gastroenteritis, one of the most common infectious diseases seen in children, is an inflammation of the stomach and intestines that accompanies numerous gastrointestinal (GI) disorders. In the United States, acute diarrhea accounts for more than 1.5 million outpatient visits, 200,000 hospitalizations, and about 300 deaths of children/year (CDC MMWR, 2003). Acute infectious gastroenteritis is caused by a variety of bacterial, viral, and parasitic pathogens. Rotavirus infection is the most common cause of gastroenteritis in infants and young children worldwide. Rotaviral gastroenteritis affects almost all children by the time they are 3 yr old, but it occurs most often between 3 and 24 mo of age.

Other common causes of infectious gastroenteritis include *Salmonella, Shigella,* and *Campylobacter* as the most common bacterial pathogens and *Giardia* and *Cryptosporidium* as the most common parasites. *Clostridium difficile* is the most common nosocomial source, and it occurs after antibiotic use.

HEALTH CARE SETTING

Primary care, with possible hospitalization depending on severity of illness

ASSESSMENT

Signs and symptoms vary widely depending on illness severity. Age, general health, and environment are factors that predispose children to gastroenteritis.

Signs and symptoms: Children usually present with some degree of the following:

- Fever
- Vomiting
- Diarrhea: Wide range of frequency and character (e.g., watery, bloody)
- Tenesmus: Painfully urgent but ineffectual attempt to urinate or defecate
- Abdominal pain
- Dehydration: Symptoms vary depending on degree of dehydration/water deficit (CDC MMWR, 2003).
  - Minimal (less than 3%): No physical signs and symptoms, possibly decreased urine output (UO).
  - Mild to moderate (3%-9%): May be alert, fatigued, restless, or irritable; thirsty, eager to drink; normal to increased heart rate (HR); normal to fast respiratory rate (RR); normal to decreased pulses; slightly sunken eyes; dry mucous membranes; prolonged capillary refill time; cool extremities; decreased UO.
  - Severe (greater than 9%): Apathetic, lethargic, or unconscious; minimal intake, may be unable to drink; tachycardia; weak, thready, or impalpable pulses; deep breathing; deeply sunken eyes; parched mucous membranes; prolonged or minimal capillary refill; cold, mottled, cyanotic extremities; minimal UO.
- Infants and children are at increased risk of dehydration due to many factors:
  - They have a greater percentage of body weight that is water than adults (e.g., a newborn has 75%-80% of body weight that is water, and 40% of that is extracellular; a preschooler has 60%-65% of body weight that is water, and 30% of that is extracellular).
  - Extracellular fluid is lost first with gastroenteritis.
  - The younger the child, the more quickly dehydration occurs.
  - Insensible water loss is also greater in infants and young children via skin and GI tract because of a proportionally greater body surface area in relation to body mass. Increased RR also increases insensible water loss as does a higher metabolic rate..

The most serious consequences of gastroenteritis are dehydration, electrolyte imbalance, and malnutrition.

DIAGNOSTIC TESTS

History is important in determining source of gastroenteritis and if there is a need for any tests. In general, laboratory tests are not performed unless the child exhibits moderate-to-severe dehydration, appears toxic, and has abdominal pain or bloody stools.

Serum electrolytes: Determine severity of electrolyte imbalance and type of fluid replacement necessary.

Complete blood count: Hematocrit is often elevated in dehydration. The differential will determine whether viral or bacterial infection is present. In a bacterial infection, the white blood cell (WBC) count is elevated with increased polymorphonuclear leukocytes or neutrophils. In a viral infection, the WBC count is slightly elevated with increased lymphocytes.

Creatinine and blood urea nitrogen: Elevated with dehydration but should return to normal with rehydration.

Blood culture: Obtained if child is acutely ill to help determine cause of illness.

Stool specimen: Examined if diarrhea lasts more than a few days to help determine cause.

Rotazyme: Rapid test to see if rotavirus is present in stool. Positive test negates need for stool culture.

Stool culture: Obtained if blood or mucus is present in stool, when symptoms are severe, or if there is history of travel to a developing country.

Stool for ova and parasites: May be used instead of culture because it is less expensive and often more reliable. A specimen is obtained 3 days in a row.

Nursing Diagnosis:

Deficient Fluid Volume

related to fluid loss secondary to fever, vomiting, diarrhea

Desired Outcome: Within 4 hr following intervention/treatment (for mild-moderate dehydration), the infant/child exhibits adequate hydration as evidenced by alertness and responsiveness, anterior fontanel soft and not sunken (in children younger than 2 yr), moist oral mucous membranes, elastic abdominal skin turgor, and age-appropriate UO (i.e., infant 2-3 ml/kg/hr, toddler and preschooler 2 ml/kg/hr, school-age child 1-2 ml/kg/hr, and adolescent 0.5-1 ml/kg/hr).

INTERVENTIONS	RATIONALES
Weigh child on admission and daily on the same scale, at same time of day, and wearing same amount of clothing (infants are weighed without any clothing). Notify health care provider if child is losing weight.	Consistency with weight measurements helps ensure more accurate results. Weight is a useful indicator of fluid balance. Weight loss indicates that child is not receiving adequate fluid replacement and adjustments need to be made.
Monitor vital signs q4h or more often if outside normal parameters. Report abnormalities to health care provider.	HR is elevated and BP is normal in compensated shock and low in uncompensated shock. Dehydration can quickly lead to shock in infants and young children in whom a falling BP is a *late* sign of shock.
Do not measure temperatures rectally.	Rectal temperature measurements stimulate stooling, which can lead to dehydration.
Administer oral rehydration solution (ORS), for example, Pedialyte, Infalyte, Rice-Lyte, Rehydralyte.	ORS replaces fluid volume in children with minimal-to-moderate dehydration.
	- To make it more palatable for child, may add 1 tsp presweetened sugar-free Kool-Aid to chilled 1-liter bottle of ORS or try flavored brands of these solutions.
	- Small amounts are given frequently, especially if child is vomiting (5 ml q5min with a gradual increase in amount consumed). This is from the 2003 guideline issued by CDC to improve health outcomes by replacing fluid and electrolytes, as well as glucose, with oral rehydration therapy (ORT). ORT includes rehydration with ORS and maintenance phase, including fluid and adequate dietary intake.
Do not give clear liquids such as apple juice, soda, gelatin, or sports drinks.	Liquids with a large amount of simple sugars can exacerbate osmotic effects associated with diarrhea and vomiting.
Do not give tea or soda with caffeine.	Caffeine can perpetuate diarrhea.
Do not give chicken or beef broth.	Broths are high in salt and low in carbohydrates.
Administer and monitor nasogastric tube (NGT) fluid replacement (for mild-moderate dehydration and vomiting) or IV fluids as prescribed for moderate-severe dehydration and vomiting.	If the child is unable to take sufficient ORS orally, use of NGT with ORS might help initial rehydration and speed up tolerance to refeeding. IV fluid and electrolyte replacement likely will be necessary if this is not successful or if the child is severely dehydrated.
Assess hydration status q4h.	Although the child may be receiving maintenance fluids, he or she may still be dehydrated because of diarrhea, vomiting, and/or insensible water losses. A dehydrated child is likely to exhibit decreasing level of consciousness, sunken fontanel, dry or sticky oral mucous membrane, tented abdominal skin, and decreasing UO.

Continued

INTERVENTIONS	RATIONALES
Ensure that child has at least minimal UO but that output is not more than intake.	This shows adequate hydration.
After child is rehydrated, calculate maintenance fluids based on child's weight.	The smaller the child, the greater the percentage of body weight is water. To meet minimal fluid requirements, the necessary volume is calculated in the following way: Up to 10 kg: 100 ml/kg/24 hr = _____ 10-20 kg: 50 ml/kg/24 hr = _____ greater than 20 kg: 20 ml/kg/24 hr = _____ = maintenance fluid requirement *For example, if child weighs 43 kg:* 10 kg × 100 ml/kg/24 hr = 1000 ml/24 hr 10 kg × 50 ml/kg/24 hr = 500 ml/24 hr 23 kg × 20 ml/kg/24 hr = 460 ml/24 hr 43 kg 1960 ml/24 hr Maintenance fluid requirement is 1960 ml/24 hr or 82 ml/hr.
Ensure that child is receiving at least maintenance fluids.	This is the minimum amount of fluid needed on a daily basis to be well hydrated if there are no unusual fluid losses (e.g., fever, diarrhea, vomiting).
Administer medications as prescribed.	For example, antibiotics are given to treat the bacterial pathogen causing the diarrhea.
After child is rehydrated, begin regular diet as tolerated.	Enteral nutrition stimulates renewal of intestinal cells, whereas fasting increases gut atrophy and permeability, which can contribute to dehydration. A regular diet is likely to comprise the following factors: low in fat, avoiding high concentrations of simple sugars, and encouraging complex carbohydrates such as starches. Examples of an appropriate diet include cereals, lean meats, yogurt, and cooked vegetables.
Instruct family members in providing ORS, monitoring intake and output, and assessing for signs of dehydration.	These instructions should improve adherence and promote optimum results.

••• **Related NIC and NOC labels:** *NIC:* Fluid/Electrolyte Management; Hypovolemia Management; Intravenous Therapy; Diarrhea Management; Vital Signs Monitoring *NOC:* Hydration

Nursing Diagnosis:

Risk for Impaired Skin Integrity

related to irritation caused by frequent stooling

Desired Outcome: Child's skin in perineal and perianal areas remains intact.

INTERVENTIONS	RATIONALES
Assess perineal and perianal areas for signs of irritation or excoriation with every diaper change.	The earlier the problem is detected, the sooner appropriate interventions can be made to ensure that skin remains intact.
Change diaper as soon as it becomes wet or soiled.	This helps keep skin clean and dry.
Cleanse buttocks gently (pat, do not rub) with water or immerse in tepid water to cleanse. Avoid using soap if possible.	Diarrheal stools are very irritating to the skin. Rubbing the skin every time the diaper is changed would irritate it further. Soap dries skin by removing normal moisturizing skin oils, thereby increasing potential for irritation and skin breakdown.

Continued

INTERVENTIONS	RATIONALES
Do not use commercial baby wipes with alcohol or perfume or baby powder on irritated or excoriated skin.	These products are painful to irritated skin.
If not contraindicated, apply protective ointments such as Vaseline, A&D, or zinc oxide when child is wearing a diaper.	This measure protects skin from irritation.
Leave diaper area open to air if possible (but not in the presence of explosive diarrhea). Reapply protective ointment before putting diaper on.	This practice facilitates drying and healing.
Instruct family members in appropriate skin care methods.	This increases likelihood of family using these techniques at home.

••• **Related NIC and NOC labels:** *NIC:* Skin Surveillance; Bathing; Skin Care: Topical Treatments; Diarrhea Management *NOC:* Tissue Integrity: Skin & Mucous Membranes

Nursing Diagnosis:

Risk for Infection

related to gastroenteritis and lack of knowledge about transmission prevention

Desired Outcome: Following intervention, family members and other children are free of indicators of gastroenteritis.

INTERVENTIONS	RATIONALES
Implement Standard Precautions as well as appropriate Transmission-Based Precautions. For more information, see Appendix A for "Infection Prevention and Control," p. 783.	Standard Precautions reduce risk of spreading infection. These include: - Good handwashing: Wash hands before and after working with child, even with appropriate gloving. - Wear gloves when changing diaper. - Wear other personal protective equipment as designated by isolation guidelines.
Dispose of linen and other soiled items per hospital protocol.	This will prevent spread of infection.
Apply diaper securely.	This prevents fecal spread.
Try to keep infants and small children from placing hands or objects in contaminated areas.	Gastroenteritis is mostly spread by the fecal-oral route. Infants and young children tend to put their hands in their mouths, and if their hands get into their diaper or stool, fecal-oral spread occurs.
Teach children, as appropriate, protective measures such as washing their hands after using the toilet.	This teaching helps prevent spread of infection.
Instruct family members and visitors in protective measures, especially handwashing and not visiting other patients.	This instruction reduces risk of spreading infection.

••• **Related NIC and NOC labels:** *NIC:* Infection Control; Infection Prevention; Communicable Disease Management *NOC:* Infection Status

Nursing Diagnosis:

Imbalanced Nutrition: Less Than Body Requirements

related to inadequate intake and fluid loss secondary to vomiting, diarrhea, and fever

Desired Outcome: Within 24-48 hr following intervention/treatment, child maintains or gains weight and exhibits no further vomiting or diarrhea.

INTERVENTIONS	RATIONALES
Assess weight on admission and daily (on same scale, at same time, wearing same clothing—no diaper on infants).	These assessments measure child's progress in attaining adequate nutrition. Consistency with weight measurements helps ensure more accurate results.
If mother is breastfeeding, encourage her to continue along with giving ORS (if child has mild-to-moderate dehydration) as described in **Deficient Fluid Volume,** earlier.	This practice tends to reduce severity and duration of illness by maintaining normal intake so that child has adequate nutrition.
Avoid BRAT (bananas, rice, apples, and toast) diet.	These foods do not provide complete caloric and protein requirements. They provide excessive carbohydrates and, overall, are also low in electrolytes. Therefore the child does not get needed nutrients.
Resume regular diet when child is rehydrated as described in **Deficient Fluid Volume,** earlier.	Enteral nutrition stimulates renewal of intestinal cells and decreases illness duration, whereas fasting increases gut atrophy and permeability.
Instruct family in appropriate diet.	This gains adherence to the treatment plan.
Monitor response to feedings.	Monitoring helps assess feeding tolerance. - Some children have increased stooling with lactose-containing milk products. - Most children do well with lactose-containing milk products, especially if they are eating foods at the same time.
Give liquids at room temperature.	Cold liquids stimulate peristalsis and hence diarrhea.
Keep room as odor free as possible.	Minimizing unpleasant or strong (perfume/aftershave) odors increases interest in eating and feeling of well-being.
Provide oral hygiene.	This enhances sense of well-being and improves chances of child eating/drinking more.

●●● **Related NIC and NOC labels:** *NIC:* Diet Staging; Nutrient Intake; Teaching: Prescribed Diet; Sustenance Support; Fluid Monitoring; Lactation Counseling *NOC:* Nutritional Status; Nutritional Status: Food & Fluid Intake; Nutritional Status: Nutrient Intake

ADDITIONAL NURSING DIAGNOSES/ PROBLEMS:

Fear	p. 87
Interrupted Family Processes related to situational crisis	p. 88
Deficient Knowledge: Patient's current health status and therapies	p. 91
"Asthma" for **Anxiety** related to illness, loss of control, and medical/nursing interventions	p. 580

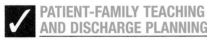

PATIENT-FAMILY TEACHING AND DISCHARGE PLANNING

When providing child-family teaching, focus on sensory information, avoid giving excessive information, and initiate a visiting nurse for follow-up teaching and assessment as needed. Stress family-centered care (viewing the family as a unit that is the "constant" in the child's life and maintaining or improving the health of the family and its members in a holistic manner). Include verbal and written information about the following (ensure that written material is at a level the reader can understand):

✓ Pathophysiology of gastroenteritis.

✓ Causes of gastroenteritis: If caused by improper food storage—address proper hygiene, formula or food preparation, handling and storage.

✓ Contagious aspect of gastroenteritis. It is important to use good handwashing technique, especially after changing a diaper. Teach children that are old enough to wash their hands after they use the toilet.

✓ Why gastroenteritis can be such a serious problem, especially for infants and young children:

• The younger the child, the greater the percentage of body weight that is water.
 Premature infant: 85%-90% of body weight is water.
 Full-term infant: 75%-80% of body weight is water.
 Preschooler: 60%-65% of body weight is water.
 Adolescents: 50%-55% of body weight is water.

• Therefore the younger the child, the quicker dehydration can occur (the child loses more fluid than is taken in).

• Problems that cause or increase severity of dehydration: fever, vomiting, diarrhea, not eating or drinking enough.

✓ Importance of checking hydration status q2-4h when child is ill with any of the previous problems (the younger the child, the more often status is reassessed):

- Is the child alert and interactive? Child would not be as alert and interactive as normal if dehydrated.
- Check the soft spot on top of head in children younger than 2 yr old: if it is sunken in, the child is dehydrated.
- No tears when crying in a child older than 6 mo old.
- Check inside the mouth, not the lips: if dry or sticky and the child is not a mouth breather, the child is dehydrated.
- Pinch skin on the abdomen: if skin sits up like a tent instead of falling down right away, the child is dehydrated.
- How many wet diapers does the child normally have per day? If the number is decreased or they are not as wet as normal, the child may be dehydrated.

✓ Feeding of child who has diarrhea:

- If child is breastfeeding, continue breastfeeding and supplement with ORS (e.g., Pedialyte, Infalyte, or Rehydralyte).
- If child is taking only formula or milk, it may not be necessary to stop that fluid as long as child is also taking ORS.
- 1 tsp presweetened sugar-free Kool-Aid can be added to a chilled 1-L bottle of ORS to improve taste or use flavored ORS.

✓ Change diaper frequently:

- Clean after stool with warm water. Pat skin; do not rub.
- Do not use soap if possible. If that is not possible, use mild, non-antiseptic soap.
- Do not use baby wipes containing alcohol or fragrances.
- Avoid powders and corn starch, which trap fluid and get caked in creases.
- Leave skin open to air if irritated (but not in the presence of explosive diarrhea).

- Put protective ointment such as Vaseline, A&D, or zinc oxide on skin.

✓ Feeding of child who is vomiting: Give small amounts of ORS frequently—amount varies depending on age and weight of child.

✓ Once child is rehydrated, begin regular diet as tolerated.

- Do not give BRAT (bananas, rice, apples, tea, or toast). This combination does not provide enough calories or protein.
- Use low-fat foods (no peanut butter, potato chips, or hot dogs).
- Give starchy foods such as cooked baby cereal, oatmeal, cream of wheat, rice, nonsugared cereals, noodles, potatoes, bread, and yogurt.
- Give fruits (not packed in syrup), vegetables without butter, and well-cooked chicken, fish, or lean meat.
- Avoid concentrated sweets such as candy or ice cream.
- Most children have no problems drinking formula or milk.

✓ Call health care provider when:

- There are signs of dehydration.
- There is blood or pus in the stool.
- The child has a fever.
- The vomiting or diarrhea lasts longer than 8-24 hr (the younger the child, the earlier the health care provider should be called).
- Child is not drinking fluids or is less alert than usual.
- Child has abdominal pain for 2 hr or more.
- Child is younger than 6 mo old and is vomiting or has diarrhea.
- Diaper area is very red or irritated and getting worse.

✓ Reinforce that child should never receive aspirin with viral illness; acetaminophen or ibuprofen should be used for fever or discomfort.

✓ Telephone numbers to call should questions or concerns about treatment or disease arise after discharge.

✓ Importance of follow-up care.

✓ Referral to community resources as necessary.

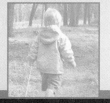

Otitis Media 85

OVERVIEW/PATHOPHYSIOLOGY

Otitis media is the most common reason for visits to the pediatrician in the first 3 yr of life, the leading cause of antibiotic use, and the most common cause of hearing loss in children. The highest incidence of otitis media occurs between 6 mo and 3 yr. With the continuing problem of overdiagnosis and the increase in drug-resistant *Streptococcus pneumoniae* (believed to be the major cause of ear infections in young children), one of the objectives of Healthy People 2010 is to reduce the number and frequency of courses of antibiotics for ear infections in young children. The American Academy of Pediatrics and the American Academy of Family Physicians (2004) recommend observation without antibiotic treatment for select children with uncomplicated acute otitis media (AOM) for 48-72 hr.

Otitis media includes several conditions ranging from acute to chronic with or without symptoms:

- **Otitis media (OM):** inflammation of the middle ear.
- **Acute otitis media (AOM):** middle ear infection with symptoms of acute illness (fever, pain, irritability) and full or bulging tympanic membrane (TM) under positive pressure that lasts 3 wk or less.
- **Otitis media with effusion (OME)** or **serous otitis media:** an inflammation of the middle ear without signs and symptoms of acute infection (other than reduced hearing), TM retracted or in neutral position under negative pressure or no pressure, and fluid in the middle ear space.
- **Chronic OM with effusion:** middle ear effusion lasting more than 3 mo.

HEALTH CARE SETTING

Primary care; possible hospitalization if OM exacerbates a chronic condition or if surgical intervention is required

ASSESSMENT

Signs and symptoms: Vary depending on type of OM and age of child.

AOM:

- *Infant or young child:* fever; possible ear drainage; crying; irritable and fussy; may tug, rub, or hold affected ear; sleep disturbances; decreased appetite; rolling head side to side; difficult to comfort; possible difficulty hearing.

- *Older child:* fever, possible ear drainage, complaints of ear hurting, crying, irritable, lethargic, decreased appetite (chewing causes increased ear pain), possible difficulty hearing.

OME: Difficulty hearing, feeling of fullness/pressure in ear, tinnitus or popping sounds, mild balance disturbances.

Physical assessment

AOM: Pneumatic otoscopy reveals bulging, red, immobile TM (or decreased mobility of TM). Crying, removal of cerumen and thereby irritating the auditory canal, and fever can cause redness of the TM without infection being present. Postauricular and cervical lymph nodes may be enlarged.

OME: Pneumatic otoscopy may show a slightly injected, dull gray membrane; obscured landmarks; and fluid visible behind the TM. There is also decreased mobility of the TM.

DIAGNOSTIC TESTS

Pneumatic otoscopy: A pneumatic attachment to the otoscope enables health care provider to introduce puffs of air into the ear. The TM does not move as well with fluid behind it. This device improves diagnostic accuracy by assessing mobility of TM, as well as visualizing it.

Tympanometry: Method of providing information about possible presence of a middle ear effusion, including the actual pressures in the middle ear space. This is a quick and simple method of assessing TM mobility.

Tympanocentesis: "Gold standard" for diagnosis of AOM, although it is not routinely used because of cost, effort, and lack of availability. It involves removal of fluid from the middle ear to identify the bacteria causing the infection. It improves diagnostic accuracy, guides treatment by finding the causative pathogen, and avoids unnecessary medical or surgical intervention. It is especially useful in AOM unresponsive to antibiotics or recurrent AOM.

Culture and sensitivity: Not routinely done, but if drainage is present or tympanocentesis is performed, it helps guide treatment in finding causative pathogen and antibiotics to which it is sensitive.

Nursing Diagnosis:

Acute Pain

related to increased pressure in the middle ear secondary to presence of fluid and/or infection

Desired Outcome: Child is free from pain or has significantly decreased pain (e.g., less than 2 on Wong-Baker FACES scale or less than 4 on FLACC [face, legs, activity, cry, consolability] or a numeric scale) within 1 hr after intervention/treatment.

INTERVENTIONS	RATIONALES
Establish appropriate pain scale for child (FLACC, Wong-Baker FACES, or numeric scale) and assess pain level at least q4h.	A pain scale appropriate for child will enable accurate assessment of pain level and help evaluate relief obtained.
Administer antipyretics/analgesics on a regular basis, for example, acetaminophen q4-6h for a maximum of 5 doses/day and/or ibuprofen q6-8h.	This protocol provides better control of fever and pain than on a prn basis. Alternating acetaminophen and ibuprofen so that child receives pain medication q3h gives maximum pain/fever control.
	Caution: Overdosage of acetaminophen can cause hepatic necrosis.
Reassess pain level and/or temperature 1 hr after administering medication.	This evaluates effectiveness of pain relief/fever control measure.
Administer antibiotics, if prescribed. Instruct parents to:	Many cases of AOM resolve in 2-3 days without antibiotics.
- Administer correct dose of medication at correct time.	This ensures optimal effectiveness of medication.
- Administer all doses (correct number/day and total number of doses prescribed).	Child may feel better after several days, and parents may stop giving medication. This may cause OM to reoccur and/or allow a more resistant bacteria to infect the child.
- Store medications appropriately.	Many antibiotics have to be refrigerated.
Use localized comfort measures based on developmental age and that which provides maximal comfort for child.	What is comforting to an infant usually is not comforting to an adolescent. Every child has specific measures that are comforting to him or her.
- Apply warm compresses to affected ear or have child lie on affected ear on a heating pad on low setting, covered with a towel to protect child from potential burns.	
- Apply wrapped ice bag over affected ear to decrease edema and pressure.	
Administer analgesic otic drops if prescribed.	These drops relieve severe pain.
Position for comfort according to type of OM.	Positioning decreases pressure on the TM.
- AOM: Position with affected ear in dependent position.	
- OME: Elevate head.	
Teach older children to open eustachian tube by yawning or performing Valsalva's maneuver.	This facilitates drainage of fluid from middle ear into the pharynx and decreases pressure on TM.

••• **Related NIC and NOC labels:** *NIC:* Medication: Administration; Pain Management; Positioning; Heat/Cold Application; Teaching: Procedure/Treatment *NOC:* Comfort Level; Pain Control

Nursing Diagnosis:

Risk for Deficient Fluid Volume

related to losses associated with fever and decreased intake

Desired Outcome: Within 24 hr of intervention, child is alert and responsive, anterior fontanel is soft and not sunken (in child younger than 2 yr), oral mucous membranes are moist, abdominal skin turgor is good, child has age/weight-appropriate urine output (e.g., infant 2-3 ml/kg/hr, toddler and preschool child 2 ml/kg/hr, school-age child 1-2 ml/kg/hr, and adolescent 0.5-1 ml/kg/hr), and child receives at least maintenance level fluids.

INTERVENTIONS	RATIONALES
Assess hydration status q4h. Instruct parent how to do this, and explain its importance.	The younger the child is and the less he or she weighs, the greater the percentage of body weight that is water. The child can become dehydrated easily. Routinely assessing for dehydration in a child who is running a fever and/or has decreased intake facilitates rapid treatment to resolve dehydration. A child who is dehydrated may have decreasing level of consciousness, sunken anterior fontanel (if younger than 2 yr old), dry or sticky oral mucous membranes, tenting abdominal skin, and decreasing urine output.
Teach parents when to call health care provider regarding dehydration.	This facilitates parent's ability to detect a problem early, thereby ensuring quicker problem resolution. Parent should call under the following conditions: - Child not as alert as usual - Anterior fontanel sunken - Inside of mouth dry or sticky if child is not a mouth breather - Skin on abdomen stays up like a tent when pinched - Fewer wet diapers than usual/voiding less than usual
Calculate maintenance fluids for the child and teach family to provide this in terms that they can understand.	Specific information enables parents to ensure that their child receives correct fluid volume. For example, if the child weighs 15 kg, maintenance fluids are 1250 ml/day (42 oz), and if the child drinks from a 6-oz "sippy" cup, that child needs to drink at least 7 sippy cupfuls of fluid a day. Calculation for minimum daily maintenance fluids: *For the child weighing 15 kg:* Up to 10 kg: 100 ml/kg/24 hr = 10 kg × 100 ml/kg/24 hr = 1000 ml/24 hr 10 to 20 kg: 50 ml/kg/24 hr = 5 kg × 50 ml/kg/24 hr = 250 ml/24 hr Greater than 20 kg: 20 ml/kg/hr = 15 kg 1250 ml/24 hr
Offer child small amounts of fluid at a time and soft food.	Sucking on a nipple or straw or chewing can increase ear pain.

••• **Related NIC and NOC labels:** *NIC:* Hypovolemia Management; Fever Treatment; Fluid Monitoring *NOC:* Hydration

Nursing Diagnosis:

Deficient Knowledge:

Disease process and prevention

Desired Outcome: Parents verbalize accurate understanding of disease process and ways to decrease/prevent future incidents of OM.

INTERVENTIONS	RATIONALES
Describe different types of OM and symptoms of each.	Knowledge and understanding improve compliance with treatment plan. - AOM: infection of middle ear; fever, pain. - OME: inflammation of middle ear with fluid behind TM without signs of acute infection; feeling of fullness in ear, difficulty hearing.
Instruct parents about importance of giving full course of antibiotics if they are prescribed and having ear rechecked when medication is finished.	Adequate treatment of AOM requires full course of antibiotics; otherwise, OM can reoccur and/or allow a more resistant bacteria to infect the child. Ear rechecks assess effectiveness of treatment.

Continued

INTERVENTIONS	RATIONALES
Discuss preventive feeding practices for infant.	Feeding practices that prevent OM in infants include the following: - Feeding infant in an upright position: facilitates drainage of middle ear. - Not putting infant in bed with a bottle: this increases incidence of ear infections. - Decreasing or eliminating use of pacifier after 6 mo old: sucking on a pacifier causes bacteria to reflux back up into the ear.
Avoid smoking around child.	Passive smoking increases incidence of OM.
Encourage gentle blowing of nose during upper respiratory infection (URI) rather than forceful nose blowing.	This decreases risk of transferring organisms from the eustachian tube to the middle ear.
Encourage blowing activities (e.g., bubbles, pinwheels) or chewing sugarless gum during a URI.	These activities help promote equalization of pressure in middle ear.
Explain prevention of ear pain during airplane travel.	Increased atmospheric pressure increases ear pain. - Health care provider may prescribe nasal mucosal shrinking spray if child has URI or chronic OME to decrease pressure on TM from edema. - Parent should offer bottle or pacifier to infant or give older child gum during descent to help equalize TM pressure.
Describe potential complications of OM.	Inadequate or nonadherence to treatment may result in the following: - Hearing loss - Perforated, scarred eardrum - Mastoiditis - Cholesteatoma (a cystic mass composed of epithelial cells and cholesterol that occurs as a result of chronic OM. It may occlude the middle ear, or enzymes produced by the cyst may destroy adjacent bones, including the ossicles.) - Intracranial infections such as meningitis

••• **Related NIC and NOC labels:** *NIC:* Teaching: Procedure/Treatment; Teaching: Disease Process; Teaching: Prescribed Medication *NOC:* Knowledge: Illness Care; Knowledge: Disease Process

ADDITIONAL NURSING DIAGNOSES/ PROBLEMS:

"Psychosocial Support for the Patient's Family and Significant Other" for relevant psychosocial nursing diagnoses   p. 87

"Asthma" for **Anxiety**   p. 580

PATIENT-FAMILY TEACHING AND DISCHARGE PLANNING

When providing child-family teaching, focus on sensory information and avoid giving excessive information. Stress family-centered care (viewing the family as a unit that is the "constant" in the child's life and maintaining or improving the health of the family and its members in a holistic manner). Include verbal and written information about the following, ensuring that written information is at a level the reader can understand:

✓ Types of ear infections, signs and symptoms, and treatment of each type.

✓ Importance of administering antibiotics as prescribed (can develop resistant strains of bacteria otherwise).

• Return demonstration of drawing up correct dose of medication and administering it to the child correctly.

• Use of a syringe or other calibrated device for administering medication to children.

• Administering doses at correct time each day and for total number of days prescribed.

• Teach five rights of medication administration:
  1. Right child
  2. Right medication
  3. Right dose (i.e., right concentration and right amount of medication)
  4. Right route (e.g., ear drops or oral medication)
  5. Right time

- Correct storage of medication (e.g., some need to be refrigerated)

✓ Method of assessing pain in child and importance of administering analgesic for pain on a regular basis.

✓ Treating fever correctly:
- Discuss at what temperature antipyretic is needed.
- Explain that fever increases ear pain.

✓ If receiving otic drops, how to administer based on child's age:
- Child younger than 3 yr old, pull earlobe down and back.
- Child older than 3 yr old, pull pinna up and back.

✓ Prevention:
- Never give infant a bottle to drink while lying down.
- Keep infant upright during feeding.
- Breastfeed as long as possible.
- Decrease the time pacifier is used or stop using after 6 mo.
- Do not smoke around child or take him or her where smoking occurs.
- If child has to go to day care, try to place with least number of children possible.
- Vaccinate child against pneumococcal and influenza infections.

✓ Signs and symptoms of dehydration:
- Child is not as alert and responsive as normal.
- Soft spot on top of head looks sunken (for children younger than 2 yr).
- Inside of mouth (not lips) is dry or sticky rather than moist (if child is not a mouth breather).
- Skin on abdomen sits up like a tent when pinched.
- Decreased number of wet diapers or same number but not as wet as normal for infant or young child or decreased number of voids/day in older child.

✓ Telephone number to call in case any questions arise about therapy or disease after office/emergency department visit.

✓ Importance of follow-up (e.g., many health care providers will do an ear recheck after child finishes medication).

✓ When to call health care provider:
- Fever or pain has not decreased after 48-72 hr while on antibiotics.
- Child is showing signs of dehydration.
- Child develops a stiff neck.
- Drainage present from child's ear canal.

✓ If child has had OME for more than 3 mo, he or she should have hearing evaluated.

✓ Referral to pediatric ear, nose, and throat specialist if OM or OME is chronic.

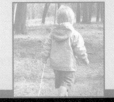

Poisoning 86

OVERVIEW/PATHOPHYSIOLOGY

Poisoning can result in death and is a leading cause of hospital visits for children. More than 89,300 children age 14 and younger were treated in hospital emergency departments for accidental poisoning in 2003. About 80% of the poison injuries were in children age 4 and younger (SAFE KIDS, 2006). Poisoning may occur through ingestion, inhalation, or contact with skin or mucous membranes and is seen most often in children younger than 5 yr old, with the greatest incidence in children younger than 2 yr old. Curiosity and natural desire to put things in their mouths put younger children at greater risk for accidental poisoning. Some of the most commonly ingested poisons in young children include cosmetics, household cleaning agents, alcohol, and medications (prescription or over the counter). Sixty percent of poisoning exposures are by nonpharmaceutical products and 40% are pharmaceuticals in children age 5 and younger (SAFE KIDS, 2006). Inhalation of carbon monoxide is a common wintertime occurrence. Adolescents also have an increased incidence of hospitalization resulting from poisoning, but it is most often intentional and frequently involves inhaling substances (e.g., glues/adhesives, nail polish remover, paint thinner, air conditioning coolant) or ingesting alcohol or drugs (e.g., marijuana or "ecstasy").

Eighty percent to 90% of all poisoning incidents occur in the home. Most homes have more than 500 toxic substances in them, and one third of these are in the kitchen. The garage is also particularly dangerous for children, with gasoline and pesticides among the toxic substances housed there. Improper storage of toxic substances and caregiver distraction are major factors of poisoning in children.

Risk factors other than developmental age:
- Male children are more likely than females to be poisoned.
- Black children younger than age 4 have a poisoning death rate nearly twice that of white children (SAFE KIDS, 2006).
- Children are more likely to suffer from elevated blood lead levels if they live in homes built before 1978, are low-income, or live in large metropolitan areas.

HEALTH CARE SETTING

Emergency department with possible hospitalization

ASSESSMENT

Varies depending on source of the poisoning.

Gastrointestinal system: Nausea, vomiting, diarrhea, abdominal pain, anorexia.

Respiratory system: Depressed or labored respirations, unexplained cyanosis.

Circulatory system: Signs of shock, including increased, weak pulse; decreased blood pressure (BP); increased, shallow respirations; pallor; cool, clammy skin.

Central nervous system: Dizziness, overstimulation, pupillary changes, sudden loss of consciousness, behavioral changes, seizures, stupor/lethargy, coma.

Integumentary system: Skin rashes; burns to mouth, esophagus, and stomach; eye inflammation; skin irritations; stains around the mouth; oral mucous membrane lesions.

Signs, Symptoms, and Basic Treatment Specific to Various Poisons

Acetaminophen ingestion: Included in many over-the-counter medications, acetaminophen is the most common drug ingestion in children. Symptoms occur in stages and are dose-dependent (e.g., child may not progress through all stages):
- Stage 1 (first 24 hr): malaise, nausea, vomiting, sweating, pallor, and weakness, or the child may be asymptomatic.
- Stage 2 (next 24-48 hr): decrease or disappearance of symptoms in stage 1 and right upper quadrant (RUQ) pain caused by liver damage and increase in liver enzymes.
- Stage 3 (3-7 days): jaundice, liver necrosis, and possible death from hepatic failure.
- Stage 4: occurs if the child does not die during the hepatic stage (stage 3) and involves gradual recovery.
- Treatment is with antidote Mucomyst.

Corrosive ingestion: Toilet and drain cleaners, bleach, ammonia, liquid dishwasher detergent, denture cleaner. Complaints of severe burning pain in mouth, throat, and stomach; whitish burns of mouth and pharynx with edema of lips, tongue, and pharynx; difficulty swallowing, which leads to drooling; respiratory distress; anxiety and agitation; and shock. Treatment involves diluting corrosive substance and avoiding emesis, which would increase damage.

Hydrocarbon ingestion: Gasoline, kerosene, paint thinner, lamp oil, turpentine, lighter fluid, some furniture polishes. Gagging, choking, coughing; nausea, vomiting; characteristic petroleum breath odor; central nervous system (CNS) depression. Respiratory symptoms of pulmonary involvement include tachypnea, cyanosis, retractions, and grunting. Treatment is symptomatic but inducing vomiting is generally contraindicated.

Lead ingestion: Paint chips from lead-based paint, lead-contaminated dust in home, soil contaminated with lead, lead solder used in plumbing and artwork, vinyl miniblinds, improperly glazed pottery, and traditional/folk remedies. Symptoms may be vague with insidious onset. Children absorb 50% of the lead they ingest and deposit it in their growing bones. Adults only absorb 10% of lead ingested.

- Gastrointestinal: anorexia, nausea, vomiting, and constipation.
- CNS: *low-dose exposure*—distractibility, impulsivity, hyperactivity, hearing impairment, mild intellectual deficits, loss of recently acquired developmental skills, and loss of coordination. *High-dose exposure*—lead encephalopathy may occur 4-6 wk following first symptoms. Mental retardation, severe ataxia, altered level of consciousness, paralysis, blindness, seizures, coma, and death all can occur.
- Cardiovascular: hypertension, bradycardia.
- Hematologic: anemia.
- Renal: glycosuria, proteinuria, possible acute or chronic renal failure, and impaired calcium function.
- Treatment depends on lead blood level.

Iron ingestion: Vitamin supplements with iron are one of most commonly ingested poisonous substances in children. Iron poisoning occurs in stages ranging from the initial stage (0.5-6 hr after ingestion) with vomiting, hematemesis, bloody stools, and abdominal pain to the hepatic injury stage (48-96 hr after the ingestion) with seizures and coma. If the child survives, pyloric or duodenal stenosis or hepatic cirrhosis may develop 2- 4 wk after ingestion. Treatment may include lavage or chelation therapy.

Carbon monoxide inhalation: Improperly ventilated heaters, wood stoves, and charcoal grills; poorly ventilated automobile.

- *Low-level exposure:* headache, stomach upset, and tiredness (similar to early "flu" symptoms).
- *High-level exposure:* Within minutes, cherry red lips and cheeks, altered level of consciousness (LOC), extreme dizziness, and coma. Cherry-red skin is a late sign most commonly noted in fatalities.
- Treatment includes administration of oxygen and symptomatic treatment.

Diagnostic Tests

History and physical examination help determine necessary tests.

Arterial blood gases: May be done if child is hypoventilating.

Serum levels: Blood levels of acetaminophen, salicylate, lead, and iron help determine if treatment with antidote is necessary.

Serum carboxyhemoglobin level: To determine degree of carbon monoxide poisoning.

Nursing Diagnosis:

Risk for Poisoning

related to inadequate parental knowledge about poison prevention

Desired Outcomes: Child does not ingest, inhale, or touch potentially toxic substances. Immediately following teaching, parents verbalize accurate understanding of how to childproof all areas (home, babysitter's home, grandparents' home) in which child lives or plays.

INTERVENTIONS	RATIONALES
Based on child's developmental age, discuss ways in which child might be exposed to poisons.	Understanding developmentally appropriate behavior enables parents to childproof home more effectively. For example, a 1-yr-old puts everything in the mouth but is not climbing yet, so any potential poison the child could reach while crawling or standing should be secured out of his or her reach.
Going room by room, discuss areas that need to be childproofed, with special emphasis on kitchen, storage areas, and bathroom.	Many poisonings involve household cleaners or medications. Knowledge of childproofing each area decreases risk of exposure to potentially toxic substances.

Continued

INTERVENTIONS	RATIONALES
Review all materials in home environment that could be poisonous.	Parents may not be aware of all the potentially poisonous substances in their home. Increased awareness likely will decrease child's exposure to poisonous substances, including the following: - Household cleaners, disinfectants - Cosmetics - Insecticides - Mouthwash with alcohol in it - Alcohol (beverages or rubbing alcohol) - Liquid dishwasher detergent - Foreign bodies and toys, such as bubble-blowing solution - Arts, crafts, and office supplies, such as pen and ink - Toxic plants - Hydrocarbons - Prescription and nonprescription medications
Describe ways to childproof home to prevent poisoning.	Guidelines enhance parents' ability to effectively and efficiently childproof home against poisoning. Examples include: - Put childproof locks on all kitchen, bathroom, and storage room cabinets. - Make sure all poisonous products are out of reach in locked cabinets. - Do not leave purse/briefcase sitting out that contains medication, cosmetics, or pens. - Buy medications with child-resistant caps but still store in a locked cabinet. - Do not store poisonous substances in food containers or water bottles; store them in the original container. - Throw away all old medications and other potential poisons that are no longer being used. Dispose of poisons out of child's reach (i.e., if poison is discarded in the kitchen trashcan and the child can reach the can, it was not disposed "out of child's reach"). Guidelines for disposing of hazardous household waste are available from the Environmental Protection Agency at *www.epa.gov/epaoswer/non-hw/muncpl/hhw.htm* and from Earth 911 at *www.earth911.org* (this website provides closest locations for disposal of hazardous materials). - Hang or install a carbon monoxide detector on each level of the home on which bedrooms are located. - If home was built before 1978, have it tested for lead-based paint.
Discuss these general guidelines to prevent poisoning. - Stay alert when using poisonous household products. - Never refer to medicine or vitamins as "candy." - Do not take medicine in front of young children.	Poisoning by ingestion or inhalation can occur in a matter of seconds. Child may think it is harmless or tastes good. Toddlers and preschoolers often imitate adult behavior.
Reinforce importance of informing family/friends of above guidelines.	Even with home childproofed by parents, visitors may bring potentially poisonous substances into the home (e.g., grandmother may visit and leave purse containing medicine bottle on the floor).
Encourage parents to childproof all residences/facilities visited by child.	Child may be safe at home but not at day care or grandparents' home.

●●● **Related NIC and NOC labels:** *NIC:* Parent Education: Childrearing Family; Environmental Management: Safety; Surveillance: Safety
NOC: Safety Behavior: Home Physical Environment; Safety Behavior: Personal; Safety Status: Physical Injury

Nursing Diagnosis:

Deficient Knowledge:

First aid for toxic ingestion/inhalation/exposure in accidental poisoning

Desired Outcome: Immediately following teaching, parents verbalize accurate knowledge of steps to take if accidental poisoning occurs.

INTERVENTIONS	RATIONALES
Teach parents the following:	
Post Poison Control Center (PCC) number on all phones. Also have emergency medical services (EMS) and pediatrician's number readily available.	It is vital to call PCC for possible ingestion of a toxic substance before administering any antidote to ensure correct treatment is implemented.
If syrup of ipecac is in the child's home, babysitter's home, or any other facility in which the child is cared for, it should be disposed of safely.	The American Academy of Pediatrics believes that ipecac should no longer be used routinely in the home as a poison treatment strategy and that any ipecac in the home should be disposed of safely (*Pediatrics* 112(5):1182-1185, 2003).
Review the following immediate action response if a child is poisoned:	Having this knowledge base enables parents to decrease absorption and provide appropriate treatment in the event of poisoning.
- If swallowed, remove any remaining poison from mouth. Call PCC immediately.	
- If poison is on the skin, remove contaminated clothing right away without touching poison and rinse skin with running water. Wash skin with soap and water and rinse well. Call PCC immediately.	
- If poison is in the eye, flush the eye with lukewarm to cool water for a full 15 min. Call PCC immediately.	
- If poison is inhaled, move child to fresh air right away. Call PCC.	
Discuss the following specific information parent should give to PCC:	Specific information enables PCC to direct treatment more appropriately.
- Child's weight and age.	
- Time poisoning occurred.	
- Amount ingested.	
- Name of poison, if possible. If medicine bottle or container is available, have it on hand when speaking with PCC.	

●●● **Related NIC and NOC labels:** *NIC:* Health Education; Teaching: Procedure/Treatment *NOC:* Knowledge: Child Safety; Knowledge: Health Resources; Knowledge: Illness Care; Knowledge: Treatment Regimen

ADDITIONAL NURSING DIAGNOSES/ PROBLEMS:

"Psychosocial Support for the Patient's Family and Significant Other" for such nursing diagnoses as **Fear** p. 87

and **Compromised Family Coping** for family whose child is being seen in emergency department or is hospitalized for life-threatening condition p. 89

"Bronchiolitis" for **Deficient Fluid Volume**. Child may be dehydrated related to effects of ingested substances, treatment for poisoning, or decreased fluid intake. p. 595

 PATIENT-FAMILY TEACHING AND DISCHARGE PLANNING

When providing child-family teaching, focus on sensory information, avoid giving excessive information, and initiate a visiting nurse referral for necessary follow-up teaching or to assess safety of home. Stress family-centered care (viewing the family as a unit that is the "constant" in the child's life and maintaining or improving the health of the family and its members). Include verbal and written information about the following (ensure that written information is at a level the reader can understand):

✓ Contributing factors to potential for poisoning for each child:

- Developmental age of child (e.g., cognitive, physical, and psychosocial)
- Environmental factors

- Behavioral problems
- Level of supervision
- ✓ Poison prevention tips:
- Keep all poisonous products out of reach in cabinets locked with safety locks.
- Know what household products are poisonous or potentially poisonous.
- Be careful and alert when using poisonous household products.
- Regularly discard old medications and other potential poisons in a safe manner.
- Keep all products in their original containers.
- Remember that many cosmetics and personal products may be poisonous (e.g., aftershave, cologne, hair spray, fingernail polish remover). Be sure to store them out of child's reach and where child cannot climb to get them.
- Buy products with child-resistant tops.
- Make sure that poisonous plants are not in the house or yard where child plays.
- Put a carbon monoxide detector on each level of the home where bedrooms are located.
- Keep all medications (prescription and nonprescription) in labeled containers and locked in a cabinet (none in purse or briefcase or on a counter or dresser).
- If home was built before 1978, have it tested for lead-based paint.
- Review sources of lead poisoning besides paint.
- Keep alcoholic beverages out of child's reach and locked up.

- ✓ Importance of having PCC, EMS, and health care provider's phone number posted by all phones. Also have home address and nearest intersection available in case babysitter or other family member needs to call EMS.
- ✓ Necessity of close supervision of infants and young children.
- ✓ Anticipatory guidance for next milestones child will achieve and childproofing for each age, including for all children in family (i.e., what is safe for a 6-mo-old is not safe for a 2-yr-old). Childproof all residences in which child stays. Reassess safety/childproofing frequently.
- ✓ Referrals to community resources, such as local and National Safe Kids Organization, safety experts, stores with a variety of materials to help childproof a home. Additional information can be obtained by contacting the following organizations:
  - National SAFE KIDS Campaign at *www.safekids.org*
  - Nationwide Poison Control Center (PCC) at (800) 222-1222
- ✓ Resources for disposal of hazardous household material:
  - EPA at *www.epa.gov/epaoswer/non-hw/muncpl/hhw.htm*
  - Earth 911 at *www.earth911.org* (lists closest location according to zip code for disposing of hazardous material)

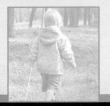

Sickle Cell Pain Crisis 87

OVERVIEW/PATHOPHYSIOLOGY

Sickle cell disease comprises a group of hereditary blood disorders in which hemoglobin S (HbS) is the dominant hemoglobin. Hemoglobin S (sickle hemoglobin) replaces normal adult hemoglobin (HbA). HbS differs from HbA in the substitution of one amino acid (valine) for another (glutamine). Under conditions of dehydration, acidosis, hypoxia, and temperature elevations, HbS changes its molecular structure and forms a crescent- or sickle-shaped red blood cell (RBC). This causes the cardinal clinical features of chronic hemolytic anemia and vasoocclusion, which result from obstruction caused by the sickled RBCs and increased RBC destruction. In most instances, the sickling response is reversible under conditions of adequate hydration and oxygenation. After repeated cycles of sickling and unsickling, the RBC remains in the sickled form. The most common form of sickle cell disease is hemoglobin SS disease, also called sickle cell anemia, in which the individual inherits a sickle cell gene from each parent.

The inheritance pattern is autosomal recessive (both parents must at least have the sickle cell trait). If both parents have the sickle cell trait, there is a 25% chance that each child will have sickle cell disease, a 25% chance that each child will have neither the trait nor the disease, and a 50% chance that each child will have the trait. Therefore a child may be asymptomatic (except under rare circumstances) with the trait or have varying degrees of symptoms with the disease. Sickle cell disease is among the most prevalent of genetic diseases in the United States, predominantly affecting African-American, African/Hispanic-Caribbean, and South American people. Approximately 1 in every 375 black infants born in the United States has sickle cell disease and 1 in 12 African Americans has sickle cell trait (London, 2007).

Pain is the leading cause of emergency department visits and hospitalizations. It can occur as early as age 4-6 mo and unpredictably throughout a lifetime. There is considerable variation in the severity, frequency, and types of pain among and within affected individuals.

HEALTH CARE SETTING

Primary care with possible hospitalization for infections or pain crisis

ASSESSMENT

Signs and symptoms: Generally do not appear in infants before 4-6 mo of age because of high levels of fetal hemoglobin. Pain is the hallmark manifestation and is caused by vasoocclusion and the resulting ischemia distal to the occlusion. Types of pain states include acute painful event, acute hand-foot syndrome (dactylitis—usually seen in children between 6 mo and 2 yr old), acute joint inflammation, acute chest syndrome (a common cause of mortality manifesting as chest pain, fever, pneumonia-like cough, and anemia), splenic sequestration (enlarged spleen with sudden drop in hemoglobin—can be life threatening), intrahepatic sickling or hepatic sequestration, abdominal and intraabdominal pain, priapism, and avascular necrosis of the femur or humerus. Stroke is another form of vasoocclusive event and has a high rate of recurrence. Children with sickle cell disease often have nonfunctional spleens due to "clogging" from the sickled RBCs, and this puts them at increased risk for sepsis. Thus, overwhelming infection/sepsis is the leading cause of death in young children with sickle cell disease.

Physical assessment: History and physical, including character, location, severity, and duration of pain, as well as at-home treatment. Information should be obtained about methods used in the past to treat pain crises effectively. Initial pain assessment should be done and repeated before and after analgesia.

DIAGNOSTIC TESTS

Hemoglobin electrophoresis, isoelectric focusing, and high-performance liquid chromatography: Enable definitive diagnosis of sickle cell disease.

Oximetry: Noninvasive method that will reveal decreased O_2 saturation if it is present.

Chest x-ray examination: Helps differentiate between acute chest syndrome and pneumonia.

Complete blood count with reticulocytes: May show increased white blood cells with infection. The life span of the normal RBC is decreased from 120 days to 10-14 days, so bone marrow compensates with increased production. Reticulocyte count gives an indication of RBC production by the bone marrow (reticulocytes are immature RBCs).

Blood culture: Infection may have triggered crisis. Sepsis is the leading cause of death in children younger than 5 yr old.

Basic metabolic panel: If signs and symptoms of dehydration are present, helps assess degree of dehydration and need for electrolyte replacement.

Nursing Diagnosis:

Acute Pain

related to tissue anoxia secondary to vasoocclusion

Desired Outcomes: For mild-to-moderate pain, child states or demonstrates that pain has decreased within 1-1½ hr of receiving oral medication. For severe pain, child states or demonstrates that pain has decreased within 24 hr of intervention/treatment. Pain is less than 2 on a 5-point scale such as Wong-Baker FACES scale or less than 4 on a 10-point scale such as FLACC or numeric scale.

INTERVENTIONS	RATIONALES
Establish pain scale appropriate for child (FLACC, Wong-Baker FACES, Oucher, Poker Chip, or numeric) and use it before and after analgesic is administered (within 10-30 min after IV medication administration and within 1-1½ hr after oral medication administration). Assess pain level q 2-4 hr unless on continuous infusion of pain medication, in which case assess qh.	A pain scale monitors degree of pain and effectiveness of pain medication.
Plan schedule of pain medication around the clock, not prn.	Consistent use lowers total amount of medication with better control. Prolonged stimulation of pain receptors results in increased sensitivity to painful stimuli and will increase the amount of drug required to relieve pain.
Do *not* administer meperidine (Demerol).	Demerol increases risk of normeperidine-induced seizures, *especially* in a child with sickle cell disease.
Carefully apply warmth to affected area.	Warmth may be soothing to child, but it should be applied judiciously because ischemic tissue is fragile.
Do *not* apply cold compresses.	Cold promotes sickling and vasoconstriction.
Assess hydration status q4h: level of consciousness (LOC), anterior fontanel if child is younger than 2 yr old, oral mucous membrane, abdominal skin turgor, and urine output.	This assessment helps detect and prevent/treat dehydration, which causes vasoocclusion/pain. A child who is dehydrated may exhibit decreased LOC, sunken anterior fontanel (if younger than 2 yr old), dry or sticky oral mucous membrane, tented abdominal skin, and decreased urine output.
Use nonpharmacologic pain control measures as appropriate for child.	Optimally, comfort measures will distract child from the pain and augment effects of pharmacologic measures. Examples include distraction (watching TV or playing games), deep breathing, relaxation exercises, music, touch, imagery, and massage.

••• **Related NIC and NOC labels:** *NIC:* Medication Management; Analgesic Administration; Presence; Simple Relaxation Therapy; Distraction; Heat Application; Music Therapy; Simple Massage; Simple Guided Imagery *NOC:* Comfort Level; Pain: Disruptive Effects

Nursing Diagnosis:

Ineffective Tissue Perfusion: Cardiopulmonary and Cerebral

related to vasoocclusion and anemia

Desired Outcomes: Within 2 hr following treatment/intervention, child's oxygen saturation is maintained at greater than 95% or at level prescribed by health care provider. There is no evidence of long-term complications from lack of oxygen.

INTERVENTIONS	RATIONALES
Assess respiratory status and mental status q2-4h and prn.	Frequent assessment ensures early detection of changes in respiratory status. Tachypnea and increased work of breathing (WOB) are early signs of hypoxia. LOC is a good indicator of oxygen perfusion to the brain.

Continued

INTERVENTIONS	RATIONALES
Monitor pulse oximetry continuously.	This is a noninvasive method of assessing oxygen saturation and noting changes promptly.
Administer oxygen as prescribed to keep oxygen saturation levels at greater than 95% or at level appropriate for individual child.	Delivering oxygen when child is hypoxic eases WOB. However, it does not reverse the sickling process, and long-term use can depress bone marrow activity and increase the anemia.
Elevate head of bed to a comfortable level for child.	This facilitates chest expansion by decreasing pressure on the diaphragm.
Ensure incentive spirometry q1-2h while child is awake.	This treatment facilitates deep breathing and decreases the incidence of acute chest syndrome.
Administer packed RBCs as prescribed.	This treatment improves tissue perfusion by correcting anemia.

••• **Related NIC and NOC labels:** *NIC:* Oxygen therapy; Respiratory Monitoring; Positioning; Blood Products Administration *NOC:* Tissue Perfusion: Pulmonary; Tissue Perfusion: Cerebral

Nursing Diagnosis:

Deficient Knowledge:

Sickle cell disease, measures to avoid vasoocclusive crisis, home management to prevent severe pain crisis, and the genetics that could result in having other children with this disease

Desired Outcome: Within 48 hr following teaching, child/family verbalizes accurate understanding of the disease process, especially pain crisis and appropriate treatment, and the genetics of disease transmission.

INTERVENTIONS	RATIONALES
Instruct older child/family in basic information about sickle cell disease and measures to minimize sickling.	Knowledge of the disease process promotes adherence to the plan of care, for example, taking prescribed medications such as penicillin and folic acid on a regular basis, staying up to date on immunizations, and avoiding precipitating factors (i.e., dehydration, exposure to individuals who are ill with infections, extreme temperatures, high elevations, excessive physical activity).
Encourage child/family to obtain medical alert bracelet/necklace and inform significant health professionals/school personnel of diagnosis.	These actions will help ensure prompt and appropriate treatment.
Explain signs of developing pain crisis, its significance, and importance of prompt treatment.	Knowledge about the signs of pain crisis and it's significance optimally will result in prompt reporting and treatment, which may avoid a severe vasoocclusive crisis. For example, in an infant or toddler, a combination of unusual behaviors such as inconsolability, decreased appetite, unexplained crying, and rapid breathing may indicate discomfort or pain. Older children may complain of mild discomfort or aching.
Discuss home treatment for mild/early symptoms of pain crisis.	The severity of pain crisis may be decreased by early/prompt treatment (e.g., resting, increasing fluid intake to 1-1.5 × maintenance fluids, and administering pain medication).
Discuss transmission of disease and refer for genetic counseling as indicated.	This information enables family to make informed reproductive decisions. See discussion in introductory data.
Encourage family members to be advocates for the child in the hospital, during appointments with the health care provider, and in day care or school setting (e.g., Individualized Education Plan [IEP] or 504 plan at school). Reinforce that they know the child best and understand what is normal or abnormal in relationship to the child.	Family members may be hesitant to ask questions or advocate for the child; however, they are the best resource. Encouraging advocacy increases likelihood that child will receive the best care and facilitates optimal development.

Continued

INTERVENTIONS	RATIONALES
Encourage inclusion of siblings with planning and providing care for the chronically ill child as appropriate.	Including siblings may help them cope with/adapt to having a brother/sister with a chronic illness.
Supply family with information about support groups, local/national sickle cell organizations, and resources for additional information.	Support systems likely will improve knowledge base about disease process and therapeutics involved as well as let them know they are not "alone."
Encourage family to have child receive follow-up visits at a sickle cell clinic on a regular basis.	Follow-up promotes continuity and quality of care.

••• **Related NIC and NOC labels:** *NIC:* Teaching: Disease Process; Risk Identification; Parent Education: Childbearing Family *NOC:* Knowledge: Treatment Regimen; Knowledge: Disease Process; Knowledge: Illness Care

Nursing Diagnosis:

Deficient Knowledge:

Precautions and side effects of prescribed medications

Desired Outcome: Within 48 hr following teaching, child/family verbalizes accurate information about prescribed medications, including precautions and side effects.

INTERVENTIONS	RATIONALES
Teach child/parent the following, depending on prescribed medication:	
Morphine Sulfate	This medication is an opioid analgesic (administered in hospital).
Monitor child for level of sedation, pain relief obtained, O_2 saturation, and respiratory and cardiac status.	This assessment helps to evaluate effectiveness of medication and possible need to adjust dosage. Morphine can cause respiratory depression, and if it occurs, O_2 saturation would decrease along with respiratory rate.
There is need to monitor for dizziness, drowsiness, itching, nausea, vomiting, constipation, urinary retention, and low blood pressure. Parent/child should notify staff or health care provider if any of these symptoms occur.	These side effects may indicate need to change dosage of medication or medication itself or to provide additional medication, such as diphenhydramine for itching or an antiemetic for nausea.
Reassure child/parents that analgesics, including opioids, are medically indicated and that high doses may be needed to relieve pain.	There is confusion about the issues of pain control and drug dependence. Children rarely become addicted, and needless suffering may occur as a result of unnecessary fears.
Acetaminophen with Codeine	This medication is a central analgesic/antipyretic with added opioid.
Monitor for and report palpitations, dizziness, drowsiness, itching, nausea, vomiting, cramping, low blood pressure, and constipation, as well as excessive sedation and respiratory depression.	These side effects may indicate need to adjust or change medication.
Assess if pain has decreased within 1-1½ hr of oral administration. If child has no relief after several doses of pain medication, parent should notify health care provider.	This assessment evaluates effectiveness of medication as this is the time of peak action. If there is no relief after several doses, health care provider may increase dosage.
Ibuprofen	This medication augments pain control when administered with morphine or acetaminophen with codeine.
Be alert to and report dizziness, drowsiness, and heartburn.	These side effects may indicate need for health care provider to adjust dosage or change medication.
Administer with food or milk.	This decreases gastrointestinal (GI) upset.
Folic Acid	This medication enhances bone marrow's ability to produce new blood cells.
Penicillin	This is a prophylactic antibiotic. Overwhelming infection/sepsis is the leading cause of death in young children with sickle cell disease.

Continued

INTERVENTIONS	RATIONALES
Importance of daily administration as prescribed at least until child is 5-6 yr old.	This reduces morbidity risks associated with pneumococcal septicemia. It may need to be continued for a longer period if child has experienced invasive pneumococcal infection, has not received pneumococcal immunizations, is on a hypertransfusion program, or is anatomically asplenic.
Monitor for and report rash, nausea, vomiting, diarrhea, black hairy tongue, and hypersensitivity reactions. Call 911 promptly if anaphylaxis occurs.	These side effects may indicate need for health care provider to adjust dosage or change medication.
Administer/take with water on an empty stomach 1 hr before meals or 2 hr after meals; may give with food to decrease GI upset.	Food or milk may decrease absorption.
Docusate	This is a stool softener.
Administer when child is taking analgesics.	Analgesics may cause constipation.
If using in liquid form, administer with a small amount of milk, fruit juice, or infant formula.	These liquids mask the bitter taste.
Ensure that child is receiving 1-1½ × maintenance fluids unless pulmonary symptoms exist. For calculation of maintenance fluids, see "Bronchiolitis," p. 595, for **Deficient Fluid Volume.**	This facilitates effectiveness of docusate and provides adequate hydration for child with sickle cell pain crisis. Increased fluids may be needed if child is dehydrated and/or has increased insensible losses (e.g., persistent fever).
Monitor for and report rash, diarrhea, abdominal cramping, or throat irritation.	These are side effects; health care provider may need to adjust dosage or change medication.
Acetaminophen	This is an analgesic.
Administer immediately for mild complaint of pain or discomfort.	This may prevent pain crisis.
Monitor for and report rash.	This side effect may indicate need for health care provider to adjust dosage or change medication.
Ensure that child is receiving therapeutic dose of acetaminophen.	This helps to provide effective pain relief while avoiding hepatic necrosis.

••• **Related NIC and NOC labels:** *NIC:* Teaching: Prescribed Medication; Analgesic Administration; Pain Management *NOC:* Knowledge: Medication

ADDITIONAL NURSING DIAGNOSES/ PROBLEMS:

Constipation can occur as a result of narcotic analgesics and decreased mobility. See "Prolonged Bedrest" for **Constipation.**   p. 67

"Psychosocial Support" for **Anticipatory Grieving/ Risk for Dysfunctional Grieving**   p. 79

"Psychosocial Support for Patient's Family and Significant Other"   p. 87

"Asthma" for **Anxiety** related to illness, loss of control, and medical/nursing interventions   p. 580

"Asthma" for **Interrupted Family Processes** related to having a child with a chronic illness   p. 581

"Bronchiolitis" for **Deficient Fluid Volume** (however, child with sickle cell pain crisis needs 1-1½ × maintenance, unless pulmonary symptoms are present, in which case then only maintenance fluids. Increased fluids may be needed if child is dehydrated and/or has increased insensible losses (e.g., persistent fever).   p. 595

Appendix A for "Infection Prevention and Control." Overwhelming infection/sepsis is the leading cause of death in young children with sickle cell disease.   p. 783

PATIENT-FAMILY TEACHING AND DISCHARGE PLANNING

When providing patient-family teaching, focus on sensory information. Avoid giving excessive instructions and institute a visiting nurse referral as necessary for follow-up teaching and assessment. Stress family-centered care (viewing the family as a unit that is the "constant" in the child's life and maintaining or improving the health of the family and its members). Include verbal and written information about the following (ensure written information is at a level the reader can understand):

✓ Basic pathophysiology about sickle disease and pain crisis.

✓ Cause of pain, including precipitating factors (e.g., dehydration, infection, fever, hot or cold temperatures, high elevations, excessive physical activity) and importance of avoiding same.

✓ For boys, priapism (prolonged erection) is possible with sickle cell disease. They need to seek medical attention if erections last more than 3 hr or occur frequently.

✓ Avoiding exposure to individuals who are ill with infections (e.g., do not go in crowded areas during flu season). Overwhelming infection/sepsis is the leading cause of death in young children with sickle cell disease.

✓ Importance of maintaining adequate oral intake to prevent dehydration and thereby prevent clumping of HbS.

✓ Signs and symptoms of early pain crisis and treatment (i.e., rest, increase fluids to 1-1½ × maintenance, and administer acetaminophen or ibuprofen first. If no relief, try prescription pain medication from the health care provider).

✓ Maintaining a pain diary, which may be beneficial in finding precipitating factors and effective pain control measures. The most effective treatment in an emergency department also should be included in the event that child is seen in another hospital.

✓ Medications, including drug name; route; purpose; dosage; precautions; drug-drug, food-drug, and herb-drug interactions; and potential side effects.

✓ Importance of taking medications at home and school as directed. Medication in the original bottle (with prescribing label) and written prescription from health care provider are needed for child to be able to take any medication at school.

✓ Nonpharmacologic methods to relieve pain:
- Psychologic strategies: distraction, imagery, education/teaching, and hypnotherapy
- Behavioral strategies: deep breathing, relaxation exercises, self-hypnosis, biofeedback, and behavior modification
- Physical strategies: careful application of heat to painful area, massage, and mild exercise, if tolerated

✓ Frequent urination, which is normal with increased fluids; enuresis may occur as a result.

✓ When to contact physician:
- Temperature 101° F or higher
- Severe pain not relieved by prescribed pain medication (usually acetaminophen with codeine)
- Child is pale, lethargic, irritable, or dehydrated
- Vomiting and/or diarrhea lasting more than a day
- Shortness of breath or other acute pulmonary symptoms

✓ Coordination of care. Parents should discuss child's illness and needs with school nurse and other adults who are in close contact with child (e.g., teachers, scout leaders, day care providers).

✓ Importance of helping siblings cope with/adapt to having a brother/sister with a chronic illness and including them in planning and/or caring for the chronically ill child depending on their age and interest.

✓ Legal rights of the child:
- Individuals with Disabilities Education Act (IDEA): Mandates federal government to provide funding to education agencies for free and appropriate education to qualifying students with disabilities, including children with sickle cell disease if the disease adversely affects school performance. School is then required to develop an Individualized Education Plan (IEP).
- IEP: A multidisciplinary team designs this plan to facilitate special education and therapeutic strategies and goals for each child. Child does not have to be in special education classes. Parents need to be involved in this process.
- Section 504 of Rehabilitation Act of 1973: Each student with a disability (physical or mental impairment) is entitled to accommodation to attend school and participate as fully as possible in school activities. This accommodation may be related to a medical condition or an educational issue. For example, child may leave the classroom to use bathroom facilities without raising his or her hand and will not be penalized for excessive absences from school that are caused by sickle cell disease. The 504 Plan may include as many accommodations as necessary for child to function well.

✓ Importance of ongoing health care management with health care provider experienced in dealing with sickle cell disease to identify and manage chronic complications:
- Receiving childhood immunizations at the appropriate age, especially pneumococcal and yearly flu vaccine
- Prompt attention to symptoms of infection (e.g., fever, sore throat)
- Regular visits with health care provider, not just when ill

✓ Telephone numbers to call in case questions or concerns arise about therapy or disease after discharge.

✓ Additional general information can be obtained by contacting the following organizations:
- The Sickle Cell Information Center at *www.scinfo.org*
- *Pain assessment and pain management in sickle cell disease: A guidebook for patients and their families*, available at *www.scinfo.org/painmgpt.htm*
- Sickle Cell Disease Association of America at *www.sicklecelldisease.org*
- *Guideline for Management of Acute and Chronic Pain in Sickle Cell Disease*, available at *www.ampainsoc.org*
- STARLIGHT-STARBRIGHT Children's Foundation, "The Sickle Cell Slime-O-Rama Game" recommended for children 6-14 yr old, available at *www.starlight.org* under "programs"

✓ Explorer Series (no charge for CD-ROM) includes the following and available at *www.sicklecellkids.org*, "A fun and educational website for children with sickle cell disease": "Spotlight on IVs" recommended for children 6-10 yr old, "Medical Imaging: Welcome to the Radiology Center" recommended for children 6-10 yr old, "Blood Tests: Exploring Our Incredible Blood" recommended for children 10-15 yr old.

NORMAL LABORATORY VALUES (PEDIATRIC PATIENTS)

TEST/SPECIMEN	AGE/GENDER/ REFERENCE	Normal Ranges			
		CONVENTIONAL UNITS		INTERNATIONAL UNITS (SI)	
ACETAMINOPHEN					
Serum or plasma	Therap. conc.	10-30 mcg/ml		66-200 μmol/L	
	Toxic conc.	More than 200 mcg/ml		More than 1300 μmol/L	
AMMONIA NITROGEN					
Plasma or serum	Newborn	90-150 mcg/dl		64-107 μmol/L	
	0-2 wk	79-129 mcg/dl		56-92 μmol/L	
	Older than 1 mo	29-70 mcg/dl		21-50 μmol/L	
ANTISTREPTOLYSIN O TITER (ASO)					
Serum	2-4 yr	Less than 160 Todd units			
	School-age children	170-330 Todd units			
BASE EXCESS					
Whole blood	Newborn	(−10) - (−2) mEq/L		(−10) - (−2) mmol/L	
	Infant	(−7) - (−1) mEq/L		(−7) - (−1) mmol/L	
	Child	(−4) - (+2) mEq/L		(−4) - (+2) mmol/L	
BICARBONATE (HCO_3)					
Serum	Arterial	21-28 mEq/L		21-28 mmol/L	
	Venous	22-29 mEq/L		22-29 mmol/L	
		Premature (mg/dl)	**Full term (mg/dl)**	**Premature (μmol/L)**	**Full term (μmol/L)**
BILIRUBIN, TOTAL					
Serum	Cord	Less than 2.0	Less than 2.0	Less than 34	Less than 34
	0-1 d	Less than 8.0	Less than 6.0	Less than 137	Less than 103
	1-2 d	Less than 12.0	Less than 8.0	Less than 205	Less than 137
	2-5 d	Less than 16.0	Less than 12.0	Less than 274	Less than 205
	Thereafter	Less than 20.0	Less than 10.0	Less than 340	Less than 171
BILIRUBIN, DIRECT (CONJUGATED)					
Serum		0.0-0.2 mg/dl		0-3.4 μmol/L	
BLEEDING TIME					
BLOOD FROM SKIN PUNCTURE					
Ivy	Normal	2-7 min		2-7 min	
	Borderline	7-11 min		7-11 min	
Simplate (G-D)		2.75-8 min		2.75-8 min	
BLOOD VOLUME					
Whole blood	Male	52-83 ml/kg		0.052-0.083 L/kg	
	Female	50-75 ml/kg		0.050-0.075 L/kg	
C-REACTIVE PROTEIN (CRP)					
Serum	Cord	52-1330 ng/ml		52-1330 mcg/L	
	2-12 yr	67-1800 ng/ml		67-1800 mcg/L	
CALCIUM, IONIZED					
Serum, plasma, or whole blood	Cord	5.0-6.0 mg/dl		1.25-1.50 mmol/L	
	Newborn, 3-24 hr	4.3-5.1 mg/dl		1.07-1.27 mmol/L	
	24-48 hr	4.0-4.7 mg/dl		1.00-1.17 mmol/L	
	Thereafter	4.8-4.92 mg/dl or 2.24-2.46 mEq/L		1.12-1.23 mmol/L	

Source: Wilson D, Hockenberry MJ: *Wong's Clinical Manual of Pediatric Nursing*, ed 7, St. Louis, 2008, Mosby. Modified from Behrman RE, Kliegman RM, Jenson HB, editors: *Nelson textbook of pediatrics*, ed 17, Philadelphia, 2004, Saunders; McMillan JA, Deangelis CD, Feigin RD, and others, editors: *Oski's pediatrics: principles and practice*, ed 3, Philadelphia, 1999, Lippincott Williams & Wilkins; and Fischbach F: *A manual of laboratory and diagnostic tests*, ed 6, Philadelphia, 2000, Lippincott Williams & Wilkins.

Continued

NORMAL LABORATORY VALUES (PEDIATRIC PATIENTS)—cont'd

TEST/SPECIMEN	AGE/GENDER/REFERENCE	Normal Ranges	
		CONVENTIONAL UNITS	INTERNATIONAL UNITS (SI)
CALCIUM, TOTAL			
Serum	Cord	9.0-11.5 mg/dl	2.25-2.88 mmol/L
	Newborn, 3-24 hr	9.0-10.6 mg/dl	2.3-2.65 mmol/L
	24-48 hr	7.0-12.0 mg/dl	1.75-3.0 mmol/L
	4-7 d	9.0-10.9 mg/dl	2.25-2.73 mmol/L
	Child	8.8-10.8 mg/dl	2.2-2.70 mmol/L
	Thereafter	8.4-10.2 mg/dl	2.1-2.55 mmol/L
CARBON DIOXIDE, PARTIAL PRESSURE (PCO_2)			
Whole blood, arterial	Newborn	27-40 mm Hg	3.6-5.3 kPa
	Infant	27-41 mm Hg	3.6-5.5 kPa
	Thereafter: Male	35-48 mm Hg	4.7-6.4 kPa
	Female	32-45 mm Hg	4.3-6.0 kPa
CARBON DIOXIDE, TOTAL (TCO_2)			
Serum or plasma	Cord	14-22 mEq/L	14-22 mmol/L
	Premature (1 wk)	14-27 mEq/L	14-27 mmol/L
	Newborn	13-22 mEq/L	13-22 mmol/L
	Infant, child	20-28 mEq/L	20-28 mmol/L
	Thereafter	23-30 mEq/L	23-30 mmol/L
CEREBROSPINAL FLUID (CSF)			
Pressure		70-180 mm H_2O	70-180 mm H_2O
Volume	Child	60-100 ml	0.06-0.10 L
CHLORIDE			
Serum or plasma	Cord	96-104 mEq/L	96-104 mmol/L
	Newborn	97-110 mEq/L	97-110 mmol/L
	Thereafter	98-106 mEq/L	98-106 mmol/L
Sweat	Normal (homozygote)	Less than 40 mEq/L	Less than 40 mmol/L
	Marginal (e.g., asthma, Addison disease, malnutrition)	45-60 mEq/L	45-60 mmol/L
	Cystic fibrosis	More than 60 mEq/L	More than 60 mmol/L
CHOLESTEROL, TOTAL			
Serum or plasma†	Acceptable	Less than 170 mg/dl	Less than 4.4 mmol/L
	Borderline	170-199 mg/dl	4.4-5.1 mmol/L
	High	≥200 mg/dl	≥5.2 mmol/L
CLOTTING TIME (LEE-WHITE)			
Whole blood		5-8 min (glass tubes)	5-8 min
		5-15 min (room temp)	5-15 min
		30 min (silicone tube)	30 min
CREATINE KINASE (CK, CPK)			
Serum	Cord	70-380 U/L	70-380 U/L
	5-8 hr	214-1175 U/L	214-1175 U/L
	24-33 hr	130-1200 U/L	130-1200 U/L
	72-100 hr	87-725 U/L	87-725 U/L
CREATININE			
Serum	Cord	0.6-1.2 mg/dl	53-106 µmol/L
	Newborn	0.3-1.0 mg/dl	27-88 µmol/L
	Infant	0.2-0.4 mg/d	18-35 µmol/L
	Child	0.3-0.7 mg/dl	27-62 µmol/L
	Adolescent	0.5-1.0 mg/dl	44-88 µmol/L
Urine, 24 hr	Premature	8.1-15.0 mg/kg/24 hr	72-133 µmol/kg/24 hr
	Full term	10.4-19.7 mg/kg/24 hr	92-174 µmol/kg/24 hr
	1.5-7 yr	10-15 mg/kg/24 hr	88-133 µmol/kg/24 hr
	7-15 yr	5.2-41 mg/kg/24 hr	46-362 mmol/kg/24 hr

†From National Cholesterol Education Program: Report of the expert panel on blood cholesterol levels in children and adolescents, *Pediatrics* 89(3 pt 2):527, 1992.

NORMAL LABORATORY VALUES (PEDIATRIC PATIENTS)—cont'd

TEST/SPECIMEN	AGE/GENDER/ REFERENCE	Normal Ranges CONVENTIONAL UNITS	INTERNATIONAL UNITS (SI)
CREATININE CLEARANCE (ENDOGENOUS)			
Serum or plasma and urine	Newborn	40-65 ml/min/1.73 m^2	
DIGOXIN			
Serum, plasma; collect at least 12 hr after dose	Therap. conc.		
	CHF	0.8-1.5 ng/ml	1.0-1.9 nmol/L
	Arrhythmias	1.5-2.0 ng/ml	1.9-2.6 nmol/L
	Toxic conc.		
	Child	More than 2.5 ng/ml	More than 3.2 nmol/L
EOSINOPHIL COUNT			
Whole blood, capillary blood		50-250 cells/mm^3 (µl)	50-250 × 10^6 cells/L
ERYTHROCYTE (RBC) COUNT			
Whole blood	Cord	3.9-5.5 million/mm^3	3.9-5.5 × 10^{12} cells/L
	1-3 d	4.0-6.6 million/mm^3	4.0-6.6 × 10^{12} cells/L
	1 wk	3.9-6.3 million/mm^3	3.9-6.3 × 10^{12} cells/L
	2 wk	3.6-6.2 million/mm^3	3.6-6.2 × 10^{12} cells/L
	1 mo	3.0-5.4 million/mm^3	3.0-5.4 × 10^{12} cells/L
	2 mo	2.7-4.9 million/mm^3	2.7-4.9 × 10^{12} cells/L
	3-6 mo	3.1-4.5 million/mm^3	3.1-4.5 × 10^{12} cells/L
	0.5-2 yr	3.7-5.3 million/mm^3	3.7-5.3 × 10^{12} cells/L
	2-6 yr	3.9-5.3 million/mm^3	3.9-5.3 × 10^{12} cells/L
	6-12 yr	4.0-5.2 million/mm^3	4.0-5.2 × 10^{12} cells/L
	12-18 yr: Male	4.5-5.3 million/mm^3	4.5-5.3 × 10^{12} cells/L
	Female	4.1-5.1 million/mm^3	4.1-5.1 × 10^{12} cells/L
ERYTHROCYTE SEDIMENTATION RATE (ESR)			
Whole blood			
Westergren (modified)	Child	0-10 mm/hr	0-10 mm/hr
Wintrobe	Child	0-13 mm/hr	0-13 mm/hr
FIBRINOGEN			
Plasma	Newborn	125-300 mg/d	1.25-3.00 g/L
	Thereafter	200-400 mg/dl	2.00-4.00 g/L
GALACTOSE			
Serum	Newborn	0-20 mg/dl	0-1.11 mmol/L
	Thereafter	Less than 5 mg/dl	Less than 0.28 mmol/L
Urine	Newborn	≤60 mg/dl	≤3.33 mmol/L
	Thereafter	Less than 14 mg/24 hr	Less than 0.08 mmol/d
GLUCOSE			
Serum	Cord	45-96 mg/dl	2.5-5.3 mmol/L
	Newborn, 1 d	40-60 mg/dl	2.2-3.3 mmol/L
	Newborn, older than 1 d	50-90 mg/dl	2.8-5.0 mmol/L
	Child	60-100 mg/dl	3.3-5.5 mmol/L
	Thereafter	70-105 mg/dl	3.9-5.8 mmol/L

GLUCOSE TOLERANCE TEST (GTT), ORAL

Serum Dosages		Normal	Diabetic	Normal	Diabetic
Child: 1.75 g/kg of ideal	60 min	120-170 mg/dl	≥200 mg/dl	6.7-9.4 mmol/L	≥11 mmol/L
weight up to maximum	90 min	100-140 mg/dl	≥200 mg/dl	5.6-7.8 mmol/L	≥11 mmol/L
of 75 g	120 min	70-120 mg/dl	≥200 mg/dl	3.9-6.7 mmol/L	≥11 mmol/L

Continued

NORMAL LABORATORY VALUES (PEDIATRIC PATIENTS)—cont'd

TEST/SPECIMEN	AGE/GENDER/REFERENCE		Normal Ranges	
			CONVENTIONAL UNITS	INTERNATIONAL UNITS (SI)
GROWTH HORMONE (GH, SOMATOTROPIN)				
Plasma	1 d		5-53 ng/ml	5-53 mcg/L
	1 wk		5-27 ng/ml	5-27 mcg/L
	1-12 mo		2-10 ng/ml	2-10 mcg/L
	Fasting child		Less than 0.7-6.0 ng/ml	Less than 0.7-6.0 mcg/L
HEMATOCRIT (HCT, HCT)				
Whole blood	1 d (cap)		48%-69%	0.48-0.69 vol fraction
	2 d		48%-75%	0.48-0.75 vol fraction
	3 d		44%-72%	0.44-0.72 vol fraction
	2 mo		28%-42%	0.28-0.42 vol fraction
	6-12 yr		35%-45%	0.35-0.45 vol fraction
	12-18 yr:	Male	37%-49%	0.37-0.49 vol fraction
		Female	36%-46%	0.36-0.46 vol fraction
HEMOGLOBIN (HB)				
Whole blood	1-3 d (cap)		14.5-22.5 g/dl	2.25-3.49 mmol/L
	2 mo		9.0-14.0 g/dl	1.40-2.17 mmol/L
	6-12 yr		11.5-15.5 g/dl	1.78-2.40 mmol/L
	12-18 yr:	Male	13.0-16.0 g/dl	2.02-2.48 mmol/L
		Female	12.0-16.0 g/dl	1.86-2.48 mmol/L
HEMOGLOBIN A				
Whole blood			More than 95% of total	More than 0.95 fraction of Hb
HEMOGLOBIN F				
Whole blood	1 d		63%-92% HbF	0.63-0.92 mass fraction HbF
	5 d		65%-88% HbF	0.65-0.88 mass fraction HbF
	3 wk		55%-85% HbF	0.55-0.85 mass fraction HbF
	6-9 wk		31%-75% HbF	0.31-0.75 mass fraction HbF
	3-4 mo		Less than 2%-59% HbF	Less than 0.02-0.59 mass fraction HbF
	6 mo		Less than 2%-9% HbF	Less than 0.02-0.09 mass fraction HbF
IMMUNOGLOBULIN A (IGA)				
Serum	Cord		1.4-3.6 mg/dl	14-36 mg/L
	1-3 mo		1.3-53 mg/dl	13-530 mg/L
	4-6 mo		4.4-84 mg/dl	44-840 mg/L
	7-12 mo		11-106 mg/dl	110-1060 mg/L
	2-5 yr		14-159 mg/dl	140-1590 mg/L
	6-10 yr		33-236 mg/dl	330-2360 mg/L
IMMUNOGLOBULIN D (IGD)				
Serum	Newborn		None detected	None detected
	Thereafter		0-8 mg/dl	0-80 mg/L
IMMUNOGLOBULIN E (IGE)				
Serum	Male		0-230 IU/ml	0-230 kIU/L
	Female		0-170 IU/ml	0-170 kIU/L
IMMUNOGLOBULIN G (IGG)				
Serum	Cord		636-1606 mg/dl	6.36-16.06 g/L
	1 mo		251-906 mg/dl	2.51-9.06 g/L
	2-4 mo		176-601 mg/dl	1.76-6.01 g/L
	5-12 mo		172-1069 mg/dl	1.72-10.69 g/L
	1-5 yr		345-1236 mg/dl	3.45-12.36 g/L
	6-10 yr		608-1572 mg/dl	6.08-15.72 g/L
IMMUNOGLOBULIN M (IGM)				
Serum	Cord		6.3-25 mg/dl	63-250 mg/L
	1-4 mo		17-105 mg/dl	170-1050 mg/L
	5-9 mo		33-126 mg/dl	330-1260 mg/L

NORMAL LABORATORY VALUES (PEDIATRIC PATIENTS)—cont'd

TEST/SPECIMEN	AGE/GENDER/ REFERENCE	Normal Ranges	
		CONVENTIONAL UNITS	INTERNATIONAL UNITS (SI)
	10-12 mo	41-173 mg/dl	410-1730 mg/L
	2-8 yr	43-207 mg/dl	430-2070 mg/L
	9-10 yr	52-242 mg/dl	520-2420 mg/L
IRON			
Serum	Newborn	100-250 mcg/dl	18-45 µmol/L
	Infant	40-100 mcg/dl	7-18 µmol/L
	Child	50-120 mcg/dl	9-22 µmol/L
	Thereafter: Male	65-170 mcg/dl	12-30 µmol/L
	Female	50-170 mcg/dl	9-30 µmol/L
	Intoxicated child	280-2550 mcg/dl	50.12-456.5 µmol/L
	Fatally poisoned child	More than 1800 mcg/dl	More than 322.2 µmol/L
IRON-BINDING CAPACITY, TOTAL (TIBC)			
Serum	Infant	100-400 mcg/dl	17.90-71.60 µmol/L
	Thereafter	250-400 mcg/dl	44.75-71.60 µmol/L
LEAD			
Whole blood	Child	Less than 10 mcg/dl	Less than 0.48 µmol/L
Urine, 24 hr		Less than 80 mcg/L	Less than 0.39 µmol/L
LEUKOCYTE COUNT (WBC COUNT)		$\times$ 1000 cells/mm^3 (µl)	$\times$ 10^9 cells/L
Whole blood	Birth	9.0-30.0	9.0-30.0
	24 hr	9.4-34.0	9.4-34.0
	1 mo	5.0-19.5	5.0-19.5
	1-3 yr	6.0-17.5	6.0-17.5
	4-7 yr	5.5-15.5	5.5-15.5
	8-13 yr	4.5-13.5	4.5-13.5
		$\times$ 1000 cells/mm^3 (µl)	$\times$ 10^6 cells/L
CSF (cell count)	Premature	0-25 mononuclear	0-25
		0-10 polymorphonuclear	0-10
		0-1000 RBC	0-1000
	Newborn	0-20 mononuclear	0-20
		0-10 polymorphonuclear	0-10
		0-800 RBC	0-800
	Neonate	0-5 mononuclear	0-5
		0-10 polymorphonuclear	0-10
		0-50 RBC	0-50
	Thereafter	0-5 mononuclear	0-5
LEUKOCYTE DIFFERENTIAL COUNT			
Whole blood	Myelocytes	0% 0 cells/mm^3 (µl)	Number fraction 0
	Neutrophils—"bands"	3%-5% 150-400 cells/mm^3 (µl)	Number fraction 0.03-0.05
	Neutrophils—"segs"	54%-62% 3000-5800 cells/mm^3 (µl)	Number fraction 0.54-0.62
	Lymphocytes	25%-33% 1500-3000 cells/mm^3 (µl)	Number fraction 0.25-0.33
	Monocytes	3%-7% 285-500 cells/mm^3 (µl)	Number fraction 0.03-0.07
	Eosinophils	1%-3% 50-250 cells/mm^3 (µl)	Number fraction 0.01-0.03
	Basophils	0%-0.75% 15-50 cells/mm^3 (µl)	Number fraction 0-0.0075
MEAN CORPUSCULAR HEMOGLOBIN (MCH)			
Whole blood	Birth	31-37 pg/cell	0.48-0.57 fmol/cell
	1-3 d (cap)	31-37 pg/cell	0.48-0.57 fmol/cel
	1 wk–1 mo	28-40 pg/cell	0.43-0.62 fmol/cell
	2 mo	26-34 pg/cell	0.40-0.53 fmol/cell
	3-6 mo	25-35 pg/cell	0.39-0.54 fmol/cell
	0.5-2 yr	23-31 pg/cell	0.36-0.48 fmol/cell
	2-6 yr	24-30 pg/cell	0.37-0.47 fmol/cell
	6-12 yr	25-33 pg/cell	0.39-0.51 fmol/cell
	12-18 yr	25-35 pg/cell	0.39-0.54 fmol/cell

Continued

NORMAL LABORATORY VALUES (PEDIATRIC PATIENTS)—cont'd

TEST/SPECIMEN	AGE/GENDER/ REFERENCE	Normal Ranges	
		CONVENTIONAL UNITS	INTERNATIONAL UNITS (SI)
MEAN CORPUSCULAR HEMOGLOBIN CONCENTRATION (MCHC)			
Whole blood	Birth	30%-36% Hb/cell or g Hb/dl RBC	4.65-5.58 mmol Hb/L RBC
	1-3 d (cap)	29%-37% Hb/cell or g Hb/dl RBC	4.50-5.74 mmol Hb/L RBC
	1-2 wk	28%-38% Hb/cell or g Hb/dl RBC	4.34-5.89 mmol Hb/L RBC
	1-2 mo	29%-37% Hb/cell or g Hb/dl RBC	4.50-5.74 mmol Hb/L RBC
	3 mo–2 yr	30%-36% Hb/cell or g Hb/dl RBC	4.65-5.58 mmol Hb/L RBC
	2-18 yr	31%-37% Hb/cell or g Hb/dl RBC	4.81-5.74 mmol Hb/L RBC
MEAN CORPUSCULAR VOLUME (MCV)			
Whole blood	1-3 d (cap)	95-121 μm^3	95-121 fl
	0.5-2 yr	70-86 μm^3	70-86 fl
	6-12 yr	77-95 μm^3	77-95 fl
	12-18 yr: Male	78-98 μm^3	78-98 fl
	Female	78-102 μm^3	78-102 fl
OSMOLALITY			
Serum	Child	275-295 mOsm/kg H_2O	
Urine, random		50-1400 mOsm/kg H_2O, depending on fluid intake; after 12-hr fluid restriction: More than 850 mOsm/kg H_2O	
Urine, 24 hr		@ 300-900 mOsm/kg H_2O	
OXYGEN, PARTIAL PRESSURE (PO$_2$)			
Whole blood, arterial	Birth	8-24 mm Hg	1.1-3.2 kPa
	5-10 min	33-75 mm Hg	4.4-10.0 kPa
	30 min	31-85 mm Hg	4.1-11.3 kPa
	Older than 1 hr	55-80 mm Hg	7.3-10.6 kPa
	1 d	54-95 mm Hg	7.2-12.6 kPa
	Thereafter (decreased with age)	83-108 mm Hg	11-14.4 kPa
OXYGEN SATURATION (SAO$_2$)			
Whole blood, arterial	Newborn	85%-90%	Fraction saturated 0.85-0.90
	Thereafter	95%-99%	Fraction saturated 0.95-0.99
PARTIAL THROMBOPLASTIN TIME (PTT)			
Whole blood (Na citrate)			
Nonactivated		60-85 s (Platelin)	60-85 s
Activated		25-35 s (differs with method)	25-35 s
PH			H+ concentration
Whole blood, arterial	Premature (48 hr)	7.35-7.50	31-44 nmol/L
Must be corrected for body	Birth, full term	7.11-7.36	43-77 nmol/L
temperature	5-10 min	7.09-7.30	50-81 nmol/L
	30 min	7.21-7.38	41-61 nmol/L
	Older than 1 hr	7.26-7.49	32-54 nmol/L
	1 d	7.29-7.45	35-51 nmol/L
	Thereafter	7.35-7.45	35-44 nmol/L
Urine, random	Newborn/neonate	5-7	0.1-10 μmol/L
	Thereafter	4.5-8 (average @6)	0.01-32 μmol/L (average @1.0 μmol/L)
Stool		7.0-7.5	31-100 nmol/L
PHENYLALANINE			
Serum	Premature	2.0-7.5 mg/dl	120-450 μmol/L
	Newborn	1.2-3.4 mg/dl	70-210 μmol/L
	Thereafter	0.8-1.8 mg/dl	50-110 μmol/L
Urine, 24 hr	10 d–2 wk	1-2 mg/d	6-12 μmol/d
	3-12 yr	4-18 mg/d	24-110 μmol/d
	Thereafter	Trace—17 mg/d	Trace—103 μmol/d

NORMAL LABORATORY VALUES (PEDIATRIC PATIENTS)—cont'd

TEST/SPECIMEN	AGE/GENDER/REFERENCE	Normal Ranges	
		CONVENTIONAL UNITS	INTERNATIONAL UNITS (SI)
PLATELET COUNT (THROMBOCYTE COUNT)			
Whole blood (EDTA)	Newborn (after 1 wk, same as adult)	84-478 × 10³/mm³ (μl)	84-478 × 10⁹/L
POTASSIUM			
Serum	Newborn	3.0-6.0 mEq/L	3.0-6.0 mmol/L
	Thereafter	3.5-5.0 mEq/L	3.5-5.0 mmol/L
Plasma (heparin)		3.4-4.5 mEq/L	3.4-4.5 mmol/L
Urine, 24 hr		2.5-125 mEq/d (varies with diet)	2.5-125 mmol/L
PROTEIN			
Serum, total	Premature	4.3-7.6 g/dl	43-76 g/L
	Newborn	4.6-7.4 g/dl	46-74 g/L
	1-7 yr	6.1-7.9 g/dl	61-79 g/L
	8-12 yr	6.4-8.1 g/dl	64-81 g/L
	13-19 yr	6.6-8.2 g/dl	66-82 g/L
Total			
Urine, 24 hr		1-14 mg/dl	10-140 mg/L
		50-80 mg/d (at rest)	50-80 mg/d
		Less than 250 mg/d (after intense exercise)	Less than 250 mg/d (after intense exercise)
CSF		Lumbar: 8-32 mg/dl	80-320 mg/L
PROTHROMBIN TIME (PT)			
One-stage (Quick)			
Whole blood (Na citrate)	In general	11-15 s (varies with type of thromboplastin)	11-15 s
Newborn	Prolonged by 2-3 s	Prolonged by 2-3 s	
Two-stage modified (Ware and Seegers)			
Whole blood (sodium citrate)		18-22 s	18-22 s
RBC COUNT: SEE ERYTHROCYTE (RBC) COUNT			
RED BLOOD CELL VOLUME			
Whole blood	Male	20-36 ml/kg	0.020-0.036 L/kg
	Female	19-31 ml/kg	0.019-0.031 L/kg
RETICULOCYTE COUNT			
Capillary	1 d	0.4%-6.0%	0.004-0.060 (number fraction)
	7 d	Less than 0.1%-1.3%	Less than 0.001-0.013 (number fraction)
	1-4 wk	Less than 0.1%-1.2%	Less than 0.001-0.012 (number fraction)
	5-6 wk	Less than 0.1%-2.4%	Less than 0.001-0.024 (number fraction)
	7-8 wk	0.1%-2.9%	0.001-0.029 (number fraction)
	9-10 wk	Less than 0.1%-2.6%	
	11-12 wk	0.1%-1.3%	
SALICYLATES			
Serum, plasma	Therap. conc.	15-30 mg/dl	1.1-2.2 mmol/L
	Toxic conc.	More than 30 mg/dl	More than 18.5 mmol/L
SEDIMENTATION RATE: SEE ERYTHROCYTE SEDIMENTATION RATE (ESR)			
SODIUM			
Serum or plasma	Newborn	134-146 mEq/L	134-146 mEq/L
	Infant	139-146 mEq/L	139-146 mEq/L
	Child	138-145 mEq/L	138-145 mEq/L
	Thereafter	136-146 mEq/L	136-146 mEq/L

Continued

NORMAL LABORATORY VALUES (PEDIATRIC PATIENTS)—cont'd

TEST/SPECIMEN	AGE/GENDER/REFERENCE	Normal Ranges CONVENTIONAL UNITS	INTERNATIONAL UNITS (SI)
Urine, 24 hr		40-220 mEq/L (diet dependent)	40-220 mEq/L
Sweat	Normal	Less than 40 mEq/L	Less than 40 mEq/L
	Indeterminate	45-60 mEq/L	45-60 mEq/L
	Cystic fibrosis	More than 60 mEq/L	More than 60 mEq/L
SPECIFIC GRAVITY			
Urine, random	After 12-hr fluid restriction	More than 1.025	More than 1.025
Urine, 24 hr		1.015-1.025	
THEOPHYLLINE			
Serum, plasma	Therap. conc.		
	Bronchodilator	10-20 mcg/ml	56-110 mmol/L
	Premature apnea	5-10 mcg/ml	28-56 mmol/L
	Toxic conc.	More than 20 mcg/ml	More than 110 mmol/L
THROMBIN TIME			
Whole blood (Na citrate)		Control time ± 2 s when control is 9-13 s	Control time ± 2 s when control is 9-13 s
THYROXINE, TOTAL (T$_4$)			
Serum	Cord	8-13 mcg/dl	103-168 nmol/L
	Newborn	11.5-24 mcg/dl (lower in low-birth-weight infants)	148-310 nmol/L
	Neonate	9-18 mcg/dl	116-232 nmol/L
	Infant	7-15 mcg/dl	90-194 nmol/L
	1-5 yr	7.3-15 mcg/dl	94-194 nmol/L
	5-10 yr	6.4-13.3 mcg/dl	83-172 nmol/L
	Thereafter	5-12 mcg/dl	65-155 nmol/L
	Newborn screen (filter paper)	6.2-22 mcg/dl	80-284 nmol/L

TRIGLYCERIDES (TG)		Male (mg/dl)	Female (mg/dl)	Male (g/L)	Female (g/L)
Serum, after ≥2-hr fast	Cord	10-98	10-98	0.10-0.98	0.10-0.98
	0-5 yr	30-86	32-99	0.30-0.86	0.32-0.99
	6-11 yr	31-108	35-114	0.31-1.08	0.35-1.14
	12-15 yr	36-138	41-138	0.36-1.38	0.41-1.38
	16-19 yr	40-163	40-128	0.40-1.63	0.40-1.28

TRIIODOTHYRONINE (T$_3$), FREE			
Serum	Cord	20-240 pg/dl	0.3-3.7 pmol/L
	1-3 d	200-610 pg/dl	3.1-9.4 pmol/L
	6 wk	240-560 pg/dl	3.7-8.6 pmol/L

TRIIODOTHYRONINE, TOTAL (T$_3$-RIA)			
Serum	Cord	30-70 ng/dl	0.46-1.08 nmol/L
	Newborn	72-260 ng/dl	1.16-4 nmol/L
	1-5 yr	100-260 ng/dl	1.54-4 nmol/L
	5-10 yr	90-240 ng/dl	1.39-3.70 nmol/L
	10-15 yr	80-210 ng/dl	1.23-3.23 nmol/L
	Thereafter	115-190 ng/dl	1.77-2.93 nmol/L

UREA NITROGEN			
Serum or plasma	Cord	21-40 mg/d	7.5-14.3 mmol/L
	Premature (1 wk)	3-25 mg/dl	1.1-9 mmol/L
	Newborn	3-12 mg/dl	1.1-4.3 mmol/L
	Infant/child	5-18 mg/dl	1.8-6.4 mmol/L
	Thereafter	7-18 mg/dl	2.5-6.4 mmol/L

URINE VOLUME			
Urine, 24 hr	Newborn	50-300 ml/d	0.05-0.3 L/d
	Infant	350-550 ml/d	0.35-0.5 L/d
	Child	500-1000 ml/d	0.5-1 L/d
	Adolescent	700-1400 ml/d	0.7-1.4 L/d

WBC: SEE LEUKOCYTE COUNT (WBC COUNT)

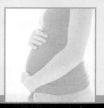

Bleeding in Pregnancy 88

OVERVIEW/PATHOPHYSIOLOGY

Bleeding in pregnancy can be minor to life threatening. Causes include implantation bleeding (bleeding after the embryo implants in the endometrium), blighted ovum (ovum does not develop because of chromosomal abnormalities of the sperm or egg), severe chromosomal abnormalities, ectopic pregnancy (implantation outside of the uterus), threatened abortion (confirmed pregnancy with vaginal bleeding), incomplete abortion (retention of some products of conception [POC]), missed abortion (fetus has died but is retained with the placenta in the uterus), inevitable spontaneous abortion (ruptured membranes or POC passed at onset of bleeding before 20 wk gestation), complete spontaneous abortion (bleeding and cramping followed by passing of tissue or POC before 20 wk gestation, followed by a marked decrease in cramping and bleeding), gestational trophoblastic disease (includes hydatidiform mole [molar pregnancy] and gestational trophoblastic tumors), cervicitis, cervical polyps, cervical dysplasia (e.g., cervical carcinoma), hyperemia of the cervix, cervical insufficiency (painless dilation of the cervix in the absence of contractions), maternal bleeding disorders, placenta previa (abnormally implanted placenta that covers or partially covers the cervix), placental abruption (premature separation from the uterine wall of a normally implanted placenta), uterine rupture (may be seen after a previous classical cesarean), cervical dilation, postcoital bleeding, and sexual assault.

HEALTH CARE SETTING

Primary care; acute care (emergency room or inpatient setting) if surgical intervention is deemed necessary

ASSESSMENT

Bleeding in the first trimester is not uncommon, inasmuch as some women are not aware they are pregnant. The bleeding can range from light pink spotting to brown discharge (indicating old blood) to bleeding like a heavy menses and may or may not be accompanied by abdominal pain. It can result in significant emotional changes from relief, concern, and ambivalence to fear. Bleeding in the second and third trimesters is of significant concern because it can affect maternal/fetal morbidity and mortality.

Early pregnancy symptoms: Amenorrhea, breast tenderness, fatigue, abdominal bloating, nausea, and vomiting. With a missed spontaneous abortion, these symptoms may no longer be present when vaginal bleeding begins.

Vaginal bleeding
- *First trimester vaginal bleeding* may be light pink, bright red, or dark brown spotting (noticed when the woman wipes her perineum or on her underpants); like a heavy menses; or bright red and saturating pads. Some women pass blood clots with or without tissue. Light vaginal spotting may be an early indication of an ectopic pregnancy or threatened abortion.
- *Second and third trimester vaginal bleeding* may be light pink, bright red, or dark brown spotting (noticed when the woman wipes her perineum or on her underpants); like a heavy menses; or bright red and saturating pads. Some women pass blood clots. Any vaginal bleeding in the second and third trimesters requires immediate evaluation and may indicate placenta previa, abruptio placentae, or antepartum rupture of a scarred uterus in patients with previous cesarean section.

Vaginal discharge (other than bleeding): If an infection is present, the woman may note a change in her vaginal discharge before the bleeding episode. Discharge may range from thick white and clumpy to thin white, yellow, or green with or without a foul odor. A malodorous discharge such as a "fishy" smell may indicate bacterial vaginosis (BV). There also may be vulvar pruritus, burning, and/or irritation.

Abdominal pain: Pain from uterine cramping may or may not be present and can range from mild to severe. In the presence of placental abruption or uterine rupture, abdominal pain is often severe, although not always. With uterine rupture, the pain may be absent to moderate or localized, and the abdomen may be tender. Shoulder pain may be present with intraabdominal accumulation of blood under the diaphragm. With placenta previa, there is usually no abdominal pain. With ectopic pregnancy, the pain may be vague and achy to sharp and colicky, may be unilateral or bilateral, and may be accompanied by nausea, vomiting, and diarrhea.

Back pain: May or may not be present with vaginal bleeding, depending on the cause. When present, it is usually described as low (lumbar), dull, and aching and may radiate around the hips and down the thighs. With abruption, the back pain may be mild to severe.

Passage of POC: Normally in the first trimester the POC appear as grainy, granular tissue that looks more like clotted blood. Some women state their bleeding and abdominal pain decrease significantly after the passage of POC.

Cardiovascular: Dizziness, lightheadedness, syncope, shortness of breath, or tachycardia if significant blood loss has occurred.

Signs—fetal: Decreased or absent fetal movement (gestation appropriate) may be present with fetal compromise or demise.

Physical assessment: Vaginal bleeding can occur at any time during pregnancy and be of varying degrees depending on its cause. Some bleeding episodes resolve on their own, and the pregnancy will continue; others lead to the spontaneous abortion of the fetus, demise of the neonate, and possible serious consequences for the mother. Maternal vital signs (VS) may be within normal limits or show postural changes (drop in blood pressure [BP] with rise in heart rate [HR], indicating fluid depletion). The woman also may be anxious, irritable, and apprehensive with significant blood loss.

Abdominal examination: Abdominal tenderness with palpation will be present with an ectopic pregnancy, placental abruption, and uterine rupture. Fetal heart tones (FHTs) may be auscultated at the appropriate gestational age or be absent in the presence of fetal demise. Uterine contractions may be palpable, depending on gestational age.

Risk factors: Previous history of spontaneous abortion, ectopic pregnancy, cervical polyps and other cervical lesions (cervical dysplasia), cervical insufficiency, bleeding in pregnancy (postpartum hemorrhage), placenta previa, molar pregnancy, or uterine myomas/leiomyomata (fibroids or smooth muscle cell tumors). Other risk factors include luteal phase defect (inadequate progesterone production by a poorly functioning corpus luteum), structural abnormalities of the uterus, antiphospholipid syndrome (autoimmune syndrome that may be associated with recurrent spontaneous abortion), chromosomal abnormalities, smoking, substance abuse (especially cocaine use), vaginal infections, abdominal trauma, previous history of abruption, and use of some chemotherapy drugs.

DIAGNOSTIC TESTS

Rapid qualitative urine or serum pregnancy test: Tests for the presence of human chorionic gonadotropin (hCG), which may be detected after implantation is complete (8-10 days after conception). A pregnancy can be diagnosed even before a menstrual period has been missed.

Serial serum qualitative and quantitative pregnancy test: Tests for the presence of hCG. After implantation is complete, hCG is detectable in serum (8-10 days after conception). Normally serum concentration of hCG doubles every 1-2 days and is helpful in determining gestational age with rising numbers or a spontaneous abortion with declining numbers.

hCG levels during pregnancy

3 wk last menstrual period (LMP)	5-50 mIU/ml
4 wk LMP	5-426 mIU/ml
5 wk LMP	18-7340 mIU/ml
6 wk LMP	1080-56,500 mIU/ml
7-8 wk LMP	7650-229,000 mIU/ml
9-12 wk LMP	25,700-288,000 mIU/ml
13-16 wk LMP	13,300-254,000 mIU/ml
17-24 wk LMP	4060-165,400 mIU/ml
25-40 wk LMP	3640-117,000 mIU/ml
Nonpregnant female	Less than 5.0 mIU/ml

Data from www.americanpregnancy.org/duringpregnancy/concernsearlydevelopment.htm

Obstetric ultrasound: Done abdominally, transvaginally, or translabially. Ultrasound detects the presence of a viable pregnancy or a fetus without cardiac activity. It locates the pregnancy as either intrauterine or ectopic and evaluates presence of a gestational sac, whether it contains a fetus or is empty, and gestational age. It also locates the position of the placenta and fetus, number of fetuses, presence of subchorionic hemorrhage (bleeding beneath the outer membrane that contains blood vessels), and abruption.

Blood Rh factor and antibody screen: Results will indicate the mother's Rh factor as either positive or negative and if there are antibodies present. Rh-negative women with negative antibodies will need Rh immune globulin (RhoGAM) administered for prevention of Rh sensitization of subsequent pregnancies.

Complete blood count: May be within normal limits unless there has been significant blood loss and anemia is present. An elevated white blood cell count is suggestive of an intrauterine infection.

Speculum examination: To examine the cervix for the presence of dilation, effacement, or evidence of POC at the cervical os or within the vaginal vault or for polyps, cervical friability, lacerations, or lesions that would contribute to the bleeding. Cultures may be taken at this time. Caution is used when performing a speculum examination on a woman with known placenta previa who has vaginal bleeding in her second or third trimester. Speculum examination also enables assessment for rupture of amniotic membranes using Nitrazine paper and ferning (microscopic crystallization of amniotic fluid when allowed to air dry on a glass slide).

Fetal monitoring: Before gestational viability, monitoring of uterine tone may be done only to elicit uterine contractions. It is used in the second and third trimesters to check for fetal well-being by eliciting FHTs and uterine tone (contractions). Normally, a reactive fetal heart rate tracing may be seen after 32 wk gestation and as early as 27 wk gestation, depending on fetal central nervous system (CNS) development. It includes a minimum of 20 min of tracing that shows a fetal heart rate baseline between 120 and 160 bpm and at least two accelerations that must rise at least 15 bpm and last at least 15 sec from onset to return to baseline. With maternal hemorrhage, as in placenta previa or abruptio placentae, fetal oxygenation is compromised because of maternal hypotension, decrease in placental surface area, and uterine hyperactivity. Nonreassuring fetal heart rate patterns that may be seen with bleeding may include the following: late decelerations, progressively severe variable decelerations, tachycardia, loss of variability, recurrent prolonged decelerations, and sinusoidal tracing. In the presence of an acute abruptio placentae, there is a rapid deceleration of the fetal heart rate, which can indicate imminent fetal demise.

Kleihauer-Betke test: Tests for the presence of fetal cells in the maternal circulation that can be seen after fetomaternal bleeding (e.g., occurring with abdominal trauma).

- *Late decelerations:* Gradual onset, ∪ shaped, start at the peak of contraction and return to baseline gradually. Generally the tracings descend 30-40 bpm below baseline. The cause is a temporary interruption of uteroplacental perfusion during peak of contractions.
- *Variable decelerations:* Onset and resolution are sharp and abrupt. Size, shape, depth, duration, and timing vary in relation to a contraction. The cause is a temporary compression of the umbilical cord.
- *Sinusoidal tracing:* A repetitive, small, wavelike pattern of the fetal heart rate. The cause is fetal anemia.

Nursing Diagnosis:

Deficient Knowledge:

Effects of bleeding on self, pregnancy, and fetus

Desired Outcome: Immediately following teaching, patient and significant other verbalize accurate knowledge about the effects of bleeding on the patient, pregnancy, and fetus and adhere to the therapy accordingly.

INTERVENTIONS	RATIONALES
Inform patient and significant other what bleeding may indicate and the effect it can have on the pregnancy, mother, and fetus.	Knowledgeable patients are more likely to adhere to therapy (e.g., bedrest, frequent clinic visits, no intercourse, stopping work, and possible hospitalizations or surgery) and understand consequences of nonadherence. Bleeding plays a major role in maternal/fetal morbidity and mortality, depending on cause and gestational age at the time of occurrence.
Teach patient the signs and symptoms of bleeding, depending on trimester.	Patient will understand that vaginal bleeding or abdominal pain in the presence of amenorrhea or a positive pregnancy test requires evaluation and that there is increased risk for maternal/fetal morbidity and mortality if bleeding occurs under these conditions. See descriptions under Assessment, earlier.
Explain that when a miscarriage is occurring there is nothing that can be done to prevent it.	More than 50% of first and second trimester spontaneous abortions occur because of chromosomal abnormalities. Understanding this may alleviate some feelings of anguish or guilt about embryo/fetus non-survival.
Teach and assist patient through the stages of grief and loss.	See **Anticipatory Grieving**, p. 677.
Teach patient how to palpate contractions that may accompany vaginal bleeding (gestation appropriate).	Palpation and awareness of contractions enable patient to be an active participant in her health care. Timely reporting of contractions to her health care provider can play a significant role in affecting outcome.

Continued

INTERVENTIONS	RATIONALES
	To palpate contractions, the patient lies comfortably on her side. She spreads her fingers apart and places one hand on the left side and the other on the right side of her abdomen. She will palpate the abdomen using her fingertips. When the uterus is relaxed, the abdomen should feel soft. In the presence of a contraction, the uterus should feel hard, tight, or firm under her fingertips. She then times the duration of the contraction from the beginning of one contraction to the beginning of the next. Any number of contractions, combined with vaginal bleeding, necessitates immediate evaluation and can prove ominous in the second and third trimesters. Contractions can increase the severity of vaginal bleeding with placenta previa and abruptio placentae. Duration of the contraction may or may not be an indication of contraction intensity. It is believed that the longer the contraction in true labor the more effective it is in progressing dilation and effacement.
Teach fetal movement counts.	Fetal movement counts are a good first-line indicator of fetal well-being and are performed as follows, beginning at 28 wk gestation: Patient lies on her side and counts "distinct fetal movements" (hiccups do not count) daily; 10 movements within a 2-hr period are reassuring. After counting 10 movements, the count is discontinued. Fewer than 10 movements signals need for fetal nonstress testing.
Teach signs and symptoms of maternal complications with vaginal bleeding.	This information promotes understanding of the need to seek medical attention in a timely manner if indicators such as saturating 1 pad/hr, passing golf-ball–size clots, dizziness, lightheadedness, syncope, shortness of breath, and tachycardia occur.
Explain how to save POC if requested by health care provider.	Proper storage and transport of POC aids in cytologic and pathologic evaluation. Each laboratory has specific requirements for transport and should be contacted accordingly.
For patients in the second and third trimesters, explain home management of placenta previa or chronic abruption and its purpose. Teach patient to decrease physical activity and avoid intercourse and insertion of anything into the vagina, including tampons.	Although some patients with placenta previa may not experience vaginal bleeding during pregnancy, vaginal bleeding with placenta previa or abruptio placentae can be serious. Patients can exsanguinate rapidly. In some patients, increased physical activity, including lifting, may decrease uterine perfusion, which increases risk of placental abruption. Intercourse and use of tampons increase risk of bleeding in the presence of placenta previa and its location over the cervical os and therefore are contraindicated.
Caution against sexual foreplay.	The uterine contractility that can occur in sexual foreplay (breast, oral, or digital stimulation) promotes release of prostaglandins, which cause uterine contractions and hence increases risk of bleeding.

••• **Related NIC and NOC labels:** *NIC:* Teaching: Disease Process; Health Education; High-Risk Pregnancy Care *NOC:* Knowledge: Pregnancy

Nursing Diagnosis:

Acute Pain

related to uterine cramping and backache that may be associated with vaginal bleeding in pregnancy

Desired Outcome: Patient reports the pain in a timely manner for appropriate evaluation and treatment and within 1-2 hr after intervention states that pain is at an acceptable level (4 or less on a 0-10 scale).

INTERVENTIONS	RATIONALES
Evaluate patient's level of abdominal pain/uterine cramping using a scale of 0-10, with 10 being the worst pain she has ever had.	Each patient experiences levels of pain differently. Baseline assessment will enable proper analgesia and help determine relief of pain obtained after subsequent evaluation.
Evaluate location and duration of pain.	Location and duration of the pain may signal different problems. For example, pain/aching under the scapula may indicate blood in the peritoneum, a sign of a ruptured ectopic pregnancy/internal bleeding.
Administer pain medications if their use is not contraindicated.	This measure provides pain relief. In some situations, however, pain is a useful indicator of a potential problem, such as a ruptured ectopic pregnancy, in which masking of symptoms is not desirable.
Provide emotional support.	Emotional support aids in decreasing anxiety, which also may decrease the level of pain.

••• **Related NIC and NOC labels:** *NIC:* Pain Management; Emotional Support; Medication Administration *NOC:* Comfort Level; Pain Control

Nursing Diagnosis:

Anticipatory Grieving

related to the potential loss of the pregnancy

Desired Outcome: Within 24 hr of this diagnosis, patient and significant other verbalize their feelings and identify and begin to use support systems to aid them in the grief process.

INTERVENTIONS	RATIONALES
Encourage patient and significant other to verbalize their feelings and concerns regarding potential or definite (e.g., ectopic) loss of the pregnancy.	This will validate their feelings and convey the message that grief is a normal and expected reaction to the potential or actual loss of the fetus. It also enables the nurse to intervene in the event of misperceptions about the bleeding.
Assess and accept patient's behavioral response.	Reactions such as disbelief, denial, guilt, anger, and depression are normal reactions to grief.
Teach the five stages of grief and explain that there is no specific time frame in which to go through this process.	This information enables the patient and family members to understand their stage in the grief process. Stages include (1) shock and numbness; (2) denial and searching-yearning; (3) anger, guilt, and sense of failure; (4) depression and disorganization; and (5) resolution.
Clarify misconceptions about the potential risk for fetal loss with vaginal bleeding.	Although they play a major role in fetal mortality, not all bleeding episodes in pregnancy lead to fetal loss. The gestational age at which the bleeding occurs and the amount of vaginal bleeding play a significant role in the outcome. This information will help the patient process information regarding bleeding in pregnancy appropriately while not being given false hope.
Involve Social Services in the care of the patient. If such services are not available, refer to a community support group if one exists.	If the patient is placed on bedrest either at home or in the hospital, the social worker will evaluate for psychologic/social/spiritual concerns and provide written material and appropriate resources and referrals for support groups.

••• **Related NIC and NOC labels:** *NIC:* Coping Enhancement; Grief Work Facilitation: Perinatal Death; Support Group; Anxiety Reduction *NOC:* Coping; Grief Resolution

Nursing Diagnosis:

Deficient Knowledge:

Purpose and potential side effects of prescribed medications

Desired Outcome: Immediately following teaching, patient and family verbalize accurate understanding of the risks and benefits of medications used.

INTERVENTIONS	RATIONALES
Teach the following about patient's prescribed medications:	A knowledgeable patient is more likely to adhere to the therapy, identify and report side effects, and recognize and report precautions that might preclude use of the prescribed drug.
Prostaglandin Synthesis Inhibitor	
Ibuprofen	Ibuprofen inhibits prostaglandin synthesis, thereby decreasing myometrial contractility/pain from cramping.
	Administration: oral.
Be alert for and report nausea, vomiting, heartburn, diarrhea, constipation, and abdominal cramps.	These are common side effects. If these symptoms persist, the medication may need to be changed, dose adjusted, or discontinued.
Take the medication with food.	This measure decreases gastrointestinal (GI) side effects.
Precaution for patients with a history of GI ulcers.	Ibuprofen may cause GI bleeding.
Explanation that in viable pregnancies, weekly monitoring of amniotic fluid volume is necessary as is discontinuation of the medication at 34 wk gestation.	Daily/routine use may cause oligohydramnios (decrease in/absence of amniotic fluid), constriction of fetal ductus arteriosus, or neonatal pulmonary hypertension (Gabbe, 2002).
Not recommended for use in patients who are taking warfarin or heparin.	Ibuprofen would further increase risk of bleeding.
Opioid Analgesics	
Percocet, Vicodin	These agents alter processes in the CNS that affect pain perception. They are used for mild to moderately severe pain.
	Administration: oral.
Be alert for and report nausea and vomiting.	These are common side effects. If these symptoms persevere, the medication may need to be discontinued or changed.
Be alert for dizziness, lightheadedness, and weakness.	These are other common side effects. Patient needs to use caution for activities that require alertness if these indicators occur.
Precautions are necessary for patients taking other CNS depressants, monoamine oxidase (MAO) inhibitors, or tricyclic antidepressants.	These drugs may potentiate CNS side effects of opioid analgesics.
Prophylactic Antibiotics	Prophylactic antibiotics prevent and reduce effects of infection and maternal morbidity. The type of antibiotic used varies and may include but is not limited to the following: ampicillins, gentamicin, and cephalosporins.
Follow complete course for all prescribed medications and take them on time.	These measures prevent development of antibiotic resistance and maintain a constant level of medication in the bloodstream.
Be alert for and report excessive and explosive diarrhea.	*Clostridium difficile* is a potentially serious side effect of antibiotic therapy in which the normal flora of the bowel are reduced and the anaerobic organism, *C. difficile,* multiplies and produces toxins causing severe diarrhea. This reaction necessitates discontinuation of the antibiotic and laboratory evaluation of a stool sample.
Uterotonic	
Prostaglandin suppository (Prostin E2)	This agent is used to produce myometrial contractions in order to evacuate the gravid uterus in a missed abortion (after 12 wk gestation) or intrauterine fetal death (up to 28 wk).
	Administration: vaginally in the hospital setting.
Use not recommended with other uterotonic drugs or in patients with history of a previous classical (vertical) uterine incision.	Uterine rupture may occur.

Continued

INTERVENTIONS	RATIONALES
Be alert for and report nausea, vomiting, diarrhea, headache, fever, chills, backache, and dizziness.	These are signs of an adverse reaction. Administration of antiemetics, analgesics, and antipyretics before administering prostaglandin may prevent or reduce these side effects.
Methylergonovine and oxytocin (Methergine and Pitocin)	These agents decrease uterine contractility and decrease uterine/vaginal bleeding after spontaneous abortion or after dilation and curettage for missed abortion.
	Administration: IV, IM, and PO after surgical procedures or delivery of fetus/neonate.
Methergine is avoided in a patient with hypertension, whether chronic or preeclamptic.	There is risk for sudden hypertension and stroke.
Carboprost (Hemabate, 15-methyl-prostaglandin F2-alpha)	This agent augments effects of uterotonics for postoperative/postpartum vaginal bleeding.
	Administration: deep IM.
Be alert for and report fever, hypertension, nausea, vomiting, diarrhea, and flushing.	These are common side effects. Because this drug is usually given in an emergent situation, premedication to reduce these side effects is usually not done.
Intravenous Infusions of Crystalloid Fluid	Crystalloids form true solutions and are capable of passing through a semipermeable membrane. They are used as a volume expander after significant blood loss.
Be alert for shortness of breath, increased pulse rate, and sacral and lower extremity edema.	These are signs of fluid overload.
IV Blood and Blood Products	They are used for blood loss/volume replacement.
Packed red blood cells (RBCs)	Packed RBCs are the most effective way to increase oxygen carrying capacity to the anemic patient after significant blood loss.
Platelets	Platelets are necessary for the initial phase of hemostasis and used in patients with disseminated intravascular coagulation, massive hemorrhage, severe preeclampsia, and idiopathic thrombocytopenic purpura.
Clotting factors (cryoprecipitate)	Cryoprecipitate is formed from warmed fresh frozen plasma, which contains clotting factors such as factor VIII, factor XIII, fibrinogen, and Von Willebrand's factor and is used to treat hypofibrinogenemia.
Whole blood	Although its use is discouraged and in some blood centers has been discontinued, it may be delivered in obstetric emergencies when there is a need to replace more than 4000 ml volume loss.
Be alert for and report severe anxiety, flushing, chest or back pain, fever, shortness of breath, dizziness, and increased pulse rate.	These are signs of a transfusion reaction, which is life threatening and must be reported promptly for immediate intervention.
Rh-Immune Globulin (Human)	
RhoGAM	This agent prevents hemolytic disease as long as the mother has not already been sensitized by the presence of Rh-positive antibodies in her bloodstream.
	Administration: IM only to nonsensitized Rh-negative women after bleeding any time during the pregnancy, after spontaneous abortion, and after delivery. It is recommended that this drug be given within 72 hr of the bleeding episode.
Patient may note discomfort at the site of injection.	This is a common side effect.

••• **Related NIC and NOC labels:** *NIC:* Teaching: Prescribed Medication; Prenatal Care *NOC:* Knowledge: Medication

ADDITIONAL NURSING DIAGNOSES/ PROBLEMS:

"Perioperative Care" for Risk for **Deficient Fluid Volume** related to bleeding/hemorrhage — p. 51

"Prolonged Bedrest" for relevant nursing diagnoses for the woman who must stay in bed, — p. 61

including **Constipation** — p. 67

"Psychosocial Support" for patients experiencing psychosocial problems, such as — p. 73

Spiritual Distress — p. 78

"Psychosocial Support for the Patient's Family and Significant Other" for such nursing diagnoses as: — p. 87

Fear — p. 87

Compromised Family Coping — p. 89

"Cervical Insufficiency" for **Sexual Dysfunction** — p. 685

"Preterm Labor" for **Caregiver Role Strain** — p. 725

 PATIENT-FAMILY TEACHING AND DISCHARGE PLANNING

Bleeding in pregnancy is an emotionally charged situation that requires both physical and psychologic management. Include verbal and written information about the following:

✓ Importance of reporting vaginal bleeding to the health care provider in a timely manner.

✓ Importance of adherence to prescribed health care and ready access to hospital and family/social support.

✓ Medications, including drug name, purpose, dosage, frequency, precautions, and potential side effects. Also discuss potential drug-drug, food-drug, and herb-drug interactions.

✓ Fetal movement counts (gestation appropriate).

✓ Palpation of contractions (gestation appropriate).

✓ Importance of complying with intercourse restrictions.

✓ Measures that help with constipation, which occurs frequently in pregnancy and is exacerbated by bedrest.

✓ Compliance with scheduled prenatal visits.

✓ Referral to local and national support organizations, including:

- Sidelines, a national support organization for women and their families experiencing complicated pregnancies, at Sidelines High Risk Pregnancy Support *www.sidelines.org*

- SHARE, a national support group for parents who have experienced loss through miscarriage, stillbirth, or newborn death, at SHARE Pregnancy & Infant Loss Support, Inc., National SHARE Office, *www.nationalshare-office.com*

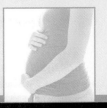

Cervical Insufficiency 89

OVERVIEW/PATHOPHYSIOLOGY

Diagnosis of cervical insufficiency is made when there is an obstetric history of recurrent, passive, and painless dilation and/or effacement of the cervix in the second or early third trimester in the absence of contractions, bleeding, infection, ruptured membranes, or fetal anomalies. This may lead to preterm premature rupture of membranes (PPROM) and preterm delivery with the possibility of fetal demise. Not all patients with a history of cervical insufficiency have a cervical cerclage placed; some may elect to monitor for cervical changes instead.

HEALTH CARE SETTING

Primary care (outpatient obstetric clinic, perinatal high-risk clinic) or acute care (inpatient antepartum unit)

ASSESSMENT

Evaluating cervical insufficiency in a patient with no previous history can be difficult. Patient may present at a routine clinic visit having acute cervical changes and complaining of vague symptoms (e.g., backache, pelvic pressure) that can be common in pregnancy.

Pelvic pressure: Patient complains of a sensation of pelvic fullness or heaviness that may or may not have been present previously during the pregnancy. Some patients relate a sensation of vaginal fullness such as that of having a large tampon in the vagina.

Increased vaginal discharge: An increase in vaginal discharge is a normal process in pregnancy. Normal vaginal discharge can be clear, white, or light yellow and thin to thick in consistency. The patient with cervical insufficiency may not note a change in consistency but a change in color such as light pink, blood-tinged, or tan. These are symptoms of possible cervical dilation as the surface vessels of the cervix break and bleed.

Backache: Although this is a very common complaint in pregnancy, any woman with a history of cervical insufficiency who complains of new-onset backache needs to be evaluated for cervical changes, especially if she describes backache as low lumbar/sacral in position, deep tissue in nature, or as a dull aching sensation that may radiate around the hips to the lower abdomen/pelvic area and down the thighs.

Contractions: Uterine tightening/contractions begin in the first trimester as the uterus enlarges and continue throughout the pregnancy. These contractions are considered Braxton-Hicks and occur at irregular intervals, usually are painless, and do not change the cervix. Some women complain of a lower pelvic aching sensation that may be detected by palpation or uterine monitoring. However, any woman with a history of cervical insufficiency who complains of new-onset contractions needs to be evaluated for cervical changes and preterm labor.

Cervical changes: Cervical insufficiency may be congenital or acquired. The cervix may dilate and then efface or efface and then dilate. Funneling of the cervix may be seen. This occurs when the internal cervical os dilates and the external os remains closed. It appears as a funnel shape when seen on ultrasound. Protrusion or bulging of the amniotic membranes may be visible through the cervical os. A normal cervical length is 3.5 cm or greater.

Complications—fetal: Prematurity and fetal/neonatal death may occur.

Physical assessment: Normally, cervical insufficiency is asymptomatic until signs of significant cervical change are present. With advanced cervical dilation, PPROM may occur, increasing fetal morbidity and mortality.

Risk factors: Previous history of cervical insufficiency or preterm birth, previous cervical trauma, cervical conization (a cone-shaped portion of the cervix is removed in the presence of cervical dysplasia), cervical biopsy, cervical length less than 3.5 cm, congenital structural anomalies, extensive cervical dilation as occurs in second-trimester pregnancy terminations, cervical laceration(s) at the time of a previous vaginal delivery, diethylstilbestrol (DES) exposure.

DIAGNOSTIC TESTS

Transvaginal or translabial ultrasound: Assessment to determine cervical length. Diagnostic ultrasound criteria of cervical insufficiency include a total cervical length between 2 and 2.5 cm, accompanied by funneling of the internal cervical os.

Digital cervical examination: A gentle digital examination of the cervix is done to evaluate the cervix for dilation, effacement, position (anterior/posterior), and consistency (firm/soft). Protrusion or bulging of the amniotic membranes through the cervical os (funneling) may be detected at this time. Of note, cervical change in the mid-to-late second trimester of 1-2 cm dilation has been seen in women who have not progressed to preterm labor and/or delivery.

Urinalysis for microscopy: Urinary tract infection (UTI) is associated with preterm labor. It is not a cause of cervical insufficiency but should be ruled out as a cofactor. If bacteria are present, including group B streptococci, antibiotic therapy should be initiated.

Obstetric ultrasound: Confirms gestational age, position of the placenta and fetus, number of fetuses, amniotic fluid volume index, presence of cervical funneling and fetal anomalies and measures cervical length and dilation. Serial ultrasound examinations can monitor the cervix for any changes. Ultrasound does not replace digital cervical exams.

Antepartum fetal monitoring: Before gestation of viability (i.e., less than 25 wk) the patient may be monitored for the presence and frequency of contractions using only the tocodynamometer. A documentation of fetal heart tones is necessary with each tracing. Once viability is reached, both the transducer and tocodynamometer are used.

Complete blood count with differential: Helps rule out chorioamnionitis, a bacterial infection of the fetal membranes. If present, white blood cell count will be elevated.

Nursing Diagnosis:

Deficient Knowledge:

Effects of cervical insufficiency on self, the pregnancy, and fetus and the treatment and expected outcome

Desired Outcome: Immediately following teaching, patient and significant other verbalize accurate knowledge about the effects of cervical insufficiency on the pregnancy and fetus and adhere to the treatment(s) accordingly.

INTERVENTIONS	RATIONALES
Explain to patient and significant other the effects cervical insufficiency may have on the mother, pregnancy, and fetus.	Information helps patients adhere to treatments and understand possible consequences of nonadherence. Cervical insufficiency may result in preterm delivery and fetal/neonatal morbidity or mortality.
Explain treatment options such as cervical cerclage placement, including benefits and risks.	A cerclage involves placement of a purse-string suture through the cervix to hold it closed until threat of miscarriage has passed. It is usually removed at around 35 wk gestation. The success of the cerclage is related to the dilation of the cervix (best when less than 2 cm) at the time of the procedure. The patient may be required to decrease physical activity or go on bedrest, decrease work hours or stop work, and avoid vaginal intercourse.
	Risks include infection, cervical injury, displacement of the cerclage, PPROM, preterm labor, and preterm delivery. The benefit is a more likely continuation of the pregnancy.
Teach signs and symptoms that may indicate cervical change and importance of reporting them promptly.	A knowledgeable patient will likely report symptoms (pelvic pressure; increased vaginal discharge; pink, bloody, or tan vaginal discharge; backache; or contractions) promptly. See introductory information for detailed signs and symptoms of cervical insufficiency. The earlier cervical insufficiency is diagnosed, the better the chance for placing a cerclage, prolonging the pregnancy, and decreasing fetal morbidity and mortality.
Teach daily fetal movement counts.	Fetal movement counts are a good first-line indicator of fetal well-being and are performed as follows beginning at 28 wk gestation: The patient lies on her side and counts "distinct fetal movements" (hiccups do not count) daily; 10 movements within a 2-hr period is reassuring. After detecting 10 movements, the count is discontinued. Fewer than 10 movements indicate need for fetal nonstress testing.

Continued

INTERVENTIONS	RATIONALES
Teach patient how to palpate contractions.	Palpation and awareness of contractions enable patient to be an active participant in her health care. Timely reporting of contractions to her health care provider can play a significant role in affecting outcome. To palpate contractions, the patient lies comfortably on her side. She spreads her fingers apart and places one hand on the left side and the other on the right side of her abdomen. She will palpate the abdomen using her fingertips. When the uterus is relaxed, the abdomen should feel soft. In the presence of a contraction, the uterus will feel hard, tight, or firm under her fingertips. She then times the duration of the contraction from the beginning of one contraction to the beginning of the next. Contractions will vary in frequency and duration. If patient experiences 4-6 contractions/hr for 1-2 hr, she should call her health care provider for further evaluation. Contractions may place tension on the cervical cerclage, cause bleeding of the cervix at the suture insertion sites, and dilate or cause funneling of the cervix above the cerclage. Duration of the contraction may or may not be an indication of contraction intensity. It is believed that the longer the contraction in true labor, the more effective it is in progressing dilation and effacement.
Question patient at each prenatal visit starting at the beginning of the second trimester if she is experiencing any cervical symptoms that may indicate cervical change. Encourage patient to report any "vague" or "subtle" symptoms no matter what time of day or night. Provide patient with written instructions and phone numbers to call accordingly.	Early recognition and reporting of cervical changes (e.g., light menstrual-like cramps, pelvic heaviness, sharp pains in the vagina or cervix, change in vaginal odor or discharge) may lead to better fetal outcome.
Instruct patient to drink at least six 8-oz glasses of water/day (48-64 fluid oz).	Patients with cervical insufficiency may also experience preterm labor. The uterus is a muscle and will respond to dehydration by cramping/ contracting. Adequate hydration is a preventive measure.

●●● **Related NIC and NOC labels**: *NIC:* High-risk Pregnancy Care; Disease Process *NOC:* Knowledge: Pregnancy; Disease Process

Nursing Diagnosis:

Ineffective Coping

related to adjustment in lifestyle to provide an optimal outcome for the pregnancy and fetus or lack of support from family, friends, and community

Desired Outcome: Within 24 hr of this diagnosis, patient begins to modify her lifestyle or behavior to provide the best pregnancy outcome for herself and the fetus.

INTERVENTIONS	RATIONALES
Assess patient's perceptions and comprehension of current health status regarding cervical incompetence.	Evaluation of perception and comprehension enables development of an individualized care plan.
Help patient identify or develop a support system.	Many people benefit from the aid and reduction of stress from outside support systems in helping them cope.
Arrange community referrals, as appropriate.	Support in the home environment promotes healthier adaptations and may avert crises.
Affirm that the necessary lifestyle adjustment (e.g., no work, bedrest, no intercourse), while it may seem austere, is for a limited time.	This information facilitates acceptance of outside support and assistance. It also reconfirms that by not making lifestyle changes, activities that cause increased pressure on an insufficient cervix with or without a cerclage increase risk of cervical dilation, preterm delivery, and possible fetal/neonatal demise.

Continued

INTERVENTIONS	RATIONALES
Provide referral sources for support groups, written material, Internet chat groups, or home help if the patient is on home bedrest or hospitalization. Also, involve Social Services in care of the patient as needed.	Communicating with others who have experienced similar circumstances may aid in developing coping mechanisms.
Offer emotional support when patient verbalizes her concerns.	This validates patient's concerns and may help her cope better.
Help patient identify previous methods of coping with life problems. Help patient focus on positive coping methods.	How patient has handled problems in the past may be a reliable predictor of how she will cope with current problems.

••• **Related NIC and NOC labels:** *NIC:* Coping Enhancement; Emotional Support; Support System Enhancement *NOC:* Coping

Nursing Diagnosis:

Caregiver Role Strain

related to care significant other, family member, or support person needs to provide not only for the patient but also possibly for other children in order for patient to adhere to treatments

Desired Outcome: Within 24 hr of this diagnosis, caregiver and patient verbalize their concerns/frustrations about caregiving responsibilities, identify at least one other support person, and recognize at least one change that would make their jobs easier.

INTERVENTIONS	RATIONALES
Encourage caregiver to relate feelings and concerns regarding added responsibilities. Help caregiver clarify the responsibilities with patient and other family members.	This validates caregiver's concerns and helps him or her understand if expectations are realistic.
Involve Social Services in support of caregiver as needed in helping to establish a plan for time-outs.	Social Services will provide caregiver with viable goals and coping mechanisms.
Encourage caregiver to identify which activities would benefit from outside assistance and assist in identifying sources of help (e.g., family members, friends, neighbors, church members).	This confirms caregiver's need to seek help. During times of stress, caregivers may know they need help, but may not know where to look for it.
Affirm that added caregiving responsibilities are for a limited time.	This information facilitates acceptance of outside support and assistance and may make current added responsibilities more tolerable.

••• **Related NIC and NOC labels:** *NIC:* Coping Enhancement; Respite Care; Support System Enhancement; Behavior Modification *NOC:* Caregiver Well-Being; Role Performance

Nursing Diagnosis:

Risk for Impaired Parent/Infant Attachment

related to disruption for bonding or interactive process secondary to fetal health risks

Desired Outcome: Patient and significant other verbalize their concerns regarding potential barriers to the parental bonding process.

INTERVENTIONS	RATIONALES
Encourage patient and significant other to verbalize concerns regarding the potential delay or loss in the bonding process.	This provides an opportunity for assessment, confirmation, and/or validation of their feelings.
If a loss occurs, allow patient and significant other time with the infant if they so desire (will depend on the appropriateness of the gestational age).	This validates their experience of loss and assists in transitioning to the grieving process.

••• **Related NIC and NOC labels:** *NIC:* Emotional Support; Coping Enhancement; Family Involvement Promotion *NOC:* Parent-Infant Attachment

Nursing Diagnosis:

Anticipatory Grieving

related to potential loss of the fetus secondary to cervical incompetence

Desired Outcome: Patient and significant other verbalize their feelings and identify and use support systems to aid them in the grief process as needed.

INTERVENTIONS	RATIONALES
Encourage patient and significant other to verbalize their feelings and concerns regarding the potential for loss of their baby.	This validates concerns and conveys the message that grief is a normal and expected reaction to the loss of a baby.
As appropriate, clarify misconceptions about the potential risk for fetal loss with cervical insufficiency.	Clarification allows patient and significant other to process the information regarding cervical insufficiency appropriately while not providing false hope.
Assess and accept patient's behavioral response.	Disbelief, denial, guilt, anger, and depression are normal reactions to grief.
Teach the five stages of grief and explain that there is no specific time frame in which to go through the process.	This information enables patient and family members to understand their stage of the grief process. Stages include (1) shock and numbness; (2) denial and searching-yearning; (3) anger, guilt, and sense of failure; (4) depression and disorganization; and (5) resolution.
Involve Social Services when available and needed or when a loss is perceived or present.	Social Services provides resources and appropriate referral services for individual counseling, support groups for bereaved parents and grandparents, and guidance through the disposition of the fetus/neonate.
If a loss occurs, provide patient and family with support if they decide to see and hold the baby (gestation appropriate) and place appropriate items in a memory/keepsake box.	These measures assist with the grieving process. Items such as footprints and lock of hair may be tucked away and not looked at right away, but it may help them to know they are there.

••• **Related NIC and NOC labels:** *NIC:* Coping Enhancement; Grief Work Facilitation: Perinatal Death; Emotional Support; Hope Instillation; Support System Enhancement *NOC:* Coping

Nursing Diagnosis:

Sexual Dysfunction

related to inability to have sexual (penile-vaginal, digital-vaginal) intercourse during the pregnancy

Desired Outcome: Immediately following teaching, patient and partner verbalize accurate understanding of the effect that intercourse may have on an incompetent cervix and the reason for abstinence.

INTERVENTIONS	RATIONALES
Teach patient and her partner the effect that sexual foreplay or sexual intercourse may have on cervical insufficiency. Explain that sexual intercourse may increase uterine contractions and promote cervical changes.	Knowledge promotes patient/partner adherence. Increased uterine activity is not uncommon after sexual intercourse. It may be caused by breast stimulation, female orgasm, or prostaglandin in male ejaculate.
Encourage patient and significant other to verbalize feelings and anxieties about sexual abstinence or having to use alternative methods (nothing per vagina) for sexual gratification. Develop strategies with patient and significant other.	These measures promote knowledge of ways to achieve sexual satisfaction while understanding need to monitor uterine activity (cramping/contractions) in response to the alternatives used (e.g., kissing, touching).

••• **Related NIC and NOC labels:** *NIC:* Sexual Counseling; Anxiety Reduction *NOC:* Sexual Functioning

ADDITIONAL NURSING DIAGNOSES/ PROBLEMS:

"Prolonged Bedrest" for applicable nursing diagnoses, including:

Deficient Diversional Activity — p. 69

Ineffective Role Performance: Dependence vs. independence — p. 70

"Psychosocial Support" for applicable nursing diagnoses, including:

Disturbed Sleep Pattern — p. 73

Anxiety — p. 74

Fear — p. 76

Ineffective Coping — p. 76

Anticipatory Grieving/Risk for Dysfunctional Grieving — p. 79

Social Isolation — p. 84

"Psychosocial Support for the Patient's Family and Significant Other" for applicable nursing diagnoses, including:

Interrupted Family Processes — p. 88

Compromised Family Coping — p. 89

"Preterm Labor" for:

Deficient Knowledge: Prescribed medications — p. 722

Constipation — p. 725

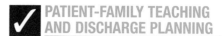

PATIENT-FAMILY TEACHING AND DISCHARGE PLANNING

Include verbal and written information about the following:

✓ Potential risk factors for cervical insufficiency that may be present at the initial prenatal visit.

✓ Monitoring for signs and symptoms that may indicate cervical changes (increased vaginal discharge, light pink, blood-tinged, or tan).

✓ Palpation of contractions.

✓ Promptly reporting signs of UTI.

✓ Importance of adequate oral hydration.

✓ Adherence to scheduled prenatal visits. Confirm date and time of next visit.

✓ Measures for coping with muscle pain, back pain, and muscle weakness that can be present with prolonged bedrest.

✓ Measures that help with constipation, which occurs frequently in pregnancy and is exacerbated by bedrest.

✓ Importance of adhering to restrictions on intercourse, heavy lifting, or prolonged (more than 90 min) standing.

✓ Medications, including drug name, purpose, dosage, frequency, precautions, potential drug reactions, and side effects. Also discuss potential drug-drug, food-drug, and herb-drug interactions.

✓ Guidelines for checking maternal pulse rate before dosing while taking terbutaline (a premature labor inhibitor).

✓ Fetal movement counts.

✓ Referral to national and local support organizations, including:

- Sidelines, a national support organization for women and their families experiencing complicated pregnancies:
- Sidelines High Risk Pregnancy Support National Office at *www.sidelines.org*
- SHARE, a national support group for parents who have experienced loss through miscarriage, stillbirth, or newborn death:
- SHARE Pregnancy & Infant Loss Support, Inc. at *www.nationalshareoffice.com*

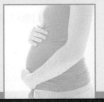

Diabetes in Pregnancy 90

OVERVIEW/PATHOPHYSIOLOGY

Diabetes mellitus (DM) is classified as either type 1 or type 2. Type 1 (insulin-deficient diabetes) is usually characterized by onset at an early age (present before pregnancy) requiring insulin injections to avoid ketoacidosis (a state of increased hepatic glucose production and decreased or absent tissue disposal of glucose that results in hyperglycemia). Type 2 (insulin-resistant diabetes) includes gestational diabetes mellitus (GDM). GDM is a carbohydrate intolerance that has its onset or is first recognized during pregnancy. There is a 50% risk of GDM turning to chronic DM within 5 yr after diagnosis if no lifestyle changes are made. Both types of diabetes pose significant risks to maternal/fetal morbidity and mortality.

HEALTH CARE SETTING

Primary care (outpatient obstetric clinic, high-risk perinatal clinic); or acute care (inpatient) when starting or adjusting insulin

ASSESSMENT

Every pregnant woman should be screened for GDM by obtaining history, clinical risk factors, or serum glucose levels. Patients with low risk factors (age younger than 25 yr, not a member of an ethnic group at risk for developing type 2 diabetes, body mass index [BMI] less than 25, no previous history of abnormal glucose tolerance, no previous history of adverse obstetric outcomes that are usually associated with GDM, and no known diabetes in a first-degree relative [mother, father, siblings]) may not need the traditional glucose tolerance test. Only 10% of the pregnant population would fall into this category, and 3% of women with GDM would not have been diagnosed using this method. Therefore many providers prefer to screen all of their patients using the 1-hr glucose tolerance test. Pregnant patients with a previous history of GDM may be screened earlier in the current pregnancy to diagnose GDM and initiate dietary changes and medications as needed to ensure better glycemic control and decrease untoward consequences to the fetus.

Type 1 DM: Increased risk of abnormal embryogenesis (growth, differentiation, and organization of fetal cellular components), spontaneous abortion, sacral agenesis or caudal dysplasia (absence or deformity of the sacrum), pyelonephritis, preterm labor/birth, polyhydramnios (abnormally high level of amniotic fluid), preeclampsia, ketoacidosis, cesarean section, fetal hypoxia, stillbirth, fetal macrosomia (birth weight 4000 g or more) or intrauterine growth restriction, birth trauma (e.g., shoulder dystocia because of macrosomia), congenital anomalies (ventral septal defect, transposition of the great vessels, anencephaly (absence of neural tissue in the cranium), open spina bifida (a defect in the closure of the neural tube), holoprosencephaly (absence of midline cerebral structures because of the incomplete division of the forebrain), respiratory distress syndrome (RDS), and neonatal hypoglycemia.

Type 2 DM/GDM: Increased risk of macrosomia or intrauterine growth restriction (depending on extent of the maternal illness and glycemic control), preeclampsia, ketoacidosis, cesarean section, hypoxia, RDS, stillbirth, birth trauma, and neonatal hypoglycemia.

Note: During pregnancy the classic symptoms of diabetes (polydipsia, polyphagia, and polyuria) cannot be used as diagnostic tools because they are normal changes of pregnancy.

Renal-urinary: Glucosuria is not a reliable sign of diabetes during pregnancy because of a lowered renal threshold that occurs at that time. If glucose (+1 or higher) appears consistently (2 times or more) in the urine, however, the patient needs to be evaluated for GDM.

Neurologic: Frequent headaches, fatigue, and drowsiness may be present as a result of maternal insulin resistance. Retinopathy is commonly seen in woman with type 1 DM (preexisting disease) caused by abnormal vasculature, capillary rupture, or hemorrhage within the retina. An ophthalmic examination during the pregnancy is recommended.

Cardiovascular: In patients with long-term diabetes, deterioration of glomerular function can lead to hypertension and superimposed preeclampsia. These women can also develop arteriosclerosis.

Other symptoms: Pregnant women with diabetes are at an increased risk of developing preeclampsia. See additional symptoms in "Preeclampsia," p. 711.

Complications—fetal:
- Miscarriage/fetal death
- Embryonic growth delay
- Congenital malformations, especially cardiac and skeletal
- Hypertrophic and congestive cardiomyopathy
- Fetal macrosomia (gigantism)
- Hypoglycemia

- RDS
- Hyperbilirubinemia
- Hypocalcemia
- Intrauterine growth restriction

Risk factors: Family history of DM, previous history of GDM, previous macrosomic infant, previous unexplained stillbirth, poor obstetric outcome, polyhydramnios (past or present), excessive weight gain or obesity, history of congenital anomalies in offspring, chronic hypertension, recurrent infections including vaginal monilial, recurrent glucosuria, and age older than 30. There is also increased risk for GDM among African Americans, Hispanics, Native Americans, Asians, and South Pacific Islanders.

DIAGNOSTIC TESTS

1-Hour glucose screening: Performed between wk 24-28 of the pregnancy or earlier, even at the initial prenatal visit. If results are negative in an earlier test, the test is repeated between 24 and 28 wk in the pregnancy if patient meets risk factors (discussed earlier). This test requires the patient to drink a 50-g glucose load, followed in 1 hr by venous plasma measurement. A value 140 mg/dl or greater is considered abnormal and indicates need for the 3-hr 100-g oral glucose tolerance test. When a 1-hr value is 190 mg/dl or greater, a fasting glucose should be done before proceeding to the 3-hr test. If the fasting value is 95 mg/dl or greater, the patient is treated for GDM.

3-Hour glucose tolerance test: After fasting for 8-12 hr and abstaining from smoking, a fasting blood sugar (FBS) is drawn after which the patient drinks 100-g glucose load followed by serum venous plasma measurements at 1, 2, and 3 hr. Two of the four values need to be abnormal to make the diagnosis of GDM. There are two diagnostic criteria for diagnosing GDM, depending on medical facility preference. They are as follows.

NATIONAL DIABETES DATA GROUP	CARPENTER AND COUSTAN
Fasting: 105	Fasting: 95
1-hr: 190	1-hr: 180
2-hr: 165	2-hr: 155
3-hr: 145	3-hr: 140

Data from ACOG, 2001

Glycosylated hemoglobin (HbA₁C): Reflects the average blood sugar levels for the 2- to 3-mo period before the test. Values may be increased in iron deficient anemia and decreased in pregnancy. Levels less than 6% are desired in pregnancy.

Home glucose monitoring: The patient at home performs glucose monitoring (obtaining whole blood from a fingerstick) at given intervals prescribed by the health care provider. Normal values during pregnancy are FBS less than 95 mg/dl and 2-hr postprandial (pp) 120 mg/dl or less. Patients with poor glucose control will have FBS well above 90-95 mg/dl and 2-hr pp well above 120 mg/dl. Careful regulation of maternal glucose levels during pregnancy leads to decreased maternal/fetal compromise and better outcomes.

Renal function studies: Normally during pregnancy creatinine clearance is increased, but it is decreased in GDM because of deterioration in glomerular function. A 24-hr urinalysis for protein is recommended early in the pregnancy that can be used as a comparison later if renal function worsens.

Obstetric ultrasound: A screening ultrasound and fetal cardiac echo are done at around 20 wk gestation to check for fetal anomalies inasmuch as incidence is increased in fetuses of mothers with diabetes. Further ultrasounds may be done at 2- to 4-wk intervals to monitor fetal growth, placental function, amniotic fluid levels, and fetal position and check for presence of polyhydramnios (excess amniotic fluid).

Antepartum fetal monitoring: Patients with GDM who are diet controlled and at low risk for intrauterine death do not routinely require antepartum fetal heart rate testing unless they have hypertension, history of prior stillbirth, or current fetal macrosomia. Any of these conditions would necessitate weekly to twice weekly testing starting at 32 wk (or sooner if necessary) to monitor fetal well-being.

Nursing Diagnosis:

Deficient Knowledge:

Effects of diabetes on self, pregnancy, and fetus

Desired Outcome: Immediately following teaching, patient verbalizes accurate knowledge about the effects of diabetes on self, the pregnancy, and fetus and adheres to the treatment accordingly.

INTERVENTIONS	RATIONALES
Explain to patient and significant other the effects diabetes may have on the mother, pregnancy, and fetus.	An informed patient is more likely to adhere to the therapeutic plan (e.g., frequent blood sugar checks, frequent clinic visits, insulin injections, dietary monitoring) and understand possible problems associated with type 1 DM and GDM and consequences of nonadherence.
Encourage adherence with prenatal appointments, testing, and dietary regimen.	Pregnant women with type 1 DM are at increased risk for maternal/fetal morbidity and mortality (see Assessment for details). Fetal death, pre-eclampsia, renal disease, cardiac disease, and retinopathy are possible. Women with GDM are at increased risk for fetal macrosomia and preeclampsia, especially when they do not adhere to the therapeutic plan. There is a 50% risk of GDM turning to chronic DM within 5 yr after diagnosis if no lifestyle changes are made.
Inform patient about probable increased need for insulin to manage glycemic control during the pregnancy.	The body's insulin requirements increase as the pregnancy advances. Insulin therapy should be considered when nutritional therapy fails to keep 1-hr pp at less than 130-140 mg/dl, 2-hr pp less than 120 mg/dl, or fasting glucose less than 95 mg/dl.
For patients with GDM, arrange for one-on-one teaching with a diabetes educator for the following: how to check blood sugars with a Glucometer, how to document blood sugars, and importance of exercise during pregnancy.	A one-on-one session with a diabetes educator experienced with GDM enables an opportunity for questions/interactions and greater patient comprehension.
Teach patient and significant other signs and symptoms of hypoglycemia, hyperglycemia, diabetic ketoacidosis, and insulin shock. For more information, see "Diabetes Mellitus," p. 377, and "Diabetic Ketoacidosis," p. 373.	A knowledgeable patient likely will report these symptoms promptly. During pregnancy the goal is for lower blood sugar levels than when not pregnant. Therefore the patient is more likely to experience hypoglycemia than hyperglycemia.
Develop a sick-day plan with the patient.	This information will help patient maintain adequate glycemic control. For example, patient should do the following: - Check blood sugar and urine for ketones q2-4h during illness. - Maintain normal insulin schedule. - Maintain normal meals when possible. Drink plenty of water and/or calorie-free liquids if unable to maintain solid foods. Consume a minimum of 150 g of carbohydrates per day, taken in small amounts over 24 hr. - Call provider if temperature is 101° F or greater (38.3° C), ketone level is moderate to high, or if vomiting and unable to keep anything down. - Patient may need to be hospitalized for IV fluids and regulation of blood sugar. - In diabetes associated with pregnancy, early detection of ketones is critical to fetal mortality because ketoacidosis is a significant factor that contributes to intrauterine death.
Encourage patient to maintain or initiate an exercise program.	Exercise improves cardiopulmonary fitness and may improve glucose metabolism.
Teach daily fetal movement counts.	Fetal movement counts are a good first-line indicator of fetal well-being and are performed as follows, beginning at 28 wk gestation: Patient lies on her side and counts "distinct fetal movements" (hiccups do not count) daily; 10 movements within a 2-hr period is reassuring. After 10 movements are noted, the count is discontinued. Fewer than 10 movements indicates need for fetal nonstress testing.

••• **Related NIC and NOC labels:** *NIC:* Teaching: Disease Process; Hyperglycemia Management; Hypoglycemia Management; Nutrition Management *NOC:* Knowledge: Diabetes Management

Nursing Diagnoses:

Imbalanced Nutrition: Less Than Body Requirements/ More Than Body Requirements

related to inability to follow prescribed dietary regimen for effective glycemic control

Desired Outcome: Patient follows prescribed dietary regimen.

INTERVENTIONS	RATIONALES
Assess patient's cultural habits surrounding diet (foods she can and cannot eat, who shops, who cooks).	Working within cultural habits aids in dietary adherence. For example, there may be high carbohydrate consumption, depending on cultural group: rice for Asian women; tortillas and rice for Hispanic women; and breads and pasta for non-Hispanic white women.
Arrange for a meeting with a nutritionist who specializes in diabetes in pregnancy.	A nutritionist is trained to answer questions regarding specific foods and meal plans that are appropriate for glycemic control and can act as a resource person for the patient. Nutritional interventions should achieve normal glucose levels and avoid ketosis while maintaining appropriate nutrition and weight gain in pregnancy.
Encourage patient to keep a daily dietary log.	A log provides a quick reference to compare blood sugars and foods eaten.
Praise patient when blood sugars are within normal limits.	Good glycemic control reduces incidence of maternal and fetal morbidity and mortality.
Inform patient of the risks to self and fetus associated with poor glycemic control related to dietary nonadherence.	Knowledge aids in adherence to the treatment plan. Dietary nonadherence can result in miscarriage, fetal anomalies, fetal macrosomia and increased risk of shoulder dystocia with a vaginal delivery, and increased potential for cesarean delivery.
Teach patient to monitor urine for ketones.	Ketones are weak acids produced when blood sugar is poorly controlled and the body burns fat instead of sugar for energy.
	Moderate to large (2-4+) ketones may signal ketoacidosis, which necessitates immediate evaluation. If untreated, prolonged ketoacidosis can result in fetal brain damage.
Develop a "sick-day plan" with patient.	See discussion in **Deficient Knowledge:** Effects of diabetes on self, pregnancy, and fetus, earlier.

●●● **Related NIC and NOC labels:** *NIC:* Nutritional Counseling; Teaching: Prescribed Diet *NOC:* Nutritional Status: Nutrient Intake

Nursing Diagnosis:

Fear

related to effects of GDM on self, pregnancy, and fetus; potential complications; and insulin injections

Desired Outcomes: Immediately following interventions, patient and significant other express fears and concerns. Within 24 hr of interventions, patient reports feeling greater psychologic comfort, understanding of the effects of diabetes on the pregnancy, and confidence in administering insulin if needed.

INTERVENTIONS	RATIONALES
Encourage and support patient and significant other in verbalizing their fears and concerns.	This validates their fears/concerns and enables development of an individualized care plan.
Acknowledge patient's fears.	Acknowledging feelings in an empathetic manner encourages communication, which optimally will reduce fear. For example, "I understand that giving yourself injections frightens you, but it is necessary to control your blood sugar."
When appropriate and if available, involve Social Services in patient management. Provide patient with a list of support groups available for patients with GDM.	Social Services can provide individual counseling and information on referrals, support groups, and Internet chat groups for patients with GDM. Some support groups are listed at the end of this care plan.
Encourage patient to ask questions and become as knowledgeable as possible about her condition and treatment.	Increasing knowledge levels about appropriate dietary intake and blood sugar control reduces/eliminates fear of the unknown and affords a sense of control.
Teach patient appropriate techniques for checking blood sugar, documenting results, and drawing up, injecting, and storing insulin (see "Diabetes Mellitus," p. 377).	This teaching provides an opportunity to assess and validate patient's knowledge and fears. Knowledge likely will help decrease fear of self-administration of insulin and aid in compliance with treatments.

••• Related NIC and NOC labels: *NIC:* Active Listening; Anxiety Reduction; Support System Enhancement; Teaching: Procedure
NOC: Fear Control

Nursing Diagnosis:

Anxiety

related to actual or perceived threat to self or fetus secondary to the effects diabetes may have on the pregnancy

Desired Outcome: Within 1-2 hr of intervention, patient states that her anxiety has lessened or resolved, and she describes appropriate coping mechanisms in managing the anxiety.

INTERVENTIONS	RATIONALES
Engage in honest communication with patient; provide empathetic understanding. Listen closely.	This establishes an atmosphere that allows free expression.
Be alert for verbal and nonverbal cues about patient's anxiety level.	These cues aid in providing appropriate assistance and support. Levels of anxiety include: - *Mild:* restlessness, irritability, increased questions, focusing on the environment. - *Moderate:* inattentiveness, expressions of concern, narrowed perceptions, insomnia, increased heart rate. - *Severe:* expression of feelings of doom, rapid speech, tremors, poor eye contact. Patient may be preoccupied with the past or unable to understand the present and may have tachycardia, nausea, and hyperventilation. - *Panic:* inability to concentrate or communicate, distortion of reality, increased motor activity, vomiting, tachypnea.
Explain that patients with poor glycemic control or who need to initiate first-time insulin use usually are admitted to the hospital for teaching and monitoring.	This offers the potential of a supportive environment that aids in decreasing anxiety and increasing patient confidence.
Encourage patient to communicate cause of anxiety, for example, dietary changes, failure to maintain adequate glycemic control, checking blood sugars, insulin injections.	This information helps determine patient's knowledge of diabetes in pregnancy and ways in which patient teaching can alleviate anxiety.

Continued

INTERVENTIONS	RATIONALES
Provide reassurance and a safe, quiet environment for patient to relax.	An anxious person has difficulty learning.
Assess at each appointment if patient has enough supplies to maintain self-care.	Having adequate supplies (e.g., Glucometer, test strips, lancets, record book, insulin, syringes, alcohol wipes, sharps disposal box) on hand may increase adherence to therapy and decrease anxiety.
Encourage patient to attend diabetes classes and support groups for patients with diabetes.	Talking with others who have or are experiencing diabetes in pregnancy aids in establishing outside support resources. Some support groups are listed at the end of this care plan.
Inform patient with GDM that although she has diabetes associated with the pregnancy, this does not mean she will have lifelong diabetes.	Having this information may alleviate anxiety and increase adherence to the therapeutic plan.
However, advise her that if she has other risk factors such as a first-line relative with history of type 1 or type 2 DM, obesity, and diet high in carbohydrates and fats, these factors can increase risk for developing chronic DM during the next 10-15 yr.	This information identifies some factors over which she has control, which optimally will decrease anxiety and encourage weight loss, dietary control, and exercise postpartum to prevent future development of chronic DM.

••• **Related NIC and NOC labels:** *NIC:* Anxiety Reduction; Active Listening; Environmental Management; Support Group *NOC:* Anxiety Control

Nursing Diagnosis:

Deficient Knowledge:

Benefits and potential side effects of prescribed medications used to treat GDM

Desired Outcome: Immediately following teaching, patient and significant other verbalize accurate understanding of the risks and benefits of medications used during the pregnancy to treat diabetes.

INTERVENTIONS	RATIONALES
Teach the following about patient's prescribed drugs:	A knowledgeable patient is more likely to adhere to the therapy, identify and report side effects, and recognize and report precautions that might preclude use of the prescribed drug.
Sulfonylureas: Second-Generation	These agents lower blood glucose by stimulating release of insulin from the pancreas.
Glyburide (Micronase, DiaBeta, Euglucon)	This is currently the only oral glycemic agent shown to be safe and effective in GDM. There is concern for teratogenicity with other oral agents. Diabetes itself is teratogenic, making it difficult to determine effects of the oral agents from those of the disease. Most patients with type 1 DM who have been managed on oral agents are changed to insulin during the pregnancy.
	Administration: oral.
Teach patient to be alert for and report shakiness, sweating, nervousness, headache, and blood sugar level less than 60 mg/dl.	These are signs of hypoglycemia.
Teach patient to be alert for and report blurred vision.	This is a side effect caused by fluctuation in blood glucose levels.
Stress importance of monitoring blood glucose levels as directed.	This helps detect hypoglycemia or hyperglycemia promptly. The usual routine in pregnancy is to monitor blood glucose fasting (first thing in the morning before breakfast or taking medications), 2 hr after eating, at bedtime, and when glucose levels have been low or high. Poor glycemic control when taking the oral agent necessitates initiation of insulin.
Teach patient to be alert for and report nausea, epigastric fullness, and heartburn.	These are adverse reactions. If these reactions occur consistently, patient may require dose adjustment or be started on insulin—whichever maintains glycemic control.

Continued

INTERVENTIONS	RATIONALES
Caution patients taking nonsteroidal antiinflammatory drugs (NSAIDs) and beta-adrenergic blocking agents to notify health care provider before taking sulfonylureas.	The hypoglycemic reaction may be potentiated by these medications.

Insulin

INTERVENTIONS	RATIONALES
Regular Humalog and lispro (rapid acting), NPH (intermediate acting), glargine (long acting)	This is a parenteral blood glucose–lowering agent that regulates glucose metabolism. Lispro has a more rapid onset of action than regular insulin and does not cross the placenta.
	Administration: Subcutaneous or by insulin pump. Some patients may be started on subcutaneous insulin as an outpatient. This choice is individualized based on patient adherence and comprehension of insulin therapy (drawing up insulin, injecting accurately, and timing doses). Inpatient setting is required for initial teaching for how to use the pump, including monitoring of glucose levels and making necessary insulin dose adjustments.
Teach patient to be alert for and report shakiness, sweating, nervousness, headache, and low blood sugar levels.	These are signs of hypoglycemia, a potential side effect. Some patients may be symptomatic between 60 and 70 mg/dl and others not until 50-60 mg/dl (or lower).
Teach patient to be alert for and report blurred vision.	This is a side effect secondary to fluctuations in blood glucose levels.
Stress importance of monitoring blood glucose levels as directed.	This aids in prompt identification of hypoglycemic reactions.
Caution patients taking NSAIDs, salicylates, and beta-adrenergic blocking agents to notify their health care provider.	Insulin requirements may be decreased when also taking drugs with hypoglycemic activity. Beta-blockers may mask the symptoms of hypoglycemia.
Caution patient taking terbutaline to notify health care provider.	This drug may alter glucose metabolism. Terbutaline is used to decrease uterine myometrial activity (contractions).

••• Related NIC and NOC labels: *NIC:* Teaching: Prescribed Medication; Hyperglycemia Management; Hypoglycemia Management
NOC: Knowledge: Medication

ADDITIONAL NURSING DIAGNOSES/ PROBLEMS:

"Psychosocial Support" for relevant nursing Diagnoses such as **Ineffective Coping**	p. 76
"Psychosocial Support for the Patient's Family and Significant Other" for such nursing diagnoses as **Compromised Family Coping**	p. 89
"Diabetic Ketoacidosis"	p. 373
"Diabetes Mellitus"	p. 377

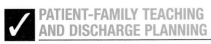

PATIENT-FAMILY TEACHING AND DISCHARGE PLANNING

Patients with GDM require close monitoring for maternal and fetal well-being. Education is the key to making the pregnancy a success. When providing patient-family teaching, avoid giving excessive information. Part of the initial assessment should include asking about existing knowledge of the disease, ability for self-management, and psychologic acceptance. Include written and verbal information about the following:

✓ Recommended glucose levels in pregnancy: Fasting, 60-90 mg/dl; before lunch, dinner, or bedtime snack, 60-105 mg/dl; 2-hr pp, 120 mg/dl or less.

✓ Reminder that stress from illness or infection can increase insulin requirements.

✓ Recognizing warning signs of both hyperglycemia and simple and advanced hypoglycemia and insulin shock, treatment, and factors that contribute to both conditions.

- *Hyperglycemia:* Possible causes include not enough insulin or increased insulin resistance (as seen with advancing gestational age), too much food, stress of illness, emotional stress, and decreased exercise. Patient should call health care provider for treatment, which may include increasing insulin dose and/or self-administering an insulin bolus.
- *Hypoglycemia:* Possible causes are too much insulin, too little food, not eating on time, vomiting, and too much exercise. (See next three items for treatment options.)
- Review "Diabetes Mellitus," p. 377, for further information.
- Foods to treat hypoglycemia such as 4-oz orange juice, 4-oz milk, 4-oz cola drink (not diet cola), 3-4 pieces of hard candy, 3-4 sugar cubes, 2-3 glucose tablets.

- How and when to take glucose tablets. Keep glucose tablets with you when away from home and available food sources. Instruct patient to use glucose tablets if becoming shaky, nauseated, nervous, headachy, drowsy, and diaphoretic and blood sugar is 60 mg/dl or less.

✓ When to call for emergency services. With advanced hypoglycemia (blood sugar 20-50 mg/dl) the patient may not be the person calling in an emergency situation; this information needs to be communicated to significant other and family members as well.

✓ Importance of carrying an identification card or wearing a bracelet or necklace that identifies patient as having diabetes in case of emergency. For patients with GDM, the necklace or bracelet may be obtained at a local pharmacy. If the patient has preexisting diabetes, the above information may be obtained by contacting the following organization: Medic Alert Foundation, 323 Colorado Avenue, Turlock, CA 96382, (209) 668-3333.

✓ Importance of adherence to prescribed health care and ready access to hospital and family/social support.

✓ Parameters and guidelines for blood sugar levels as recommended by health care provider.

✓ Nutritional regimen as recommended by health care provider. Adequate nutrition and controlled calories are essential to maintaining normoglycemia and appropriate fetal growth.

✓ Medications, including drug name, purpose, dosage, frequency, precautions, administration, and potential side effects. Also discuss potential drug-drug, food-drug, and herb-drug interactions.

✓ How to monitor urine for ketones.

✓ Fetal movement counts (gestational age appropriate).

✓ Referrals to local and national support organizations, including:

- American Diabetes Association (ADA) at *www.diabetes.org*
- Sidelines, a national support organization for women and their families experiencing complicated pregnancies, at Sidelines High Risk Pregnancy Support National Office, *www.sidelines.org*
- Joslin Diabetes Center at *www.joslin.harvard.edu*

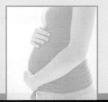

Hyperemesis Gravidarum 91

OVERVIEW/PATHOPHYSIOLOGY

Nausea and vomiting are common symptoms of unknown cause in the first trimester of pregnancy. Hyperemesis is excessive vomiting in pregnancy that can interfere with hydration, electrolytes, acid-base balance, and nutritional status and may last throughout the entire pregnancy. Theories regarding cause include rising estrogen and human chorionic gonadotropin levels (hCG), relaxation of the smooth muscles of the abdomen caused by an increase in progesterone, decrease in motilin levels, and psychogenic factors.

HEALTH CARE SETTING

Some hyperemesis patients may be treated on an outpatient basis with oral medications or home IV infusion therapy given to replace fluids and electrolytes, and some may receive total parenteral nutrition. Others require hospitalization.

ASSESSMENT

Patients with nausea and vomiting in pregnancy who can no longer retain solids or liquids need to be evaluated for dehydration, weight loss, and electrolyte imbalances. They may exhibit a low-grade fever, weakness, dry skin, and poor skin turgor. Patients may appear extremely fatigued and listless with cracked, dry lips and may have lost 5%-10% of total body weight; be constipated as a result of dehydration; and have a markedly decreased urinary output with ketonemia (presence of ketones in the blood). Women with diabetes who have hyperemesis need to be monitored closely to maintain glycemic control and avoid ketoacidosis. See "Diabetes in Pregnancy," p. 687.

Gastrointestinal: Gastrointestinal (GI) motility is reduced because of increased progesterone and decreased motilin levels. "Normal" nausea and vomiting of pregnancy usually has an onset between 4 and 6 wk, peaks at about 12 wk, and optimally resolves at around 20 wk. Nausea and vomiting with hyperemesis may extend beyond this period, possibly throughout the entire pregnancy.

Fluid and electrolyte imbalance: With the inability to maintain adequate fluids for hydration and solids for fuel, the body experiences an imbalance of the elements necessary for health maintenance, which can lead to maternal ketosis.

Cardiopulmonary: The patient may experience one or all of the following: tachycardia, hypotension, postural changes, and tachypnea.

Renal: Possible presence of oliguria and ketonuria.

Complications—fetal: With prolonged dehydration and maternal weight loss, fetal intrauterine growth restriction (IUGR) and low birth weight may be seen.

Physical assessment: The pregnant patient with hyperemesis looks and is ill, appearing extremely fatigued and pale. A thorough assessment is needed to rule out other causes of severe nausea and vomiting, such as gastroenteritis, cholecystitis, pyelonephritis, GI ulcers, or a molar pregnancy (intrauterine neoplastic mass of grapelike enlarged chorionic villi).

Risk factors: Previous history of hyperemesis, molar pregnancy, multiple gestation, emotional/psychologic stress, gastroesophageal reflux, primigravida, uncontrolled thyroid disease, increased body weight/obesity.

DIAGNOSTIC TESTS

Complete blood count (CBC): With dehydration, there likely will be evidence of hemoconcentration (i.e., elevated red blood cell and hematocrit levels).

Serum chemistry: Azotemia (increased blood urea nitrogen) is seen with salt and water depletion. Serum creatinine will be elevated because of changes in renal function caused by the dehydration. Hyponatremia and hypokalemia also may be present because of fluid loss.

Liver enzymes: Slight elevations of aspartate aminotransferase and alanine aminotransferase, which reverse with IV fluid hydration, adequate nutrition, and cessation of vomiting.

Urine chemistry: The urine may be "dipped" (or sent for microscopy) for the presence of ketones, which are seen in dehydration/prolonged vomiting.

Obstetric ultrasound: Ultrasound is used to evaluate a normal intrauterine pregnancy vs. a molar pregnancy, presence of multiple gestation, and fetal growth for IUGR and amniotic fluid volume/amniotic fluid index (AFI).

Nursing Diagnosis:

Imbalanced Nutrition: Less Than Body Requirements

related to inability to ingest and maintain sufficient calories secondary to the nausea and vomiting of hyperemesis gravidarum

Desired Outcome: Within 1 wk of this diagnosis, patient increases her nutritional intake and demonstrates improvement in her acid-base balance and electrolyte and nutritional status.

INTERVENTIONS	RATIONALES
Suggest frequent small meals, six or more per day.	This measure helps reduce feeling of a distended stomach and hence the potential for nausea and vomiting.
Suggest eating meals with the highest protein/calorie intake when the nausea is the least problematic, possibly after taking medication for nausea and vomiting.	The meal providing the most nutrition would be consumed at the time the patient is most likely to retain it.
Suggest that patient use high-protein supplemental drinks.	Liquids may be easier to tolerate than solid foods.
Suggest that patient avoid food odors and foods that are greasy, highly spiced, rich, or overly sweet.	These measures prevent stimulating the gag reflex or increasing acid reflux. However, because some patients prefer salty and spicy foods, patient should try anything that is appealing and that she believes she will be able to keep down.
Administer IV hydration as needed.	This will aid in resolving dehydration and improving electrolyte balance.
Administer parenteral nutrition as needed. Secure assistance of the hyperalimentation team to manage patient's parenteral nutrition.	This will improve nutritional status and thereby help ensure adequate fetal growth.
Encourage patient to take approximately 100 ml of liquid between meals and avoid fluids with meals.	This measure prevents dehydration between meals and overdistention of the stomach during meals, allowing more space for caloric foods.
Encourage patient to stay upright for 2 hr after eating.	This prevents esophageal spasms that can be caused by reflux of acid and food into the esophagus. Gravity aids in facilitating movement of food through the esophagus to the stomach and into the small intestine.

••• **Related NIC and NOC labels:** *NIC:* Fluid Management; Intravenous Therapy; Total Parenteral Nutrition Administration; Sustenance Support *NOC:* Nutritional Status: Food & Fluid Intake

Nursing Diagnosis:

Anxiety

related to actual or perceived threat to self and fetus because of inadequate nutritional status

Desired Outcome: Within 1-2 hr of intervention, patient verbalizes her anxieties, assesses her support system(s), and uses appropriate coping mechanisms for management.

INTERVENTIONS	RATIONALES
Engage in honest communication with patient; provide empathetic understanding. Listen closely.	This establishes an atmosphere that promotes free expression.
Encourage patient to communicate cause(s) of her anxiety.	This information aids in developing a care plan specific to patient's needs, such as whether home or hospital treatment will be more helpful. Examples of causes that may be contributing to patient's anxiety include weight loss, frustration with constant nausea and vomiting, ambivalence about the pregnancy, lack of support from significant other and family, inability to care for self or others, and loss of income if unable to work.

Continued

INTERVENTIONS	RATIONALES
	Patients with severe nausea and vomiting who demonstrate changes in laboratory values and weight loss should be admitted to the hospital for hydration, nutritional supplementation, medications, and monitoring of weight loss or gain. This will provide a supportive environment that aids in decreasing anxiety and increasing patient comfort.
Be alert for verbal and nonverbal cues about patient's anxiety level.	These cues aid in providing appropriate assistance and support. Levels of anxiety include: - *Mild:* restlessness, irritability, increased questions, focusing on the environment. - *Moderate:* inattentiveness, expressions of concern, narrowed perceptions, insomnia, increased heart rate. - *Severe:* expression of feelings of doom, rapid speech, tremors, and poor eye contact. Patient may be preoccupied with the past or unable to understand the present and may have tachycardia, increased nausea and vomiting, and hyperventilation. - *Panic:* inability to concentrate or communicate, distortion of reality, increased motor activity, increased vomiting and tachypnea.
Involve assistance of Social Services when available.	Social Services provides counseling, support, and resources for written material and internet chat groups with others who have experienced similar circumstances.
Involve assistance of a psychologist as needed.	A psychologist enables evaluation for possible psychologic factors that may be contributing to the anxiety and hyperemesis.
Involve assistance of spiritual advisor if patient desires.	Pastoral care and sharing of concerns with a spiritual advisor may decrease anxiety.
Encourage patient to obtain as much rest as possible.	Rest enhances coping mechanisms by decreasing physical and psychologic stress.

••• **Related NIC and NOC labels:** *NIC:* Anxiety Reduction; Active Listening; Coping Enhancement; Counseling *NOC:* Anxiety Control; Coping

Nursing Diagnosis:

Ineffective Coping

related to loss of control over maintaining adequate nutritional intake secondary to the nausea and vomiting of pregnancy

Desired Outcome: Within the 24-hr period after this diagnosis is made, patient verbalizes her concerns, fears, strengths, and weaknesses and identifies personal coping mechanisms and support systems.

INTERVENTIONS	RATIONALES
Assess patient's perceptions and ability to understand current health status.	Evaluation of patient's perceptions and comprehension level enables development of an individualized care plan.
Establish honest and empathetic communication with patient.	Empathy and honesty promote effective communication. For example, "Please tell me what I can do to help you through this difficult time in your pregnancy."
Help patient identify previous methods of coping with life problems.	How patient has handled problems in the past may be a reliable predictor of how she will cope with current problems.
Identify patient's support systems. If possible, observe their interactions with the patient.	Knowing the family unit's strengths and weaknesses aids in planning patient's care and, optimally, reducing stress and promoting effective coping.

Continued

INTERVENTIONS	RATIONALES
Enlist assistance from social workers, nutritional services, and spiritual care as needed.	These services provide emotional support, education, and appropriate referrals as needed.
Teach patient how to effectively use her time when she feels well (e.g., performing activities of daily living or running errands).	This information will give patient some sense of control over her situation.
Teach possible treatment methods for hyperemesis.	Knowledge that there are viable treatments aids in improving coping mechanisms and treatment compliance. For examples of treatments, see next two care plans.

••• **Related NIC and NOC labels:** *NIC:* Coping Enhancement; Support System Enhancement; Emotional Support *NOC:* Coping

Nursing Diagnosis:

Deficient Knowledge:

Effects hyperemesis has on self, the pregnancy, and fetus and the treatment and expected outcome

Desired Outcome: Immediately following teaching, patient and significant other verbalize accurate knowledge about hyperemesis, its treatment, and the expected outcome.

INTERVENTIONS	RATIONALES
Explain to patient and family the effect hyperemesis has on the patient and the fetus.	Hyperemesis causes decreased maternal-fetal placental transfer of nutrients and IUGR. Information helps patient adhere to treatments and understand possible consequences of nonadherence.
Explain the various treatment options.	Treatments may include IV hydration, medications (IV, IM, PO), total parenteral nutrition, home care, and hospitalization.
	Explanation of treatment options aids patient and provider in deciding on a care plan that is most beneficial to patient and fetus.
Teach signs and symptoms that may indicate worsening hyperemesis and dehydration.	A knowledgeable patient likely will report symptoms (inability to keep solids or liquids down for previous 12 hr, dizziness, extreme fatigue, poor skin turgor, caramel-colored urine, and weight loss) promptly. Early evaluation and treatment may decrease severity of symptoms.
Explain expected outcome that adequate fluid and nutritional intake will have on fetal development: increases maternal fetal placental transfer of nutrients and ensures intrauterine fetal growth.	This information reinforces need for patient's adherence to possible hospitalization or home infusion, IV fluids, or parenteral nutrition.
Encourage patient to avoid brushing her teeth within 1-2 hr after meals or on arising in the morning.	This action stimulates the gag reflex and aggravates vomiting in women who are pregnant.
Encourage good oral hygiene.	This prevents dental decay that may accompany contact with the acids present in emesis and for some may help decrease nausea. For example, patient may use mouthwash and brush and floss teeth when she feels the least nauseated.

••• **Related NIC and NOC labels:** *NIC:* Teaching: Disease Process; Teaching: Procedure/Treatment *NOC:* Knowledge: Disease Process; Knowledge: Treatment Procedures

Nursing Diagnosis:

Deficient Knowledge:

Purpose, potential side effects, and safety of prescribed medications and nonprescribed devices used during hyperemesis gravidarum

Desired Outcome: Immediately following teaching, patient verbalizes accurate understanding of the risks, benefits, and precautions of medications used during pregnancy in the treatment of hyperemesis.

INTERVENTIONS	RATIONALES
Teach the following about patient's prescribed medications:	A knowledgeable patient is more likely to adhere to the therapy, identify and report side effects, and recognize and report precautions that might preclude use of the prescribed drug.
Metoclopramide Hydrochloride (Reglan)	This is an antiemetic that works on the chemoreceptor trigger zone in the brain to decrease nausea and vomiting. It helps move food through the GI tract, counteracting the effects of progesterone produced in the pregnancy that slow down the GI tract. It may be given inpatient or outpatient.
	Administration: PO/IM/IV.
Be alert for and report twitching of the eyelids or muscles surrounding the eyes, hands, or legs.	These are extrapyramidal reactions seen with high IV doses.
Be alert for and report involuntary repetitious movements of the muscles of the face, limbs, and trunk.	This is a sign of tardive dyskinesia (a syndrome of potentially irreversible involuntary repetitious movements) and a serious side effect seen with long-term use.
Be alert for and report drowsiness, agitation, seizures, hallucinations, lactation, constipation, and diarrhea.	These are common side effects.
Caution is necessary in patients with seizure disorders.	This drug may lower the seizure threshold.
Caution is necessary in patients taking this medication with sedatives, narcotics, and tranquilizers.	Additive sedative effects may occur.
Pantoprazole (Protonix)	Antiulcer/proton pump inhibitor
	Administration: PO/IV
Be alert for and report diarrhea, stomach pain, loss of appetite, headache, heartburn, muscle pain, skin rash, and drowsiness.	These are possible side effects. Patients should avoid activities that require alertness until the drug's effect on the central nervous system (CNS) is known.
Be alert for and report weakness, sore throat, fever, sores on mouth, unusual bruising, cloudy or bloody urine, difficult or painful urination.	These are rare but serious side effects that necessitate discontinuance of medication.
Caution is necessary in patients taking anticoagulants.	This drug increases their anticoagulant effect.
Promethazine (Phenergan)	Antiemetic/antihistamine/tranquilizer.
	Administration: PO/IV/IM/rectal.
Be alert for and report sedation, blurred vision, fatigue, ringing in the ears, nervousness, insomnia, and tremors.	These are common side effects. Patient should avoid activities that require alertness until the drug's effect on the CNS is known.
Precautions are needed for patients taking other CNS depressants such as opioids.	Drug interactions can occur, necessitating a lower dose of opioids.
Be alert for and report involuntary movements and decreased blood pressure (BP).	Extrapyramidal reactions (involuntary movements) and hypotension are seen with rapid IV administration.
Be alert for and report dry mouth and blurred vision.	These are anticholinergic side effects.
Caution is necessary in patients taking monoamine oxidase (MAO) inhibitors.	Drug interaction can occur, causing increased incidence of extrapyramidal reactions.

Continued

INTERVENTIONS	RATIONALES
Prochlorperazine (Compazine)	Antiemetic.
	Administration: PO/IM/IV/rectal.
Be alert for and report blurred vision, fatigue, ringing in the ears, nervousness, insomnia, and tremors.	These are common CNS side effects. Patient should avoid activities that require alertness until the drug's effect on the CNS is known.
Precautions are needed for patients taking other CNS depressants such as narcotics.	Drug interactions can occur, necessitating decreasing the opioid dose by half.
Be alert for and report involuntary movements and decreased BP.	Extrapyramidal reactions and hypotension are seen with IV administration.
Be alert for and report heart palpitations, seizures, dry mouth, constipation, and urinary retention.	These are less common side effects.
Ondansetron (Zofran)	Antiemetic.
	Administration: PO/IM/IV.
Be alert for and report pain, redness, and burning at the site of injection.	These signs can occur as a local reaction with IM injection or IV infiltration.
Be alert for and report headache, fever, constipation, and diarrhea.	These are common side effects.
Be alert for and report involuntary movements.	Extrapyramidal reactions are rare CNS side effects.
Be alert for and report rapid heart rate, dizziness, feeling faint, and chest pain.	These are cardiac side effects.
Caution is necessary in patients with liver disease.	Liver clearance of this drug is reduced in patients with hepatic impairment.
Doxylamine (Unisom Nighttime Sleep Aid)	Antihistamine. It may be used as an antiemetic with mild symptoms of nausea and vomiting caused by pregnancy. It is often used in combination with pyridoxine (Vitamin B$_6$).
	Administration: PO.
Be alert for and report sedation.	This is a common side effect. Patient needs to avoid activities that require alertness until the drug's effect on the CNS is known.
Pyridoxine (Vitamin B$_6$)	It may be used as an antiemetic for mild symptoms of nausea and vomiting in pregnancy. It is often used in combination with doxylamine (Unisom).
	Administration: oral
Be alert for and report nausea, headache, and numbness or tingling in hands or feet.	This is a rare but serious side effect and necessitates discontinuance of medication.
Motion Sickness Bands	This is a motion sickness device worn on both wrists that applies gentle pressure to acupressure points on the wrists and is available without a prescription. They come in various brands; some are battery operated.

••• **Related NIC and NOC labels:** *NIC:* Teaching: Prescribed Medication *NOC:* Knowledge: Medication

ADDITIONAL NURSING DIAGNOSES/ PROBLEMS:

"Prolonged Bedrest" for relevant nursing diagnoses   p. 61
    (The patient may be on self-imposed bedrest for
    comfort reasons.)

"Psychosocial Support" for relevant nursing diagnoses
    such as:

Disturbed Sleep Pattern   p. 73

Anxiety   p. 74

Disturbed Body Image   p. 80

Social Isolation   p. 84

"Psychosocial Support for the Patient's Family and Signif-
    icant Other" for relevant nursing diagnoses such as:

Interrupted Family Processes   p. 88

"Cervical Insufficiency" for **Caregiver Role Strain**   p. 684

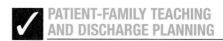

PATIENT-FAMILY TEACHING AND DISCHARGE PLANNING

Include verbal and written information about the following:

✓ Possible causes and effect hyperemesis has on the pregnancy and fetus.

✓ Signs and symptoms patient should report to her health care provider.

✓ Treatment of hyperemesis.

✓ Importance of attaining as much rest as possible.

✓ Nutritional options that would be most beneficial to patient.

✓ Importance of eating small, frequent meals during the day.

✓ Importance of oral hydration.

✓ Importance of avoiding lying down or reclining for 2 hr after eating.

✓ If parenteral nutrition is needed, the importance of maintaining insertion site and reporting any signs of site infection and pump malfunction.

✓ Importance of frequent clinic visits if being monitored on an outpatient basis and the date and time of next clinic visit.

✓ Importance of informing health care provider of any physical and emotional changes that may exacerbate the hyperemesis.

✓ Medications, including drug name, purpose, dosage, frequency, precautions, and potential side effects. Also discuss potential drug-drug, food-drug, and herb-drug interactions.

✓ Referral to local and national support organizations, including Sidelines, a national support organization for women and their families experiencing complicated pregnancies, at *www.sidelines.org*

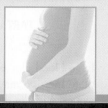

Postpartum Wound Infection 92

OVERVIEW/PATHOPHYSIOLOGY

Abdominal wound infection after cesarean section is not uncommon and can be caused by endogenous or exogenous bacteria. The incidence increases when amniotic membranes have been ruptured for 6 hours or more before delivery. Two determining factors are the amount of bacterial contamination present and resistance of the patient in warding off infection. *Episiotomy infections* can occur but are less common. Sepsis (septic shock), though rare, is associated with *Staphylococcus aureus* at the wound site. A patient who persistently has a fever and does not respond to multiple antibiotic therapies may have *septic pelvic thrombophlebitis*. Patients with this condition do not generally appear ill and may have minimal to no pain. The only variance is the wide swing in temperature. These patients are treated with subcutaneous heparin and normally have rapid improvement within 48-72 hours. This condition occurs more often after cesarean section than after vaginal birth. Prompt evaluation and treatment of these infections help alleviate need for lengthy hospitalizations and home therapy.

When there is little to no improvement in wound site infection with first choice antibiotics, methicillin-resistant *Staphylococcus aureus* (MRSA) infection must be considered and treated appropriately and aggressively.

HEALTH CARE SETTING

Primary care (outpatient clinic), acute care (hospital), or home care

ASSESSMENT

Early-onset infections occur within the first 48 hr after surgery and are seen as a discoloration, usually pink to light red, of the skin surrounding the incision (cellulitis), warm to the touch, and may be accompanied with a fever. This should be caught early with daily inspection of the wound site or episiotomy while the patient is in the hospital. Late-onset infections are usually seen 6-8 days after surgery. Indicators include fever and a swollen, erythematous, and draining wound.

Cardiopulmonary: Tachycardia, hypotension, tachypnea, or syncope may be seen in the acutely ill patient when sepsis is present.

Fever: Temperature may be 101° F (38.3° C) or higher. With mild infection the patient may remain afebrile. Headache and overall "body aches" may accompany fever.

Chills: Patient may feel she cannot get warm even in the presence of an elevated temperature. Body shakes may accompany the chills. An overall flulike feeling may be present.

Malaise: A feeling of uneasiness, general discomfort, and fatigue may be present.

Pain: Pain may be present with light or deep external palpation of the abdomen or bimanual palpation of the uterus. Cervical motion tenderness on bimanual exam also may be present with a uterine infection. With an episiotomy infection, pain may be localized (throbbing, aching, or sharp) and deep tissue in nature. Some women complain of a sensation of vaginal pressure or "fullness."

Vaginal discharge: With an episiotomy infection, discharge may be purulent, and it may be foul smelling if endometritis (intrauterine infection) coexists with the infected episiotomy.

Abdominal surgical incision: In early-onset infection, the skin around the incision is erythematous and warm to the touch. In late-onset infection, the incision is swollen, may have a "woody" appearance, and appears erythematous. If the wound is not already open and draining bloody, serosanguineous, or purulent discharge, it may be probed with a cotton-tipped applicator to promote drainage. Dehiscence may or may not have occurred.

Episiotomy or perineal laceration: Localized edema, erythema, and exudate. Dehiscence of the episiotomy may or may not have occurred. Any episiotomy, whether infected or not, causes interruption of tissue integrity that can lead to stress incontinence, pelvic floor prolapse, anal incontinence, and pelvic floor muscle dysfunction.

Complications—neonatal: If the maternal infection is caused by an antepartum uterine infection (chorioamnionitis), the neonate is at increased risk for infection or sepsis and should be monitored carefully. When the infection appears within the first week of life and most likely within the first 48 hr of life, rapid deterioration and a high mortality rate are possible for the neonate.

Physical assessment: Not every patient with a wound infection looks or feels acutely ill. Some mild infections, such as cellulitis, respond well to early oral antibiotic coverage. Others will require IV antibiotic administration, wound débridement, or daily wound packing that allows the open incision to heal from the inside out via secondary intention (tissue granulation). In some instances, as in the case when there is a large blood clot behind the incision, reopening of the complete incision may be necessary, which then requires use of a wound vacuum device or secondary surgical closure using retention sutures and extended hospitalization.

Early assessment and treatment are critical in reducing maternal morbidity/mortality. Sepsis is rare but can occur.

Risk factors: Advanced maternal age, type 1 diabetes, low socioeconomic status, positive group B streptococci culture, malnutrition, obesity, anemia, prolonged preoperative hospitalization, extended duration of ruptured membranes before delivery, long labor, frequent vaginal examinations during labor, corticosteroid therapy, immunosuppressed state, duration of the surgery (cesarean section or postpartum tubal ligation), razor shaving the operative site, use of electrosurgical knife, use of open drains (e.g., Jackson Pratt, Penrose), closure technique (suture vs. staples), and emergency surgery (e.g., fetal distress).

DIAGNOSTIC TESTS

Complete blood count with differential: Leukocytes (white blood cells) will be elevated in the presence of an infection. The differential lists the five types of leukocytes, which all perform a special function. The type of leukocyte elevation will depend on the type of infection present (e.g., monocytes = severe infection by phagocytosis; lymphocytes = viral infections).

Blood cultures: During acute febrile illness, blood cultures identify the source of bacteria causing the infection, and sensitivity analysis determines the most effective antibiotic coverage.

Gram stain and culture of foul-smelling lochia: Helps in identifying clostridia, anaerobes, and *Chlamydia* and indicates the sensitivity analysis for the most effective antibiotic to use.

Urinalysis for microscopy: Detects presence of a urinary tract infection (UTI), which may be seen postoperatively after removal of an indwelling urinary catheter.

Pelvic ultrasound: Detects and locates possible abscesses and hematomas.

CT scan and MRI scan: In patients who do not respond to antibiotic coverage and have a negative ultrasound examination, this study can detect obscure pelvic abscesses and pelvic thrombi.

Nursing Diagnosis:

Impaired Skin Integrity

related to wound infection and/or dehiscence

Desired Outcome: Patient's wound heals within an acceptable time frame (2-3 wk).

INTERVENTIONS	RATIONALES
Teach patient how to monitor abdominal surgical site or episiotomy for suture integrity and signs and symptoms of infection.	A knowledgeable patient is likely to report infection indicators promptly. Prompt medical intervention reduces maternal morbidity and possibly hospitalization and length of treatment.
	- *Abdominal surgical site:* redness surrounding incision, abdomen warm to touch, drainage from incision, wound dehiscence (incision partially or fully open), and evisceration (protrusion of an organ, usually bowel, through open surgical wound).
	- *Episiotomy:* extreme pain in any position but especially sitting, foul vaginal odor in the absence of abdominal tenderness, drainage of pus, or dehiscence of sutures. Patient should use a mirror for self-examination or ask a family member to examine her perineum.
Assess patient's and significant other's level of acceptance/confidence in caring for the wound on an outpatient basis.	This evaluates their comfort level for home wound care. Subsequent teaching/reassurance, if need is determined, will provide an opportunity for patient to take control of her own care.
As needed, provide patient with a home nursing care referral.	This measure decreases stress when patient or family members are unable to care for the wound because of work commitments or uneasiness in self-management of a surgical wound. Home care also enables patient to be home and decreases medical costs.
Teach patient or significant other aseptic techniques in caring for the wound, such as thorough handwashing, wearing gloves (nonsterile acceptable), disposing of soiled dressings in plastic bags, maintaining a clean field for irrigation and packing, and alternatives to tapes for holding dressings in place. See Appendix A for "Infection Prevention and Control," p. 783, for more information.	These measures decrease risk of introducing additional microorganisms into the wound.
	Dressings with body fluids are considered hazardous waste.
	Tape can cause skin reactions and break down sensitive tissue.

Continued

INTERVENTIONS	RATIONALES
Encourage patient to eat a well-balanced diet that includes protein, carbohydrates, fruits, vegetables, and adequate fluid intake.	Adequate diet provides nutrients and a positive nitrogen state, which in turn promote wound healing. Adequate hydration also promotes wound healing.
Encourage patient to keep medical appointments.	Adherence to appointments enables evaluation of the wound's healing process and changes in care as needed.
Provide patient with abdominal support/binder after a cesarean section or bilateral tubal ligation.	This provides support and decreases stretching/tension on muscles/surrounding tissue of the wound to promote healing.

••• **Related NIC and NOC labels:** *NIC:* Incision Site Care; Perineal Care; Wound Irrigation; Wound Care; Skin Care: Topical Treatments; Nutrition Management; Infection Protection *NOC:* Tissue Integrity: Skin & Mucous Membranes

Nursing Diagnosis:

Deficient Knowledge:

Purpose for and potential side effects of prescribed medications used to treat wound infections

Desired Outcome: Immediately following teaching, patient and family verbalize accurate understanding of the risks and benefits of medications used in treating postpartum wound infections.

INTERVENTIONS	RATIONALES
Teach the following about patient's prescribed drugs:	A knowledgeable patient is more likely to adhere to the therapy, identify and report side effects, and recognize and report precautions that might preclude use of the prescribed drug.
Antimicrobials	These agents may be used as a perioperative prophylaxis, treating potential wound cellulitis/infection.
Cephalosporins: cefazolin (Ancef, Kefzol), cefoxitin (Mefoxin), cefotetan (Cefotan), cefoperazone (Cefobid), cephalexin (Keflex)	Administration: IV, PO, IM.
Teach patients who are breastfeeding that this drug will be present in low concentrations in breast milk.	Patients can breastfeed without it causing a problem to the infant.
Explain caution necessary for patients with sensitivity to penicillins.	Cross-sensitivity with penicillins is possible. Serious and possible fatal reactions can occur.
Teach importance of following complete course for all prescribed medications and taking them on time.	These measures reduce risk of reinfection, prevent development of antibiotic resistance, and maintain a constant level of medication in the bloodstream.
Teach patient to be alert for and report diarrhea, nausea, vomiting, stomach cramps, and anorexia.	These are possible side effects.
Advise patient to be alert for and report excessive and explosive diarrhea.	*Clostridium difficile* infection is a potentially serious side effect in which the normal flora of the bowel are reduced by antibiotic therapy and the anaerobic organism *C. difficile* multiplies and produces its toxins, causing severe diarrhea. This problem necessitates discontinuation of the antibiotic and laboratory evaluation of a stool sample.
Caution patient to be alert for a rash and pruritus.	These may be signs of an allergic reaction.
Penicillins: penicillin, amoxicillin, amoxicillin/clavulanate potassium (Augmentin), ampicillin-sulbactam (Unasyn)	Administration: IV/IM/PO.
	Breastfeeding: okay with amoxicillin.
Caution patient that the drug is not to be used if allergic to penicillins.	Serious and possible fatal reactions can occur.
Caution use in patients with a sensitivity to cephalosporins.	Possible cross-sensitivity can lead to serious and sometimes fatal reactions.

Continued

INTERVENTIONS	RATIONALES
Advise patient to follow complete course for all prescribed medications and take them on time.	These measures reduce risk of reinfection, prevent development of antibiotic resistance, and maintain a constant level of medication in the bloodstream.
Teach patient to be alert for and report nausea, indigestion, and vomiting.	These are possible side effects.
Teach patient to monitor for and report itching, rash, and shortness of breath.	These indicators may signal an allergic reaction.
Teach patient to be alert for and report excessive and explosive diarrhea.	See discussion of *C. difficile,* earlier.
Aminoglycosides: gentamicin (Garamycin)	Gentamicin is not administered during pregnancy because it crosses the placenta and can cause total irreversible bilateral congenital deafness.
	Administration: IM/IV.
	Breastfeeding: unknown.
Teach patient to be alert for and report lethargy, confusion, respiratory depression, visual disturbances, depression, weight loss, hypotension or hypertension, decreased appetite, rash, itching, headache, nausea, vomiting, and hearing loss.	These are potential adverse and allergic reactions.
Teach patient to be alert for and report excessive and explosive diarrhea.	See discussion of *C. difficile,* earlier.
Caution use in patients with neuromuscular disorders.	This drug may lead to neurotoxicity.
Caution use in patients with impaired renal function.	This drug may lead to nephrotoxicity.
Clindamycin (Cleocin)	Administration: IV/IM/PO.
	Breastfeeding: not recommended.
Teach patient to monitor for and report itching and rash.	These signs can occur with allergic reactions.
Teach patient to be alert for and report diarrhea, nausea, vomiting, stomach cramps, and anorexia.	These are possible adverse reactions.
Advise patient to follow complete course for all prescribed medications and take them on time.	These measures reduce risk of reinfection, prevent development of antibiotic resistance, and maintain a constant level of medication in the bloodstream.
Advise patient to be alert for and report excessive and explosive diarrhea.	See discussion of *C. difficile,* earlier.
Caution use in patients with a history of colitis.	This drug may exacerbate the colitis.
Teach patient to be alert for and report redness, swelling, and pain at IV insertion site.	Thrombophlebitis can occur after IV infusion of clindamycin.
Caution use in patients with renal disease.	The injectable drug is potentially nephrotoxic.
Linezolid (ZYVOX)	This antibiotic is used to treat complicated skin and skin structure infections caused by MRSA.
	Administration: IV, PO
Caution use in patients with hypertension.	This drug may increase preexisting hypertension.
Teach patients who are breastfeeding that caution should be used when taking this drug.	It is unknown whether linezolid is excreted in breast milk.
Teach patient to be alert for and report diarrhea, headache, nausea, vomiting, insomnia, constipation, rash, dizziness, and fever.	These are possible side effects.
Teach patient to be alert for and report cognitive dysfunction, hyperpyrexia, hyperreflexia, and incoordination.	Serotonin syndrome can be associated with the coadministration of ZYVOX and selective serotonin reuptake inhibitors.
Teach patient to be alert for, and immediately report visual blurring, changes in color vision, or loss of vision.	Peripheral and optic neuropathy may be associated with the drug when it is used beyond the recommended treatment (more than 28 days).
Teach patient to be alert for and immediately report repeated episodes of nausea and vomiting.	Lactic acidosis is a possible side effect.
Teach patient to be alert for and report excessive and explosive diarrhea.	See discussion of *C. difficile,* earlier.

Continued

INTERVENTIONS

INTERVENTIONS	RATIONALES
Teach patients to avoid ingesting excessive amounts of foods or beverages with high tyramine content while taking this drug.	Foods with greater than 100 mg of tyramine (e.g., red wine, aged cheese) may enhance the pressor response of this drug and increase blood pressure (BP).
Teach patient to avoid medications containing pseudophedrine HCL or phenylpropanolamine HCL.	The drug enhances the increases in systolic BP caused by pseudophedrine HCL or phenylpropanolamine HCL.

Analgesics

INTERVENTIONS	RATIONALES
Meperidine (Demerol)	This is an opioid analgesic used in the treatment of moderate-to-severe pain.
	Administration: IM/IV (poor oral absorption/efficacy).
	Breastfeeding: not recommended.
Teach patient to be alert for and report dry mouth, blurring vision, and dizziness.	These are side effects.
Teach patient to be alert for and report itching and rash.	These are signs of a possible allergic reaction.
Caution patient to be alert for and report weakness, headache, restlessness, agitation, hallucinations, and disorientation.	These are potential adverse reactions.
Advise patient to be alert for and report shortness of breath.	This is an adverse reaction that may indicate overdose.
Caution patient to arise slowly from a supine position or have assistance with ambulating after receiving this medication. Caution patient to avoid activities that require alertness until the drug's effect on the central nervous system (CNS) is known.	Meperidine is a CNS depressant. It may impair mental and/or physical abilities and cause hypotension. Drowsiness is a common side effect.
Caution use with other CNS depressants.	This drug can potentiate the CNS effects of other depressants.
Morphine	This opioid is used in the treatment of moderate-to-severe pain.
	Administration: IV/IM/PO.
	Breastfeeding: generally accepted as safe.
Teach patient to be alert for and report itching and rash.	These are possible allergic reactions.
Teach patient to be alert for and report weakness, headache, restlessness, agitation, hallucinations, and disorientation.	These are possible adverse reactions.
Teach patient to be alert for and report shortness of breath.	This is a possible adverse reaction that may indicate overdose.
Caution patient to arise slowly from a supine position or have assistance with ambulating after receiving this medication.	Morphine is a CNS depressant. It may impair mental and/or physical abilities and cause hypotension.
Caution patient to avoid activities that require alertness until the drug's effect on the CNS is known.	Drowsiness is a common side effect.
Caution use with other CNS depressants.	Morphine can potentiate CNS effects of these drugs.
Caution use in patients with seizure disorder.	Seizures may result from high doses.
Caution use in patients with renal/hepatic insufficiency.	Morphine's active metabolite may accumulate and potentiate the sedative effects.
Oxycodone with acetaminophen (Percocet) and hydrocodone with acetaminophen (Vicodin)	These are opioid analgesics used to treat moderate to moderately severe pain.
	Administration: oral.
Teach patient to be alert for and report itching, rash, nausea, and vomiting.	These are signs of a possible allergic reaction.
Teach patient to be alert for and report dizziness and headache.	These are common adverse reactions.
Teach patient to be alert for and report shortness of breath.	This adverse reaction may indicate overdose.
Caution patient to arise slowly from a supine position or have assistance with ambulating after taking this medication.	These drugs are CNS depressants. They may impair mental and/or physical abilities and cause hypotension.
Caution patient to avoid activities that require alertness until the drug's effect on the CNS is known.	Drowsiness is a common side effect.

Continued

INTERVENTIONS	RATIONALES
Anticoagulant	
Heparin	Heparin inhibits the reaction that leads to clotting of blood and formation of fibrin clots. It is used in treating septic pelvic thrombophlebitis.
	Administration: subcutaneous/IV. IM not recommended.
Teach patient to be alert for and report increase in vaginal bleeding (saturating one regular-size sanitary pad/hr and/or passing golf-ball–sized clots).	Hemorrhage can occur at any site in patients receiving heparin.
Caution patient about using aspirin or aspirin-containing products and nonsteroidal antiinflammatory drugs (NSAIDs; e.g., ibuprofen) or NSAID-containing products while taking heparin.	Aspirin and NSAIDs are platelet aggregation (clotting) inhibitors that can lead to increased bleeding.
Inform patient that bleeding and bruising at the site of injection is not unusual.	Heparin can lead to bleeding and bruising. The tendency for bleeding at the injection site will necessitate prolonged compression over injection site.
Teach patient to be alert for and report redness, pain, swelling, and firmness at injection site.	These are signs of local irritation that may indicate injection site cellulitis.
Advise patient to take a calcium supplement while receiving heparin.	Heparin affects bone density and may lead to osteoporosis.

••• **Related NIC and NOC labels:** *NIC:* Teaching: Prescribed Medication *NOC:* Knowledge: Medication

Nursing Diagnosis:

Deficient Knowledge:

Effects of postpartum wound infection (either abdominal or episiotomy) on self and neonate and the importance of following the treatment course

Desired Outcome: Immediately following teaching, patient and significant other verbalize accurate knowledge about the effects of postpartum wound infections on the patient and neonate and the treatment involved.

INTERVENTIONS	RATIONALES
Teach patient, significant other, and family about the effect a postpartum wound infection may have on the mother and neonate and the likely treatments for the infection.	Information helps patient adhere to treatments, report symptoms in a timely manner, and understand consequences of nonadherence. Effects an infection may have on the mother include pain, fever, chills, wound dehiscence, sepsis, and increased morbidity/mortality. For the neonate, effects include fever and possible rapid deterioration and increased morbidity/mortality. Likely treatments include IV antibiotics and fluids, wound packing, secondary wound closure, and possible lengthy hospitalization or home treatments.
Teach signs and symptoms of worsening wound infection.	A knowledgeable patient will be more likely to report these symptoms (increasing fever, foul-smelling vaginal discharge, spreading abdominal cellulitis, severe pain, vaginal bleeding, wound drainage) in a timely manner. Early evaluation and treatment result in decreased maternal morbidity.
Explain potential for complications with wound infections.	Explanation of potential complications (e.g., cellulitis, seroma, hematoma, dehiscence, secondary closure, necrotizing fasciitis, bacteremia, and disseminated intravascular coagulation) provides knowledge that optimally will promote adherence to the therapeutic regimen.
Explain treatment options such as daily wound packing or secondary wound closure and IV or PO antibiotics in treating the infection and decreasing risk for further infection.	Once the acute infection has been treated with antibiotics, the patient may be treated at home. If a secondary wound closure is done, it requires readmittance to the hospital (or an extended stay if the infection occurs before hospital discharge). Daily wound care consists of inspecting, irrigating, débridement, packing, and applying dressings. (See "Managing Wound Care," p. 559, for more information.)

Continued

INTERVENTIONS	RATIONALES
Explain to patient and partner that intercourse is not recommended during the process of wound healing, especially in the presence of wound dehiscence.	Usually intercourse is not recommended until 6 wk postpartum. This time frame allows the cervix to close, bleeding to stop, and incisions to heal without risk of introducing bacteria and potential risk for infection.

••• **Related NIC and NOC labels:** *NIC:* Teaching: Individual; Infection Control; Teaching: Procedure/ Treatment *NOC:* Knowledge: Illness Care

Nursing Diagnosis:

Ineffective Coping

related to needed adjustment in lifestyle to provide an optimal environment for wound healing or lack of support from family, friends, and community

Desired Outcome: Optimally within 24 hr of this diagnosis, patient modifies her lifestyle or behavior to promote wound healing.

INTERVENTIONS	RATIONALES
Assess patient's perceptions and ability to understand current health status.	Evaluation of patient's perceptions and comprehension enables development of an individualized care plan.
Establish empathetic communication with patient.	Honesty and empathy promote effective therapeutic communication. For example, "I know this is difficult to deal with while caring for a newborn. Tell me what I can do to help you."
Help patient identify previous methods of coping with life problems.	How patient has handled problems in the past may be a reliable predictor of how she will cope with current problems.
Help patient identify or develop a support system.	Many people benefit from outside support systems in helping them cope. Patient may need assistance with personal and homemaking tasks in order to modify her lifestyle so that wound healing can occur.
Arrange community referrals such as visiting nurse service, as appropriate.	Support in the home environment is likely to promote healthier adaptations.
Affirm that lifestyle adjustment (e.g., increased rest, dressing changes, frequent clinic visits, taking medications) is for a limited time.	This information facilitates acceptance of outside support and assistance while reinforcing understanding of the healing process of an infected wound.
Explain diagnostic tests (e.g., blood work to monitor for further infection, ultrasound to check for abscess) and procedures (e.g., wound packing, secondary wound closure).	Explanations of what to expect enable patient to initiate her coping mechanisms.

••• **Related NIC and NOC labels:** *NIC:* Coping Enhancement; Counseling; Support System Enhancement; Behavior Modification; Health Education *NOC:* Coping; Role Performance

ADDITIONAL NURSING DIAGNOSES/ PROBLEMS:

"Prolonged Bedrest" for relevant nursing diagnoses   p. 61

"Psychosocial Support" for nursing diagnoses such as **Anxiety**   p. 74

"Psychosocial Support for the Patient's Family and Significant Other" for such nursing diagnoses as:

Fear   p. 87

Interrupted Family Processes   p. 88

Compromised Family Coping   p. 89

"Managing Wound Care"   p. 559

"Preeclampsia" for:

Caregiver Role Strain   p. 717

Risk for Impaired Parent/Infant Attachment   p. 717

 PATIENT-FAMILY TEACHING AND DISCHARGE PLANNING

Wound infections place a great deal of strain on the patient and family dynamics. Any form of information or patient education that can be provided optimally will decrease the level of anxiety. Referral to a wound care specialist may be necessary at any time during the assessment/healing process. Include verbal and written information about the following:

✓ Signs and symptoms of a wound infection.

✓ Wound care (cleansing, packing, and dressing); instructions will vary depending on facility and provider preference. Check with health care provider for specific instructions. Also see care plans in "Managing Wound Care," p. 559.

✓ Importance of good handwashing.

✓ Where to obtain dressing materials for home care (prescriptions for supplies that may be acquired via a pharmacy or medical supply store).

✓ Importance of adequate rest, nutrition, and oral hydration for effective wound healing.

✓ Importance of compliance with prescribed health care regimen and ready access to hospital and family/social support.

✓ Medications, including drug name, purpose, dosage, frequency, precautions, potential drug reactions, and side effects. Also discuss potential drug-drug, food-drug, and herb-drug interactions.

✓ Referral to local and national support organizations, including Sidelines, a national support organization for women and their families experiencing complicated pregnancies, at *www.sidelines.org*

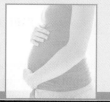

Preeclampsia 93

OVERVIEW/PATHOPHYSIOLOGY

Preeclampsia, characterized primarily by the onset of acute hypertension, is a multiorgan disease process with onset usually after 20 wk of gestation except in the case of gestational trophoblastic disease (includes hydatidiform mole and gestational trophoblastic tumors). Preeclampsia can affect the cardiovascular, neurologic, renal, hepatic, and hematologic systems. The cause is unknown, and clinical manifestations can be mild to severe, thereby affecting maternal/fetal morbidity and mortality. It complicates approximately 5%-7% of pregnancies (Wagner, 2004).

Blood pressure (BP) in mild preeclampsia is at least 140 mm Hg systolic or at least 90 mm Hg diastolic. Severe preeclampsia is defined as a BP of at least 160 mm Hg systolic or at least 110 mm Hg diastolic on at least two occasions 6 hr apart with the patient on bedrest (ACOG, 2002).

A pregnant woman with a blood pressure of 140/90 mm Hg or more before 20 weeks' gestation with none or a trace of protein in her urine is considered to have chronic hypertension. If the same woman develops proteinuria of 1+ or greater with increasing blood pressure, she is considered to have preeclampsia superimposed on her chronic hypertension.

A pregnant woman with a blood pressure of 140/90 mm Hg or more after 20 weeks' gestation and 1+ or greater proteinuria is considered to have preeclampsia. If there is no proteinuria or just a trace, she is considered to have gestational hypertension.

Individuals with severe preeclampsia may show evidence of HELLP syndrome (*h*emolysis of red blood cells, *e*levated *l*iver enzymes, and *l*ow *p*latelet count). HELLP syndrome may be present even in the absence of severe hypertension and is most common in Caucasian women. HELLP syndrome can occur at any time during the second and third trimesters.

Individuals with preexisting hypertension or chronic hypertension are at an increased risk of developing preeclampsia. Patients with preeclampsia whose blood pressure does not return to normal postpartum may then have chronic hypertension.

HEALTH CARE SETTING

Primary care, including obstetric or high-risk perinatal clinic, or acute care antepartum/intrapartum unit

ASSESSMENT

Preeclampsia is one of the most common medical complications in pregnancy. It may have a gradual or rapid onset depending on the organ system involved.

HELLP syndrome: Epigastric or right upper quadrant (RUQ) pain, nausea and vomiting, body aches, malaise, edema, and weight gain. Some of these symptoms overlap with preeclampsia; therefore laboratory values become the deciding diagnostic factor.

Cardiovascular: Normally during pregnancy, plasma volume and cardiac output increase approximately 40%. Blood pressure 140/90 mm Hg or higher on at least two occasions taken a minimum of 4 hr apart, along with proteinuria (see Renal), are diagnostic of preeclampsia.

Vasospasm is a major pathophysiologic change of this disease process, along with activation of the coagulation system and abnormal hemostasis, and plays a major role in end-organ effects. It results in increased peripheral vascular resistance with decreased perfusion to tissues and vital organs. Maternal signs and symptoms vary depending on which blood vessels are affected.

Neurologic: *Hyperreflexia* with or without clonus (abnormal pattern of rapidly alternating involuntary contraction and relaxation of skeletal muscle) reflects the effects of the disease on upper motor neurons and central nervous system (CNS). Although deep tendon reflexes (DTRs) may be increased before a seizure, seizures can occur without hyperreflexia.

Headaches, typically frontal or occipital and unrelieved by analgesics, usually are related to vasoconstriction, cerebral edema, or cerebral ischemia.

Other cerebral symptoms may include dizziness, drowsiness, and tinnitus.

Visual disturbances usually are described as flashing lights, "seeing spots," "floaters," blurring of vision, diplopia, or scotomata (an area of depressed vision within the visual field surrounded by an area of less depressed or of normal vision). Occasionally, blindness may result. These symptoms are the result of retinal arteriolar spasm, ischemia, and edema or, on rare occasion, retinal detachment.

Eclampsia: Presence of convulsions (seizures) or coma that is not related to other cerebral conditions and occurs in the presence of the signs and symptoms of preeclampsia. The seizures may occur antepartum, intrapartum, or postpartum (usually within 48 hr). Other associated symptoms are presence of 2+ or more proteinuria, headache, visual disturbances, and RUQ pain. The cause of seizure activity during preeclampsia is not known.

Renal: Sodium retention leads to nondependent edema of the face, hands, and lower extremities. Edema also may be caused by damage to the endothelial lining of the blood vessels, which enables fluid to leak into the interstitial space. Vasospasm and glomerular capillary endothelial swelling lead to a reduction in the glomerular filtration rate. Protein concentrations of 0.1 g/L in two random urine specimens collected 4 hr apart or 0.3 g in a 24-hr period are indicative of preeclampsia. Oliguria (urine output less than 500 ml in 24 hr) can be seen in severe preeclampsia.

Hepatic: Epigastric/RUQ pain may occur because of stretching of the hepatic capsule as a result of hepatic edema or hemorrhage. This causes feelings of indigestion or heartburn that are unrelieved with antacids. Nausea and vomiting may be seen.

Complications—fetal:

- *Intrauterine growth restriction (IUGR):* an abnormally restricted symmetric or asymmetric growth of the fetus.
- *Oligohydramnios:* abnormally low volume of amniotic fluid.
- *Risk of placental abruption:* premature separation of a normally situated placenta from the wall of the uterus.
- *Risk of preterm delivery (often iatrogenic):* delivery before 37 wk gestation.

Physical assessment:

- Rapid weight gain of 5 lb or more in 1 wk with generalized edema or edema of the face, hands, and lower extremities (edema need not be present to make the diagnosis of preeclampsia)
- Gradual or rapid increase in BP prenatally, antenatally, and postpartum
- Headache, mental confusion, hyperreflexia, epigastric pain (substernal that may radiate to the right side and back), nausea and vomiting, and shortness of breath
- Decreased fetal movement
- Oliguria (urine output less than 500 ml in 24 hr)
- Proteinuria

Risk factors: Nulliparity (status of a woman who has not given birth to a viable infant), African-American race, history of preeclampsia, renal disease, diabetes mellitus, age younger than 20 yr or older than 40 yr, family history of preeclampsia (mother/sister), chronic hypertension, thrombophilias (antiphospholipid syndrome, proteins C and S, antithrombin deficiency, factor V Leiden), multifetal pregnancy, oocyte donation or donor insemination, urinary tract infections, obesity, gestational trophoblastic disease (molar pregnancy) (Gabbe, 2002, Wagner, 2004).

DIAGNOSTIC TESTS

Complete blood count: May be within normal limits unless anemia is present or there is evidence of hemoconcentration in which the hematocrit (Hct) rises and the platelets drop. Thrombocytopenia may be evident.

Liver function tests: In mild preeclampsia, serum aspartate aminotransferase (AST; serum glutamic-oxaloacetic transaminase [SGOT]) and serum alanine aminotransferase (ALT; serum glutamic-pyruvic transaminase [SGPT]) are usually within normal limits or slightly elevated. In severe preeclampsia and HELLP syndrome, AST will be increased.

Coagulation studies: The most common hematologic abnormality in preeclampsia is thrombocytopenia (platelet count less than 150,000 mm^3). The degree to which platelets are decreased is indicative of disease severity and is dependent on coexistence of abruptio placentae. The platelet count, fibrinogen, prothrombin time, and partial thromboplastin time are usually normal in mild preeclampsia or begin to show a slight decline in values.

Urine/renal function studies: Proteinuria is present in preeclampsia with a minimum of 300 mg in a 24-hr urine analysis. Proteinuria, along with hypertension, is an indicator of fetal risk. In mild preeclampsia, blood urea nitrogen (BUN) and creatinine are usually within normal limits to slightly elevated. Uric acid is the most sensitive indicator and increases as the severity of preeclampsia increases. In severe preeclampsia with HELLP syndrome, the BUN and creatinine are significantly elevated.

Obstetric ultrasound: May be prescribed q2-3wk to follow fetal growth trend in a case of mild preeclampsia that is being monitored closely. IUGR can become evident with significant uteroplacental insufficiency caused by vasospasm.

Antepartum fetal monitoring: Weekly to twice weekly fetal nonstress testing is done to monitor fetal well-being. This also may include weekly amniotic fluid index checks and biophysical profiles.

Nursing Diagnosis:

Deficient Knowledge:

Effects of preeclampsia on patient, the pregnancy, and fetus

Desired Outcome: Immediately after teaching, patient and significant other verbalize accurate knowledge about the effects of preeclampsia on the patient, pregnancy, and fetus and adhere to the treatment accordingly.

INTERVENTIONS	RATIONALES
Inform patient and family/significant other about the effect preeclampsia may have on the pregnancy, mother, and fetus.	An informed patient is more likely to adhere to the prescribed therapy and understand the consequences of nonadherence. Examples of effects preeclampsia may have on the pregnancy, mother, and fetus include uteroplacental insufficiency (alteration in uteroplacental blood flow and oxygenation), IUGR (abnormally restricted symmetric or asymmetric growth of the fetus), oligohydramnios (abnormally low volume of amniotic fluid), preterm delivery (delivery before 37 wk gestation), and placental abruption (premature separation of a normally situated placenta from the wall of the uterus). Likely therapies include bedrest, taking medications, stopping work, frequent clinic visits, and possible lengthy hospitalizations.
Teach patient to lie on either her right or left side when on bedrest and avoid the supine position.	These positions increase uteroplacental blood flow and oxygenation to the fetus by eliminating compression of the maternal aorta by the enlarging uterus and fetus as would occur while in the supine position.
Teach daily fetal movement counts.	Fetal movement counts are a good first-line indicator of fetal well-being and are performed beginning at 28 wk gestation, as follows: Patient lies on her side and counts "distinct fetal movements" (hiccups do not count) daily; 10 movements within a 2-hr period is reassuring. After 10 movements are counted, the assessment is discontinued. Fewer than 10 movements indicates need for fetal nonstress testing.
Teach patient how to palpate contractions.	Palpation and awareness of contractions enable patient to be an active participant in her health care. Timely reporting of contractions to her health care provider can play a significant role in affecting outcome.
	To palpate contractions, the patient lies comfortably on her side. She spreads her fingers apart and places one hand on the left side and the other on the right side of her abdomen. She will palpate the abdomen using her fingertips. When the uterus is relaxed, the abdomen should feel soft. In the presence of a contraction, the uterus will feel hard, tight, or firm under her fingertips. She then times the duration of the contraction from the beginning of one contraction to the beginning of the next. Contractions will vary in frequency and duration. See "Preterm Labor," p. 719, if contractions occur at less than 35 wk gestation. Contractions in a patient with preexisting preeclampsia can raise maternal BP even higher and therefore require close monitoring. If the patient experiences 4-6 painful contractions over a 1-2-hr period, she needs to call her primary provider for evaluation.
	Duration of the contraction may or may not be an indication of contraction intensity. It is believed that the longer the contraction in true labor, the more effective it is in progressing dilation and effacement.
Teach signs and symptoms that indicate worsening preeclampsia.	Onset of preeclampsia may be slow with minimal symptoms or rapid with severe symptoms. A knowledgeable patient will likely report these symptoms promptly, including headache; visual changes such as blurred vision, spots, or flashing lights; epigastric/RUQ pain; nausea; vomiting; rapid weight gain (5 lb/wk or more); increasing edema (face, hands, feet); and decreased fetal movements (see above).

Continued

INTERVENTIONS	RATIONALES
Explain that urine and blood work will be evaluated on a daily basis, especially if patient is hospitalized.	Urine and blood analysis monitor for worsening preeclampsia or onset of HELLP syndrome. The following values are diagnostic:
	- Oliguria: 400 ml or less urine output in 24 hr
	- Urinary dipstick for protein: 3+ or more
	- Total urine protein: 5 g/24 hr or more
	- Hct: greater than 35%
	- Platelet count: less than 150,000/mm^3
	- Serum creatinine: 0.9 mg/dl or more
	- Serum uric acid: 6.6 mg/dl or more
	- Creatinine clearance: 100 ml/min or more
	- AST: more than 50 U/L
	- ALT: more than 50 U/L
	Platelets: The following classes are used to predict rapidity of recovery postpartum, maternal-perinatal outcome, and need for plasmapheresis.
	Class I platelets: less than 50,000/mm^3—Patient is at extreme risk for hemorrhage, is unable to receive regional anesthesia (e.g., epidural, spinal, caudal), and may require plasmapheresis.
	Class II platelets: 50,000-100,000/mm^3—Patient is at a moderately increased risk for hemorrhage and, at the anesthesiologist's discretion, may not be able to receive regional anesthesia.
	Class III platelets: 100,000-150,000/mm^3—Patient is at risk of increased postpartum bleeding but should be able to receive regional anesthesia.
With the diagnosis of severe preeclampsia (including HELLP syndrome), inform patient of the seriousness of the diagnosis and that conservative management (e.g., stopping work and home bedrest) is not usually effective.	Development of severe preeclampsia is an indication to proceed with delivery. Severe preeclampsia increases need for maternal blood transfusions and risk for renal failure, pulmonary edema, ascites (abnormal intraperitoneal accumulation of fluid), pleural effusions (abnormal accumulation of fluid in the intrapleural spaces of the lungs), hepatic rupture, placenta abruption, and disseminated intravascular coagulation (hypercoagulability followed by a deficiency in clotting). Explanation aids the family in understanding the possibility of an early delivery and mode of management.

••• **Related NIC and NOC labels:** *NIC:* Teaching: Individual; Teaching: Procedure/Treatment; High-Risk Pregnancy Care *NOC:* Knowledge: Illness Care; Knowledge: Pregnancy

Nursing Diagnosis:

Deficient Knowledge:

Purpose and potential side effects of prescribed medications

Desired Outcome: Immediately following teaching, patient and family verbalize accurate understanding of the risks and benefits of medications used during the pregnancy to aid in treatment of preeclampsia.

INTERVENTIONS	RATIONALES
Teach the following about patient's prescribed medications:	A knowledgeable patient is more likely to adhere to the therapeutic regimen, identify and report side effects, and recognize and report precautions that might preclude use of the prescribed drug.

Continued

INTERVENTIONS	RATIONALES
Magnesium Sulfate (MgSO₄)	This agent is used to decrease the CNS irritability seen with preeclampsia in preventing seizure activity. Therapeutic level is 4-8 mg/dl. It is used inpatient only.
	Administration: IV. It is never used with nifedipine because their combined use could lead to pulmonary edema.
Teach patient to be alert for and report headaches, hot flashes, nausea, vomiting, and dizziness.	These are common side effects.
Teach patient to be alert for and report shortness of breath, coughing, and lethargy.	Pulmonary edema is a serious side effect of this drug. For this reason, it is used with caution in patients who have received a large amount of IV fluid hydration.
Explain that BP, heart rate (HR), respiratory rate, deep tendon reflexes (DTRs), urinary output, and level of consciousness will be monitored at frequent intervals.	This drug has potentially serious side effects. Levels outside therapeutic range can cause toxicity:
	- Loss of DTRs: 9-12 mg/dl
	- Respiratory arrest: more than 15 mg/dl
	- Cardiac arrest: more than 25-30 mg/dl
Advise patient that use is contraindicated in maternal renal failure and hypocalcemia, and serum values of calcium will be monitored.	MgSO₄ is excreted via the kidneys; therefore increases in maternal serum magnesium may result in maternal hypocalcemia because magnesium opposes the action of calcium in the body.
Calcium Channel Blocker **Nifedipine (Procardia)**	This drug vasodilates and reduces peripheral resistance of the blood vessels without reducing cardiac output. Usually it is used to treat the chronic hypertension present before onset of preeclampsia. No adverse maternal/fetal side effects have been reported. It may be used outpatient.
	It is never used in combination with MgSO₄ because their combined use could lead to pulmonary edema.
	Administration: oral route.
Teach patient to be alert for and report lightheadedness and dizziness. Instruct patient to rise slowly from a supine position.	There is potential for hypotension with this drug.
Explain that patient may notice transient headaches and flushing for the first few days of taking this drug.	These are common side effects.
Advise that this drug is used with caution in patients with hepatic disease.	Nifedipine is primarily metabolized and excreted by the liver; therefore with hepatic disease these two processes may be delayed, causing an increase in serum nifedipine levels.
Beta-Blockers **Labetalol (Normodyne) and Atenolol (Tenormin)**	These drugs decrease blood pressure and maternal heart rate without significantly decreasing cardiac output. Usually they are used to treat chronic hypertension present before onset of preeclampsia.
	Administration: oral route. It may be given IV on an inpatient basis only.
Advise that patient may notice transient paresthesias or scalp tingling.	These are possible mild side effects seen at onset of treatment.
Teach patient to be alert for and report dizziness, fatigue, nausea, vomiting, and shortness of breath.	These are adverse reactions.
Caution patients with diabetes of need for vigilance regarding checking blood glucose levels when taking these drugs.	These drugs reduce the release of insulin in response to hyperglycemia.
Advise patients with bronchial asthma and systemic lupus erythematosus (SLE) of the need to use caution when taking these drugs.	These drugs may exacerbate symptoms of asthma and SLE.
Advise patients taking tricyclic antidepressants of the need to use caution when taking beta-blockers.	Beta-blockers may cause tremors when used along with tricyclic antidepressants.
Teach importance of serial ultrasounds to monitor fetal growth when taking this drug.	These drugs have been associated with fetal growth restriction.

Continued

INTERVENTIONS	RATIONALES
Antenatal Glucocorticoid **Betamethasone or dexamethasone**	Antenatal glucocorticoid aids in reducing effects of respiratory distress syndrome (RDS), intraventricular hemorrhage, and necrotizing enterocolitis on preterm neonate when preterm delivery is anticipated. These drugs also accelerate maturation of fetal organs, including cardiovascular, and the CNS. - Betamethasone: 2 doses of 12 mg given 24 hr apart. - Dexamethasone: 4 doses of 6 mg given 12 hr apart. They are usually administered when a preterm delivery is anticipated and after gestation of viability (25 wk). Maximum benefit is 48 hr after administration.
Explain that patients with diabetes need to monitor glucose levels and inform provider of abnormal levels: fasting greater than 90 mg/dl, 2 hr postprandial (pp) greater than 120 mg/dl, and at bedtime greater than 120 mg/dl.	A side effect of these drugs is impaired glucose tolerance. Women with borderline gestational diabetes may develop true gestational diabetes. A rise in blood glucose is usually seen for approximately 48-96 hr after administration, and it may require IV insulin.
Aspirin **Low-dose aspirin (81 mg)**	During pregnancy aspirin decreases platelet aggregation and increases vasodilation. It is given to women with autoimmune disease to prevent fetal wastage. Its use as a preventive measure for preeclampsia is controversial. Administration: oral.
Teach patient to be alert for and report nausea, vomiting, and epigastric pain.	These are possible side effects. However, they are also symptoms of worsening preeclampsia.
Advise of the need for caution in patients with a history of gastrointestinal (GI) ulcers.	Aspirin may cause GI bleeding.

••• **Related NIC and NOC labels:** *NIC:* Teaching: Prescribed Medication *NOC:* Knowledge: Medication

Nursing Diagnosis:

Ineffective Coping

related to needed adjustment in lifestyle to provide an optimal outcome for the pregnancy and fetus or lack of support from family, friends, and community

Desired Outcome: Within 24 hr of this diagnosis, patient modifies her lifestyle or behavior to provide the best pregnancy outcome for both herself and the fetus.

INTERVENTIONS	RATIONALES
Assess patient's perceptions and ability to understand current health status.	Evaluation of patient's comprehension and perceptions enables development of an individualized care plan.
Help patient identify support systems (e.g., family members, neighbors, church members, coworkers). Observe their interaction with the patient.	Understanding strengths and weaknesses of patient's support systems will aid in planning patient's overall care; eliciting support from available and positive support systems optimally will help reduce patient's stress and facilitate coping.
Affirm that lifestyle adjustments (e.g., bedrest and cessation of work, cooking, cleaning, shopping), while austere, are for a limited time.	This information likely will facilitate acceptance of outside support and assistance and reconfirms for patient that activities could increase her blood pressure, as well as risk of maternal/fetal morbidity and mortality.
Provide patient with referral sources for support groups, written material, Internet chat groups, or home help if patient is on home bedrest or hospitalization is required. Involve Social Services in the care of patient if indicated.	Talking with others who have experienced similar circumstances may aid in developing coping mechanisms.

••• **Related NIC and NOC labels:** *NIC:* Coping Enhancement; Support Group Enhancement *NOC:* Coping

Nursing Diagnosis:

Caregiver Role Strain

related to care the significant other, family member, or support person needs to provide not only to the patient but also possibly to other children in order for the patient to remain compliant and thereby prolong the gestational period

Desired Outcome: Within 24 hr of this diagnosis, caregiver verbalizes concerns/frustrations about caregiving responsibilities, identifies at least one other support person, and recognizes at least one change that would make his or her job easier.

INTERVENTIONS	RATIONALES
Encourage caregiver to relate feelings and concerns regarding added responsibilities. Help caregiver clarify responsibilities with patient and other family members.	This validates caregiver's concerns and helps him or her understand if expectations are realistic.
Encourage caregiver to identify which activities would benefit from outside assistance.	This confirms caregiver's need to seek help and facilitates that help.
Involve Social Services in support of the caregiver establishing a plan for time-outs or for referrals to community support groups.	This also confirms need to seek help and provides caregiver with coping mechanisms. During times of stress, caregivers may know they need help but may not know where to find it.

••• **Related NIC and NOC labels:** *NIC:* Caregiver Support; Respite Care; Coping Enhancement *NOC:* Caregiver Well-Being

Nursing Diagnosis:

Risk for Impaired Parent/Infant Attachment

related to disruption for bonding or interactive process secondary to maternal/fetal health risks

Desired Outcome: Within 24 hr of this diagnosis, patient and family members verbalize their concerns regarding the parental bonding process and barriers present and participate in care of mother and infant when possible.

INTERVENTIONS	RATIONALES
Encourage patient and family to verbalize feelings and concerns regarding the labor, delivery, and postpartum experience and the effect it will have on parental bonding.	This provides an opportunity for reassessment, confirmation, and validation of patient's/family's feelings and concerns.
If the infant is in the neonatal intensive care unit (NICU) and the mother is unable to visit because of her medical condition, arrange for significant other or family to visit and provide her with updates on baby's condition and items such as photos and footprints.	These measures provide for one form of maternal bonding.
Encourage mother to speak with her infant's caregivers for updates.	This enables her to participate in care and well-being of her infant.
When possible, encourage mother to visit NICU as soon as possible.	This promotes the bonding process.
Assist mother with breast pumping.	This enables the bonding process and fetal nutrition.
If it is necessary for the infant to be transferred to another facility, provide opportunity for parents and family to see and touch the infant before transport.	This measure assists in the bonding process.

••• **Related NIC and NOC labels:** *NIC:* Attachment Promotion; Anticipatory Guidance; Breastfeeding Assistance; Family Involvement Promotion *NOC:* Parent-Infant Attachment

ADDITIONAL NURSING DIAGNOSES/ PROBLEMS:

"Prolonged Bedrest" as indicated   p. 61

"Psychosocial Support" for **Anxiety**   p. 74

"Psychosocial Support for the Patient's Family and Signifi-   p. 88
cant Other" for **Interrupted Family Processes**

✔ PATIENT-FAMILY TEACHING AND DISCHARGE PLANNING

Preeclampsia is a progressive disease in which monitoring for maternal and fetal changes is of critical importance. Include verbal and written information about the following:

✓ Signs and symptoms of worsening preeclampsia (headache, increased edema, oliguria, RUQ pain, decreased fetal movement, nausea, and vomiting) and importance of contacting health care provider promptly should they occur.

✓ Seizure precautions.

✓ Medications, including drug name, purpose, dosage, frequency, precautions, potential drug reactions, and side effects. Also discuss potential drug-drug, food-drug, and herb-drug interactions.

✓ Importance of adherence to the prescribed health care and ready access to hospital and family/social support.

✓ Parameters and guidelines for home bedrest.

✓ Measures that help with constipation, which occurs frequently in pregnancy and can be exacerbated with bedrest.

✓ Measures for coping with muscle pain, back pain, and muscle weakness that can be present with prolonged bedrest.

✓ Fetal movement counts.

✓ Referrals to national and local support agencies, including:

- Sidelines, a national support organization for women and their families experiencing complicated pregnancies, at *www.sidelines.org*
- SHARE, a national support group for parents who have experienced loss through miscarriage, stillbirth, or newborn death, at *www.nationalshareoffice.com*

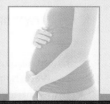

Preterm Labor 94

OVERVIEW/PATHOPHYSIOLOGY

Preterm labor (PTL) is labor occurring after 20 wk gestation and before completion of the 37th wk. Preterm labor leading to preterm delivery plays a major role in neonatal morbidity and mortality, although infants born at 34 wk gestation usually do fine, barring major preexisting medical complications. PTL is a major medical concern. Spontaneous labor involves a series of interactions among hormones, enzymes, and cells between the fetus and mother. It is unclear whether the mechanisms associated with labor in a term pregnancy are the same as those with PTL. Surviving preterm infants may suffer from neurodevelopmental handicaps, chronic respiratory disease, and long-term mental and physical impairment.

HEALTH CARE SETTING

Some patients may be managed via primary care on an outpatient basis with frequent clinic evaluation or in a high-risk perinatal clinic. Others may receive acute care in an inpatient antepartum setting.

ASSESSMENT

Symptoms may range from the obvious to subtle—from light menstrual-like cramping to strong, palpable contractions. There may be an increase in normal vaginal discharge, low dull backache to an intense aching that may radiate to the hips and down the thighs, and no bleeding to light pink vaginal spotting or bright red vaginal bleeding. The mother may feel that the baby is "balling up" in her abdomen and describe a "heavy" feeling in the perineum or pelvic pressure. Many symptoms of PTL do not cause pain, and it does not present in the same way as labor at term.

Contractions/uterine tightening: As the pregnancy progresses, so does the frequency of uterine activity. Uterine tightening/contractions begin in the first trimester as the uterus enlarges and continue throughout the pregnancy. These contractions are considered Braxton-Hicks and occur at irregular intervals, usually are painless, and do not change the cervix. PTL is diagnosed when uterine contractions are persistent and accompanied by cervical change, either dilation or effacement.

Backache: Although this is a very common complaint in pregnancy, any woman with a history of preterm labor/delivery who complains of new-onset backache needs to be evaluated for cervical changes, especially if she describes the backache as low lumbar/sacral in position, deep tissue in nature, or a dull aching sensation that radiates around the hips to the lower abdomen/pelvic area and down the thighs.

Pelvic pressure: May be described as "heaviness" or a sensation of "fullness," either constant or intermittent. The mother may state that she feels the "baby has dropped."

Abdominal cramping: Gastrointestinal (GI) symptoms such as increased flatus or diarrhea may be present. The abdomen may be tender to palpate, as is seen with chorioamnionitis (inflammatory reaction in the amniotic membranes caused by bacteria or virus).

Vaginal discharge: An increase in vaginal discharge is normal during pregnancy. It can be clear, thick, or thin and "milky white" or light yellow. It may become watery in nature as with preterm premature ruptured membranes (PPROM) or bloody as with placental abruption or when the cervix dilates and its surface vessels break. Vaginal itching or burning or a foul odor may indicate an infection.

Fever: Temperature may range from 98.6° F (37° C) to 101° F (38.3° C) or higher if an infection is present.

General complaints: Other symptoms may include a feeling of unease and body aches. The woman may state, "I just feel different."

Physical assessment: Even with vague symptoms, cervical changes may be taking place. Therefore it is important not to underestimate reported symptoms. Early evaluation and treatment are critical in attempting to stop PTL and preventing fetal morbidity and mortality.

Risk factors: Abdominal surgery during current pregnancy, chronic urinary tract infections (UTIs), polyhydramnios (excess amniotic fluid), poor weight gain after 20 wk, prepregnancy weight less than 100 lb, multiple gestation, previous preterm delivery, smoking, substance abuse, poor prenatal care, uterine/cervical anomalies, cervical incompetence, maternal infection, age younger than 18 or older than 35, history of cervical conization, low socioeconomic status, non-Caucasian, the patient herself was a preterm infant, strenuous work, previous second trimester abortion, uterine infections, abruptio placentae, psychologic stress, and domestic violence leading to physical or emotional abuse.

Complications—fetal:
- Preterm delivery
- Respiratory distress syndrome (RDS)

- Patent ductus arteriosus (PDA; an abnormal opening between the pulmonary artery and aorta)
- Intraventricular hemorrhage (IVH)
- Sepsis
- Necrotizing enterocolitis (ischemic, inflammatory bowel disorder that can lead to perforation and peritonitis)
- Hyperbilirubinemia
- Hypoglycemia
- Impaired/immature immunologic system
- Neonatal death

DIAGNOSTIC TESTS

Cervical evaluation: Digital cervical examinations are done to evaluate cervical dilation (centimeters [cm] dilated), effacement (percentage of thinning), consistency (e.g., soft, firm), and position (e.g., anterior vs. posterior position in the vaginal vault) to confirm the diagnosis of PTL. During a nonsterile speculum examination, cultures may be done to evaluate for the presence of *Chlamydia trachomatis*, herpes simplex virus, group B streptococci, *Gardnerella vaginalis*, and other anaerobes.

External uterine and fetal monitoring: External uterine monitoring is done to evaluate fetal well-being and the presence, frequency, and duration of uterine contractions. Abnormal fetal heart rate patterns (decreased variability, moderate-to-severe variable decelerations and late decelerations) are suggestive of fetal compromise, which uteroplacental insufficiency, umbilical cord compression, cord prolapse or infection can cause. This is an important diagnostic tool because some women are not aware of contractions when they are clearly documented on monitoring.

Urinalysis for microscopy: UTIs are associated with PTL. A clean-catch urine specimen should be obtained when attempting to rule out PTL, even when the patient is asymptomatic. When a UTI is present, antibiotic therapy will be initiated.

Sterile speculum examination to rule out rupture of membranes: This examination is not routinely done in patients with PTL; it is performed only if there is reason to suspect that membranes may have ruptured. A sterile speculum is inserted into the vagina to visualize leaking of amniotic fluid coming from the cervical os or observe pooling of amniotic fluid in the vagina. Vaginal fluid pH is tested with Nitrazine paper. A positive test is noted when the paper turns from yellow to blue (the pH is greater than 6.0). False-positive results can be seen in the presence of semen, blood, vaginal infections, or alkaline antiseptics. Vaginal fluid is examined under the microscope for the presence of a ferning pattern that amniotic fluid makes when it dries on a slide. A digital examination of the cervix is not recommended in a patient with suspected PPROM who is not in labor because of the risk of introducing an infection.

Ultrasound: Abdominal ultrasound is used to confirm gestational age, calculate amniotic fluid index and biophysical profile, rule out multiple gestation, and determine placental location and fetal presentation. Transvaginal or translabial ultrasound is used to evaluate cervical length, dilation, effacement, and the presence of funneling (see discussion in "Cervical Insufficiency") of the internal cervical os. The shorter the cervix, the greater the risk of PTL. The shortest acceptable cervical length is 3 cm. A cervical length of 2.5 cm or less is associated with increased PTL risk. Cervical length determination by ultrasound should not take the place of digital examinations.

Blood Rh factor and antibody screen: Some patients' first prenatal visit may be at the onset of preterm labor and will require this testing. See p. 674 for detailed information.

Fetal fibronectin enzyme immunoassay: Fetal fibronectin (fFN) is an extracellular matrix protein, a gluelike substance that is present between fetal membranes and the uterine decidua. It is usually seen after 37 wk gestation. Its presence between 22 and 37 wk may have a predictive value for pending PTL. It is obtained from secretions present in the posterior vaginal vault, but only if the amniotic membranes are intact, cervical dilation is less than 3 cm, and the gestational age is between 24 and 35 wk. This test is best used as a negative predictor. In other words, if fFN is not present between 22 and 37 wk gestation, chances are great the woman will not deliver prematurely. In symptomatic patients at less than 34 wk gestation, fFN showed 76%-98% sensitivity and 83%-88% specificity for PTD within 7 days of sample collection (Kim, 2000). The use of this test varies between providers and institutions.

Amniocentesis: To determine fetal lung maturity as a predictor for fetal RDS, as well as to check for chorioamnionitis.

Nursing Diagnosis:

Deficient Knowledge:

Effects of preterm labor on self and the fetus

Desired Outcome: Patient and significant other verbalize accurate knowledge about the effects of preterm labor on the patient, pregnancy, and fetus and adhere to the treatment accordingly.

INTERVENTIONS

INTERVENTIONS	RATIONALES
Inform patient and significant other about treatments for PTL and the effects preterm labor and delivery can have on the fetus.	Information about the effects preterm labor and delivery can have on the fetus (i.e., RDS, hypoglycemia, IVH, sepsis, necrotizing enterocolitis, hyperbilirubinemia, and neonatal death) is likely to promote adherence to the therapeutic regimen (e.g., bedrest, adequate hydration, decreasing activity, stopping work, frequent clinic visits, no intercourse, taking medications, possible lengthy hospitalizations).
Explain importance of access to a specialized facility.	Delivering a preterm infant at a facility with perinatal and neonatal specialists and neonatal intensive care unit (NICU) provides the greatest opportunity for infant survival.
Teach signs and symptoms of PTL to *all* pregnant women.	An informed patient likely will report these symptoms promptly. See introductory information for detailed signs and symptoms of preterm labor. Barring the presence of chorioamnionitis, the earlier PTL is diagnosed, the better the chance for prolonging the pregnancy and decreasing fetal morbidity and mortality.
Question patient at each prenatal visit, starting at the beginning of the second trimester, if she is experiencing any signs or symptoms of preterm labor/contractions.	Early recognition of PTL (see signs and symptoms in the introductory data) may lead to prolonging the gestational period and decreasing fetal morbidity and mortality.
Encourage patient to report even vague or subtle symptoms no matter the time of day or night. Provide written instructions and telephone numbers to call should concerns or changes arise.	Uterine contractions may be painless. Fewer than 50% of patients in PTL are aware of their contractions. Incidence of PTL is approximately 10%, and preterm birth accounts for almost 85% of all neonatal mortality not caused by congenital anomalies (Chin, 2001).
Teach daily fetal movement counts.	Fetal movement counts done twice a day are a good first-line indicator of fetal well-being and are performed as follows, beginning at 28 wk gestation: Patient lies on her side and counts "distinct fetal movements" (hiccups do not count); 10 movements within a 2-hr period is considered reassuring. After 10 movements are discerned, the count is discontinued. Fewer than 10 movements in a 2-hr period signals need for fetal nonstress testing.
Teach patient how to palpate contractions.	Timely reporting of preterm contractions to her health care provider can play a significant role in affecting outcome. Palpation and awareness of contractions enable patient to be an active participant in her health care.
	To palpate contractions, the patient lies comfortably on her side. She spreads her fingers apart and places one hand on the left side and the other on the right side of her abdomen. She will palpate the abdomen using her fingertips. When the uterus is relaxed, the abdomen should feel soft.
	In the presence of a contraction, the uterus should feel hard, tight, or firm under her fingertips. She then times the duration of the contraction from the beginning of one contraction to the beginning of the next. Contractions will vary in frequency and duration. If the patient experiences 4-6 contractions for 1-2 hr, she needs to call her primary provider. Contractions may be mild to severe in intensity and difficult for a gravida I (first pregnancy) mother to discern as PTL.
Instruct patient to drink at least six 8-oz glasses of water per day (48-64 fluid oz).	The uterus is a muscle and will respond to dehydration by cramping/contracting. Adequate oral hydration is a preventative measure for PTL.
Teach patient and her partner the effect that sexual foreplay or intercourse may have on PTL. Advise patient to avoid all forms of sexual stimulation.	This information promotes patient/partner understanding and adherence. Sexual intercourse may increase uterine contractions and promote cervical change. Increased uterine activity also may be caused by breast stimulation, female orgasm, and prostaglandin in male ejaculate.

••• **Related NIC and NOC labels:** *NIC:* Teaching: Individual; Teaching: Disease Process; High-Risk Pregnancy Care *NOC:* Knowledge: Medication; Knowledge: Pregnancy

Nursing Diagnosis:

Deficient Knowledge:

Purpose and potential side effects of prescribed medications

Desired Outcome: Immediately following teaching, patient and family relate accurate understanding of the risks and benefits of medications used during the pregnancy to aid in managing PTL.

INTERVENTIONS	RATIONALES
Teach patient and family the following about prescribed fluids and medications:	A knowledgeable patient is more likely to adhere to therapy, identify and report side effects, and recognize and report precautions that might preclude use of the prescribed drug.
Intravenous Fluid Hydration Type of IV fluids varies among providers.	In the dehydrated patient, IV fluids may be useful in treating PTL. They have not been shown to be beneficial in treating the hydrated patient.
Caution is necessary when used with tocolytic drugs.	IV fluid overload can lead to pulmonary edema when used with tocolytic drugs. A tocolytic drug is any agent used to suppress PTL. Examples include indomethacin (Indocin), magnesium sulfate ($MgSO_4$), nifedipine (Procardia), and terbutaline (Brethine).
Prostaglandin Synthesis Inhibitor **Ibuprofen**	Ibuprofen inhibits prostaglandin synthesis, thereby decreasing myometrial contractility (contractions).
	Administration: Oral.
Be alert for and report nausea and vomiting, heartburn, diarrhea, constipation, and abdominal cramps.	These are common side effects. If these symptoms persist, the medication may need to be changed, dose adjusted, or discontinued.
Avoid use of this drug after 34-35 wk.	This drug can decrease amniotic fluid volume (oligohydramnios) and prevent closure of PDA (an abnormal opening between the pulmonary artery and aorta).
Caution is necessary for patients with GI ulcers and renal disease.	Ibuprofen may cause gastric bleeding, fluid retention, and renal toxicity.
Take these drugs with food.	This will decrease GI side effects.
Avoid use if taking warfarin or heparin.	Ibuprofen increases risk of bleeding.
Indomethacin (Short-Term Use Only)	Indomethacin inhibits prostaglandin synthesis, thereby decreasing myometrial contractility (contractions). It is used as a second- or third-line agent for tocolysis (an agent that suppresses uterine contractions).
	Pregnancy: safety unknown or controversial.
	Not used for more than 48 hr.
	Administration: oral or rectal suppository.
Be alert for and report nausea and vomiting, drowsiness, dizziness, depression, psychosis, and headaches.	These are possible maternal side effects. If these symptoms occur, the medication should be discontinued.
Take this medication with food.	This will decrease GI symptoms.
Avoid taking this drug after 34-35 wk.	This drug can decrease amniotic fluid volume (oligohydramnios) and prevent closure of PDA (an abnormal opening between the pulmonary artery and aorta).
Avoid this drug if also taking warfarin or heparin.	This drug may increase risk of bleeding.
Caution is necessary in patients with asthma.	This drug may exacerbate asthmatic symptoms.
Caution is necessary in patients with renal disease.	This drug may cause renal toxicity.
Calcium Channel Blocker **Nifedipine**	Nifedipine inhibits smooth muscle contractility, thus decreasing or eliminating uterine contractions. It may be used outpatient.
	Administration: oral route.
	No adverse maternal/fetal effects have been reported.
	It is never used with $MgSO_4$ because their combined use could lead to pulmonary edema.

Continued

INTERVENTIONS	RATIONALES
Patient may notice transient headaches and flushing for the first 24-72 hr of taking this drug.	These are common side effects; symptoms resolve after this time.
Rise slowly from a supine position.	There is potential for hypotension (especially in a normotensive woman).
Be alert for and report nausea, flushing, and nervousness.	These are common side effects. If these symptoms persist, the dose of the medication may need to be changed or dose adjusted.
Caution is necessary for patients with hepatic disease.	Nifedipine is primarily metabolized and excreted by the liver; therefore with hepatic disease these two processes may be delayed, causing an increase in serum nifedipine levels.
Caution is necessary for patients taking cimetidine (Tagamet).	Cimetidine causes increase in peak nifedipine plasma levels (higher drug concentration).
Beta-Adrenergic Agonist	This drug decreases uterine myometrial activity (contractions).
Terbutaline (Brethine)	Administration: IM, subcutaneous, PO.
Be alert for and report rapid heart rate, restlessness, agitation, nausea, and vomiting.	These are common side effects. If these symptoms persist, the dose of the medication may need to be changed or discontinued.
Be alert for and report shortness of breath.	There is potential for pulmonary edema, which is the most common maternal side effect and can occur between 30 and 60 hr after IV administration of the first dose.
Rise slowly from a supine position.	There is potential for hypotension with this drug.
This drug is contraindicated with maternal cardiac dysrhythmias, diabetes mellitus, maternal cardiac disease, uncontrolled hypertension, and thyrotoxicosis (Graves' disease/hyperthyroidism).	Significant cardiac side effects are seen in patients without cardiac disease who take this drug.
Magnesium Sulfate (MgSO₄)	$MgSO_4$ decreases uterine myometrial activity (contractions) at a therapeutic serum magnesium level of 4-8 mg/dl.
	Administration: IV infusion.
	Used on an inpatient basis only.
	It is never used with nifedipine because their combined use could lead to pulmonary edema.
Be alert for and report headaches, hot flashes, nausea, vomiting, and dizziness.	These are common side effects.
Be alert for and report shortness of breath, coughing, and lethargy.	Pulmonary edema is a serious side effect that can occur in patients taking this drug who have received large amounts of IV fluid hydration.
Blood pressure, heart rate, respiratory rate, deep tendon reflexes (DTRs), and urinary output will be monitored at frequent intervals.	This drug has potentially serious side effects. Levels outside therapeutic range can cause toxicity: - Loss of DTRs: 9-12 mg/dl - Respiratory arrest: 15 mg/dl - Cardiac arrest: 25-30 mg/dl
Use is contraindicated with maternal renal failure and hypocalcemia.	$MgSO_4$ is excreted via the kidneys; increases in maternal serum magnesium can result in maternal hypocalcemia because magnesium opposes the action of calcium in the body.
Antenatal Glucocorticoid **Betamethasone or dexamethasone**	These drugs aid in reducing the effects of RDS, IVH, and necrotizing enterocolitis on the preterm neonate. They also accelerate the maturation of the central nervous system and fetal organs, including cardiovascular. They are usually administered when a preterm delivery is anticipated after the gestation of viability. Maximum benefit is 48 hr after administration. - Betamethasone: 2 doses of 12 mg given 24 hr apart. - Dexamethasone: 4 doses of 6 mg given 12 hr apart.

Continued

INTERVENTIONS	RATIONALES
Be alert for and report signs of infection (elevated temperature, chills, body aches) and elevated maternal glucose levels.	Possible side effects of this medication are reduced maternal/fetal resistance to infection, impaired glucose tolerance (people with borderline gestational diabetes may develop true gestational diabetes), and suppression of maternal or neonatal adrenal function. Usually a rise in blood glucose is seen for approximately 48-96 hr after administration, and it may require IV insulin. Individuals with diabetes need to monitor glucose levels closely and inform provider of abnormal levels (fasting more than 90 mg/dl, 2-hr postprandial more than 120 mg/dl, and at bedtime more than 120 mg/dl) and decrease in fetal movement.

••• **Related NIC and NOC labels:** *NIC:* Teaching: Prescribed Medication *NOC:* Knowledge: Medication

Nursing Diagnosis:

Ineffective Coping

related to adjustment in lifestyle to provide an optimal environment for the fetus or lack of support from family, friends, and community

Desired Outcome: Within the 24-hr period after this diagnosis is made, patient verbalizes feelings and identifies strengths and coping behaviors to provide the best pregnancy outcome for herself and fetus.

INTERVENTIONS	RATIONALES
Assess patient's perceptions and ability to understand current health status regarding PTL.	Evaluation of patient's perceptions and comprehension enables development of an individualized care plan.
Provide referral sources for support groups, written material, Internet chat groups, or home help if patient is on home bedrest or hospitalization. Involve Social Services in care of patient as needed.	Communicating with or learning about others who have experienced similar circumstances may aid in the development of positive coping mechanisms.
Help patient identify or develop a support system.	Having a support system will aid in patient's overall care and reduction of stress to promote positive coping behaviors.
Arrange community referrals as appropriate or at the request of the patient.	Support in the home environment promotes healthier adaptations and may avert crises.
Offer realistic hope for continuing the pregnancy to a safe gestation. Help patient and family develop realistic expectations for the future if a preterm delivery occurs and to identify support persons or systems that will assist them with planning for the future.	These measures foster realistic expectations about a preterm neonate's health status (in the absence of congenital anomalies) and promotes adaptation to possible changes in family dynamics.
Teach patient and family that hospitalization and medical interventions in preventing a preterm birth may not always be effective or wise.	Medications, bedrest, and hydration are not always successful in stopping PTL. In some instances an early delivery may be in the best interest of the mother, fetus, or both, as would be the case in the presence of infection, nonreassuring fetal heart rate tracings, severe oligohydramnios (abnormally low amount of amniotic fluid), anhydramnios (no amniotic fluid), and congenital anomalies.
Affirm that lifestyle adjustment (e.g., no work, bedrest, no intercourse) is for a limited time.	This information facilitates acceptance of outside support and assistance and reinforces knowledge that routine or increased activity with PTL may increase risk of cervical change and possible preterm delivery.

••• **Related NIC and NOC labels:** *NIC:* Coping Enhancement; Anxiety Reduction; Counseling; Emotional Support; Support System Enhancement; Family Involvement Enhancement *NOC:* Coping; Social Support

Nursing Diagnosis:

Caregiver Role Strain

related to the care significant other, family member, or support person needs to provide not only to the patient but also possibly to other family members in order for patient to remain compliant and prolong the gestational period

Desired Outcome: Within 24 hr from this diagnosis, caregiver verbalizes concerns/frustrations about caregiving responsibilities, identifies at least one other support person, and recognizes at least one change that would make his or her job easier.

INTERVENTIONS	RATIONALES
Encourage caregiver and patient to relate their feelings and concerns regarding their roles.	This validates concerns and helps them understand if expectations are realistic.
Acknowledge caregiver's role in patient care; identify and praise strengths.	This reinforces positive ways of dealing with current health crisis and promotes a sense of involvement and appreciation.
Involve Social Services in support of the caregiver in helping establish a plan for time-outs.	Social Services can provide caregiver with a weekly viable goal and coping mechanisms and validate need to seek help.
Provide patient and caregiver with status reports on effectiveness of patient's bedrest, decreased activity, stopping work, or inability to participate in routine household activities.	Reassuring patient and caregiver that the support and assistance are positively affecting patient's health likely will promote more of the same.
Affirm that this is for a limited time.	This information facilitates patient's and caregiver's acceptance in receiving and giving support and assistance.
Encourage diversional activities (e.g., time alone away from home or hospital and other children) and interaction with support persons or systems outside the family.	Promoting respite enhances coping and assists family members in remaining focused and supportive of patient. For example, "I know this must be a difficult time and you want to stay with your wife, but I will call you if any changes occur."

••• **Related NIC and NOC labels:** *NIC:* Caregiver Support; Coping Enhancement; Respite Care; Family Involvement Promotion; Support System Enhancement *NOC:* Caregiver Lifestyle Disruption; Caregiver Well-Being

Nursing Diagnosis:

Constipation

related to decreased peristalsis secondary to immobility, stress, lack of exercise, and prolonged bedrest

Desired Outcome: Patient has normal bowel movements and minimal discomfort from gas and hard stooling within 2-3 days of interventions, thereby reducing the risk of preterm contractions.

INTERVENTIONS	RATIONALES
Identify patient's normal bowel status and whether she requires laxatives or stool softeners on a routine basis.	This assessment identifies if constipation is playing a role in PTL. Constipation is a normal symptom of pregnancy because the descending colon vies for space with the uterus as it enlarges and because progesterone, one of the hormones produced in pregnancy, decreases gastric motility. However, in a patient prone to PTL who is on bedrest, constipation can be exacerbated because of the decrease in peristalsis associated with inactivity.
Explain effects of constipation in a patient prone to PTL.	Constipation or gastric irritability can increase uterine irritability in the form of contractions. This would increase risk of PTL.
Encourage daily intake of at least 8-10 glasses of water/day and increasing dietary fiber or adding a fiber laxative or stool softener to her daily regimen.	These measures provide bulk and aid in keeping the stool soft to promote evacuation.

••• **Related NIC and NOC labels:** *NIC:* Constipation Management; Fluid Management *NOC:* Bowel Elimination; Hydration; Symptom Control

Nursing Diagnosis:

Risk for Impaired Parent/Infant Attachment

related to disruption for bonding or interactive process secondary to maternal/fetal health risks

Desired Outcome: Patient and family members verbalize their concerns regarding the parental bonding process and barriers present and participate in the care of both mother and infant when possible.

INTERVENTIONS	RATIONALES
Encourage mother and family to take a guided tour of the NICU (time permitting) if a preterm delivery is expected or necessary.	A guided tour decreases fear of the unknown and facilitates questions and answers.
Encourage patient and family to verbalize feelings and concerns regarding the labor, delivery, and postpartum experience.	This provides for an opportunity of reassessment, confirmation, and/or validation of their concerns and feelings.
When possible, encourage mother to visit baby in NICU as soon as possible after the delivery. Provide the mother with written information on care provided in the NICU.	These measures promote the bonding process, encourage communication with baby's care providers, and provide an opportunity to have questions answered.
Encourage mother to breastfeed or express milk for later feeding of the infant.	In the preterm infant, it is not always possible or recommended to feed at the breast. However, either method promotes psychologic benefits for the mother by involving her in the infant's daily care and reinforcing importance her breast milk has to the health of her infant.
Explain benefits of breast milk for the preterm infant.	For the preterm infant, breast milk decreases incidences of infectious complications and metabolic disturbances. Maternal antibodies in breast milk also promote immunologic health inasmuch as the infant's immune system is immature.
	Infants fed breast milk will gain the same weight at the same rate as if they were fed formula. Breast milk also helps establish nonpathogenic bacterial flora in the newborn intestinal tract and stimulates passage of stool.

Continued

INTERVENTIONS	RATIONALES
If the mother chooses to breastfeed by expressing milk for later infant feeding, assist her with breast pump operation and arrange for rental of a breast pump for home use as needed.	A breast pump aids in producing/sustaining breast milk for later infant feeding.
If it is necessary for the infant to be transferred to another facility, provide the opportunity for parents and family to see and touch the infant before transport.	This measure assists in the bonding process. Some facilities transport the mother along with the preterm infant.

••• **Related NIC and NOC labels:** *NIC:* Attachment Promotion; Environmental Management: Attachment Process; Breastfeeding; Assistance Infant Care; Family Involvement Promotion *NOC:* Parent-Infant Attachment

Nursing Diagnosis:

Ineffective Breastfeeding

related to interruption in the normal process resulting from a premature and/or ill infant

Desired Outcome: Patient produces breast milk using a breast pump or makes an informed decision regarding which method of feeding most benefits the infant's needs and her own emotional/physical state of well-being.

INTERVENTIONS	RATIONALES
Encourage mother to verbalize her concerns.	This validates her concerns and evaluates possible obstacles preventing her from producing adequate milk supply.
Teach patient the physical process of lactation after birth.	This information assists in decreasing her anxiety about "not having enough milk" and helps her understand the importance of breast stimulation via actual breastfeeding or pumping.
	Delivery of the placenta causes a fall in progesterone and a rise in prolactin, the hormone that stimulates lactogenesis (milk production). Prolactin is released from the anterior pituitary gland during breastfeeding, which in turn stimulates milk production. Oxytocin is released from the posterior pituitary gland at the same time and causes the milk ejection reflex, or milk "let down." During the course of breastfeeding, these hormones are released and regulated on a supply and demand basis.
Provide support to the mother through lactation specialists available within the hospital or as outside consultants.	Lactation instructors assist the mother in proper use of a breast pump or in actual infant breastfeeding, positioning the infant for comfort and ease of nursing, and use of various breast shields as needed and teach how to manage engorgement, inverted or flat nipples, milk supply problems, plugged ducts, sore nipples, and infant sucking problems.
Teach use of a breast pump and manual expression, storage, and transport of milk.	These measures aid in the success of producing milk and the safety of its storage.
Teach importance of adequate oral hydration, nutrition, and rest.	Adequate maternal caloric intake, oral hydration, and rest help meet the periods of increased demand for breast milk during infant's growth spurts and maintain a consistent supply of breast milk.
See **Risk for Impaired Parent/Infant Attachment** for other interventions and details.	

••• **Related NIC and NOC labels:** *NIC:* Breastfeeding Assistance; Lactation Counseling; Fluid Management; Nutritional Counseling *NOC:* Breastfeeding Establishment: Maternal

ADDITIONAL NURSING DIAGNOSES/ PROBLEMS:

"Psychosocial Support" for relevant nursing diagnoses such as:

Disturbed Sleep Pattern	p. 73
Anxiety	p. 74
Fear	p. 76
Spiritual Distress	p. 78
Anticipatory Grieving/Risk for Dysfunctional Grieving	p. 79
Disturbed Body Image	p. 80
Social Isolation	p. 84

"Psychosocial Support for the Patient's Family and Significant Other" for such nursing diagnoses as:

Interrupted Family Process	p. 88
Compromised Family Coping	p. 89

PATIENT-FAMILY TEACHING AND DISCHARGE PLANNING

Preterm labor and birth can have lifelong effects on the child and family. Early diagnosis and treatment are imperative. Educating each patient about signs and symptoms of PTL should be a part of every woman's prenatal care. Include verbal and written information about the following:

✓ Potential risk factors for PTL that may be present early in prenatal care.

✓ Signs and symptoms of PTL.

✓ Palpation of contractions.

✓ Promptly reporting any signs of UTI.

✓ Importance of adequate oral hydration during the pregnancy.

✓ Importance of compliance with routine prenatal care.

✓ Medications, including drug name, purpose, dosage, frequency, precautions, potential drug reactions, and potential side effects. Also discuss potential drug-drug, food-drug, and herb-drug interactions.

✓ Measures that help with constipation, which occurs frequently in pregnancy and can be exacerbated with bedrest.

✓ Measures for coping with muscle pain, back pain, and muscle weakness that can be present with prolonged bedrest.

✓ Fetal movement counts.

✓ Referral to local and national support organizations, including:

- Sidelines, a national support organization for women and their families experiencing complicated pregnancies, at *www.sidelines.org*
- SHARE, a national support group for parents who have experienced loss through miscarriage, stillbirth, or newborn death, at *www.nationalshareoffice.com*
- La Leche League at *www.lalecheleague.org*

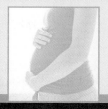

Preterm Premature Rupture of Membranes 95

PATHOPHYSIOLOGY

Preterm premature rupture of membranes (PPROM) is the leakage of amniotic fluid before the 37th week of gestation. The balance of amniotic fluid is maintained by the production of fetal lung fluid and urine and is reabsorbed by fetal swallowing. The fetal lungs secrete approximately 300-400 ml/day at term. Fetal urine is the main source of amniotic fluid, with an output averaging 400-1200 ml/day at term. Amniotic fluid volume at term has a wide range from approximately 500-1500 ml. Amniotic fluid provides an environment that protects the fetus from trauma and injury, provides even distribution of temperature, and enables a medium in which the fetus can move. It also plays a major role in fetal development of the lungs and kidneys. Although its cause is unknown, PPROM plays a major role in the morbidity and mortality of the neonate, depending on gestational age. The risk for a preterm birth is high. The majority of patients with PPROM deliver from within 24 hr to 2 wk of onset.

HEALTH CARE SETTING

The woman may be evaluated in the health care provider's clinic and then managed by obstetricians or perinatologists as an outpatient or inpatient, depending on week of gestation. Hospital sites may vary depending on gestational age and ability of the hospital to provide care for a high-risk pregnancy and neonate. Some patients with PPROM before gestational viability (25 weeks) may be managed at home.

ASSESSMENT

Patients may have difficulty determining presence of ruptured membranes, and symptoms may be obvious or subtle. Some women liken the sensation of leaking amniotic fluid to that of leaking urine. Therein lies the difficulty in determining PPROM from subjective data alone and the necessity of hands-on evaluation. On some occasions, leakage of amniotic fluid may stop, or it may reaccumulate without signs of infection.

Vaginal discharge: Patients may experience a "sudden gush" or sensation that something "popped" followed by a constant slow leakage of clear, watery fluid from the vagina. The fluid may be blood-tinged or meconium-stained. Patient may state that her underwear is wet or that she needs to wear a sanitary pad. Vaginal bleeding may accompany PPROM and range from light pink spotting to bleeding as with a heavy menses.

Backache: May or may not be present with PPROM. In the presence of infection, the patient may complain of a low lumbar/sacral pain that is deep tissue in nature or a dull, aching sensation that may radiate around the hips to the lower abdomen/pelvic area. If abruptio placentae is present with PPROM, the back pain may be mild to severe.

Abdominal pain/cramping or uterine cramping contractions: There may be a feeling of pelvic pressure or fullness or menstrual-like cramping or contractions. Some women state that their thighs ache when experiencing uterine cramping. In the presence of infection, the patient may complain of abdominal/uterine tenderness or pain. If abruptio placentae accompanies PPROM, the pain may be mild to severe.

Fever: May occur in the presence of an infection and temperature may be 101° F (38.3° C) or higher.

Complications—fetal: The risk to the fetus depends on the gestational age at the time of PPROM, the severity of PPROM (the amount of amniotic fluid remaining, if any), and the presence of infection.

- Prematurity
- Fetal infections/sepsis
- Hypoxia and asphyxia caused by umbilical cord compression/prolapse
- Fetal deformities with PPROM at an early gestational age (i.e., hypoplastic lungs)
- Amniotic band syndrome (an abnormal condition characterized by development of fibrous bands within the uterus that entangle the fetus, leading to deformities in fetal structure and function)
- Abruptio placentae
- Fetal death

Physical assessment: In most cases, the cause of PPROM is unknown and there is no forewarning. Therefore it is important to evaluate changes in vaginal discharge. A timely diagnosis of PPROM is critical to optimum fetal outcome.

Risk factors: Genital tract infections such as *Chlamydia trachomatis*, gonorrhea, bacterial vaginosis, or trichomoniasis; low socioeconomic status; smoking; multiple gestation; incompetent cervix (painless cervical dilation before term without contractions); previous history of PPROM; diethylstilbestrol (DES) exposure; amniocentesis; chorionic villi sampling (CVS); coitus; group B streptococci; poor nutrition; bleeding in pregnancy; polyhydramnios (excess of amniotic fluid); cervical cerclage (a suture used for holding the cervix closed during a pregnancy); previous cervical laceration or surgery; placental abruption (abnormal separation of the placenta from the wall of the uterus before delivery); chorioamnionitis (intraamniotic infection); history of midtrimester pregnancy loss; cocaine use; hypertension; diabetes; and Ehlers-Danlos syndrome (a group of heritable connective tissue diseases).

DIAGNOSTIC TESTS

Sterile speculum examination: A sterile speculum is inserted into the vagina to visualize leaking of amniotic fluid coming from the cervical os or pooling of amniotic fluid in the vagina. This fluid is tested with Nitrazine paper. If positive for amniotic fluid, the paper will turn from yellow to dark blue, and the pH will be greater than 6.0. False-positive results may be seen in the presence of semen, blood, vaginal infections, or alkaline antiseptics. Using a cotton swab, a sample of vaginal fluid is taken from the posterior vaginal fornix (the posterior space below the cervix) and examined under the microscope for the presence of a ferning pattern that amniotic fluid makes when it dries on a slide. A digital examination of the cervix is not recommended in a patient with suspected PPROM who is not in labor to avoid the risk of introducing an infection.

External uterine and fetal monitoring: External uterine monitoring is done to evaluate fetal well-being and presence,

frequency, and duration of uterine contractions. Abnormal fetal heart rate patterns (decreased variability, moderate-to-severe variable decelerations, and late decelerations) are suggestive of fetal compromise, which can be caused by umbilical cord compression, cord prolapse, or infection that can accompany PPROM.

Obstetric ultrasound: Abdominal ultrasound is used to confirm gestational age, calculate amniotic fluid index (AFI) and biophysical profile (BPP), rule out multiple gestation, and determine placental location and fetal presentation. A normal value for the AFI is between 10 and 20 ml of amniotic fluid. A normal rating on the BPP is 6-8 out of 10.

Amniocentesis: Transabdominal aspiration of remaining amniotic fluid to test for fetal lung maturity and the presence of chorioamnionitis.

Intrauterine dye test: Done only if other tests are inconclusive in determining PPROM or to document that the membranes have sealed over. Resealing is rare, but it can occur. Under ultrasound guidance a diluted solution of indigo carmine dye is inserted with a spinal needle transabdominally into the uterus. The patient is observed for passage of blue fluid from the vagina that would indicate rupture of membranes.

Blood Rh factor and antibody screen: This test should be a part of the routine prenatal screening. In patients with no prenatal care who have PPROM, this laboratory test needs to be performed on admittance to determine need for Rh-immune globulin in an Rh-negative patient.

Nursing Diagnosis:

Deficient Knowledge:

Signs and symptoms of PPROM, its effects on the pregnancy and fetus, and guidelines to follow for an optimal outcome

Desired Outcome: Immediately following teaching, patient and significant other verbalize accurate knowledge about the effects of PPROM on the patient and fetus, as well as its signs and symptoms and treatment guidelines for an optimal outcome.

INTERVENTIONS	RATIONALES
Teach patient and significant other signs and symptoms of PPROM and chorioamnionitis (intraamniotic infection), which may be present after PPROM.	A knowledgeable patient likely will report symptoms promptly and understand consequences of nonadherence. PPROM plays a major factor in the morbidity and mortality of the neonate, depending on gestational age. See introductory information for signs and symptoms of PPROM. Indicators of chorioamnionitis include abdominal pain, uterine tenderness, fever, chills, foul vaginal odor, and contractions.
Inform patient and significant other about the effects PPROM can have on patient and fetus.	Information facilitates adherence to the treatment regimen. Amniotic fluid is critical to fetal development. PPROM increases risk of preterm delivery and neonatal pulmonary hypoplasia. PPROM also increases risk of chorioamnionitis (see above symptoms) for the mother and subsequently poses a postpartum risk of endometritis (inflammation of the endometrial lining of the uterus) following delivery. Maternal death from sepsis is rare, but it can occur.

Continued

INTERVENTIONS	RATIONALES
Discuss risks/benefits of conservative management (delaying delivery and monitoring mother for signs of infection and fetus for signs of distress) vs. active delivery with the possibility of a preterm infant with respiratory distress syndrome (RDS), infection, and neonatal death but enabling ability to monitor and support baby more safely in an extrauterine environment.	When there are no signs of maternal infection or cervical change and the intrauterine environment is safe for both mother and fetus, conservative management may buy time for fetal lung maturation. In the presence of a uterine infection, however, labor should not be stopped. Treating the mother postpartum and the fetus in an extrauterine environment improves maternal/fetal well-being.
Teach daily fetal movement counts.	Fetal movement counts are a good first-line indicator of fetal well-being and are performed as follows, beginning at 28 weeks' gestation: Patient lies on her side and counts "distinct fetal movement" (hiccups do not count) daily; 10 movements within a 2-hr period is reassuring. After 10 movements, the count is discontinued. Fewer than 10 movements indicates need for fetal nonstress testing.
Teach patient palpation of contractions, which may accompany PPROM (gestation appropriate).	A knowledgeable patient likely will report an increase in contractions promptly: for a singleton pregnancy, 4 contractions/hr or more; for a multiple pregnancy, 6 contractions/hr or more. Palpation and awareness of contractions enable patient to be an active participant in her health care. Timely reporting of contractions can play a significant role in optimum maternal/fetal outcome. Although contraction frequency alone is insufficient in diagnosing preterm labor, it can serve as a helpful guideline.
	Patient lies comfortably on her side. She will spread her fingers apart and place one hand on the left side and the other on the right side of the abdomen. Palpation is done with the fingertips of both hands. When the uterus is relaxed, the abdomen should feel soft. When a contraction occurs, the uterus will feel hard, tight, or firm under the fingertips. She will time the duration from the beginning of one contraction to the beginning of the next. Duration of the contraction may or may not be an indication of contraction intensity. It is believed that the longer the contraction in true labor, the more effective it is in progressing dilation and effacement.

••• **Related NIC and NOC labels:** *NIC:* Teaching: Disease Process; Teaching: Individual; High-Risk Pregnancy Care; Prenatal Care
NOC: Knowledge: Illness Care; Knowledge: Pregnancy

Nursing Diagnosis:

Ineffective Coping

related to health crisis, sense of vulnerability, inadequate support systems, and needed adjustment in lifestyle to provide an optimal environment for the fetus and prolong the gestational period

Desired Outcome: Within 24 hr of this diagnosis, patient verbalizes feelings, identifies strengths, exhibits positive coping behaviors, and modifies her lifestyle to provide the best pregnancy outcome for her fetus.

INTERVENTIONS	RATIONALES
Assess patient's perceptions and ability to understand current health status of herself and fetus.	Evaluation of patient's comprehension enables development of an individualized care plan.
Help patient identify previous methods of coping with life problems.	How patient has handled problems in the past may be a reliable predictor of how she will cope with current problems.
Provide patient with resources for support groups, written information, Internet chat groups, or home helpers.	Talking with others who have experienced similar circumstances may aid in development of coping mechanisms. A home helper, for example, likely will decrease pressure on patient and thereby promote coping abilities.

Continued

INTERVENTIONS	RATIONALES
Affirm that lifestyle adjustments and need for support systems will be necessary only for a limited time.	This knowledge may facilitate acceptance of outside support and assistance and facilitate coping accordingly.
Acknowledge patient's cultural beliefs regarding coping during pregnancy.	This shows respect for the patient and a willingness to understand and work with her emotional state and coping skills. You might ask, "In your home country a high-risk pregnancy must be very difficult to deal with. Could you tell me how you and your family are coping with this pregnancy?"
	Different cultures perceive pregnancy in various ways. Some patients come from countries in which maternal/fetal mortality rate is high and daily survival is the major focus. Their method of coping may be emotional detachment from the fetus. The current pregnancy may not seem as important as the children and family that are already at home and need care. In the Hmong culture, for example, women and their families do not appear to bond with their infant after birth. They believe to do so would be prideful and welcome evil spirits who would take the infant away (infant death).
Involve assistance of Social Services when available.	Social Services provides counseling and makes recommendations for referrals.
Provide patient and family with information regarding effectiveness of hospitalization bedrest vs. home bedrest.	This information helps patient and her health care provider decide the best method of management. Before gestation of viability (25 wk), when fetal survival rates are lower, home management of bedrest in the absence of signs of maternal/fetal infection may be assumed. Patients undergoing home bedrest must be able to remain in bed in alternating side-lying positions (occasionally sitting up propped with pillows) and avoid doing housework, laundry, cooking, or shopping. The side-lying position improves uteroplacental blood flow and oxygenation, which in turn improves the chance of reaccumulation of amniotic fluid. After gestation of viability, hospitalization is usually recommended to monitor for signs of maternal/fetal infection, fetal distress, preterm labor, and worsening oligohydramnios (abnormally low volume of amniotic fluid) or anhydramnios (absence of amniotic fluid).
	Both home management and hospitalization may require outside assistance to care for family members or pets at home.
Encourage patient and family to verbalize their concerns in a supportive environment.	This will help alleviate stress, anxiety, and misconceptions. See **Anxiety,** p. 74.

••• **Related NIC and NOC labels:** *NIC:* Coping Enhancement; Counseling; Support Group; Support System Enhancement; Family Involvement Promotion *NOC:* Coping; Role Performance

Nursing Diagnosis:

Deficient Knowledge:

Purpose and potential side effects of prescribed medications for managing PPROM

Desired Outcome: Immediately following teaching, patient and family relate accurate understanding of the risks and benefits of medications used to manage PPROM.

INTERVENTIONS	RATIONALES
Teach the following about patient's prescribed medications:	A knowledgeable patient is more likely to adhere to therapy, identify and report side effects, and recognize and report precautions that might preclude use of the prescribed drug.

Antenatal Glucocorticoids

Betamethasone or dexamethasone

These drugs aid in reducing effects of RDS, intraventricular hemorrhage, and necrotizing enterocolitis on preterm neonate when delivery is anticipated to be preterm and after the gestation of viability. They also accelerate maturation of the central nervous system (CNS) and fetal organs, including cardiovascular.

- Betamethasone: two doses of 12 mg given 24 hr apart.
- Dexamethasone: four doses of 6 mg given 12 hr apart.
- Maximum benefit is 48 hr after administration.

Be alert and report signs of infection (elevated fever, chills, body aches), decrease in fetal movement (gestation appropriate), and elevated maternal glucose levels in patients with diabetes.

Possible side effects of medication include reduced maternal-fetal resistance to infection, impaired glucose tolerance (people with borderline gestational diabetes may develop true gestational diabetes), and suppression of maternal or neonatal adrenal function. Usually a rise in blood glucose is seen for approximately 48-96 hr after administration, and it may necessitate IV insulin.

Prophylactic Antibiotics

The type of antibiotic used varies and may include but is not limited to the following: ampicillin, erythromycin, gentamicin, and cephalosporins.

Prophylactic antibiotics prevent or reduce effects of maternal-fetal infections and may reduce morbidity and prolong the pregnancy.

Caution patient to follow complete course for all prescribed medications and take them on time.

These measures prevent development of antibiotic resistance and maintain a constant level of medication in the bloodstream.

Teach patient to be alert for and report excessive and explosive diarrhea.

Clostridium difficile is a potentially serious side effect in which the normal flora of the bowel are reduced by antibiotic therapy and the anaerobic organism *C. difficile* multiplies and produces its toxins, causing severe diarrhea. This problem necessitates discontinuation of the antibiotic and laboratory evaluation of a stool sample.

Magnesium Sulfate (MgSO$_4$)

This agent decreases uterine myometrial activity (contractions) at a therapeutic serum magnesium level of 4-8 mg/dl. It is used inpatient only.

Administration: IV. It is never used with nifedipine because their combined use could lead to pulmonary edema.

Teach patient to be alert for and report headaches, hot flashes, nausea, vomiting, and dizziness.

These are common side effects.

Explain that this drug is used with caution in patients who have received large amounts of IV fluid hydration. Patient should be alert for and report shortness of breath, coughing, and lethargy.

Pulmonary edema is a serious side effect.

Advise patient that blood pressure (BP), heart rate (HR), respiratory rate (RR), deep tendon reflexes (DTRs), and urinary output will be monitored at frequent intervals.

Levels outside the therapeutic range of this drug can cause toxicity

- Loss of DTRs: 9-12 mg/dl
- Respiratory arrest: more than 15 mg/dl
- Cardiac arrest: more than 25-30 mg/dl

Caution patient that use is contraindicated in maternal renal failure and hypocalcemia.

MgSO$_4$ is excreted via the kidneys; therefore increases in maternal serum magnesium may result in maternal hypocalcemia.

Continued

INTERVENTIONS	RATIONALES
Calcium Channel Blocker	
Nifedipine	This drug inhibits smooth muscle contractility, thereby decreasing or eliminating uterine contractions.
	No adverse maternal/fetal side effects have been reported.
	Administration: oral route
	It may be used on an outpatient basis. It is never to be used with MgSO$_4$ because their combined use could lead to pulmonary edema.
Teach patient to be alert for and report lightheadedness and dizziness. Instruct patient to rise slowly from a supine position.	There is potential for hypotension with this drug.
Explain that patient may notice transient headaches and flushing for the first few days of taking this drug.	These are common side effects.
Caution patients with hepatic disease about using this drug.	Nifedipine is primarily metabolized and excreted by the liver; therefore with hepatic disease these two processes may be delayed, causing an increase in serum nifedipine levels.
β-Adrenergic Agonist	
Terbutaline (Brethine)	This drug decreases uterine myometrial activity (contraction). With PPROM it is used only on a short-term basis (24-26 wk) to allow for the antenatal glucocorticoids (earlier) and antibiotics to become effective.
	Administration: subcutaneous, IM, PO.
	It may be used on an outpatient basis.
Teach patient to be alert for increased heart rate, restlessness, nervousness, tremor (shaking hands), nausea, and vomiting.	These are common side effects. They are usually transient in nature and do not require intervention.
Teach patient to be alert for and report shortness of breath and chest pain.	These indicators may signal pulmonary edema and myocardial ischemia, conditions that would warrant discontinuation of the medication.
Advise patient to rise slowly from a supine position.	There is potential for hypotension.
Explain that the drug is contraindicated in patients with maternal cardiac dysrhythmias, diabetes mellitus, and maternal cardiac disease.	The drug has significant cardiac side effects in patients without cardiac disease and can increase maternal blood sugar.
Rh-Immune Globulin (human)	
RhoGAM	This agent prevents hemolytic disease as long as the mother has not already been sensitized by the presence of Rh-positive antibodies in her bloodstream.
	Administration: IM only to nonsensitized Rh-negative women after bleeding any time during the pregnancy, after spontaneous abortion, or after delivery. Recommended administration is within 72 hr after the bleeding episode.
Advise that patient may note discomfort at the site of injection.	This is a common side effect.

••• **Related NIC and NOC labels:** *NIC:* Teaching: Prescribed Medication *NOC:* Knowledge: Medication

Nursing Diagnosis:

Deficient Knowledge:

Muscle weakness, back pain, and decreased circulation that can occur with prolonged bedrest

Desired Outcome: Within 24 hr of this diagnosis, patient verbalizes understanding of and demonstrates measures to reduce or relieve back pain and improve circulation.

INTERVENTIONS	RATIONALES
Teach patient to recognize signs and symptoms of back pain related to bedrest vs. back pain associated with contraction activity.	A knowledgeable patient optimally will discern the different causes of back pain and report these symptoms accordingly. Back pain related to bedrest is usually thoracic to lumbar in location and superficial in nature and will be improved by position change or massage to promote circulation. Back pain related to contraction activity is usually lumbar/sacral in position and deep tissue in nature, and it may radiate to the hips and low abdominal/pelvic area. Position change and massage may decrease intensity.
Teach patient the probable causes of muscle pain, weakness, and back pain.	This information aids in patient understanding and optimally in adherence to therapeutic management. For example, probable causes include lack of use of certain muscles, delay in change of positioning, increasing weight of the uterus, and dehydration, which can lead to the buildup of lactic acid in the muscles and cause pain.
Teach patient leg exercises for period in which she is on bedrest.	Leg exercises promote peripheral tissue perfusion and decrease risk of deep vein thrombosis (DVT) and muscle wasting. Calf-pumping (ankle dorsiflexion–plantar flexion) and ankle-circling exercises are examples of leg exercises. Patient should repeat each movement 10 times, performing each exercise hourly during extended periods of immobility, provided patient is free of symptoms of DVT. Passive and active range-of-motion (ROM) exercises are other options.
Encourage patient to change positions frequently in bed, from alternating side-lying positions to sitting propped up with pillows. Teach patient to use pillows between knees to prevent pressure on the back.	Changing position at frequent intervals (i.e., q2h) promotes circulation and decreases pressure and hence discomfort on tissues, joints, and muscles. Pillows provide support and decrease strain on muscles and promote comfort.
Caution patient to *avoid* the supine position.	The supine position places pressure on the aorta by the enlarging fetus. This could result in a vasovagal response, which would decrease maternal blood pressure and cause diaphoresis, nausea, dizziness, and decreased uteroplacental perfusion.
Provide patient with referral for physical or massage therapy for back pain related to prolonged bedrest.	Professional interventions likely will aid in promoting circulation and patient comfort.

••• **Related NIC and NOC labels:** *NIC:* Teaching: Individual; Teaching: Disease Process; High-Risk Pregnancy Care *NOC:* Knowledge: Disease Process; Knowledge: Pregnancy

Nursing Diagnosis:

Anticipatory Grieving

related to potential fetal loss secondary to PPROM

Desired Outcome: Patient and significant other verbalize their feelings and identify and use support systems to aid them in the grief process within 24 hr of this diagnosis.

INTERVENTIONS	RATIONALES
Encourage patient and significant other to verbalize their feelings and concerns regarding the potential for loss of their baby.	This measure validates concerns and conveys message that grief is a normal and expected reaction to the potential loss of a baby.
Assess and accept patient's behavioral response.	Disbelief, denial, guilt, anger, and depression are normal reactions to grief.
Teach patient the stages of grief and explain that there is no specific time frame in which to go through the process.	This information enables patient to understand where she or her family members may be in the grief process. Stages include (1) shock and numbness; (2) denial and searching-yearning; (3) anger, guilt, and sense of failure; (4) depression and disorganization; and (5) resolution.

Continued

INTERVENTIONS	RATIONALES
Clarify misconceptions about the potential risk for fetal loss with PPROM.	This allows patient and significant other to process the information regarding PPROM appropriately while not providing false hope. The gestational age at which the PPROM occurs plays a significant role in the outcome. The earlier the gestational age at delivery, the higher the risk of fetal loss. A gestational age of 25 wk is considered viable, but with each passing day and week, there is better opportunity for fetal survival and decreased morbidity barring preexisting fetal complications such as cardiac, respiratory, and CNS problems.
If available, involve Social Services when a loss is perceived or present.	Social Services provides resources and referrals for individual counseling and support groups for bereaved parents and grandparents, which may help the participants feel less isolated. Social Services also can guide the family through the disposition of the infant should the death occur.
If a loss occurs, provide patient and family with support if they decide to see and hold the baby and place appropriate items in a memory/keepsake box.	These measures assist with the grieving process by enabling parents/grandparents to spend time with and affirm their baby. Such items as footprints and a lock of hair may be tucked away and not looked at right away, but it may help to know they are there.

••• **Related NIC and NOC labels:** *NIC:* Coping Enhancement; Grief Work Facilitation: Perinatal Death; Anxiety Reduction; Emotional Support; Family Support; Support Group Enhancement; Hope Instillation *NOC:* Coping; Family Coping; Grief Resolution

ADDITIONAL NURSING DIAGNOSES/ PROBLEMS:

"Prolonged Bedrest" for such nursing diagnoses as **Constipation**

"Psychosocial Support" for such nursing diagnoses as:	p. 67
Disturbed Sleep Pattern	p. 73
Anxiety	p. 74
Fear	p. 76
Ineffective Coping	p. 76
Anticipatory Grieving/Risk for Dysfunctional Grieving	p. 79
Spiritual Distress	p. 78
Social Isolation	p. 84
"Psychosocial Support for the Patient's Family and Significant Other" for such nursing diagnoses as:	
Interrupted Family Processes	p. 88
Compromised Family Coping	p. 89

✔ PATIENT-FAMILY TEACHING AND DISCHARGE PLANNING

PPROM is potentially life threatening to the fetus, depending on gestational age at the time of occurrence. When reviewing the symptoms of PPROM and the importance of patient adhering to the therapeutic regimen with the hope of decreasing fetal morbidity and mortality, include verbal and written information about the following:

✓ Signs and symptoms of ruptured membranes and the importance of contacting health care provider in a timely manner.

✓ Signs and symptoms of preterm labor (see p. 719) because it may precede or follow PPROM.

✓ Palpation of contractions.

✓ Importance of adherence to prenatal care.

✓ Potential risk factors for PPROM that may be present early in the pregnancy.

✓ Measures for muscle pain, back pain, and muscle weakness that can be present with prolonged bedrest. See **Deficient Knowledge,** earlier.

✓ Measures that help with constipation, which occurs frequently in pregnancy and can be exacerbated with bedrest.

✓ Availability of Social Services and spiritual care.

✓ Medications, including drug name, purpose, dosage, frequency, precautions, and potential side effects. Also discuss potential drug-drug, food-drug, and herb-drug interactions.

✓ Fetal movement counts.

✓ Referral to local and national support organizations, including:

• Sidelines, a national support organization for women and their families experiencing complicated pregnancies, at *www.sidelines.org*

• SHARE, a national support group for parents who have experienced loss through miscarriage, stillbirth, or newborn death, at *www.nationalshareoffice.com*

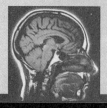

Anxiety Disorders 96

OVERVIEW/PATHOPHYSIOLOGY

Anxiety is a diffuse response to a vague threat, as opposed to fear, which is an acute response to a clear-cut external threat. Anxiety often precedes significant changes, for example, beginning new employment. When it is prolonged or excessive, crippling physical or psychologic symptoms may develop. The anxiety disorders are a group of conditions characterized by anxiety symptoms and behavioral efforts to avoid these symptoms. They are the most common psychiatric disorders in the United States, affecting more than 23 million people. Acute anxiety creates physical sensations of arousal (fight or flight), an emotional state of panic, decreased cognitive problem-solving ability, and altered spiritual state with hopelessness and/or helplessness. Anxiety is considered abnormal when reasons for it are not evident or when manifestations are excessive in intensity and duration. Psychologic *stress* refers to the response of an individual appraising the environment and concluding that it exceeds his or her resources and jeopardizes well-being. Some stressors are universal, whereas others are person specific because of highly individual interpretations of events.

Anxiety is always part of the stress response and has four levels, ranging from mild to panic. Normally, a person experiencing mild-to-moderate anxiety uses voluntary behaviors called *coping skills*, that is, distraction, deliberate avoidance, and information seeking. Another common response is use of unconscious defense mechanisms, including repression, suppression, projection, introjection, reaction formation, undoing, displacement, denial, and regression. If stress continues at an unbearable level or if the individual lacks sufficient biologic mechanisms for coping, an anxiety disorder may develop. There are eight major categories:

Generalized anxiety disorder: Characterized by excessive, uncontrollable worrying over a period of at least 6 months. Symptoms include motor tension (trembling; shakiness; muscle tension, aches, soreness; easy fatigue), autonomic hyperactivity (shortness of breath, palpitations, sweating, dry mouth, dizziness, nausea, diarrhea, frequent urination), and scanning behavior (feeling on edge, having an exaggerated startle response, difficulty concentrating, sleep disturbance, irritability).

Panic disorder: Characterized by a specific period of intense fear or discomfort with at least four of the following symptoms: palpitations or pounding heart, sweating, trembling or shaking, sensations of smothering or difficulty breathing, feeling of choking, chest pain, nausea, feeling dizzy or faint, feeling of unreality or losing control, numbness, and chills or flushes.

Phobias: Characterized by a persistent and severe fear of a clearly identifiable object or situation despite awareness that the fear is unreasonable. There are two types, specific and social. Specific phobias are subdivided into five types: animals, natural environment (e.g., lightning), blood-injection-injury type, situational (e.g., flying), and other (situations that could lead to choking or contracting an illness). Social phobia relates to profound fear of social or performance situations in which embarrassment could occur.

Obsessive-compulsive disorder (OCD): Characterized by a preoccupation with recurrent, ritualistic thoughts or actions. Obsessions are persistent thoughts, ideas, impulses, or images that are intrusive and cause marked anxiety. Compulsions are repetitive acts that follow an obsession, are performed according to strict rules, and are aimed at decreasing the feeling of distress/anxiety caused by the obsessions.

Posttraumatic stress disorder: Results from a pathologic response to a devastating event such as war, natural disaster, or rape. The person continues to reexperience the event through intrusive thoughts or nightmares. Memories of the trauma occur randomly, or symptoms may emerge when the person is exposed to situations that resemble or symbolize the original trauma. Fear and persistent states of arousal lead to difficulty falling asleep or remaining asleep. Hypervigilance with an exaggerated startle response may occur, resulting in problems concentrating and completing tasks. The duration of the symptoms is at least 1 month, and the syndrome may emerge many months after the event. On the other hand, some victims may have no memories of the trauma for a period of time. They may complain of feeling detached or separate from others and lose the ability to enjoy pleasurable events, reflecting "psychic numbing." In both cases, anger, sadness, rage, depression, or stoicism may be demonstrated.

Acute stress disorder: Like posttraumatic stress disorder (PTSD), the problem begins with exposure to a traumatic event, with a response of intense fear, helplessness, or horror. In addition, the person shows dissociative symptoms, that is, subjective sense of numbing, feeling "in a daze," depersonalization, or amnesia and clearly tries to avoid stimuli that arouse recollection of the trauma. But just like PTSD, the

victim reexperiences the trauma and shows functional impairment in social, occupational, and problem-solving skills. The key difference is that this syndrome occurs within 4 wk of the traumatic event and only lasts 2 days to 4 wk.

Anxiety disorder caused by medical condition: May be characterized by severe anxiety, panic attacks, or obsessions or compulsions, but the cause is clearly related to a medical problem, excluding delirium. History, physical examination, and laboratory findings support a specific diagnosis, for example, hypoglycemia, pheochromocytoma, or thyroid disease.

Anxiety disorder not otherwise specified: Describes individuals with significant anxiety or phobic avoidance but not enough symptoms to meet the criteria for a particular anxiety or adjustment disorder diagnosis. The patient may show a mixed anxiety-depressive picture or demonstrate social phobic symptoms related to having another medical problem, for example, Parkinson's disease, or present with insufficient data to rule out a general medical condition or substance abuse.

HEALTH CARE SETTING

Depends on the type of anxiety disorder. Primary (outpatient) care is likely for most categories, and possibly emergency department care for panic disorders. If the patient has developed panic disorder with agoraphobia, psychiatric home care may be the best care option. Some patients may be hospitalized for physiologic problems.

ASSESSMENT

Physical indicators: Dry mouth, elevated vital signs, diarrhea, increased urination, nausea, diaphoresis, hyperventilation, fatigue, insomnia, sexual dysfunction, irritability, tenseness.

Emotional indicators: Fear, sense of impending doom, helplessness, insecurity, low self-confidence, anger, guilt.

Cognitive indicators: Mild anxiety produces increased awareness and problem-solving skills. Higher levels produce narrowed perceptual field, missed details, diminished problem-solving skills, and deteriorated logical thinking.

Social indicators: Marital and parental functioning may be adversely affected by anxiety and therefore should be assessed.

Spiritual indicators: Patient may exhibit hopelessness/helplessness, feeling of being cut off from God, anger at God for allowing anxiety.

Suicidality: Suicide assessment is critical with anxious patients, especially those with panic disorder. For patients suffering dual diagnoses of depression and substance abuse or even other anxiety disorders, risk of self-injury is even greater. Suicidal assessment includes questions to determine presence of suicidal ideation and the lethality of any plan. Essential questions to ask include:

- Have you thought of hurting yourself?
- Are you presently thinking about hurting yourself?
- If you have been thinking about suicide, do you have a plan?
- What is the plan?
- Have you thought about what life would be like if you were no longer a part of it?

A previous history of suicide attempts combined with depression places the patient at high risk in the present. A patient whose depression is lifting is at higher risk for suicide than a severely depressed individual. The improvement may result in an increase in energy. This increased energy is not enough to make the patient feel well or hopeful, but it is enough to carry out a suicidal plan.

DIAGNOSTIC TESTS

There is no specific diagnostic test for anxiety disorders. The diagnosis of anxiety is made through history, interview of patient and family, and observation of verbal and nonverbal behaviors. A number of effective scales are available to quantify the degree of anxiety, such as the Yale-Brown Obsessive Scale, the Maudsley Obsessional-Compulsive Inventory, the Leyton Obsessional Inventory, Hamilton Rating Scale for Anxiety, Panic Attack Cognitions Questionnaire, State-Trait Anxiety Inventory, Sheehan Patient Rated Anxiety Inventory, and the Beck Anxiety Inventory.

Nursing Diagnosis:

Deficient Knowledge:

Causes, signs and symptoms, and treatment of anxiety or specific anxiety disorder

Desired Outcome: By discharge (if inpatient) or after 2 wk of outpatient treatment, patient and/or significant other verbalize accurate information about at least two of the possible causes of anxiety, four of the signs and symptoms of the specific anxiety disorder, and the available treatment options.

INTERVENTIONS	RATIONALES
Inform patient and significant other that anxiety disorders are physiologic disorders caused by the interplay of many factors, such as stress, imbalance in brain chemistry, psychodynamic factors, faulty learning, and genetics.	Many people who suffer from anxiety disorders accept that they are just "nervous worriers" and lack the knowledge that anxiety disorders represent a complex interplay of treatable biologic, genetic, and environmental factors.
Inform patient and significant other about the holistic nature of anxiety, which produces physical, emotional, cognitive, social, and spiritual symptoms.	Many people believe that anxiety equates with nervousness and fail to recognize the many other signs and symptoms that make this a holistic disorder.
Inform patient and significant other that anxiety disorders are treatable.	Medications are usually indicated for treatment of these disorders and may include antidepressants and anxiolytics or a combination of medications. In addition, other interventions are useful, including dietary interventions (e.g., elimination of caffeinated products), breathing control, exercise program, relaxation techniques, and psychologic interventions (i.e., distraction, positive self-talk, psychoeducation, exposure therapy, systematic desensitization, implosive therapy, social interventions, cognitive therapy, stress and time management interventions).

●●● **Related NIC and NOC labels:** *NIC* Teaching: Individual; Teaching: Procedure/Treatment; Teaching: Disease Process *NOC*: Knowledge: Illness Care

Nursing Diagnosis:

Anxiety

related to recurring panic attacks

Desired Outcome: Within 24 hr of treatment/intervention, patient verbalizes methods for dealing with panic attacks and understanding that panic attacks are not life threatening and that they are time limited and demonstrates this knowledge accordingly.

INTERVENTIONS	RATIONALES
Administer medication as prescribed for panic attacks.	Panic attacks are neurobiologic events that respond to medications.
Teach patient to reduce or eliminate dietary substances that may promote anxiety and panic, such as caffeine, food coloring, and monosodium glutamate (MSG).	Caffeine increases feelings of anxiety. However, caffeine withdrawal symptoms also can stimulate panic. Therefore the plan should include focus on reducing consumption first, followed by elimination from the diet. Some individuals are sensitive to food colorings and MSG. This sensitivity is experienced as increased anxiety.
Teach patient relaxation techniques; assist with practicing imagery, deep breathing, progressive relaxation, and use of relaxation tapes. See **Health-Seeking Behaviors:** Relaxation technique effective for stress reduction and control, p. 172.	Relaxation is effective in reducing anxiety. The patient's ability to master relaxation techniques provides a sense of control and enhances self-care ability.
Stay with patient during panic attacks. Use short, simple directions. Encourage patient to use relaxation, remind patient that attack is time limited, and reduce environmental stimulation. ***Remain calm.***	During a panic attack, ability to refocus is limited. The patient needs reassurance that he or she is not dying and that this will pass. Therefore, it is important that the nurse remain calm and not respond to patient's anxiety with anxiety.
Teach patient to self-administer anxiolytic medication when first signs and symptoms of a panic attack start.	This information empowers the patient by providing a strategy to deal with panic attacks.

●●● **Related NIC and NOC labels:** *NIC*: Anxiety Reduction; Behavior Management; Calming Technique; Medication Administration; Presence; Simple Relaxation Therapy; Simple Guided Imagery; Progressive Muscle Relaxation *NOC*: Anxiety Control

Nursing Diagnosis:

Social Isolation

related to agoraphobia

Desired Outcome: By discharge (if inpatient) or after 4 wk of outpatient treatment, patient demonstrates behavior consistent with increased social interaction.

INTERVENTIONS	RATIONALES
Assist patient in graded exposure plan to gradually increase independent functions and interactions with others.	Gradual exposure is effective in treating agoraphobia.
Assist patient with practicing relaxation techniques.	Relaxation helps mitigate impending panic attacks.
Discuss alternatives for social interaction.	Patient may need assistance with developing activity plans.

••• **Related NIC and NOC labels:** *NIC:* Socialization Enhancement; Coping Enhancement *NOC:* Well-Being; Social Support; Social Involvement

Nursing Diagnosis:

Ineffective Coping

related to anxiety

Desired Outcome: Within 24 hr of intervention/treatment, patient identifies ineffective coping behaviors and consequences, expresses feelings appropriately, identifies options and uses resources effectively, and uses effective problem-solving techniques.

INTERVENTIONS	RATIONALES
Identify previous methods of coping with life problems.	How patient has handled problems in the past is a reliable predictor of how current problems will be handled.
Determine use of substances (alcohol, other drugs, smoking and eating patterns).	Patient may have used substances as coping mechanisms to control anxiety. This pattern can interfere with ability to deal with the current situation.
Provide information regarding different ways to deal with situations that promote anxious feelings, for example, identification and appropriate expression of feelings and problem-solving skills.	This information provides patient with an opportunity to learn new coping skills.
Role-play and rehearse new skills.	Role-playing promotes skill acquisition in a nonthreatening environment.
Encourage and support patient in evaluating lifestyle and identifying activities and stresses of family, work, and social situations.	These measures enable patient to examine areas of life that may contribute to anxiety and make decisions about how to engender changes gradually without adding undue anxiety.
Assist patient with identifying some short- and long-term goals focused on making life changes and decreasing anxiety.	Goals help provide direction in making necessary changes.
Teach patient how to break responsibilities into manageable units.	Small steps enhance success and avoid the anxiety that comes from facing a huge task and feeling overwhelmed.
Suggest incorporating stress management techniques (e.g., relaxation) into normal day.	This encourages patient to take care of self, take control, and decrease stress.
Teach importance of balance in life.	A life out of balance adds tremendously to stress and anxiety. Changes such as getting adequate sleep, nutrition, exercise, quiet time, work time, family time, and spiritual time enhance quality of life, decrease anxiety, and increase sense of power and control.
Refer to outside resources, including support groups, psychotherapy, religious resources, and community recreation resources.	Many people benefit from the support of other people and resources to help keep life in balance and monitor stress level.

••• **Related NIC and NOC labels:** *NIC:* Coping Enhancement; Decision-Making Support; Anxiety Reduction; Sleep Enhancement; Support Group; Spiritual Support; Simple Relaxation Therapy; Mutual Goal Setting; Behavior Modification *NOC:* Coping

Nursing Diagnosis:

Compromised Family Coping

related to family disorganization and role changes

Desired Outcome: Within 24 hr of this diagnosis, family members identify resources within themselves to deal with the situation; interact appropriately with patient, providing support and assistance as needed; recognize own needs for support; seek assistance; and use resources effectively.

INTERVENTIONS	RATIONALES
Assess level of information available to and understood by family.	Lack of understanding about patient's anxiety disorder can lead to unhealthy interaction patterns and contribute to anxiety felt by family members.
Identify role of patient and current family roles, and discuss how illness has changed the family organization.	The patient's disability (e.g., resulting in inability to go to work or maintain the household) interferes with performance of usual family role and can substantially contribute to family stress and disorganization.
Help family identify other factors besides patient's illness that affect ability to provide support to each other.	This takes focus off of the patient as "the problem" and helps family members examine each of their individual responsibilities and behaviors.
Discuss reasons for patient's behaviors.	This helps the family understand and accept behaviors that may be very difficult to handle.
Help family and patient recognize to whom the problem belongs and who is responsible for resolution of the problem.	This recognition promotes self-responsibility for owning and fixing a problem. The individual with the problem can seek support and ask for help, but it is not the responsibility of the family to rescue that person or to solve the person's problem.
Teach the family constructive problem solving skills.	These skills help the family learn new ways to deal with conflicts and reduce anxiety-provoking situations.
Refer family to appropriate community resources.	The family may need additional assistance (e.g., from counselors, psychotherapy, Social Services, financial advisors, and spiritual advisor) to work through family issues and remain intact.

●●● **Related NIC and NOC labels:** *NIC:* Coping Enhancement; Support Group; Family Integrity Promotion; Role Enhancement; Spiritual Support; Normalization Promotion *NOC:* Family Coping; Family Normalization

Nursing Diagnosis:

Deficient Knowledge:

Prescribed medications, their purpose, and their potential side effects

Desired Outcome: By discharge (if inpatient) or after 4 wk of outpatient treatment, the patient verbalizes accurate information about the prescribed medications and their side effects.

INTERVENTIONS	RATIONALES
Teach the physiologic action of anxiolytics and/or antidepressants and how they alleviate symptoms of patient's anxiety disorder.	Anxiety disorders are neurobiologic occurrences that respond to both anxiolytics and antidepressants. Many people who suffer from anxiety are fearful of taking medication because they fear drug dependence and view taking it as a sign of weakness.
Explain importance of taking antidepressant medication as prescribed.	These medications require certain blood levels to be therapeutic; therefore patient needs to take them at the dose and time interval prescribed.

Continued

INTERVENTIONS	RATIONALES
Teach the side effect profile and its management of the patient's prescribed drugs that follow:	The anxiolytic medications, as well as each class of antidepressants, carry specific side-effect profiles. Knowledge about expected side effects, ways to manage these side effects, and how long these side effects last is important for ensuring therapy adherence.
Tricyclic antidepressants: amitriptyline (Elavil), desipramine (Norpramin), doxepin (Sinequan), imipramine (Tofranil), nortriptyline (Pamelor), protriptyline (Vivactil), and trimipramine (Surmontil)	Imipramine and desipramine are very effective in anxiety disorders and are used in higher doses than would be used for depressive disorders.
Monitor for anticholinergic effects, sedation, decreased blood pressure, and weight gain.	These are common side effects.
Drink at least 8 glasses of water a day and add high-fiber foods to diet.	Water and high-fiber foods combat constipation, a potential anticholinergic effect.
Rise from sitting position slowly. Discuss risks of falling related to dizziness associated with hypotension.	Orthostatic hypotension is a potential side effect.
Suck on sugar-free candy or mints or use sugar-free chewing gum.	These products combat dry mouth, a potential anticholinergic effect.
Establish sleep routine and regular exercise.	Regular sleep and exercise combat feelings of fatigue associated with these drugs.
Limit intake of refined sugars and carbohydrates.	Eating sugar and carbohydrates can cause weight gain and carbohydrate cravings.
Be aware of seizure potential.	Tricyclic antidepressants lower the seizure threshold. Caution is needed for patients with epilepsy or other seizure disorder.
Be alert for and report signs of cardiac toxicity. Patients older than 40 yr of age need an electrocardiogram evaluation before treatment and periodically thereafter.	These drugs may decrease vagal influence on the heart secondary to muscarinic blockade and by acting directly on the bundle of His to slow conduction. Both effects increase risk of dysrhythmias.
Discuss possible drug interactions.	The combination of tricyclics with monoamine oxidase (MAO) inhibitors can cause severe hypertension. The combination of tricyclics with central nervous system (CNS) depressants, such as alcohol, antihistamines, opioids, and barbiturates, can cause severe CNS depression. Because of the anticholinergic effects of tricyclics, any other anticholinergic drug, including over-the-counter antihistamines and sleeping aids, should be avoided.
MAO inhibitors: isocarboxazid (Marplan), phenelzine (Nardil), and tranylcypromine (Parnate)	Phenelzine and tranylcypromine are used in anxiety disorders in doses higher than those for treating depressive disorders and are useful for patients who have not responded to other drugs.
There is potential for mild sedation and hypotension.	These are common side effects.
Discuss MAO inhibitor restrictions.	MAO inhibitors combined with dietary tyramine can cause a life-threatening hypertensive crisis. Dietary restrictions include avocados; fermented bean curd; fermented soybean; soybean paste; figs; bananas; fermented, smoked, or aged meats; liver; bologna, pepperoni, and salami; dried, cured, fermented, or smoked fish; practically all cheeses; yeast extract; some imported beers; Chianti wine; protein dietary supplements; soups that contain protein extract; shrimp paste; and soy sauce. Large amounts of chocolate, fava beans, ginseng, and caffeine may cause a reaction.
Explain possible drug interactions and the need to avoid all prescription and over-the-counter drugs unless health care provider has specifically approved them.	MAO inhibitors can interact with many drugs to cause potentially serious results. Use of ephedrine or amphetamines can lead to hypertensive crisis. The interaction of tricyclic antidepressants with MAO inhibitors is discussed above. Selective serotonin reuptake inhibitors (SSRIs) should not be used with MAO inhibitors. Antihypertensive drugs combined with MAO inhibitors may result in excessive lowering of blood pressure. MAO inhibitors with meperidine (Demerol) can cause hyperpyrexia (excessive elevation of temperature).

Continued

INTERVENTIONS	RATIONALES
SSRIs: fluoxetine (Prozac), fluvoxamine maleate (Luvox), sertraline (Zoloft), paroxetine (Paxil), citalopram (Celexa), and escitalopram (Lexapro)	SSRIs are helpful not only for patients with obsessive-compulsive symptoms but for patients with panic and anxiety disorders as well.
Be alert for nausea, headache, nervousness, insomnia, anxiety, agitation, sexual dysfunction, dizziness, fatigue, rash, diarrhea, excessive sweating, and anorexia with weight loss.	These are reported side effects. Because these drugs can increase anxiety, it is recommended that treatment be started at very low doses and increased gradually.
Discuss possible drug interactions.	Interaction with MAO inhibitors can cause serotonin syndrome, a potentially life-threatening event. Symptoms include anxiety, diaphoresis, rigidity, hyperthermia, autonomic hyperactivity, and coma. Because of this possibility, MAO inhibitors should be withdrawn at least 14 days before starting an SSRI, and when an SSRI is discontinued, at least 5 wk should elapse before an MAO inhibitor is given.
Benzodiazepines: diazepam (Valium), chlordiazepoxide (Librium), clorazepate (Tranxene), prazepam (Centrax), flurazepam (Dalmane), lorazepam (Ativan), oxazepam (Serax), temazepam (Restoril), triazolam (Halcion), alprazolam (Xanax), halazepam (Paxipam), and clonazepam (Klonopin)	All except for alprazolam are used for generalized anxiety disorder. Alprazolam is used for panic disorder.
Explain that drowsiness, impairment of intellectual function, impairment of memory, ataxia, and reduced motor coordination can occur.	These are common side effects that subside as tolerance to the drug develops.
For patients who use these medications for sleep, there may daytime fatigue, drowsiness, and cognitive impairments that can continue while person is awake.	These are common side effects that subside as tolerance to the drug develops.
A gradual tapering is recommended when being taken off the drug.	Abrupt discontinuation of the benzodiazepines can result in a recurrence of target symptoms such as anxiety.
Nausea, vomiting, impaired appetite, dry mouth, and constipation may occur.	These are gastrointestinal (GI) symptoms associated with this drug.
Take the drug with food.	Taking the drug with food may ease GI distress.
Monitor for worsening of depression symptoms.	This effect may occur in patients who are both depressed and anxious.
Older adults should take the smallest possible therapeutic dose.	Older adults taking this drug are at increased risk for incontinence, memory disturbances, dizziness, and falls.
Pregnant women and nursing mothers should avoid using benzodiazepines.	Benzodiazepines are excreted in breast milk of nursing mothers. They also cross the placenta and are associated with increased risk of certain birth defects.
Decrease or stop smoking altogether.	Nicotine decreases effectiveness of benzodiazepines.
Nonbenzodiazepines: buspirone	Buspirone is indicated in treatment of generalized anxiety disorder. It does not add to depression, so it is a good choice when anxiety and depression coexist. It is not effective in treating other anxiety disorders.
Take buspirone on a continual dosing schedule tid.	Buspirone has a short half-life.
Cardiac patients should avoid this drug.	Buspirone can cause digoxin toxicity.
This drug can cause liver and kidney toxicity. Patients with kidney or liver impairment must be monitored for this adverse effect.	Buspirone is metabolized in the liver and excreted predominantly by the kidneys.
Be alert for dizziness, drowsiness, nausea, excitement, and headache.	These are common side effects.

••• **Related NIC and NOC labels:** *NIC*: Teaching: Prescribed Medication *NOC*: Knowledge: Medication

ADDITIONAL NURSING DIAGNOSES/ PROBLEMS:

"Major Depression" for:

Hopelessness	p. 763
Risk for Suicide	p. 763
Self-Esteem: Chronic low	p. 765

✔ PATIENT-FAMILY TEACHING AND DISCHARGE PLANNING

The patient with an anxiety disorder experiences a wide variety of symptoms that affect ability to learn and retain information. Teaching must be geared to a time when medication has begun to calm the person and improve abilities to concentrate and learn; otherwise, it is wasted effort. Verbal teaching should be simple and supplemented with reading materials to which the patient and/or significant other and family can refer at a later time. Ensure that follow-up treatment is scheduled and that patient and/or significant other and family understand need to get prescriptions filled and to take medication as prescribed. Psychiatric home care might be a valuable part of the discharge planning to facilitate compliance with the discharge plan. In addition, provide verbal and written information about the following issues:

✔ Medications, including drug name; purpose; dosage; frequency; precautions; drug-drug, food-drug, and herb-drug interactions; and potential side effects.

✔ Thought-stopping techniques to deal with negativism.

✔ Importance of maintaining a healthy lifestyle—balanced diet, minimal to no caffeine, decrease or stop smoking, exercise, and regular adequate sleep patterns—for remaining in remission.

✔ Importance of continuing medication use long after symptoms have gone.

✔ Importance of social support and strategies to obtain it.

✔ Importance of using constructive coping skills to deal with stress.

✔ Importance of using relaxation techniques to minimize stress.

✔ Importance of maintaining or achieving spiritual well-being.

✔ Importance of follow-up care, including day treatment programs, appointments with psychiatrist and therapists, and vocational rehabilitation program if indicated.

✔ Referrals to community resources for support and education. Additional information can be obtained by contacting the following organizations:

- Anxiety Disorders Association of America (ADAA) at *www.adaa.org*
- National Alliance for the Mentally Ill (NAMI) for information on panic disorders at *www.nimh.nih.gov/ healthinformation/panicmenu.cfm*
- National Institute of Mental Health (NIMH) for information on anxiety disorders at *www.nimh.nih.gov/ healthinformation/anxietymenu.cfm*

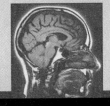

Bipolar Disorder 97
(Manic Component)

OVERVIEW/PATHOPHYSIOLOGY

Bipolar disorder is a mood disorder characterized by episodes of major depression and mania or hypomania. (See the care plan on "Major Depression," p. 761, for specifics regarding depression.) *Mania* is characterized by a period in which there is a dramatic change in mood; the individual is either elated and expansive or irritable. For the diagnosis to be made, this change in mood must last 1 wk (less if hospitalization is required). At least three other symptoms from the following list must be present: inflated self-esteem or grandiosity, decreased need for sleep, pressured speech, flight of ideas, distractibility, increased involvement in goal-directed activities or psychomotor agitation, and overinvolvement in pleasurable activities with potentially damaging consequences, for example, hypersexuality, impulsive spending, and reckless and dangerous behavior.

Hypomania is characterized by at least 4 days of abnormally and persistently elevated, expansive, or irritable mood accompanied by at least three additional symptoms seen in a manic episode.

About 25% of the first episodes of bipolar disorder occur before age 20. Hormonal factors may account for a greater rate of rapid cycling (meaning highs and lows in a short period) by women, but, in general, women and men are equally affected with this disorder. There is no difference in prevalence rates by race or ethnicity. Bipolar disorder is a chronic, relapsing, and episodic disease. In individuals 40 yr of age or older who experience a first episode of mania, it is most likely related to medical conditions such as substance abuse or a cerebrovascular disorder. About 50% of bipolar patients have concurrent substance abuse disorders. Theories that explain causation of bipolar disorder include disorders in brain function or structure, sleep deprivation, and genetic factors.

HEALTH CARE SETTING

Primary (outpatient) care for most patients, except for those who are at high risk for suicide, represent a danger to others, or are experiencing a psychotic mania. Acute care (inpatient) stays are brief and focus on restabilization. Patients with bipolar disorder require long-term medication management, intensive psychosocial support to function within the community, and possibly individual, group, and family therapy.

ASSESSMENT

Similar to depression, the assessment of mania involves much more than an assessment of mood. This is a holistic disorder that results in changes in self-attitude (feelings of self-worth), as well as vital sense (sense of physical well-being) and spiritual sense. Depression diminishes self-worth, self-attitude, and vital sense, whereas mania increases these perceptions.

Feelings, attitudes, and knowledge: During manic episodes, patients express inflated views of themselves. Many manic patients state that they enjoyed being high and because of this refused medications. After the mania has subsided, the patient is confronted with the consequences of behaviors and actions engaged in while manic. Being faced with the reality of those behaviors and their consequences produces negative feelings expressed as shame, humiliation, denial, anger, fear of experiencing a relapse, fear of passing the disorder onto children, and fear of completing the bipolar cycle with an episode of depression.

Elevated mood or irritability: Patients may be excessively cheerful and unusually elated or display irritability over the smallest matters. This irritability increases when others attempt to reason with them. A manic person may display a haughty or superior attitude toward others. He or she may display overt anger, particularly if his or her requests or behaviors are curtailed.

Increased self-attitude: Patients may express and act in unusually optimistic fashion, engaging in behaviors that reflect poor judgment. The manic person is overconfident and energetic. Unfortunately the excess energy is channeled into inappropriate, dangerous, or indiscreet behaviors. A normally conservative person may engage in sexual indiscretions or speak in overly critical or judgmental terms, often at inappropriate times and about sensitive subjects.

Increased vital sense: The person with mania has increased energy and may appear tireless in the face of physical and mental efforts that would greatly tax unaffected individuals. He or she may feel completely refreshed after only a few minutes or hours of sleep.

Spiritual issues: Bipolar disorder mania carries with it many negative experiences—such as marital and family problems, divorce, legal difficulties, financial ruin, and unemployment—that contribute to the downward spiral of self-appraisals. Bipolar disorder can lead to a crisis in faith in self, others, life, and ultimately God. This loss of faith and hope contributes significantly to the risk of suicide.

Additional signs: Manic individuals may experience a voracious appetite or may be too busy to eat. A change in sleep pattern is characteristic of mania, with many individuals feeling less need for sleep, so sleep is usually decreased. An increase in sexual interest and activity is characteristic of manic individuals.

Suicidality: Suicide assessment is critical with manic patients. The presence of psychotic thinking, hyperactivity, impulsiveness, and possible substance abuse increases suicide risk significantly. It is important to ask questions to determine the presence of suicidal ideation and the lethality of any plan. Essential questions to ask include:

- Have you thought of hurting yourself?
- Are you presently thinking about hurting yourself?
- If you have been thinking about suicide, do you have a plan? What is the plan?
- Have you thought about what life would be like if you were no longer a part of it?

A previous history of suicide attempts places the patient at high risk for attempting suicide.

DIAGNOSTIC TESTS

There are no diagnostic tests to diagnose bipolar disorder-mania. Diagnosis is made through history, interview of patient and family, and observation of verbal and nonverbal behaviors. The Young Mania Scale is an effective instrument to quantify the degree of mania.

Nursing Diagnosis:

Risk for Other-Directed Violence

related to manic excitement

Desired Outcome: By the time of discharge from an inpatient setting, patient demonstrates self-control and decreased hyperactivity.

INTERVENTIONS	RATIONALES
Decrease environmental stimuli, avoid exposure to situations of predictable high stimulation, and remove patient from area if he or she becomes agitated.	Patient may be unable to focus attention on relevant stimuli and will be reacting/responding to all environmental stimuli.
Continually evaluate patient's response to frustration or difficult situations.	This enables early intervention and helps patient manage situation independently, if possible.
Ensure that environment is safe. Remove objects that could be dangerous and rearrange room to decrease environmental risks to prevent accidental/purposeful injury to self or others.	Hyperactive behavior and grandiose thinking can lead to destructive actions with possible harm to self or others.
Intervene at earliest signs of agitation. Use direct verbal interventions prompting appropriate behavior, redirect or remove patient from difficult situation, establish voluntary time-out or move to a quiet room, use physical control (e.g., hold patient).	Early intervention assists patient in regaining control, defuses a difficult situation, prevents violence, and enables treatment to continue in least restrictive manner.
Until patient is calm, avoid analyzing or problem solving regarding prevention of violence or collecting information about precipitating events or provoking stimuli.	Any questioning will only add to agitation. Analyze and problem solve when patient is calm.
Communicate rationale for taking action using a concrete, direct, and simple approach.	People are unable to process complicated communication when they are agitated or upset.
When patient is ready to leave quiet area or time-out location, allow gradual reentry to area of greater stimulation.	Patient has diminished tolerance for environmental stimuli; gradual reentry fosters coping skills.
Do not argue with patient who verbalizes put-downs or unrealistic or grandiose ideas.	Arguing only increases agitation and reinforces undesirable behavior.
Ignore and minimize attention given to bizarre dress or use of profanity, while placing clear limits on destructive behavior.	This avoids reinforcing negative behavior while providing controls for potentially dangerous behavior.
Avoid unnecessary delay of gratification when patient makes a request. If refusal is necessary, make sure that rationale is given in nonjudgmental and concrete manner.	Patients in a hyperactive state do not tolerate waiting or delays that add to frustration or agitation level. Any unnecessary delays could trigger aggressive behavior.

Continued

INTERVENTIONS	RATIONALES
Offer alternatives when available.	This uses patient's distractibility to decrease the frustration of having request refused. For example, "I don't have any soda. Would you like a glass of juice?"
When patient is less agitated and labile, provide information about alternative problem-solving strategies.	When calm, patient is able to hear and retain information.
When patient is calm, help to examine the antecedents/precipitants to agitation.	This promotes early recognition of the developing problem, enabling patient to plan for alternative responses and intervene in a timely fashion.
Collaborate with patient to identify alternative behaviors that are acceptable to both patient and staff. Role-play how to use these behaviors if appropriate.	Patient is more apt to follow through if the alternatives are mutually agreed on. This practice enables patient to "try on" new behaviors while calm and ready to learn.
Give positive reinforcement when patient attempts to deal with difficult situations without violence.	Praise increases patient's sense of success and increases likelihood that desired behaviors will be repeated.
Administer the following medications as prescribed:	
Antimanic medications: lithium carbonate (Lithobid, Eskalith), divalproex sodium (Depakote), carbamazepine (Tegretol), gabapentin (Neurontin), topiramate (Topamax), and lamotrigine (Lamictal).	Lithium is the drug of choice for mania and is indicated for alleviation of hyperactive symptoms. Some patients are lithium nonresponders and may need either divalproex, carbamazepine, gabapentin, topiramate, or lamotrigine.
Antipsychotic medications: chlorpromazine (Thorazine), haloperidol (Haldol), or clonazepam (Klonopin), a benzodiazepine.	These drugs are useful in decreasing extreme hyperactivity and improving an accompanying thought disorder until therapeutic level of lithium is achieved or when lithium is ineffective.
Atypical antipsychotics with mood stabilizing effects: olanzapine (Zyprexa) and quetiapine (Seroquel).	Olanzapine is better tolerated and prevents relapse more effectively than lithium. Quetiapine is also effective in treating the anxiety symptoms in bipolar depression.
Provide restraint or seclusion per agency policy.	These measures may be necessary for brief periods to protect patient, staff, and others.
Prepare patient for electroconvulsive therapy (ECT) if indicated.	In severely manic episode, ECT may be necessary.

••• Related NIC and NOC labels: *NIC:* Environmental Management: Safety; Behavior Management; Counseling; Impulse Control Training; Medication Management; Physical Restraint; Seclusion *NOC:* Impulse Control

Nursing Diagnosis:

Deficient Knowledge:

Causes, signs and symptoms, and treatment of bipolar disorder mania

Desired Outcome: Within 24 hr of teaching, patient and/or significant other, verbalize accurate information about at least two possible causes of bipolar disorder, four signs and symptoms of the disorder, and available treatment options.

INTERVENTIONS	RATIONALES
Inform patient and significant other that bipolar disorder is a physiologic disorder caused by the interplay of many factors, such as imbalance in brain function and structure, sleep deprivation, psychodynamic factors, and genetics.	Providing education about the physical basis for the disorder increases understanding and acceptance and decreases blaming behavior.
Inform patient and significant other that there are treatments available for bipolar disorder.	Medications are essential to stabilize and maintain mood. However, they are not enough. Comprehensive treatment involves intensive outpatient programs, frequent office visits, crisis telephone calls, family involvement, and psychosocial interventions including psychoeducation, suicide prevention, psychotherapy for depression, and limit setting in mania and hypomania. Management of bipolar disorders is a lifelong commitment.

••• Related NIC and NOC labels: *NIC:* Teaching: Individual; Teaching: Procedure/Treatment *NOC:* Knowledge: Illness Care

Nursing Diagnosis:

Imbalanced Nutrition: Less Than Body Requirements

related to inadequate intake in relation to metabolic expenditures

Desired Outcome: Immediately following interventions, patient displays increased attention to eating behaviors.

INTERVENTIONS	RATIONALES
Establish a baseline regarding nutritional and fluid intake, as well as activity level.	This assessment is necessary to quantify deficits, needs, and progress toward goals.
Weigh patient daily.	This is another form of quantification that provides information about therapeutic needs and effectiveness of interventions.
Serve meals in a setting with minimal distractions.	This encourages patient to focus on eating and prevents other distractions from interfering with food intake.
Stay with patient during mealtime, even if this means walking with patient.	This provides support and encouragement for patient to take in adequate nutrition and does not set unrealistic expectation that patient must sit during mealtime.
Provide finger foods, snacks, and juices.	Patient will most likely eat small frequent meals on the move and this allows a reasonable accommodation for this behavior.
Enable patient to choose food when he or she is able to make choices.	Encouraging choices before patient is ready may add to confusion. However, if patient is able to handle choices, this increases sense of control.
Refer to dietitian as indicated.	It may be useful to involve an expert in determining patient's nutritional needs and the most appropriate options for meeting these needs.
Administer vitamins and mineral supplements as prescribed.	Supplements correct dietary deficiencies and improve nutritional status.

••• **Related NIC and NOC labels:** *NIC:* Nutrition Management: Nutritional Monitoring *NOC:* Nutritional Status

Nursing Diagnosis:

Self-Care Deficit

related to impulsivity and lack of concern

Desired Outcome: Immediately following interventions, patient performs self-care activities within level of ability.

INTERVENTIONS	RATIONALES
Assess current level of functioning; reevaluate daily.	Patient's abilities for self-care may change daily. This information is needed to plan or modify care.
Provide physical assistance, supervision, simple directions, reminders, encouragement, and support as needed.	This helps patient focus on the task. Providing only required assistance fosters independence.
If possible, use patient's clothing and toiletries.	Patient may have been disorganized entering the hospital or was hospitalized as an emergency measure, so own belongings were left at home. Having own clothes and supplies supports autonomy and self-esteem.
As appropriate, limit choices regarding clothing.	During periods of extreme hyperactivity and distractibility, patient may be unable to make appropriate choices or to care for personal belongings.
Monitor patient's ability to manage money and valuables, as well as other personal effects.	Manic patients may give away possessions, spend money extravagantly, or become involved in grandiose plans, necessitating intervention.

Continued

INTERVENTIONS	RATIONALES
Intervene to protect patient from own impulsivity and exploitation from others.	This intervention protects patient from negative consequences of impulsiveness.
As condition improves, set goals to establish minimum standards for self-care, for example, take a bath every other day.	Setting goals promotes the idea that patient is responsible for self and enhances sense of self-worth.

••• **Related NIC and NOC labels:** *NIC:* Self-Care Assistance; Self-Responsibility Facilitation; Behavior Modification *NOC:* Self-Care: Activities of Daily Living

Nursing Diagnosis:

Deficient Knowledge:

Medication use, including purpose and potential side effects of prescribed medications

Desired Outcome: Immediately following teaching interventions, patient verbalizes accurate information about the prescribed medications.

INTERVENTIONS	RATIONALES
Teach physiologic action of mood stabilizers.	Bipolar disorder mania responds to mood stabilizers, with lithium carbonate being the drug of choice.
Teach importance of taking medication as prescribed and the need for follow-up blood tests to monitor drug serum level.	The medication requires certain blood levels to be therapeutic, and therefore patient needs to take it at the dose and time interval prescribed. The scheduled serum evaluations ensure that the medication level remains within therapeutic range.
Antimanic drugs for adults: lithium carbonate (Lithobid, Eskalith, Duralith) or lithium citrate (Cibalith)	Lithium provides mood stability and prevents dangerous highs and despairing lows experienced in bipolar disorder.
Teach patient the following:	
Monitor for swelling of feet or hands, fine hand tremor, mild diarrhea, muscle weakness, fatigue, memory and concentration difficulties, metallic taste, nausea or abdominal discomfort, polydipsia, polyuria.	These are common side effects.
Importance of monitoring intake and output, sodium intake, and weight and how to elevate legs when sitting or lying down.	These are interventions for edema of the feet and hands.
Importance of notifying health care provider if urinary output decreases.	This may be a sign of increasing serum level of lithium.
Patient should notify prescriber if tremors interfere with work.	A drug that interferes with work may result in compliance issues. Smaller, more frequent doses may help. In addition, tremors worsen when patient is anxious.
Take lithium with meals and replace fluids lost with diarrhea.	These are interventions for mild diarrhea.
Notify prescriber if diarrhea becomes severe.	Prescriber may need to change patient's medication.
If muscle weakness, fatigue, and memory and concentration difficulties occur, patient should avoid driving or operating hazardous equipment during this period and should use reminders and cues for memory.	These are interventions for muscle weakness, fatigue, and memory and concentration difficulties, which if they occur are short-lasting.
Notify prescriber if muscle weakness, fatigue, and memory and concentration problems become severe.	Prescriber may change patient's medication.
Use sugarless candies or throat lozenges and engage in frequent oral hygiene.	These are interventions for metallic taste.
Take medication with meals.	This is an intervention for nausea or abdominal discomfort.
Drinking large amounts of fluids is a normal mechanism for coping with the side effect of increased urine.	This information provides reassurance for polydipsia.
Have laboratory work done as prescribed.	This helps ensure that serum drug level is maintained between 0.6 and 1.2 mEq/L. Usually once stabilization is achieved, laboratory work is done q1-2 wk during first 2 mo and q3-6 mo during long-term maintenance.

Continued

INTERVENTIONS	RATIONALES
Avoid alcohol or other central nervous system (CNS) depressant drugs.	These substances may increase serum lithium level.
Notify prescriber if pregnant or planning to become pregnant. Do not breastfeed while taking this medication.	Safe use during pregnancy and breastfeeding has not been established.
Notify prescriber before taking any other prescription or over the-counter (OTC) medication.	Many other drugs interact with lithium to either increase or decrease the serum level.
Do not abruptly discontinue this drug.	This could lead to exacerbation of manic symptoms.
Antiseizure medications with mood-stabilizing effects: divalproex sodium or valproic acid (Depakote or Depakene), carbamazepine (Tegretol), gabapentin (Neurontin), topiramate (Topamax), and lamotrigine (Lamictal).	These medications are generally used when lithium does not work or when side effects from lithium are intolerable to the patient.
Atypical antipsychotics with mood stabilizing effects: olanzapine (Zyprexa) and quetiapine (Seroquel)	Olanzapine is better tolerated and prevents relapse more effectively than lithium. Quetiapine is also effective in treating the anxiety symptoms in bipolar depression.
Teach patient to be alert for anorexia, nausea, vomiting, drowsiness (most common), and tremor.	These are common side effects.

ADDITIONAL NURSING DIAGNOSES/PROBLEMS:

"Major Depression" for:

Hopelessness	p. 763
Risk for Suicide	p. 763
Self-Esteem: Chronic low	p. 765

PATIENT-FAMILY TEACHING AND DISCHARGE PLANNING

The patient with a bipolar disorder mania experiences a wide variety of symptoms that affect the ability to learn and retain information. Teaching must be geared to a time when medication has begun to decrease hyperactive symptoms and improve abilities to concentrate and learn; otherwise, it is a wasted effort. Verbal teaching should be simple and supplemented with reading materials the patient and/or significant other and family can refer to at a later time. Ensure that follow-up treatment is scheduled and that patient and/or significant other and family understand need to get prescriptions filled and importance of taking medication as prescribed. Consider whether or not patient has transportation available to get to follow-up treatment. Psychiatric home care might be a valuable part of the discharge planning to facilitate compliance with the discharge plan. In addition, provide patient and/or significant other/family with verbal and written information about the following issues:

✓ Medications, including drug name; purpose; dosage; frequency; precautions; drug-drug, food-drug, and herb-drug interactions; and potential side effects.

✓ Importance of laboratory follow-up tests for serum lithium levels.

✓ Importance of maintaining a healthy lifestyle—balanced diet, minimal to no caffeine or alcohol, exercise, and regular adequate sleep patterns—to ensure remaining in remission.

✓ Importance of continuing medication use probably for a lifetime.

✓ Importance of social support and strategies for obtaining it.

✓ Importance of using community follow-up resources, for example, psychiatrist, psychiatric nurse, intensive outpatient, support groups, family counseling.

✓ Importance of maintaining or achieving spiritual well-being.

✓ Referrals to community resources for support and education. Additional information can be obtained by contacting the following organizations:

- Depression and Related Affective Disorders Association (DRADA) at *www.drada.org*. This nonprofit organization is composed of individuals with mood disorders, family members, and mental health professionals. It offers information, education, referral, and support services to people nationwide. DRADA sponsors a nationally renowned training program for group leaders.
- Depression Awareness, Recognition, and Treatment Program (D/ART), 5600 Fishers Lane, Suite 10-85, Rockville, MD 20857, (301) 443-4140, Fax: (301) 443-4045. D/ART is a national self-help clearinghouse. It provides a list of resources throughout the United States that can help in networking and providing consultative assistance.
- Depression and Bipolar Support Alliance (DBSA) at *www.dbsalliance.org*. The DBSA provides education as well as support to individuals and families impacted by depression and bipolar illnesses.

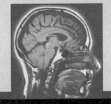

Dementia—Alzheimer's Type 98

OVERVIEW/PATHOPHYSIOLOGY

Dementia is a chronic cognitive disorder that is part of a category of psychiatric disorders classified as *Delirium, Dementia,* and other *Cognitive Disorders.* These disorders are divided into two categories: *Acute Cognitive Disorders,* which includes delirium, and *Chronic Cognitive Disorders,* which includes the various types of dementia. There are five types of dementia: primary, dementia with extrapyramidal symptoms (EPS), dementia resulting from brain lesions, vascular dementia, and dementia associated with other physical conditions.

The most common form is Alzheimer's disease, a primary dementia accounting for 60% to 80% of dementia cases, and it is the focus of this care plan. Although Alzheimer's disease is age related, it does not represent the normal process of aging. It occurs with distinctive brain lesions without any known physiologic basis. The brain lesions are neurofibrillary tangles and neuritic plaques that take up space in the brain, replacing normal tissue in the cell body of the neuron. There are multiple theories to explain the occurrence of Alzheimer's disease, including genetic transmission, a decrease in acetylcholine, beta-amyloid activity, impact of head injury, ministrokes, lack of estrogen, immunologic factors, effects of a slow-acting virus, and environmental factors.

Alzheimer's disease affects more than 4 million people, making it the most common neuropsychiatric illness in older adults. The actual course of the disorder follows a predictable pattern of early, middle, and late stages, each displaying characteristic behaviors and requiring a different focus of treatment. The early stage is frequently referred to as the *amnestic stage,* the middle stage as the *dementia stage,* and the late stage as the *vegetative stage.* As the disease progresses, patients lose control over their bladder and bowel functions and later over swallowing. Seizures are common. Death inevitably occurs as a result of neurologic complications imposed by the brain lesions.

Alzheimer's disease represents the clinical prototype for chronic cognitive disorders. The care required by the Alzheimer's patient, especially in the middle and late stages of the disorder, is essentially the same care required by all dementia patients regardless of type. The cognitive symptoms of dementia involve serious memory impairment, as well as significant alterations in language and perceptual acuity and abilities to abstract, problem solve, and make appropriate judgments. Patients ultimately experience loss of all memory and aphasia (loss of meaningful verbal communication). Noncognitive behavioral symptoms can be just as profound. These include significant personality changes, purposeless movements, agitation and aggression, overreaction to situations, irritating behavior, and emotional disinhibition.

HEALTH CARE SETTING

In the early stage of Alzheimer's disease, care takes place in the home and primary care setting. By the end of the early stage of the disease, additional services such as home care and use of adult day care are needed to maintain the patient at home. At the end of the early stage and moving into the middle stage, the decision regarding where to place the patient begins. Patient is generally moved into residential care in the middle stage, and during the late stage, care is provided in a skilled nursing facility.

ASSESSMENT

Psychiatric Assessment

Involves assessment of primary and secondary psychiatric manifestations of Alzheimer's disease and differential diagnosis from psychosis, depression, anxiety, and phobias.

Family history: Dementing illness, psychiatric disease, neurologic disease, substance abuse.

Social history: Education, past level of functioning per occupational history, close relationships, current living situation.

Medical history: All past and present medical illnesses, past surgeries, past trauma especially to the head, allergies, and medication.

Psychiatric history: Psychotic illness, depressive illness, other psychiatric illnesses, psychiatric symptoms, past and current treatments, hospitalizations, suicide ideation, violence.

Present illness: Length of cognitive loss and degree of memory loss:
- Is short-term memory loss so significant that patient is no longer able to remember activities of daily living (ADL)?
- Other presenting problems, physical symptoms, functional deficits, psychiatric symptoms.
- Personality changes, including low tolerance for normal frustrations, oversensitivity to remarks of others, lack of initiative, decreased attention span, diminished emotional presence, emotional lability, restlessness.
- Difficulty with word finding and comprehension; thought blocking.

Mental status examination: Appearance, behavior, speech, mood, hallucinations, delusions, anxiety, phobias, cognition, insight and judgment, behavioral disturbances such as agitation, combativeness, screaming, catastrophic reactions.

Physical Assessment

Psychomotor functioning: Difficulty carrying out new or complex motor tasks is apparent in the early stages; difficulty carrying out activities such as dressing, eating, and walking becomes apparent in the middle stages. Unsteadiness of gait and a listing posture pose a significant risk for falls during the middle stages. In addition, marked psychomotor agitation is common. Restlessness, agitation, and aimless pacing replace normal motion.

Nutrition and elimination: Eating difficulties may present in early stages. Patient may forget that he or she has just eaten, exhibit lax table manners, fail to know it is mealtime without prompting, experience changes in taste and appetite, express denial of hunger or need to eat, and experience weight loss. As disease progresses, patient does not respond to need for elimination, which necessitates the caregiver to plan regular bathroom breaks. Constipation and incontinence of urine and feces become problems.

Activity and rest: Fatigue increases severity of symptoms, especially as evening approaches. Patient may reverse days and nights, with wakefulness and aimless wandering at night and disturbance of sleep rhythms. Patient may be content to sit and watch others. Main activity may be hoarding inanimate objects, hiding articles, wandering, or engaging in repetitive motions.

Hygiene: As disease progresses, so does dependence on caregiver to meet basic hygiene needs. Appearance may be disheveled, and patient may have body odor. Clothing may be inappropriate for situation or weather conditions. Patient may forget to go to the bathroom and the steps involved in toileting.

Social assessment: Patient may ignore rules of social conduct and exhibit inappropriate behavior. Speech may be fragmented; family roles may be altered/reversed as patient becomes more dependent.

Spiritual Assessment

An assessment of patient's faith tradition, practices, level of commitment, and connection to a faith community is critical. In the early stage of Alzheimer's disease, the patient may have full awareness of the journey that lies ahead, and spirituality may offer support and comfort in ways that nothing else can. As the disease progresses and deficits become greater, it is difficult to assess the patient's spiritual needs. However, because long-term memory remains intact long after the short-term memory is gone, patient may still be comforted by spiritual traditions such as worship services, prayers, and hymns that are a vivid part of his or her history. Moreover, care of the Alzheimer's patient is so demanding that spiritual needs of the caregiver must be assessed and support provided. A faith community may provide invaluable assistance in the actual care of the patient, providing caregiver with respite and help with day-to-day activities.

DIAGNOSTIC TESTS

Obtaining an accurate differential diagnosis of dementia is essential. Alzheimer's disease is basically a rule-out disorder; that is, the diagnosis is made after family history, laboratory tests, and brain imaging eliminate other disorders with similar cognitive deficits. Sources of information needed to make a differential diagnosis of dementia include a full neurologic assessment, laboratory tests to rule out metabolic factors, and family history of patient's past behavior and symptom progression. Mini-Mental State Examination and functional assessment of ADL provide necessary information. A computerized axial tomography (CT) scan identifies structural deficits. Brain imaging with positron emission tomography provides the clinician with information about changes in the metabolic activity and neurochemical characteristics associated with dementia. Typically, testing of patients in the early stage of Alzheimer's disease reveals a normal electroencephalogram, CT scan, and magnetic resonance imaging (MRI) study, and generally laboratory tests are within normal range. Comprehensive psychiatric assessment provides additional information.

Nursing Diagnosis:

Deficient Knowledge:

Disease progression and care of the dementia patient

Desired Outcome: By the time the diagnosis of Alzheimer's disease is confirmed, significant other/family relay accurate information about the course of the disease and the role they will play in the care of their loved one.

INTERVENTIONS	RATIONALES
Provide significant other/family information about the staging of the disease and changes to expect in their loved one.	The significant other and family play integral roles in the care of their loved one. Initially, they are the informants, providing information that facilitates diagnosis; they move into role of advocate, then primary caregivers, and finally patient supporter. Staging is discussed in introductory data.
Provide written information regarding educational resources, such as *The Thirty-Six Hour Day* (1999) by Mace and Rabins, and support groups.	The cited book presents a compilation of family experiences with the disorder at different stages. Although there are other helpful books, this one remains the definitive resource for family caregivers. Support groups for family members offer an ongoing, practical socioeducational source, even in the early stage. They provide a safe place to explore issues such as whether or not the patient should stop driving; whether other people should be told about the diagnosis; whether the patient should wear an ID bracelet or carry a card indicating a dementia diagnosis; what the healthy spouse should do to handle the sexual desires of the affected spouse when the unaffected spouse no longer feels as though he or she has an adult relationship anymore.
Coach the family to use all their senses and past memories in talking with their loved one.	Families feel more comfortable and are more likely to continue to interact with the patient if they know that reduced animation in the patient's face is part of the disease. Conversation may have noticeable pauses with less spontaneous speech; conversations should be short and simple. Reassuring the patient decreases overconcern about minor matters; touch continues to be important; and sharing important memories from the past helps maintain links to patient even if the response is minimal.
Teach about safety issues.	Safety issues become the responsibility of the caregiver early in the disorder. The Alzheimer's patient needs room to pace and fails to notice scatter rugs, spills on the floor, and changes in floor elevations, which make falls more likely. Other safety concerns deal with wandering, forgetting the stove is turned on, and using toxic substances inappropriately.
Provide information about legal matters.	Decisions about durable power of attorney need to be decided in the early stage of the disease when the patient is still competent. Legal counsel may be desirable for decisions regarding financial matters.
Provide information about health care resources.	The job of the family caregiver is overwhelming. Family members need to consider use of adult day care centers and varieties of respite care, even in the early stage of the illness. Use of home health services also may be of assistance to the caregiver.
Teach strategies to deal with behavioral issues such as wandering, rummaging, incontinence, difficulty following directions, and profound memory loss.	The more knowledge the family has regarding strategies to deal with these various behaviors, the better they will be able to care for the patient.

••• **Related NIC and NOC labels:** *NIC:* Teaching: Disease Process; Teaching: Procedure/Treatment *NOC:* Knowledge: Illness Care; Knowledge: Disease Process

Nursing Diagnosis:

Risk for Injury

related to impaired judgment and inability to recognize danger in the environment

Desired Outcome: Patient remains free of signs and symptoms of injury.

INTERVENTIONS	RATIONALES
Assess degree of impairment in patient's ability. Assist caregiver to identify risks and potential hazards that may cause harm in patient's environment and the necessary interventions that must be made to ensure patient's safety.	Patients with impulsive behavior are at increased risk for harm because they are less able to control their own behaviors. Patients may have visual/perceptual deficits that increase risk of falls. Caregivers need heightened awareness of potential risks in the environment and need to take appropriate action.
Eliminate or minimize identified environmental risks.	Because a person with a cognitive deficit is unable to take responsibility for basic safety needs, the caregiver must eliminate as many risks as possible: take knobs off of stove, remove scatter rugs, place a safety gate at the top and bottom of stairs, and make sure doors to outside are locked.
Routinely monitor patient's behavior. Initiate interventions to prevent negative behaviors from escalating.	Close observation of patient's behavior allows early identification of problematic behaviors (e.g., increasing agitation) and enables early intervention.
Use distraction or redirection of patient's attention when agitated or dangerous behavior such as climbing out of bed occurs.	Using patient's distractibility avoids confrontation and maintains safety.
Ensure that patient wears an ID bracelet providing name, phone number, and diagnosis. Do not allow patient to have access to stairways or exits.	Because of memory deficits and confusion, these patients may not be able to provide this basic identifying information. The ID bracelet facilitates patient's safe return.
Ensure that doors to outside are locked. Make sure there is supervision and/or activities if patient is regularly awake at night.	Taking appropriate preventive measures facilitates safety without constant supervision. Activities keep patient occupied and limit wandering.
Ensure that patient is dressed appropriately for weather/physical environment and individual need.	Patients with cognitive disorders many times experience seasonal disorientation. In addition, Alzheimer's disease affects the hypothalamic gland, making the person feel cold. The patient is not able to make appropriate choices regarding dress.
Inspect patient's skin during care activities.	Identification of rashes, lacerations, and areas of ecchymosis enables necessary treatment and signals need for closer monitoring and protective interventions.
Attend to nonverbal expression of physiologic discomfort.	Patient may lack ability to express needs clearly but may give clue of a problem by grimacing, sweating, doubling over, or panting.
Monitor for medication side effects; signs of overmedication, for example, gastrointestinal (GI) upset; extrapyramidal symptoms; and orthostatic hypotension.	Drugs easily build up to toxic levels in older adults, and patient may not be able to report any signs or symptoms that would indicate drug toxicity.

●●● **Related NIC and NOC labels:** *NIC:* Environmental Management: Safety; Surveillance: Safety; Fire-Setting Precautions; Risk Identification; Security Enhancement; Fall Prevention *NOC:* Safety Behavior: Home Physical Environment; Safety Status: Falls Occurrence

Nursing Diagnosis:

Disturbed Thought Processes

related to physiologic changes secondary to progressive course of Alzheimer's disease

Desired Outcome: Patient remains calm and displays fewer undesirable behaviors.

INTERVENTIONS	RATIONALES
Provide a predictable environment with orientation cues.	A calm environment with scheduled activities, adequate lighting, low noise level, calendars, clocks, and frequent verbal orientation helps maintain patient's sense of calm and security.
Always address patient by name.	Patients may respond to own name long after they no longer recognize their significant others. Names are an integral part of self-identity; using a person's name is a part of reality orientation.

Continued

INTERVENTIONS	RATIONALES
Communicate with patient using a low voice, slow speech, and eye contact.	Deliberate communication techniques such as these increase patient's attention and chance for comprehension. Calm begets calm.
Break directions into a simple step-by-step process, giving one direction at a time and using simple and clear words.	As the disease progresses, patient's ability to comprehend complex directions and interactions diminishes greatly. Simplicity is the key to effective communication.
Encourage patient's response, allow pauses in interaction, and use open-ended comments and phrases.	These interventions invite a verbal response.
Listen carefully to the content of patient's speech even if it is incomprehensible.	The patient may be having difficulty processing and decoding messages. However, listeners need to continue to show interest and encouragement to keep communication going.
Offer interpretations regarding patient's statements, meanings, and words. If patient struggles to find a word, supply the word if possible.	Assisting patient in processing words promotes continuing communication efforts and decreases frustration.
Avoid negative comments, taking argumentative stands, confrontations, and criticism.	These aggressive responses only serve to increase frustration, agitation, and inappropriate behaviors. Cognitively impaired patients have no internal controls over their thinking and communications.
Engage patient in conversation about real events and real people.	Patients who are encouraged and allowed to ruminate about people and events that are not real will experience greater disorientation.
Monitor for presence of hallucinations. Observe patient for verbal and nonverbal cues of responding to hallucinations. Validate patient's hallucinatory experiences.	Validating that patient is hearing voices allows some discussion of fears associated with the experience and permits assurance that the experience is part of the illness.
Allow patient to hoard safe objects.	This provides patient with a sense of security.
Provide useful and productive outlets for patient to engage in repetitive activities, for example, folding and unfolding laundry, collecting junk mail, dusting, and sweeping floors.	This measure acknowledges that repetitive activities are a normal expression of illness but channels these activities in a way that increases patient's self-esteem and may decrease restlessness.

••• **Related NIC and NOC labels:** *NIC:* Dementia Management: Hallucination Management; Anxiety Reduction; Environmental Management: Safety; Active Listening *NOC:* Distorted Thought Control

Nursing Diagnosis:

Disturbed Sensory Perceptions: Visual or Auditory

related to altered sensory reception, transmission, and/or integration

Desired Outcomes: Patient demonstrates improved response to stimuli. Caregiver identifies and controls external factors that contribute to sensory/perceptual disturbances.

INTERVENTIONS	RATIONALES
Encourage use of assistive devices, corrective lenses, and hearing aids.	This measure enhances sensory input and reduces misinterpretation of stimuli.
Ensure that interpersonal communication and environment are geared to reality orientation.	Reality cues (e.g., calendars, clocks, notes, cards, signs, seasonal cues) are necessary in the environment. Interpersonal communication must include verbal reminders of time, place, and person in order to reduce confusion and promote coping with frustrating struggles of misperception and being disoriented and confused. Visual clues provide concrete reminders that promote recognition and may help with memory gaps, increasing independence.
Ensure that the environment is quiet, calm, and visually nondistracting.	These qualities help to avoid visual/auditory overload.
Provide touch to patient in a caring way.	Touch enhances perception of self and body boundaries, as well as communicates caring.

Continued

INTERVENTIONS	RATIONALES
Involve patient in activities that enable use of remaining skills.	Activities such as folding laundry, clearing the table, and watering plants provide outlets for the patient that support dignity and provide pleasure and satisfaction.
Use reminiscence therapy with props such as photo albums, old music, historic events, and mementos. Encourage patient to talk about memories and feelings attached to these items.	This measure aids in preservation of self by recalling past accomplishments and events, increases patient's sense of security, and encourages sharing that keeps patient linked to others socially.
Encourage intellectual activity such as word games, discussion of current events, and story telling.	This provides patient with normalcy and connection to others and the world and stimulates remaining cognitive abilities.
Advise caregiver to facilitate spiritual activities, including Bible study, participation in worship services, singing hymns, visitation by clergy or church members, or televised church services.	Spiritual needs remain important. There is no certainty that because cognitive decline occurs, spirituality in anyway declines in awareness and importance.
Suggest that caregiver accompany patient on short outings in the car, taking walks, and going shopping.	This decreases sense of isolation, increases physical stamina, and provides sensory pleasure.
Advise caregiver to involve patient in social activities as tolerated.	Social activities involving crafts, family parties, socialization groups at day care center, and involvement with pets help maintain some level of social contact and sensory pleasure.

••• **Related NIC and NOC labels:** *NIC:* Dementia Management; Environmental Management; Reminiscence Therapy; Surveillance: Safety; Reality Orientation; Communication Enhancement: Visual Deficit; Recreation Therapy; Communication Enhancement: Hearing Deficit
NOC: Cognitive Orientation; Distorted Thought Control

Nursing Diagnosis:

Anticipatory Grieving

related to awareness on part of patient and significant other/family that something is seriously wrong as changes in memory and behaviors are increasingly evident

Desired Outcome: Patient and family discuss loss and participate in planning for the future.

INTERVENTIONS	RATIONALES
Encourage patient and family to discuss feelings associated with anticipated losses.	This conveys the message that grief is a normal and expected reaction to the diagnosis of Alzheimer's disease.
Acknowledge expressions of anger and statements of despair and hopelessness, such as, "I and my family would be better off if I were dead."	Feelings of anger may be patient's way of dealing with underlying feelings of despair. Despairing and hopeless statements may be indicative of suicidal ideation. These should be explored and appropriate action taken to protect patient from self-directed violence (see **Risk for Suicide,** p. 763, in "Major Depression").
Provide honest answers and do not give false reassurances or gloomy predictions.	Honesty promotes a trusting relationship and open communication. False reassurances or predictions of gloom are not helpful.
Discuss with patient and significant other/family ways they can plan for the future.	Participation in problem solving increases patient's and family's sense of control.
Emphasize that this is a disease in which research is active and ongoing, as well as the possibility the disease will progress slowly.	Real hope may exist for the future.
Assist patient/significant other/family to identify strengths they see in themselves, each other, and in available support systems.	This emphasizes that there are supports and resources to help work through grief.
Encourage family to participate in a support group for caregivers of Alzheimer's patients.	Support groups not only provide valuable information but also communicate to caregivers that they are not alone as they struggle to manage the illness.

••• **Related NIC and NOC labels:** *NIC:* Coping Enhancement; Anticipatory Guidance; Caregiver Support; Family Support; Hope Instillation; Support System Enhancements; Decision-Making Support

Nursing Diagnosis:

Risk for Caregiver Role Strain

related to severity of patient's illness, duration of care required, and complexity and number of caregiving tasks required

Desired Outcome: Caregiver exhibits behaviors consistent with a healthy lifestyle.

INTERVENTIONS	RATIONALES
Assess caregiver's physical/emotional/spiritual condition and the caregiving demands that are present.	This assessment helps to determine individual care needs of caregiver.
Determine caregiver's level of responsibility, involvement in, and anticipated duration of care involved.	This helps caregiver realistically assess what is involved in a commitment to providing care.
Identify strengths of caregiver and patient.	This identifies positive aspects of each so that they may be incorporated into daily activities.
Encourage caregiver to discuss personal perspective and views about the situation.	This allows venting of concerns and provides opportunity for validation and acceptance of caregiver's issues.
Explore available supports and resources.	This enables evaluation of adequacy of current resources. For example, "What is currently used? Is it effective? What else is needed?"
Encourage and offer to facilitate family conference to develop plan for family involvement in care activities.	The more people that are involved in care, the less risk that one person will become overwhelmed.
Identify additional resources, including financial, legal, and respite care.	These issues of concern can add to the burden of caregiving if not resolved.
Identify equipment needs/resources and other environmental adaptations.	Appropriate equipment and environmental modifications promote patient safety and ease the care burden on the primary caregiver.
Teach caregiver/family techniques and strategies to deal with acting out and disoriented behaviors, as well as incontinence and other physical challenges.	This increases sense of control and competency of caregiver and family.
Teach caregiver the importance of continuing own activities.	Risk of caregiver burden, burnout, and stress is greatly diminished if caregiver takes time for self, for example, continuing a hobby, pursuing social activities, and taking care of personal needs.
Encourage and help caregiver/family to plan for changes that may be necessary, such as home care services, use of adult day care, and eventual placement in a long-term facility.	Planning is essential for these eventualities. As the disease progresses, the burden of care outstrips the resources of the caregiver.

••• Related NIC and NOC labels: *NIC:* Caregiver Support; Coping Enhancement; Respite Care; Decision-Making Support; Family Support; Support System Enhancement; Family Involvement Promotion; Home Maintenance Assistance; Anticipatory Guidance *NOC:* Caregiver Lifestyle Disruption; Caregiver Well-Being

Nursing Diagnosis:

Deficient Knowledge:

Rationale, potential side effects, and interventions for side effects of prescribed medications

Desired Outcome: Immediately following teaching, caregiver and/or family verbalize accurate information about the rationale for use of certain medications, their common side effects, and methods for dealing with those side effects.

INTERVENTIONS	RATIONALES
Describe the physiologic action of cholinesterase inhibitors and how they improve cognition.	There are four cholinesterase inhibitors. Tacrine (Cognex) was the first to be developed and is no longer prescribed. The three others in this category including donepezil (Aricept), rivastigmine tartrate (Exelon), and galantine (Razadyne, formerly Reminyl) do not cure Alzheimer's disease. Instead, they slow cognitive decline by slowing breakdown of acetylcholine released by intact cholinergic neurons.
Advise patient, caregiver, and family that these drugs will return patient's function to the level that was present 6-12 mo before the medication was started.	This is a significant improvement and may delay nursing home placement for as much as a year.
Teach the side-effect profile of the specific prescribed medication and methods for dealing with those effects as follows:	Knowledge about expected side effects and adverse effects is important for promoting adherence to the therapeutic regimen.
- Be alert for headache, fatigue, dizziness, confusion, nausea, vomiting, diarrhea, upset stomach, poor appetite, abdominal pain, rhinitis, and skin rash.	These are common side effects, which, if severe, should be reported to prescriber for possible decrease in dosage or gradual discontinuation.
- Take drug exactly as prescribed around the clock and on an empty stomach.	This helps ensure medication effectiveness.
- If GI upset occurs, administer with meals.	A full stomach may decrease gastric upset.
- Maintain appointments for regular blood work and medical follow-up while adjusting to drug.	This is especially important if patient has preexisting medical conditions, such as renal, liver, or cardiac disease, because these drugs may affect these organs.
- Do not abruptly discontinue drug.	This can cause cognitive disorder.
- Avoid use in pregnancy.	Safety is not established.
- Caution is necessary for patients with renal and hepatic disease, seizures, sick sinus syndrome, and GI bleeding.	These drugs can worsen these conditions.
- Avoid concomitant use with nonsteroidal antiinflammatory drugs.	Concomitant use may increase effects and risk of toxicity.
- Concomitant use with anticholinergic agents may decrease available acetylcholine in the brain and lead to increased confusion.	The action of cholinesterase inhibitors is to inhibit action of cholinesterase, thus elevating acetylcholine levels in the cortex.
Describe the physiologic effects of memantine (Namenda).	Memantine targets the N-methyl-D-aspartate receptors, another chemical and structural system involved in memory. It is the first drug to be developed that targets symptoms during the moderate to severe stages of Alzheimer's disease.
See care plans for "Major Depression," p. 761, "Anxiety Disorders," p. 737, and "Schizophrenia," p. 769, for a review of antidepressants, anxiolytics, and antipsychotic medications.	Patients with Alzheimer's disease may also suffer from depression, anxiety, and psychosis.

••• **Related NIC and NOC labels:** *NIC:* Teaching: Prescribed Medication *NOC:* Knowledge: Medication

ADDITIONAL NURSING DIAGNOSES/PROBLEMS:

"Prolonged Bedrest" for **Constipation**   p. 67

"Psychosocial Support" for nursing diagnoses   p. 73
    as appropriate

"Psychosocial Support for the Patient's Family   p. 87
    and Significant Other" for nursing diagnoses
    as appropriate

"Anxiety Disorders" for **Compromised Family**   p. 741
    Coping

"Bipolar Disorder" for **Imbalanced Nutrition:**   p. 748
    Less Than Body Requirements

Self-Care Deficit   p. 748

✓ PATIENT-FAMILY TEACHING AND DISCHARGE PLANNING

The patient with dementia—Alzheimer's type progresses through predictable stages, each with characteristic symptoms and behaviors that directly affect the ability to effectively process and use new information. As the disease progresses, the patient requires increasing amounts of physical care, and the caregiver/family require information and support. Dementia is a family disease.

As soon as the diagnosis is made, education of the family begins. They need information on the nature and expected progress of the disease and use of memory triggers; establishment of a schedule for basic activities, such as bathing, toileting, meals, and naps; monitoring for intake and output, weight, and skin status; recognition of nonverbal indications of needs and problems; use of redirection and distraction to reduce difficult behaviors; identification of new symptoms or changes; physical and mental activities; necessary environmental modifications, safety measures, and legal issues; sources of information and support; and community resources for caregiving assistance and respite.

Teaching must be geared to a time when medication has begun to lift mood and clear thinking processes; otherwise, it is a wasted effort. Verbal teaching should be simple and supplemented with reading materials the patient and/or significant other and family can refer to at a later time. Ensure that follow-up treatment is scheduled and that patient and/or significant other and family understand the need to get prescriptions filled and to take medication as prescribed. Consider whether or not patient has transportation available to get to follow-up treatment. Psychiatric home care might be a valuable part of the discharge planning to facilitate compliance with the discharge plan. In addition, provide patient and/or significant other/ family with verbal and written information about the following issues:

✓ Nature and expected course of Alzheimer's disease.

✓ Medications, including drug name; purpose; dosage; frequency; precautions; drug-drug, food-drug, and herb-drug interactions; and potential side effects.

✓ Strategies to deal with difficult behaviors.

✓ Strategies to maintain patient safety.

✓ Importance of self-care for the caregiver.

✓ Importance of using all available supports to aid in caregiving.

✓ Importance of caregiver and family engaging in honest expression of feelings and confronting negative emotions.

✓ Importance of caregiver using relaxation techniques to minimize stress.

✓ Importance of maintaining or achieving spiritual well-being for patient and caregiver.

✓ Referrals to community resources for support and education. Additional information can be obtained by contacting the following organizations:

- Alzheimer's Association at *www.alz.org*. It provides a 24-hour hotline, free publications, and information for local chapters. *Worship Services for People with Alzheimer's Disease and Their Families: A Handbook* is also available through this organization.
- American Association of Retired Persons (AARP) at *www.aarp.org*. This is an advocacy group for elderly; it also provides (for a reasonable fee) training materials associated with reminiscence therapy.
- National Institute on Aging (NIA) at *www.nia.nih.gov*. Alzheimer's Disease Education and Reference Center (ADEAR) is available through NIA.

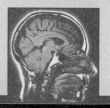

Major Depression 99

OVERVIEW/PATHOPHYSIOLOGY

Major depression is one of the mood disorders, a category of disorders characterized by profound sadness or apathy, irritability, or elation. These disorders rank among the most serious and poorly diagnosed and treated of the health problems in the United States. Major depression is defined as an illness characterized by either depression or the loss of interest in nearly all activities. The symptoms must be present for at least 2 wk. At least four other symptoms must be present from the following list: changes in appetite or weight, sleep, and psychomotor activity; feelings of worthlessness and guilt; difficulty concentrating or making decisions; and recurrent thoughts of death or suicidal ideation, plans, or attempts.

Major depression affects emotional, cognitive, behavioral, and spiritual dimensions. Depression may range from mild-to-moderate states to severe states with or without psychotic features. Major depression can begin at any age, although it usually begins in the mid-20s and 30s. The risk factors for depression include prior history of depression, family history of depression, prior suicide attempts, female gender, age of onset younger than 40 yr of age, postpartum period, medical comorbidity, lack of social support, stressful life events, personal history of sexual abuse, and current substance abuse. There are many theories to explain causation of depression. Research supports influence of the following factors: sleep disturbance; effects of pharmacologic substances, including many of the antihypertensive, steroidal, cardiovascular, and antipsychotic medications; neuronal factors that involve injury or malfunction of the brain, such as stroke, Parkinson's disease, and deficiencies in neurotransmitters; endocrinologic factors, such as thyroid dysfunction; genetic factors; and psychodynamic factors.

HEALTH CARE SETTING

Primarily primary care settings, that is, offices of private psychiatrist, psychologist, or psychiatric nurse practitioner or clinics with occasional brief acute care hospitalization for very severe depression, especially if there is serious suicide threat.

ASSESSMENT

The assessment of major depression involves much more than an assessment of mood. It is a holistic disorder that results in changes in self-attitude (feelings of self-worth), as well as vital sense (sense of physical well-being) and spiritual sense.

Feelings, attitudes, and knowledge: Negative feelings expressed include sadness, lack of joy and happiness about anything, shame, humiliation, fear of reprisals if others find out about depression, denial, anger, fear of experiencing a relapse, and fear of passing the disorder on to children.

Signs of low mood: Withdrawal from activities that once provided pleasure, as well as from social interactions; negativism expressed in excessive skepticism and stubborn resistance to suggestions, orders, or instructions from others; and unhappiness expressed in persistent sadness or frequent crying.

Signs of lowered self-attitude: Self-deprecating, guilty, or self-blaming comments are common, as well as expressions of hopelessness.

Signs of decreased vital sense: A depressed person may neglect personal appearance or let assignments, tasks, and projects slide. Decreased energy is very common, with the depressed person complaining of fatigue and difficulty getting activities started, especially in the early morning hours. A decreased ability to concentrate makes it difficult for individuals to think through a problem. The inability to make choices becomes apparent even with simple decisions that were previously made routinely.

Spiritual issues: Depression carries with it many negative experiences, such as marital and family problems, divorce, and unemployment, which contribute to the downward spiral of self-appraisals. Depression can lead to a crisis in faith in self, others, life, and ultimately God. This loss of faith and hope contributes significantly to the risk of suicide.

Additional signs: Some depressed individuals experience decreased appetite leading to weight loss. Others experience an increase in appetite and weight. A change in sleep pattern is characteristic of depression, with many depressed individuals awakening in the early morning hours between 2 AM and 6 AM, whereas others experience a need for excessive sleep and have difficulty awakening. A decline in sexual interest and activity is characteristic of depressed individuals.

Suicidality: Suicide assessment is critical with depressed patients and includes questions to determine the presence of suicidal ideation and the lethality of any plan. Essential questions to ask include:

- Have you thought of hurting yourself?
- Are you presently thinking about hurting yourself?
- If you have been thinking about suicide, do you have a plan?

- What is the plan?
- Have you thought about what life would be like if you were no longer a part of it?

A previous history of suicide attempts combined with depression places the patient at high risk in the present for attempting suicide. A patient whose depression is lifting is at higher risk for suicide than a severely depressed individual. The improvement may result in an increase in energy. This increased energy is not enough to make the patient feel good or hopeful, but it is enough to carry out a suicidal plan.

DIAGNOSTIC TESTS

Although there are physical changes such as abnormal sleep electroencephalograms (EEGs) that coincide with sleep disturbances, sleep EEGs are not used to diagnose depression. The diagnosis of depression is made through history, interview of patient and family, and observation of verbal and nonverbal behaviors. A number of effective scales are available to quantify the degree of depression, such as the Zung Self-Rating Depression Scale, the Beck Depression Inventory, and the Geriatric Depression Scale.

Nursing Diagnosis:

Deficient Knowledge:

Causes, signs and symptoms, and treatment of depression

Desired Outcome: By discharge (if inpatient) or after 4 wk of outpatient treatment, patient and significant other verbalize accurate information about at least two of the possible causes of depression, four of the signs and symptoms of depression, and use of medications, psychotherapy, and/or electroconvulsive therapy (ECT) as treatment.

INTERVENTIONS	RATIONALES
Inform patient and significant other that depression is a physiologic disorder caused by the interplay of many factors such as stress, loss, imbalance in brain chemistry, and genetics.	Many people believe that depression is caused by character weakness. This belief contributes to the stigma experienced by the person suffering with depression and interferes with seeking treatment.
Inform patient and significant other about the major symptoms of depression.	Many people believe depression equates with sadness and fail to recognize the many other signs and symptoms that make this a holistic disorder. These include sadness and loss of interest in normal activities, plus at least four of the following: changes in appetite or weight, sleep, or psychomotor activity; feelings of worthlessness and guilt; difficulty concentrating or making decisions; recurrent thoughts of death or suicidal ideation, plans, or attempts. If the depressed individual displays sadness through irritability, the conclusion that depression is present may be missed, and consequently, necessary treatment may be delayed or avoided entirely.
Inform patient and significant other that depression is treatable.	Medications are usually indicated for treatment. They do not solve the stressors or problems that may have precipitated the depression, but they provide the energy to deal with these issues. Antidepressants or psychotherapy or a combination of both generally relieves the symptoms of depression in weeks.
Inform patient and significant other about ECT if this is appropriate.	Many antidepressant drugs take 3 wk or more to lift the mood. In the meantime, ECT may be used to achieve more rapid results and may provide necessary protection for the suicidal patient. Patient and significant other/family may fear ECT. This intervention provides an opportunity for education that presents ECT as a positive treatment alternative.

••• **Related NIC and NOC labels:** *NIC:* Teaching: Disease Process; Teaching: Procedures/Treatment *NOC:* Knowledge: Illness Care; Knowledge: Disease Process

Nursing Diagnosis:

Hopelessness

related to losses, stresses, and basic symptoms of depression

Desired Outcome: By discharge (if inpatient) or by the end of 4 wk of outpatient treatment, patient verbalizes feelings and acceptance of life situations over which he or she has no control, demonstrates independent problem-solving techniques to take control over life, and does not demonstrate or verbalize suicidality.

INTERVENTIONS	RATIONALES
Identify unhealthy behaviors used to cope with feelings.	Patient may have tried to overcome feelings of hopelessness with harmful and ineffective behaviors (e.g., withdrawal, substance abuse, avoidance). Recognizing these behaviors provides an opportunity for change.
Encourage patient to identify and verbalize feelings and perceptions.	The process of identifying feelings that underlie and drive behaviors enables patients to begin taking control of their lives.
Identify individual signs of hopelessness.	This helps focus attention on areas of individual need. These signs may include decreased physical activity and social withdrawal.
Express hope to patient in a low-key manner.	Patient may feel hopeless, but it is helpful to hear positive expressions from others.
Help patient identify areas of life that are under his or her control.	Patient's emotional state may interfere with problem solving. Assistance may be required to identify areas that are under his or her control and to have clarity about options for taking control.
Encourage patient to assume responsibility for own self-care, for example, setting realistic goals, scheduling activities, and making independent decisions.	Helping patient set realistic goals increases feelings of control and provides satisfaction when goals are achieved, thereby decreasing feelings of hopelessness.
Help patient identify areas of life situation that are not within his or her ability to control. Discuss feelings associated with this lack of control.	Patient needs to recognize and resolve feelings associated with inability to control certain life situations before acceptance can be achieved and hopefulness becomes possible.
Encourage patient to examine spiritual supports that may provide hope.	Many people find that spiritual beliefs and practices are a great source of hope.
Conduct a suicide assessment to determine level of suicide risk.	High risk will necessitate hospitalization.
Ask patient to enter into a "No Harm Contract" whereby he or she makes a commitment not to harm self.	Unwillingness to enter into a "No Harm Contract" is indication for hospitalization. The rationale for the contract is that people usually honor commitments they make. In addition, agreeing with a nurse or physician not to harm self communicates an awareness that the nurse and/or physician cares about patient's safety.
Administer antidepressant medication or teach importance of taking medication as prescribed (for additional interventions, see **Risk for Suicide**).	Suicidal thinking is a symptom of depression that is ameliorated through appropriate medication.

••• Related NIC and NOC labels: *NIC:* Crisis Intervention; Hope Installation; Spiritual Support; Suicide Prevention; Decision-Making Support; Patient Contracting; Self-Modification Assistance *NOC:* Mood Equilibrium; Decision Making; Depression Control

Nursing Diagnosis:

Risk for Suicide

related to depressed mood and feelings of worthlessness

Desired Outcome: By discharge (if inpatient) or by the end of 4 wk (if outpatient), patient expresses and demonstrates that he or she is free of suicidal thinking.

INTERVENTIONS	RATIONALES
Complete an initial suicide assessment (see specific questions under "Assessment").	The degree of hopelessness expressed by the patient is important in assessing risk for suicide. The more the patient has thought out the plan, the greater the risk. Risk for suicide is increased if the patient has a history of a previous attempt or there is family history of suicide and depression. Patients who display impulsive behaviors are more likely to attempt suicide without giving clues. Patients who are experiencing psychotic thinking, especially when there are "voices" that encourage self-harm, are at great risk. Use of alcohol/substance abuse in the presence of any of the above risk factors increases the overall risk for a suicide attempt. A high risk for suicide should prompt hospitalization.
Reassess for suicidality, especially during times of change.	Changes such as patient's mood improving, medication regimen being altered, discharge planning being initiated, and increasing withdrawal are all signals to reassess suicidality. Suicide risk is greatest in the first few weeks after treatment is begun. The patient may be feeling a little better but not well enough to feel hopeful and may have regained enough energy to actually act on what seemed to be just suicidal thoughts.
Ask patient to enter into a "No Harm Contract" whereby he or she makes a commitment not to harm self.	This contract is signed by patient and nurse. It may also include other information such as telephone numbers of crisis hotlines, police, or other emergency personnel for patient to call if suicidal thinking becomes more intense and patient doubts his or her ability to honor the "No Harm Contract." Unwillingness to enter into a "No Harm Contract" is indication for hospitalization. The rationale for the contract is that people usually honor commitments they make. In addition, agreeing with a nurse or physician not to harm self communicates an awareness that the nurse and/or physician care about patient's safety.
Administer antidepressant medication or instruct patient regarding importance of taking medication as prescribed.	Suicidal thinking is a symptom of depression, which is ameliorated through appropriate medication.
Teach significant other safety precautions and to be alert for changes in patient's behavior and/or verbalization that would indicate an increase in suicidal thinking.	Using available support provides a safety net for patient and communicates that he or she is not alone but that others are concerned and involved in care.
If patient is hospitalized:	
Monitor q15min for moderate risk or provide constant one-on-one observation for serious risk. Place in room close to nurses' station. Do not assign to a single room. Accompany patient to all off-unit activities. Ask patient to remain in view of staff at all times.	Providing close observation may prevent suicidal attempts.
Remove items such as belts, scarves, razor blades, shoelaces, scissors—anything that could be used for self-harm. Check all items brought into unit by patients. Instruct family members to avoid bringing into the unit any hazardous items.	This provides environmental safety and removes potential suicide weapons.
Provide supervision when patient is in bathroom—door must remain open with staff member outside.	It is important to remove all opportunities to engage in self-harmful behaviors.
Make sure that patient swallows medications that are administered.	This prevents saving up medications to overdose or discarding and not taking.
Ensure that nursing rounds are made at frequent but irregular intervals, especially at times that are predictably busy for the staff, that is, change of shift, toward early morning.	It is important that staff surveillance not be predictable; otherwise, patient would be able to identify a possible suicide time. In addition, it is essential to maintain awareness of patient's location at all times.
Routinely check environment for hazards and ensure environmental safety.	Minimizing opportunities for self-harm (e.g., keeping doors, windows, and access to stairways and roof locked and monitoring cleaning, chemical, and repair supplies) is an ongoing concern requiring constant vigilance.

••• **Related NIC and NOC labels:** *NIC:* Area Restriction; Behavior Management: Self-Harm; Environmental Management: Safety; Patient Contracting; Risk Identification; Security Enhancement; Surveillance: Safety; Suicide Prevention *NOC:* Impulse Control; Suicide Self-Restraint

Nursing Diagnosis:

Dysfunctional Grieving

related to actual or perceived loss

Desired Outcome: By discharge (if inpatient) or by the end of 4 wk of outpatient treatment, patient demonstrates progress in dealing with stages of grief at own pace, participates in work/self-care activities at own pace, and verbalizes a sense of progress toward resolution of grief and hope for the future.

INTERVENTIONS	RATIONALES
Assess losses that have occurred in the patient's life. Discuss the meaning these losses have had for patient.	Many people deny the importance/impact of a loss. They fail to recognize, acknowledge, or talk about their pain and act as if everything is fine. This, then, has a cumulative effect on the individual. Denial requires physical and psychic energy. When individuals become clinically depressed, they likely do so in a physically and emotionally depleted state.
Discuss cultural practices and religious beliefs and ways in which patient has dealt with past losses.	Cultural practices and religious beliefs influence how people express and accept the grieving process.
Encourage patient to identify and verbalize feelings and examine the relationship between feelings and event/stressor.	Verbalizing feelings in a nonthreatening environment can help patient deal with unrecognized/unresolved issues that may be contributing to depression. It also helps patient connect the response (feeling) to the stressor or precipitating event.
Discuss healthy ways to identify and cope with underlying feelings of hurt, rejection, and anger.	This helps expand patient's repertoire of coping strategies. The presentation of choices for behaving differently can often decrease feeling of being stuck.
If indicated, tell stories of how others have coped with similar situations.	This not only provides possible solutions but also suggests that the problem is manageable.
Teach normal stages of grief and acknowledge the reality of associated feelings, that is, guilt, anger, powerlessness.	This information helps the patient realize the normalcy of feelings and may alleviate some of the guilt generated by these feelings.
Assist patient with naming the problem, identifying need to address the problem differently, and fully describing all aspects of the problem.	Before patient can agree to change, he or she needs clarity about what the problem is.
Help patient identify and recognize early signs of depression and plan ways to alleviate these signs. Assist with formulating a plan that recognizes need for outside support if symptoms continue and/or worsen.	This actively involves patient and conveys the message that patient is not powerless but rather options are available.

••• **Related NIC and NOC labels:** *NIC:* Coping Enhancement; Counseling; Grief Work Facilitation; Emotional Support; Support System Enhancement; Active Listening *NOC:* Coping; Grief Resolution

Nursing Diagnosis:

Self-Esteem: Chronic Low

related to the negative self-appraisal that is symptomatic of depression

Desired Outcome: By discharge (if inpatient) or after 4 wk of outpatient treatment, patient demonstrates behaviors consistent with increased self-esteem.

INTERVENTIONS	RATIONALES
Encourage patient to engage in self-care grooming activities.	Attending to grooming is often an initial step in feeling better about oneself.
Provide positive reinforcement for all observable accomplishments.	Patients with low self-esteem do not benefit from flattery or insincere praise. Honest, positive feedback enhances self-esteem.
Encourage patient to participate in simple recreational activities or art projects, proceeding to more complex activities in a group setting.	Initially patient may be too overwhelmed to engage in activities that involve more than one person.
If patient persists in negativism about self, place a limit on length of time you will listen to negativity.	Time limits allow patient a safe time and place to vent negative feelings and demonstrate thought stopping, the conscious interruption of negative thoughts. For example, agree to 10 min of negativity followed by 10 min of positive comments.
Teach thought-stopping techniques.	Many depressed people engage in self-critical thinking and need to be taught to consciously stop that type of thinking and substitute positive thinking in its place.
Explore patient's personal strengths and suggest making a list to use as a reminder when negative thoughts return.	Having a written list to review can help patient during difficult times.

●●● **Related NIC and NOC labels:** *NIC:* Self-Esteem Enhancement; Cognitive Restructuring; Self-Awareness Enhancement; Socialization Enhancement *NOC:* Self-Esteem

Nursing Diagnosis:

Deficient Knowledge:

Medication use in depression, including potential side effects

Desired Outcome: By discharge (if inpatient) or after 4 wk of outpatient treatment, patient verbalizes accurate information about prescribed medications and their potential side effects.

INTERVENTIONS	RATIONALES
Teach physiologic action of antidepressant and how it alleviates symptoms of depression.	Many depressed patients resist taking medications because they fear becoming "addicted" to the drug. However, the antidepressants are not addictive drugs. Providing the patient with information about the drug's physiologic action helps with adherence.
Caution patient about importance of taking medication at prescribed dose and time interval.	These medications require certain blood levels to be therapeutic; therefore patient needs to take the medication at the dose and time prescribed.
Teach the side-effect profile of the specific prescribed medication, including interventions to combat these effects, for the following drugs.	Each class of antidepressants carries with it a specific side-effect profile. Knowledge about expected side effects, ways to manage these side effects, and the length of time these side effects last is important in ensuring adherence.
Tricyclic antidepressants: amitriptyline (Elavil), desipramine (Norpramin), doxepin (Sinequan), imipramine (Tofranil), nortriptyline (Pamelor), protriptyline (Vivactil), and trimipramine (Surmontil)	These older antidepressant medications are effective in decreasing signs and symptoms of depression but can produce some troublesome side effects, such as anticholinergic effects, fatigue, weight gain, and orthostatic changes.
- Watch for potential for anticholinergic effects, sedation, hypotension, and weight gain.	These are common side effects.
- Drink at least 8 glasses of water a day and add high-fiber foods to diet.	These measures combat constipation, an anticholinergic effect.
- Rise from a sitting position slowly.	Orthostatic hypotension is a potential side effect.
- Suck on sugar-free candy or mints or use sugar-free chewing gum.	These measures combat dry mouth, an anticholinergic effect.

Continued

INTERVENTIONS	RATIONALES
- Establish sleep routine and regular exercise.	Regular sleep and exercise combat feelings of fatigue.
- Limit refined sugars and carbohydrates.	This measure combats weight gain and controls carbohydrate cravings.
- Patients with seizure history need to be monitored for seizures.	Tricyclics lower the seizure threshold.
- Watch for signs of cardiac toxicity. Patients older than 40 yr of age need an electrocardiogram (ECG) evaluation before treatment and periodically thereafter.	These drugs may decrease the vagal influence on the heart secondary to muscarinic blockade and by acting directly on bundle of His to slow conduction. Both effects increase risk of dysrhythmias.
- Watch for possible drug interactions.	The combination of tricyclics with monoamine oxidase (MAO) inhibitors can cause severe hypertension. The combination of tricyclics with central nervous system (CNS) depressants such as alcohol, antihistamines, opioids, and barbiturates can cause severe CNS depression. Because of the anticholinergic effects of tricyclics, any other anticholinergic drug, including over-the-counter antihistamines and sleeping aids, should be avoided.
MAO inhibitors: isocarboxazid (Marplan), phenelzine (Nardil), and tranylcypromine (Parnate)	MAO inhibitors are used when patient has not responded to other antidepressants. When MAO activity is reduced in the CNS, there is increased dopamine, serotonin, norepinephrine, and epinephrine at the receptor sites, thereby promoting an antidepressant effect.
- Watch for potential for mild sedation and hypotension.	These are common side effects.
- Enforce MAO inhibitor restrictions.	MAO inhibitors combined with dietary tyramine can cause a life-threatening hypertensive crisis. Dietary restrictions include avocados; fermented bean curd; fermented soybean; soybean paste; figs; bananas; fermented, smoked, or aged meats; liver; bologna, pepperoni, and salami; dried, cured, fermented, or smoked fish; practically all cheeses; yeast extract; some imported beers; Chianti wine; protein dietary supplements; soups that contain protein extract; shrimp paste; and soy sauce. Large amounts of chocolate, fava beans, ginseng, and caffeine may cause a reaction.
- Watch for possible drug interactions and need to avoid all prescription and over-the-counter drugs unless they have been specifically approved by provider.	MAO inhibitors can interact with many drugs to cause potentially serious results. Use of ephedrine or amphetamines can lead to hypertensive crisis. The interaction of tricyclic antidepressants with MAO inhibitors is discussed above. Selective serotonin reuptake inhibitors (SSRIs) should not be used with MAO inhibitors (see rationale, below). Antihypertensive drugs combined with MAO inhibitors may result in excessive lowering of blood pressure. MAO inhibitors with meperidine (Demerol) can cause hyperpyrexia (excessive elevation of temperature).
SSRIs: fluoxetine (Prozac), fluvoxamine maleate (Luvox), sertraline HCl (Zoloft), paroxetine (Paxil), citalopram (Celexa), and escitalopram (Lexapro)	SSRIs are as effective as tricyclic antidepressants but have a better safety profile and are better tolerated. These agents enhance serotonergic function by inhibiting serotonin uptake, which in turn promotes an anti-depression effect.
- Watch for nausea, headache, nervousness, insomnia, anxiety, agitation, sexual dysfunction, dizziness, fatigue, rash, diarrhea, excessive sweating, and anorexia with weight loss.	These are reported side effects.
- Watch for possible drug interactions.	Interaction with MAO inhibitors can cause serotonin syndrome, a potentially life-threatening event. Symptoms include anxiety, diaphoresis, rigidity, hyperthermia, autonomic hyperactivity, and coma. Because of this possibility, MAO inhibitors should be withdrawn at least 14 days before starting an SSRI, and when an SSRI is discontinued, at least 5 wk should elapse before an MAO inhibitor is given.
Dual-mechanism drugs: venlafaxine (Effexor), nefazodone HCl (Serzone), mirtazapine (Remeron), and duloxetine (Cymbalta)	These drugs inhibit both norepinephrine and serotonin uptake and are used when tricyclics and SSRIs fail to improve symptoms.
- Watch for nausea, somnolence, dizziness, dry mouth, and sweating.	These are common side effects.
- Teach importance of frequent blood pressure (BP) measurements for patients taking venlafaxine.	At doses greater than 200 mg/day, venlafaxine causes an increase in BP.

Continued

INTERVENTIONS	RATIONALES
Selective Norepinephrine Reuptake Inhibitor: reboxetine (Vestra)	
- Watch for anticholinergic side effects, decreased libido, potential for drug interactions.	These are common side effects.
Miscellaneous antidepressants: trazodone (Desyrel), amoxapine (Asendin), bupropion (Wellbutrin), and maprotiline (Ludiomil)	
- Watch for anticholinergic effects (except trazodone), sedation, hypotension, and risks of falling related to dizziness associated with hypotension.	These are common side effects.
- Be aware of risk for seizures.	Risk is moderate with trazodone and increases with amoxapine, bupropion, and maprotiline.
- Be aware of risk of cardiac toxicity. Patients older than 40 yr of age need an ECG evaluation before treatment and periodically thereafter.	Risk is minimal with amoxapine, bupropion, and trazodone. There is significant risk with maprotiline.

••• **Related NIC and NOC labels:** *NIC:* Teaching: Prescribed Medication *NOC:* Knowledge: Medication

---

ADDITIONAL NURSING DIAGNOSES/ PROBLEMS:

"Anxiety" for **Social Isolation**   p. 739

"Bipolar Disorder" for:

    Imbalanced Nutrition: Less Than Body Requirements   p. 748

    Self-Care Deficit   p. 748

"Substance Abuse" for **Interrupted Family Processes**   p. 777

✔ PATIENT-FAMILY TEACHING AND DISCHARGE PLANNING

The patient with major depression experiences a wide variety of symptoms that affect the ability to learn and retain information. Teaching must be geared to a time when medication has begun to lift mood and clear thinking processes; otherwise, it is a wasted effort. Verbal teaching should be simple and supplemented with reading materials the patient and/or significant other and family can refer to at a later time. Ensure that follow-up treatment is scheduled and that patient and/or significant other and family understand the need to get prescriptions filled and importance of taking medication as prescribed. Consider whether or not patient has transportation available to get to follow-up treatment. Psychiatric home care might be a valuable part of the discharge planning to facilitate compliance with the discharge plan. In addition, provide patient and/or significant other/family verbal and written information about the following issues:

✔ Remission/exacerbation aspects of depression.

✔ Medications, including drug name; purpose; dosage; frequency; precautions; drug-drug, food-drug, and herb-drug interactions; and potential side effects.

✔ Thought-stopping techniques for dealing with negativism.

✔ Importance of maintaining a healthy lifestyle—balanced diet, exercise, and regular adequate sleep patterns—to facilitate remaining in remission.

✔ Importance of continuing medication use long after depressive symptoms have gone.

✔ Importance of social support and strategies for obtaining it.

✔ Importance of using constructive coping skills to deal with stress.

✔ Importance of honest expression of feelings and confronting of negative emotions.

✔ Importance of using relaxation techniques to minimize stress.

✔ Importance of maintaining or achieving spiritual well-being.

✔ Importance of follow-up care, including day treatment programs, appointments with psychiatrist and therapists, and vocational rehabilitation program if indicated.

✔ Referrals to community resources for support and education. Additional information can be obtained by contacting the following organizations:

- Depression and Related Affective Disorders Association (DRADA) at *www.drada.org*. This nonprofit organization is composed of individuals with mood disorders, family members, and mental health professionals. It offers information, education, referral, and support services to people nationwide. DRADA sponsors a nationally renowned training program for group leaders.

- Depression Awareness, Recognition, and Treatment Program (D/ART) at (301) 443-4140. D/ART is a national self-help clearinghouse. It provides a list of resources throughout the United States that can help in networking and providing consultative assistance.

- Depression and Bipolar Support Alliance (DBSA) at *www.dbsalliance.org*. The DBSA provides education as well as support to individuals and families impacted by depression and bipolar illnesses.

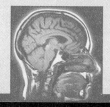

Schizophrenia 100

OVERVIEW/PATHOPHYSIOLOGY

Schizophrenia is a neurobiologic disorder of the brain categorized as a thought disorder with disturbances in thinking, feeling, perceiving, and relating to others and the environment. Schizophrenia is a mixture of both positive and negative symptoms that are present for a significant part of a 1-mo period but with continuous signs of disturbance persisting for at least 6 mo. Positive symptoms are those that exist but should not be present including delusions, hallucinations, thought disorder, disorganized speech, and disorganized or catatonic behavior. Negative symptoms refer to behaviors that should be present but are not, including restriction or flattening in the range and intensity of emotion, reduced fluency and productivity of thought and speech, withdrawal and inability to initiate and persist in goal-directed activity, and inability to experience pleasure. Schizophrenia is considered the most disabling of the major mental disorders, with an estimated 2 million Americans afflicted. Risk factors include being unmarried and younger than 45 years of age for both men and women, having been the product of a difficult birth during the winter, and living in an industrialized urban area as a member of the lower socioeconomic class. Theories of causation include genetics, infectious autoimmune factors, neuroanatomic changes, the dopamine hypothesis, and psychologic factors. There are several subtypes of schizophrenia, including paranoid, disorganized, catatonic, undifferentiated, and residual.

HEALTH CARE SETTING

Most patients with schizophrenia receive treatment across a variety of settings, including inpatient and partial hospitalization, day treatment, psychiatric home care, and crisis stabilization. Community services include assertive community treatment, outpatient therapy, case management, and psychosocial rehabilitation.

ASSESSMENT

Schizophrenia affects all aspects of a person's being. How the individual looks, feels, thinks, interacts with others, and moves in the world are all drastically affected by this disorder. A thorough assessment focuses not only on the bizarre behaviors characteristic of the disease but on the whole person—his or her physical, emotional, social, and spiritual dimensions.

Biologic: A thorough history and physical are essential to rule out medical illness or substance abuse that could cause

the psychiatric symptoms. It is essential to screen for comorbid treatable medical illnesses. People with schizophrenia have a higher mortality rate from physical illness and often have smoking-related illnesses such as emphysema and other pulmonary and cardiac disorders. The patient may appear awkward and uncoordinated, with poor motor skills and abnormalities in eye tracking. It is important before any medications are begun to have a baseline regarding abnormal movements. Use of a standardized assessment of abnormal movement disorders such as the Abnormal Involuntary Movement Scale (AIMS) or the Simpson-Angus Rating Scale is recommended.

Psychologic: Many patients report prodromal symptoms of tension and nervousness, lack of interest in eating, difficulty concentrating, disturbed sleep, decreased enjoyment and loss of interest, restlessness, forgetfulness, depression, social withdrawal from friends, feeling that others are laughing at them, feeling bad for no reason, thinking about religion more, hearing voices or seeing things, and feeling too excited. Most of these symptoms are negative ones.

Appearance: Patient may appear in bizarre and eccentric dress, be disheveled, and have poor hygiene.

Objective behaviors: Patient may display stereotypy (idiosyncratic, repetitive, purposeless movements), echopraxia (involuntary imitation of another's movements), and waxy flexibility (posture held in odd or unusual fixed position for extended periods). Patients may display altered mood states ranging from heightened emotional activity to severely limited emotional responses. Affect, the outward expression of mood, may be described as flat, blunted, or full range, or it may be described as inappropriate. Other common emotional symptoms include affective lability, ambivalence, and apathy.

Delusions: Delusions are beliefs that are held despite clear contradictory evidence. Sometimes they are nonbizarre and plausible; at other times the delusions expressed are bizarre, implausible, and not derived from ordinary life experiences. Delusions of persecution are the most common type. Delusions of grandeur are also commonly expressed. Ideas of reference are delusional ideas in which these patients believe actions of others are directed toward them. Two other forms of delusional thinking include thought broadcasting—the belief that one's thoughts can be heard by others—and thought insertion—the belief that thoughts of others can be inserted into one's mind. It is important to assess content of the delusion; the degree of conviction with which the delusion is held; how extensively other aspects of the patient's life are incorporated into the delusion; the degree of internal consistency, organization, and logic evidenced in the delusion; and the impact exerted on the patient's life by this delusion.

Hallucinations: A hallucination is an alteration in sensory stimulation. Although hallucinations can be experienced in all sensory modalities, auditory hallucinations are the most frequent in schizophrenia. Patients may not spontaneously share their hallucinations, and in order to assess for them, nurses may need to rely on observations of the patient's behavior, including pauses in a conversation during which the patient seems to be preoccupied or appears to be listening to someone other than the interviewer, looking toward the perceived source of a voice, or responding to the voices in some manner.

Disorganized communication: Both speech content and patterns are important to assess. Abrupt shifts in conversational focus are typical of disorganized communication and are referred to as loose association. The most severe shifts may occur after only one or two words, referred to as *word salad*—a jumble of unrelated words; a less severe shift may occur after one or two phrases, referred to as *flight of ideas*; the least severe shift in the focus occurs when a new topic is repeatedly suggested and pursued from the current topic, referred to as *tangentiality*. In addition to these abrupt shifts from one topic to another, the person with schizophrenia experiences thought blocking in which thoughts and psychic activity unexpectedly cease. Language may be difficult to understand and may begin to serve as a tool of self-expression rather than a tool of communication. Sometimes the person creates completely new words, referred to as *neologisms*.

Cognitive impairments: Although cognitive impairments vary widely from patient to patient, several problems are consistent across most patients; these include hypervigilance (increased and sustained attention on external stimuli over an extended time), a diminished ability to distinguish relevant from irrelevant stimuli, familiar cues going unrecognized or being improperly interpreted, and diminished information processing leading to inappropriate or illogical conclusions from available observations and information.

- *Memory and orientation:* Individuals with schizophrenia display impairments in memory and abstract thinking. Although orientation to time, place, and person remains relatively intact unless the person is preoccupied with delusions and hallucinations, all aspects of memory are affected in schizophrenia. Patients experience diminished ability to recall within seconds newly learned information. Short- and long-term memory are affected.

- *Insight and judgment:* Insight and judgment depend on cognitive functions that are frequently impaired in people with schizophrenia.

Social issues: As the disorder progresses, individuals become increasingly socially isolated. People with schizophrenia have difficulty connecting with others on a one-to-one basis. Emotional blunting, inability to form emotional attachments, problems with face and affect recognition, inability to recall past interactions, problems making decisions and using appropriate judgment in difficult situations, and poverty of speech and language all serve to separate and isolate the individual.

Spiritual issues: Persons with schizophrenia may experience delusions and hallucinations with religious content, and some health care providers tend to dismiss all religious verbalizations as psychotic expressions. However, the contrary is true. Religion and spirituality can be a source of comfort to patients dealing with a terrible disease. It is important to assess religious commitment, religious practices, and spiritual issues such as the meaning of the illness to the individual, the role of God, and sources of hope and support.

Suicidality: Suicide assessment is critical in schizophrenia. The presence of psychotic thinking and command hallucinations, coupled with possible substance abuse, increases the suicide risk significantly. It is important to ask questions to determine the presence of suicidal ideation and the lethality of any plan. Essential questions to ask include:
- Have you thought of hurting yourself?
- Are you presently thinking about hurting yourself?
- If you have been thinking about suicide, do you have a plan? What is the plan?
- Have you thought about what life would be like if you were no longer a part of it?

DIAGNOSTIC TESTS

There are no specific tests to diagnose schizophrenia. Diagnosis is made using the diagnostic criteria put forth in *The Diagnostic and Statistical Manual IV* (American Psychiatric Association, 1994) through history, interview of patient and family, and observation of verbal and nonverbal behaviors. There are several reliable rating scales that are useful in the diagnosis of schizophrenia. These include the Scale for the Assessment of Negative Symptoms (SANS), Scale for the Assessment of Positive Symptoms (SAPS), Abnormal Involuntary Movement Scale (AIMS), Brief Psychiatric Rating Scale (BPRS), and Simpson-Angus Rating Scale.

Nursing Diagnosis:

Deficient Knowledge:

Causes, signs and symptoms, and treatment of schizophrenia

Desired Outcome: Before discharge from care facility or after 4 wk of outpatient treatment, patient and/or significant other verbalize accurate information about at least two of the possible causes of schizophrenia, four of the signs and symptoms of the disorder, and the available treatment options.

INTERVENTIONS	RATIONALES
Explain that schizophrenia is a physiologic disorder caused by the interplay of many factors such as stress, genetics, infectious-autoimmune factors, neuroanatomic changes, the dopamine hypothesis, and psychologic factors.	Providing education about the physical basis for the disorder increases understanding and acceptance and decreases blaming behavior. Signs and symptoms are discussed under Assessment.
Inform patient and significant other that there are treatments available for schizophrenia.	Medications are essential to stabilize and maintain patients with schizophrenia. They decrease psychotic thinking, hallucinations, and delusions. Some, but not all, drugs target negative symptoms. However, medications are not enough. Comprehensive treatment involves inpatient and partial hospitalization, day treatment, psychiatric home care, and crisis stabilization. Community services include assertive community treatment, outpatient therapy, case management, and psychosocial rehabilitation.

••• **Related NIC and NOC labels:** *NIC:* Teaching: Disease Process; Teaching: Procedure/Treatment *NOC:* Knowledge: Illness Care; Knowledge: Disease Process

Nursing Diagnosis:

Disturbed Sensory Perception: Auditory

related to disturbance in thought and perception

Desired Outcome: Before discharge from care facility or after 4 wk of outpatient treatment, patient defines and tests reality and recognizes that hallucinations are not part of reality.

INTERVENTIONS	RATIONALES
Evaluate and observe for hallucinations. Redirect back to reality by distracting patient with conversation.	Early assessment enables evaluation of patient's responses to hallucinations and how much time patient focuses on them. It also enables the nurse to assess if hallucinations place patient or others at risk and permits early intervention to protect patient, as well as others.
Ask what the voices are telling the patient.	It is essential to know if "voices" are command hallucinations that tell the patient to harm self or others. This question also communicates that the nurse does not hear the voices while at the same time validates presence of the voices in the patient's reality.
Assure patient that you will provide safety for him or her regardless of what the voices say will happen.	This provides an anchor to reality and decreases patient's fear that harm will occur based on what the voices say.
Avoid touching the patient.	Distortion of reality may lead patient to misinterpret physical touch, which along with excessive environmental stimuli can increase anxiety and precipitate hallucinations or aggressive response.
Determine when anxiety increases. Stay with patient to ensure safety.	Increasing anxiety often precedes hallucinations.
Administer antipsychotic medications as prescribed.	Antipsychotic medications reduce psychotic symptoms, including hallucinations.

Continued

INTERVENTIONS	RATIONALES
Assist patient with increasing social interaction gradually, starting first with one-on-one interaction and progressing to small groups. Be available in a consistent, no-demand, supportive relationship.	Social isolation and lack of interpersonal relationships contribute to use of hallucinations as a substitute for human interaction. A slow, gradual approach to interaction with others based on reality enables some desensitization because interpersonal contacts often precipitate anxiety.
Investigate with patient sources of stress and explain the relationship of anxiety and stress to hallucinations.	Providing information about the relationship of anxiety and stress to hallucinations gives the patient increased control over the occurrence of hallucinations.
Teach patient to verbalize fears and describe methods for managing anxiety and stress constructively.	Verbalization of fears is one method of reducing anxiety. Alternative methods may also prove effective.

●●● **Related NIC and NOC labels:** *NIC:* Hallucination Management; Reality Orientation; Active Listening; Environmental Management; Anxiety Reduction *NOC:* Distorted Thought Control

Nursing Diagnosis:

Deficient Knowledge:

Medications used in schizophrenia, including purpose and potential side effects

Desired Outcome: Before discharge from care facility or after 4 wk of outpatient treatment, patient verbalizes accurate information about the prescribed medications.

INTERVENTIONS	RATIONALES
Teach patient about the physiologic action of antipsychotic medications.	Antipsychotics work by blocking dopamine receptors. People with schizophrenia appear to have excessive dopamine levels. Blocking dopamine decreases hallucinations, delusions, and confusion and improves disorganized speech, behavior, and perceptions.
Teach the following side-effect profiles of the specific prescribed medication, as well as interventions to mitigate the effects.	A knowledgeable patient is likely to report adverse symptoms and know how to intervene properly for others, which optimally will promote adherence.
Traditional antipsychotics: chlorpromazine (Thorazine), thioridazine (Mellaril), mesoridazine (Serentil), acetophenazine (Tindal), loxapine (Loxitane), molindone (Moban), perphenazine (Trilafon), trifluoperazine (Stelazine), thiothixene (Navane), fluphenazine (Prolixin), haloperidol (Haldol), and pimozide (Orap)	Traditional antipsychotics block all dopamine receptors in the central nervous system (CNS) and can produce serious movement disorders, referred to as extrapyramidal side effects (EPS).
Explain that sedation, orthostatic hypotension, and anticholinergic effects can occur.	These are common side effects of traditional antipsychotic drugs.
Teach the patient to be alert for EPS, including acute dystonia (impaired muscle tone), parkinsonism, akathisia (restlessness, agitation), and tardive dyskinesia (involuntary movements of the face, trunk, and limbs) using the AIMS.	These are adverse effects of traditional antipsychotic drugs, with tardive dyskinesia being the most serious. Use of AIMS enables objective quantification of changes in movements and permits early intervention before the appearance of tardive dyskinesia.
Explain the potential for neuroleptic malignant syndrome (NMS).	This is an idiosyncratic hypersensitivity to antipsychotics that is believed to affect the body's thermoregulatory mechanism. It is a rare but serious reaction that carries with it a 4% risk of mortality.
Caution patient that there is a risk for seizures.	Antipsychotics can reduce the seizure threshold and should be used with caution for patients with epilepsy or other seizure disorder.

Continued

INTERVENTIONS	RATIONALES
Teach the importance of avoiding all drugs with anticholinergic actions, including antihistamines and specific over-the-counter sleeping aids.	Drugs with anticholinergic properties intensify the anticholinergic responses to antipsychotic drugs, including dry mouth, constipation, blurred vision, urinary hesitancy, and tachycardia.
Explain the importance of avoiding alcohol and other drugs with CNS-depressant actions, for example, antihistamines, opioids, and barbiturates.	Antipsychotics can intensify CNS depression caused by other drugs.
For patients taking Thorazine, Vesprin, Serentil, Mellaril, Tindal, Prolixin, Trilafon, or Stelazine, teach the importance of avoiding excessive exposure to sunlight, using sunscreen, and wearing protective clothing.	These drugs belong to the phenothiazine class that causes sensitization of the skin to ultraviolet light, thus increasing the chance of severe sunburn.
Teach the patient that sexual dysfunction is a possible side effect and should be reported to the prescriber.	It is important that the patient not just stop the medication but rather report it so that the prescriber can intervene accordingly.
Atypical antipsychotic agents: clozapine (Clozaril), risperidone (Risperdal), olanzapine (Zyprexa), quetiapine (Seroquel), ziprasidone (Geodon), and aripiprazole (Abilify)	Atypical antipsychotics are more selective in blocking specific dopamine receptors. Because of this, they have less risk of EPS.
Patients taking clozapine should be alert for drowsiness and sedation, hypersalivation, tachycardia, constipation, and postural hypotension.	These are common side effects.
Patients taking clozapine need weekly hematologic monitoring for first 6 mo of treatment, and after 6 mo, monitoring is monthly. Advise patient that clozapine will not be dispensed if the monthly blood test is not done.	Agranulocytosis occurs in 1%-2% of patients, with an overall risk of death of about 1 in 5000. Agranulocytosis usually occurs in the first 6 mo.
Patients taking clozapine, especially those with seizure disorder, are at risk for seizures.	Generalized tonic-clonic seizures occur in 3% of patients, and the risk is dose related, with higher incidence in patients receiving doses greater than 600 mg. Patients who have experienced a seizure should be warned not to drive a car or participate in other potentially hazardous activities while on this medication.
Patients taking clozapine should avoid drugs that can suppress bone marrow function such as carbamazepine (Tegretol) and many cancer drugs. Cimetidine and erythromycin increase levels of clozapine, leading to toxicity. Smoking, Tegretol, and phenytoin can decrease levels of clozapine, diminishing its efficacy.	These are drug interactions that can occur with clozapine.
Patients taking risperidone are at risk for insomnia, agitation, anxiety, constipation, nausea, dyspepsia, vomiting, dizziness, and sedation.	These are common side effects.
Patients taking risperidone should be alert for EPS.	This is an adverse effect that is dose related (reported in doses greater than 10 mg/day).
Patients taking olanzapine should be alert for headache, insomnia, constipation, weight gain, akathisia, and tremor.	These are common side effects.
Patients taking quetiapine should be alert for headache, somnolence, constipation, and weight gain.	These are common side effects.
Patients taking ziprasidone (Geodon) who have a history of cardiac disease, low electrolyte levels, or family history of QT prolongation are at risk for electrocardiogram changes, specifically QT prolongation.	These are common side effects.

••• **Related NIC and NOC labels:** *NIC:* Teaching: Prescribed Medication *NOC:* Knowledge: Medication

ADDITIONAL NURSING DIAGNOSES/ PROBLEMS:

"Anxiety Disorders" for:

Ineffective Coping	p. 740
Compromised Family Coping	p. 741

"Bipolar Disorder" for **Self-Care Deficit**   p. 748

"Major Depression" for:

Hopelessness	p. 763
Risk for Suicide	p. 763
Self-Esteem: Chronic Low	p. 765

✔ PATIENT-FAMILY TEACHING AND DISCHARGE PLANNING

The patient with schizophrenia experiences a wide variety of symptoms that affect the ability to learn and retain information. Teaching must be geared to a time when medication has begun to decrease the psychotic symptoms, thoughts are more organized, and communication is more effective. Verbal teaching should be simple and supplemented with reading materials that the patient and/or significant other and family can refer to at a later time.

Most patients with schizophrenia experience memory deficits, so retention of new information does not come easily. Repetition and attention to clarity and simplicity of teaching approaches and materials facilitate learning. Ensure that follow-up treatment is scheduled and that patient and/or significant other and family understand the need to get prescriptions filled and to take medication as prescribed. Consider whether or not patient has transportation available to get to follow-up treatment. Psychiatric home care might be a valuable part of the discharge planning to facilitate adherence to the discharge plan. In addition, provide patient and/or significant other/family with verbal and written information about the following issues:

✔ Medications, including drug name; purpose; dosage; frequency; precautions; drug-drug, food-drug, and herb-drug interactions; and potential side effects.

✔ Importance of laboratory follow-up tests if patient is taking Clozaril.

✔ Importance of maintaining a healthy lifestyle—balanced diet, minimal to no caffeine or alcohol, exercise, and regular adequate sleep patterns—to facilitate remaining in remission.

✔ Importance of continuing medication use probably for a lifetime.

✔ Importance of social support and strategies to obtain it.

✔ Importance of using community follow-up resources, for example, psychiatrist, psychiatric nurse, intensive outpatient, support groups, family counseling, psychosocial programs including club houses, and other patient-run support groups.

✔ Importance of following up with medical care, as well as psychiatric care.

✔ Importance of maintaining or achieving spiritual well-being.

✔ Referrals to community resources for support and education. Additional information can be obtained by contacting the following organizations:

- Person to Person (free Consumer and Family Support Service) at P.O. Box 21510, Boulder, CO, 80308-4510, (800) 376-8282. This organization provides free educational and support services for people taking Risperdal (risperidone) and was developed by Janssen Pharmaceutic Inc., Titusville, NJ, 08560.

- Lilly Cares Patient Assistance Program, at Eli Lilly and Company, Lilly Corporate Center, Indianapolis, IN, 46285, (800) 545-6962. This program was designed to assist providers, patients, and patient caregivers through reimbursement support and temporary provision of Zyprexa and other drugs at no charge to eligible patients.

- National Alliance for the Mentally Ill (NAMI) at *www.nami.org*. Contact NAMI chapter in local state for information and schedule or contact national office of NAMI. The NAMI Family to Family Education Program is a 12-session comprehensive course for families of people with serious mental illnesses.

- NAMI for patients and families who are dealing with schizophrenia to seek educational and support opportunities: *www.nami.org/template.cfm?section*=schizophrenia.

- Mental Illness Education Project, Inc., at *www.miepvideos.org* has a new videotape for families and mental health professionals entitled, "Families Coping with Mental Illness."

- MedicAlert Foundation at *www.medicalert.org* provide a simple tool to ensure that people with schizophrenia receive proper care in an emergency department or to help family members find a loved one who has stopped taking medication and is experiencing behavioral problems in public. To order a MedicAlert bracelet or necklace costs $35.00 for a 1-year membership. MedicAlert also has a program for people who cannot afford the fees.

- National Institute of Mental Health, NIMH Public Inquiries at *www.nimh.nih.gov* has a booklet prepared by the Schizophrenia Research Branch, NIMH entitled, "Schizophrenia: Questions and Answers" (DHHS Publication No. ADM 90-1457).

- National Alliance for Research on Schizophrenia and Depression (NARSAD) at *www.narsad.org*.

- Schizophrenia Society of Canada at *www.schizophrenia.ca*.

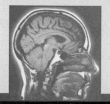

Substance Abuse Disorders 101

OVERVIEW/PATHOPHYSIOLOGY

Substance abuse is one of the major health issues in the United States. The connection between substance use and social and health problems is well documented and includes such issues as an increase in illegal and violent activities associated with the sale and distribution of illegal drugs, major health problems including the spread of human immunodeficiency virus (HIV) and other communicable diseases among IV drug users, developmental problems of babies born to addicted mothers, the epidemic of "crack babies," fetal alcohol syndrome babies, low-birth-weight babies, and the increase in domestic violence and child abuse/neglect. Deaths caused by motor vehicular accidents are directly linked to alcohol consumption. In addition, there are a full range of medical complications that are a direct result of alcohol dependence, including cardiovascular, respiratory, hematologic, nervous, digestive, endocrine, metabolic, skin, musculoskeletal, and genitourinary problems, as well as nutritional deficiencies.

The *Diagnostic and Statistical Manual IV (DSM-IV)* defines a substance abuse disorder as the nontherapeutic use of psychoactive agents or illicit use of a prescribed drug on a regular, binge, or episodic basis. The distinction between substance abuse and substance dependence is that the latter involves physical dependence and withdrawal symptoms. The rationale for classifying psychoactive substance disorders within a generic category of either substance use or substance dependence relates to commonalities in psychologic behavior patterns across drug classifications. Knowing the specific drug(s) abused is essential for treating toxicity and withdrawal. However, it is the outcome of psychoactive drug use, shared in common by all drug classifications, that is most likely to account for the problems associated with the disorder. These properties include acute and chronic structural and functional changes in the brain associated with drug intake; variable effects on the person taking the drugs; the concepts of dependence, tolerance, and reinforcing properties that are unique characteristics of most psychoactive substances and are not found in other pharmacologic classifications; and the concepts of recovery and relapse prevention after cessation of drug intake.

HEALTH CARE SETTING

Treatment of substance abuse disorders occurs over the full range of the health care continuum. Acute detoxification usually takes place in an acute care facility. However, long-term care takes place in various community settings, including support groups like Alcoholics Anonymous (AA), Narcotics Anonymous (NA), outpatient therapy, vocational supports, family therapy, residential programs such as Phoenix House, Synanon, and Odyssey House, and employee assistance programs.

ASSESSMENT (ALCOHOLISM)

Assessment focuses on alcoholism because it constitutes the most frequently used and abused psychoactive substance in the United States.

Major symptoms supportive of a diagnosis of alcohol dependency:

- Withdrawal symptoms and significant interference with psychosocial functioning in family and job relationships.
- Tolerance, as evidenced by ability to consume the equivalent of a fifth of liquor or having a blood alcohol level of 100 dl or more.
- Indiscriminate or regular drinking despite social or medical contraindications.
- Arrests for driving while under the influence of alcohol.

Assessment interview: Family history, history of drug use, and a description of behavior patterns described above. It is important to ask about preexisting mental disorders, metabolic conditions, cardiac and gas exchange problems, prescribed medications, and head injuries, all of which have symptoms that sometimes mimic acute intoxication or withdrawal symptoms.

Psychologic symptoms and behavior patterns: Patient uses denial to insist that she or he does not have a problem despite concrete evidence to the contrary. Rationalization appears in the form of self-imposed rules that explain the person's drinking habits as legitimate. Statements may be made such as, "I only drink on weekends" or "I limit myself to a beer, none of the hard stuff for me." Projection is evidenced in the blaming of external forces for stimulating the need to drink, for example, a nagging wife or a stressful job. Blackouts occur when there is a neuronal irritability that erases the alcoholic's memory of self-destructive behaviors while under the influence.

Physical indicators/examination:

- **Activity/rest:** Difficulty sleeping, not feeling well rested.
- **Cardiovascular:** Peripheral pulses weak, irregular, or rapid; hypertension common in early withdrawal stage from alcohol

but may become labile and progress to hypotension as withdrawal progresses; tachycardia common in early withdrawal; numerous dysrhythmias may be identified; other abnormalities depend on underlying heart disease/concurrent drug use.

- **Elimination:** Diarrhea, varied bowel sounds resulting from gastric complications such as gastric hemorrhage or distention.
- **Nutrition and fluid intake:** Nausea, vomiting, and food intolerance; difficulty chewing and swallowing food; muscle wasting; dry, dull hair; swollen salivary glands, inflamed buccal cavity, capillary fragility (malnutrition); possible generalized tissue edema resulting from protein deficiency; gastric distention, ascites, liver enlargement (seen in cirrhosis with long-term use).
- **Pain/discomfort:** Possible constant upper abdominal pain and tenderness radiating to the back (pancreatic inflammation).
- **Respiratory:** History of smoking; recurrent/chronic respiratory problems; tachypnea (with hyperactive state of alcohol withdrawal); diminished breath sounds.
- **Neurosensory:** Internal shakes, headache, dizziness, blurred vision, blackouts.
- **Psychiatric:** Possible dual diagnoses, for example, paranoid schizophrenia, bipolar disorder, major depression.
- **Level of consciousness/orientation:** Confusion, stupor, hyperactivity, distorted thought processes, slurred/incoherent speech.
- **Affect/mood/behavior:** May be fearful, anxious, easily startled, inappropriate, irritable, physically/verbally abusive, depressed, or paranoid.

Withdrawal assessment:
- **Stage I:** Mild. Temperature, pulse, respirations (TPR) and systolic blood pressure (SBP) elevated; slight diaphoresis; oriented × 3; mild anxiety and restlessness; restless sleep; hand tremors; decreased appetite; nausea.

- **Stage II:** Moderate. Pulse 100-120 bpm; increased temperature; increased SBP; obvious diaphoresis; intermittent confusion; transient visual and auditory hallucinations, primarily at night; increased anxiety and motor restlessness; insomnia; nightmares; nausea, vomiting, anorexia.
- **Stage III:** Severe. Pulse 120-140 bpm; increased temperature; increased diastolic blood pressure (DBP) and SBP; marked diaphoresis; marked disorientation and confusion; frightening visual, auditory, and tactile hallucinations; illusions (misinterpretation of objects); delusions; delirium tremens; disturbances in consciousness; agitation, panic states; inability to sleep; gross uncontrollable tremors, convulsions; inability to ingest any oral fluids or foods.

Safety assessment: History of recurrent accidents, such as falls, fractures, lacerations, burns, blackouts, or automobile accidents.

Suicidal assessment: Alcoholic suicide attempts may be as much as 30% higher than the national average.

Social assessment: Dysfunctional family system; problems in current relationships; frequent sick days off work/school; history of arrests because of fighting with others, disorderly conduct, or automobile accidents.

Spiritual assessment: It is important to assess for spiritual beliefs, practices, faith tradition, and commitment to that tradition. Many alcoholics and others addicted to substances find recovery through the spiritual model of AA and NA. Spiritual beliefs may provide the anchor that prevents an addicted individual from turning to suicide as a way out.

DIAGNOSTIC TESTS

Blood alcohol and drug levels can be obtained. However, diagnosis is generally made through interview history and physical examination. The diagnosis is made by confirmation of the presence of the four major symptoms of alcoholism listed above. Two of the most common assessment tools used to establish a definitive diagnosis are the Michigan Alcohol Screening Test (MAST) and the CAGE-AID questionnaire.

Nursing Diagnosis:

Risk for Injury

related to altered cerebral function (with risk for seizures) secondary to alcohol withdrawal

Desired Outcome: Patient does not exhibit evidence of physical injuries caused by alcohol withdrawal.

INTERVENTIONS	RATIONALES
Identify stage of alcohol withdrawal and severity of symptoms. Monitor vital signs, gait and motor coordination, presence and severity of tremors, mental status, and electrolyte status.	The greater the severity of symptoms, the more likely the patient will experience increasing disorientation, confusion, and restlessness. As the withdrawal moves from stage I (mild) to stage III (severe), the risk for a fall or injury increases significantly.
Monitor for seizure activity; institute seizure precautions: bed in lowest position with side rails padded, oral airway at the bedside.	Withdrawal seizures usually occur within 48 hr following last drink.

Continued

INTERVENTIONS	RATIONALES
Keep communication simple.	As the disease progresses, patient's ability to comprehend complex directions and interactions diminishes greatly. Simplicity is the key to effective communication.
Stay with patient and provide emotional support and encouragement.	Risk of seizures is higher if patient is alone and has no one to keep him or her grounded in reality.
Continue to orient patient to surroundings and call light.	As blood alcohol level drops, disorientation increases and can last several days.
Maintain a calm, quiet environment.	Controlling the amount of external stimulation and keeping it at a minimal level promotes calm in the patient.
Administer IV/PO fluids with caution as indicated.	Careful fluid replacement corrects dehydration and facilitates renal clearance of toxins. Excessive alcohol use damages the cardiac muscle and/or conduction system. Overhydration poses significant risk to cardiac functioning.
Administer medications as prescribed and be alert for side effects.	
- Benzodiazepines: clonazepam (Klonopin), diazepam (Valium), or chlordiazepoxide (Librium)	These medications are commonly used to control neuronal activity as alcohol is detoxified from the body. Either IV or PO route is preferred. These drugs produce muscle relaxation, which is effective in controlling the "shakes," trembling, and ataxic movements. They are usually initiated at a high dose and tapered and discontinued within 96 hr. They must be used cautiously in patients with hepatic disease because they are metabolized by the liver.
- Oxazepam (Serax)	This may be the drug of choice for patients with liver disease. Although it does not produce quite the dramatic effects of controlling withdrawal symptoms, it has a shorter half-life, so it is safer in the presence of hepatic disease.
- Phenobarbital	This drug is highly effective in suppressing withdrawal symptoms and is an effective anticonvulsant. Use must be monitored to prevent exacerbation of respiratory depression.

••• **Related NIC and NOC labels:** *NIC:* Surveillance: Safety; Environmental Management: Safety; Risk Identification; Seizure Management
NOC: Safety Status: Physical Injury

Nursing Diagnosis:

Interrupted Family Processes

related to long-term pattern of alcoholism and use of denial, rationalization, and projection

Desired Outcome: Before patient is discharged from care facility or after 4 wk if patient is outpatient, family members verbalize the dysfunctional behavioral dynamics present within the family system, the difference between caring and enabling, and the available services and treatment options that would help them.

INTERVENTIONS	RATIONALES
Provide family members with an opportunity to discuss their experiences of living with the disabling effects of alcoholism.	This validates their experience and encourages open discussion of the problem.
Educate family members about the effects of alcoholism on the family system.	This information enables recognition that the dynamics in their family, although dysfunctional, is a predictable response to having a family member addicted to alcohol. It also encourages engagement in realistic appraisal of the family's dynamics.

Continued

INTERVENTIONS	RATIONALES
Provide family members with a list of services and treatment options available.	This validates that the dysfunction within the family is serious and requires support of professionals to correct the patterns.
Define the term *enabling* for family members. Encourage each of them to identify at least one time when he or she enabled the patient. Offer family members alternative choices to enabling behaviors. Have them practice what they will do and say when a situation arises.	It is important to reframe helping behavior as enabling behavior in order for family members to recognize the pattern. It is also important for them to realize that changing these patterns requires practice and feedback. During times of anxiety, it is normal to fall back on previous patterns of behaving.
Encourage the couple to consider marital therapy to begin to discuss regrets and resentments that have occurred as a result of alcoholism.	After many years of denial, it is important to begin to talk about feelings that have been buried. This process should be undertaken with a professional who can act as a mediator and teach the couple how to communicate without blaming, a common dynamic in a marriage affected by alcoholism.
Explain how roles have changed within the family as a result of alcoholism.	Teaching may have to be repeated frequently based on the family's readiness to learn. Alcoholism produces dramatic role shifts that families are unaware of when they are in the midst of the problem. Presenting this emotionally charged information in a concrete, didactic manner increases family members' ability to hear.
Encourage family members to tell one another their needs and that caring about them is different from enabling.	Social and emotional isolation and denial of needs are common in alcoholic families. Enabling behaviors are frequently intended to be caring.
Encourage family to attend an Al-Anon meeting.	Significant change will require long-term commitment and support.

••• **Related NIC and NOC labels:** *NIC:* Coping Enhancement; Family Support; Counseling; Family Therapy; Support Group; Support Group Enhancement; Role Enhancement; Behavior Modification *NOC:* Family Coping; Family Functioning

Nursing Diagnosis:

Ineffective Denial

related to minimization of the symptoms and effects of alcoholism

Desired Outcome: Before discharge from care facility or after 4 wk if patient is outpatient, patient acknowledges that his or her drinking is out of control and his or her life has become unmanageable.

INTERVENTIONS	RATIONALES
Encourage patient to self-admit to an alcohol treatment program.	Self-admittance is preferred because the element of denial has been addressed to a certain degree.
Assure patient that alcoholism is a physiologic problem and not a moral one.	This demonstrates a nonjudgmental attitude; it is easier to accept treatment for an illness than it is for what may be perceived as a moral weakness or flaw.
Encourage patient to compile a written list of the deleterious consequences of excessive alcohol use experienced over the time he or she has been drinking. Ask patient to show the list to another nurse or peer.	These interventions help break through the process of denial.
Ask patient to compile a list of situations that influenced excessive drinking and discuss ways to respond to these situations that do not involve drinking.	To help avoid relapse, it is important to know which situations triggered excessive drinking in the past.

••• **Related NIC and NOC labels:** *NIC:* Counseling; Decision-Making Support; Self-Awareness Enhancement; Self-Responsibility Facilitation; Behavior Modification *NOC:* Acceptance: Health Status; Symptom Control

Nursing Diagnosis:

Disturbed Sensory Perception: Visual, Auditory, or Tactile

related to sudden cessation of alcohol consumption

Desired Outcome: Optimally, hallucinations do not occur, but if they do, patient's response is calm and controlled.

INTERVENTIONS	RATIONALES
Assess level of consciousness (LOC) and ability to communicate and respond to stimuli and commands.	Speech may be slurred, confused, or garbled. Response to commands may indicate inability to concentrate, impaired judgment, or muscle coordination deficits.
Monitor for disorientation, hyperactivity, confusion, restlessness, irritability, and sleeplessness.	Sleeplessness is common with loss of sedating effect of alcohol "nightcap." Sleep deprivation aggravates disorientation and confusion. Hyperactivity related to central nervous system (CNS) disturbances may show rapid escalation. Progression of these symptoms may signal impending hallucinations (common in stage II of alcohol withdrawal) or delirium tremens (seen in stage III of alcohol withdrawal).
Monitor for onset of hallucinations. Document as auditory, visual, or tactile.	Auditory hallucinations can be very frightening and threatening to the patient. Visual hallucinations include insects, animals, or faces of friends or enemies. The patient may yell for help from perceived threat. A tactile hallucination may include, for example, the sense that insects are crawling under the skin.
If hallucinations occur, stay with patient and speak in a calm, reassuring voice. Reassure patient that the voices and visions are not real and that he or she is safe.	Calm begets calm.
Turn off radio and/or TV; regulate lighting.	These measures reduce external stimuli when patient is hyperactive. Some patients become more agitated in a darkened room; others respond better to a quiet, darkened room.
Maintain consistency in care providers as much as possible; try to remain with patient as much as possible.	Consistency promotes a sense of security; being with patient reduces fear.
Make sure environment is safe: bed in lowest position, bed rails padded, call light within reach, articles removed that could harm patient, doors in full open position, ongoing patient monitoring.	In addition to hallucinations, patient may experience reality distortion that could produce fear or suicidal ideation. Protection from self-harm is essential.
Administer medications as prescribed: see previous care plan, **Risk for Injury.**	It may be necessary to provide calming effect and decrease symptoms of withdrawal.

••• Related NIC and NOC labels: *NIC:* Hallucination Management; Anxiety Reduction; Medication Management; Environmental Management; Reality Orientation; Substance Use Treatment *NOC:* Cognitive Orientation

Nursing Diagnosis:

Imbalanced Nutrition: Less Than Body Requirements

related to poor dietary intake

Desired Outcome: Within 24 hr of this diagnosis, patient verbalizes accurate understanding of the effects of alcohol and reduced dietary intake on nutritional status and demonstrates nutritional intake adequate for his or her needs.

INTERVENTIONS	RATIONALES
Assess for abdominal distention, tenderness, and presence and quality of bowel sounds.	Excessive alcohol intake may irritate gastric mucosa and result in epigastric pain and hyperactive bowel sounds. Other more serious gastrointestinal (GI) effects may occur secondary to hepatitis and cirrhosis.
Note presence of nausea/vomiting and diarrhea.	These signs are frequently among the first indicators of alcohol withdrawal and may interfere with establishing adequate nutritional intake.
Assess patient's ability to feed self.	A number of factors, including tremors, mental status changes, and hallucinations, may interfere with independent feeding and signal need for assistance.
Provide small, easily digested, and frequent feedings/snacks as desired; increase as tolerated.	Small feedings may enhance intake and toleration of nutrients by limiting gastric distress. As appetite and ability to tolerate food increase, adjustments are made to diet to ensure that adequate calories and nutrition are supplied for tissue repair and healing and restoration of energy and vitality.
Review liver function tests.	Liver function status influences choice of diet and need for/effectiveness of supplemental therapy.
Refer to dietitian as indicated.	Expert advice may be necessary to coordinate patient's nutritional regimen.
Provide diet high in protein with about 50% of calories supplied by carbohydrates.	This diet provides for energy needs and tissue healing while stabilizing blood sugar levels.
Administer medications as prescribed:	
- Antacids, antiemetics, and antidiarrheals	These medications reduce gastric irritation.
- Thiamine and vitamins	All substance abusers should receive thiamine and vitamins because most have these deficiencies.
Keep patient NPO (nothing by mouth) if indicated.	It may be necessary to reduce gastric/pancreatic stimulation in the presence of GI bleeding or excessive vomiting.

••• **Related NIC and NOC labels:** *NIC:* Nutrition Monitoring; Self-Care Assistance: Feeding; Nutritional Counseling; Medication Management; Laboratory Data Interpretation *NOC:* Nutritional Status: Food and Fluid Intake; Nutritional Status: Nutrient Intake

Nursing Diagnosis:

Deficient Knowledge:

Prescribed medications, rationale for use, and potential side effects

Desired Outcome: Patient verbalizes accurate information about prescribed medication, including rationale for use and common side effects.

INTERVENTIONS	RATIONALES
Teach patient about the two medications that are sometimes used as adjuncts to alcohol dependence treatment:	
Disulfiram (Antabuse)	This agonist medication is used as a deterrent to impulsive drinking.
Teach risks of drinking while taking Antabuse.	Response of taking alcohol while on Antabuse includes the following: severe nausea, vomiting, hypotension, headache, cardiovascular collapse, heart palpitations, seizures, or death.
Inform patient both verbally and in writing of serious side effects that occur when ingesting alcohol or other substances containing alcohol such as cough syrups or cold remedies.	Potential side effects are so serious that informed consent is essential.
Teach patient:	
- Do not take any form of alcohol (beer, wine, liquor, vinegars, cough medicines, sauces, aftershave lotions, liniments, or cologne).	Doing so may cause a severe, even life-threatening reaction.
- Take the drug daily (at bedtime if it produces fatigue or dizziness). Crush or mix tablet with liquid if necessary.	
- Wear or carry medical identification with you at all times.	This alerts any medical emergency personnel that patient is taking Antabuse.
- Keep appointments for follow-up laboratory tests.	Disulfiram may worsen coexisting conditions such as diabetes mellitus, hypothyroidism, chronic and acute nephritis, and hepatic disease. It also increases prothrombin time. When these conditions exist, blood sugar monitoring, kidney and liver function tests, thyroid tests, and prothrombin times need scheduled follow-up evaluations.
- The metallic aftertaste is temporary and will disappear after the drug is discontinued.	
- Avoid driving or performing tasks that require alertness.	Drowsiness, fatigue, or blurred vision may occur.
Naltrexone (Trexan)	This is a narcotic antagonist originally used as a treatment for heroin abuse but has now been approved for treatment of alcoholism. The drug reduces the cravings for alcohol.
Teach patient about adverse effects: difficulty sleeping, anxiety, nervousness, headache, low energy, abdominal pain, cramps, nausea, vomiting, delayed ejaculations, decreased potency, skin rash, chills, increased thirst, and joint and muscle pain.	These common adverse effects should be reported to prescriber.
Teach patient:	
- This drug will make it easier for patient not to drink and it blocks the effects of narcotics.	
- Wear a medical identification tag. Notify other health professionals that you are taking this drug.	This alerts emergency medical personnel that patient is taking this drug.
- Avoid use of heroin or other opiate drugs.	Small doses may have no effect, but large doses can cause death, serious injury, or coma.
- Report any signs and symptoms of adverse effects.	
- Keep appointments for follow-up blood tests and treatment program.	

••• **Related NIC and NOC labels:** *NIC:* Teaching: Prescribed Medication *NOC:* Knowledge: Medication

ADDITIONAL NURSING DIAGNOSES/ PROBLEMS:

"Psychosocial Support" for relevant nursing diagnoses in the care of the patient — p. 73

"Psychosocial Support for the Patient's Family and Significant Other" for relevant nursing diagnoses for patient's family/significant other — p. 87

"Anxiety Disorders" for:

Anxiety — p. 739

Social Isolation — p. 740

Ineffective Coping — p. 740

Compromised Family Coping — p. 741

"Bipolar Disorder" for:

Risk for Other-Directed Violence — p. 746

Self-Care Deficit — p. 748

"Major Depression" for:

Hopelessness — p. 763

Dysfunctional Grieving — p. 765

 ## PATIENT-FAMILY TEACHING AND DISCHARGE PLANNING

The patient with a substance abuse disorder suffers from a problem that can and will affect every area of his/her life. To remain free of substances, the patient will probably require lifelong support through AA or NA. The patient and family need to recognize that substance abuse disorders become family problems and professional counseling may be necessary and that alcoholism is a relentlessly progressive disease with profound medical, psychologic, social, and spiritual implications. Provide patient and family with verbal and written information about the following issues:

✓ Nature and expected course of alcoholism/substance abuse disorder.

✓ Medications, including drug name; purpose; dosage; frequency; precautions; drug-drug, food-drug, and herb-drug interactions; and potential side effects.

✓ Withdrawal process—what to expect.

✓ Nutrition issues.

✓ Emergency measures.

✓ Importance of social support and strategies to obtain it; importance of changing social support if that support promotes drug use.

✓ Importance of using relaxation techniques to minimize stress.

✓ Importance of maintaining or achieving spiritual well-being.

✓ Importance of lifestyle issues such as benefits of exercise.

✓ Importance of group support for continued healing through AA or NA. Additional information can be obtained by contacting the following organizations:

- National Clearinghouse for Alcohol and Drug Information (NCADI) at *http://ncadi.samhsa.gov*
- National Institute on Alcohol Abuse and Alcoholism (NIAAA) at *www.niaaa.nih.gov*
- National Institute on Drug Abuse (NIDA) at *www. nida.nih.gov*
- Online Alcoholics Anonymous (AA) Recovery Resources at *www.recovery.org/aa*
- Research Institute on Addictions at *www.ria.buffalo. edu*

For several decades, infection prevention and control efforts have focused on the use of barriers (e.g., gloves, gowns, masks) to interrupt transmission of organisms among and between patients and health care workers. These barriers are a major component of various systems of transmission precautions.

SYSTEMS OF TRANSMISSION PRECAUTIONS

Many different systems of transmission precautions have been used in hospitals over the years and are commonly called isolation precautions. These recommendations are updated periodically, with the most recent revisions (2006 and 2007) by the Centers for Disease Control and Prevention (CDC) intended to reflect evidence-based practices and current knowledge. The purpose of these techniques and procedures, which is to interrupt transmission of organisms, adheres to five guiding principles: (1) to provide infection control recommendations for all components of the health care delivery system, including hospitals, long-term care facilities, ambulatory care, and home care and hospice; (2) to reaffirm Standard Precautions as the foundation for preventing transmission during patient care in all health care settings; (3) to reaffirm the importance of implementing transmission-based precautions based on clinical presentation or syndrome and likely pathogens until the infectious etiology has been determined; (4) to provide epidemiologically sound and, whenever possible, evidence-based recommendations; and (5) to provide a unified infection control approach to multidrug-resistant organisms (MDROs). Specific recommendations for MDROs were published in December of 2006 by the CDC. The 2007 guideline contains two tiers of precautions (Table A-1): Standard Precautions, which are designed for the care of all patients in any health care setting, regardless of diagnosis or presumed infection status, and Transmission-Based Precautions, which are used for patients known to be or suspected of being infected or colonized with epidemiologically important pathogens that can be transmitted by airborne or droplet transmission or by contact with dry skin or contaminated surfaces. A new type of Transmission-Based Precautions also has been added, the Protective Environment, which is specifically for patients receiving hematopoietic stem cell transplantation (HSCT) who are at particular risk for infections with airborne fungi.

The 2006 and 2007 guidelines replace the 1996 guideline for isolation precautions in hospitals. The 1996 Standard Precautions system synthesized the major features of Universal Precautions and Body Substance Isolation and applied to (1) blood, (2) all body fluids, secretions, and excretions, except sweat, regardless of whether they contain visible blood, (3) nonintact skin, and (4) mucous membranes. In addition, Standard Precautions were designed to reduce risks of transmission of microorganisms from both recognized and unrecognized sources of infectious agents. The 2006 and 2007 guidelines continue these same principles of Standard Precautions and apply them to a broader range of situations and care settings. The 1996 Transmission-Based Precautions were designed for patients documented to be or suspected of being infected or colonized with organisms transmitted by the airborne route, by droplets, and by contact where extra precautions were necessary to interrupt transmission. As always, the CDC offers hospitals and other types of health care settings the option of modifying the recommendations according to their needs and circumstances and as directed by federal, state, or local regulations. For example, the Occupational Safety and Health Administration (OSHA) Bloodborne Pathogens Standard (1991; revised 2001) is still operable, and all facilities are required to comply with its provisions. The CDC's 2007 Standard Precautions incorporate all requirements of the OSHA Bloodborne Pathogens Standard.

TRANSMISSION PRECAUTIONS FOR PATIENTS WITH PULMONARY OR LARYNGEAL TUBERCULOSIS

Airborne Infection Isolation Precautions are for persons diagnosed with or suspected of having pulmonary or laryngeal tuberculosis (TB) that can be transmitted to others via the airborne route. These guidelines focus on early identification and treatment of persons with a diagnosis or suspected diagnosis of active TB. In addition, the CDC defined requirements for special ventilation and use of respiratory protection masks that provide better filtration and a tighter fit than standard surgical masks. Masks of this type are called *particulate respira-*

Text continued on p. 792

Table A-1
Recommendations for Isolation Precautions in Health Care Settings, 2007

	Standard Precautions	Transmission-Based Precautions: Airborne Infection Isolation	Transmission-Based Precautions: Droplet	Transmission-Based Precautions: Contact	Transmission-Based Precautions: Protective Environment
When to use	For care of all patients in all health care settings.	For patients known or suspected to be infected with microorganisms transmitted person-to-person by airborne droplet nuclei that remain suspended in the air and that can be dispersed widely by air currents.	For patients known or suspected to be infected with microorganisms transmitted by respiratory droplets (more than 5 micrometers in size) generated by patient when coughing, sneezing, talking, or during performance of cough-inducing procedures.	For patients with known or suspected infections or evidence of syndromes that represent increased risk for contact transmission. If the patient is known or suspected of being colonized or infected with multidrug-resistant organisms, follow specific recommendations in the 2006 CDC guideline Management of multi-drug organisms in health care settings, 2006.**	For allogeneic hematopoietic stem cell transplantation (HSCT) patients to minimize fungal spore counts in the air. Specific requirements for the Protective Environment were defined by the CDC in 2000.*
Hand hygiene 1. When hands are visibly dirty or contaminated with proteinaceous material or visibly soiled with blood or other body fluids, wash hands with either a non-antimicrobial soap and water or an antimicrobial soap and water. 2. If hands are not visibly soiled, use an alcohol-based handrub for routinely decontaminating hands in all other clinical situations; alternatively, wash hands with an antimicrobial soap and water.	Decontaminate hands in the following circumstances: before having direct contact with patients; after contact with blood, body fluids or excretions, mucous membranes, nonintact skin, or wound dressings; after contact with a patient's intact skin (e.g., when taking a pulse or blood pressure or lifting a patient); if hands will be moving from a contaminated body site to a clean body site; after contact with inanimate objects in the immediate vicinity of the patient; after removing gloves.				

Gloves

Wear gloves when it can be reasonably anticipated that contact with blood or other potentially infectious materials, mucous membranes, nonintact skin, or potentially contaminated intact skin could occur. Wear gloves with fit and durability appropriate to the task; wear disposable medical examination gloves for providing direct patient care; wear disposable medical examination gloves or reusable utility gloves for cleaning the environment or medical equipment.

Remove gloves after contact with patient and/or surrounding environment (including medical equipment), using proper technique to prevent hand contamination. Do not wear same pair of gloves for care of more than one patient. Change gloves during patient care if hands will move from a contaminated body site to a clean body site.

Wear gloves as indicated according to Standard Precautions and whenever touching patient's intact skin or surfaces and articles in close proximity to patient (e.g., medical equipment or bed rails). Don gloves upon entry into the room.

Modified from Siegel J, Strausbaugh L, Jackson M, Rhinehart E, Chiarello L, and the Healthcare Infection Control Practices Advisory Committee (HICPAC): Guideline for Isolation Precautions: preventing transmission of infectious agents in healthcare settings, to be published by the Centers for Disease Control and Prevention in 2007.

NOTE: *This table was developed when this publication was in DRAFT form; therefore the final version may differ slightly from what is published here.*

*CDC: Guidelines for preventing opportunistic infections among hematopoietic stem cell transplant recipients: recommendations of CDC, the Infectious Disease Society of America, and the American Society of Blood and Marrow Transplantation, MMWR 49(RR-10):1-125, 2000.

**Siegel JD, Rhinehart E, Jackson M, Chiarello L, and the Healthcare Infection Control Practices Advisory Committee (HICPAC). Management of multidrug-resistant organisms in healthcare settings, 2006. Available from: *www.cdc.gov/ncidod/dhap/pdf/ar/mdroGuideline2006.pdf.*

Centers for Disease Control and Prevention. Guidelines for preventing the transmission of *Mycobacterium tuberculosis* in health-care settings, 2005. *Morbidity and Mortality Weekly Report* (MMWR), December 2005, Vol.54 (No. RR-17, 1-141).

Continued

Table A-1
Recommendations for Isolation Precautions in Health Care Settings, 2007—cont'd

	Standard Precautions	Transmission-Based Precautions: Airborne Infection Isolation	Transmission-Based Precautions: Droplet	Transmission-Based Precautions: Contact	Transmission-Based Precautions: Protective Environment
Mouth, nose, eye, and respiratory protection	Wear a mask and eye protection or a face shield to protect mucous membranes of eyes, nose, and mouth during procedures and patient care activities that are likely to generate splashes or sprays of blood, body fluids, secretions, and excretions. Select masks, goggles, face shields, and combinations of each according to the task performed.	Restrict susceptible health care personnel from entering rooms of patients known or suspected to have measles (rubeola), varicella (chickenpox), zoster, or smallpox if other immune health care personnel are available. Wear fit-tested National Institute for Occupational Safety and Health–approved N95 or higher respirator for respiratory protection when entering room or home of a patient when the following diseases are suspected or confirmed: Infectious pulmonary or laryngeal tuberculosis or draining tuberculous skin lesions, smallpox, severe acute respiratory syndrome (SARS), avian influenza.	Wear a mask for close patient contact (e.g., within 3 ft). Use of eye protection should follow pathogen-specific recommendations in the CDC isolation guideline (2007).		During periods of construction, to prevent inhalation of respirable particles that could contain infectious spores, provide respiratory protection (e.g., N95 respirator) to patients who are medically fit enough to tolerate a respirator when they are required to leave the Protective Environment. Ensure that patients are instructed on respirator use. In the absence of construction, the CDC makes no recommendation for use of particulate respirators when leaving the Protective Environment.

Respiratory Hygiene/Cough Etiquette	Educate staff on importance of source control measures to contain respiratory secretions and prevent droplet and fomite transmission of respiratory pathogens, especially during seasonal outbreaks of viral respiratory tract infections.	Post signs in ambulatory and in-patient settings with instructions to patients and other persons to inform them to cover mouths/noses when coughing or sneezing, use and dispose of tissues, and perform hand hygiene after hands have been in contact with respiratory secretions. The health care facility should provide tissues and no-touch receptacles for disposal of used tissues as well as conveniently located dispensers of alcohol-based hand rubs, and where sinks are available, supplies for hand-washing. Although this is most important during periods of increased rates of respiratory infections in the community, some facilities may find it logistically easier to institute these recommendations year-round as a standard practice.

Modified from Siegel J, Strausbaugh L, Jackson M, Rhinehart E, Chiarello L, and the Healthcare Infection Control Practices Advisory Committee (HICPAC): Guideline for Isolation Precautions: preventing transmission of infectious agents in healthcare settings, to be published by the Centers for Disease Control and Prevention in 2007.

NOTE: *This table was developed when this publication was in DRAFT form; therefore the final version may differ slightly from what is published here.*

*CDC: Guidelines for preventing opportunistic infections among hematopoietic stem cell transplant recipients: recommendations of CDC, the Infectious Disease Society of America, and the American Society of Blood and Marrow Transplantation, MMWR 49(RR-10):1-125, 2000.

**Siegel JD, Rhinehart E, Jackson M, Chiarello L, and the Healthcare Infection Control Practices Advisory Committee (HICPAC). Management of multidrug-resistant organisms in healthcare settings, 2006. Available from: *www.cdc.gov/ncidod/dhap/pdf/ar/mdroGuideline2006.pdf.*

Centers for Disease Control and Prevention. Guidelines for preventing the transmission of Mycobacterium tuberculosis in health-care settings, 2005. *Morbidity and Mortality Weekly Report* (MMWR), December 2005, Vol.54 (No. RR-17, 1-141).

Continued

Table A-1
Recommendations for Isolation Precautions in Health Care Settings, 2007—cont'd

	Standard Precautions	Transmission-Based Precautions: Airborne Infection Isolation	Transmission-Based Precautions: Droplet	Transmission-Based Precautions: Contact	Transmission-Based Precautions: Protective Environment
Gowns	Wear a gown or other personal protective equipment (PPE) attire that is appropriate to the task, to protect skin and prevent soiling of clothing during procedures and patient-care activities when contact with blood, body fluids, secretions, or excretions is anticipated. Wear a gown for direct patient contact if patient has uncontained secretions or excretions. Remove gown and other PPE attire and perform hand hygiene before leaving patient's environment.			Wear a gown whenever anticipating that clothing will have direct contact with patient or potentially contaminated environmental surfaces or items in patient's room. Don gown upon entry into the room. Remove gown and observe hand hygiene before leaving patient's environment. After gown removal, ensure that clothing and skin do not contact potentially contaminated environmental surfaces to avoid transfer of microorganisms to other patients or environmental surfaces.	

Patient placement	Include the potential for transmission of infectious agents when making patient placement decisions.	In acute care hospitals or residential settings, place patient in a single-patient Airborne Infection Isolation Room (AIIR) that has been constructed in accordance with current guidelines; keep AIIR door closed when not required for entry and exit. If appropriate AIIR room is not available, consult facility's ICP for alternatives. Discontinue Airborne Precautions after signs and symptoms have resolved or according to pathogen-specific recommendations in the CDC isolation guideline (2007).	In acute care settings, place patients in a single patient room when available. If single patient rooms are in short supply, prioritize patients who have excessive cough and sputum production for single-patient room placement because of their risk of transmission. Avoid placing patients who require Droplet Precautions in same room with patients who are at increased risk for infection or adverse outcomes associated with infection (e.g., immunocompromised or have anticipated prolonged length of stay). Place together (cohort) in same room patients who are infected with same organism or are suitable roommates. In other situations or care settings, consult facility's ICP for alternatives.	In acute care settings, place patients who may require Contact Precautions in a single patient room when available. If single patient rooms are in short supply, prioritize patients with conditions that may facilitate transmission (e.g., uncontained drainage, stool incontinence) for single-patient room placement. Place together (cohort) in same room patients who are infected or colonized with the same pathogen and are suitable roommates. Ensure that patients are physically separated (i.e., more than 3 ft) from each other. Draw privacy curtain between beds to minimize opportunity for direct contact. Change protective attire and perform hand hygiene between patients. For patient placement in other situations or care settings, consult facility's ICP.

Modified from Siegel J, Strausbaugh L, Jackson M, Rhinehart E, Chiarello L, and the Healthcare Infection Control Practices Advisory Committee (HICPAC): Guideline for Isolation Precautions: preventing transmission of infectious agents in healthcare settings, to be published by the Centers for Disease Control and Prevention in 2007.

NOTE: *This table was developed when this publication was in DRAFT form; therefore the final version may differ slightly from what is published here.*

*CDC: Guidelines for preventing opportunistic infections among hematopoietic stem cell transplant recipients: recommendations of CDC, the Infectious Disease Society of America, and the American Society of Blood and Marrow Transplantation, MMWR 49(RR-10):1-125, 2000.

**Siegel JD, Rhinehart E, Jackson M, Chiarello L, and the Healthcare Infection Control Practices Advisory Committee (HICPAC). Management of multidrug-resistant organisms in healthcare settings, 2006. Available from: *www.cdc.gov/ncidod/dhap/pdf/ar/mdroGuideline2006.pdf*.

Centers for Disease Control and Prevention. Guidelines for preventing the transmission of *Mycobacterium tuberculosis* in health-care settings, 2005. *Morbidity and Mortality Weekly Report* (MMWR), December 2005, Vol.54 (No. RR-17, 1-141).

Continued

Table A-1
Recommendations for Isolation Precautions in Health Care Settings, 2007—cont'd

	Standard Precautions	Transmission-Based Precautions: Airborne Infection Isolation	Transmission-Based Precautions: Droplet	Transmission-Based Precautions: Contact	Transmission-Based Precautions: Protective Environment
Patient transport		In inpatient and residential settings, limit movement and transport of patients who require Airborne Precautions to medically necessary purposes. If transport or movement outside Airborne Infection Isolation Room is necessary, instruct patient to wear a mask. Instruct patients who cannot tolerate wearing masks because of medical conditions to observe Respiratory Hygiene/Cough Etiquette procedures. Discontinue Airborne Precautions after signs and symptoms have resolved or according to pathogen-specific recommendations in the CDC isolation guideline (2007).	Limit movement and transport of patient to medically necessary purposes. Instruct patient to wear a mask and follow Respiratory Hygiene/Cough Etiquette during transport. No mask is required for persons who are transporting patient. Discontinue Droplet Precautions after signs and symptoms have resolved or according to pathogen-specific recommendations in the CDC isolation guideline (2007).	Limit transport and movement of patients to outside the room to medically necessary purposes. When transport is required, ensure that infected or colonized areas of the patient are contained and covered. Remove contaminated PPE and perform hand hygiene prior to transporting patient on Contact Precautions. Don clean PPE to handle patient when transport destination has been reached.	
Patient care equipment	Follow established policies and procedures for containing, transporting, and handling patient care equipment that may be contaminated with blood or body fluids; always clean patient care equipment to remove organic material before disinfection and sterilization processes are used.			Manage patient care equipment according to Standard Precautions. Use disposable patient care items (e.g., blood pressure cuffs) whenever possible or implement patient-dedicated use of noncritical equipment to avoid sharing between patients. If use of common equipment or items is unavoidable, clean and disinfect them before use on another patient.	

Care of the environment	Follow established policies and procedures for cleaning and maintaining environmental surfaces as appropriate for level of patient contact and degree of soiling.
	Ensure that rooms of patients on Contact Precautions are given cleaning priority with a focus on frequent (e.g., at least daily) cleaning and disinfection of high touch surfaces (e.g., bed rails, bedside commodes, faucet handles, doorknobs, carts, charts) and equipment in immediate vicinity of the patient.
Textiles, laundry	Handle used textiles and fabrics with minimum agitation to avoid contamination of air, surfaces, and persons.
Workers' safety	Adhere to federal and state requirements for protection of health care personnel from exposure to bloodborne pathogens.

Modified from Siegel J, Strausbaugh L, Jackson M, Rhinehart E, Chiarello L, and the Healthcare Infection Control Practices Advisory Committee (HICPAC): Guideline for Isolation Precautions: preventing transmission of infectious agents in healthcare settings, to be published by the Centers for Disease Control and Prevention in 2007.

NOTE: *This table was developed when this publication was in DRAFT form; therefore the final version may differ slightly from what is published here.*

*CDC: Guidelines for preventing opportunistic infections among hematopoietic stem cell transplant recipients: recommendations of CDC, the Infectious Disease Society of America, and the American Society of Blood and Marrow Transplantation, MMWR 49(RR-10):1-125, 2000.

**Siegel JD, Rhinehart E, Jackson M, Chiarello L, and the Healthcare Infection Control Practices Advisory Committee (HICPAC). Management of multidrug-resistant organisms in healthcare settings, 2006. Available from: *www.cdc.gov/ncidod/dhqp/pdf/ar/mdroGuideline2006.pdf.*

Centers for Disease Control and Prevention. Guidelines for preventing the transmission of *Mycobacterium tuberculosis* in health-care settings, 2005. *Morbidity and Mortality Weekly Report (MMWR)*, December 2005, Vol.54 (No. RR-17, 1-141).

tors (PRs), and the specific type of PR for TB protection is called an *N95 respirator*. This type of respiratory protection is also appropriate for susceptible persons caring for patients known or suspected of having measles (rubeola), varicella (chickenpox), or smallpox. Of course, the best protection for any of the vaccine-preventable infectious diseases is for all caregivers to be immunized, then respiratory protection masks are not necessary.

MANAGEMENT OF DEVICES AND PROCEDURES TO REDUCE RISK OF NOSOCOMIAL INFECTION

Use of barriers is but one of many strategies that can reduce the risk of nosocomial infection among patients and personnel. In fact, studies from the CDC show that significant gains can be made in reducing infection risks by focusing on the management of devices and procedures commonly used in patient care. For example, many patients need intravascular devices that deliver therapeutic medications, but they are put at risk for site infections and bacteremias when these devices are used. It is well known that rotating the access site at appropriate intervals reduces these risks to the patient, and catheter materials that are more "vein friendly" also reduce

trauma to the vascular system. In addition, use of needles to deliver medications and fluids to patients through these intravascular devices can put the health care worker at risk for puncture injury. Needleless or needle-free IV access devices are used to access line ports so that it is not necessary to use needles once the intravascular catheter has entered the vascular system. Thus the use of newer and safer intravascular devices and procedures can benefit both the patient and health care worker by reducing their risk of health care–associated infection. Research studies of interventions to reduce health care–associated infection risks are published in general and specialty journals and presented at professional meetings each year. Infection control professionals (ICPs) and hospital epidemiologists use these studies to make recommendations about changes in nursing and medical practice. The Joint Commission (TJC) requires that all accredited facilities have a person qualified to provide infection surveillance, prevention, and control services. The national associations for these professionals are the Association for Professionals in Infection Control and Epidemiology, Inc. (APIC), which publishes the *American Journal of Infection Control*, and the Society for Healthcare Epidemiology of America (SHEA), which publishes the journal *Infection Control and Hospital Epidemiology*.

Appendix B
Laboratory Tests Discussed in This Manual: Normal Values

Table B-1
Complete Blood Count (CBC)

	Adult Normal Values* (Traditional—U.S.)	SI Adult Normal Values* (International System)
Hemoglobin (Hgb)	Male: 14-18 g/dl	Male: 135-170 g/L
	Female: 120-160 g/L	Female: 12-16 g/dl
Hematocrit (Hct)	Male: 40%-54%	Male: 0.400-0.500 L/L
	Female: 37%-47%	Female: 0.370-0.490 L/L
Red blood cell (RBC) count	Male: 4.7-6.1 $\times$ 10^6/microL	Male: 4.50-6.00 $\times$ 10^{12}/L
	Female: 4.2-5.4 $\times$ 10^6/microL	Female: 4.00-5.50 $\times$10^{12}/L
RBC indices		
Mean corpuscular volume	80-95 mm^3	80-100 fl
Mean corpuscular hemoglobin	27-31 pg	27-31 pg
Mean corpuscular hemoglobin concentration	32-36 g/dl	320-360 g/L
White blood cell (WBC) count	4500-11,000/mm^3	4-11 $\times$ 10^9/L
Neutrophils	54%-75%	2.5-7.5 $\times$ 10^9/L
Band neutrophils	3%-8%	2% $\pm$ 4
Lymphocytes	20%-40%	1-4 $\times$ 10^9/L
Monocytes	2%-8%	0-1 $\times$ 10^9/L
Eosinophils	1%-4%	0-0.7 $\times$ 10^9/L
Basophils	0.5%-1.0%	0-0.3 $\times$ 10^9/L
Platelet count	150,000-400,000/mm^3	150-400 $\times$ 10^9/L

*Normal values may vary significantly with different laboratory methods of testing.

Table B-2
Serum, Plasma, and Whole Blood Chemistry

	Adult Normal Values* (Traditional—U.S.)	SI Adult Normal Values* (International System)
Adrenocorticotropic hormone (ACTH)	8-10 AM, Less than 100 pg/ml	0-16 pmol/L
Antidiuretic hormone (ADH; vasopressin)	1-5 pg/ml	0-10 ng/L
Albumin	3.5-5.0 g/dl	35-50 g/L
Aldosterone	Male: 6-22 ng/dl	140-415 pmol/L
	Female: 4-31 ng/dl	
Alanine aminotransferase (ALT)	5-35 units/L	Male: less than 40 units/L
		Female: less than 31 units/L
Ammonia	10-80 mcg/dl	6-47 μmol/L
Amylase	60-180 Somogyi units/dl	Less than 125 units/L

*Normal values may vary significantly with different laboratory methods of testing.

Continued

Table B-2
Serum, Plasma, and Whole Blood Chemistry—cont'd

	Adult Normal Values* (Traditional—U.S.)	SI Adult Normal Values* (International System)
Aspartate aminotransferase (AST)	8-20 units/L (values slightly higher in older adults than in younger adults and slightly lower in females than in males)	Male: less than 37 units/L Female: less than 31 units/L
Bicarbonate	22-26 mEq/L	22-26 mEq/L
Bilirubin	Total: 0.3-1.4 mg/dl	Total: 2-17 μmol/L
Blood gases, arterial		
pH	7.35-7.45	7.35-7.45
$Paco_2$	35-45 mm Hg	35-45 mm Hg
Pao_2	80-100 mm Hg	80-100 mm Hg
O_2 saturation (Sao_2)	95%-99%	95%-99%
Blood urea nitrogen (BUN)	6-20 mg/dl	3-7 mmol/L
CA-125 cancer marker	0-35 units/ml	0-35 units/mol
Calcitonin	Less than 100 pg/ml	0-100 ng/L
Calcium	8.5-10.5 mg/dl; 4.3-5.3 mEq/L	2.2-2.6 mmol/L
Carcinoembryonic antigen (CEA)	Less than 5 ng/ml	0-4.6 mcg/L
Chloride (Cl^-)	95-108 mEq/L	95-108 mmol/L
Cortisol		
8-10 AM	5-25 mcg/dl	140-500 nmol/L
4 pm-midnight	2-18 mcg/dl	83-441 nmol/L
CO_2 content (total CO_2)	22-28 mEq/L	22-30 mmol/L
C-reactive protein (CRP)	Less than 1 mg/dl	Less than 10 mg/L
Creatinine	0.6-1.5 mg/dl	50-110 μmol/L
Creatinine clearance	Male: 107-141 ml/min Female: 87-132 ml/min	1.5-2.2 ml/sec
Creatinine phosphokinase (CPK)	Male: 55-170 units/L Female: 30-135 units/L	Male: 130-150 IU/L Female: 20-115 IU/L
CPK isoenzyme (MB)	5% total CPK activity	Less than 5% total CPK activity
D-dimer	Less than 0.5 mg/ml	Less than 0.5 mg/L
Erythrocyte sedimentation rate (ESR)	0-10 mm/hr	
Westergren method	Male: up to 15 mm/hr Female: up to 20 mm/hr	
Fibrin split products (FSPs, FDPs)	Less than 10 mcg/ml	Less than 400 mcg/L
Folic acid (folate)	5-25 ng/mL	11-57 mmol/L
Follicle-stimulating hormone (FSH, follitropin)		
Adult female		Follicular less than 16 IU/L
	Premenopausal 4-30 mU/ml Postmenopausal 40-250 mU/ml	Luteal less than 12 units/L Postmenopausal 23-167 units/L
Adult male	4-25 mU/ml	Less than 18 units/L
Globulins, total	1.5-3.5 g/dl	27-36 g/L
Glucose, fasting	True glucose: 60-120 mg/dl All sugars: 80-120 mg/dl	4-6 mmol/L
Glucose, random	Less than 145 mg/dl	
Glucose tolerance, oral		
Fasting:	60-120 mg/dl	3.3-6.0 mmol/L
1 hr:	Less than 165 mg/dl	3.3-11.1 mmol/L
2 hr:	Less than 120 mg/dl	3.3-7.8 mmol/L
Glycosylated hemoglobin (glycohemoglobin [GHb])	4%-8%	0.040-0.066
Growth hormone (GH)	Less than 10 ng/ml	0-7 mcg/L
Homocysteine (Hcy)	4-14 μmol/L	
Insulin	11-240 μU/ml 4-24 μU/ml	Fasting: 0-215 pmol/L
Iron	Total: 60-200 mcg/dl	10-30 μmol/L
Iron	Male, average: 125 mcg/dl Female, average: 100 mcg/dl Older adult: 60-80 mcg/dl	

Table B-2
Serum, Plasma, and Whole Blood Chemistry—cont'd

	Adult Normal Values* (Traditional—U.S.)	SI Adult Normal Values* (International System)
Total iron-binding capacity	25-420 mcg/dl	45-80 μmol/L
Ketone bodies	2-4 mcg/dl	Negative
Lactic acid	Arterial: 3-7 mg/dL	0.5-2.0 mmol/L
	Venous: 5-20 mg/dL	
Lactic dehydrogenase	45-90 units/L	100-250 units/L
Lipase	0-110 units/L	0-110 units/L
Magnesium	1.3-2.1 mEq/L	0.7-1.1 mmol/L
Osmolality	280-300 mOsm/kg H_2O	280-300 mmol/kg
Partial thromboplastin time (PTT)	60-70 sec	25.5-35.0 sec
On anticoagulant therapy	1.5-2.5 $\times$ control value	
Phosphatase, acid	0-1.1 units/ml (Bodansky)	Total: 0-6 units/L
	1-4 units/ml (King-Armstrong)	
	0.13-0.63 units/ml (Bessey-Lowery)	
Phosphatase, alkaline	1.5-4.5 units/dl (Bodansky)	30-110 units/L
	4-13 units/dl (King-Armstrong)	
	0.8-2.3 units/ml (Bessey-Lowery)	
Phosphorus	2.5-4.5 mg/dl; 1.7-2.6 mEq/L	0.80-1.45 mmol/L
Potassium (K^+)	3.5-5.0 mEq/L	3.5-5.0 mmol/L
Prolactin	Male: 0-20 ng/mL	Male: 0-20 mcg/L
	Female: 0-25 ng/mL	Female: 0-25 mcg/L
Prothrombin time (PT)	11-12.5 sec	INR: 0.81-1.2
Renin		
Normal sodium intake		
Supine	4-6 hr: 0.5-1.6 ng/ml/hr	Overnight or 6 hr: 6.4-23.8 ng/L/sec
Sitting	4 hr: 1.8-3.6 ng/ml/hr	2 hr: 9.3-43.4 ng/L/sec
Sitting		2 hr plus diuretic: 12.3-80.5 ng/L/sec
Low sodium intake		
Supine	4-6 hr: 2.2-4.4 ng/ml/hr	Overnight or 6 hr: less than 10.2 ng/L/sec
Sitting	4 hr: 4.0-8.1 ng/ml/hr	2 hr: 5.8-20.2 ng/L/sec
Reticulocyte count	0.5%-2% of total erythrocytes	40-80 $\times$ 10^9/L
Reticulocyte index	1.0	1.0
Sodium (Na^+)	137-147 mEq/L	137-147 mmol/L
Thyroid screen		
Free thyroxine index (FTI)	0.9-2.4 ng/dl	12-22 pmol/L
Free thyroxine (free T_4)		0.27-4.2 μmol/L
Thyroid-stimulating hormone	2-10 mU/L	
Thyroxine-binding prealbumin	20-30 mg/dl	
Triiodothyronine (T_3)	110-230 ng/dl	1.2-3.2 nmol/L
Thyroxine uptake (T uptake)		0.75-1.25 nmol/L
Transferrin	200-400 mg/dl	1.7-3.9 g/L
Urea clearance, serum/24 hr urine		
Maximum	64-99 ml/min	64-99 ml/min
Standard	41-65 ml/min	41-65 ml/min
Uric acid	Male: 4.0-8.5 mg/dl	Male: 0.24-.51 mmol/L
	Female: 2.7-7.3 mg/dL	Female: 0.16-0.43 mmol/L

*Normal values may vary significantly with different laboratory methods of testing.

Table B-3
Urine Chemistry

	Adult Normal Values* (Traditional—U.S.)	SI Adult Normal Values* (International System)
Albumin		
Random	Negative	Negative
24 hr	10-150 mg	150 mg
Amylase	Up to 5000 Somogyi units/24 hours	6.5-48.1 units/hour
Bilirubin (random)	Negative	Negative
Calcium (CA^{2+})		
Random	1+; less than 40 mg/dl	
24 hr	50-300 mg	2.5-6.3 mmol/L
Creatine (24 hr)	Male: 20-26 mg/kg	7.0-22 mmol/day
	Female: 14-22 mg/kg	
Creatine clearance	Male: 107-141 ml/min/1.73 m²	1.5-2.2 ml/sec
	Female: 87-132 ml/min/1.73 m²	
Glucose		
Random	Negative	Negative
24 hr	Less than 0.5 g/day	Less than 2.78 mmol/day
Ketone (random)	Negative	Negative
Microalbumin		
Random		Less than 20 mg/L
Night collection		7 ± 2 mcg/min
24 hr		10 ± 3 mg/day
Microalbumin/creatine ratio		
Male		Less than 2.0 mg/mmol
Female		Less than 2.8 mg/mmol
Osmolality		
Random	350-700 mOsm/kg H_2O	
24 hr	300-900 mOsm/kg H_2O	
Physiologic range	50-1400 mOsm/kg H_2O	
pH	4.6-8.0	4.6-8.0
Phosphorous (24 hr)	0.9-1.3 g; 0.2-0.6 mEq/L	16.1-48.4 mmol/day
Protein		
Random	Negative: 2-8 mg/dl	Negative
24 hr	40-150 mg	150 mg/day
Sodium (Na^+)		
Random	50-130 mEq/L	
24 hr	40-220 mEq/L	40-220 mmol/day
Specific gravity		
Random	1.010-1.020	1.003-1.035
After fluid restriction	1.025-1.035	
Sugar (random)	Negative	Negative
Urea clearance (24 hr)		
Maximum	64-99 ml/min	64-99 ml/min
Standard	41-65 ml/min	41-65 ml/min

*Normal values may vary significantly with different laboratory methods of testing.

Table B-4
Cerebrospinal Fluid (CSF)

	Adult Normal Values* (Traditional—U.S.)	SI Adult Normal Values* (International System)
Albumin	11-48 mg/dl	0.11-0.48 g/L
Blood	Not present	Not present
Cell count	0-5 mononuclear cells/μL	0-5 $\times$ 10^6 cells/L
Culture and sensitivity	No organisms present	No organisms present
Cytology	No malignant cells present	No malignant cells present
Glucose	50-75 mg/dl	2.8-4.2 mmol/L
Pressure	70-180 mm H_2O	70-180 mm H_2O
Protein	15-45 mg/dl	0.15-0.45 g/L

*Normal values may vary significantly with different laboratory methods of testing.

Selected Bibliography

GENERAL CARE PLANS

A legacy to remember (website): *www.alegacytoremember.com*

Acute Pain Management Guideline Panel: *Acute pain management: operative or medical procedures and trauma—clinical practices guideline*, AHCPR pub. no. 92-0032, Rockville, Md, 1992, Agency for Health Care Policy and Research, Public Health Service, U.S. Department of Health and Human Services.

Agency for Health Care Policy and Research: *Clinical practice guideline: management of cancer pain*, AHCPR pub. no. 94-0592, Rockville, Md, 1994, U.S. Department of Health and Human Services, Public Health Service, Agency for Health Care Policy and Research.

American Association of Cardiovascular and Pulmonary Rehabilitation: *Guidelines for cardiac rehabilitation and secondary prevention programs*, ed 4, Champaign, Ill, 2004, Human Kinetic Publishers.

American Cancer Society: *A cancer source book for nurses*, ed 8, Sudbury, Mass, 2004, Jones & Bartlett.

American Cancer Society: *Facts and figures 2006* Atlanta, GA, 2006, American Cancer Society.

American College of Sports Medicine: *ACSM's guidelines for exercise testing and prescription*, ed 6, Philadelphia, 2000, Lippincott, Williams & Wilkins.

American Nurses Association & American Society for Pain Management in Nursing (2005): Pain management nursing: scope & standards of practice, Silver Spring, Md (website): *www.nursesbooks.org.*

American Pain Society: *Principles of analgesic use in the treatment of acute and cancer pain*, ed 5, Glenview, Ill, 2003, The Society.

American Pharmaceutical Association, Semla TP, Beizer JL, Higbee MD: *Geriatric dosage handbook*, ed 11, Hudson, Ohio, 2006, Lexicomp.

Bailes BK: Perioperative care of the elderly surgical patient, *AORN* 72(2):186-207, 2000.

Beers M, Berkow R, editors: *Merck manual of geriatrics*, ed 3, Whitehouse Station, NJ, 2000, Merck Research Lab.

Belin de Chantemele E, Blanc S, Pellet N et al.: Does resistance exercise prevent body fluid changes after a 90-day bed rest? *Eur J Appl Physiol* 92(4-5):555-564, 2004.

Bieri D, Reeve RA, Champion GD et al.: The Faces Pain Scale for the self-assessment of the severity of pain experienced by children: development, initial validation, and preliminary investigation for ratio scale properties, *Pain* 41(2):139-150, 1990.

Bleeker MW, De Groot PC, Poelkens F et al.: Vascular adaptation to 4 wk of deconditioning by unilateral lower limb suspension, *Am J Physiol Heart Circ Physiol* 288(4):1H747-1755, 2005.

Borg GA: Psychophysical bases of perceived exertion, *Med Sci Sports Exerc* 14(5):377-381, 1982.

Brant JM, Wickham RS, editors: *Statement on the scope and standards of oncology nursing practice*, Washington, DC, 2004, American Nurses Publishing.

Byock I: *The four things that matter most*, New York, 2004, Free Press.

Camp-Sorrell D: *Access device guidelines: recommendations for nursing practice and education*, ed 2, Pittsburgh, 2004, Oncology Nursing Society.

Cao P, Kimura S, Macias BR et al.: Exercise within lower body negative pressure partially counteracts lumbar spine deconditioning associated with 28-day bed rest, *J Appl Physiol* 99(1):39-44, 2005.

Center to Advance Palliative Care: *How to establish a palliative care program: primary, secondary, tertiary model of palliative care delivery*, 2004 (website): *www.capc.org.*

Chan D, Brennan NJ: Delirium: making the diagnosis, improving the prognosis, *Geriatrics* 54(3):28-42, 1999.

Chochinov HM: Dignity-conserving care—a new model for palliative care: helping the patient feel valued, *JAMA* 287(17):2253-2260, 2002.

Dartmouth Demonstration Project to Improve Pain Management Funded by the Mayday Fund: *Pain pocket card*, Lebanon, NH, April 2005, revised by P&T, Pain and Palliative Care.

Department of Pain Medicine & Palliative Care at Beth Israel Medical Center: 2004 (website): *www.stoppain.org.*

Doyle D, Hanks G, Cherny N, Calman K: *Oxford textbook of palliative medicine*, ed 3, Oxford, England, 2005, Oxford University Press.

Edwards N: Differentiating the three D's: delirium, dementia, depression, *Med Surg Nurs* 12(6):347-357, 2003.

Ferrell BR, Coyle N: *Textbook of palliative nursing*, ed 2, Oxford, England, 2005, Oxford University Press.

Fishman M et al.: *Cancer chemotherapy guidelines and recommendations for practice*, ed 2, Pittsburgh, 1999, Oncology Nursing Press.

Five Wishes—an advance directive document available from The Commission on Aging with Dignity: 1-888-5-WISHES or (website): *www.agingwithdignity.org.*

Hanley C: Delirium in the acute setting, *Med Surg Nurs* 13(4):217-225, 2004.

Herr KA; Mobily PR, Kohout FJ, Wagenaar D et al.: Evaluation of the Faces Pain Scale for use with the elderly, *Clin J Pain* 14(1):29-38, 1998.

Institute for Safe Medication Practices: Safety issues with patient-controlled analgesia. Part I, How errors occur, *ISMP Medication Safety Alert* 8(14), 2003 (website): *www.ismp.org*.

Institute for Safe Medication Practices: Safety issues with patient-controlled analgesia. Part II, How to prevent error, *ISMP Medication Safety Alert* 8(15), 2003 (website): *www.ismp.org*.

Institute for Safe Medication Practices: Safety issues with patient-controlled analgesia. Part I, *ISMP Medication Safety Alert Nurse Advise—ERR* 3(1), 2003 (website): *www.ismp.org*.

Institute for Safe Medication Practices: Safety issues with patient-controlled analgesia. Part II, *ISMP Medication Safety Alert Nurse Advise—ERR* 3(2), 2003 (website): *www.ismp.org*.

Institute of Medicine, Cassel CK, Field MJ, editors: *Approaching death: improving care at the end of life*, Washington, DC, 1997, National Academy Press.

Johnson M, Bulechek G, Butcher H et al.: *NANDA, NOC, and NIC linkages: nursing diagnoses, outcomes, and interventions*, ed 2, St. Louis, 2006, Mosby.

Joint Commission on Accreditation of Healthcare Organizations: *Patient's rights standard*, Oakbrook Terrace, Ill, 2004, TMJ (website): *www.jointcommission.org*.

Joint Commission on Accreditation of Healthcare Organizations: *Ambulatory care national patient safety goals*, Oakbrook Terrace, Ill, 2005, TMJ, (website): *www.jointcommission.org*.

Joint Commission on Accreditation of Healthcare Organizations: *Universal protocol for preventing wrong site, wrong procedure, wrong person surgery*, Oakbrook Terrace, Ill, 2003, TMJ, (website): *www.jointcommission.org*.

Kirkwood JM: *Current cancer therapeutics*, ed 4, Philadelphia, 2001, Churchill Livingstone.

Last acts: means to a better end: a report on dying in America today, Washington, DC, 2002, Last Acts National Program Office.

Letizia M, Shenk J, Jones TD: Intermittent subcutaneous injections for symptom control in hospice care: a retrospective investigation, *Hospice J* 15(2):1-11, 2000.

Logan P: *Principles of practice for the acute care nurse practitioner*, Boston, 2000, Prentice Hall.

Longnecker DE, Murphy FL: *Dripps, Eckenhoff Vandam—introduction to anesthesia*, ed 9, Philadelphia, 1997, Saunders.

Martinez J, Wagner S: Hospice and palliative care. In Yarbro C, Henson Frogge M, Goodman M, Groenwald S, editors: *Cancer nursing: principles and practice*, ed 5, Sudbury, Mass, 2000, Jones & Bartlett.

McCaffrey M, Pasero C: *Pain: clinical manual*, ed 2, St. Louis, 1999, Mosby.

National Concensus Project for Quality Palliative Care (NCP) (website): *www.nationalconsensusproject.org*.

National Institute for Occupational Safety and Health: *Preventing occupational exposure to antineoplastic and other hazardous drugs in health care settings*, Washington, DC, 2004, NIOSH (website): *www.cdc.gov/niosh/docs/2004-165/#sum*.

North American Nursing Diagnosis Association: *NANDA-I nursing diagnoses: definitions and classification, 2007-2008*, Philadelphia, 2007, NANDA International.

Oncology Nursing Society, Itano JK, Taoka KN: *Core curriculum for oncology nursing*, ed 4, Philadelphia, 2005, Saunders.

Oyama K: When delirium takes hold, *RN* 68(5):52-56, 2005.

Polovich M, White J, Kelleher L: *Chemotherapy and biotherapy guidelines and recommendations for practice*, ed 2, Pittsburgh, 2005, Oncology Nursing Press, Inc.

Quill TE: Terri Schiavo—a tragedy compounded, *N Engl J Med* 352(16):1630-1633, 2005.

Rieger PT: *Biotherapy: a comprehensive overview*, ed 2, Sudbury, Mass, 2001, Jones & Bartlett.

Schuster JL Jr: Delirium, confusion, and agitation at the end of life, *J Palliat Med* 1(2):177-186, 1998.

Spaak J, Montmerle S, Sundblad P, Linnarsson D: Long-term bed rest–induced reductions in stroke volume during rest and exercise: cardiac dysfunction vs. volume depletion, *J Appl Physiol* 98(2):648-654, 2005.

Taylor LJ, Herr K: Pain intensity assessment: a comparison of selected pain intensity scales for use in cognitively intact and cognitively impaired minority elders, poster presentation, Phoenix, Ariz, 2001, 20th Annual Scientific Meeting of the American Pain Society (APS).

Waller A, Caroline NL: *Handbook of palliative care in cancer*, ed 2, Boston, 2000, Butterworth-Heinemann.

Wallis MA: Looking at depression through bifocal lenses, *Nursing* 30(9):58-61, 2000.

Wilkes GM, Barton Burke M: *2005 Oncology nursing drug handbook*, Sudbury, Mass, 2005, Jones & Bartlett.

World Health Organization: *Palliative care: what is it?* Geneva, Switzerland, 1990, World Health Organization (website): *www.who.int/hiv/topics/palliative/care/en/print.htm*.

World Health Organization: Cancer pain relief with a guide to opioid availability, ed 2, Report of the WHO Expert Committee Technical Report Series No. 804, Geneva, Switzerland, 1996, World Health Organization.

Yarbro C, Hansen Frogge M, Goodman M, editors: *Cancer nursing: principles and practice*, ed 6, Sudbury, Mass, 2005, Jones & Bartlett.

Yurk R, Morgan D, Franey S et al.: Understanding the continuum of palliative care for patients and their caregivers, *J Pain Symptom Manage* 24(5):459-470, 2002.

Respiratory Care Plans

Altman EE: Update on COPD. Today's strategies improve quality of life. *Adv Nurse Pract* 12(3):49-54, 2004.

Barnett M: Supported discharge for patients with COPD. *Nursing Stand* 18(45):33-37, 2004.

Bartlett JG, Dowell SF: Practice guidelines for the management of community acquired pneumonia in adults, *Clin Infect Disease* 31:347-382, 2000.

Bernard GR, Artigas A: The American-European consensus conference on ARDS. Definitions, mechanisms, relevant outcomes, and clinical trial coordination, *Am J Respiratory Care Med* 143(3):818-824, 2001.

Blank-Reid C, Reid PC: Taking the tension out of traumatic pneumothoraxes, *Nursing* 29(4):41-47, 1999.

Booker R: Chronic obstructive pulmonary disease: non-pharmacological approaches, *Br J Nurs* 14(1):14-18, 2005.

Booker R: Chronic obstructive pulmonary disease and the NICE guidelines, *Nurs Stand* 19(22):43-52, 2005.

Carroll P: Exploring chest drain options, *RN* 63(10):50-58, 2000.

Celi BR, MacNee W: Standards for the diagnosis and treatment of patients with COPD: a summary of the ATS/ERS position paper, *Eur Respir J* 23(6):932-946, 2004.

Centers for Disease Control and Prevention: Guidelines for preventing the transmission of *Mycobacterium tuberculosis* in health-care settings, 2005. *Morbid and Mortality Wkly Rpt (MMWR)*, December, 2005, Vol.54 (No. RR-17, 1-141).

Ferguson GT: Recommendations for the management of COPD, *Chest* 117:23S-28S, 2000.

Fine, MJ, Stone RA et al.: Processes and outcomes of care for patients with community acquired pneumonia: results from the pneumonia patient outcome research team (PORT) cohort study, *Arch Intern Med* 159:970-80, 1999.

Frazier SC: Implications of the GOLD report for chronic obstructive lung disease for the home care clinician, *Home Heatlhcare Nurse* 23(2):109-114, 2005.

Gibbar-Clements T, Shirrell D, Dooley R et al.: The challenge of warfarin therapy, *Am J Nurs* 100(3):38-40, 2000.

Global Initiative for Chronic Obstructive Lung Disease (GOLD): Executive summary: global strategy for the diagnosis, management, and prevention of chronic obstructive pulmonary disease, 2005 (website): *www.goldcopd.com*.

Guidelines for the management of adult with community-acquired pneumonia, diagnosis, assessment of severity, antimicrobial therapy, and prevention, *Am J Respiratory Crit Care Med* 163:1730-1754, 2001.

Jackson MM. Viewpoint: delayed diagnosis: the tuberculosis tragedy, *Am J Nurs* 106(4):13, 2006.

Johnson M, Bulechek G, Butcher H et al.: *NANDA, NOC, and NIC linkages: nursing diagnoses, outcomes, and interventions*, ed 2, St. Louis, 2006, Mosby.

Koschel MJ: Pulmonary embolism: quick diagnosis can save a patient's life, *Am J Nurs* 104(6):46-50, 2004.

Mathews PJ, Roark-Sample B, Schmidt J, Brooks K: The latest in respiratory care, *Nurs Manager* Suppl 20:22-24, 2004.

Milner D: The physiological effects of smoking on the respiratory system, *Nursing Times* 100(24):56-59, 2004.

Myrianthefs PM, Kalafati M, Samara I, Baltopoulos GJ: Nosocomial pneumonia, *Crit Care Nurs* 27(3):241-257, 2004.

North American Nursing Diagnosis Association: NANDA-I nursing diagnoses: definitions and classification, 2007-2008, Philadelphia, 2007, NANDA International.

O'Hanlon-Nicholas T: Clinical savvy. Commonly asked questions about chest tubes, *Am J Nursing* 95(5):60-64, 1996.

Opperwall B: Asthma, allergy, and upper airway disease, *Nurs Clin North Am* 38(4):697-711, 2003.

Reid E: Pulmonary embolism: an overview of treatment and nursing issues, *Br J Nurs* 11-24(20):1373-1378, 1999.

Reigle J: Evaluating patients with chest pain, *J CV Nurs* 20(4):225, 2005.

Ruffolo DC: Pulmonary embolism. Intervene quickly to halt the great masquerader, *Adv Nurse Pract* 12(6):30-34, 2004.

Schleder BJ: Taking charge of hospital-acquired pneumonia, *Nurse Pract* 29(3):50-53, 2004.

Seventh ACCP Conference on Antithrombotic and Thrombolytic Therapy: Evidence based guidelines, *CHEST* 127:335-371, 2005.

Sieggreen M: Venous disorders: overview of current practice, *J Vascular Nurs* 23(1):33-35, 2005.

Simmons P, Simmons M: Informed nursing practice: the administration of oxygen to patients with COPD, *Med Surg Nurs* 13(2):82-85, 2004.

Smith T: Oxygen therapy for older people, *Nurs Older People* 16(5):22-28, 2004.

United States Department of Health and Human Services, Centers for Disease Control and Prevention: Guideline for isolation precautions: preventing transmission of infectious agents in healthcare settings 2007. *Morbid Mortal Wkly Rpt* (to be published later in 2007).

Ware LB, Matthay MA: The acute respiratory distress syndrome, *N Engl J Med* 342(18):1334-1349, 2000.

Cardiovascular Care Plans

Albert NM, Eastwood CA, Edwards ML: Evidence-based practice for acute decompensated heart failure, *Crit Care Nurse* 24(6):14-16, 18-25, 26-29, 2004.

American College of Cardiology Foundation/American Heart Association Task Force on Practice Guidelines: *ACC/AHA 2004 guideline update for coronary artery bypass graft surgery* (website): *www.acc.org/clinical/guidelines/cabg/index.pdf*.

Apple MS: Common cardiovascular disorders. In Morton P, Fontaine D, Hudak C, Gallo B, editors: *Critical care nursing: a holistic approach*, ed 8, Philadelphia, 2004, Lippincott Williams & Wilkins.

Aronow WS, Fleg JL: *Cardiovascular disease in the elderly*, ed 3, New York, 2004, Marcel Dekker.

Bernstein AD, Daubert JC, Fletcher RD et al., North American Society of Pacing and Electrophysiology/British Pacing and Electrophysiology Group: The revised NASPE/BPEG generic code for antibradycardia, adaptive-rate, and multisite pacing, *Pacing Clin Electrophysiol* 25(2):260-264, 2002.

Boden WE, Pepine CJ: Introduction to "optimizing management of non-ST-segment elevation acute coronary syndromes," *J Am Coll Cardiol* 41(4 Suppl):1S-6S, 2003.

Braunwald E, Goldman L: *Primary cardiology*, ed 2, Philadelphia, 2003, Saunders.

Braunwald E, Antman EM, Beasley JW et al.: ACC/AHA 2002 guideline update for the management of patients with unstable angina and non-ST-segment elevation myocardial infarction, American College of Cardiology Foundation/American Heart Association (website): *www.acc. org/clinical/guidelines/unstable/update_explantext.htm.*

Brinker JA: *Interventional catheterization and interventional cardiology,* American College of Cardiology Self-Assessment Program (ACCSAP V) Bethesda, Md, February 2002, American College of Cardiology Foundation (website): *www.cardiosource.com.*

Cannon CP: *Unstable angina,* American College of Cardiology Self-Assessment Program (ACCSAP V), Bethesda, Md, March 2002, American College of Cardiology Foundation (website): *www.cardiosource.com.*

DeVon HA, Ryan CJ: Chest pain and associated symptoms of acute coronary syndromes, *J Cardiovasc Nurs* 20(4): 232-238. 2005.

Fahey VA: *Vascular nursing,* ed 4, St. Louis, 2004, Saunders.

Fonarow GC, Adams KF Jr, Abraham WT et al.: Risk stratification for in-hospital mortality in acutely decompensated heart failure: classification and regression tree analysis, *JAMA* 293(5):572-580, 2005.

Fonarow GC, Weber JE, editors: Rapid clinical assessment of hemodynamic profiles and targeted treatment of patients with acutely decompensated heart failure, *Clin Cardiol (Supp V)* 27:1-20, 2004.

Fox KA: Management of acute coronary syndromes: an update, *Heart* 90(6):698-706, 2004.

Hallett JW Jr, Brewster DC, Rasmussen TE: *Handbook of patient care in vascular diseases,* ed 4, Philadelphia, 2001, Lippincott Williams & Wilkins.

Hunt SA, Abraham WT, Chin MH et al.: ACC/AHA 2005 guideline update for the diagnosis and management of chronic heart failure in the adult—summary article, *Circulation* 112(12):1825-1852, 2005.

Johnson M, Bulechek G, Butcher H et al.: *NANDA, NOC, and NIC linkages: nursing diagnoses, outcomes, and interventions,* ed 2, St. Louis, 2006, Mosby.

Katz SD: Mechanisms and treatment of anemia in chronic heart failure, *Congest Heart Fail* 10(5):243-247, 2004.

Mueller C, Scholer A, Laule-Kilian K et al.: Use of B-type natriuretic peptide in the evaluation and management of acute dyspnea, *N Engl J Med* 350(7):647-654, 2004.

National Heart, Lung, and Blood Institute, Department of Health and Human Services, National Institute of Health: Seventh report of the Joint National Committee on Prevention, Detection, Evaluation, and Treatment of High Blood Pressure (JNC 7), Pub No. 04-5230, Washington, DC, 2003, NHLBI, DHHS, NIH (website): *www.nhlbi.nih. gov/guidelines/hypertension/jnc7full.htm.*

Nettina SM, editor: *The Lippincott manual of nursing practice,* ed 8, Philadelphia, 2005, Lippincott, Williams & Wilkins.

Rubin LJ, American College of Chest Physicians: Diagnosis and management of pulmonary arterial hypertension: ACCP evidence-based clinical practice guidelines, *Chest* 126(1 Suppl):4S-6S, 2004.

Runge MS, Ohman M, editors: *Netter's cardiology,* Teterboro, NJ, 2004, Icon Learning Systems.

Steinbis S: What you should know about pulmonary hypertension, *Nurs Pract* 29(4):8-15, 19, 2004.

Urden LD, Stacy KM, Lough ME: *Thelan's critical care nursing: diagnosis and management,* ed 5, St. Louis, 2006, Mosby.

Theroux P: *Acute coronary syndromes: a companion to Braunwald's heart disease,* Philadelphia, 2003, Saunders.

Weaver DW: *Acute myocardial infarction,* American College of Cardiology Self-Assessment Program (ACCSAP V), Bethesda. Md, 2004, American College of Cardiology Foundation (website): *www.cardiosource.com.*

Wiegand DL: Advances in cardiac surgery: valve repair, *Crit Care Nurse* 23(2):72-91, 2003.

Wingate S: *Presentations in focus: reports and expert commentary: updates, trends, and issues in heart failure treatment—a nursing perspective,* New York, 2004, Rogers Medical Intelligence Solutions.

Woods SL, Froelicher ES. Motzer SA, Bridges EJ: *Cardiac nursing,* ed 5, Philadelphia, 2004, Lippincott Williams & Wilkins.

Young JB, Mills RM: *Clinical management of heart failure,* ed 2, West Islip, NY, 2004, Professional Communications.

Renal-Urinary Care Plans

American Nephrology Nurses' Association (ANNA) Transplantation Special Interest Group: *ANNA transplantation fact sheet* (website): *www.annanurse.org.*

Beers MH, Berkow R, editors: *Merck manual of geriatrics,* ed 3, Whitehouse Station, 2000, Merck Research Lab.

Beitz JM: Continent diversions: the new gold standards of ileoanal reservoir and neobladder, *Ostomy Wound Manage* 50(9):26-35, 2004.

Boyd L: Intravesical Basillus Calmette-Guerin for treating bladder cancer, *Urology Nurs* 23(3):189-191, 199, 2003.

Burrows L, Prowant BF: Peritoneal dialysis. In Parker J, editor: *Contemporary nephrology nursing,* ed 3, Pitman, NJ, 1998, American Nephrology Nurses' Association.

Burrows-Hudson S, Prowant BF: *ANNA nephrology nursing standards of practice and guidelines for care,* Pitman, NJ, 2005, American Nephrology Nurses' Association.

Carlson SL: Prostate disease, *RN* 67(9):54-59, 2004.

Chambers A: Transurethral resection syndrome: it does not have to be a mystery, *AORN J* 75(1):156-164, 166, 168-170, 2002.

Churchill DN, Blake PG, Jindal KK et al.: Clinical practice guidelines for initiation of dialysis. Canadian Society of Nephrology, *J Am Soc Nephrol* 10(S13):S289-S291, 1999.

Danovich GM, editor: *Handbook of kidney transplantation,* ed 3, Philadelphia, 2001, Lippincott Williams & Wilkins.

Eknoyan G, Levin A, Levin NW et al., National Kidney Foundation: K/DOQI clinical practice guidelines for bone metabolism and disease in chronic kidney disease, *Am J Kidney Dis* 42(4 Suppl 3):S1-S201, 2003.

Gilchrist K: Benign prostatic hyperplasia: is it a precursor to prostate cancer? *Nurse Pract* 29(6):30-37, 2004.

Gray M: Assessment and management of urinary incontinence, *Nurse Pract* 30(7):32-33, 36-43, 2005.

Huizinga R: Update in immunosuppression, *Nephrol Nurs J* 29(3):261-267, 2002.

Johnson M, Bulechek G, Butcher H et al.: *NANDA, NOC, and NIC linkages: nursing diagnoses, outcomes, and interventions*, ed 2, St. Louis, 2006, Mosby.

Kurella M, Bennett WM, Chertow GM: Analgesia in patients with ESRD: a review of available evidence, *Am J Kidney Dis* 42(2):217-228, 2003.

Lancaster L, editor: *Core curriculum for nephrology nursing*, ed 4, Pitman, NJ, 2001, American Nephrology Nurses' Association.

Levey AS, Rocco MV, Anderson S et al.: K/DOQI clinical practice guidelines on hypertension and antihypertensive agents in chronic kidney disease, *Am J Kidney Dis* 43 (5 Suppl 1):S1-S290, 2004.

Little C: Renovascular hypertension, *Am J Nurs* 100(2): 46-51, 2000.

Maloney-Monaghan C, Cafiero M: Male bladder control problems: a guide to assessment, *Ostomy Wound Manage* 50(12):42-48, 2004.

Mauk KL: Conservative therapy for urinary incontinence can help older adults, *Nursing* 35(8):20-21, 2005.

Mitzel H, Snyders M: Anonymous donation: a transplant center's experience, *Nephrol Nurs J* 29(3):275-277, 2002.

Kaiske B, Cosio FG, Beto J et al., National Kidney Foundation: Clinical practice guidelines for managing dyslipidemias in kidney transplant patients: a report from the Managing Dyslipidemias in Chronic Kidney Disease Work Group of the National Kidney Foundation Kidney Disease Outcomes Quality Initiative, *Am J Transplant* 4(Suppl 7):13-53, 2004.

National Kidney Foundation: K/DOQI clinical practice guidelines for managing dyslipidemias in chronic kidney disease, *Am J Kidney Dis* 41(Suppl 3):S1-S92, 2003.

National Kidney Foundation: K/DODI clinical practice guidelines for vascular access: update 2000, *Am J Kidney Dis* 37(1 Suppl 1):S137-S181, 2001.

NFK-K/DOQI Anemia Work Group: NFK-K/DOQI clinical practice guidelines for anemia of chronic kidney disease: update 2000, *Am J Kidney Dis* 37(1 Suppl 1):S182-S238, 2001.

NFK-K/DOQI Chronic Kidney Disease Working Group: Clinical practice guidelines for chronic kidney disease, *Am J Kidney Dis* 39(2 Suppl 1):2002.

North American Nursing Diagnosis Association: NANDA-I nursing diagnoses: definitions and classification, 2007-2008, Philadelphia, 2007, NANDA International.

Parker KP: Acute and chronic renal failure. In Parker J, editor: *Contemporary nephrology nursing*, ed 3, Pitman, NJ, 1998, American Nephrology Nurses' Association.

Preisig P, Chmielewski C, Keen M et al.: Renal physiology. In Parker J, editor: *Contemporary nephrology nursing*, ed 3, Pitman, NJ, 1998, American Nephrology Nurses' Association.

Price CA: Continuous renal replacement therapy. In Parker J, editor: *Contemporary nephrology nursing*, ed 3, Pitman, NJ, 1998, American Nephrology Nurses' Association.

Salai PB: Hemodialysis. In Parker J, ed: *Contemporary nephrology nursing*, ed 3, Pitman, NJ, 1998, American Nephrology Nurses' Association.

Neurologic Care Plans

Adam H, Adams R, Del Zoppo G, Goldstein LB: Guidelines for the early management of patients with ischemic stroke, AHA/ASA scientific statement 2005 guidelines update, a scientific statement from the stroke council of the American Heart Association/American Stroke Association, *Stroke* 36 (4): 916-923, 2005.

Adams HP: *Handbook of cerebrovascular diseases*, ed 2, New York, 2005, Marcel Dekker.

Albano C, Comandante L, Nolan S: Innovations in the management of cerebral injury, *Crit Care Nurs Q* 28(2):135-149, 2005.

Arbour R: Intracranial hypertension: monitoring and nursing assessment, *Crit Care Nurse* 24(5):19-32, 2004.

Bader MK, Littlejohns LR, American Association of Neuroscience Nurses: *AANN core curriculum for neuroscience nursing*, ed 4, Philadelphia, 2004, Saunders.

Baird MS, Keen JH, Swearingen PL: *Manual of critical care nursing: nursing interventions and collaborative management*, ed 5, St. Louis, 2005, Mosby.

Barker E: *Neuroscience nursing: a spectrum of care*, ed 2, St. Louis, 2002, Mosby.

Barker E: New hope for stroke patients, *RN* 68(2):38-42, 2005.

Barker E: SCI patients take a big step forward, *RN* 68(7): 30-34, 2005.

Barker E, Saulino MF: First-ever guidelines for spinal cord injuries, *RN* 65(10):32-37, 2002.

Benevento BT, Sipski ML: Neurogenic bladder, neurogenic bowel and sexual dysfunction in people with spinal cord injury, *Phys Ther* 82(6):601-612, 2002.

Bhatia S, Gupta A: Impairments in activities of daily living in Parkinson's disease: implications for management, *NeuroRehabilitation* 18(3):209-214, 2003.

Capezuti E: Minimizing the use of restrictive devices in dementia patients at risk for falling, *Nurs Clin North Am* 39(3):625-647, 2004.

Cook NF: Subarachnoid haemorrhage and vasospasm: using physiological theory to generate nursing interventions, *Intens Crit Care Nurs* 20(3):163-173, 2004.

D'Arcy Y: Conquering pain: have you tried these new techniques? *Nursing* 35(3):36-41, 2005.

DeLisser HM: Guillain-Barré syndrome in adults. In Rose BD, editor: *UpToDate*, Wellesley, Mass, 2005, UpToDate.

Dooling E, Winkelman C: Hyponatremia in the patient with subarachnoid hemorrhage, *J Neurosci Nurs* 36(3):130-135, 2004.

Estep M: Meningococcal meningitis in critical care: an overview, new treatments/prevention, and a case study, *Crit Care Nurs Q* 28(2):111-121, 2005.

Fan JY: Effect of backrest position on intracranial pressure and cerebral perfusion pressure in individuals with brain injury: a systematic review, *J Neurosci Nurs* 36(5):278-288, 2004.

Finesilver C: Defenses gone awry: multiple sclerosis, *RN* 66(4):36-43, 2003.

Fries JM: Critical rehabilitation of the patient with spinal cord injury, *Crit Care Nurs Q* 28(2):179-187, 2005.

Krause P, Straube A: Reduction of spastic tone increase induced by peripheral repetitive magnetic stimulation is frequency-independent, *NeuroRehabilitation* 20(1):63-65, 2005.

Gambrell M, Flynn N: Seizures 101, *Nursing 2004* 34(8): 36-41, 2004.

Haslam C: Managing bladder symptoms in people with multiple sclerosis, *Nursing Times* 101(2):48-50, 52, 2005.

Hickey JV: *The clinical practice of neurological and neurosurgical nursing*, ed 5, Philadelphia, 2003, Lippincott Williams & Wilkins.

Holland NJ, Madonna M: Nursing grand rounds: multiple sclerosis, *J Neurosci Nurs* 37(1):15-19, 2005.

Hommes OR, Comi G: *Early indicators, early treatments, neuroprotection in multiple sclerosis*, Milan, Italy, 2004, Springer-Verlag.

Horgas AL, Ellioll AF: Pain assessment and management in persons with dementia, *Nurs Clin North Am* 39(3): 593-606, 2004.

Johnson M, Bulechek G, Butcher H et al.: *NANDA, NOC, and NIC linkages: nursing diagnoses, outcomes, and interventions*, ed 2, St. Louis, 2006, Mosby.

Kieseier BC, Hemmer B, Hartung HP et al.: Multiple sclerosis: novel insights and new therapeutic strategies, *Curr Opin Neurol* 18(3):211-220, 2005.

Kosty T: Cerebral vasospasm after subarachnoid hemorrhage: an update, *Crit Care Nurs Q* 28(2):122-134, 2005.

Lausten G: Menactra for prevention of meningococcal disease, *Nurse Pract* 30(5):52-53, 2005.

Littlejohns LR, Bader MK, March K: Brain tissue oxygen monitoring in severe brain injury, I: reasearch and usefulness in critical care, *Crit Care Nurse* 23(4):17-25, 2003.

Liverman CT, Altevogt BM, Joy JE, Johnson RT, editors, Committee on Spinal Cord Injury, Institute of Medicine: *Spinal cord injury: progress, promise, and priorities*, Washington, DC, 2005, National Academies Press.

McCarter-Bayer A, Bayer F, Hall K: Preventing falls in acute care: an innovative approach, *J Gerontol Nurs* 31(3):25-33, 2005.

Medscape Medical News: French physical therapy technique effective in patients with refractory chronic back pain. AAN 57th Annual Meeting: Abstract S51.003, presented April 14, 2005.

Meinzer M, Djundja D, Barthel G et al.: Long-term stability of improved language functions in chronic aphasia after constraint-induced aphasia therapy, *Stroke* 36(7):1462-1466, 2005.

Miller J, Elmore S: Call a stroke code! *Nursing* 35(3):58-63, 2005.

Nolan S: Traumatic brain injury: a review, *Crit Care Nurs Q* 28(2):188-194, 2005.

Nowlin A: The promise of stem cells, *RN* 68(4):48-52, 2005.

Ogden JA: *Fractured minds: a case-study approach to clinical neuropsychology*, ed 2, Oxford, England, 2005, Oxford University Press.

Oliveira-Filho J, Koroshetz WJ: Thrombolytic therapy for acute ischemic stroke. In Rose BD, editor: *UpToDate*, Wellesley, Mass, 2005, UpToDate.

Oyama K, Criddle L: Vasospasm after aneurysmal subarachnoid hemorrhage, *Crit Care Nurse* 24(5):58-67, 2004.

Paolino AS, Garner KM: Effects of hyperglycemia on neurologic outcome in stroke patients, *J Neurosci Nurs* 37(3):130-135, 2005.

Pryor J: What cues do nurses use to predict aggression in people with acquired brain injury? *J Neurosci Nurs* 37(2):117-121, 2005.

Rawlins PK: Intrathecal baclofen therapy over 10 years, *J Neuroscience Nurs* 36(6):322-327, 2004.

Schacter SC: Pharmacology of antiepileptic drugs. In Rose BD, editor: *UpToDate*, Wellesley, Mass, 2005, UpToDate.

Shorvon SO, Fish DR, Dosdon WE, Perucca E: *The treatment of epilepsy*, ed 2, Malden, Mass, 2004, Blackwell.

Smith ER, Amin-Hanjani S: Evaluation and management of elevated intracranial pressure in adults. In Rose BD, editor: *UpToDate*, Wellesley, Mass, 2005, UpToDate.

Taub E, Uswatte G, Morris DM: Improved motor recovery after stroke and massive cortical reorganization following Constraint-Induced Movement therapy, *Phys Med Rehabil Clin N Am* 14(1 Suppl):S77-S91, 2003.

Varelas PN: *Seizures in critical care: a guide to diagnosis and therapeutics*, Totowa, NJ, 2005, Humana Press.

Vollmer T, Key L, Durkalski V et al.: Oral simvastatin treatment in relapsing-remitting multiple sclerosis, *Lancet* 363(9421):1607-1608, 2004.

Ward C: Neuroleptic malignant syndrome in a patient with Parkinson's disease: a case study, *J Neurosci Nurs* 37(3):160-162, 2005.

Endocrine Care Plans

AACE Thyroid Task Force: American Association of Clinical Endocrinologists medical guidelines for clinical practice for the evaluation and treatment of hyperthyroidism and hypothyroidism, *Endocr Pract* 8(6):457-469, 2002.

American Association of Clinical Endocrinologists: Inpatient diabetes and metabolic control: conference proceedings, *Endocr Pract* 10(Suppl 2):1-108, 2004.

American Diabetes Association: Standards of medical care in diabetes, *Diabetes Care* 28(Suppl 1):S4-S36, 2005.

American Diabetes Association: Diagnosis and classification of diabetes mellitus, *Diabetes Care* 28(Suppl 1):S37-S42, 2005.

Bailes BK: Hyperthyroidism in elderly patients, *AORN J* 69(1):254-258, 1999.

Berant CF, editor: *Medical management of type 2 diabetes*, Alexandria, Va, 2004, American Diabetes Association.

Bode BW, editor: *Medical management of type 1 diabetes*. Alexandria, Va, 2004, American Diabetes Association.

Braithwaite SS: Thyroid disorders. In Parrillo JE, Dellinger RP: *Critical care medicine: principles of diagnosis and management in the adult*, ed 2, St. Louis, 2002, Mosby.

Cohen AS, Ayello EA: Diabetes has taken a toll on your patient's vision: how can you help? *Nursing* 35(5):44-45, 2005.

De letter EA, Piette MH, Lambert WE, De Leenheer AP: Medico-legal implications of hidden thyroid dysfunction: a study of two cases, *Med Sci Law* 40(3):251-257, 2000.

Diehl-Oplinger L, Kaminski MF: Choosing the right fluid to counter hypovolemic shock, *Nursing* 34(3):52-57, 2004.

Fain JA: Unlock the mysteries of insulin therapy, *Nursing* 34(3):41-43, 2004.

Fitzgerald P: Endocrinology. In Tierney LM Jr, McPhee SJ, Papadakis MA: *Current medical diagnosis and treatment*, ed 43, New York, 2004, Lange Medical Books/McGraw-Hill.

Funnell MM, Barlage DL: Diabetes update, part 1: Managing diabetes with "agent oral," *Nursing* 34(3):36-40, 2004.

Garber AJ, Moghissi ES: *Consensus development conference on inpatient diabetes and metabolic control: position statement*, December 16, 2003, Washington, DC, American College of Endocrinology.

Genuth S et al.: The Expert Committee on the Diagnosis and Classification of Diabetes Mellitus: Follow-up report on the diagnosis of diabetes mellitus, *Diabetes Care* 26(11):3160-3167, 2003.

Johnson M, Bulechek G, Butcher H et al.: *NANDA, NOC, and NIC linkages: nursing diagnoses, outcomes, and interventions*, ed 2, St. Louis, 2006, Mosby.

North American Nursing Diagnosis Association: NANDA-I nursing diagnoses: definitions and classification, 2007-2008, Philadelphia, 2007, NANDA International.

Pittas AG, Siegel RD, Lau J: Insulin therapy for critically ill hospitalized patients: a meta-analysis of randomized controlled trials, *Arch Intern Med* 164(18):2005-2011, 2004.

Stoller WA, Massone T: Acute diabetic emergencies and hypoglycemia. In Parrillo JE, Dellinger RP: *Critical care medicine: principles of diagnosis and management in the adult*, ed 2, St. Louis, 2002, Mosby.

Van den Berghe G, Wouters P, Weekers F et al.: Intensive insulin therapy in critically ill patients, *N Engl J Med* 345(19):1359-1367, 2001.

Waltman PA, Brewer JM, Lobert S: Thyroid storm during pregnancy, *Crit Care Nurse* 24(2):74-79, 2004.

Gastrointestinal Care Plans

Afdhal NH: Diseases of the gallbladder and bile ducts. In Goldman L, Ausiello D, editors: *Cecil Textbook of Medicine*, ed 22, Philadelphia, 2004, Saunders.

American Gastroenterological Association: American Gastroenterological Association Medical Position Statement: Treatment of pain in chronic pancreatitis, *Gastroenterology* 115(3):763-764, 1998.

Auld RM: Medical therapy of inflammatory bowel disease, Inflammatory Bowel Disease Workshop, Santa Rosa, Calif, June 1, 2005, Crohn's and Colitis Foundation of America.

Beckingham IJ, Bornman PC: ABC of diseases of liver, pancreas, and biliary system: acute pancreatitis, *BMJ* 322(7286):595-598, 2001.

Bornman PC, Beckingham IJ: ABC of diseases of liver, pancreas, and biliary system: chronic pancreatitis, *BMJ* 322(7287):660-663, 2001.

Blank-Reid C: Abdominal trauma: dealing with the damage, *Nursing* 34(9):36-41, 2004.

Broadwell DC, Jackson BS: *Principles of ostomy care*, St. Louis, 1982, Mosby.

Brown A: Predicting severity in acute pancreatitis: in search of a perfect marker, *J Clin Gastroenterol* 36(3):195-197, 2003.

Brozenec SA: Assessment of the hepatic system. In Phipps WJ, Monahan FD, Marek JE et al., editors: *Medical-surgical nursing: health and illness perspectives*, ed 7, Philadelphia, 2003, Mosby.

Colwell JC, Goldberg MT, Carmel JE: *Fecal and urinary diversions: management principles*, St. Louis, 2004, Mosby.

Drugs Information Online (website): *www.drugs.com.*

Friedman LS: Liver, biliary tract, & pancreas. In Tierney LM et al.: *Current Medical Diagnosis & Treatment*, ed 43, New York, 2004, Lange Medical/McGraw-Hill.

Friedman SL, Schiano TD: Cirrhosis and its sequelae. In Goldman L, Ausiello D, editors: *Cecil textbook of medicine*, ed 22, Philadelphia, 2004, Saunders.

Graham DY: Peptic ulcer disease. In Goldman L, Ausiello D, editors: *Cecil textbook of medicine*, ed 22, Philadelphia, 2004, Saunders.

Gavaghan M: The pancreas—hermit of the abdomen, *AORN J* 75(6):1110-1138, 2002.

Goldsmith C, Stover SE: Abdominal trauma: a major cause of morbidity and mortality, *Emergency Nurses Specialty Guide* 66-69, 2004.

Hemminger LL, Wolfsen HC: Photodynamic therapy for Barrett's esophagus and high grade dysplasia: results of a patient satisfaction survey, *Gastroenterol Nurs* 25(4):139-141, 2002.

Hoofnagle JH, Lindsay KL: Acute viral hepatitis. In Goldman L, Ausiello D, eds: *Cecil textbook of medicine*, ed 22, Philadelphia, 2004, Saunders.

Khoo RE: Surgery for inflammatory bowel disease, Inflammatory Bowel Disease Workshop, Santa Rosa, Calif, June 1, 2005, Crohn's and Colitis Foundation of America.

Lucey MR: Diseases of the peritoneum, mesentery, and omentum. In Goldman L, Ausiello D, editors: *Cecil textbook of medicine*, ed 22, Philadelphia, 2004, Saunders.

McQuaid KR: Alimentary tract. In Tierney LM, McPhee SJ, Papadakis MA, editors: *Current medical diagnosis and treatment 2006*, ed 45, New York, 2006, McGraw-Hill.

Medline Plus, a service of the U.S. National Library of Medicine and the National Institutes of Health (website): *www.nlm.nih.gov/medlineplus/druginformation.html.*

Nathens AB, Curtis JR, Beale RJ et al.: Management of the critically ill patient with severe acute pancreatitis, *Crit Care Med* 32(12):2524-2536, 2004.

North American Nursing Diagnosis Association: NANDA-I nursing diagnoses: definitions and classification, 2007-2008, Philadelphia, 2007, NANDA International.

Orloff S, Debas H: Peptic ulcer disease: surgical therapy. In Goldman L, Ausiello D, eds: *Cecil textbook of medicine*, ed 22, Philadelphia, 2004, Saunders.

Owyang C: Pancreatitis. In Goldman L, Ausiello D, editors: *Cecil textbook of medicine*, ed 22, Philadelphia, 2004, Saunders.

Pagana KD, Pagana TJ: *Mosby's diagnostics and laboratory test reference*, ed 7, St. Louis, 2005, Mosby.

Ray SW, Secrest J, Ch'ien AP, Corey RS: Managing gastroesophageal reflux disease, *Nurse Pract* 27(5):36-53, 2002.

Rockey AD: What you need to know about Barrett's esophagus, *Gastroenterol Nurs* 25(6):237-240, 2002.

Rothstein RD: Dysphagia and esophageal obstruction. In Rakel RE, Bope ET, editors: *Conn's current therapy 2006*, Philadelphia, 2006, Saunders.

Sands, JK: Gastrointestinal problems. In Phipps WJ, Monahan FD, Marek JE et al., eds: *Medical-surgical nursing: health and illness perspectives*, ed 7, Philadelphia, 2004, Mosby.

Sands JK: Gallbladder and exocrine pancreatic problems. In Phipps WJ, Monahan FD, Marek JE et al, editors: *Medical-surgical nursing: health and illness perspectives*, ed 7, Philadelphia, 2004, Mosby.

Semrad CE, Powell DW: Approach to the patient with diarrhea and malabsorption. In Goldman L, Ausiello D, editors: *Cecil textbook of medicine*, ed 22, Philadelphia, 2004, Saunders.

Smotkin J, Tenner S: Laboratory diagnostic tests in acute pancreatitis, *J Clin Gastroenterol* 34(4):459-462, 2002.

Spechler SJ, American Gastroenterological Association: American Gastroenterological Association Medical Position Statement on treatment of patients with dysphagia caused by benign disorders of the distal esophagus, *Gastroenterology* 117(1):229-233, 1999.

Spechler SJ: Barrett's esophagus and esophageal adenocarcinoma: pathogenesis, diagnosis, and therapy, *Med Clin N Am* 86(6):1423-1445, 2002.

Tintinalli JE, Kelen GD, Stapczynski JS: *Emergency medicine: a comprehensive study guide*, ed 6, New York, 2004, McGraw-Hill.

Wilcox CM: Appendicitis, diverticulitis, and miscellaneous intestinal inflammatory conditions. In Goldman L, Ausiello D, editors: *Cecil textbook of medicine*, ed 22, Philadelphia, 2004, Saunders.

Hematologic Care Plans

Beers M, Berkow R et al., editors: Anemias. In Beers M, Berkow R, editors: *The Merck manual of diagnosis and therapy*, ed 17, West Point, NY, 1999, Merck.

Brecher M, editor: *American Association of Blood Banks technical manual*, ed 14, Bethesda, Md, 2002, American Association of Blood Banks.

Cines DB, Blanchette VS: Immune thrombocytopenic purpura, *N Engl J Med*, 346(13):995-1008, 2002.

Coutre S: Heparin-induced thrombocytopenia (website): *www.uptodate.com*, version 13.1.

Embury S, Vichinsky E: Overview of the clinical manifestations of sickle cell disease (website): *www.uptodate.com*, version 13.1.

Golden C: Polycythemia vera: a review, *Clin J Oncol Nurs* 7(5); 553-556, 2003.

Johnson M, Bulechek G, Butcher H et al.: *NANDA, NOC, and NIC linkages: nursing diagnoses, outcomes, and interventions*, ed 2, St. Louis, 2006, Mosby.

Kline N: Alterations of hematologic function in children. In McCance K, Huether S, editors: *Pathophysiology: the biologic basis for disease in adults and children*, ed 4, St. Louis, 2002, Mosby.

Linker CA: Blood. In Tierney L, Papadakis M, McPhee S, editors: *STAT!Ref Online Electronic Medical Library*, New York, 2005, McGraw-Hill (website): *http://online.Statref.com*.

Mansen T, McCance K: Alterations of leukocyte, lymphoid, and hemostatic function. In McCance K, Huether S, editors: *Pathophysiology: the biologic basis for disease in adults and children*, ed 4, St. Louis, 2002, Mosby.

North American Nursing Diagnosis Association: NANDA-I nursing diagnoses: definitions and classification, 2007-2008, Philadelphia, 2007, NANDA International.

Ohene-Frempong K: Sickle cell disease. In Rudolph AM, Rudolph CD, editors: *Rudolph's pediatrics*, ed 21, New York, 2002, McGraw-Hill.

Peason H: Thalassemia. In Rudolph AM, Rudolph CD, editors: *STAT!Ref Rudolph's pediatrics*, ed 21, New York, 2002, McGraw-Hill (website): *www.statref.com/ourProducts/libraries/disciplines.htm*.

Spratto G, Woods L: PDR nurse's drug handbook 2005 edition, Clifton Park, NJ, 2005, Thomson Delmar Learning.

Musculoskeletal Care Plans

AlloSource: *About allografts*, 2005 (website): *www.allosource.org/aboutallografts.html*.

American Academy of Orthopaedic Surgeons (AAOS) and American Association of Tissue Banks (AATB): *What can you tell me about bone and tissue transplantation?* 2005 (website): *www.aatb.org/aaosinfo.htm*.

American College of Rheumatology: *Exercise and arthritis*, 2003 (website): *www.rheumatology.org/public/factsheets/exercise.asp?aud=pat*.

American College of Rheumatology: *Rheumatoid arthritis*, 2004 (website): *www.rheumatology.org/public/factsheets/ra_new.asp?aud5pat*.

Arthritis Foundation: *The facts about arthritis*, 2004 (website): *www.arthritis.org/resources/gettingstarted/default.asp*.

Arthritis Foundation: *Delivering on the promise in rheumatoid arthritis: new therapies* (website): *www.arthritis.org/research/Research_Program/RA/new_therapies.asp*.

Arthritis Foundation: *Arthritis Today's drug guide 2005* (website): *www.arthritis.org/conditions/DrugGuide/about_analgesics.asp*.

Arthritis Foundation, Association of State and Territorial Health Officials, and Centers for Disease Control and Prevention: *National arthritis action plan: a public health strategy*, Atlanta, 1999, Arthritis Foundation.

Burkus JK: *New bone graft techniques and applications in the spine*, 2002 (website): *www.medscape.com/viewprogram/2073*.

Childs SG: Athletic performance and injury. In Maher AB, Salmond SW, Pellino TA, editors: *Orthopaedic nursing*, ed 3, Philadelphia, 2002, Saunders.

Dunkin MA: *Guide to lab tests*, 2004 (website): *www.arthritis.org/conditions/Lab_Tests/labtestmain.asp*.

Ehde DM, Czerniecki JM, Smith DG et al.: Chronic phantom sensations, phantom pain, residual limb pain, and other regional pain after lower limb amputation, *Arch Phys Med Rehab* 81(8):1039-1044, 2000.

Food and Drug Administration (FDA): *FDA approves teriparatide to treat osteoporosis*, 2002 (website): *www.fda.gov/bbs/topics/ANSWERS/2002/ANS01176.html*.

Institute of Medicine: *Dietary reference intakes for calcium, phosphorus, magnesium, vitamin D, and fluoride*, 1997 (website): *http://books.nap.edu/openbook/0309063507/html/index.html*.

Johnson M, Bulechek G, Butcher H et al.: *NANDA, NOC, and NIC linkages: nursing diagnoses, outcomes, and interventions*, ed 2, St. Louis, 2006, Mosby.

Klippel JH, editor: *Primer on the rheumatic diseases*, ed 12, Atlanta, 2001, Arthritis Foundation.

Kunkler CE: Fractures. In Maher AB, Salmond SW, Pellino TA, editors: *Orthopaedic nursing*, ed 3, Philadelphia, 2002, Saunders.

Mahawald ML: Infections of bones and joints. In Beers MH, Berkow R, editors: *Merck manual of diagnosis and therapy*, ed 17, Whitehouse Station, NJ, 1999, Merck.

North American Nursing Diagnosis Association: *NANDA-I nursing diagnoses: definitions and classification, 2007-2008*, Philadelphia, 2007, NANDA International.

National Osteoporosis Foundation: *Boning up on osteoporosis*, Washington, DC, 2000, National Osteoporosis Foundation.

National Osteoporosis Foundation: *Osteoporosis: fast facts*, 2004 (website): *www.nof.org/osteoporosis/diseasefacts.htm*.

Pellino TA, Preston MAS, Bell N et al.: Complications of orthopaedic disorders and orthopaedic surgery. In Maher AB, Salmond SW, Pellino TA, editors: *Orthopaedic nursing*, ed 3, Philadelphia, 2002, Saunders.

Redemann S: Modalities for immobilization. In Maher AB, Salmond SW, Pellino TA, editors: *Orthopaedic nursing*, ed 3, Philadelphia, 2002, Saunders.

Roberts D: Management of clients with musculoskeletal trauma or overuse. In Black JM, editor: *Medical-surgical nursing: clinical management for positive outcomes*, ed 7, Philadelphia, 2005, Saunders.

Roberts D: Nursing management: arthritis and connective tissue diseases. In Lewis SM, Heitkemper MM, Dirksen SR, editors: *Medical-surgical nursing: assessment and management of clinical problems*, ed 6, St. Louis, 2004, Mosby.

Roberts D: Care of the patient with hip problems. In Mosher C: *An introduction to orthopaedic nursing*, ed 3, Chicago, 2004, NAON.

Roberts D: Degenerative disorders. In Maher AB, Salmond SW, Pellino TA, editors: *Orthopaedic nursing*, ed 3, Philadelphia, 2002, Saunders.

Roberts D: Arthritic and connective tissue disorders. In Schoen D, editor: *Core curriculum for orthopaedic nursing*, ed 4, Pitman, NJ, 2001, NAON.

Roberts D, Lappe J: Management of clients with musculoskeletal disorders. In Black JM, editor: *Medical-surgical nursing: clinical management for positive outcomes*, ed 7, Philadelphia, 2005, Saunders.

Russell T, Palmieri A: Fractures of the pelvis, acetabulum and lower extremity. In Brotzman SB, Wilk KE, editors: *Clinical orthopaedic rehabilitation*, ed 2, St. Louis, 2003, Mosby.

Sedlak CA, Doheny MO: Metabolic conditions. In Maher AB, Salmond SW, Pellino TA, editors: *Orthopaedic nursing*, ed 3, Philadelphia, 2002, Saunders.

Sharkey NA, Williams NI, Guerin JB: The role of exercise in the prevention and treatment of osteoporosis and osteoarthritis, *Nurs Clin North Am* 35(1):209-221, 2000.

Simon LS: Osteoporosis. In Beers MH, Berkow R, editors: *Merck manual of diagnosis and therapy*, ed 17, Whitehouse Station, NJ, 1999, Merck.

Welland D: *Arthritis Today's 2002—2003 supplement guide*, Atlanta, 2002, Arthritis Foundation.

Williamson V: Amputation. In Maher AB, Salmond SW, Pellino TA, editors: *Orthopaedic nursing*, ed 3, Philadelphia, 2002, Saunders.

Women's Health Initiative (WHI): *Advice about postmenopausal hormone therapy*, 2002 (website): *www.nhlbi.nih.gov/health/women/pht_facts.htm#advice*.

Special Needs Care Plans

Ayello EA. Conquer chronic wounds with wound bed preparation, *Nurse Pract* 29(3):8-25; quiz 26-27, 2004.

Ayello EA, Dowsett C, Schultz GS et al.: TIME heals all wounds, *Nursing* 34(4):36-42, 2004.

Bartlett, JG: *The Johns Hopkins Hospital 2005-2006 Guide to Medical Care of Patients with HIV Infection*, ed 12, Philadelphia, 2005, Lippincott Williams & Wilkins.

Bradley-Springer L: *2004 HIV Symptom Management*, Akron, 2004, Association of Nurses in AIDS Care.

Braden Scale for Predicting Pressure Sore Risk (website): *www.bradenscale.com/braden.PDF*.

Centers for Disease Control and Prevention: Advancing HIV prevention: new strategies for a changing epidemic-United States, 2003, *MMWR* 52(15):329-332, 2003.

CDC, HRSA, NIH, HIV Medicine Association of the Infectious Diseases Society of America, HIV Prevention in Clinical Care Working Group: Recommendation for incorporating human immunodeficiency virus (HIV) prevention into the medical care of persons living with HIV, *CID* 38(1):104-121, 2004.

Centers for Disease Control and Prevention: Antiretroviral postexposure prophylaxis after sexual, injection-drug use, or other nonoccupational exposure to HIV in the United States: recommendations from the U.S. Department of Health and Human Services, *MMWR* 54(No. RR-2):[1-17], 2005.

Centers for Disease Control and Prevention: Revised guidelines for HIV counseling, testing and referral: technical expert panel review of CDC HIV counseling, testing and referral guidelines, *MMWR* 50(No. RR-19):[1-58], 2001.

Centers for Disease Control and Prevention: Treating opportunistic infections among HIV-infected adults and adolescents: recommendations from CDC, the National Institutes of Health, and the HIV Medicine Association/Infectious Diseases Society of America, *MMWR* 53(No. RR-15):[1-112], 2004.

Centers for Disease Control and Prevention: Updated U.S. Public Health Service guidelines for the management of occupational exposures to HIV and recommendations for postexposure prophylaxis, *MMWR* 54(No. RR-9):[1-11], 2005.

Centers for Disease Control and Prevention: Incorporating HIV prevention into the medical care of persons living with HIV: recommendations of CDC, Health Resources and Services Administration, the National Institutes of Health, and the HIV Medicine Association of the Infectious Diseases Society of America, *MMWR* 52(12):1-24, 2003.

Charney P: Enteral nutrition: indications, options, and formulations. In Holcombe BJ, Gottschlich MM, editors: *The Science and practice of nutrition support: a case-based core curriculum*, Dubuque, Iowa, 2000, Kendall/Hunt.

Franch-Arcas G: The meaning of hypoalbuminaemia in clinical practice. *Clin Nutr* 20:265-269, 2001.

Franks L: Caring for patients with human immunodeficiency virus disease. In Swearingen PL: *Manual of medical-surgical nursing care*, ed 6, St. Louis, 2007, Mosby.

Fuhrman MP, Charney P, Mueller C: Hepatic proteins and nutrition assessment, *J Am Diet Assoc* 104:1258-1264, 2004.

Gopal S, Carr B, Nelson P: Does microalbuminuria predict illness severity in critically ill patients on the intensive care unit? A systemic review. *Crit Care Med* 34:1805-1810, 2006.

Gupta S, Baharestani M, Baranoski S et al.: Guidelines for managing pressure ulcers with negative pressure wound therapy, *Adv Skin Wound Care* Suppl 2:1-16, 2004.

Johnson M, Bulechek G, Butcher H et al.: *NANDA, NOC, and NIC linkages: nursing diagnoses, outcomes, and interventions*, ed 2, St. Louis, 2006, Mosby.

Lansdown AB: Nutrition 2: a vital consideration in the management of skin wounds, *Br J Nurs* 13(20):1199-1210, 2004.

Mangram AJ, Horan TC, Pearson ML et al.: Guideline for prevention of surgical site infection, 1999, Centers for Disease Control and Prevention (CDC) Hospital Infection Control Practices Advisory Committee, *Am J Infect Control* 27(2):97-134, 1999.

Marik PE, Zaloga GP: Gastric versus post-pyloric feeding: a systematic review, *Crit Care* 7(3):R46-51, 2003.

McMahon MM: Management of parenteral nutrition in acutely ill patients with hyperglycemia, *Nutr Clin Pract* 19(2):120-128, 2004.

Metheny NA, Meert KL: Monitoring feeding tube placement, *Nutr Clin Pract* 19(5):487-495, 2004.

Nassar, NN, Keiser P, Gregg CR: *Parkland Pocket Guide to HIV Care*, ed 3, Dallas, 2004, Texas/Oklahoma AIDS Education and Training Center and Parkland Health and Hospital System.

National Pressure Ulcer Advisory Panel: New stage I definition, *Adv Wound Care* 11(2):59, 1998.

North American Nursing Diagnosis Association: NANDA-I nursing diagnoses: definitions and classification, 2007-2008, Philadelphia, 2007, NANDA International.

Panel on Clinical Practices for Treatment of HIV Infection convened by the Department of Health and Human Services (DHHS): *Guidelines for the use of antiretroviral agents in HIV-1-infected adults and adolescents*, October 6, 2005 (website) *http://AIDSinfo.nih.gov.*

Panel on the Treatment of Pressure Ulcers: *Treatment of pressure ulcers: clinical practice guideline*, no. 15, pub no. 95-0652, Rockville, Md, 1994, USDHHS, Agency for Health Care Policy Research.

Parker CM, Heyland DK: Aspiration and the risk of ventilator-associated pneumonia, *Nutr Clin Pract* 19(6):597-609, 2004.

Public Health Service Task Force: Recommendations for use of antiretroviral drugs in pregnant HIV-1-infected women for maternal health and interventions to reduce perinatal HIV-1 transmission in the United States, February 24, 2005 (website:) *http://AIDSinfo.nih.gov.*

Russell MK et al., ASPEN Board of Directors: Standards for specialized nutrition support: adult hospitalized patients, *Nutr Clin Pract* 17(6):384-391, 2002.

Stotts NA: Impaired wound healing. In Carrieri-Kohlman V, West CM, Lindsey AM, editors: *Pathophysiological phenomena in nursing: human response to illness*, ed 3, St. Louis, 2003, Saunders.

Vanek VW: Ins and outs of enteral access. Part 1: Short-term enteral access, *Nutr Clin Pract* 17(5):275-283, 2002.

Vanek VW: Ins and outs of enteral access. Part 2: Long-term access—esophagostomy and gastrostomy, *Nutr Clin Pract* 18(1):50-74, 2003.

Vanek VW: Ins and outs of enteral access. Part 3: Long-term access—jejunostomy, *Nutr Clin Pract* 18:210-220, 2003.

Whitmire SF: Fluid and electrolytes. In Holcombe BJ, Gottschlich MM, editors: *The science and practice of nutrition support: a case-based core curriculum*, Dubuque, Iowa, 2001, Kendall/Hunt.

Whitney JD. Overview: acute and chronic wounds. *Nurs Clin North Am* 40(2):191-205, 2005.

Part II: Pediatric Nursing Care Plans

Administration for Children and Families, U.S. Department of Health and Human Services: Chapter 3—Victims, child maltreatment, 2003 (website): *www.acf.hhs.gov/programs/cb/pubs/cm03/chapterthree.htm*.

Alberti G et al.: Type 2 diabetes in the young: the evolving epidemic, *Diabetes Care* 27:1798-1811, 2004, (website): *www.care.diabetesjournals.org/cgi/content/extract/27/7/1798?maxtoshow =&HITS=10&hits=10&RESULTFORMAT=&fulltext=*.

American Academy of Pediatrics: Committee on Child Abuse and Neglect: Shaken baby syndrome: rotational cranial injuries—technical report, *Pediatrics* 108(1):206-210, 2001.

American Academy of Pediatrics: Diagnosis and evaluation of the child with attention-deficit/hyperactivity disorder (AC0002), *Pediatrics* 105(5):1158-1170, 2000.

American Academy of Pediatrics: Clinical practice guideline: treatment of the school-aged child with attention-deficit/hyperactivity disorder, *Pediatrics* 108(4):1033-1042, 2001.

American Academy of Pediatrics: *Pediatric clinical practice guidelines & policies*: American Academy of Pediatrics and American Academy of Family Physicians: Diagnosis and management of acute otitis media, 141-155, 2004, book published 2006.

American Diabetes Association Position Statement: Diabetes care in the school and day care setting, *Diabetes Care* 29:S49-S55, 2006 (website): *www.care.diabetesjournals.org/cgi/content/full/29/suppl_1/s49*.

American Lung Association: Lung Disease Data: 2006, Asthma, 13-18 (website): *www.lungusa.org*.

Betz CL: Editorial—attention deficit hyperactivity disorder: nurses are important members of the team, *J Pediatr Nursing: Nursing Care Child Fam* 21(3):171-174, 2006.

Betz CL: Use of 504 plans for children and youth with disabilities: nursing applications, *Pediatr Nurs* 27(4):347-352, 2001.

Bindler R, Howry L: *Prentice Hall pediatric drug guide with nursing implications*, Upper Saddle River, 2005, Pearson Education, Inc.

Broderick M: Pediatric poisoning, *RN* 67(9):37, 38, 40-43, 2004.

Castiglia PT: Growth and development: shaken baby syndrome, *J Pediatr Health Care* 15(2):78-80, 2001.

Center for Disease Control and Prevention: Managing acute gastroenteritis among children: oral rehydration, maintenance, and nutritional therapy, *MMWR* 52(RR16):1-16, 2003 (website): *www.cdc.gov/mmwr/preview/mmwrhtml/rr5216la1.htm*.

Chase HP: *Understanding insulin dependent diabetes*, ed 11, Denver, 2006, Barbara Davis Center for Childhood Diabetes at Denver.

Childhelp: National child abuse statistics, 2006 (website): *www.childhelpusa.org/resources/learning-center/statistics*.

Cystic Fibrosis Foundation: *Cystic fibrosis-related diabetes*, created by Washington University School of Medicine Adult Cystic Fibrosis Team June 2005 (website): *www.cff.org/UploadedFiles/living_with_cf/Files/Final%20CFRD%20brochure%20v2.pdf*.

Cystic Fibrosis Foundation: What is cystic fibrosis? New statistics show CF patients living longer, July 5, 2006 (website): *www.cf.org*.

Elkin MK, Perry AG, Potter PA: *Nursing interventions and clinical skills*, ed 3, St. Louis, 2004, Mosby.

Hockenberry MJ: *Wong's clinical manual of pediatric nursing*, ed 6, St. Louis, 2003, Mosby.

Hockenberry MJ et al., editors: *Wong's nursing care of infants and children*, ed 7, St. Louis, 2004, Mosby.

Keep Kids Healthy.com: Rectal prolapse, July 5, 2006 (website): *www.keepkidshealthy.com/cgi-bin/MasterPFP.cgi*.

Lane PA et al.: Sickle cell disease in children and adolescents: diagnosis, guidelines for comprehensive care paths and protocols for management of acute and chronic complications, July 20, 2006 (website): *www.scinfo.org/protchildindex.htm*, last update January 2003.

Lauts NM: RSV: protecting the littlest patients, *RN* 68(12):46-51, 2005.

London ML, Ladewig PW, Ball JW, Bindler RC: *Maternal & child nursing care*, ed 2, Upper Saddle River, 2007, Pearson Education, Inc.

Manworren RCB, Hyman LS: Clinical validation of FLACC: Preverbal patient pain scale, *Pediatr Nurs* 29(2):140-146, 2003.

March of Dimes: Professional and researchers: cerebral palsy, July 2, 2006 (website): *www.marchofdimes.com/professionals/14332_1208.asp*.

Meleski DD: Families with chronically ill children, *Am J Nurs* 102(5):47-54, 2002.

Mulryan K: Helping abuse victims, part 3: How to recognize and respond to child abuse, *Nursing* 34(10):52-55, 2004.

National Asthma Education and Prevention Program: NAEPP expert panel report.Guidelines for the diagnosis and management of asthma: updates on selected topics, National Heart, Lung, and Blood Institute. NIH publication 02-5075.2002 (website): *www.nhlbi.nih.gov/guidelines/asthma/astupdt.htm*.

National Child Abuse Statistics, 2006 (website): *www.childhelpusa.org/resources/learning-center/statistics*.

National Diabetes Education Program: Overview of diabetes in children and adolescents: a fact sheet, January 2006 (website): *www.ndep.nih.gov/diabetes/pubs/Youth_FactSheet.pdf*.

National Institutes of Health, National Heart, Lung, and Blood Institute: Management of sickle cell disease, NIH Publication No. 02-2117, ed 4, 2002 (website): *www.scinfo.org/nihnewcontents.htm*.

NICHCY: Attention-deficit/hyperactivity disorder, fact sheet 19 (FS19), 2004 (website): *www.nichcy.org/pubs/factshe/ fs19txt.htm.*

Pagana KD, Pagana TJ: *Mosby's diagnostic and laboratory test reference*, ed 7, St. Louis, 2005, Mosby.

Redstone F, West J: The importance of postural control for feeding, *Pediatr Nurs* 30(2):97-100, 2004.

Robertson J, Shilkofski N, editors: *The Harriet Lane handbook: a manual for pediatric house officers*, ed. 17, Philadelphia, 2005, Elsevier.

Safe Kids: Facts about childhood burns, June 3, 2006 (website): *www.safekids.org.*

Safe Kids: Facts about childhood poisoning, June 10, 2006 (website): *www.safekids.org.*

Silverstein J et al.: Care of children and adolescents with type 1 diabetes, *Diabetes Care* 28:186-212, 2005 (website): *www.care.diabetesjournals.org/cgi/content/full/28/1/186.*

Taketoma CK, Hodding JH, Kraus DM: *Pediatric dosage handbook*, ed 13, Cleveland, 2006, American Pharmaceutical Association, Lexi-Comp.

Thompson Micromedex Healthcare Series: DRUGDEX Drug Point: atomoxetine hydrochloride, July 23, 2006 (website): *www.thomsonhc.com.*

Torpy JM, Lynn C, Glass R: Inflicted brain injury in children, *JAMA* 290(5):698, 2003.

Travis LB: *An instructional aid on insulin-dependent diabetes mellitus*, ed 12, Austin, 2003, Designer's Ink.

United Cerebral Palsy Foundation: Cerebral palsy—facts and figures, July 2, 2006 (website): *www.ucp.org/ucp_general-doc.cfm/1/9/37/37-37/447*, updated October 2001.

Vlam SL: Attention-deficit/hyperactivity disorder: diagnostic assessment methods used by advanced practice registered nurses, *Pediatr Nurs* 32(1):18-24, 2006.

Part III: Maternity Nursing Care Plans

American College of Obstetricians and Gynecologists: Premature rupture of membranes, Washington, DC, 1998, The Association (Technical Bulletin No. 1).

American College of Obstetricians and Gynecologists: Cervical insufficiency, Washington, DC, 2003, The Association (Technical Bulletin No. 48).

American College of Obstetricians and Gynecologists: Gestational diabetes, Washington, DC, 2001, The Association (Technical Bulletin No. 30).

American College of Obstetricians and Gynecologists: Diagnosis and management of preeclampsia and eclampsia, Washington, DC, 2002, The Association (Technical Bulletin No. 33).

American Pregnancy: Guidelines to hCG levels during pregnancy, March 13, 2006 (website): *www.americanpregnancy. org/duringpregnancy/concersearlydevelopment.htm.*

Gabbe SG, Neibyl JR, Simpson JL: *Obstetrics, normal and problem pregnancies*, ed 4, New York, 2002, Churchill Livingstone.

Griffith HW: *Complete guide to prescription and nonprescription drugs*. New York, 2003, The Berkley Publishing Group.

Johnson M, Bulechek G, Butcher H et al.: *NANDA, NOC, and NIC linkages: nursing diagnoses, outcomes, and interventions*, ed 2, St. Louis, 2006, Mosby.

Kim WJ: Fetal fibronectin, 2000, April 1, 2006 (website): *www.dlslab.com/dls/page_server.*

Pfizer: ZYVOX is a clear choice to treat infections caused by MRSA, April 2, 2006 (website): *www.zyvox.com/about. asp?hcp=true.*

Quintero JC, Jeanty P: Cervical incompetence, 2001, April 1, 2006 (website): *www.thefetus.net/page.php?id5274.*

Star WL et al.: *Ambulatory obstetrics*, ed 3, San Francisco, 1999, UCSF Nursing Press.

Wagner LK: Diagnosis and management of preeclampsia. *American Family Physician* 70(12) (website): *www.aafp.org.*

Part IV: Psychiatric Nursing Care Plans

American Nurses Association: *Statement on the scope and standards of psychiatric-mental health nursing practice*, Washington, DC, 2000, American Nurses Publishing.

American Psychiatric Association: *Diagnostic and statistical manual of mental disorders TR (4th ed Text Revised)*, Washington, DC, 2000, American Psychiatric Association.

American Psychiatric Association: *Practice guidelines for the treatment of psychiatric disorders: compendium 2000*. Washington, DC, 2000, American Psychiatric Association.

Anxiety Disorders Association of America: Statistics and facts about anxiety disorders, 2003 (website): *www.adaa. org/mediaroom/index.cfm.*

Bauer MS: Mood disorders: bipolar (manic depression) disorders. In Tasman A, Kay J, Lieberman JA, editors: *Psychiatry*, ed 2, West Sussex, England, 2003, John Wiley & Sons.

Beck AT, Rush AJ: Cognitive therapy. In Kaplan HI, Sadock BJ, editors: *Comprehensive textbook of psychiatry IV*, Vol. 2, Baltimore, 1995, Williams & Wilkins.

Becker KL, Walton-Moss B: Detecting and addressing alcohol abuse in women, *Nurse Pract* 26(10), 13-16, 19-23; quiz 24-15, 2001.

Beng-Choon H, Black DW, Andreasen NC: Schizophrenia and other psychotic disorders. In Hales RE, Yudofsky SC, editors: *Essentials of clinical psychiatry*, ed 2, Washington, DC, 2004, American Psychiatric Publishing.

Blairy S et al.: Social adjustment and self-esteem of bipolar patients: a multicentric study, *J Affect Disord* 79:97-103, 2004.

Cornelius J, Bukstein O, Salloum I, Clark D: Alcohol and psychiatric comorbidity, *Rec Dev Alcohol* 16:361-374, 2003.

Dubovsky SL, Davies R, Dubovsky AN: Mood disorders. In Hales RE, Yudofsky SC, editors: *Essentials of clinical psychiatry*, ed 2, Washington, DC, 2004, American Psychiatric Publishing.

Freeman MP, Wiegand C, Gelenberg AJ: Lithium. In Schatzberg AF, Nemeroff CB, editors: *The American Psychiatric Publishing textbook of psychopharmacology*, ed 3, Washington, DC, 2004, American Psychiatric Press.

Golden RN, Bebchuk J, Leatherman ME: Trazodone and other antidepressants. In Schatzberg AF, Nemeroff CB, editors: *The American Psychiatric Press textbook of psychopharmacology*, Washington, DC, 2003, American Psychiatric Press.

Gorman JM: Anxiety disorders: introduction and overview. In Sadock BJ, Sadock VA, editors: *Comprehensive textbook of psychiatry*, ed 7, Vol. 1, Philadelphia, 2000, Lippincott Williams & Wilkins.

Gruenberg AM, Goldstein RD: Mood disorders: depression. In Tasman A, Kay J, Lieberman JA, editors: *Psychiatry*, ed 4, Sussex, England, 2003, John Wiley & Sons.

Halter MJ: Stigma and help seeking related to depression: a study of nursing students. *J Psychosocial Nursing and Mental Health Services* 42(2):42-51, 2004.

Hambrick JP, Turk CL, Heimberg RG, Schneier FR, Liebowitz RG: Cognitive-behavioral therapy for social anxiety disorder: supporting evidence and future directions, *CNS Spectrums* 8(5):373-381, 2003.

Hopkins HS, Gelenberg AJ: Mood stabilizers. In Lieberman JA, Tasman A, editors: *Psychiatric drugs*, Philadelphia, 2000, WB Saunders.

Johnson H, Maas M, Meriden M, Moorehead S: *Nursing outcomes classification*, ed 2, St. Louis, 2004, Mosby.

Johnson M, Bulechek G, Butcher H et al.: *NANDA, NOC, and NIC linkages: nursing diagnoses, outcomes, and interventions*, ed 2, St. Louis, 2006, Mosby.

Kaplan BJ, Kaplan VA: *Kaplan & Sadock's concise textbook of clinical psychiatry*, ed 2, Philadelphia, 2004, Lippincott Williams & Wilkins.

Keltner NL Zielinshi AL, Hardin MS: Drugs used for the cognitive symptoms of Alzheimer's disease, *Persp Psychiatric Care* 37(1):31-34, 2001.

Lehne RA: *Pharmacology for nursing care*, ed 6, Philadelphia, 2006, WB Saunders.

Lenze EJ: Comorbidity of depression and anxiety in the elderly, *Curr Psychiatric Rep* 5:62-67, 2003.

Lieberman JA, Mendelowitz AJ: Antipsychotic drugs. In Lieberman JA, Tassman A, editors: *Psychiatric drugs*, Philadelphia, 2000, WB Saunders.

Marangell LB, Silver JM, Goff DC, Yudofsky SC: Psychopharmacology and electroconvulsive therapy. In Hales RE, Yudofsky SC, Talbott JA, editors: *Textbook of psychiatry*, ed 2, Washington, DC, 2004, American Psychiatric Press.

Maxmen JS, Ward NG: *Psychotropic drugs: fast facts*, ed 3, New York, 2002, W.W. Norton.

Mills J: Dealing with voices and strange thoughts. In Gamble C, Brennan G, editors: *Working with serious mental illness: a manual for clinical practice*, London, 2000, Bailliere Tindall.

Minkoff K: Dual diagnoses. In Tasman A, Kay J, Lieberman JA, editors: *Psychiatry*, ed 2, Vol. 2, Sussex, England, 2003, John Wiley & Sons.

Moorhead S, Johnson M, Maas M: *Nursing outcomes classification (NOC)*, ed 3, St. Louis, 2004, Mosby.

Moller MD, Murphy MF: *Recovering from psychosis: a wellness approach*, ed 15, Nine Mile Falls, Wash, 2002, Psychiatric Resource Network, Inc.

National Institutes of Mental Health: *Older adults: depression and suicide facts*. NIH publication No. 03-4593, Bethesda, Md, 2003.

Patel JK et al.: Schizophrenia and other psychoses. In Tasman A, Kay J, Lieberman JA, editors: *Psychiatry*, ed 2, West Sussex, England, 2003, John Wiley & Sons.

Resnick B, Perry D, Applebaum G, Armstrong L, Cotterman M, Dillman S et al.: The impact of alcohol use in community-dwelling older adults, *J Commun Health Nurs* 20(3):135-145, 2003.

Resick PA, Nishith P, Griffin MG: How well does cognitive-behavioral therapy treat symptoms of complex PTSD? *CNS Spectrums* 8(15):340-342, 351-355, 2003.

Sabbagh MN: Alzheimer's disease diagnosis and treatment: past, present and future. Proceedings from the 12th Annual Caregiver Conference, *Visions of Hope: Living Today, Planning Tomorrow*. Alzheimer's Association Desert Southwest Chapter, Central Arizona Region, March 21, 2003.

Serby M, Yu M: There is good news about depression in the elderly, *The Clinical Advisor*, September 25, 2003, pp. 64-75.

Stuart DE: Physical symptoms of depression: emerging needs in special populations, *J Clinical Psychiatry* 64(7):12-16, 2003.

Sutherland JE, Sutherland SJ, Hoehns JD: Achieving the best outcome in treatment of depression, *J Fam Pract* 52:3), 201-209, 2003.

Tsung-Ung WW, Zimmet SV, Wojcik JD, Canuso CM, Green AI: Treatment of schizophrenia. In Schatzberg AF, Nemeroff CB, editors: *The American Psychiatric Publishing Textbook of Psychopharmacology*, ed 3, Washington, DC, 2004, American Psychiatric Publishing.

Tuttle J, Melnyk BM, Loveland-Cherry C, Becker KL, Walton-Moss B, Shoultz J, et al.: Adolescent drug and alcohol use. Strategies for assessment, intervention, and prevention, *Nurs Clin North Am* 37(3):443-460, ix, 2002.

Varcarolis EM, Carson VB, Shoemaker NC: *Foundations of psychiatric mental health nursing: a clinical approach*, ed 5, St. Louis, 2006, Elsevier.

Wilkaitis J, Mulvihill T, Nasrallah HA: In Schatzberg AF, Nemeroff CB: *The American Psychiatric Publishing textbook of psychopharmacology*, ed 3, Washington, DC, 2004, American Psychiatric Publishing.

Appendix A

Boyce JM, Pittet D: Guideline for hand hygiene in health-care settings: recommendations of the Healthcare Infection Control Practices Advisory Committee and the HICPAC/SHEA/APIC/IDSA Hand Hygiene Task Force, Society for Healthcare Epidemiology of America/Association for Professionals in Infection Control/Infectious Diseases Society of America, *MMWR* 51(RR-16):1-45, quiz CE1-4, 2002.

Garner JS, Hospital Infection Control Practices Advisory Committee (HICPAC), Centers for Disease Control Practices and Prevention: Guidelines for isolation precautions in hospitals, *Infect Control Hosp Epidemiol* 17(1):53-80, 1996.

OSHA, Department of Labor: Occupational Safety and Health Administration: occupational exposure to blood-borne pathogens: final rule, 29 CFR Part 1910:1030, *Federal Register* 56:64003-64182, 1991; CFR 66:5317-25, revised 2001.

Siegel J, Strausbaugh L, Jackson M, Rhinehart E, Chiarello L, and the Healthcare Infection Control Practices Advisory Committee (HICPAC): DRAFT: Guideline for Isolation Precautions: preventing transmission of infectious agents in healthcare settings, revised 2007.

Siegel JD, Rhinehart E, Jackson M, Chiarello L, and the Healthcare Infection Control Practices Advisory Committee (HICPAC): Management of multidrug-resistant organisms in healthcare settings, 2006 (website): *www.cdc.gov/ncidod/dhap/pdf/ar/mdroGuideline2006.pdf*.

A

AA (Alcoholics Anonymous), 775, 782
AAAs (abdominal aortic aneurysms), 149. *See also* Aneurysms.
AAFA (Asthma and Allergy Foundation of America), 584
AANMA (Allergy and Asthma Network of Mothers of Asthmatics), 584
AAP (American Academy of Pediatrics), 585, 615
AARP (American Association of Retired Persons), 759
Abdominal postpartum wound infection, 703. *See also* Postpartum wound infection.
Abdominal trauma, 419-428
  assessments for, 419-420
  diagnoses and interventions for, 421-427
    additional considerations for, 427
    breathing patterns, ineffective, 421
    fluid volume, deficient, 421-422
    imbalanced nutrition, less than body requirements, 425-426
    ineffective tissue perfusion, gastrointestinal, 424-425
    infection risks, 423-424
    pain, acute, 422-423
    post-trauma syndrome, 426-427
    skin integrity, impaired, 425
  diagnostic tests for, 420
  discharge planning for, 427
  fundamentals of, 419
  health care settings for, 419
  pathophysiology of, 419
  patient-family education for, 427
Abdominal x-rays, 149
ABG (arterial blood gas) levels, 117-118, 124, 131-132, 138, 147-148, 178, 183, 196, 577-578, 593, 600, 654
ABI (ankle-brachial index), 151, 509
Abnormal Movement Scale. *See* AIMS (Abnormal Movement Scale).
Absence seizures, generalized, 324. *See also* Seizures and epilepsy.
Abuse and neglect, child, 615-620
  assessments for, 616
  child maltreatment, 615
  diagnoses and interventions for, 616-619
    anxiety, 618-619
    fear, 618-619
    injury risks, 616-617
    parenting, impaired, 618
  diagnostic tests for, 616
  discharge planning for, 619
  emotional abuse and neglect, 615-616
  fundamentals of, 615
  health care settings for, 616
  medical care neglect, 615
  Munchausen syndrome by proxy, 615-616
  pathophysiology of, 615
  patient-family education for, 619
  physical abuse and neglect, 615-616
  SBS, 615-616
  sexual abuse, 615-616
ACE (angiotensin-converting enzyme) inhibitors, 231

Acetaminophen
  with codeine, 662-663
  with oxycodone, 707
Acid-fast stains and cultures, 124, 143-144
Acquired immunodeficiency syndrome. *See* HIV/AIDS (human immunodeficiency virus/acquired immuno-deficiency syndrome).
ACS (acute coronary syndrome), 165. *See also* CAD (coronary artery disease).
ACS (American Cancer Society), 1-3, 256
Activity intolerance
  anemia of chronic disease and, 495-496
  bedrest, prolonged and, 61-63
  CAD and, 168
  cancer care and, 17
  cardiac surgeries and, 162
  CD and, 450
  COPD and, 120
  HF and, 187-188
  HIV/AIDS and, 554
  hypothyroidism and, 409
  joint replacement surgeries and, 526
  pulmonary hypertension and, 197-198
Acute confusion
  BPH and, 208-215
  older adult care and, 93-95
Acute coronary syndrome. *See* ACS (acute coronary syndrome).
Acute decompensated heart failure. *See* ADHF (acute decompensated heart failure).
Acute otitis media. *See* AOM (acute otitis media).
Acute pain. *See also* Pain management care.
  abdominal trauma, 422-423
  amputations and, 510
  appendicitis and, 430-431
  bacterial meningitis, 283
  bleeding in pregnancy and, 676-677
  BPH and, 211
  burns and, 602
  cancer care and, 4-6
  CD and, 449
  cholelithiasis, cholecystitis, and cholangitis, 434-435
  vs. chronic pain, 39-43. *See also* Chronic pain.
  fractures and, 515-516, 638
  GBS and, 292
  general neurologic care and, 273-274
  HIV/AIDS and, 553-554
  hyperthyroidism and, 404
  OA and, 530-531
  OM and, 648
  palliative and end-of-life care and, 107
  pancreatitis and, 471-472
  peritonitis and, 482
  pneumothorax and hemothorax and, 134-135
  TBIs and, 367
  thrombocytopenia and, 508
  UC and, 490-491
  ureteral calculi and, 244
  urinary tract obstructions and, 259
  venous thrombosis and thrombophlebitis and, 202-203
Acute pancreatitis, 469. *See also* Pancreatitis.

Acute pulmonary edema, 182. *See also* HF (heart failure).
Acute renal failure. *See* ARF (acute renal failure).
Acute respiratory distress syndrome. *See* ARDS (acute respiratory distress syndrome).
Acute respiratory failure. *See* ARF (acute respiratory failure).
Acute stress disorder, 737-738. *See also* Anxiety disorders.
Acute tubular necrosis. *See* ATN (acute tubular necrosis).
AD (autonomic dysreflexia), 335-336
ADA (American Diabetes Association), 378, 386, 629-630, 694
ADAA (Anxiety Disorders Association of America), 744
ADEAR (Alzheimer's Disease Education and Reference Center), 759
ADHD (attention deficit-hyperactivity disorder), 585-592
  assessments for, 585
  CP and, 609. *See also* CP (cerebral palsy).
  deficient knowledge issues for, 587-590
  diagnoses and interventions for, 586-590
    family coping, compromised, 590
    injury risks, 587
    low self-esteem, chronic, 586
    thought processes, disturbed, 586
  diagnostic tests for, 585
  discharge planning for, 591
  fundamentals of, 585
  health care settings for, 585
  pathophysiology of, 585
  patient-family education for, 591
ADHF (acute decompensated heart failure), 181-182. *See also* HF (heart failure).
ADLs (activities of daily living)
  ADHD and, 586
  dementia (Alzheimer's type) and, 751-752
  GBS and, 287
  MS and, 307-310
AEDs (antiepileptic drugs), 328-330
Aerosolized antibiotics, 625
Aerosolized mucolytic enzymes, 625-626
Agency for Health Care Policy and Research. *See* AHCPR (Agency for Health Care Policy and Research).
Aging-related care, 93-104
  diagnoses and interventions for, 93-104
    aspiration risks, 96-97
    confusion, acute, 93-95
    constipation, 102-103
    fluid volume, deficient, 98
    gas exchange, impaired, 95-96
    hopelessness, 103-104
    hypothermia risks, 100
    infection risks, 98-99
    powerlessness, 104
    skin integrity, impaired, 100-101
    sleep patterns, disturbed, 101-102
  fundamentals of, 93
AHCPR (Agency for Health Care Policy and Research), 39-41, 129, 176

Entries followed by *t* indicate tables.

AIDS. *See* HIV/AIDS (human immunodeficiency virus/ acquired immunodeficiency syndrome).
AIMS (Abnormal Movement Scale), 769-770
Airborne Infection Isolation, 144-145, 783-792, 784t-791t
Airway clearance, ineffective
  asthma and, 578-579
  bronchiolitis and, 593-594
  CF and, 622-623
  palliative and end-of-life care and, 108-109
  perioperative care and, 48-49
  pneumonia and, 125-126
  SCIs and, 337
Albuterol, 579, 625
Alcoholic cirrhosis, 437-444. *See also* Cirrhosis.
Alcoholic hepatitis, 463-468. *See also* Hepatitis.
Alcoholics Anonymous. *See* AA (Alcoholics Anonymous).
Alcoholism, 775-782. *See also* Substance abuse disorders.
Allergen skin testing, 578
Allergy and Asthma Network of Mothers of Asthmatics. *See* AANMA (Allergy and Asthma Network of Mothers of Asthmatics).
Alpha-1 antitrypsin deficiency screens, 117-118
Alveolar hypoventilation, 147-148
Alzheimer's Association, 759
Alzheimer's type dementia, 751-760
  assessments for, 751-752
  deficient knowledge issues for, 752-753, 757-758
    disease progression, 752-753
    medication impacts, 757-758
  diagnoses and interventions for, 752-759
    additional considerations for, 759
    anticipatory grieving, 756
    caregiver role strain, 756
    injury risks, 753-754
    sensory perceptions, disturbed, 755-756
    thought processes, disturbed, 754-755
Ambulatory monitoring, 166, 177-178
American Academy of Pediatrics. *See* AAP (American Academy of Pediatrics).
American Association of Retired Persons. *See* AARP (American Association of Retired Persons).
American Cancer Society. *See* ACS (American Cancer Society).
American Diabetes Association. *See* ADA (American Diabetes Association).
American Epilepsy Society, 331
American Gastroenterological Association, 436
American Heart Association, 176, 194, 386
American Liver Foundation, 443
American Lung Association, 577, 584, 597
American Nurses Association. *See* ANA (American Nurses Association).
American Pain Society. *See* APS (American Pain Society).
American Parkinson Disease Association, 322
American Urological Association. *See* AUA (American Urological Association).
American with Disabilities Act, 331
Amniocentesis, 720, 730
Amputations, 509-514
  assessments for, 509
  deficient knowledge issues for, 512-513
    pressure necrosis, 512-513
    protheses care, 512-513
    residual limb care, 512-513
    skin irritation, 512-513
  diagnoses and interventions for, 510-513
    additional considerations for, 513
    body image, disturbed, 511-512
    disuse syndrome, 511
    pain, acute *vs.* chronic, 510
    role performance, ineffective, 511-512
  diagnostic tests for, 509
  discharge planning for, 513-514

Amputations (*Continued*)
  fundamentals of, 509
  health care settings for, 509
  pathophysiology of, 509
  patient-family education for, 513-514
Amputee Resource Foundation, 514
ANA (American Nurses Association), 40-41
Analgesics, 40-43, 707
Analgesics, opioid, 41-43, 678
Anaphylactic shock, 157. *See also* Shock (cardiac *vs.* noncardiac).
Anemia of chronic disease, 495-496
  activity intolerance and, 495-496
  assessments for, 495
  diagnoses and interventions for, 495-496
  diagnostic tests for, 495
  discharge planning for, 496
  fundamentals of, 495
  health care settings for, 495
  pathophysiology of, 495
  patient-family education and, 496
Aneurysms, 149-150
  AAAs, 149
  assessments for, 149
  diagnoses and interventions for, 150
  diagnostic tests for, 149
  discharge planning for, 150
  femoral, 149
  fundamentals of, 149-150
  health care settings for, 149
  pathophysiology of, 149
  patient-family education for, 150
  thoracic, 149
  tissue perfusion, ineffective, 150
Angina, 167-168. *See also* CAD (coronary artery disease).
Angiographic studies, 138, 151, 363, 420, 438
Angiotensin-converting enzyme inhibitors. *See* ACE (angiotensin-converting enzyme) inhibitors.
Ankle-brachial index. *See* ABI (ankle-brachial index).
Antenatal glucocorticoids, 716, 723-724, 733-734
Antepartum fetal monitoring, 682, 688, 712
Anthropometric data, 566
Antiandrogen therapy, 14-15
Antibiotics, 283-284, 625-626, 678, 733-734
  aerosolized, 625
  prophylactic, 678, 733-734
Anticholinergic medication side effects, 319-320
Anticipatory grieving. *See also* Grieving.
  bleeding in pregnancy and, 677
  cervical insufficiency and, 685
  dementia (Alzheimer's type) and, 756
  palliative and end of life care and, 115-116
  PPROM and, 735-736
Anticoagulants, 141-142, 708
Antidepressants, tricyclic, 589, 742-743, 766-767
Antiepileptic drugs. *See* AEDs (antiepileptic drugs).
Antihypertensive therapy, 193-194, 221-222
Antimanics, 747, 749
Antimicrobials, 705-706
Antiparkinson drugs, 316-320
Antipsychotics, 747, 750, 772-773
Antiviral agents, 318-320
Anxiety disorders, 737-744
  acute stress disorder, 737-738
  assessments for, 738
  caused by medical conditions, 738
    asthma and, 580
    child abuse and neglect and, 618-619
    death, 113
    GBS and, 290
    HIV/AIDS and, 556
    hyperemesis gravidarum, 696-697
    hyperthyroidism and, 402
    palliative and end-of-life care and, 112-113

Anxiety disorders (*Continued*)
    psychosocial support and, 74-75
    urinary diversions and, 249-250
  death anxiety, 113
  deficient knowledge issues for, 738-739, 741-743
    causes, signs, and symptoms, 738-739
    medication effects, 741-743
  diagnoses and interventions for, 738-744
    additional considerations for, 744
    coping, ineffective, 740
    family coping, compromised, 740
    panic attacks, 739-740
    social isolation, 740
  diagnostic tests for, 738
  discharge planning for, 744
  fundamentals of, 737
  GDM and, 691-692
  generalized anxiety disorder, 737
  health care settings for, 738
  not otherwise specified, 738
  OCD, 737
  panic disorder, 737
  pathophysiology of, 737-738
  patient-family education for, 744
  phobias, 737
  PTSD, 737-738
Anxiety Disorders Association of America. *See* ADAA (Anxiety Disorders Association of America).
AOM (acute otitis media), 647. *See also* OM (otitis media).
Appendicitis, 429-432
  assessments for, 429
  diagnoses and interventions for, 430-431
    additional considerations for, 431
    infection risks, 430
    nausea, 430-431
    pain, acute, 430-431
  diagnostic tests for, 429
  discharge planning for, 431
  fundamentals of, 429
  health care settings for, 429
  pathophysiology of, 429
  patient-family education for, 431
APS (American Pain Society), 39-41
ARDS (acute respiratory distress syndrome), 123
ARF (acute renal failure), 231-238
  assessments for, 231
  ATN and, 231
  diagnoses and interventions for, 232-237
    additional considerations for, 237
    fluid volume, deficient, 236
    fluid volume, excess, 234-235
    imbalanced nutrition, less than body requirements, 236-237
    infection risks, 232
    protection, ineffective, 232-234
  diagnostic tests for, 231-232
  discharge planning for, 237
  fundamentals of, 231
  health care settings for, 231
  pathophysiology of, 231
  patient-family education for, 237
  prerenal *vs.* postrenal failure, 231
ARF (acute respiratory failure), 147-148
  additional considerations for, 147-148
  assessments for, 147
  diagnoses and interventions for, 147-148
  diagnostic tests for, 147
  discharge planning for, 148
  fundamentals of, 147
  health care settings for, 147
  pathophysiology of, 147
  patient-family education for, 148
Arterial blood gas levels. *See* ABG (arterial blood gas) levels.
Arteriography, contrast, 149

Artery disease, coronary. See CAD (coronary artery disease).
Arthritis, 529-534, 541-546
  OA, 529-534
    assessments for, 529-530
    deficient knowledge issues for, 532
    diagnoses and interventions for, 530-533
    diagnostic tests for, 530
    discharge planning for, 533
    fundamentals of, 529
    health care settings for, 529
    idiopathic vs. secondary, 529
    pathophysiology of, 529
    patient-family education for, 533
  RA, 541-546
    assessments for, 541
    deficient knowledge issues for, 542-543
    diagnoses and interventions for, 542-546
    diagnostic tests for, 541
    discharge planning for, 546
    fundamentals of, 541
    health care settings for, 541
    pathophysiology of, 541
    patient-family education for, 546
Arthroplasty, total hip vs. total knee. See Joint replacement surgeries.
Ascending colostomy, 455-456. See also Fecal diversions (colostomy, ileostomy, and IPAA).
ASIA (American Spinal Injury Association) impairment scale for, 333-335
Aspiration risks
  general neurologic care and, 266-267
  nutritional support and, 571-572
  older adult care and, 96-97
  perioperative care and, 49-50
Aspirin, 41, 716
Assessments. See also Diagnostic tests.
  for cardiovascular care, 149, 151, 177, 182, 195, 201
    aneurysms, 149
    atherosclerotic arterial occlusive disease, 151
    CAD, 165
    dysrhythmias and conduction disturbances, 177
    HF, 182
    pulmonary hypertension, 195
    venous thrombosis and thrombophlebitis, 201
  for endocrine care, 373-374, 378, 387-390, 395-396, 399, 407, 415
    DI, 373-374
    DKA, 387-390
    DM, 378
    HHNK syndrome, 395-396
    hyperthyroidism, 399
    hypothyroidism, 407
    SIADH, 415
  for GI care, 419-420, 429, 433-434, 437-439, 445-446, 463-464, 469-470, 477-478, 481, 487-488
    abdominal trauma, 419-420
    appendicitis, 429
    CD, 445-446
    cholelithiasis, cholecystitis, and cholangitis, 433-434
    cirrhosis, 437-439
    hepatitis, 463-464
    pancreatitis, 469-470
    peptic ulcers, 477-478
    peritonitis, 481
    UC, 487-488
  for hematologic care, 495, 497, 501, 505
    anemia of chronic disease, 495
    DIC, 497
    polycythemia, 501
    thrombocytopenia, 505
  for maternity care, 673-674, 681-682, 687-688, 695, 703, 711-712, 719-720, 729-730
    bleeding in pregnancy, 673-674
    cervical insufficiency, 681-682
    GDM, 687-688

Assessments (Continued)
    hyperemesis gravidarum, 695
    postpartum wound infection, 703
    PPROM, 729-730
    preeclampsia, 711-712
    PTL, 719-720
  for musculoskeletal care, 509, 515, 529-530, 535, 541
    amputations, 509
    fractures, 515
    OA, 529-530
    osteoporosis, 535
    RA, 541
  for neurologic care, 281, 287-288, 295-296, 305-306, 313-314, 323-325, 333-335, 350-351, 361-363
    bacterial meningitis, 281
    GBS, 287-288
    intervertebral disk disease, 295-296
    MS, 305-306
    PD, 313-314
    SCIs, 333-335
    seizures and epilepsy, 323-325
    stroke, 350-351
    TBIs, 361-363
  for pediatric care, 577-578, 585, 593, 600, 609, 616, 621, 629, 637, 641, 647, 653, 659
    ADHD, 585
    asthma, 577-578
    bronchiolitis, 593
    burns, 600
    CF, 621
    child abuse and neglect, 616
    CP, 609
    DM, 629
    fractures, 637
    gastroenteritis, 641
    OM, 647
    poisoning, 653
    sickle cell pain crisis, 659
  for psychiatric care, 737, 745-746, 751-752, 761-762, 769, 775-776
    anxiety disorders, 737
    bipolar disorder (manic component), 745-746
    dementia (Alzheimer's type), 751-752
    depression, major, 761-762
    schizophrenia, 769
    substance abuse disorders, 775-776
  for renal-urinary care, 207, 217, 231, 243, 257-258
    ARF, 231
    BPH, 207
    CKD, 217
    ureteral calculi, 243
    urinary tract obstructions, 257-258
  for respiratory care, 117, 131, 137, 147
    ARF, 147
    COPD, 117
    PE, 137
    pneumothorax and hemothorax, 131
  for special needs care, 548-549, 559, 561-562, 565-568
    HIV/AIDS, 548-549
    nutritional support, 565-568
    wound management, 559, 561-562
Asthma, 577-584
  assessments for, 577-578
  deficient knowledge issues for, 581-583
  diagnoses and interventions for, 578-583
    airway clearance, ineffective, 578-579
    anxiety, 580
    family processes, interrupted, 581
    fatigue, 579-580
  diagnostic tests for, 577-578
  discharge planning for, 583-584
  fundamentals of, 577
  health care settings for, 577
  pathophysiology of, 577
  patient-family education for, 583-584

Asthma and Allergy Foundation of America. See AAFA (Asthma and Allergy Foundation of America).
Ataxic CP (cerebral palsy), 609. See also CP (cerebral palsy).
Atherosclerosis. See Atherosclerotic arterial occlusive disease.
Atherosclerotic arterial occlusive disease, 151-156
  assessments for, 151
  deficient knowledge issues for, 153-154
    infection risks, 153-154
    tissue integrity, impaired, 153-154
  diagnoses and interventions for, 152-155
    additional considerations for, 155, 583
    pain, chronic, 152-153
    peripheral tissue perfusion, ineffective, 154-155
    tissue integrity, impaired, 152
  diagnostic tests for, 151
  discharge planning for, 156, 583-584
  fundamentals of, 151
  health care settings for, 151
  pathophysiology and, 151
  patient-family education for, 156, 583-584
Athetoid CP (cerebral palsy), 609. See also CP (cerebral palsy).
ATN (acute tubular necrosis), 231
Attention deficit-hyperactivity disorder. See ADHD (attention deficit-hyperactivity disorder).
AUA (American Urological Association), 207
Auditory perception, disturbed. See Sensory perception, disturbed.
Automaticity disturbances, 177. See also Conduction disturbances and dysrhythmias.
Autonomic dysreflexia. See AD (autonomic dysreflexia).

B
Bacterial meningitis, 281-286
  assessments for, 281
  deficient knowledge issues for, 282-284
    antibiotics, 283-284
    Transmission-Based Precautions (Droplet), 283
  diagnoses and interventions for, 282-285
    additional considerations for, 285
    pain, acute, 283
  diagnostic tests for, 281-282
  discharge planning for, 286
  fundamentals of, 281
  health care settings for, 281
  pathophysiology of, 281
  patient-family education and, 286
Barium enema and upper GI series, 446
Barium swallow, 438, 478
Basic metabolic panels, 630, 659
Beck Anxiety Inventory, 738, 746
Beck Depression Inventory, 762
Bedrest, prolonged, 61-71
  diagnoses and interventions for, 61-71
    activity intolerance risks, 61-63
    additional considerations, 71
    constipation, 67-68
    dependence vs. independence, 70-71
    disuse syndrome risks, 63-65
    diversional activity, deficient, 69
    ineffective tissue perfusion, cerebral, 66-67
    ineffective tissue perfusion, peripheral, 65-66
    role performance, ineffective, 70-71
    sexuality patterns, ineffective, 70
  fundamentals of, 61
  pathophysiology of, 61
  PPROM and, 734-735. See also PPROM (preterm premature rupture of membranes).
Benign prostatic hypertrophy. See BPH (benign prostatic hypertrophy).
Benzodiazepines, 743
Beta-andrenergics, 734
Beta-blockers, 169-170, 715-716

Beta$_2$-agonists, 582-583
Bibliographies, 799-812
Bilateral orchiectomy, 14-15
Biliary cirrhosis, 437-444. *See also* Cirrhosis.
Biochemical data, 566
Biomarkers, cardiac, 166
Biopsies, 182-183, 218
Bipolar disorder (manic component), 745-750
    assessments for, 745-746
    deficient knowledge issues for, 747-750
        causes, signs, and symptoms, 747-748
        medication impacts, 749-750
    diagnoses and interventions for, 746-750
        additional considerations for, 750
        imbalanced nutrition, less than body requirements, 747
        other-directed violence risks, 746-747
        self-care deficits, 747-748
    diagnostic tests for, 746
    discharge planning for, 750
    fundamentals of, 745
    health care settings for, 745
    hypomania *vs.* mania, 745
    pathophysiology of, 745
    patient-family education for, 750
Bleeding in pregnancy, 673-680
    assessments for, 673-674
    deficient knowledge issues for, 675-676, 678-679
        bleeding effects, 675-676
        medication impacts, 678-679
    diagnoses and interventions, 675-680
        additional considerations for, 680
        grieving, anticipatory, 677
        pain, acute, 676-677
    diagnostic tests for, 674-675
    discharge planning for, 680
    fundamentals of, 673
    health care settings for, 673
    pathophysiology of, 673
    patient-family education for, 680
Blood
    bleeding in pregnancy. *See* Bleeding in pregnancy.
    blood-urea-nitrogen levels. *See* BUN (blood-urea-nitrogen) levels.
    Bloodborne Pathogens Standard, 783
    cultures, 642, 659, 704
    glucose monitoring, 630-631
    pressure checks. *See* BP (blood pressure) checks.
    products, IV, 679
    Rh factor and antibody screens, 674, 720, 730
Blot tests, Western, 548-549
Body image, disturbed
    amputations and, 511-512
    burns and, 605-606
    cancer care and, 36
    fecal diversions and, 459-460
    HIV/AIDS and, 557
    hyperthyroidism and, 403
    psychosocial support and, 80-81
    RA and, 545
Body temperature, imbalanced, 274-275
Bone
    marrow aspiration, 501
    scans, 616, 637
Bowel incontinence, 458-459
BP (blood pressure) checks, 193-194, 221-222
BPH (benign prostatic hypertrophy), 207-216
    assessments for, 207
    deficient knowledge issues for, 212-214
        Kegel exercise programs, 214
        postsurgical sexual function, 212
    diagnoses and interventions for, 208-215
        additional considerations for, 214
        confusion, acute, 208-215
        constipation, 212
        fluid volume, deficient, 209-210

BPH (*Continued*)
        fluid volume, excess, 210
        pain, acute, 211
        skin integrity, impaired, 211
        urinary incontinence, stress, 213-214
        urinary incontinence, urge, 213
    diagnostic tests for, 207
    discharge planning for, 215
    fundamentals of, 207
    health care settings for, 207
    pathophysiology of, 207
    patient-family education for, 215
BPRS (Brief Psychiatric Rating Scale), 770
Brain
    attacks, 349-350. *See also* Stroke.
    death, 363
    herniation, 363
    injuries, traumatic. *See* TBIs (traumatic brain injuries).
    lacerations, 362
Breastfeeding, ineffective, 727
Breathing patterns, ineffective
    abdominal trauma and, 421
    cancer care and, 4
    COPD and, 118
    GBS and, 288-289
    hypothyroidism and, 408
    palliative and end-of-life care and, 107-108
    perioperative care and, 50-51
    pneumothorax and hemothorax and, 132-133
Brief Psychiatric Rating Scale. *See* BPRS (Brief Psychiatric Rating Scale).
Bronchiolitis, 593-598
    assessments for, 593
    diagnoses and interventions for, 593-596
        additional considerations for, 596
        airway clearance, ineffective, 593-594
        fluid volume, deficient, 595-596
        gas exchange, impaired, 594-595
    diagnostic tests for, 593
    discharge planning for, 596
    fundamentals of, 593
    health care settings for, 593
    pathophysiology of, 593
    patient-family education for, 596
Bronchodilators, 625
Brooke ileostomy, 455-456. *See also* Fecal diversions (colostomy, ileostomy, and IPAA).
Buckle fractures, 637. *See also* Fractures.
BUN (blood-urea-nitrogen) levels, 183, 207, 217-218, 231-232, 243, 257, 600, 641-642
Burns, 599-608
    assessments for, 600
    diagnoses and interventions for, 600-606
        additional considerations for, 606
        body image, disturbed, 605-606
        fluid volume, deficient, 600-601
        imbalanced nutrition, less than body requirements, 604-605
        infection risks, 603-604
        pain, acute, 602
        skin integrity, impaired, 602-603
        tissue integrity, impaired, 602-603
    diagnostic tests for, 600
    discharge planning for, 606-608
    full-thickness, 600
    fundamentals of, 599
    health care settings for, 600
    partial-thickness, 600
    pathophysiology of, 599-600
    patient-family education for, 606-608
    rule of nines, modified, 599
    superficial, 600
    TBSA and, 599

C
CABG (coronary artery bypass grafting), 161
CAD (coronary artery disease), 165-176
    ACS and, 165
    assessments for, 165
    deficient knowledge issues for, 169-173
        beta-blocker impacts, 170
        catheterization procedures, 172-173
        disease process, 170-171
        lifestyle impacts, 170-171
        nitrate impacts, 169-170
    diagnoses and interventions for, 167-176
        activity intolerance, 168
        additional considerations for, 175
        angina, 167-168
        fluid volume, deficient, 174
        health-seeking behaviors, 172
        ineffective tissue perfusion, cardiopulmonary, 173
        ineffective tissue perfusion, cerebral, 173
        ineffective tissue perfusion, peripheral, 173-174
        ineffective tissue perfusion, renal, 175
        nutrition, imbalanced, 169
        pain, acute, 167-168
    diagnostic tests for, 165-166
    discharge planning for, 176
    fundamentals of, 165
    health care settings for, 165
    pathophysiology of, 165
    patient-family education for, 176
    STEMI *vs.* NSTEMI, 165
CAGE-AID questionnaire, 776
Calcium channel blockers, 715-716, 722, 734
Calculi, ureteral, 243-248
    deficient knowledge issues for, 246-247
        calculi formation, 246-247
        dietary impacts, 246-247
    diagnoses and interventions for
        additional considerations for, 247
        pain, acute, 244
        skin integrity, impaired, 245-246
        urinary elimination, impaired, 244-245
    diagnostic tests for, 243
    discharge planning for, 247
    fundamentals of, 243
    health care settings for, 243
    pathophysiology of, 243
    patient-family education for, 247
Canadian Diabetes Association, 386
Cancer care, 1-38
    ACS recommendations for, 1-2
    antiandrogen therapy, 14-15
    auditory perception, disturbed, 37
    body image, disturbed, 36
    breathing patterns, ineffective, 4
    chemotherapy, 34
    deficient knowledge issues for, 14-15, 31-35
        antiandrogen therapy, 14-15
        chemotherapy, 34
        external beam radiation therapy, 33
        immunotherapy, 35
        orchiectomy, bilateral, 14-15
        radiation implants, 31-32
        VADs, 12-14
    diagnoses and interventions for, 4-37
        activity intolerance, 17
        auditory perception, disturbed, 37
        body image, disturbed, 36
        breathing patterns, ineffective, 4
        chemotherapy, 15-16
        constipation, 9
        diarrhea, 9
        disuse syndrome, 12
        gas exchange, impaired, 4
        imbalanced nutrition, less than body requirements, 26-27

Cancer care (Continued)
immunotherapy, 15-16
ineffective protection, 17-19
ineffective tissue perfusion, cardiopulmonary, 7
ineffective tissue perfusion, peripheral, 6
injury risks, 23-25
kinesthetic perception, disturbed, 37
oral mucous membranes, impaired, 28
pain management and, acute vs. chronic, 4-6. See also Pain management care.
physical mobility, impaired, 7
radiation therapy, 15-16
sensory perception, disturbed, 37
sexual dysfunction, 10-11
skin integrity, impaired, 7-9, 19-22
stress, 10
swallowing, impaired, 28-29
tactile perception, disturbed, 37
tissue integrity, impaired, 19-23
urinary elimination, impaired, 29-30
urinary incontinence, 10
fundamentals of, 1
genitourinary cancers, 3
GI malignancies, 1-2. See also GI (gastrointestinal) care.
head and neck cancers, 2
health care settings for, 1
hematopoietic system, neoplastic diseases of, 2
lung cancer, 1
nervous system tumors, 1
pathophysiology of, 1
sensory perception, disturbed, 37
Cancer screenings, 1-3
CAPD (continuous ambulatory peritoneal dialysis), 227-230. See also Dialysis.
Carboprost, 679
Cardiac biomarkers, 166
Cardiac catheterization, 182-183
Cardiac output, decreased, 178-179, 186-187
Cardiac shock. See Shock (cardiac vs. noncardiac).
Cardiac surgeries, 161-164
deficient knowledge issues for, 161-162
diagnoses and interventions for, 161-163
activity intolerance, 162
additional considerations for, 163
discharge planning for, 163
fundamentals of, 161
health care settings for, 161
pathophysiology of, 161
patient-family education for, 163
Cardiogenic shock, 157. See also Shock (cardiac vs. noncardiac).
Cardiomyopathies, 181-182. See also HF (heart failure).
dilated, 181
hypertrophic, 181-182
restrictive, 182
Cardiopulmonary tissue perfusion, ineffective. See also Tissue perfusion, ineffective.
CAD and, 173
cancer care and, 6-7
circulatory failure and, 157-159
DIC and, 498
GBS and, 289
HF and, 185-186
polycythemia and, 504
SCIs and, 338-339
sickle cell pain crisis and, 660-661
venous thrombosis and thrombophlebitis and, 202
Cardiovascular care, 149-206, 801-802
aneurysms, 149-150
atherosclerotic arterial occlusive disease, 151-156
CAD, 165-176
cardiac surgeries, 161-164
circulatory failure, 157-160
dysrhythmias and conduction disturbances, 177-180
HF, 181-192

Cardiovascular care (Continued)
hypertension, 193-195
hypertension, pulmonary, 195-200
reference resources for, 801-802
venous thrombosis and thrombophlebitis, 201-205
Care plans
infection prevention and control, 783-796
APIC and, 792
CDC, Standard Precautions, 783-792, 784t-791t
ICPs and, 792
isolation precaution recommendations, 784t-791t
MDROs and, 783
nosocomial infection reduction, 792
OSHA, Bloodborne Pathogens Standard, 783
SHEA and, 792
TJC and, 792
Transmission-Based Precautions (Airborne Infection Isolation), 783-792, 784t-791t
Transmission-Based Precautions (Contact), 783-792, 784t-791t
Transmission-Based Precautions (Droplet), 783-792, 784t-791t
Transmission-Based Precautions (Protective Environment), 783-792, 784t-791t
laboratory tests (normal values), 665-672, 793-798
adult, 793-798
pediatric patients, 665-672
maternity, 673-736
bleeding in pregnancy, 673-680
cervical insufficiency, 681-686
GDM, 687-694
hyperemesis gravidarum, 695-702
PPROM, 729-736
preeclampsia, 711-718
PTL, 719-736
wound infection, postpartum, 703-710
medical-surgical, 1-572
cardiovascular, 149-206
endocrine, 373-418
general, 1-116
GI, 419-494
hematologic, 495-508
musculoskeletal, 509-546
neurologic, 261-372
renal-urinary, 207-260
respiratory, 117-148
special needs, 541-576
pediatric, 577-672
ADHD, 585-592
asthma, 577-584
bronchiolitis, 593-598
burns, 599-608
CF, 621-628
child abuse and neglect, 615-620
CP, 609-614
DM, 629-636
fractures, 637-640
gastroenteritis, 641-646
normal laboratory values, pediatric, 665-672
OM, 647-652
poisoning, 653-658
sickle cell pain crisis, 659-664
psychiatric, 737-782
anxiety disorders, 737-744
bipolar disorder (manic component), 745-750
dementia (Alzheimer's type), 751-760
depression, major, 761-768
schizophrenia, 769-774
substance abuse disorders, 775-783
reference resources for, 799-812
Care settings. See Health care settings.
CareFirst, 627
Caregiver role considerations
cervical insufficiency and, 684
dementia (Alzheimer's type) and, 756
palliative and end-of-life care and, 114-115

Caregiver role considerations (Continued)
preeclampsia and, 717
PTL and, 725
TBIs and, 364
Carotid angioplasty/stent procedures, 357-358
Carotid endarterectomy procedures, 357-358
Catheters
CAD and, 172-173, 182-183
ureteral, 245
CBC (complete blood count), 131-132, 183, 196, 501, 578, 593, 616, 621-622, 641-642, 674, 695
CBC with differential, 682
CCPD (continuous cycling peritoneal dialysis), 227-230. See also Dialysis.
CD (Crohn's disease), 445-454
assessments for, 445-446
deficient knowledge issues for, 451-452
diagnoses and interventions for, 447-453
activity intolerance, 450
additional considerations for, 453
diarrhea, 449-450
fluid volume, deficient, 447
infection risks, 448-449
nausea, 449
pain, acute, 449
protection, ineffective, 448-449
diagnostic tests for, 446
discharge planning for, 453
fundamentals of, 445
health care settings for, 445
IBD and, 445
pathophysiology of, 445
patient-family education for, 453
vs. UC, 445. See also UC (ulcerative colitis).
CDC (Centers for Disease Control and Prevention)
diabetes data of, 629
gastroenteritis data, 641
Standard Precautions, 783-792, 784t-791t
Cecostomy, 455-456. See also Fecal diversions (colostomy, ileostomy, and IPAA).
Cerebral blood vessel rupture, 362-363. See also TBIs (traumatic brain injuries).
Cerebral palsy. See CP (cerebral palsy).
Cerebral tissue perfusion, ineffective, 66-67, 157-159, 173, 185-186, 498
bedrest, prolonged and, 66-67
CAD and, 173
circulatory failure and, 157-159
DIC and, 498
GBS and, 289
HF and, 185-186
polycythemia and, 502-503
SCIs and, 338
sickle cell pain crisis and, 660-661
thrombocytopenia and, 507
Cerebrospinal fluid analyses. See CSF (cerebrospinal fluid) analyses.
Cerebrovascular accident. See Stroke.
Cervical insufficiency, 681-686
assessments for, 681-682
deficient knowledge issues for, 682-683
diagnoses and interventions for, 682-686
additional considerations for, 686
caregiver role strain, 684
coping, ineffective, 683-684
grieving, anticipatory, 685
parent-child attachment, impaired, 684
sexual dysfunction, 685
diagnostic tests for, 681-682
discharge planning for, 686
fundamentals of, 681
health care settings for, 681
pathophysiology of, 681
patient-family education for, 686
CF (cystic fibrosis), 621-628
assessments for, 621
deficient knowledge issues for, 625-626

CF (Continued)
  diagnoses and interventions for, 622-627
    additional considerations for, 626
    airway clearance, ineffective, 622-623
    gas exchange, impaired, 623-624
    imbalanced nutrition, less than body requirements, 624
  diagnostic tests for, 621-622
  discharge planning for, 626-627
  fundamentals of, 621
  health care settings for, 621
  pancreatic enzyme deficiency and, 621
  pathophysiology of, 621
  patient-family education for, 626-627
  progressive chronic obstructive lung disease and, 621
  sweat gland dysfunction and, 621
CFF (Cystic Fibrosis Foundation), 621, 627
CHADD (Children and Adults with Attention-Deficit/Hyperactivity Disorder), 591
Chemotherapy, 1-38
Chest x-rays, 117-118, 123-124, 131-132, 138, 143-144, 147-148, 166, 182-183, 195, 282, 578, 593, 621-622, 659
Child abuse and neglect, 615-620
  assessments for, 616
  child maltreatment, 615
  diagnoses and interventions for, 616-619
    anxiety, 618-619
    fear, 618-619
    injury risks, 616-617
    parenting, impaired, 618
  diagnostic tests for, 616
  discharge planning for, 619
  emotional abuse and neglect, 615-616
  fundamentals of, 615
  health care settings for, 616
  medical care neglect, 615
  Munchausen syndrome by proxy, 615-616
  pathophysiology of, 615-616
  patient-family education for, 619
  physical abuse and neglect, 615-616
  SBS, 615-616
  sexual abuse, 615-616
Children and Adults with Attention-Deficit/Hyperactivity Disorder. See CHADD (Children and Adults with Attention-Deficit/Hyperactivity Disorder).
Cholelithiasis, cholecystitis, and cholangitis, 433-436
  assessments for, 433-434
  diagnoses and interventions for, 434-436
    additional considerations for, 436
    injury risks, 435-436
    nausea, 434-435
    pain, acute, 434-435
  diagnostic tests for, 434
  discharge planning for, 436
  fundamentals of, 433
  health care settings for, 433
  pathophysiology of, 433
  patient-family interventions for, 436
Christopher Reeve Paralysis Foundation, 348
Chronic disease, anemia of, 495-496
  activity intolerance and, 495-496
  assessments for, 495
  diagnoses and interventions for, 495-496
  diagnostic tests for, 495
  discharge planning for, 496
  fundamentals of, 495
  health care settings for, 495
  pathophysiology of, 495
  patient-family education and, 496
Chronic hepatitis, 463-468. See also Hepatitis.
Chronic kidney disease. See CKD (chronic kidney disease).
Chronic low self-esteem
  ADHD and, 586
  major depression and, 764-765

Chronic obstructive pulmonary disease. See COPD (chronic obstructive pulmonary disease).
Chronic OM (otitis media), 647. See also OM (otitis media).
Chronic pain. See also Pain management care.
  vs. acute pain, 39-43
  amputations and, 510
  arthritis and, 530-531
  atherosclerotic arterial occlusive disease and, 152-153
  HIV/AIDS and, 553-554
  MS and, 310
Chronic pancreatitis, 469. See also Pancreatitis.
Chronic spasms, 310
Circulatory failure (cardiac vs. noncardiac shock), 157-160
  anaphylactic shock, 157
  cardiogenic shock, 157
  diagnoses and interventions for, 157-160
    additional considerations for, 160
    ineffective tissue perfusion, cardiopulmonary, 157-159
    ineffective tissue perfusion, cerebral, 157-159
    ineffective tissue perfusion, peripheral, 157-159
    ineffective tissue perfusion, renal, 157-159
  diagnostic tests for, 157
  discharge planning for, 160
  fundamentals of, 157
  gas exchange, impaired, 160
  health care settings for, 157
  hypovolemic shock, 157
  neurogenic shock, 157
  pathophysiology of, 157
  patient-family education for, 160
  septic shock, 157
Cirrhosis, 437-444
  alcoholic (Laennec's), 437-444
  assessments for, 437-439
  biliary, 437-444
  diagnoses and interventions for, 439-443
    additional considerations for, 443
    fluid volume, excess, 442-443
    gas exchange, impaired, 440
    imbalanced nutrition, less than body requirements, 439
    protection, ineffective, 440-441
    sensory perception disturbed, 441-442
  diagnostic tests for, 437-439
  discharge planning for, 443
  fundamentals of, 437
  health care settings for, 437
  pathophysiology of, 437
  patient-family education for, 443
  postnecrotic, 437-444
Cisternograms, 363
CKD (chronic kidney disease), 217-222
  acute complications of, 217
  assessments for, 217
  deficient knowledge issues for, 221-222
    antihypertensive therapy, 221-222
    BP checks, 221-222
    insulin requirement changes, 221-222
  diagnoses and interventions for, 218-222
    activity intolerance, 218-219
    additional considerations for, 222
    discharge planning for, 222
    imbalanced nutrition, less than body requirements, 220
    skin integrity, impaired, 220-221
  diagnostic tests for, 217-218
  discharge planning for, 222
  fundamentals of, 217
  health care settings for, 217
  pathophysiology of, 217
  patient-family education for, 222
Clearance, airway
  asthma and, 578-579
  bronchiolitis and, 593-594

Clearance, airway (Continued)
  CF and, 622-623
  palliative and end-of-life care and, 108-109
  perioperative care and, 48-49
  pneumonia and, 125-126
  SCIs and, 337
Clindamycin, 706
Clonidine, 590
Closed pneumothorax, 131-132. See also Pneumothorax and hemothorax.
Closures, wound, 559-564. See also Wound management care.
  by primary intention, 559-560
  by secondary intention (surgical or traumatic), 561-564
Co-analgesics, 42-43
Coagulation tests and studies, 282, 438, 505, 616, 712
Code strokes, 349-350. See also Stroke.
Codeine, 662-663
Codeine with acetaminophen, 662-663
Colitis
  granulomatous and transmural. See CD (Crohn's disease).
  UC, 445, 487-494
    vs. CD, 445
    deficient knowledge issues for, 492-493
    diagnoses and interventions for, 488-489
Colostomy, 455-462. See also Fecal diversions (colostomy, ileostomy, and IPAA).
Coma, myxedema, 412
Communication, impaired
  CP and, 613
  general neurologic care and, 275-276
  psychosocial support and, 81-82
  stroke and, 353-354
Community-acquired pneumonia, 123. See also Pneumonia.
Complete blood count. See CBC (complete blood count).
Complete fractures, 637. See also Fractures.
Compromised family coping, 590. See also Family coping.
Computed tomography scans. See CT (computed tomography) scans.
Concussions, 361, 364. See also TBIs (traumatic brain injuries).
Conduction disturbances and dysrhythmias, 177-180
  assessments for, 177
  automaticity disturbances and, 177
  cardiac output, decreased, 178-179
  deficient knowledge issues for, 179-180
    dysrhythmia mechanisms, 179-180
    lifestyle impacts, 179-180
  diagnoses and interventions for, 178-180
  diagnostic tests for, 177-178
  discharge planning for, 180
  fundamentals of, 177
  health care settings for, 177
  pathophysiology of, 177
  patient-family education for, 180
Confusion, acute
  BPH and, 208-215
  older adult care and, 93-95
Constipation
  bedrest, prolonged and, 67-68
  BPH and, 212
  cancer care and, 9
  fractures and, 519
  general neurologic care, 277
  hypothyroidism and, 410-411
  nutritional support and, 573
  older adult care and, 102-103
  perioperative care and, 56-57
  PTL and, 725-726
  SCIs and, 342
Contact (Transmission-Based Precautions), 783-792, 784t-791t
Continent urinary diversions, 249. See also Urinary diversions.

Continuous ambulatory peritoneal dialysis. *See* CAPD (continuous ambulatory peritoneal dialysis).

Continuous cycling peritoneal dialysis. *See* CCPD (continuous cycling peritoneal dialysis).

Continuous passive movement exercises. *See* CPM (continuous passive movement) exercises.

Continuous venovenous hemodiafiltration. *See* CVVHD (continuous venovenous hemodiafiltration).

Contrast arteriography, 149

Contusions, brain, 361-362. *See also* TBIs (traumatic brain injuries).

Conventional ileostomy, 455-456. *See also* Fecal diversions (colostomy, ileostomy, and IPAA).

COPD (chronic obstructive pulmonary disease), 117-121

  assessments of, 117

  diagnoses and interventions for, 118-121

    activity intolerance, 120

    additional considerations for, 121

    breathing patterns, ineffective, 118

    gas exchange, impaired, 118-119

    imbalanced nutrition, less than body requirements, 119-120

  diagnostic tests for, 117

  discharge planning for, 121

  education, patient-family and, 121

  fundamentals of, 117

  health care settings for, 117

  pathophysiology of, 117

Coping

  family, 89-91, 740

    anxiety disorders and, 740

    compromised, 740

    disabled, 90-91

    enhanced, 91

    impaired, 89-90

  ineffective, 76-77, 683-684, 697-698, 709, 716, 724, 731-732, 740

    anxiety disorders and, 737, 740

    cervical insufficiency and, 683-684

    hyperemesis gravidarum and, 697-698

    postpartum wound infection and, 709

    PPROM and, 731-732

    preeclampsia and, 716

    psychosocial support and, 76-77

    PTL and, 724

  skills, 737

Corneal tissue integrity, impaired, 402-403

Coronary artery bypass grafting. *See* CABG (coronary artery bypass grafting).

Coronary artery disease. *See* CAD (coronary artery disease).

Corticosteroids, 582-583

CP (cerebral palsy), 609-614

  ADHD and, 609. *See also* ADHD (attention deficit-hyperactivity disorder).

  assessments for, 609

  ataxic, 609

  diagnoses and interventions for, 610-614

    additional considerations for, 614

    imbalanced nutrition, less than body requirements, 610

    injury risks, 611

    physical mobility, impaired, 611-612

    self-care deficits, 612-613

    verbal communication, impaired, 613

  diagnostic tests for, 609

  discharge planning for, 614

  dyskinetic/athetoid, 609

  fundamentals of, 609

  health care settings for, 609

  mixed, 609

  pathophysiology of, 609

  patient-family education for, 614

  spastic, 609

CPM (continuous passive movement) exercises, 527

Craniotomy procedures, 367-369

Creatinine levels and clearance, 183, 207, 217-218, 231-232, 243, 257, 378, 600, 641-642

Crohn's disease. *See* CD (Crohn's disease).

Cromolyn sodium/nedocromil sodium, 582-583

CSF (cerebrospinal fluid) analyses, 287-288, 363, 667, 793-795

CT (computed tomography) scans, 138, 149, 166, 195, 232, 243, 282, 296, 324-325, 351, 616, 637, 704, 752

Current health status concerns, 84-85, 91-92

CVA (cerebrovascular accident). *See* Stroke.

CVVHD (continuous venovenous hemodiafiltration), 223-226. *See also* Hemodialysis.

Cystic fibrosis. *See* CF (cystic fibrosis).

Cystic Fibrosis Foundation. *See* CFF (Cystic Fibrosis Foundation).

Cystoscopy, 207, 258

Cytologic studies, 609

D

D/ART (Depression Awareness, Recognition, and Treatment) Program, 750

D-dimer tests, 138, 201-202, 497

DAIs (diffuse axonal injuries), 361. *See also* TBIs (traumatic brain injuries).

DBSA (Depression and Bipolar Support Alliance), 750

DDAVP challenge tests, 373-374

Death anxiety, 113. *See also* Anxiety disorders.

Decompensated heart failure, acute. *See* ADHF (acute decompensated heart failure).

Decreased cardiac output, 178-179, 186-187

Decreased intracranial adaptive capacity, 261-264

Deep brain stimulation, 321-322

Deficient diversional activity, 69

Deficient fluid volume. *See also* Fluid volume, imbalanced.

  bronchiolitis and, 595-596

  burns and, 600-601

  gastroenteritis, 642-643

  OM and, 648-649

  pancreatitis and, 470-471

Deficient knowledge issues

  for cardiovascular care, 153-154, 161-162, 169-173, 179-180, 189-191, 193-194, 198-199, 204

    atherosclerotic arterial occlusive disease, 153-154

    CAD, 169-173

    cardiac surgeries, 161-162

    dysrhythmias and conduction disturbances, 179-180

    HF, 189-191

    hypertension, 193-194

    pulmonary hypertension, 198-199

    venous thrombosis and thrombophlebitis, 204

  for endocrine care, 382-384, 392-394, 396-397, 403-404

    DKA, 392-394

    DM, 382-384

    HHNK syndrome, 396-397

    hyperthyroidism, 403-404

  for general care, 14-15, 31-35, 45-47, 84-85, 91-92, 105-116

    cancer, 14-15, 31-35

    palliative and end-of-life, 105-116

    perioperative, 45-47

    psychosocial support, family, 91-92

    psychosocial support, patient, 84-85

  for GI care, 451-452, 460-461, 464-465, 492-493

    CD, 451-452

    fecal diversions, 460-461

    hepatitis, 464-465

    UC, 492-493

  for HIV/AIDS care, 555-556

  for maternity care, 675-676, 678-679, 682-683, 688-689, 692-693, 698-700, 705-709, 713-716, 720-724, 732-735

    bleeding in pregnancy, 675-676, 678-679

    cervical insufficiency, 682-683

    GDM, 688-689, 692-693

Deficient knowledge issues *(Continued)*

    hyperemesis gravidarum, 698-700

    postpartum wound infection, 705-709

    PPROM, 732-735

    preeclampsia, 713-716

    PTL, 720-724

  for musculoskeletal care, 512-513, 520-521, 526-527, 532, 542-543

    amputations, 512-513

    fractures, 520-521

    joint replacement surgeries, 526-527

    OA, 532

    RA, 542-543

  for neurologic care, 282-284, 291-292, 298-303, 306-310, 316-322, 327-330, 357-358, 364, 367-371

    bacterial meningitis, 282-284

    GBS, 291-292

    intervertebral disk disease, 298-303

    MS, 306-310

    PD, 316-322

    seizures and epilepsy, 327-330

    stroke, 357-358

    TBIs, 364, 367-371

  for pediatric care, 581-583, 587-590, 625-626, 630-634, 649-650, 656, 661-663

    ADHD, 587-590

    asthma, 581-583

    CF, 625-626

    DM, 630-634

    OM, 649-650

    poisoning, 656

    sickle cell pain crisis, 661-663

  for psychiatric care, 738-739, 741-743, 747-750, 752-753, 757-758, 762-763, 766-767, 771-773, 780-781

    anxiety disorders, 738-739, 741-743

    bipolar disorder (manic component), 747-750

    dementia (Alzheimer's type), 752-753, 757-758

    depression, major, 762-763, 766-767

    schizophrenia, 771-773

    substance abuse disorders, 780-781

  for renal-urinary care, 212-214, 221-222, 240-241, 246-247, 255-256

    BPH, 212-214

    CKD, 221-222

    renal transplants, 240-241

    ureteral calculi, 246-247

    urinary diversions, 255-256

  for respiratory care, 141-142, 144-145

    PE, 141-142

    TB, 144-145

  for special needs care, 555-556

Dehydration *vs.* edema, 110. *See also* Fluid volume, imbalanced.

Delirium, 109-110. *See also* Thought processes, disturbed.

Dementia (Alzheimer's type), 751-760

  assessments for, 751-752

  deficient knowledge issues for, 752-753, 757-758

    disease progression, 752-753

    medication impacts, 757-758

  diagnoses and interventions for, 752-759

    additional considerations for, 759

    anticipatory grieving, 756

    caregiver role strain, 756

    injury risks, 753-754

    sensory perceptions, disturbed, 755-756

    thought processes, disturbed, 754-755

  diagnostic tests for, 752

  discharge planning for, 759

  fundamentals of, 751

  health care settings for, 751

  pathophysiology of, 751

  patient-family education for, 759

Denial, ineffective, 778

Dependence *vs.* independence issues, 70-71

Depression, major, 761-768
  assessments for, 761-762
  deficient knowledge issues for, 762-763, 766-767
    causes, signs, and symptoms, 762-763
    medication impacts, 766-767
  diagnoses and interventions for, 762-768
    additional considerations for, 768
    dysfunctional grieving, 764
    hopelessness, 763
    low self-esteem, chronic, 764-765
    suicide risks, 763-764
  diagnostic tests for, 762
  discharge planning for, 768
  fundamentals of, 761
  health care settings for, 761
  pathophysiology of, 761
  patient-family education for, 768

Depression and Bipolar Support Alliance. *See* DBSA
  (Depression and Bipolar Support Alliance).

Depression and Related Affective Disorders Association.
  See DRADA (Depression and Related Affective
  Disorders Association).

Depression Awareness, Recognition, and Treatment
  Program, D/ART (Depression Awareness, and
  Treatment) Program, Recognition

Descending colostomy, 455-456. *See also* Fecal diversions
  (colostomy, ileostomy, and IPAA).

Descriptive pain scales, 39-40

DI (diabetes insipidus), 373-376. *See also* Diabetes-
  related care.
  assessments for, 373-374
  diagnoses and interventions for, 374-375
    fluid volume, deficient, 374
    protection, ineffective, 375
  diagnostic tests for, 373-374
  discharge planning for, 375
  fundamentals of, 373
  health care settings for, 373
  pathophysiology of, 373
  patient-family education for, 375

Diabetes Insipidus Foundation, 375

Diabetes-related care
  DI, 373-376
    assessments for, 373-374
    diagnoses and interventions for, 374-375
    diagnostic tests for, 373-374
    discharge planning for, 375
    fundamentals of, 373
    health care settings for, 373
    pathophysiology of, 373
    patient-family education for, 375
  DKA, 387-394
    assessments for, 387-390
    deficient knowledge issues for, 392-394
    diagnoses and interventions for, 389-394
    diagnostic tests for, 387-390
    discharge planning for, 394
    fundamentals of, 387
    health care settings for, 387
    vs. HHNK syndrome, 387-388
    vs. hypoglycemia, 387-388
    pathophysiology of, 387
    patient-family education for, 394
  DM, 377-386, 629-636
    assessments for, 378
    complications of, 378-379
    deficient knowledge issues for, 382-384
    diagnoses and interventions for, 379-384
    diagnostic tests for, 379
    discharge planning for, 385-386
    fundamentals of, 377
    health care settings for, 378
    pathophysiology of, 377-378
    patient-family education for, 385-386
    pediatric care and, 629-636. *See also* Pediatric care.
    types of, 377-378

Diabetes-related care (*Continued*)
  GDM, 687-694. *See also* Maternity care.
    assessments for, 687-688
    deficient knowledge issues for, 688-689, 692-693
    diagnoses and interventions for, 688-694
    diagnostic tests for, 688
    discharge planning for, 693-694
    fundamentals of, 687
    health care settings for, 687
    pathophysiology of, 687
    patient-family education for, 693-694

Diabetic ketoacidosis. *See* DKA (diabetic ketoacidosis).

Diagnoses and interventions
  for cardiovascular care, 150, 152-155, 157-163, 167-176,
    178-180, 183-192, 194, 196-199, 201-205
    aneurysms, 150
    atherosclerotic arterial occlusive disease, 152-155
    CAD, 167-176
    cardiac surgeries, 161-163
    circulatory failure, 157-160
    dysrhythmias and conduction disturbances, 178-180
    HF, 183-192
    hypertension, 194
    pulmonary hypertension, 196-199
    venous thrombosis and thrombophlebitis, 201-205
  for endocrine care, 374-375, 379-384, 389-394, 396-397,
    400-405, 408-412, 415-418
    DI, 374-375
    DKA, 389-394
    DM, 379-384
    HHNK syndrome, 396-397
    hyperthyroidism, 400-405
    hypothyroidism, 408-412
    SIADH, 415-418
  for general care plans, 4-37, 39-43, 45-71, 73-85,
    87-104, 107-116
    bedrest, prolonged, 61-71
    cancer care, 4-37
    older adult, 93-104
    pain management, 39-43
    palliative and end-of-life, 107-116
    perioperative care, 45-60
    psychosocial support, family, 87-92
    psychosocial support, patient, 73-85
  for GI care, 421-427, 430-431, 434-436, 439-443,
    447-453, 456-461, 464-467, 470-475, 478-480,
    482-485, 488-489
    abdominal trauma, 421-427
    appendicitis, 430-431
    CD, 447-453
    cholelithiasis, cholecystitis, and cholangitis,
      434-436
    cirrhosis, 439-443
    fecal diversions, 456-461
    hepatitis, 464-467
    pancreatitis, 470-475
    peptic ulcers, 478-480
    peritonitis, 482-485
    UC, 488-489
  for hematologic care, 495-504, 506-508
    anemia of chronic disease, 495-496
    DIC, 497-500
    polycythemia, 501-504
    thrombocytopenia, 506-508
  for maternity care, 675-680, 682-686, 688-694,
    696-701, 704-710, 713-718, 720-728, 730-736
    bleeding in pregnancy, 675-680
    cervical insufficiency, 682-686
    GDM, 688-694
    hyperemesis gravidarum, 696-701
    postpartum wound infection, 704-710
    PPROM, 730-736
    preeclampsia, 713-718
    PTL, 720-728

Diagnoses and interventions (*Continued*)
  for musculoskeletal care, 510-513, 515-521, 524-528,
    536-539, 542-546
    amputations, 510-513
    fractures, 515-521
    joint replacement surgeries, 524-528
    osteoporosis, 536-539
    RA, 542-546
  for neurologic care, 261-280, 282-285, 288-293,
    296-304, 306-311, 314-322, 325-331, 335-348,
    351-359, 364-372
    bacterial meningitis, 282-285
    GBS, 288-293
    general, 261-280
    intervertebral disk disease, 296-304
    MS, 306-311
    PD, 314-322
    SCIs, 335-348
    seizures and epilepsy, 325-331
    stroke, 351-359
    TBIs, 364-372
  for pediatric care, 578-583, 586-590, 593-596,
    600-606, 610-614, 616-619, 622-627, 629-634,
    638-640, 642-645, 648-651, 654-656, 660-663
    ADHD, 586-590
    asthma, 578-583
    bronchiolitis, 593-596
    burns, 600-606
    CF, 622-627
    child abuse and neglect, 616-619
    CP, 610-614
    DM, 630-634
    fractures, 638-640
    gastroenteritis, 642-645
    OM, 648-651
    poisoning, 654-656
    sickle cell pain crisis, 660-663
  for psychiatric care, 738-744, 746-750, 752-759,
    762-768, 771-774, 776-782
    anxiety disorders, 738-744
    bipolar disorder (manic component), 746-750
    dementia (Alzheimer's type), 752-759
    depression, major, 762-768
    schizophrenia, 771-774
    substance abuse disorders, 776-782
  for renal-urinary care, 208-215, 218-226, 228-230,
    232-237, 239-242, 244-247, 249-256, 258-259
    ARF, 232-237
    BPH, 208-215
    CKD, 218-222
    hemodialysis, 223-226
    peritoneal dialysis, 228-230
    renal transplants, 239-242
    ureteral calculi, 244-247
    urinary diversions, 249-256
    urinary tract obstructions, 258-259
  for respiratory care, 118-121, 124-127, 132-135,
    138-142, 144-145, 147-148
    ARF, 147-148
    COPD, 118-121
    PE, 138-142
    pneumonia, 124-127
    pneumothorax and hemothorax, 132-135
    TB, 144-145
  for special needs care, 549-564, 568-576
    HIV/AIDS, 549-558
    nutritional support, 568-576
    wound management, 559-564

Diagnostic and Statistical Manual-IV. *See* DSM-IV
  (Diagnostic and Statistical Manual-IV) criteria.

Diagnostic tests
  ABG levels, 117-118, 124, 131-132, 138, 147-148,
    178, 183, 196, 577-578, 593, 600, 654
  ABI, 151, 509
  acid-fast stains and cultures, 124, 143-144
  allergen skin testing, 578

Diagnostic tests (*Continued*)
alpha-1 antitrypsin deficiency screens, 117-118
ambulatory monitoring, 166, 177-178
amniocentesis, 720, 730
angiographic studies, 138, 151, 363, 420, 438
antepartum fetal monitoring, 682, 688, 712
arteriography, contrast, 149
barium enema and upper GI series, 446
barium swallow, 438, 478
basic metabolic panels, 630, 659
biomarkers, cardiac, 166
biopsies, 182-183, 218
blood cultures, 642, 659, 704
blood Rh factor and antibody screens, 674, 720, 730
bone marrow aspiration, 501
bone scans, 616, 637
BUN levels, 183, 207, 217-218, 231-232, 243, 257, 600, 641-642
cancer screenings, 1-3
for cardiovascular care, 149, 151, 157, 165-166, 177-178, 182-183, 195-196, 201
aneurysms, 149
atherosclerotic arterial occlusive disease, 151
CAD, 165-166
circulatory failure, 157
dysrhythmias and conduction disturbances, 177-178
HF, 182-183
pulmonary hypertension, 195-196
venous thrombosis and thrombophlebitis, 201
catheterization, cardiac, 182-183
CBC, 131-132, 183, 196, 501, 578, 593, 616, 621-622, 641-642, 674, 695, 793
CBC with differential, 682, 704
cervical evaluations, 720
chemistries, 600, 793-795
cisternograms, 363
coagulation tests and studies, 282, 438, 505, 616, 712
colonoscopy, 446
creatinine levels and clearance, 183, 207, 217-218, 231-232, 243, 257, 378, 600, 641-642
CSF analyses, 287-288, 363, 667, 793-795
CT scans, 138, 149, 166, 195, 232, 243, 282, 296, 324-325, 351, 616, 637, 704, 752
cystoscopy, 207, 258
cytologic studies, 609
D-dimer tests, 138, 201-202, 497
DDAVP challenge tests, 373-374
digoxin levels, 183
diskography, 296
DNA analyses, 622
Doppler flow studies, 151
duplex imaging, 201-202
ECGs, 165-166, 177-178, 182-183, 195
EEGs, 609, 762
electrolyte levels, 609
electromyography, 288, 296
electrophysiologic studies, 177-178
ELISA tests, 548-549
for endocrine care, 373-374, 379, 387-390, 395-396, 399, 407, 415
DI, 373-374
DKA, 387-390
DM, 379
HHNK syndrome, 395-396
hyperthyroidism, 399
hypothyroidism, 407
SIADH, 415
endoscopy, 477-478
EP studies, 288, 296, 306, 351, 363
erythropoietin levels, 501
esophagoscopy, 438
FAST, 420
fasting lipid profiles, 378
fasting plasma glucose, 378, 630
fFN enzyme immunoassays, 720
fMRI studies, 324-325

Diagnostic tests (*Continued*)
for GI care, 420, 429, 434, 446, 463-464, 470, 477-478, 481-482, 488
abdominal trauma, 420
appendicitis, 429
CD, 446
cholelithiasis, cholecystitis, and cholangitis, 434
hepatitis, 463-464
pancreatitis, 470
peptic ulcers, 477-478
peritonitis, 481-482
UC, 488
glucose levels, 600, 667-688
glycosylated hemoglobin, 630
gram stain cultures, 281-282
for hematologic care, 495, 497, 501, 505-506
anemia of chronic disease, 495
DIC, 497
polycythemia, 501
thrombocytopenia, 505-506
high-performance liquid chromatography, 659
IGRA, 143-144
immunoglobulin levels, 668-669
immunoreactive trypsinogen test, 622
impedance plethysmography, 201-202
intrauterine dye tests, 730
isoelectric focusing, 659
ketone levels, 630
Kleihauer-Betke test, 65
laparoscopy, 438
laparotomy, 420
lipid panels, 166, 630
liver enzyme levels, 695
liver function tests, 420
lumbar punctures, 287-288, 314, 351
malabsorption tests, 446
for maternity care, 674-675, 681-682, 688, 695, 704, 712, 720, 730
bleeding in pregnancy, 674-675
cervical insufficiency, 681-682
GDM, 688
hyperemesis gravidarum, 695
postpartum wound infection, 704
PPROM, 730
preeclampsia, 712
PTL, 720
measurement instruments and scales. *See* Measurement instruments and scales.
metabolic studies, 609
MRI studies, 151, 282, 296, 306, 324-325, 351, 616, 637, 704, 752
for musculoskeletal care, 509, 515, 523, 530, 535, 541
amputations, 509
fractures, 515
joint replacement surgeries, 523
OA, 530
osteoporosis, 535
RA, 541
myelograms, 296
nerve conduction velocity tests, 218
for neurologic care, 281-282, 287-288, 296, 306, 314, 324-325, 334-335, 350-351, 363
bacterial meningitis, 281-282
GBS, 287-288
intervertebral disk disease, 296
MS, 306
PD, 314
SCIs, 334-335
seizures and epilepsy, 324-325
stroke, 350-351
TBIs, 363
normal values for, 665-672, 793-798
adult, 793-798
pediatric patients, 665-672
nuclear imaging modalities, cardiac, 166

Diagnostic tests (*Continued*)
oximetry, 117-118, 124, 131-132, 178, 183, 196, 578, 593, 621-622, 659
p24 antigen tests, 548-549
for pediatric care, 577-578, 585, 593, 600, 609, 616, 621-622, 629-630, 637, 641-642, 647, 654, 659
ADHD, 585
asthma, 577-578
bronchiolitis, 593
burns, 600
CF, 621-622
child abuse and neglect, 616
CP, 609
DM, 629-630
fractures, 637
gastroenteritis, 641-642
OM, 647
poisoning, 654
sickle cell pain crisis, 659
PEFRs, 578
perfusion scans, 195
peritoneoscopy, 438
PET studies, 306, 314, 324-325, 351
pilocarpine iontophoresis, 621-622
plasma chemistries, 793-795
plasma marker tests, 201-202
platelet counts, 420, 505, 671
PPD injection tests, 144
pregnancy tests, 674
PSA tests, 207
for psychiatric care, 738, 746, 752, 762, 770-771, 776
anxiety disorders, 738
bipolar disorder (manic component), 746
dementia (Alzheimer's type), 752
depression, major, 762
schizophrenia, 770-771
substance abuse disorders, 776
psychometric tests, 439
pulmonary function tests, 578, 622
QuantiFERON-TB Gold test, 143-144
quantitative sweat chloride test, 621-622
radiographs, 616
radiologic studies, 438
radionuclide imaging, 195
rapid HIV tests, 549
RBC counts, 671
renal function studies, 688, 712
renal scans, 232
for renal-urinary care, 207, 231-232, 243
ARF, 231-232
BPH, 207
ureteral calculi, 243
for respiratory care, 117, 123-124, 131-132, 144, 147
ARF, 147
COPD, 117
pneumonia, 123-124
pneumothorax and hemothorax, 131-132
TB, 144
retrograde urography, 232
Rotazyme tests, 642
RSV washing, 593
scintigraphy, thyroid, 379
serum chemistries, 218, 695, 793-795
serum electrolyte levels, 177-178, 641-642
serum osmolality, 373-374, 671
sigmoidoscopy, 446
sleep studies, 196
for special needs care, 548-549, 559, 562
HIV/AIDS, 548-549
wound management, 559, 562
spirometry, 117-118
sputum cultures, 117-118, 578, 622
sterile speculum examinations, 720, 730
stool cultures, 642
stool fat analyses, 622
stress tests, 166, 178, 182-183, 196

Diagnostic tests (Continued)
thyroid-stimulating hormone levels, 630
thyrotropin levels, 379
thyroxine levels, 630
tremor studies, 314
tuberculin skin tests, 144
tympanocentesis, 647
tympanometry, 647
ultrasound, 166, 201-202, 207, 218, 232, 243, 379, 407, 509, 674, 681-682, 688, 695, 704, 712, 720, 730
Doppler, 201-202, 379, 407, 509, 720
intravascular, 166
obstetric, 674, 682, 688, 695, 712, 730
pelvic, 704
renal, 218, 232, 243
translabial, 681
transrectal, 207
transvaginal, 681
urinalysis, 138, 207, 231-232, 243, 314, 378, 439, 671-672, 682, 704, 720
urinary osmolality, 231-232
urine chemistries, 671-672, 695, 793-795
urine cultures and sensitivity, 207, 243
urine function studies, 712
urine osmolality, 373-374
uterine monitoring, external, 720, 730
vasopressin challenge tests, 373-374
ventilation-perfusion scans, pulmonary, 138
viral load testing, 549
viral resistance testing, 549
water deprivation tests, 373-374
WBC counts, 124, 420, 439, 669
Western blot tests, 548-549
whole blood chemistries, 793-795
x-rays, 117-118, 123-124, 131-132, 138, 143-144, 147-149, 166, 182-183, 195, 218, 282, 334-335, 578, 593, 621-622, 637, 659
abdominal, 149
chest, 117-118, 123-124, 131-132, 138, 143-144, 147-148, 166, 182-183, 195, 282, 578, 593, 621-622, 659
KUB, 218
sinus, 282
skull, 282
spine, 334-335
xenon-133 studies, 509
Dialysis, 223-230
hemodialysis, 223-226
components of, 223
diagnoses and interventions for, 223-226
discharge planning for, 226
fundamentals of, 223
health care settings for, 223
pathophysiology of, 223
patient-family education for, 226
peritoneal, 227-230
components of, 227
diagnoses and interventions for, 228-230
discharge planning for, 230
fundamentals of, 227
health care settings for, 227
pathophysiology of, 227
patient-family education for, 230
types of, 227
Diarrhea
cancer care and, 9
CD and, 449-450
HIV/AIDS and, 551
UC and, 491
Diastolic dysfunction, 181-182. See also HF (heart failure).
DIC (disseminated intravascular coagulation), 497-500
assessments for, 497
diagnoses and interventions for, 497-500
additional considerations for, 500
ineffective tissue perfusion, cardiopulmonary, 498

DIC (Continued)
ineffective tissue perfusion, cerebral, 498
ineffective tissue perfusion, peripheral, 498
ineffective tissue perfusion, renal, 498
protection, ineffective, 499
skin integrity, impaired, 500
diagnostic tests for, 497
discharge planning for, 500
fundamentals of, 497
health care settings for, 497
pathophysiology of, 497
patient-family education for, 500
thrombocytopenia and, 505. See also Thrombocytopenia.
Diet-related support and impacts. See Nutritional support.
Dietary histories, 565
Dietary-related considerations. See Nutritional support.
Diffuse axonal injuries. See DAIs (diffuse axonal injuries).
Digoxin, 183, 190
Dilated cardiomyopathy, 181. See also HF (heart failure).
Disabled family coping, 90-91. See also Family coping.
Discharge planning
for cardiovascular care, 150, 156, 160, 163, 176, 180, 192, 194, 199, 205
aneurysms, 150
atherosclerotic arterial occlusive disease, 156
CAD, 176
cardiac surgeries, 163
circulatory failure, 160
dysrhythmias and conduction disturbances, 180
HF, 192
hypertension, 194
pulmonary hypertension, 199
venous thrombosis and thrombophlebitis, 205
for endocrine care, 375, 385-386, 394, 397, 405, 413, 418
DI, 375
DKA, 394
DM, 385-386
HHNK syndrome, 397
hyperthyroidism, 405
hypothyroidism, 413
SIADH, 418
for GI care, 427, 431, 436, 453, 461, 467, 475, 480, 485, 493
abdominal trauma, 427
appendicitis, 431
CD, 453
cholelithiasis, cholecystitis, and cholangitis, 436
fecal diversions, 461
hepatitis, 467
pancreatitis, 475
peptic ulcers, 480
peritonitis, 485
UC, 493
for hematologic care, 496, 500, 504, 508
anemia of chronic disease, 496
DIC, 500
polycythemia, 504
thrombocytopenia, 508
for maternity care, 680, 686, 693-694, 701, 710, 718, 728, 736
bleeding in pregnancy, 680
cervical insufficiency, 686
GDM, 693-694
hyperemesis gravidarum, 701
postpartum wound infection, 710
PPROM, 736
preeclampsia, 718
PTL, 728
for musculoskeletal care, 513-514, 521, 528, 533, 539-540, 546
amputations, 513-514
fractures, 521
joint replacement surgeries, 528

Discharge planning (Continued)
OA, 533
osteoporosis, 539-540
RA, 546
for neurologic care, 286, 294, 304, 311, 322, 331, 348, 358, 372
bacterial meningitis, 286
GBS, 294
intervertebral disk disease, 304
MS, 311
PD, 322
SCIs, 348
seizures and epilepsy, 331
stroke, 358
TBIs, 372
for pediatric care, 583-584, 591, 596, 606-608, 614, 619, 626-627, 634-636, 639, 645-646, 650-651, 655-656, 663-664
ADHD, 591
asthma, 583-584
bronchiolitis, 596
burns, 606-608
CF, 626-627
child abuse and neglect, 619
CP, 614
DM, 634-636
fractures, 639
gastroenteritis, 645-646
OM, 650-651
poisoning, 655-656
sickle cell pain crisis, 663-664
for psychiatric care, 744, 750, 759, 768, 774, 782
anxiety disorders, 744
bipolar disorder (manic component), 750
dementia (Alzheimer's type), 759
depression, major, 768
schizophrenia, 774
substance abuse disorders, 782
for renal-urinary care, 215, 222, 226, 230, 237, 242, 247, 256, 260
ARF, 237
BPH, 215
CKD, 222
hemodialysis, 226
peritoneal dialysis, 230
renal transplants, 242
ureteral calculi, 247
urinary diversions, 256
urinary tract obstructions, 260
for respiratory care, 121, 135, 145, 148
ARF, 148
COPD, 121
pneumothorax and hemothorax, 135
TB, 145
for special needs care, 558, 560, 562, 564
HIV/AIDS, 558
wound management, 560, 562, 564
Disease management choices, 105-106
Disease processes, progressive, 106
Disk disease, intervertebral, 295-304
assessments for, 295-296
deficient knowledge issues for, 298-303
diskectomy with laminectomy procedures, 300-303
fusion procedures, 300-303
pain management, 298-299
diagnoses and interventions for, 296-304
additional considerations for, 304
health-seeking behaviors, 296-297
swallowing, impaired, 303-304
diagnostic tests for, 296
discharge planning for, 304
fundamentals of, 295
health care settings for, 295
pathophysiology of, 295
patient-family education for, 304
Diskectomy with laminectomy procedures, 300-303

Diskography, 296
Disseminated intravascular coagulation. *See* DIC (disseminated intravascular coagulation).
Distress, spiritual, 114
Disturbances, conduction. *See* Conduction disturbances and dysrhythmias.
Disturbed auditory perception. *See* Sensory perception, disturbed.
Disturbed body image
  amputations and, 511-512
  burns and, 605-606
  cancer care and, 36
  fecal diversion and, 459-460
  HIV/AIDS and, 557
  hyperthyroidism and, 403
  psychosocial support and, 80-81
  RA and, 545
Disturbed kinesthetic perception, 37
Disturbed sensory perception
  cancer care and, 37
  dementia (Alzheimer's type) and, 755-756
  general neurologic care and, 280
  hypothyroidism and, 410-411
  schizophrenia and, 771-772
  stroke and, 355-356
Disturbed sleep patterns
  hyperthyroidism and, 401-402
  older adult care and, 101-102
  perioperative care and, 57-58
  psychosocial support and, 73-74
Disturbed tactile perception. *See* Disturbed sensory perception.
Disturbed thought processes
  ADHD and, 586
  dementia (Alzheimer's type) and, 754-755
  palliative and end-of-life care and, 109-110
Disturbed visual perception. *See* Sensory perception, disturbed.
Disulfiram, 781
Disuse syndrome
  amputations and, 511
  bedrest, prolonged and, 63-65
  cancer care and, 12
  SCIs and, 343-344
Diuretics, 189-190
Diversional activity, deficient, 69
Diversions
  fecal, 455-462
    colostomy, 455
    deficient knowledge issues for, 460-461
    diagnoses and interventions for, 456-461
    discharge planning for, 461
    fundamentals of, 455
    health care settings for, 455
    ileostomy, 455-456
    IPAA, 456
    pathophysiology of, 455
    patient-family education for, 461
  urinary, 249-256
    continent, 249
    deficient knowledge issues for, 255-256
    diagnoses and interventions for, 249-256
    discharge planning for, 256
    fundamentals of, 249
    health care settings for, 249
    intestinal (ileal conduit), 249
    orthotopic neobladder, 249
    pathophysiology of, 249
    patient-family education for, 256
DKA (diabetic ketoacidosis), 387-394. *See also* Diabetes-related care.
  assessments for, 387-390
  deficient knowledge issues for, 392-394
  diagnoses and interventions for, 389-394
    additional considerations for, 394
    fluid volume, deficient, 389-390

DKA (*Continued*)
    ineffective tissue perfusion, peripheral, 392
    infection risks, 390-391
    injury risks, 391
  diagnostic tests for, 387-390
  discharge planning for, 394
  fundamentals of, 387
  health care settings for, 387
  vs. HHNK syndrome, 387-388
  vs. hypoglycemia, 387
  pathophysiology of, 387
  patient-family education for, 394
DM (diabetes mellitus), 377-386, 629-636. *See also* Diabetes-related care.
  assessments for, 378
  complications of, 378-379
  deficient knowledge issues for, 382-384
    exercise, 382-384
    insulin administration and impacts, 382-384
    nutrition precautions, 382-384
  diagnoses and interventions for, 379-384
    additional considerations for, 384
    infection risks, 381
    skin integrity, impaired, 382
    unstable glucose levels, 379-381
  diagnostic tests for, 379
  discharge planning for, 385-386
  fundamentals of, 377
  GDM, 687-694. *See also* Maternity care.
    assessments for, 687-688
    deficient knowledge issues for, 688-689, 692-693
    diagnoses and interventions for, 688-694
    diagnostic tests for, 688
    discharge planning for, 693-694
    fundamentals of, 687
    health care settings for, 687
    pathophysiology of, 687
    patient-family education for, 693-694
  health care settings for, 378
  pathophysiology of, 377
  patient-family education for, 385-386
  pediatric care and, 629-636. *See also* Pediatric care.
    additional considerations for, 634
    assessments for, 629
    blood glucose monitoring and, 630-631
    complications of, 629
    deficient knowledge issues for, 630-634
    diagnoses and interventions for, 630-634
    diagnostic tests for, 629-630
    discharge planning for, 634-636
    fundamentals of, 629
    health care settings for, 629
    hyperglycemia and, 632-633
    hypoglycemia and, 632-633
    meal planning and, 633-634
    pathophysiology of, 629
    patient-family education for, 634-636
  types of, 377-378
DNA analyses, 622
Dopamine replacement therapy, 318-320
Doppler flow studies, 151
Doppler ultrasound, 201-202, 379, 407, 509, 720
Doxylamine, 700
DRADA (Depression and Related Affective Disorders Association), 750
Droplet (Transmission-Based Precautions), 283, 783-792, 784t-791t
Drug-related impacts
  anxiety disorders and, 741-743
  bipolar disorder (manic component) and, 749-750
  bleeding in pregnancy and, 678-679
  chemotherapy, 1-3
  dementia (Alzheimer's type) and, 757-758
  GDM and, 688-689, 692-693
  hyperemesis gravidarum and, 699-700
  major depression and, 766-767

Drug-related impacts (*Continued*)
  MS and, 307-310
  PE and, 141-142
  postpartum wound infection and, 705-708
  PPROM and, 732-733
  preeclampsia and, 714-716
  PTL and, 722-724
  RA and, 545
  schizophrenia and, 772-773
  of specific drugs and drug classes. *See also under specific drugs and drug classes.*
    ACE inhibitors, 231
    acetaminophen with codeine, 662-663
    acetaminophen with oxycodone, 707
    AEDs, 328-330
    albuterol, 579, 625
    analgesics, 40-43, 707
    analgesics, opioid, 41-43, 678
    antenatal glucocorticoids, 716, 723-724, 733-734
    antibiotics, 283-284, 626
    antibiotics, aerosolized, 625
    antibiotics, prophylactic, 678, 733-734
    anticoagulants, 141, 708
    antidepressants, tricyclic, 589, 742-743, 766-767
    antimanics, 747, 749
    antimicrobials, 705-706
    antiparkinson drugs, 316-320
    antipsychotics, 747, 750, 772-773
    antiviral agents, 318-320
    aspirin, 41, 716
    benzodiazepines, 743
    beta-andrenergics, 734
    beta-blockers, 169-170, 715-716
    beta$_2$-agonists, 582-583
    blood products, IV, 679
    bronchodilators, 625
    calcium channel blockers, 715-716, 722, 734
    carboprost, 679
    clindamycin, 706
    clonidine, 590
    co-analgesics, 42-43
    corticosteroids, 582-583
    cromolyn sodium/nedocromil sodium, 582-583
    digoxin, 190
    disulfiram, 781
    diuretics, 189-190
    dopamine replacement therapy, 318-320
    doxylamine, 700
    dual-mechanism drugs, 767-768
    folic acid, 662-663
    heparin, 138-139, 708
    hydration, IV, 722
    ibuprofen, 662-663, 678
    immunosuppressive agents, 240-241
    insulin, 373-386
    leukotriene modifiers, 582-583
    linezolid, 706
    LMWH, 138-139, 708
    magnesium sulfate, 715-716, 722, 733-734
    MAO inhibitors, 589, 742-743, 767
    meperidine, 707
    methylergonovine, 679
    methylxanthines, 583
    metoclopramide hydrochloride, 699
    morphine, 662-663, 707
    mucolytic enzymes, aerosolized, 625-626
    naltrexone, 781
    nitrates, 169-170
    nitroglycerin, 165-176
    nonbenzodiazepines, 743
    NSAIDs, 41, 231
    ondansetron, 700
    opioid analgesics, 41-43, 678
    oxycodone with acetaminophen, 707
    oxytocin, 679
    pancreatic enzymes, 625-626

Drug-related impacts *(Continued)*
  pantoprazole, 699
  penicillins, 662-663
  promethazine, 699-700
  prostaglandin synthesis inhibitors, 678, 722
  pyridoxine, 700
  Rh-immune globulin, 679, 734
  SNRIs, 589, 768
  SSRIs, 743, 767
  steroids, 582-583
  stimulants, 588-589
  sulfonylureas, second-generation, 692-693
  uterotonics, 678-679
  vaccines, pneumococcal, 283-284, 286
  vasodilators, 183-185
  vitamin and mineral supplements, 626
  substance abuse disorders and, 780-781
Dry mouth, 111. *See also* Oral mucous membranes,
    impaired.
DSM-IV (Diagnostic and Statistical Manual-IV)
    criteria, 585, 770, 775
Dual-mechanism drugs, 767-768
Duplex imaging, 201-202
Dysfunction, sexual
  BPH and, 207-216
  cervical insufficiency and, 685
Dysfunctional grieving, 764. *See also* Grieving.
Dyskinetic/athetoid CP (cerebral palsy), 609. *See also*
    CP (cerebral palsy).
Dyspnea, 107-108. *See also* Breathing patterns, ineffective.
Dysreflexia, autonomic, 335-336
Dysrhythmias and conduction disturbances, 177-180
  assessments for, 177
  automaticity disturbances and, 177
  cardiac output, decreased, 178-179
  deficient knowledge issues for, 179-180
    dysrhythmia mechanisms, 179-180
    lifestyle impacts, 179-180
  diagnoses and interventions for, 178-180
  diagnostic tests for, 177-178
  discharge planning for, 180
  fundamentals of, 177
  health care settings for, 177
  pathophysiology of, 177
  patient-family education for, 180
Dysuria, 244-245

E

Eater Seals Disability Services, 614
ECGs (echocardiograms), 165-166, 177-178, 182-183,
    195
Echocardiograms. *See* ECGs (echocardiograms).
Edema *vs.* dehydration, 110. *See also* Fluid volume,
    imbalanced.
Education, patient-family
  for cardiovascular care, 150, 156, 160, 163, 176, 180,
      192, 194, 199, 205
    aneurysms, 150
    atherosclerotic arterial occlusive disease, 156
    CAD, 176
    cardiac surgeries, 163
    circulatory failure (cardiac *vs.* noncardiac shock), 160
    dysrhythmias and conduction disturbances, 180
    HF, 192
    hypertension, 194
    pulmonary hypertension, 199
    venous thrombosis and thrombophlebitis, 205
  for endocrine care, 375, 385-386, 394, 397, 405, 413,
      418
    DI, 375
    DKA, 394
    DM, 385-386
    HHNK syndrome, 397
    hyperthyroidism, 405
    hypothyroidism, 413
    SIADH, 418

Education, patient-family *(Continued)*
  for GI care, 427, 431, 436, 453, 461, 467, 475, 480,
      485, 493
    abdominal trauma, 427
    appendicitis, 431
    CD, 453
    cholelithiasis, cholecystitis, and cholangitis, 436
    fecal diversions, 461
    hepatitis, 467
    pancreatitis, 475
    peptic ulcers, 480
    peritonitis, 485
    UC, 493
  for hematologic care, 496, 500, 504, 508
    anemia of chronic disease, 496
    DIC, 500
    polycythemia, 504
    thrombocytopenia, 508
  IEPs, 591, 614, 636, 664
  for maternity care, 680, 686, 693-694, 701, 710, 718,
      728, 736
    bleeding in pregnancy, 680
    cervical insufficiency, 686
    GDM, 693-694
    hyperemesis gravidarum, 701
    postpartum wound infection, 710
    PPROM, 736
    preeclampsia, 718
    PTL, 728
  for musculoskeletal care, 513-514, 521, 528, 539-540,
      546
    amputations, 513-514
    fractures, 521
    joint replacement surgeries, 528
    OA, 533
    osteoporosis, 539-540
    RA, 546
  for neurologic care, 286, 294, 304, 311, 322, 331, 348,
      372
    bacterial meningitis, 286
    GBS, 294
    intervertebral disk disease, 304
    MS, 311
    PD and, 322
    SCIs and, 348
    seizures and epilepsy, 331
    TBIs and, 372
  for pediatric care, 583-584, 591, 596, 606-608, 614,
      619, 626-627, 634-636, 639, 645-646, 650-651,
      655-656, 663-664
    ADHD, 591
    asthma, 583-584
    bronchiolitis, 596
    burns, 606-608
    CF and, 626-627
    child abuse and neglect, 619
    CP, 614
    DM, 634-636
    fractures, 639
    gastroenteritis, 645-646
    OM, 650-651
    poisoning, 655-656
    sickle cell pain crisis, 663-664
  for psychiatric care, 744, 750, 759, 768, 774, 782
    anxiety disorders, 744
    bipolar disorder (manic component), 750
    dementia (Alzheimer's type), 759
    depression, major, 768
    schizophrenia, 774
    substance abuse disorders, 782
  for renal-urinary care, 215, 222, 226, 230, 237, 242,
      247, 256, 260
    ARF, 237
    BPH, 215
    CKD, 222
    hemodialysis, 226

Education, patient-family *(Continued)*
    peritoneal dialysis, 230
    renal transplants, 242
    ureteral calculi, 247
    urinary diversions, 256
    urinary tract obstructions, 260
  for respiratory care, 128, 135, 148
    ARF, 148
    COPD, 121
    pneumonia, 128
    pneumothorax and hemothorax, 135
    TB, 145
  for special needs care, 558, 560, 562
    HIV/AIDS, 558
    wound management, 560, 562
EEGs (electroencephalograms), 609, 762
Electrolyte levels, 177-178, 609, 641-642
Electromyography, 288, 296
Electrophysiologic studies, 177-178
Elimination urinary, impaired
  cancer care and, 29-30
  ureteral calculi and, 244-245
  urinary diversions and, 250-251
ELISA tests, 548-549
Embolus, pulmonary, 137-142. *See also* PE (pulmonary
    embolus).
Emotional abuse and neglect, 615-616. *See also* Child
    abuse and neglect.
End-of-life and palliative care, 105-116
  deficient knowledge issues for, 105-116
    disease management choices, 105-106
    expectations, 106
    progressive disease processes, 106
  diagnoses and interventions for, 107-116
    airway clearance, ineffective, 108-109
    breathing patterns, ineffective, 107-108
    fluid volume, imbalanced, 110
    imbalanced nutrition, less than body requirements,
        111-112
    oral mucous membranes, impaired, 111
    pain, acute *vs.* chronic, 107
    thought processes, disturbed, 109-110
  psychosocial diagnoses and interventions, 112-116.
      See also Psychosocial support.
    additional considerations, 116
    anticipatory grieving, 115-116
    anxiety, 112-133
    caregiver role strain risks, 114-115
    death anxiety, 113
    fear, feelings of, 112
    powerlessness, feelings of, 113-114
    spiritual distress, 114
End-stage renal disease. *See* ESRD (end-stage renal
    disease).
Endocrine care, 373-418, 804-805
  diabetes, 373-394
    DI, 373-376
    DKA, 387-394
    DM, 377-386
  HHNK syndrome, 395-398
  reference resources for, 804-805
  SIADH, 415-418
  thyroid disorders, 399-414
    hyperthyroidism, 399-406
    hypothyroidism, 407-414
Endoscopy, 477-478
Enhanced family coping, 91. *See also* Family coping.
Enteritis, regional. *See* CD (Crohn's disease).
Environmental Protection Agency. *See* EPA (Environ-
    mental Protection Agency).
EP (evoked potential) studies, 288, 296, 306, 351, 363
EPA (Environmental Protection Agency), 657
Epilepsy and seizures, 323-332
  assessments for, 323-325
  deficient knowledge issues for, 327-330
    AED side effects, 328-330
    life-threatening environmental factors, 327-328
    preventive measures, 327-328

Epilepsy and seizures (Continued)
  diagnoses and interventions for, 325-331
    additional considerations for, 331
    therapy noncompliance, 330-331
    trauma risks, 325-327
  diagnostic tests for, 324-325
  discharge planning for, 331
  epileptic syndromes, 324
  fundamentals of, 323
  generalized absence (petit mal) seizures, 324
  generalized myoclonic seizures, 324
  generalized tonic-clonic (grand mal) seizures, 323-324
  health care settings for, 323
  partial complex (psychomotor) seizures, 324
  partial simple (focal) motor seizures, 324
  pathophysiology of, 323
  patient-family education for, 331
  SE, 323
  temporal lobe seizures, 324
Epilepsy Foundation, 331
Episiotomy infections, 703. See also Postpartum wound infection.
Erythropoietin levels, 501
Esophagoscopy, 438
ESRD (end-stage renal disease), 223-226
Estimations, nutritional requirements, 566-567
Evaluations. See also Diagnostic tests.
  for cardiovascular care, 149, 151, 177, 182, 195, 201
    aneurysms, 149
    atherosclerotic arterial occlusive disease, 151
    CAD, 165
    dysrhythmias and conduction disturbances, 177
    HF, 182
    pulmonary hypertension, 195
    venous thrombosis and thrombophlebitis, 201
  for endocrine care, 373-374, 378, 387-390, 395-396, 399, 407, 415
    DI, 373-374
    DKA, 387-390
    DM, 378
    HHNK syndrome, 395-396
    hyperthyroidism, 399
    hypothyroidism, 407
    SIADH, 415
  for GI care, 419-420, 429, 433-434, 437-439, 445-446, 463-464, 469-470, 477-478, 481, 487-488
    abdominal trauma, 419-420
    appendicitis, 429
    CD, 445-446
    cholelithiasis, cholecystitis, and cholangitis, 433-434
    cirrhosis, 437-439
    hepatitis, 463-464
    pancreatitis, 469-470
    peptic ulcers, 477-478
    peritonitis, 481
    UC, 487-488
  for hematologic care, 495, 497, 501, 505
    anemia of chronic disease, 495
    DIC, 497
    polycythemia, 501
    thrombocytopenia, 505
  for maternity care, 673-674, 681-682, 687-688, 695, 703, 711-712, 719-720, 729-730
    bleeding in pregnancy, 673-674
    cervical insufficiency, 681-682
    GDM, 687-688
    hyperemesis gravidarum, 695
    postpartum wound infection, 703
    PPROM, 729-730
    preeclampsia, 711-712
    PTL, 719-720
  for musculoskeletal care, 509, 515, 529-530, 535, 541
    amputations, 509
    fractures, 515
    OA, 529-530
    osteoporosis, 535
    RA, 541

Evaluations (Continued)
  for neurologic care, 281, 287-288, 295-296, 305-306, 313-314, 323-325, 333-335, 350-351, 361-363
    bacterial meningitis, 281
    GBS, 287-288
    intervertebral disk disease, 295-296
    MS, 305-306
    PD, 313-314
    SCIs, 333-335
    seizures and epilepsy, 323-325
    stroke, 350-351
    TBIs, 361-363
  for pediatric care, 577-578, 585, 593, 600, 609, 616, 621, 629, 637, 641, 647, 653, 659
    ADHD, 585
    asthma, 577-578
    bronchiolitis, 593
    burns, 600
    CF, 621
    child abuse and neglect, 616
    CP, 609
    DM, 629
    fractures, 637
    gastroenteritis, 641
    OM, 647
    poisoning, 653
    sickle cell pain crisis, 659
  for psychiatric care, 737, 745-746, 751-752, 761-762, 769, 775-776
    anxiety disorders, 737
    bipolar disorder (manic component), 745-746
    dementia (Alzheimer's type), 751-752
    depression, major, 761-762
    schizophrenia, 769
    substance abuse disorders, 775-776
  for renal-urinary care, 207, 217, 231, 243, 257-258
    ARF, 231
    BPH, 207
    CKD, 217
    ureteral calculi, 243
    urinary tract obstructions, 257-258
  for respiratory care, 117, 131, 137, 147
    ARF, 147
    COPD, 117
    PE, 137
    pneumothorax and hemothorax, 131
  for special needs care, 548-549, 559, 561-562, 565-568
    HIV/AIDS, 548-549
    nutritional support, 565-568
    wound management, 559, 561-562
Evoked potential studies. See EP (evoked potential) studies.
Excess fluid volume. See also Fluid volume, imbalanced.
  ARF and, 234-235
  BPH and, 210
  cirrhosis and, 442-443
  HF and, 184-185
  hypothyroidism and, 408-409
  perioperative care and, 53-54
  SIADH and, 415-416
  TBIs and, 366-367
Exchange, gas. See Gas exchange, impaired.
Exercise impacts, 382-384
External beam radiation therapy, 33
External fixation function and care, 520-521. See also Fractures.
External uterine monitoring, 720, 730

F
Faces Pain Scale, 39-40
Failure, circulatory. See Circulatory failure (cardiac vs. noncardiac shock).
Failure to thrive. See FFT (failure to thrive).
Fall risks
  general neurologic care and, 265-266
  PD and, 314-315

Family coping. See also Coping.
  ADHD and, 590
  anxiety disorders and, 740
  compromised, 590, 740
  disabled, 90-91
  enhanced, 91
  impaired, 89-90
Family education. See Education, patient-family.
Family processes, interrupted
  asthma, 581
  family psychosocial support and, 88-89
  substance abuse disorders and, 777-778
Family psychosocial support, 87-92. See also Psychosocial support.
  deficient knowledge issues for, 91-92
    current health status, 91-92
    prescribed therapies, 91-92
  diagnoses and interventions for, 87-92
    family coping, compromised, 89-90
    family coping, disabled, 90-91
    family coping, enhanced, 91
    family processes, interrupted, 88-89
    fear, 87-88
  fundamentals of, 87
  HIPAA and, 87
FAST (Focused Assessment Sonogram for Trauma), 420
Fasting lipid profiles, 378
Fatigue
  asthma and, 579-580
  hepatitis and, 464-465
  RA and, 544-545
Fear
  child abuse and neglect and, 618-619
  GDM and, 690-691
  HF and, 188-189
  palliative and end-of-life care and, 112
  psychosocial support and, 76, 87-88
    family, 87-88
    patient, 76
Fecal diversions (colostomy, ileostomy, and IPAA), 455-462
  deficient knowledge issues for, 460-461
  diagnoses and interventions for, 456-461
    additional considerations for, 461
    body image, disturbed, 459-460
    incontinence, bowel, 458-459
    skin integrity, impaired, 456-457
    tissue integrity, impaired, 456-457
  discharge planning for, 461
  fundamentals of, 455
  health care settings for, 455
  pathophysiology of, 455
  patient-family education for, 461
  surgical interventions, 455-456
    colostomy, 455
    ileostomy, 455-456
    IPAA, 456
Fecal impaction, 342
Feedings, transitional, 568. See also Nutritional support.
Femoral aneurysms, 149. See also Aneurysms.
Fetal monitoring, antepartum, 682, 688, 712
fFN (fetal fibronectin) enzyme immunoassays, 720
FFT (failure to thrive), 616
Flow studies, Doppler, 151
Fluid volume, imbalanced
  ARF and, 234-236
  BPH and, 209-210
  bronchiolitis and, 595-596
  burns and, 600-601
  CAD and, 174
  CD and, 447
  cirrhosis and, 442-443
  deficient, 174, 209-210, 236, 258-259, 271-272, 374, 389-390, 447, 470-471, 488-489, 525, 595-596, 600-601, 642-643, 648-649
  dehydration vs. edema, 53-54, 98, 110, 126-127

Fluid volume, imbalanced (*Continued*)
   diabetes and, 374, 389-390
      DI, 374
      DKA, 389-390
   dialysis and, 223-224, 228-229
      hemodialysis, 223-224
      peritoneal, 228-229
   excess, 53-54, 184-185, 210, 234-235, 366-367,
      408-409, 415-416, 442-443. *See also* Excess fluid
      volume.
   gastroenteritis, 642-643
   general neurologic care, 271-272
   hypothyroidism and, 408-409
   joint replacement surgeries and, 525
   nutritional support and, 575-576. *See also* Nutritional
      support.
   older adult care and, 98
   OM and, 648-649
   pancreatitis and, 470-471
   perioperative care and, 51-54
   pneumonia and, 126-127
   SIADH and, 415-416
   TBIs and, 366-367
   UC and, 488-489
   urinary tract obstructions and, 258-259
FLUTTER mucus clearance devices, 626-627
fMRI (functional MRI) studies, 324-325
Focal motor seizures, 324
Focused Assessment Sonogram for Trauma. *See* FAST
   (Focused Assessment Sonogram for Trauma).
Folic acid, 662-663
Food-related considerations. *See* Nutritional support.
Fractures, 515-522
   assessments for, 515
   deficient knowledge issues for, 520-521
      external fixation function and care, 520-521
      infection risks, 520-521
      pin function and care, 520-521
   diagnoses and interventions for, 515-521
      constipation, 519
      pain, acute, 515-516
      peripheral neurovascular dysfunction, 516-517
      physical mobility, impaired, 517-518
      self-care deficits, 519-520
      skin integrity, impaired, 518-519
   diagnostic tests for, 515
   discharge planning for, 521
   fundamentals of, 515
   health care settings for, 515
   pathophysiology of, 515
   patient-family education for, 521
   in pediatric patients, 637-640. *See also* Pediatric care.
      additional considerations for, 639
      assessments for, 637
      diagnoses and interventions for, 638-640
      diagnostic tests for, 637
      discharge planning for, 639
      fundamentals of, 637
      health care settings for, 637
      ineffective tissue perfusion, peripheral, 638-639
      pain, acute, 638
      pathophysiology of, 637
      patient-family education for, 639
      skin integrity, impaired, 639
   skull, 362. *See also* TBIs (traumatic brain injuries).
Frequency, 244-245
Full-thickness burns, 600. *See also* Burns.
Functional MRI studies. *See* fMRI (functional MRI)
   studies.
Fundamental concepts
   of cardiovascular care, 149, 151, 157, 161, 165, 177,
      181, 195, 201
      aneurysms, 149
      atherosclerotic arterial occlusive disease, 151
      CAD, 165
      cardiac surgery, 161

Fundamental concepts (*Continued*)
      circulatory failure, 157
      dysrhythmias and conduction disturbances, 177
      HF, 181
      hypertension, 195
      pulmonary hypertension, 195
      venous thrombosis and thrombophlebitis, 201
   of endocrine care, 373, 377, 387, 395, 399, 407, 415
      DI, 373
      DKA, 387
      DM, 377
      HHNK syndrome, 395
      hyperthyroidism, 399
      hypothyroidism, 407
      SIADH, 415
   of general care plans, 1, 39, 45, 61, 87, 93
      bedrest, prolonged, 61
      cancer care, 1
      older adult, 93
      pain management, 39
      perioperative, 45
      psychosocial support, family, 87
   of GI care, 419, 429, 433, 445, 455, 463, 469, 477,
      481, 487
      abdominal trauma, 419
      appendicitis, 429
      CD, 445
      cholelithiasis, cholecystitis, and cholangitis, 433
      fecal diversions, 455
      hepatitis, 463
      pancreatitis, 469
      peptic ulcers, 477
      peritonitis, 481
      UC, 487
   of hematologic care, 495, 497, 501, 505
      anemia of chronic disease, 495
      DIC, 497
      polycythemia, 501
      thrombocytopenia, 505
   of maternity care, 70, 673, 681, 687, 695, 711, 719, 729
      bleeding in pregnancy, 673
      cervical insufficiency, 681
      GDM, 687
      hyperemesis gravidarum, 695
      postpartum wound infection, 70
      PPROM, 729
      preeclampsia, 711
      PTL, 719
   of musculoskeletal care, 509, 515, 523, 529, 535, 541
      amputations, 509
      fractures, 515
      joint replacement surgeries, 523
      OA, 529
      osteoporosis, 535
      RA, 541
   of neurologic care, 281, 287, 295, 305, 313, 323, 333,
      349-350, 361
      bacterial meningitis, 281
      GBS, 287
      intervertebral disk disease, 295
      MS, 305
      PD, 313
      SCIs, 333
      seizures and epilepsy, 323
      stroke, 349-350
      TBIs, 361
   of pediatric care, 577, 585, 593, 599, 609, 615, 621,
      629, 637, 641, 647, 653, 659
      ADHD, 585
      asthma, 577
      bronchiolitis, 593
      burns, 599
      CF and, 621
      child abuse and neglect, 615
      CP, 609
      DM, 629

Fundamental concepts (*Continued*)
      fractures, 637
      gastroenteritis, 641
      OM, 647
      poisoning, 653
      sickle cell pain crisis, 659
   of psychiatric care, 737, 745, 751, 761, 769, 775
      anxiety disorders, 737
      bipolar disorder (manic component), 745
      dementia (Alzheimer's type), 751
      depression, major, 761
      schizophrenia, 769
      substance abuse disorders, 775
   of renal-urinary care, 207, 217, 223, 227, 231, 239,
      243, 249, 257
      ARF, 231
      BPH, 207
      CKD, 217
      hemodialysis, 223
      peritoneal dialysis, 227
      renal transplants, 239
      ureteral calculi, 243
      urinary diversions, 249
      urinary tract obstructions, 257
   of respiratory care, 117, 123, 131, 137, 143, 147
      ARF, 147
      COPD, 117
      PE, 137
      pneumonia, 123
      pneumothorax and hemothorax, 131
      TB, 143
   of special needs care, 547, 559, 565
      HIV/AIDS, 547
      nutritional support, 565
      wound management, 559
Fusion procedures, 300-303

G
Gas exchange, impaired
   bronchiolitis and, 594-595
   cancer care and, 4
   CF and, 623-624
   circulatory failure and, 160
   COPD and, 118-119
   HF and, 183-184
   HIV/AIDS and, 549-550
   older adult care and, 95-96
   pancreatitis and, 473
   PE and, 139
   peritonitis and, 483
   pneumonia and, 124-125
   pneumothorax and hemothorax and, 133-134
   pulmonary hypertension and, 196-197
Gastroenteritis, 641-646
   assessments for, 641
   diagnoses and interventions for, 642-645
      additional considerations for, 645
      fluid volume, deficient, 642-643
      imbalanced nutrition, less than body requirements,
         644-645
      infection risks, 644
      skin integrity, impaired, 643-644
   diagnostic tests for, 641-642
   discharge planning for, 645-646
   fundamentals of, 641
   health care settings for, 641
   pathophysiology of, 641
   patient-family education for, 645-646
Gastrointestinal care. *See* GI (gastrointestinal) care.
GBS (Guillain-Barre syndrome), 287-294
   assessments for, 287-288
   deficient knowledge issues for, 291-292
   diagnoses and interventions for, 288-293
      additional considerations for, 293
      anxiety, 290
      breathing patterns, ineffective, 288-289

GBS (Guillain-Barre syndrome) (Continued)
  imbalanced nutrition, less than body requirements, 289-290
  ineffective tissue perfusion, cardiopulmonary, 289
  ineffective tissue perfusion, cerebral, 289
  pain, acute, 292
  plasma exchange procedures, 291-292
  diagnostic tests for, 287-288
  discharge planning for, 294
  fundamentals of, 287
  health care settings for, 287
  pathophysiology of, 287
  patient-family education for, 294
GDM (gestational diabetes mellitus), 687-694. See also
    DM (diabetes mellitus).
  assessments for, 687-688
  deficient knowledge issues for, 688-689, 692-693
    diabetes effects, 688-689
    medication impacts, 692-693
  diagnoses and interventions for, 688-694
    additional considerations for, 693
    anxiety, 691-692
    fear, 690-691
    imbalanced nutrition, less than body requirements, 690
    imbalanced nutrition, more than body require-ments, 690
  diagnostic tests for, 688
  discharge planning for, 693-694
  fundamentals of, 687
  health care settings for, 687
  pathophysiology of, 687
  patient-family education for, 693-694
General care, 1-116, 261-280, 799-800
  bedrest, prolonged, 61-71
  cancer, 1-38
  for neurologic disorders, 261-280. See also Neurologic
      care.
    aspiration risks, 266-267
    body temperature, imbalanced, 274-275
    constipation, 277
    fall risks, 265-266
    fluid volume, deficient, 271-272
    IICP, 261-264
    imbalanced nutrition, less than body requirements, 273-274
    impaired tissue integrity, corneal, 270-271
    infection risks, 264-265
    injury risks, 269-270
    intracranial adaptive capacity, decreased, 261-264
    pain, acute, 273-274
    self-care deficits, 277-280
    sensory perception, disturbed, 280
    swallowing, impaired, 267-269
    verbal communication, impaired, 275-276
  older adult, 93-104
  pain management, 39-44
  palliative and end-of-life, 105-116
  perioperative, 45-60
  psychosocial support, 73-92
    family and significant other, 87-92
    patient, 73-86
  reference resources for, 799-800
Generalized absence (petit mal) seizures, 324
Generalized anxiety disorder, 737. See also Anxiety
    disorders.
Generalized myoclonic seizures, 324
Generalized tonic-clonic (grand mal) seizures, 323-324
Genitourinary cancers, 3
Geriatric care, 93-104
  diagnoses and interventions for, 93-104
    aspiration risks, 96-97
    confusion, acute, 93-95
    constipation, 102-103
    fluid volume, deficient, 98
    gas exchange, impaired, 95-96

Geriatric care (Continued)
  hopelessness, feelings of, 103-104
  hypothermia risks, 100
  infection risks, 98-99
  powerlessness, feelings of, 104
  skin integrity, impaired, 100-101
  sleep patterns, disturbed, 101-102
  fundamentals of, 93
Geriatric Depression Scale, 762
GI (gastrointestinal) care, 419-494, 805-806
  abdominal trauma, 419-428
  appendicitis, 429-432
  CD, 445-454
  cholelithiasis, cholecystitis, and cholangitis, 433-436
  cirrhosis, 437-444
  fecal diversions, 455-462
  hepatitis, 463-468
  malignancies, 1-2. See also Cancer care.
  pancreatitis, 469-476
  peptic ulcers, 477-480
  peritonitis, 481-486
  reference resources for, 805-806
  UC, 487-494
Globulin, Rh-immune, 679, 734
Glucocorticoids, antenatal, 716, 723-724, 733-734
Glucose levels, 600, 667-688
Glucose levels, unstable, 379-381
Glycosylated hemoglobin, 630
Grafting, bypass, 161
Gram stain cultures, 281-282
Grand mal seizures, 323-324
Granulomatous colitis. See CD (Crohn's disease).
Greensticks, 637. See also Fractures.
Grieving
  anticipatory, 79-80, 115-116, 677, 685, 735-736, 756
  bleeding in pregnancy and, 677
  cervical insufficiency and, 685
  dementia (Alzheimer's type) and, 756
  dysfunctional, 79-80
  dysfunctional grieving, 764
  major depression and, 764
  palliative and end-of-life care and, 115-116
  PPROM and, 735-736
  psychosocial support and, 79-80
Guillain-Barre syndrome. See GBS (Guillain-Barre
    syndrome).

H
Hamilton Rating Scale for Anxiety, 738, 746
HAV, HBV, HCV, HDV, HEV, and HGV, 463-468. See
    also Hepatitis.
Head and neck cancers, 2
Health care settings
  cancer care and, 1
  for cardiovascular care, 149, 151, 157, 161, 165, 177,
      182, 195, 201
    aneurysms, 149
    atherosclerotic arterial occlusive disease, 151
    CAD, 165
    cardiac surgeries, 161
    circulatory failure (cardiac vs. noncardiac shock),
        157
    dysrhythmias and conduction disturbances, 177
    HF, 182
    pulmonary hypertension, 195
    venous thrombosis and thrombophlebitis, 201
  for endocrine care, 373, 378, 387, 395, 399, 407, 415
    DI, 373
    DKA, 387
    DM, 378
    HHNK syndrome, 395
    hyperthyroidism, 399
    hypothyroidism, 407
    SIADH, 415

Health care settings (Continued)
  for GI care, 419, 429, 433, 445, 455, 463, 469, 477,
      481, 487
    abdominal trauma, 419
    appendicitis, 429
    CD, 445
    cholelithiasis, cholecystitis, and cholangitis, 433
    fecal diversions, 455
    hepatitis, 463
    pancreatitis, 469
    peptic ulcers, 477
    peritonitis, 481
    UC, 487
  for hematologic care, 495, 497, 501, 505
    anemia of chronic disease, 495
    DIC, 497
    polycythemia, 501
    thrombocytopenia, 505
  for maternity care, 673, 681, 687, 695, 703, 711, 719,
      729
    bleeding in pregnancy, 673
    cervical insufficiency, 681
    GDM, 687
    hyperemesis gravidarum, 695
    postpartum wound infection, 703
    PPROM, 729
    preeclampsia, 711
    PTL, 719
  for musculoskeletal care, 509, 515, 523, 529, 535, 541
    amputations, 509
    fractures, 515
    joint replacement surgeries, 523
    OA, 529
    osteoporosis, 535
    RA, 541
  for neurologic care, 295, 305, 313, 323, 333, 350, 361
    bacterial meningitis, 281
    GBS, 287
    intervertebral disk disease, 295
    MS, 305
    PD, 313
    SCIs, 333
    seizures and epilepsy, 323
    stroke, 350
    TBIs, 361
  of neurologic care, 281
    bacterial meningitis, 281
  for pediatric care, 577, 585, 593, 600, 609, 616, 621,
      629, 637, 641, 647, 653-654, 659
    ADHD, 585
    asthma, 577
    bronchiolitis, 593
    burns, 600
    CF, 621
    child abuse and neglect, 616
    CP, 609
    DM, 629
    fractures, 637
    gastroenteritis, 641
    OM, 647
    poisoning, 653-654
    sickle cell pain crisis, 659
  for psychiatric care, 738, 745, 751, 761, 769, 775
    anxiety disorders, 738
    bipolar disorder (manic component), 745
    dementia (Alzheimer's type), 751
    depression, major, 761
    schizophrenia, 769
    substance abuse disorders, 775
  for renal-urinary care, 207, 217, 223, 227, 231, 239,
      243, 249, 257
    ARF, 231
    BPH, 207
    CKD, 217
    hemodialysis, 223
    peritoneal dialysis, 227

Health care settings (Continued)
  renal transplants, 239
  ureteral calculi, 243
  urinary calculi, 243
  urinary diversions, 249
  urinary tract obstructions, 257
  for respiratory care, 117, 131, 137, 143, 147
    ARF, 147
    COPD, 117
    PE, 137
    pneumothorax and hemothorax, 131
    TB, 143
  for special needs care, 547, 559, 561-562, 565
    HIV/AIDS, 547
    nutritional support, 565
    wound management, 559, 561-562
Health Insurance Portability and Accountability Act.
    See HIPAA (Health Insurance Portability and
    Accountability Act of 1996).
Health-seeking behaviors
  CAD and, 172
  intervertebral disk disease and, 296-297
  osteoporosis and, 536-537
  PD and, 320-321
Heart failure. See HF (heart failure).
HELLP syndrome, 711-712. See also Preeclampsia.
Hematologic care, 495-508
  anemia of chronic disease, 495-496
  DIC, 497-500
  polycythemia, 501-504
  reference resources for, 806
  thrombocytopenia, 505-508
Hematopoietic system, neoplastic diseases of, 2
Hemodialysis, 223-226. See also Dialysis.
  components of, 223
  diagnoses and interventions for, 223-226
    fluid volume, imbalanced, 223-225
    ineffective tissue perfusion, peripheral, 224-225
    infection risks, 224-225
  discharge planning for, 226
  fundamentals of, 223
  health care settings for, 223
  pathophysiology of, 223
  patient-family education for, 226
Hemodynamic alterations, 181-182
Hemolytic hepatitis, 463-468. See also Hepatitis.
Hemorrhagic stroke, 349-350. See also Stroke.
Hemothorax and pneumothorax, 131-136
  assessments for, 131
  diagnoses and interventions for, 132-135
    additional considerations for, 135
    breathing patterns, ineffective, 132-133
    pain, acute, 134-135
  diagnostic tests for, 131-132
  discharge planning for, 135
  fundamentals of, 131
  health care settings for, 131
  pathophysiology of, 131
  patient-family education for, 135
Heparin, 138-139, 708
Heparin-induced thrombocytopenia. See HIT (heparin-
    induced thrombocytopenia).
Hepatic (hepatocellular) hepatitis, 463-468. See also
    Hepatitis.
Hepatitis, 463-468
  alcoholic, 463-468
  assessments for, 463-464
  chronic, 463-468
  deficient knowledge issues for, 464-465
  diagnoses and interventions for, 464-467
    additional considerations for, 466
    fatigue, 464-465
    protection, ineffective, 466
    skin integrity, impaired, 465
  diagnostic tests for, 463-464
  discharge planning for, 467

Hepatitis (Continued)
  fundamentals of, 463
  HAV, HBV, HCV, HDV, HEV, and HGV, 463-468
  health care settings for, 463
  hepatic (hepatocellular), 463-468
  pathophysiology of, 463
  patient-family education for, 467
  posthepatic (obstructive), 463-468
  prehepatic (hemolytic), 463-468
Hepatocellular hepatitis, 463-468. See also Hepatitis.
Herniation, brain, 363. See also TBIs (traumatic brain
    injuries).
HF (heart failure), 181-192
  acute pulmonary edema, 182
  ADHF, 181-182
  assessments for, 182
  cardiomyopathies, 181-182
    dilated, 181
    hypertrophic, 181-182
    restrictive, 182
  deficient knowledge issues for, 189-191
    additional considerations for, 191
    digoxin therapy, 190
    diuretic therapies, 189-190
    vasodilation, 190-191
  diagnoses and interventions for, 183-192
    activity intolerance, 187-188
    cardiac output, decreased, 186-187
    fear, feelings of, 188-189
    fluid volume, excess, 184-185
    gas exchange, impaired, 183-184
    ineffective tissue perfusion, cardiopulmonary,
      185-186
    ineffective tissue perfusion, cerebral, 185-186
    ineffective tissue perfusion, peripheral, 185-186
  diagnostic tests for, 182-183
  diastolic dysfunction, 181-182
  discharge planning for, 192
  fundamentals of, 181
  health care settings for, 182
  hemodynamic alterations, 181-182
  neurohormonal activation, increased, 181-182
  pathophysiology of, 181-182
  patient-family education for, 192
  remodeling, 181-182
  systolic dysfunction, 181-182
HHNK (hyperosmolar hyperglycemic nonketonic)
    syndrome, 395-398
  additional considerations for, 397
  assessments for, 395-396
  deficient knowledge issues for, 396-397
  diagnoses and interventions for, 396-397
  diagnostic tests for, 395-396
  discharge planning for, 397
  vs. DKA, 387-388. See also DKA (diabetic
    ketoacidosis).
  fundamentals of, 395
  health care settings for, 395
  pathophysiology of, 395
  patient-family education for, 397
High-performance liquid chromatography, 659
HIPAA (Health Insurance Portability and Accountabil-
    ity Act of 1996), 87
HIT (heparin-induced thrombocytopenia), 505. See also
    Thrombocytopenia.
HIV/AIDS (human immunodeficiency virus/acquired
    immunodeficiency syndrome), 547-558
  assessments for, 548-549
  deficient knowledge issues for, 555-556
    disease processes, 555-556
    lifestyle impacts, 555-556
    treatment plans, 555-556
  diagnoses and interventions for, 549-558
    activity intolerance, 554
    additional considerations for, 558
    anxiety, 556

HIV/AIDS (Continued)
    body image, disturbed, 557
    diarrhea, 551
    gas exchange, impaired, 549-550
    imbalanced nutrition, less than body requirements,
      552
    impaired environmental interpretation syndrome,
      555
    pain, acute vs. chronic, 553-554
    social isolation, 557
    tissue integrity, impaired, 553
  diagnostic tests for, 548-549
  discharge planning for, 558
  fundamentals of, 547
  health care settings for, 547
  monitoring of, 549
  pathophysiology of, 547
  patient-family education for, 558
  pneumonia and, 123. See also Pneumonia.
Hopelessness
  major depression and, 763
  older adult care and, 103-104
Hospital-associated pneumonia, 123. See also Pneumonia.
Hydration, IV, 722
Hyperemesis gravidarum, 695-702
  assessments for, 695
  deficient knowledge issues for, 698-700
    expected outcomes, 698
    medication impacts, 699-700
  diagnoses and interventions for, 696-701
    additional considerations for, 701
    anxiety, 696-697
    coping, ineffective, 697-698
    imbalanced nutrition, less than body requirements,
      696
  diagnostic tests for, 695
  discharge planning for, 701
  fundamentals of, 695
  health care settings for, 695
  pathophysiology of, 695
  patient-family education for, 701
Hyperosmolar hyperglycemic nonketonic syndrome. See
    HHNK (hyperosmolar hyperglycemic nonketonic)
    syndrome.
Hypertension, 193-195
  additional considerations for, 194
  deficient knowledge issues for, 193-194
    antihypertensive therapy, 193-194
    BP (blood pressure) checks, 193-194
    lifestyle impacts, 193-194
  diagnoses and interventions for, 194
  discharge planning for, 194
  fundamentals of, 193
  health care settings for, 193
  JNC VII and, 193
  pathophysiology of, 193
  patient-family education for, 194
  pulmonary, 195-200. See also Pulmonary hypertension.
Hyperthyroidism, 399-406. See also Thyroid disorders.
  assessments for, 399
  deficient knowledge issues for, 403-404
    iodide impacts, 403-404
    thioamide impacts, 403-404
  diagnoses and interventions for, 400-405
    additional considerations for, 405
    anxiety, 402
    body image, disturbed, 403
    imbalanced nutrition, less than body requirements,
      401
    impaired tissue integrity, corneal, 402-403
    pain, acute, 404
    protection, ineffective, 400-401
    sleep patterns, disturbed, 401-402
    swallowing, impaired, 405
  diagnostic tests for, 399
  discharge planning for, 405

Hyperthyroidism (Continued)
    fundamentals of, 399
    health care settings for, 399
    pathophysiology of, 399
Hypertrophic cardiomyopathy, 181-182. See also HF
    (heart failure).
Hypoglycemia
    vs. DKA, 387
    pediatric care and, 632-633
Hypomania, 745. See also Bipolar disorder (manic component).
Hypomania vs. mania, 745
Hypothermia risks, 100
Hypothyroidism, 407-414. See also Thyroid disorders.
    assessments for, 407
    diagnoses and interventions for, 408-412
        activity intolerance, 409
        breathing patterns, ineffective, 408
        constipation, 410-411
        fluid volume, excess, 408-409
        imbalanced nutrition, more than body
          requirements, 410
        infection risks, 409-410
        myxedema coma, 412
        protection, ineffective, 412
        sensory perception, disturbed, 410-411
    diagnostic tests for, 407
    discharge planning for, 413
    fundamentals of, 407
    health care settings for, 407
    pathophysiology of, 407
    patient-family education for, 413
    primary vs. secondary vs. tertiary, 407
Hypovolemic shock, 157. See also Shock (cardiac vs.
    noncardiac).

I
IBD (inflammatory bowel disease), 445
Ibuprofen, 662-663, 678
ICPs (infection control professionals), 792
IDDM (insulin-dependent diabetes). See DM (diabetes
    mellitus).
IDEA (Individuals with Disabilities Education Act),
    591, 635-636
Idiopathic OA (osteoarthritis), 529. See also OA (osteo-
    arthritis).
Idiopathic thrombocytopenic purpura. See ITP (idio-
    pathic thrombocytopenic purpura).
IEPs (individualized education plans), 591, 614, 636,
    664
IGRA (interferon gamma release assay), 143-144
IICP (increased intracranial pressure), 261-264, 362-363
Ileal conduit urinary diversions, 249. See also Urinary di-
    versions.
Ileal pouch anal anastomosis. See IPAA (ileal pouch
    anal anastomosis).
Ileostomy, 455-462. See also Fecal diversions (colostomy,
    ileostomy, and IPAA).
Image, body. See Body image, disturbed.
Imbalanced body temperature
    deficient, 600-601
    general neurologic care and, 274-275
Imbalanced fluid volume
    ARF and, 234-236
    BPH and, 209-210
    bronchiolitis and, 595-596
    burns and, 600-601
    CAD and, 174
    CD and, 447
    cirrhosis and, 442-443
    deficient, 174, 209-210, 236, 258-259, 271-272, 374,
      389-390, 447, 470-471, 488-489, 525, 595-596,
      600-601, 642-643, 648-649
    dehydration vs. edema, 53-54, 98, 110, 126-127
    DI, 374
    diabetes and, 374, 389-390

Imbalanced fluid volume (Continued)
    DI, 374
    DKA, 389-390
    dialysis and, 223-224, 228-229
      hemodialysis, 223-224
      peritoneal, 228-229
    DKA and, 389-390
    excess, 53-54, 184-185, 210, 234-235, 366-367, 408-
      409, 415-416, 442-443. See also Excess fluid
      volume.
    gastroenteritis, 642-643
    general neurologic care and, 271-272
    hypothyroidism and, 408-409
    joint replacement surgeries and, 525
    nutritional support and, 575-576. See also Nutritional
      support.
    older adult care and, 98
    OM and, 648-649
    pancreatitis and, 470-471
    perioperative care and, 51-54
    pneumonia and, 126-127
    SIADH and, 415-416
    TBIs and, 366-367
    UC and, 488-489
    urinary tract obstructions and, 258-259
Imbalanced nutrition. See also Nutritional support.
    CAD and, 169
    less than body requirements, 26-27, 111-112, 119-120,
      220, 229-230, 236-237, 401, 474-475, 503, 552,
      624, 644-645, 690, 747, 779-780
      abdominal trauma and, 425-426
      ARF (acute renal failure) and, 236-237
      bipolar disorder (manic component) and, 747
      burns and, 604-605
      cancer care and, 26-27
      CF and, 624
      CKD and, 220
      COPD and, 119-120
      CP and, 610
      gastroenteritis, 644-645
      GBS and, 289-290
      GDM and, 690
      general neurologic care, 273-274
      HIV/AIDS and, 552
      hyperemesis gravidarum and, 696
      hyperthyroidism and, 401
      osteoporosis and, 538-539
      palliative and end-of-life care and, 111-112
      pancreatitis, 474-475
      peritoneal dialysis and, 229-230
      peritonitis and, 484-485
      polycythemia and, 503
      substance abuse disorders and, 779-780
    more than body requirements, 690
Immunoglobulin levels, 668-669
Immunoreactive trypsinogen test, 622
Immunosuppressive agents, 240-241
Immunotherapy, 15-16, 35
Impaction, fecal, 342
Impaired elimination, urinary
    cancer care and, 29-30
    ureteral calculi and, 244-245
    urinary diversions and, 250-251
Impaired environmental interpretation syndrome, 555
Impaired family coping, 89-90. See also Family coping.
Impaired gas exchange
    bronchiolitis and, 594-595
    cancer care and, 4
    CF and, 623-624
    circulatory failure and, 160
    COPD and, 118-119
    HF and, 183-184
    HIV/AIDS and, 549-550
    older adult care and, 95-96
    pancreatitis and, 473
    PE and, 139

Impaired gas exchange (Continued)
    peritonitis and, 483
    pneumonia and, 124-125
    pneumothorax and hemothorax and, 133-134
    pulmonary hypertension and, 196-197
Impaired oral mucous membranes
    cancer care and, 28
    palliative and end-of-life care and, 111
    perioperative care and, 60
Impaired parent-child attachment
    cervical insufficiency and, 684
    preeclampsia and, 717
    PTL and, 726-727
Impaired parenting, 618
Impaired physical mobility
    cancer care and, 7
    CP and, 611-612
    fractures and, 517-518
    joint replacement surgeries and, 527
    OA and, 531-532
    PD and, 315-316
    perioperative care and, 58
    stroke and, 351-352
Impaired skin integrity
    abdominal trauma and, 425
    BPH and, 211
    burns and, 602-603
    cancer care and, 7-9, 19-22
    CKD and, 220-221
    DM and, 382
    fecal diversions and, 456-457
    fractures and, 518-519, 639
    gastroenteritis and, 643-644
    hepatitis and, 465
    older adult care and, 100-101
    perioperative care and, 59-60
    SCIs and, 345-346
    UC and, 492
    ureteral calculi and, 245-246
    urinary diversions and, 253-254
Impaired stomal tissue perfusion, 254-255
Impaired swallowing
    cancer care and, 28-29
    general neurologic care and, 267-269
    hyperthyroidism and, 405
    intervertebral disk disease and, 303-304
    nutritional support and, 574
Impaired tissue integrity
    atherosclerotic arterial occlusive disease and, 152-154
    burns and, 602-603
    corneal, 270-271, 402-403
    fecal diversions (colostomy, ileostomy, and IPAA)
      and, 456-457
    general neurologic care and, 270-271
    HIV/AIDS and, 553
    hyperthyroidism and, 402-403
    peptic ulcers and, 479-480
    wound management and, 559-564
Impaired verbal communication
    CP and, 613
    general neurologic care and, 275-276
    psychosocial support and, 81-82
    stroke and, 353-354
Impedance plethysmography, 201-202
Implanted venous access ports, 13
Incontinence
    bowel, 458-459
    urinary, 339-341
Increased intracranial pressure. See IICP (increased
    intracranial pressure).
Increased neurohormonal activation, 181-182
Independence vs. dependence issues, 70-71
Indiana pouches, 249
Individualized education plans, IEPs (individualized
    education plans)

Individuals with Disabilities Education Act. *See* IDEA (Individuals with Disabilities Education Act).
Ineffective airway clearance
    asthma and, 578-579
    bronchiolitis and, 593-594
    CF and, 622-623
    palliative and end-of-life care and, 108-109
    perioperative care and, 48-49
    pneumonia and, 125-126
    SCIs and, 337
Ineffective breastfeeding, 727
Ineffective breathing patterns
    abdominal trauma and, 421
    cancer care and, 4
    COPD and, 118
    GBS and, 288-289
    hypothyroidism and, 408
    palliative and end-of-life care and, 107-108
    perioperative care and, 50-51
    pneumothorax and hemothorax, 132-133
Ineffective coping
    anxiety disorders and, 740
    cervical insufficiency and, 683-684
    hyperemesis gravidarum and, 697-698
    postpartum wound infection and, 709
    PPROM and, 731-732
    preeclampsia and, 716
    PTL and, 724
Ineffective denial, 778
Ineffective protection
    ARF and, 232-234
    CD and, 448-449
    DI and, 375
    hepatitis and, 466
    hypothyroidism and, 412
    PE and, 139
    peptic ulcers and, 478-479
    SIADH and, 416-417
    thrombocytopenia and, 506-507
    thyroid disorders and
        hyperthyroidism, 400-401
        hypothyroidism, 412
    urinary diversions and, 252-253
Ineffective role performance
    amputations and, 511-512
    bedrest, prolonged and, 70-71
Ineffective sexuality patterns, 70
Ineffective tissue perfusion
    aneurysms and, 150
    cardiopulmonary, 6-7, 157-169, 173, 185-186, 202, 289, 338-339, 498, 504, 660-661
        CAD and, 173
        cancer care and, 6-7
        circulatory failure and, 157-159
        DIC and, 498
        GBS and, 289
        HF and, 185-186
        polycythemia and, 504
        SCIs and, 338-339
        sickle cell pain crisis, 660-661
        venous thrombosis and thrombophlebitis and, 202
    cerebral, 66-67, 157-159, 173, 185-186, 289, 338, 498, 502-503, 507, 660-661
        bedrest, prolonged and, 66-67
        CAD and, 173
        circulatory failure and, 157-159
        DIC and, 498
        GBS and, 289
        HF and, 185-186
        polycythemia and, 502-503
        SCIs and, 338
        sickle cell pain crisis, 660-661
        thrombocytopenia and, 507
    gastrointestinal, 424-425
    impaired stomal, 254-255
    joint replacement surgeries and, 524-525

Ineffective tissue perfusion (*Continued*)
    peripheral, 6, 65-66, 154-159, 173-174, 185-186, 202-203, 224-225, 338-339, 392, 489, 502-503, 507, 638-639
        atherosclerotic arterial occlusive disease and, 154-155
        bedrest, prolonged and, 65-66
        CAD and, 173-174
        cancer care and, 6
        circulatory failure and, 157-159
        DIC and, 498
        DKA and, 392
        fractures and, 638-639
        hemodialysis and, 224-225
        HF and, 185-186
        polycythemia and, 502-503
        SCIs and, 338-339
        thrombocytopenia and, 507
        venous thrombosis and thrombophlebitis and, 202-203
    renal, 157-159, 175, 254-255, 498, 502-503, 507
        CAD and, 175
        circulatory failure and, 157-159
        DIC and, 498
        polycythemia and, 502-503
        thrombocytopenia, 507
        urinary diversions and, 254-255
Infection control professionals. *See* ICPs (infection control professionals).
Infection prevention and control, 783-796, 811-812. *See also* Infection risks.
    APIC and, 792
    CDC, Standard Precautions, 783-792, 784t-791t
    ICPs and, 792
    isolation precaution recommendations, 784t-791t
    MDROs and, 783
    nosocomial infection reduction, 792
    OSHA, Bloodborne Pathogens Standard, 783
    reference resources for, 811-812
    SHEA and, 792
    TJC and, 792
    Transmission-Based Precautions (Airborne Infection Isolation), 144-145, 783-792, 784t-791t
    Transmission-Based Precautions (Droplet), 283, 783-792, 784t-791t
    Transmission-Based Precautions (Protective Environment), 783-792, 784t-791t
Infection risks. *See also* Infection prevention and control.
    abdominal trauma and, 423-424
    appendicitis and, 430
    ARF and, 232
    atherosclerotic arterial occlusive disease and, 153-154
    burns and, 603-604
    CD and, 448-449
    dialysis and, 224-225, 228
        hemodialysis, 224-225
        peritoneal dialysis, 228
    DKA and, 390-391
    DM and, 381
    gastroenteritis and, 644
    general neurologic care and, 264-265
    hypothyroidism and, 409-410
    nutritional support and, 574-575
    older adult care and, 98-99
    pancreatitis and, 474
    perioperative care and, 54-56
    peritonitis and, 483-484
    pneumonia and, 127-128
    postpartum wounds, 703-710. *See also* Postpartum wound infection.
    renal transplants and, 239-240
    TBIs and, 364-366
    UC and, 489-490
    urinary diversions and, 252
    UTIs, 257

Inflammatory bowel disease. *See* IBD (inflammatory bowel disease).
Injury risks
    ADHD and, 587
    cancer care and, 23-25
    child abuse and neglect and, 616-617
    cholelithiasis, cholecystitis, and cholangitis, 435-436
    CP and, 611
    dementia (Alzheimer's type) and, 753-754
    DKA and, 391
    osteoporosis and, 538
    PE and, 138-139
    perioperative care and, 47-48
    peritonitis and, 483-484
    SCIs and, 344-345
    substance abuse disorders and, 776-777
    UC and, 489-490
Instruments and scales. *See* Measurement instruments and scales.
Insufficiency, cervical. *See* Cervical insufficiency.
Insulin-dependent diabetes. *See* DM (diabetes mellitus).
Insulin impacts, 221-222, 373-386
Integrity, skin
    cancer care and, 7-9, 19-22
    older adult care and, 100-101
    perioperative care and, 59-60
Interferon gamma release assay. *See* IGRA (interferon gamma release assay).
Intermittent peritoneal dialysis. *See* IPD (intermittent peritoneal dialysis).
International Transplant Nurses Society, 242
Interrupted family processes
    asthma and, 581
    family psychosocial support and, 88-89
    substance abuse disorders and, 777-778
Interventions and diagnoses
    for cardiovascular care, 150, 152-155, 157-163, 167-176, 178-180, 183-192, 194, 196-199, 201-205
        aneurysms, 150
        atherosclerotic arterial occlusive disease, 152-155
        CAD, 167-176
        cardiac surgeries, 161-163
        circulatory failure, 157-160
        dysrhythmias and conduction disturbances, 178-180
        HF, 183-192
        hypertension, 194
        pulmonary hypertension, 196-199
        venous thrombosis and thrombophlebitis, 201-205
    for endocrine care, 374-375, 379-384, 396-397, 400-405, 408-412, 415-418
        DI, 374-375
        DM, 379-384
        HHNK syndrome, 396-397
        hyperthyroidism, 400-405
        hypothyroidism, 408-412
        SIADH, 415-418
    for general care plans, 4-37, 45-71, 73-85, 87-104, 107-116
        bedrest, prolonged, 61-71
        cancer care, 4-37
        older adult, 93-104
        pain management, 39-43
        palliative and end-of-life, 107-116
        perioperative, 45-60
        psychosocial support, family, 87-92
        psychosocial support, patient, 73-85
    for GI care, 421-427, 434-436, 447-453, 456-461, 464-467, 470-475, 478-480, 482-485, 488-489
        abdominal trauma, 421-427
        CD, 447-453
        cholelithiasis, cholecystitis, and cholangitis, 434-436
        fecal diversions, 456-461
        hepatitis, 464-467
        pancreatitis, 470-475

Interventions and diagnoses (Continued)
   peptic ulcers, 478-480
   peritonitis, 482-485
   UC, 488-489
  for hematologic care, 495-500, 506-508
   anemia of chronic disease, 495-496
   DIC, 497-500
   thrombocytopenia, 506-508
  for maternity care, 675-680, 682-686, 688-694,
    696-701, 704-710, 720-728
   bleeding in pregnancy, 675-680
   cervical insufficiency, 682-686
   GDM, 688-694
   hyperemesis gravidarum, 696-701
   postpartum wound infection, 704-710
   PPROM, 730-736
   PTL, 720-728
  for musculoskeletal care, 510-513, 515-521, 524-528,
    536-539, 542-546
   amputations, 510-513
   fractures, 515-521
   joint replacement surgeries, 524-528
   osteoporosis, 536-539
   RA, 542-546
  for neurologic care, 261-280, 282-285, 288-293,
    296-304, 314-322
   bacterial meningitis, 282-285
   GBS, 288-293
   general, 261-280
   intervertebral disk disease, 296-304
   PD, 314-322
  for pediatric care, 578-583, 600-606, 610-614,
    616-619, 630-634, 638-640, 642-645, 648-651,
    654-656, 660-663
   asthma, 578-583
   burns, 600-606
   child abuse and neglect, 616-619
   CP, 610-614
   DM, 630-634
   fractures, 638-640
   gastroenteritis, 642-645
   OM, 648-651
   poisoning, 654-656
   sickle cell pain crisis, 660-663
  for psychiatric care, 738-744, 746-750, 752-759,
    762-768, 776-782
   anxiety disorders, 738-744
   bipolar disorder (manic component), 746-750
   dementia (Alzheimer's type), 752-759
   depression, major, 762-768
   substance abuse disorders, 776-782
  for renal-urinary care, 208-215, 218-226, 228-230,
    232-237, 239-242, 244-247, 258-259
   ARF, 232-237
   BPH, 208-215
   CKD, 218-222
   hemodialysis, 223-226
   peritoneal dialysis, 228-230
   renal transplants, 239-242
   ureteral calculi, 244-247
   urinary tract obstructions, 258-259
  for respiratory care, 118-121, 124-127, 132-135,
    138-142, 144-145, 147-148
   ARF, 147-148
   COPD, 118-121
   PE, 138-142
   pneumonia, 124-127
   pneumothorax and hemothorax, 132-135
   TB, 144-145
  for special needs care, 549-564, 568-576
   HIV/AIDS, 549-558
   nutritional support, 568-576
   wound management, 559-564
Intervertebral disk disease, 295-304
  assessments for, 295-296
  deficient knowledge issues for, 298-303

Intervertebral disk disease (Continued)
   diskectomy with laminectomy procedures, 300-303
   fusion procedures, 300-303
   pain management, 298-299
  diagnoses and interventions for, 296-304
   additional considerations for, 304
   health-seeking behaviors, 296-297
   swallowing, impaired, 303-304
  diagnostic tests for, 296
  discharge planning for, 304
  fundamentals of, 295
  health care settings for, 295
  pathophysiology of, 295
  patient-family education for, 304
Intestinal (ileal conduit) urinary diversions, 249. See also
   Urinary diversions.
Intolerance, activity
  anemia of chronic disease and, 495-496
  bedrest, prolonged and, 61-63
  CAD and, 168
  cancer care and, 17
  cardiac surgeries and, 162
  CD and, 450
  COPD and, 120
  HF and, 187-188
  HIV/AIDS and, 554
  hypothyroidism and, 409
  joint replacement surgeries and, 526
  pulmonary hypertension and, 197-198
Intracranial adaptive capacity, decreased, 261-264
Intrauterine dye tests, 730
Intravascular ultrasound, 166
Iodide impacts, 403-404
IPAA (ileal pouch anal anastomosis), 455-462. See also
   Fecal diversions (colostomy, ileostomy, and IPAA).
IPD (intermittent peritoneal dialysis), 227-230. See also
   Dialysis.
Ischemic stroke, 349-350. See also Stroke.
Isoelectric focusing, 659
Isolation precaution recommendations, 784t-791t. See
   also Infection prevention and control.
ITP (idiopathic thrombocytopenic purpura), 505. See
   also Thrombocytopenia.
IV blood products, 679
IV hydration, 722

J

JDRF (Juvenile Diabetes Research Foundation), 636
JNC (Joint National Committee) VII, 193
Joint Commission, The. See TJC (The Joint Commission).
Joint National Committee. See JNC (Joint National
   Committee) VII.
Joint replacement surgeries, 523-528
  deficient knowledge issues for, 526-527
   activity precautions, 526
   CPM exercises, 527
  diagnoses and interventions for, 524-528
   additional considerations for, 528
   fluid volume, deficit, 525
   ineffective tissue perfusion, 524-525
   peripheral neurovascular dysfunction, 524
   physical mobility, impaired, 527
  diagnostic tests for, 523
  discharge planning for, 528
  fundamentals of, 523
  health care settings for, 523
  pathophysiology of, 523
  patient-family education for, 528
  THA, 523-528
  TKA, 523-528
Joslin Diabetes Center, 386, 694

K

Kegel exercise programs, 214
Ketone levels, 630

Kidney disease, chronic. See CKD (chronic kidney
   disease).
Kinesthetic perception, disturbed, 37
Kleihauer-Betke test, 65
Knowledge deficiency issues. See Deficient knowledge
   issues.
Kock pouches, 249
KUB x-rays, 218

L

La Leche League, 726
Labor, preterm, 719-728
  assessments for, 719-720
  deficient knowledge issues for, 720-724
   medication impacts, 722-724
   PTL effects, 720-721
  diagnoses and interventions for, 720-728
   additional considerations for, 728
   breastfeeding, ineffective, 727
   caregiver role strain, 725
   constipation, 725-726
   coping, ineffective, 724
   parent-child attachment, impaired, 726-727
  diagnostic tests for, 720
  discharge planning for, 728
  fundamentals of, 719
  health care settings for, 719
  pathophysiology of, 719
  patient-family education for, 728
Laboratory tests
  ABG levels, 117-118, 124, 131-132, 138, 147-148,
    178, 183, 196, 577-578, 593, 600, 654
  ABI, 151, 509
  acid-fast stains and cultures, 124, 143-144
  allergen skin testing, 578
  alpha-1 antitrypsin deficiency screens, 117-118
  ambulatory monitoring, 166, 177-178
  amniocentesis, 720, 730
  angiographic studies, 138, 151, 363, 420, 438
  anteparturm fetal monitoring, 682, 688, 712
  arteriography, contrast, 149
  barium enema and upper GI series, 446
  barium swallow, 438, 478
  basic metabolic panels, 630, 659
  biomarkers, cardiac, 166
  biopsies, 182-183, 218
  biopsy, 182-183, 218
  blood cultures, 642, 659, 704
  blood Rh factor and antibody screens, 674, 720, 730
  bone marrow aspiration, 501
  bone scans, 616, 637
  BUN levels, 183, 207, 217-218, 231-232, 243, 257,
    600, 641-642
  cancer screenings, 1-3
  for cardiovascular care, 149, 151, 157, 165-166,
    177-178, 182-183, 195-196, 201
   aneurysms, 149
   atherosclerotic arterial occlusive disease, 151
   CAD, 165-166
   circulatory failure, 157
   dysrhythmias and conduction disturbances, 177-178
   HF, 182-183
   pulmonary hypertension, 195-196
   venous thrombosis and thrombophlebitis, 201
  catheterization, cardiac, 182-183
  CBC, 131-132, 183, 196, 501, 578, 593, 616,
    621-622, 641-642, 674, 695
  CBC with differential, 682
  cervical evaluations, 720
  chemistries, 600
  cisternograms, 363
  creatinine levels and clearance, 183, 207, 217-218,
    231-232, 243, 257, 378, 600, 641-642
  CSF analyses, 287-288, 363, 667, 793-795
  CT scans, 138, 149, 166, 195, 232, 243, 282, 296,
    324-325, 351, 616, 637, 704, 752

Laboratory tests (*Continued*)
 cystoscopy, 207, 258
 cytologic studies, 609
 D-dimer tests, 138, 201-202, 497
 DDAVP challenge tests, 373-374
 digoxin levels, 183
 diskography, 296
 DNA analyses, 622
 Doppler flow studies, 151
 duplex imaging, 201-202
 ECGs, 165-166, 177-178, 182-183, 195
 EEGs, 609, 762
 electrolyte levels, 609
 electromyography, 288, 296
 electrophysiologic studies, 177-178
 ELISA tests, 548-549
 for endocrine care, 373-374, 379, 387-390, 395-396,
   399, 407, 415
  DI, 373-374
  DKA, 387-390
  DM, 379
  HHNK syndrome, 395-396
  hyperthyroidism, 399
  hypothyroidism, 407
  SIADH, 415
 endoscopy, 477-478
 EP studies, 288, 296, 306, 351, 363
 erythropoietin levels, 501
 esophagoscopy, 438
 FAST, 420
 fasting lipid profiles, 378
 fFN enzyme immunoassays, 720
 fMRI studies, 324-325
 for GI care, 420, 429, 434, 446, 463-464, 470, 477-
   478, 481-482, 488
  abdominal trauma, 420
  appendicitis, 429
  CD, 446
  cholelithiasis, cholecystitis, and cholangitis, 434
  hepatitis, 463-464
  pancreatitis, 470
  peptic ulcers, 477-478
  peritonitis, 481-482
  UC, 488
 glucose levels, 600, 667-688
 glycosylated hemoglobin, 630
 gram stain cultures, 281-282
 for hematologic care, 495, 497, 501, 505-506
  anemia of chronic disease, 495
  DIC, 497
  polycythemia, 501
  thrombocytopenia, 505-506
 high-performance liquid chromatography, 659
 IGRA, 143-144
 immunoglobulin levels, 668-669
 immunoreactive trypsinogen test, 622
 impedance plethysmography, 201-202
 intrauterine dye tests, 730
 isoelectric focusing, 659
 ketone levels, 630
 Kleihauer-Betke test, 65
 laparoscopy, 438
 laparotomy, 420
 lipid panels, 166, 630
 liver enzyme levels, 695
 liver function tests, 420
 lumbar punctures, 287-288, 314, 351
 malabsorption tests, 446
 for maternity care, 674-675, 681-682, 688, 695, 704,
   712, 720, 730
  bleeding in pregnancy, 674-675
  cervical insufficiency, 681-682
  GDM, 688
  hyperemesis gravidarum, 695
  postpartum wound infection, 704
  PPROM, 730

Laboratory tests (*Continued*)
  preeclampsia, 712
  PTL, 720
 measurement instruments and scales. *See* Measurement instruments and scales.
 metabolic studies, 609
 MRI studies, 151, 282, 296, 306, 324-325, 351, 616,
   637, 704, 752
 for musculoskeletal care, 509, 515, 523, 530, 535, 541
  amputations, 509
  fractures, 515
  joint replacement surgeries, 523
  OA, 530
  osteoporosis, 535
  RA, 541
 myelograms, 296
 nerve conduction velocity tests, 218
 for neurologic care, 281-282, 287-288, 296, 306, 314,
   324-325, 334-335, 350-351, 363
  bacterial meningitis, 281-282
  GBS, 287-288
  intervertebral disk disease, 296
  MS, 306
  PD, 314
  SCIs, 334-335
  seizures and epilepsy, 324-325
  stroke, 350-351
  TBIs, 363
 normal values for, 665-672, 793-798
  adult, 793-798
  CBC
  CSF
  pediatric patients, 665-672
  serum, plasma, and whole blood chemistry
  urine chemistry
 nuclear imaging modalities, cardiac, 166
 oximetry, 117-118, 124, 131-132, 178, 183, 196, 578,
   593, 621-622, 659
 p24 antigen tests, 548-549
 for pediatric care, 577-578, 585, 593, 600, 609, 616,
   621-622, 629-630, 637, 641-642, 647, 654, 659
  ADHD, 585
  asthma, 577-578
  bronchiolitis, 593
  burns, 600
  CF, 621-622
  child abuse and neglect, 616
  CP, 609
  DM, 629-630
  fractures, 637
  gastroenteritis, 641-642
  OM, 647
  poisoning, 654
  sickle cell pain crisis, 659
 PEFRs, 578
 perfusion scans, 195
 peritoneoscopy, 438
 PET studies, 306, 314, 324-325, 351
 pilocarpine iontophoresis, 621-622
 plasma chemistries, 793-795
 plasma marker tests, 201-202
 platelet counts, 420, 505, 671
 PPD injection tests, 144
 pregnancy tests, 674
 PSA tests, 207
 for psychiatric care, 738, 746, 752, 762, 770-771, 776
  anxiety disorders, 738
  bipolar disorder (manic component), 746
  dementia (Alzheimer's type), 752
  depression, major, 762
  schizophrenia, 770-771
  substance abuse disorders, 776
 psychometric tests, 439
 pulmonary function tests, 578, 622
 QuantiFERON-TB Gold test, 143-144
 quantitative sweat chloride test, 621-622

Laboratory tests (*Continued*)
  radiographs, 616
  radiologic studies, 438
  radionuclide imaging, 195
  rapid HIV tests, 549
  RBC counts, 671
  renal function studies, 688, 712
  renal scans, 232
  for renal-urinary care, 207, 231-232, 243
   ARF, 231-232
   BPH, 207
   ureteral calculi, 243
  for respiratory care, 117, 123-124, 131-132, 144, 147
   ARF, 147
   COPD, 117
   pneumonia, 123-124
   pneumothorax and hemothorax, 131-132
   TB, 144
  retrograde urography, 232
  Rotazyme tests, 642
  RSV washing, 593
  scintigraphy, thyroid, 379
  serum chemistries, 218, 695, 793-795
  serum electrolyte levels, 177-178, 641-642
  serum osmolality, 373-374, 671
  sigmoidoscopy, 446
  sleep studies, 196
  for special needs care, 548-549, 559, 562
   HIV/AIDS, 548-549
   wound management, 559, 562
  spirometry, 117-118
  sputum cultures, 117-118, 578, 622
  sterile speculum examinations, 720, 730
  stool cultures, 642
  stool fat analyses, 622
  stress tests, 166, 178, 196m 182-183
  thyroid-stimulating hormone levels, 630
  thyrotropin levels, 379
  thyroxine levels, 630
  tremor studies, 314
  tuberculin skin tests, 144
  tympanocentesis, 647
  tympanometry, 647
  ultrasound, 166, 201-202, 207, 218, 232, 243, 379,
   407, 509, 674, 681-682, 688, 695, 704, 712, 720,
   730
   Doppler, 201-202, 379, 407, 509, 720
   intravascular, 166
   obstetric, 674, 682, 688, 695, 712, 730
   pelvic, 704
   renal, 218, 232, 243
   translabial, 681
   transrectal, 207
   transvaginal, 681
  urinalysis, 138, 207, 231-232, 243, 314, 378, 439, 671-
   672, 682, 704, 720
  urine chemistries, 671-672, 695, 793-795
  urine cultures and sensitivity, 207, 243
  urine function studies, 712
  urine osmolality, 373-374
  uterine monitoring, external, 720, 730
  vasopressin challenge tests, 373-374
  ventilation-perfusion scans, pulmonary, 138
  viral load testing, 549
  viral resistance testing, 549
  water deprivation tests, 373-374
  WBC counts, 124, 420, 439, 669
  Western blot tests, 548-549
  whole blood chemistries, 793-795
  x-rays, 117-118, 123-124, 131-132, 138, 143-144,
   147-149, 166, 182-183, 195, 218, 282, 334-335,
   578, 593, 621-622, 637, 659
   abdominal, 149
   chest, 117-118, 123-124, 131-132, 138, 143-144,
    147-148, 166, 182-183, 195, 282, 578, 593,
    621-622, 659

Laboratory tests (*Continued*)
    KUB, 218
    sinus, 282
    skull, 282
    spine, 334-335
    xenon-133 studies, 509
Lacerations, brain, 362. *See also* TBIs (traumatic brain injuries).
Lacunar stroke, 349-350. *See also* Stroke.
Ladder, analgesic, 40-41
Laennec's cirrhosis, 437-444. *See also* Cirrhosis.
Laparoscopy, 438
Laparotomy, 420
LBTIs (latent tuberculosis infections), 143-146. *See also* TB (pulmonary tuberculosis).
Less than body nutritional requirements. *See* Imbalanced nutrition.
Leukotriene modifiers, 582-583
Leyton Obsessional Inventory, 738, 746
Life-threatening environmental factors, 327-328
Lifestyle impacts
    CAD and, 170-171
    dysrhythmias and conduction disturbances and, 179-180
    HIV/AIDS and, 555-556
    hypertension and, 193-194
Lilly Cares Patient Assistance Program, 774
Linezolid, 706
Lipid
    panels, 166, 630
    profiles, fasting, 378
Liquid chromatography, high-performance, 659
Liver enzyme levels, 695
Liver function tests, 420
LMWH (low-molecular weight heparin), 138-139, 708
Low-dose aspirin, 41, 716
Low-molecular weight heparin. *See* LMWH (low-molecular weight heparin).
Low self-esteem, chronic
    ADHD and, 586
    major depression and, 764-765
LTBIs (latent tuberculosis infections), 143. *See also* TB (pulmonary tuberculosis).
Lumbar punctures, 287-288, 314, 351
Lung cancer, 1

M
Magnesium sulfate, 715-716, 722, 733-734
Magnetic resonance imaging studies. *See* MRI (magnetic resonance imaging) studies.
Major depression, 761-768
    assessments for, 761-762
    deficient knowledge issues for, 762-763, 766-767
        causes, signs, and symptoms, 762-763
        medication impacts, 766-767
    diagnoses and interventions for, 762-768
        additional considerations for, 768
        dysfunctional grieving, 764
        hopelessness, 763
        low self-esteem, chronic, 764-765
        suicide risks, 763-764
    diagnostic tests for, 762
    discharge planning for, 768
    fundamentals of, 761
    health care settings for, 761
    pathophysiology of, 761
    patient-family education for, 768
Malabsorption tests, 446
Maltreatment, child, 615. *See also* Child abuse and neglect.
Manic component, bipolar disorder, 745-750
    assessments for, 745-746
    deficient knowledge issues for, 747-750
        causes, signs, and symptoms, 747-748
        medication impacts, 749-750
    diagnoses and interventions for, 746-750

Manic component (*Continued*)
        additional considerations for, 750
        imbalanced nutrition, less than body requirements, 747
        other-directed violence risks, 746-747
        self-care deficits, 747-748
    diagnostic tests for, 746
    discharge planning for, 750
    fundamentals of, 745
    health care settings for, 745
    hypomania and, 745
    hypomania vs. mania, 745
    mania and, 745
    pathophysiology of, 745
    patient-family education for, 750
MAO inhibitors, 589, 742-743, 767
March of Dimes, 597
MAST (Michigan Alcohol Screening Test), 776
Maternity care, 673-736, 810
    bleeding in pregnancy, 673-680
    cervical insufficiency, 681-686
    DM and, 687-694. *See also* DM (diabetes mellitus).
    hyperemesis gravidarum, 695-702
    PPROM, 729-736
    preeclampsia, 711-718
    PTL, 719-728
    reference resources for, 810
    wound infection, postpartum, 702-710
Mature-onset of diabetes in youth. *See* MODY (mature-onset diabetes of youth).
Maudsley Obsessional-Compulsive Inventory, 746
MDR TB (multidrug-resistant tuberculosis), 143. *See also* TB (pulmonary tuberculosis).
MDROs (multidrug-resistant organisms), 783
Meal planning, 633-634
Measurement instruments and scales
    AIMS, 769-770
    Beck Anxiety Inventory, 746
    Beck Depression Inventory, 762
    BPRS, 770
    CAGE-AID questionnaire, 776
    DSM-IV criteria, 585, 770, 775
    Geriatric Depression Scale, 762
    Hamilton Rating Scale for Anxiety, 746
    Leyton Obsessional Inventory, 746
    MAST, 776
    Maudsley Obsessional-Compulsive Inventory, 746
    pain scales, 39-43
    Panic Attack Cognitions Questionnaire, 746
    SANS, 770
    SAPS, 770
    Sheehan Patient Rated Anxiety Inventory, 746
    Simpson-Angus Rating Scale, 770
    State-Trait Anxiety Inventory, 746
    Yale-Brown Obsessive Scale, 746
    Young Mania Scale, 746
    Zung Self-Rating Depression Scale, 762
Mechanical ventilation, 127
Medical care neglect, child, 615. *See also* Child abuse and neglect.
Medical-surgical care plans, 1-572
    cardiovascular, 149-206
        aneurysms, 149-150
        atherosclerotic arterial occlusive disease, 151-156
        CAD, 165-176
        cardiac surgeries, 161-164
        circulatory failure, 157-160
        dysrhythmias and conduction disturbances, 177-180
        HF, 181-192
        hypertension, 193-195
        hypertension, pulmonary, 195-200
        venous thrombosis and thrombophlebitis, 201-205
    endocrine, 373-418
        diabetes, DI, 373-376
        diabetes, DKA, 387-394
        diabetes, DM, 377-386

Medical-surgical care plans (*Continued*)
        HHNK syndrome, 395-398
        hyperthyroidism, 399-406
        hypothyroidism, 407-414
        SIADH, 415-418
    general, 1-116
        bedrest, prolonged, 61-71
        cancer, 1-38
        older adult, 93-104
        pain management, 39-44
        palliative and end-of-life, 105-116
        perioperative, 45-60
        psychosocial support, family and significant other, 87-92
        psychosocial support, patient, 73-86
    GI, 419-494
        abdominal trauma, 419-428
        appendicitis, 429-432
        CD, 445-454
        cholelithiasis, cholecystitis, and cholangitis, 433-436
        cirrhosis, 437-444
        fecal diversions, 455-462
        hepatitis, 463-468
        pancreatitis, 469-476
        peptic ulcers, 477-480
        peritonitis, 481-486
        UC, 487-494
    hematologic, 495-508
        anemia of chronic disease, 495-496
        DIC, 497-500
        polycythemia, 501-504
        thrombocytopenia, 505-508
    musculoskeletal, 509-546
        amputations, 509-514
        arthritis, OA, 529-534
        arthritis, RA, 541-546
        fractures, 515-522
        joint replacement surgeries, 523-528
        osteoporosis, 535-540
    neurologic, 261-372
        GBS, 287-294
        general, 261-264
        intervertebral disk disease, 295-304
        meningitis, bacterial, 281-286
        MS, 305-312
        PD, 313-322
        SCIs, 333-348
        seizures and epilepsy, 323-332
        stroke, 349-360
        TBIs, 361-372
    reference resources for, 799-812
    renal-urinary, 207-260
        ARF, 231-238
        BPH, 207-216
        calculi, ureteral, 243-248
        CKD, 217-222
        dialysis, hemodialysis, 223-226
        dialysis, peritoneal, 227-230
        diversions, urinary, 249-256
        transplants, renal, 239-242
        urinary tract obstructions, 257-260
    respiratory, 117-148
        ARF, 147-148
        COPD, 117-121
        PE, 137-142
        pneumonia, 123-129
        pneumothorax and hemothorax, 131-136
        TB, 143-146
    special needs, 547-576
        HIV/AIDS, 547-558
        nutritional support, 565-576
        wound management, 559-564
MedicAlert Foundation, 694, 774

Medication-related impacts
  anxiety disorders and, 741-743
  bipolar disorder (manic component) and, 749-750
  bleeding in pregnancy and, 678-679
  chemotherapy, 1-3
  dementia (Alzheimer's type) and, 757-758
  GDM and, 688-689, 692-693
  hyperemesis gravidarum and, 699-700
  major depression and, 766-767
  MS and, 307-310
  PE and, 141-142
  postpartum wound infection and, 705-708
  PPROM and, 732-733
  preeclampsia and, 714-716
  PTL and, 722-724
  RA and, 545
  schizophrenia and, 772-773
  of specific drugs and drug classes. See also under specific
      drugs and drug classes.
    ACE inhibitors, 231
    acetaminophen with codeine, 662-663
    acetaminophen with oxycodone, 707
    AEDs, 328-330
    albuterol, 579, 625
    analgesics, 40-43, 707
    analgesics, opioid, 41-43, 678
    antenatal glucocorticoids, 716, 723-724, 733-734
    antibiotics, 283-284, 626
    antibiotics, aerosolized, 625
    antibiotics, prophylactic, 678, 733-734
    anticoagulants, 141, 708
    antidepressants, tricyclic, 589, 742-743, 766-767
    antimanics, 747, 749
    antimicrobials, 705-706
    antiparkinson drugs, 316-320
    antipsychotics, 747, 750, 772-773
    antiviral agents, 318-320
    aspirin, 41, 716
    benzodiazepines, 743
    beta-andrenergics, 734
    beta-blockers, 169-170, 715-716
    beta$_2$-agonists, 582-583
    blood products, IV, 679
    bronchodilators, 625
    calcium channel blockers, 715-716, 722, 734
    carboprost, 679
    chemotherapy, 1-38
    clindamycin, 706
    clonidine, 590
    co-analgesics, 42-43
    corticosteroids, 582-583
    cromolyn sodium/nedocromil sodium, 582-583
    digoxin, 190
    disulfiram, 781
    diuretics, 189-190
    dopamine replacement therapy, 318-320
    doxylamine, 700
    dual-mechanism drugs, 767-768
    folic acid, 662-663
    heparin, 138-139, 708
    hydration, IV, 722
    ibuprofen, 662-663, 678
    immunosuppressive agents, 240-241
    insulin, 373-386
    leukotriene modifiers, 582-583
    linezolid, 706
    LMWH, 138-139, 708
    magnesium sulfate, 715-716, 722, 733-734
    MAO inhibitors, 589, 742-743, 767
    meperidine, 707
    methylergonovine, 679
    methylxanthines, 583
    metoclopramide hydrochloride, 699
    morphine, 662-663, 707
    mucolytic enzymes, aerosolized, 625-626
    naltrexone, 781

Medication-related impacts (Continued)
    nitrates, 169-170
    nitroglycerin, 165-176
    nonbenzodiazepines, 743
    NSAIDs, 41, 231
    ondansetron, 700
    opioid analgesics, 41-43, 678
    oxycodone with acetaminophen, 707
    oxytocin, 679
    pancreatic enzymes, 625-626
    pantoprazole, 699
    penicillins, 662-663
    promethazine, 699-700
    prostaglandin synthesis inhibitors, 678, 722
    pyridoxine, 700
    Rh-immune globulin, 679, 734
    SNRIs, 589, 768
    SSRIs, 743, 767
    steroids, 582-583
    stimulants, 588-589
    sulfonylureas, second-generation, 692-693
    uterotonics, 678-679
    vaccines, pneumococcal, 283-284, 286
    vasodilators, 183-185
    vitamin and mineral supplements, 626
  substance abuse disorders and, 780-781
Meningitis, bacterial, 281-286
  assessments for, 281
  deficient knowledge issues for, 282-284
    antibiotics, 283-284
    transmission-based precautions, droplet, 283
  diagnoses and interventions for, 282-285
    additional considerations for, 285
    pain, acute, 283
  diagnostic tests for, 281-282
  discharge planning for, 286
  fundamentals of, 281
  health care settings of, 281
  pathophysiology of, 281
  patient-family education and, 286
Meningitis Foundation of America, 286
Mental Illness Education Project, 774
Meperidine, 707
Metabolic disorder care, 373-418
  diabetes, 373-394. See also Diabetes-related care.
    DI, 373-376
    DKA, 387-394
    DM, 377-386
  hyperthyroidism, 399-406
  hypothyroidism, 407-414
  SIADH, 415-418
Metabolic studies, 609
Methylergonovine, 679
Methylxanthines, 583
Metoclopramide hydrochloride, 699
MI (myocardial infarction), 165
Michigan Alcohol Screening Test. See MAST (Michi-
    gan Alcohol Screening Test).
Mineral and vitamin supplements, 626
Mixed CP (cerebral palsy), 609. See also CP (cerebral
    palsy).
Mobility, impaired
  cancer care and, 7
  perioperative care and, 58
Modalities, nutritional support, 567-568. See also Nutri-
    tional support.
Modified rule of nines, 599
MODY (mature-onset diabetes of youth), 629. See also
    DM (diabetes mellitus).
Monoamine inhibitors. See MAO inhibitors.
Morphine, 662-663, 707
MRI (magnetic resonance imaging) studies, 151, 282,
    296, 306, 324-325, 351, 616, 637, 704, 752
MS (multiple sclerosis), 305-312
  assessments for, 305-306
  deficient knowledge issues for, 306-310

MS (Continued)
    medication side effects, 307-310
    symptom exacerbation, 306-307
  diagnoses and interventions for, 306-311
    additional considerations for, 311
    pain, chronic, 310
    spasms, chronic, 310
  diagnostic tests for, 306
  discharge planning for, 311
  fundamentals of, 305
  health care settings for, 305
  pathophysiology of, 305
  patient-family education for, 311
Mucolytic enzymes, aerosolized, 625-626
Mucous membranes (oral), impaired
  cancer care and, 28
  palliative and end-of-life care and, 111
  perioperative care and, 60
Multidrug-resistant organisms. See MDROs (multidrug-
    resistant organisms).
Multidrug-resistant tuberculosis. See MDR TB
    (multidrug-resistant tuberculosis).
Multiple sclerosis. See MS (multiple sclerosis).
Multiple Sclerosis Association of America, 311
Multiple Sclerosis Foundation, 311
Munchausen syndrome by proxy, 615-616. See also Child
    abuse and neglect.
Musculoskeletal care, 509-546, 806-807
  amputations, 509-514
  arthritis, 529-546
    OA, 529-534
    RA, 541-546
  fractures, 515-522
  joint replacement surgeries, 523-528
  osteoporosis, 535-540
  reference resources for, 806-807
Myelograms, 296
Myocardial infarction. See MI (myocardial infarction).
Myoclonic seizures, generalized, 324
Myxedema coma, 412

N
N95 respirators, 783, 792
NA (Narcotics Anonymous), 775, 782
Naltrexone, 781
NAMI (National Alliance for the Mentally Ill), 744,
    774
Narcotics Anonymous. See NA (Narcotics Anonymous).
NARSAD (National Alliance for Research on Schizo-
    phrenia and Depression), 774
National Alliance for Research on Schizophrenia and
    Depression. See NARSAD (National Alliance for
    Research on Schizophrenia and Depression).
National Alliance for the Mentally Ill. See NAMI (Na-
    tional Alliance for the Mentally Ill).
National Asthma Education and Prevention Program
    Expert Panel, 578
National Cancer Institute, 176, 256
National Center on Shaken Baby Syndrome, 620
National Child Abuse Hotline, 620
National Clearinghouse for Alcohol and Drug Informa-
    tion. See NCADI (National Clearinghouse for Al-
    cohol and Drug Information).
National Diabetes Education Program. See NDEP (Na-
    tional Diabetes Education Program).
National Institute of Diabetes and Digestive and Kidney
    Diseases, 436
National Institute of Mental Health. See NIMH (Na-
    tional Institute of Mental Health).
National Institute of Neurological Disorders. See NINDS
    (National Institute of Neurological Disorders).
National Institute on Aging. See NIA (National Insti-
    tute on Aging).
National Institute on Alcohol Abuse and Alcoholism.
    See NIAAA (National Institute on Alcohol Abuse
    and Alcoholism).

National Institute on Drug Abuse. *See* NIDA (National Institute on Drug Abuse).
National Institutes of Health. *See* NIH (National Institutes of Health).
National Kidney and Urologic Diseases Information Clearinghouse, 226, 230, 237
National Kidney Foundation, 222, 226, 237, 242
National Library of Medicine. *See* NLM (National Library of Medicine).
National Multiple Sclerosis Society, 311
National Parkinson Foundation, 322
National Spinal Cord Injury Association, 348
Nausea
    appendicitis and, 430-431
    CD and, 449
    cholelithiasis, cholecystitis, and cholangitis, 434-435
    nutritional support and, 572-573
    peritonitis and, 482
    UC and, 490-491
NCADI (National Clearinghouse for Alcohol and Drug Information), 782
NDEP (National Diabetes Education Program), 629
Neck and head cancers, 2
Necrosis, pressure, 512-513
Nedocromil sodium, 582-583
Neglect
    child neglect and abuse, 615-620
        assessments for, 616
        child maltreatment, 615
        diagnoses and interventions for, 616-619
        diagnostic tests for, 616
        discharge planning for, 619
        emotional abuse and neglect, 615-616
        fundamentals of, 615
        health care settings for, 616
        medical care neglect, 615
        Munchausen syndrome by proxy, 615-616
        pathophysiology of, 615
        patient-family education for, 619
        physical abuse and neglect, 615-616
        SBS, 615-616
        sexual abuse, 615-616
    unilateral, 354-355
Nerve conduction velocity tests, 218
Nervous system tumors, 1
Neurogenic shock, 157. *See also* Shock (cardiac *vs.* noncardiac).
Neurohormonal activation, increased, 181-182
Neurologic care, 261-372
    GBS, 287-294
    general, 261-280. *See also* General care.
        aspiration risks, 266-267
        body temperature, imbalanced, 274-275
        constipation, 277
        fall risks, 265-266
        fluid volume, deficient, 271-272
        IICP, 261-264
        imbalanced nutrition, less than body requirements, 273-274
        impaired tissue integrity, corneal, 270-271
        infection risks, 264-265
        intracranial adaptive capacity, decreased, 261-264
        pain, acute, 273-274
        self-care deficits, 277-279
        sensory perception, disturbed, 280
        swallowing, impaired, 267-269
        verbal communication, impaired, 275-276
    intervertebral disk disease, 295-304
    meningitis, bacterial, 281-286
    MS, 305-312
    PD, 313-322
    reference resources for, 803-804
    SCIs, 333-348
    seizures and epilepsy, 323-332
    stroke, 349-360
    TBIs, 361-372

Neurovascular dysfunction, peripheral. *See* Peripheral neurovascular dysfunction.
NIA (National Institute on Aging), 759
NIAAA (National Institute on Alcohol Abuse and Alcoholism), 782
NICHCY (National Information Center for Children and Youth with Disabilities), 591
NIDA (National Institute on Drug Abuse), 782
NIH (National Institutes of Health), 782
NIMH (National Institute of Mental Health), 744, 774
NINDS (National Institute of Neurological Disorders), 359
Nitrates, 169-170
Nitroglycerin, 165-176
NLM (National Library of Medicine), 584
Nonbenzodiazepines, 743
Noncardiac shock. *See* Shock (cardiac *vs.* noncardiac).
Noncompliance considerations, 330-331
NonST-elevation myocardial infarction. *See* NSTEMI (nonST-elevation myocardial infarction).
Nonsteroidal antiinflammatory drugs. *See* NSAIDs (nonsteroidal antiinflammatory drugs).
Nontunneled catheters, 13
Normal values, laboratory tests, 665-672, 793-798
    adult, 793-798
    pediatric patients, 665-672
Nosocomial infection reduction, 792
Nosocomial pneumonia, 123. *See also* Pneumonia.
NSAIDs (nonsteroidal antiinflammatory drugs), 41, 231, 532
NSTEMI (nonST-elevation myocardial infarction), 165
Nuclear imaging modalities, cardiac, 166
Nursing care plans
    infection prevention and control, 783-792
        APIC and, 792
        CDC, Standard Precautions, 783-792, 784t-791t
        ICPs and, 792
        isolation precaution recommendations, 784t-791t
        MDROs and, 783
        nosocomial infection reduction, 792
        OSHA, Bloodborne Pathogens Standard, 783
        SHEA and, 792
        TJC and, 792
        Transmission-Based Precautions (Airborne Infection Isolation), 783-792, 784t-791t
        Transmission-Based Precautions (Droplet), 783-792, 784t-791t
        Transmission-Based Precautions (Protective Environment), 783-792, 784t-791t
    laboratory tests (normal values), 665-672, 793-798
        adult, 793-798
        pediatric patients, 665-672
    maternity, 673-736
        bleeding in pregnancy, 673-680
        cervical insufficiency, 681-686
        DM and, 687-694
        hyperemesis gravidarum, 695-702
        PPROM, 729-736
        preeclampsia, 711-718
        PTL, 719-728
        wound infection, postpartum, 703-710
    medical-surgical, 1-572
        cardiovascular, 149-206
        endocrine, 373-418
        general, 1-116
        GI, 419-494
        hematologic, 495-508
        renal-urinary, 207-260
        respiratory, 117-148
        special needs, 541-576
    pediatric, 577-672
        ADHD, 585-592
        asthma, 577-584
        bronchiolitis, 593-598
        burns, 599-608
        CF, 621-628

Nursing care plans (*Continued*)
        child abuse and neglect, 615-620
        CP, 609-614
        DM, 629-636
        fractures, 637-640
        gastroenteritis, 641-646
        normal laboratory values, 665-672
        OM, 647-652
        poisoning, 653-658
        sickle cell pain crisis, 659-664
    psychiatric, 737-782
        anxiety disorders, 737-744
        bipolar disorder (manic component), 745-750
        dementia (Alzheimer's type), 751-760
        depression, major, 761-768
        schizophrenia, 769-774
        substance abuse disorders, 775-782
    reference resources for, 799-812
Nutritional support, 565-576
    assessments for, 565-568
        anthropometric data, 566
        biochemical data, 566
        dietary histories, 565
        nutritional requirement estimations, 566-567
        physical, 565-568
    diagnoses and interventions for, 568-576
        additional considerations for, 576
        aspiration risks, 571-572
        constipation, 573
        fluid volume, imbalanced, 575-576. *See also* Imbalanced fluid volume.
        infection risks, 574-575
        nausea, 572-573
        swallowing, impaired, 574
    DM and, 382-384
    fundamentals of, 565
    health care settings for, 565
    imbalanced nutrition, 26-27, 111-112, 119-120, 141-142, 169, 246-247, 401
        abdominal trauma and, 425-426
        bipolar disorder (manic component) and, 747
        burns and, 604-605
        CAD and, 169
        cancer care and, 26-27
        CF and, 624
        CKD and, 220
        COPD and, 119-120
        CP and, 610
        gastroenteritis and, 644-645
        GBS and, 289-290
        GDM and, 690
        general neurologic care and, 273-274
        hyperemesis gravidarum and, 696
        hyperthyroidism and, 401
        less than body requirements, 26-27, 111-112, 119-120, 273-274, 289-290, 401, 425-426, 484-485, 538-539, 568-570, 604-605, 610, 624, 644-645, 690, 696, 747, 779-780
        more than body requirements, 690
        osteoporosis and, 538-539
        palliative and end-of-life care and, 111-112
        PE and, 141-142
        peritonitis and, 484-485
        substance abuse disorders and, 779-780
        ureteral calculi and, 246-247
    modalities for, 567-568
    TPN, 567-568
    transitional feedings, 568

O

OA (osteoarthritis), 529-534. *See also* Arthritis.
    assessments for, 529-530
    deficient knowledge issues for, 532
    diagnoses and interventions for, 530-533
        pain, chronic *vs.* acute, 530-531
        physical mobility, impaired, 531-532
        sexual dysfunction, 532-533

OA (Continued)
  diagnostic tests for, 530
  discharge planning for, 533
  fundamentals of, 529
  health care settings for, 529
  herbal product interactions, 532
  idiopathic vs. secondary, 529
  NSAID interactions, 532
  pathophysiology of, 529
  patient-family education for, 533
Obsessive-compulsive disorder. See OCD (obsessive-compulsive disorder).
Obstetric ultrasound, 674, 682, 688, 695, 712, 730
Obstructions, urinary tract, 257-260
  diagnoses and interventions for, 258-259
    additional considerations for, 259
    fluid volume, deficient, 258-259
    pain, acute, 259
  discharge planning for, 260
  fundamentals of, 257
  health care settings for, 257
  pathophysiology of, 257
  UTIs and, 257
Obstructive hepatitis, 463-468. See also Hepatitis.
Occlusive disease, atherosclerotic arterial, 151-156
  assessments for, 151
  deficient knowledge issues for, 153-154
    infection risks, 153-154
    tissue integrity, impaired, 153-154
  diagnoses and interventions for, 152-155
    additional considerations for, 155
    pain, chronic, 152-153
    peripheral tissue perfusion, ineffective, 154-155
    tissue integrity, impaired, 152
  diagnostic tests for, 151
  discharge planning for, 156
  fundamentals of, 151
  health care settings for, 151
  pathophysiology and, 151
  patient-family education for, 156
Occupational Safety and Health Administration. See OSHA (Occupational Safety and Health Administration), Bloodborne Pathogens Standard.
OCD (obsessive-compulsive disorder), 737. See also Anxiety disorders.
Older adult care, 93-104
  diagnoses and interventions for, 93-104
    aspiration risks, 96-97
    confusion, acute, 93-95
    constipation, 102-103
    fluid volume, deficient, 98
    gas exchange, impaired, 95-96
    hopelessness, feelings of, 103-104
    hypothermia risks, 100
    infection risks, 98-99
    powerlessness, feelings of, 104
    skin integrity, impaired, 100-101
    sleep patterns, disturbed, 101-102
  fundamentals of, 93
OM (otitis media), 647-652
  AOM, 647
  assessments for, 647
  chronic, 647
  deficient knowledge issues for, 649-650
  diagnoses and interventions for, 648-651
    additional considerations for, 650
    fluid volume, deficient, 648-649
    pain, acute, 648
  diagnostic tests for, 647
  discharge planning for, 650-651
  fundamentals of, 647
  health care settings for, 647
  OME, 647
  pathophysiology of, 647
  patient-family education for, 650-651

OME (otitis media with effusion), 647. See also OM (otitis media).
Oncology-related care, 1-38
  ACS recommendations for, 1-2
  deficient knowledge issues for, 14-15, 31-35
    antiandrogen therapy, 14-15
    chemotherapy, 34
    external beam radiation therapy, 33
    immunotherapy, 35
    orchiectomy, bilateral, 14-15
    radiation implants, 31-32
    VADs, 12-14
  diagnoses and interventions for, 4-37
    activity intolerance, 17
    auditory perception, disturbed, 37
    body image, disturbed, 36
    breathing patterns, ineffective, 4
    chemotherapy, 15-16
    constipation, 9
    diarrhea, 9
    disuse syndrome risks, 12
    gas exchange, impaired, 4
    imbalanced nutrition, less than body requirements, 26-27
    incontinence, urinary, 10
    ineffective protection, 17-19
    ineffective tissue perfusion, cardiopulmonary, 7
    ineffective tissue perfusion, peripheral, 6
    injury risks, 23-25
    kinesthetic perception, disturbed, 37
    oral mucous membranes, impaired, 28
    pain, acute, 4
    pain, chronic, 4-6
    pain management and, acute vs. chronic, 4-6. See also Pain management care.
    physical mobility, impaired, 7
    radiation therapy, 15-16
    sensory perception, disturbed, 37
    sexual dysfunction, 10-11
    skin integrity, impaired, 7-9, 19-22
    stress, 10
    swallowing, impaired, 28-29
    tactile perception, disturbed, 37
    tissue integrity, impaired, 19-23
    urinary elimination, impaired, 29-30
Ondansetron, 700
Operative-medical care plans
  cardiovascular, 149-206
    aneurysms, 149-150
    atherosclerotic arterial occlusive disease, 151-156
    CAD, 165-176
    cardiac surgeries, 161-164
    circulatory failure, 157-160
    dysrhythmias and conduction disturbances, 177-180
    HF, 181-192
    hypertension, 193-195
    hypertension, pulmonary, 195-200
    venous thrombosis and thrombophlebitis, 201-205
  endocrine, 373-418
    diabetes, DI, 373-376
    diabetes, DKA, 387-394
    diabetes, DM, 377-386
    HHNK syndrome, 395-398
    hyperthyroidism, 399-406
    hypothyroidism, 407-414
    SIADH, 415-418
  general, 1-116
    bedrest, prolonged, 61-71
    cancer, 1-38
    older adult, 93-104
    pain management, 39-44
    palliative and end-of-life, 105-116
    perioperative, 45-60
    psychosocial support, family and significant other, 87-92
    psychosocial support, patient, 73-86

Operative-medical care plans (Continued)
  GI, 419-494
    abdominal trauma, 419-428
    appendicitis, 429-432
    CD, 445-454
    cholelithiasis, cholecystitis, and cholangitis, 433-436
    cirrhosis, 437-444
    fecal diversions, 455-462
    pancreatitis, 469-476
    peptic ulcers, 477-480
    UC, 487-494
  GI care
    hepatitis, 463-468
    peritonitis, 481-486
  hematologic, 495-508
    anemia of chronic disease, 495-496
    DIC, 497-500
    polycythemia, 501-504
    thrombocytopenia, 505-508
  musculoskeletal, 509-546
    amputations, 509-514
    arthritis, OA, 529-534
    arthritis, RA, 541-546
    fractures, 515-522
    joint replacement surgeries, 523-528
    osteoporosis, 535-540
  neurologic, 261-372
    GBS, 287-294
    general, 261-264
    intervertebral disk disease, 295-304
    meningitis, bacterial, 281-286
    MS, 305-312
    PD, 313-322
    SCIs, 333-348
    seizures and epilepsy, 323-332
    stroke, 349-360
    TBIs, 361-372
  reference resources for, 799-812
  renal-urinary, 207-260
    ARF, 231-238
    BPH, 207-216
    calculi, ureteral, 243-248
    CKD, 217-222
    dialysis, hemodialysis, 223-226
    dialysis, peritoneal, 227-230
    diversions, urinary, 249-256
    transplants, renal, 239-242
    urinary tract obstructions, 257-260
  respiratory, 117-148
    ARF, 147-148
    COPD, 117-121
    PE, 137-142
    pneumonia, 123-129
    pneumothorax and hemothorax, 131-136
    TB, 143-146
  special needs, 547-576
    HIV/AIDS, 547-558
    nutritional support, 565-576
    wound management, 559-564
Opioid analgesics, 41-43, 678
Oral anticoagulation therapy, 141-142
Oral mucous membranes, impaired
  cancer care and, 28
  palliative and end-of-life care and, 111
  perioperative care, 60
Orchiectomy, bilateral, 14-15
Orthotopic neobladder urinary diversions, 249. See also Urinary diversions.
OSHA (Occupational Safety and Health Administration), Bloodborne Pathogens Standard, 24, 783
Osmolality, serum, 373-374, 671
Osteoarthritis. See OA (osteoarthritis).

Osteoporosis, 535-540
  assessments for, 535
  diagnoses and interventions for, 536-539
    additional considerations for, 539
    health-seeking behaviors, 536-537
    imbalanced nutrition, less than body requirements, 538-539
    injury risks, 538
  diagnostic tests for, 535
  discharge planning for, 539-540
  fundamentals of, 535
  health care settings for, 535
  pathophysiology of, 535
  patient-family education for, 539-540
  postmenopausal, 535-549
  secondary, 535-549
  senile, 535-549
Other-directed violence risks, 746-747
Otitis media. See OM (otitis media).
Outcome measurements and scales. See Measurement instruments and scales.
Output, cardiac, 178-179
Oximetry, 117-118, 124, 131-132, 178, 183, 196, 578, 593, 621-622, 659
Oxycodone with acetaminophen, 707
Oxytocin, 679

P
p24 antigen tests, 548-549
Pain management care, 39-44
  acute pain. See also Acute pain.
    abdominal trauma and, 422-423
    amputations and, 510
    appendicitis and, 430-431
    atherosclerotic arterial occlusive disease and, 152-153
    bacterial meningitis and, 283
    bleeding in pregnancy and, 676-677
    BPH and, 211
    burns and, 602
    CAD and, 167-168
    cancer care and, 4-6
    CD and, 449
    cholelithiasis, cholecystitis, and cholangitis and, 434-435
    fractures and, 515-516, 638
    GBS and, 292
    general neurologic care and, 273-274
    hemothorax and pneumothorax and, 134-135
    HIV/AIDS and, 553-554
    hyperthyroidism and, 404
    intervertebral disk disease and, 298-299
    MS and, 310
    neurologic care (general) and, 273-274
    OA and, 530-531
    OM and, 648
    palliative and end-of-life care and, 107
    pancreatitis and, 471-472
    peritonitis and, 482
    pneumothorax and hemothorax care and, 134-135
    polycythemia and, 501-502
    TBIs and, 367
    thrombocytopenia, 508
    thrombophlebitis and venous thrombosis and, 202-203
    UC and, 490-491
    ureteral calculi and, 244
    urinary tract obstructions and, 259
    venous thrombosis and thrombophlebitis and, 202-203
  chronic pain. See also Chronic pain.
    amputations and, 510
    atherosclerotic arterial occlusive disease and, 152-153
    cancer care and, 4-6
    HIV/AIDS and, 553-554

Pain management care (Continued)
    MS and, 310
    palliative care and end-of-life care, 107
  diagnoses and interventions for, 39-43, 530-531
    acute vs. chronic pain, 39-43
    AHCPR guidelines, 39-41
    ANA Standard of Pain Management Nursing Practice, 40-41
    APS and, 39-41
    descriptive pain scales, 39-40
    VASs and, 39-40
    WHO analgesic ladder and, 40-41
    Wong-Baker Faces Pain Scale and, 39-40
  fundamentals of, 39
  sickle cell pain crisis and, 659-664
Palliative and end-of-life care, 105-116
  deficient knowledge issues for, 105-116
    disease management choices, 105-106
    expectations, 106
    progressive disease processes, 106
  diagnoses and interventions for, 107-116
    airway clearance, ineffective, 108-109
    breathing patterns, ineffective, 107-108
    fluid volume, imbalanced, 110
    imbalanced nutrition, less than body requirements, 111-112
    oral mucous membranes, impaired, 111
    pain, acute vs. chronic, 107
    thought processes, disturbed, 109-110
  psychosocial diagnoses and interventions, 112-116.
      See also Psychosocial support.
    additional considerations for, 116
    anticipatory grieving, 115-116
    anxiety, 112-113
    caregiver role strain risks, 114-115
    death anxiety, 113
    fear, feelings of, 112
    powerlessness, feelings of, 113-114
    spiritual distress, 114
Palsy, cerebral. See CP (cerebral palsy).
Pancreatic enzymes, 621-626
Pancreatitis, 469-476
  acute vs. chronic, 469
  assessments for, 469-470
  diagnoses and interventions for, 470-475
    additional considerations for, 475
    fluid volume, deficient, 470-471
    gas exchange, impaired, 473
    imbalanced nutrition, less than body requirements, 474-475
    infection risks, 474
    pain, acute, 471-472
  diagnostic tests for, 470
  discharge planning for, 475
  fundamentals of, 469
  health care settings for, 469
  pathophysiology of, 469
  patient-family education for, 475
Panic Attack Cognitions Questionnaire, 738, 746
Panic attacks, 737-740. See also Anxiety disorders.
Paralyzed Veterans of America, 348
Parent-child attachment, impaired
  cervical insufficiency and, 684
  preeclampsia and, 717
  PTL and, 726-727
Parenting, impaired, 618
Parents Anonymous, 620
Parkinson's disease. See PD (Parkinson's disease).
Parkinson's Disease Foundation, 322
Partial complex seizures, 324
Partial simple motor seizures, 324
Partial-thickness burns, 600. See also Burns.
Particulate respirators, 783, 792
Pathophysiology
  cardiovascular care and, 149, 151, 157, 161, 165, 177, 181-182, 193, 195, 201
    aneurysms, 149

Pathophysiology (Continued)
    atherosclerotic arterial occlusive disease, 151
    CAD, 165
    cardiac surgeries, 161
    circulatory failure, 157
    dysrhythmias and conduction disturbances, 177
    HF, 181-182
    hypertension, 193
    pulmonary hypertension, 195
    venous thrombosis and thrombophlebitis, 201
  endocrine care and, 373, 377, 387, 395, 399, 407, 415
    DI, 373
    DKA, 387
    DM, 377
    HHNK syndrome, 395
    hyperthyroidism, 399
    hypothyroidism, 407
    SIADH, 415
  general care plans and, 1, 61
    bedrest, prolonged, 61
    cancer, 1
  GI care and, 419, 429, 433, 445, 455, 463, 469, 477, 481, 487
    abdominal trauma, 419
    appendicitis, 429
    CD, 445
    cholelithiasis, cholecystitis, and cholangitis, 433
    fecal diversions, 455
    hepatitis, 463
    pancreatitis, 469
    peptic ulcers, 477
    peritonitis, 481
    UC, 487
  hematologic care and, 495, 497, 501, 505
    anemia of chronic disease, 495
    DIC, 497
    polycythemia, 501
    thrombocytopenia, 505
  maternity care and, 70, 673, 681, 687, 695, 711, 719, 729
    bleeding in pregnancy, 673
    cervical insufficiency, 681
    GDM, 687
    hyperemesis gravidarum, 695
    postpartum wound infection, 70
    PPROM, 729
    preeclampsia, 711
    PTL, 719
  musculoskeletal care and, 509, 515, 523, 529, 535, 541
    amputations, 509
    fractures, 515
    joint replacement surgeries, 523
    OA, 529
    osteoporosis, 535
    RA, 541
  neurologic care and, 281, 287, 295, 305, 313, 323, 333, 349-350, 361
    bacterial meningitis, 281
    GBS, 287
    intervertebral disk disease, 295
    MS, 305
    PD, 313
    SCIs, 333
    seizures and epilepsy, 323
    stroke, 349-350
    TBIs, 361
  pediatric care and, 577, 585, 593, 599, 609, 615, 621, 629, 637, 641, 647, 653, 659
    ADHD, 585
    asthma, 577
    bronchiolitis, 593
    burns, 599
    CF and, 621
    child abuse and neglect, 615
    CP, 609

Pathophysiology (*Continued*)
DM, 629
fractures, 637
gastroenteritis, 641
OM, 647
poisoning, 653
sickle cell pain crisis, 659
psychiatric care and, 737-738, 745, 751, 761, 769, 775
anxiety disorders, 737-738
bipolar disorder (manic component), 745
dementia (Alzheimer's type), 751
depression, major, 761
schizophrenia, 769
substance abuse disorders, 775
renal-urinary care and, 207, 217, 223, 227, 231, 239, 243, 249, 257
ARF, 231
BPH, 207
CKD, 217
hemodialysis, 223
peritoneal dialysis, 227
renal transplants, 239
ureteral calculi, 243
urinary diversions, 249
urinary tract obstructions, 257
respiratory care and, 117, 131, 137, 143, 147
ARF, 147
COPD, 117
PE, 137
pneumothorax and hemothorax, 131
TB, 143
special needs care and, 547
HIV/AIDS, 547
Patient-family education. *See* Education, patient-family.
Patient psychosocial support, 73-86. *See also* Psychosocial support.
additional considerations for, 85
deficient knowledge issues for, 83-85
current health status, 83-85
prescribed therapies, 83-85
diagnoses and interventions for, 73-85
anxiety, 74-75
body image, disturbed, 80-81
coping, ineffective, 76-77
fatigue, 73
fear, 76
grieving, anticipatory *vs.* dysfunctional, 79-80
powerlessness, 77-78
sensory perception, disturbed, 82-83
sleep patterns, disturbed, 73-74
social isolation, 84
spiritual distress, 78-79
verbal communication, impaired, 81-82
fundamentals of, 73
Patterns, breathing. *See* Breathing patterns, ineffective.
PCC (Poison Control Center), 656-657
PD (Parkinson's disease), 313-322
assessments for, 313-314
deficient knowledge issues for, 316-322
anticholinergic medication side effects, 319-320
antiparkinson drugs, 316-317
antiviral agent side effects, 318-319
deep brain stimulation, 321-322
dopamine replacement therapy side effects, 318
diagnoses and interventions for, 314-322
additional considerations for, 322
fall risks, 314-315
health-seeking behaviors, 320-321
physical mobility, impaired, 315-316
diagnostic tests for, 314
discharge planning for, 322
fundamentals of, 313
health care settings for, 313
pathophysiology of, 313
patient-family education for, 322

PE (pulmonary embolus), 137-142
assessments for, 137
deficient knowledge issues for, 141-142
food-related impacts, 141-142
medication-related impacts, 141-142
oral anticoagulation therapy side effects, 141-142
diagnoses and interventions for, 138-142
additional considerations for, 140
gas exchange, impaired, 139
injury risks, 138-139
protection, ineffective, 139
fundamentals of, 137
health care settings for, 137
histories and, 137-138
pathophysiology of, 137
risk factors for, 137-142
Peak expiratory flow rates. *See* PEFRs (peak expiratory flow rates).
Pediatric care, 577-672, 809-810
ADHD, 585-592
asthma, 577-584
bronchiolitis, 593-598
burns, 599-608
CF, 621-628
child abuse and neglect, 615-620
CP, 609-614
DM, 629-636
fractures, 637-640
gastroenteritis, 641-646
normal laboratory values, 665-672
OM, 647-652
poisoning, 653-658
reference resources for, 809-810
sickle cell pain crisis, 659-664
PEEP (positive end expiratory pressure), 131
PEFRs (peak expiratory flow rates), 578
Pelvic ultrasound, 704
Penicillins, 662-663
Peptic ulcers, 477-480
assessments for, 477-478
diagnoses and interventions for, 478-480
additional considerations for, 480
protection, ineffective, 478-479
tissue integrity, impaired, 479-480
diagnostic tests for, 477-478
discharge planning for, 480
fundamentals of, 477
health care settings for, 477
pathophysiology of, 477
patient-family education for, 480
Perception, kinesthetic, 37
Perfusion, tissue. *See* Tissue perfusion, ineffective.
Perfusion scans, 195
Perioperative care, 45-60
deficient knowledge issues for, 45-47
postoperative care, 45-47
preoperative routines, 45-47
surgical procedures, 45-47
diagnoses and interventions for, 45-60
additional considerations, 60
airway clearance, ineffective, 48-49
aspiration risks, 49-50
breathing patterns, ineffective, 50-51
constipation, 56-57
fluid volume, deficient, 51-53
fluid volume, excess, 53-54
infection risks, 54-56
injury risks, 47-48
oral mucous membranes, impaired, 60
physical mobility, impaired, 58
skin integrity, impaired, 59-60
sleep patterns, disturbed, 57-58
trauma risks, 59
fundamentals of, 45

Peripheral neurovascular dysfunction
fractures and, 516-517
joint replacement surgeries and, 524
Peripheral tissue perfusion, ineffective
atherosclerotic arterial occlusive disease and, 154-155
bedrest, prolonged and, 65-66
CAD and, 173-174
cancer care and, 6
circulatory failure and, 157-159
DIC and, 498
DKA and, 392
fractures and, 638-639
hemodialysis and, 224-225
HF and, 185-186
polycythemia and, 502-503
SCIs and, 338-339
thrombocytopenia and, 507
venous thrombosis and thrombophlebitis and, 202-203
Peritoneal dialysis, 227-230. *See also* Dialysis.
components of, 227
diagnoses and interventions for, 228-230
additional considerations for, 230
fluid volume, imbalanced, 228-229
imbalanced nutrition, less than body requirements, 229-230
infection risks, 228
discharge planning for, 230
fundamentals of, 227
health care settings for, 227
pathophysiology of, 227
patient-family education for, 230
types of, 227
Peritoneoscopy, 438
Peritonitis, 481-486
assessments for, 481
diagnoses and interventions for, 482-485
additional considerations, 485
gas exchange, impaired, 483
imbalanced nutrition, less than body requirements, 484-485
infection risks, 483-484
injury risks, 483-484
nausea, 482
pain, acute, 482
diagnostic tests for, 481-482
discharge planning for, 485
fundamentals of, 481
health care settings for, 481
pathophysiology of, 481
patient-family education for, 485
Person to Person, 774
PET (positron emission tomography) studies, 306, 314, 324-325, 351
Petit mal seizures, 324
Pharmaceutical-related impacts
anxiety disorders and, 741-743
bipolar disorder (manic component) and, 749-750
bleeding in pregnancy and, 678-679
chemotherapy, 1-3
dementia (Alzheimer's type) and, 757-758
GDM and, 688-689, 692-693
hyperemesis gravidarum and, 699-700
major depression and, 766-767
MS and, 307-310
PE and, 141-142
postpartum wound infection and, 705-708
PPROM and, 732-733
preeclampsia and, 714-716
PTL and, 722-724
RA and, 545
schizophrenia and, 772-773
of specific drugs and drug classes. *See also under specific drugs and drug classes.*
ACE inhibitors, 231
acetaminophen with codeine, 662-663

Pharmaceutical-related impacts (Continued)
acetaminophen with oxycodone, 707
AEDs, 328-330
albuterol, 579, 625
analgesics, 40-43, 707
analgesics, opioid, 41-43, 678
antenatal glucocorticoids, 716, 723-724, 733-734
antibiotics, 283-284, 626
antibiotics, aerosolized, 625
antibiotics, prophylactic, 678, 733-734
anticoagulants, 141, 708
antidepressants, tricyclic, 589, 742-743, 766-767
antimanics, 747, 749
antimicrobials, 705-706
antiparkinson drugs, 316-320
antipsychotics, 747, 750, 772-773
antiviral agents, 318-320
aspirin, 41, 716
benzodiazepines, 743
beta-andrenergics, 734
beta-blockers, 169-170, 715-716
beta₂-agonists, 582-583
blood products, IV, 679
bronchodilators, 625
calcium channel blockers, 715-716, 722, 734
carboprost, 679
clindamycin, 706
clonidine, 590
co-analgesics, 42-43
corticosteroids, 582-583
cromolyn sodium/nedocromil sodium, 582-583
digoxin, 190
disulfiram, 781
diuretics, 189-190
dopamine replacement therapy, 318-320
doxylamine, 700
dual-mechanism drugs, 767-768
folic acid, 662-663
heparin, 138-139, 708
hydration, IV, 722
ibuprofen, 662-663, 678
immunosuppressive agents, 240-241
insulin, 373-386
leukotriene modifiers, 582-583
linezolid, 706
LMWH, 138-139, 708
magnesium sulfate, 715-716, 722, 733-734
MAO inhibitors, 589, 742-743, 767
meperidine, 707
methylergonovine, 679
methylxanthines, 583
metoclopramide hydrochloride, 699
morphine, 662-663, 707
mucolytic enzymes, aerosolized, 625-626
naltrexone, 781
nitrates, 169-170
nitroglycerin, 165-176
nonbenzodiazepines, 743
NSAIDs, 41, 231
ondansetron, 700
opioid analgesics, 41-43, 678
oxycodone with acetaminophen, 707
oxytocin, 679
pancreatic enzymes, 625-626
pantoprazole, 699
penicillins, 662-663
promethazine, 699-700
prostaglandin synthesis inhibitors, 678, 722
pyridoxine, 700
Rh-immune globulin, 679, 734
SNRIs, 589, 768
SSRIs, 743, 767
steroids, 582-583
sulfonylureas, second-generation, 692-693
uterotonics, 678-679
vaccines, pneumococcal, 283-284, 286

Pharmaceutical-related impacts (Continued)
vasodilators, 183-185
vitamin and mineral supplements, 626
substance abuse disorders and, 780-781
Phobias, 737. See also Anxiety disorders.
Physical abuse and neglect, child, 615-616. See also
Child abuse and neglect.
Physical mobility, impaired
cancer care and, 7
CP and, 611-612
fractures and, 517-518
joint replacement surgeries and, 527
OA and, 531-532
PD and, 315-316
perioperative care and, 58
stroke and, 351-352
Pilocarpine iontophoresis, 621-622
Pin function and care, 520-521. See also Fractures.
Plans for nursing care
infection prevention and control, 783-796
APIC and, 792
CDC, Standard Precautions, 783-792, 784t-791t
ICPs and, 792
isolation precaution recommendations, 784t-791t
MDROs and, 783
nosocomial infection reduction, 792
OSHA, Bloodborne Pathogens Standard, 783
SHEA and, 792
TJC and, 792
Transmission-Based Precautions (Airborne Infection Isolation), 783-792, 784t-791t
Transmission-Based Precautions (Droplet),
783-792, 784t-791t
Transmission-Based Precautions (Protective
Environment), 783-792, 784t-791t
laboratory tests (normal values), 665-672, 793-798
adult, 793-798
pediatric patients, 665-672
maternity, 673-736
bleeding in pregnancy, 673-680
cervical insufficiency, 681-686
DM, 687-694
hyperemesis gravidarum, 695-702
PPROM, 729-736
preeclampsia, 711-718
PTL, 719-728
wound infection, postpartum, 703-710
medical-surgical, 1-572
cardiovascular, 149-206
endocrine, 373-418
general, 1-116
GI, 419-494
hematologic, 495-508
musculoskeletal, 509-546
neurologic, 261-372
renal-urinary, 207-260
respiratory, 117-148
special needs, 541-576
pediatric, 577-672
ADHD, 585-592
asthma, 577-584
bronchiolitis, 593-598
burns, 599-608
CF, 621-628
child abuse and neglect, 615-620
CP, 609-614
DM, 629-636
fractures, 637-640
gastroenteritis, 641-646
OM, 647-652
poisoning, 653-658
sickle cell pain crisis, 659-664
psychiatric, 737-782
anxiety disorders, 737-744
bipolar disorder (manic component), 745-750
dementia (Alzheimer's type), 751-760

Plans for nursing care (Continued)
depression, major, 761-768
schizophrenia, 769-774
substance abuse disorders, 775-782
reference resources for, 799-812
Plasma
chemistries, 793-795
exchange procedures, 291-292
marker tests, 201-202
Plastic deformations, 637. See also Fractures.
Platelet counts, 420, 505, 671
Plethysmography, impedance, 201-202
Pneumococcal vaccines, 283-284, 286
Pneumonia, 123-129
assessments of, 123-124
community acquired, 123
diagnoses and interventions for, 124-127
additional considerations for, 127
airway clearance, ineffective, 125-126
fluid volume, deficient, 126-127
gas exchange, impaired, 124-125
infection risks, 127-128
mechanical ventilation and, 127
diagnostic tests for, 123-124
discharge planning for, 128
education, patient-family and, 128
fundamentals of, 123
health care settings for, 123
hospital-associated (nosocomial), 123
in immunocompromised patients, 123
pathophysiology of, 123
Pneumothorax and hemothorax, 131-136
assessments for, 131
diagnoses and interventions for, 132-135
additional considerations for, 135
breathing patterns, ineffective, 132-133
gas exchange, impaired, 133-134
pain, acute, 134-135
diagnostic tests for, 131-132
discharge planning for, 135
fundamentals of, 131
health care settings for, 131
pathophysiology of, 131
patient-family education for, 135
pneumothorax, 131-132
spontaneous (closed), 131-132
tension, 131-132
traumatic, 131-132
Poison Control Center. See PCC (Poison Control
Center).
Poisoning, 653-658
assessments for, 653-654
deficient knowledge issues for, 656
diagnoses and interventions for, 654-656
additional considerations for, 655
risk factors, 654-655
diagnostic tests for, 654
discharge planning for, 655-656
fundamentals of, 653
health care settings for, 653-654
pathophysiology of, 653
patient-family education for, 655-656
signs, symptoms, and basic treatments for, 653-654
acetaminophen ingestion, 653
carbon monoxide ingestion, 654
corrosive ingestion, 653-654
hydrocarbon ingestion, 654
iron ingestion, 654
lead ingestion, 654
Polycythemia, 501-504
assessments for, 501
diagnoses and interventions for, 501-504
imbalanced nutrition, less than body requirements,
503
ineffective tissue perfusion, cardiopulmonary, 504
ineffective tissue perfusion, cerebral, 502-504

Polycythemia (*Continued*)
    ineffective tissue perfusion, peripheral, 502-503
    ineffective tissue perfusion, renal, 502-503
    pain, acute, 501-502
  diagnostic tests for, 501
  discharge planning for, 504
  fundamentals of, 501
  health care settings for, 501
  pathophysiology of, 501
  patient-family education for, 504
Positive end expiratory pressure. *See* PEEP (positive end expiratory pressure).
Positron emission tomography studies. *See* PET (positron emission tomography) studies.
Post-trauma syndrome, 426-427
Posthepatic (obstructive) hepatitis, 463-468. *See also* Hepatitis.
Postmenopausal osteoporosis, 535-549. *See also* Osteoporosis.
Postoperative care, 45-47. *See also* Perioperative care.
Postpartum wound infection, 703-710
  abdominal, 703
  assessments for, 703-704
  deficient knowledge issues for, 705-709
    infection impacts, 708-709
    medication impacts, 705-708
    treatment impacts, 705-708
  diagnoses and interventions for, 704-710
    additional considerations for, 709
    coping, ineffective, 709
  diagnostic tests for, 704
  discharge planning for, 710
  episiotomy, 703
  fundamentals of, 70
  health care settings for, 703
  pathophysiology of, 70
  patient-family education for, 710
  sepsis, 703
  septic pelvic thrombophlebitis, 703
Postrenal *vs.* prenal failure, 231. *See also* ARF (acute renal failure).
Postsurgical sexual function, 212
Posttraumatic stress disorder. *See* PTSD (posttraumatic stress disorder).
Pouches, Indiana *vs.* Kock, 249
Powerlessness
  older adult care and, 104
  palliative and end-of-life care and, 113-114
  psychosocial support and, 77-78
PPD (purified protein derivative) injection tests, 144
PPROM (preterm premature rupture of membranes), 729-736
  assessments for, 729-730
  deficient knowledge issues for, 732-735
    bedrest, prolonged, 734-735
    medication impacts, 732-733
    signs, symptoms, and outcomes, 730-731
  diagnoses and interventions for, 730-736
    additional considerations for, 736
    coping, ineffective, 731-732
    grieving, anticipatory, 735-736
  diagnostic tests for, 730
  discharge planning for, 736
  fundamentals of, 729
  health care settings for, 729
  pathophysiology of, 729
  patient-family education for, 736
Preeclampsia, 711-718
  assessments for, 711-712
  deficient knowledge issues of, 713-716
    medication effects, 714-716
    preeclampsia effects, 713-714
  diagnoses and interventions for, 713-718
    additional considerations for, 718
    caregiver role strain, 717
    coping, ineffective, 716
    parent-child attachment, impaired, 717

Preeclampsia (*Continued*)
  diagnostic tests for, 712
  discharge planning for, 718
  fundamentals of, 711
  health care settings for, 711
  HELLP syndrome, 711-712
  pathophysiology of, 711
  patient-family education for, 718
Pregnancy-related care, 673-736, 810
  bleeding in pregnancy, 673-680
  cervical insufficiency, 681-686
  GDM and, 687-694. *See also* DM (diabetes mellitus).
  hyperemesis gravidarum, 695-702
  PPROM, 729-736
  preeclampsia, 711-718
  PTL, 719-728
  reference resources for, 810
  wound infection, postpartum, 702-710
Pregnancy tests, 674
Prehepatic (hemolytic) hepatitis, 463-468. *See also* Hepatitis.
Premature membrane rupture, preterm. *See* PPROM (preterm premature rupture of membranes).
Preoperative routines, 45-47. *See also* Perioperative care.
Prenal *vs.* postrenal failure, 231. *See also* ARF (acute renal failure).
Pressure necrosis, 512-513
Pressure ulcers, 562-564. *See also* Wound management care.
Preterm premature membrane rupture. *See* PPROM (preterm premature rupture of membranes).
Primary hypothyroidism, 407. *See also* Hypothyroidism.
Procedures, surgical, 45-47. *See also* Perioperative care.
Progressive chronic obstructive lung disease, 621
Progressive disease processes, 106
Prolonged bedrest, 61-71
  diagnoses and interventions for, 61-71
    activity intolerance risks, 61-63
    additional problems, 71
    constipation, 67-68
    dependence *vs.* independence, 70-71
    disuse syndrome risks, 63-65
    diversional activity, deficient, 69
    ineffective tissue perfusion, cerebral, 66-67
    ineffective tissue perfusion, peripheral, 65-66
    role performance, ineffective, 70-71
    sexuality patterns, ineffective, 70
  fundamentals of, 61
  pathophysiology of, 61
  PPROM and, 734-735
Promethazine, 699-700
Prophylactic antibiotics, 678, 733-734
Prostaglandin synthesis inhibitors, 678, 722
Prostate-specific antigen tests. *See* PSA (prostate-specific antigen) tests.
Protection, ineffective
  ARF and, 232-234
  CD and, 448-449
  DI and, 375
  hepatitis and, 466
  hypothyroidism and, 412
  PE and, 139
  peptic ulcers and, 478-479
  SIADH and, 416-417
  thrombocytopenia and, 506-507
  thyroid disorders and
    hyperthyroidism, 400-401
    hypothyroidism, 412
  urinary diversions and, 252-253
Protective Environment (Transmission-Based Precautions), 783-792, 784t-791t
Protheses care, 512-513
PSA (prostate-specific antigen) tests, 207
Psychiatric care, 737-783, 810-811
  anxiety disorders, 745-750
  bipolar disorder (manic component), 745-750
  dementia (Alzheimer's type), 751-760

Psychiatric care (*Continued*)
  depression, major, 761-768
  reference resources for, 810-811
  schizophrenia, 769-774
  substance abuse disorders, 775-782
Psychometric tests, 439
Psychomotor seizures, 324
Psychosocial support, 73-92
  family, 87-92
    current health status, patient, 91-92
    deficient knowledge issues and, 91-92
    diagnoses and interventions for, 87-92
    family coping, disabled, 90-91
    family coping, enhanced, 91
    family coping, impaired, 89-90
    family processes, interrupted, 88-89
    fear, feelings of, 87-88
    fundamentals of, 87
    HIPAA and, 87
    prescribed therapies, patient, 91-92
  for palliative and end-of-life care, 112-116. *See also* Palliative and end-of-life care.
  patient, 73-86
    additional considerations for, 85
    anxiety, 74-75
    body image, disturbed, 80-81
    coping, ineffective, 76-77
    current health status, 84-85
    deficient knowledge issues for, 84-85
    diagnoses and interventions for, 73-85
    fear, feelings of, 76
    fundamentals of, 73
    grieving, anticipatory *vs.* dysfunctional, 79-80
    powerlessness, feelings of, 77-78
    prescribed therapies, 84-85
    sensory perception, disturbed, 82-83
    sleep patterns, disturbed, 73-74
    social isolation, 84
    spiritual distress, 78-79
    verbal communication, impaired, 81-82
PTL (preterm labor), 719-728
  assessments for, 719-720
  deficient knowledge issues for, 720-724
    medication impacts, 722-724
    PTL effects, 720-721
  diagnoses and interventions for, 720-728
    additional considerations for, 728
    breastfeeding, ineffective, 727
    caregiver role strain, 725
    constipation, 725-726
    coping, ineffective, 724
    parent-child attachment, impaired, 726-727
  diagnostic tests for, 720
  discharge planning for, 728
  fundamentals of, 719
  health care settings for, 719
  pathophysiology of, 719
  patient-family education for, 728
PTSD (posttraumatic stress disorder), 737-738. *See also* Anxiety disorders.
Pulmonary edema, acute. *See* HF (heart failure).
Pulmonary embolus. *See* PE (pulmonary embolus).
Pulmonary function tests, 578, 622
Pulmonary hypertension, 195-200. *See also* Hypertension.
  assessments for, 195
  deficient knowledge issues for, 198-199
  diagnoses and interventions for, 196-199
    activity intolerance, 197-198
    additional considerations for, 199
    gas exchange, impaired, 196-197
  diagnostic tests for, 195-196
  discharge planning for, 199
  fundamentals of, 195
  health care settings for, 195
  pathophysiology of, 195
  patient-family education for, 199

Pulmonary tuberculosis, 143-146
   airborne infection isolation procedures and, 144-145
   assessments for, 143-144
   deficient knowledge issues for, 144-145
   diagnoses and interventions for, 144-145
   diagnostic tests for, 144
   discharge planning for, 145
   fundamentals of, 143
   health care settings for, 143
   LTBIs, 143
   MDR, 143
   pathophysiology of, 143
   patient-family education for, 145
Pulse oximetry. See Oximetry.
Pyridoxine, 700

Q
QuantiFERON-TB Gold test, 143-144
Quantitative sweat chloride test, 621-622

R
RA (rheumatoid arthritis), 541-546. See also Arthritis.
   assessments for, 541
   deficient knowledge issues for, 542-543
   diagnoses and interventions for, 542-546
      additional considerations for, 545
      body image, disturbed, 545
      fatigue, 544-545
      self-care deficits, 543-544
   diagnostic tests for, 541
   discharge planning for, 546
   fundamentals of, 541
   health care settings for, 541
   medication impacts and, 542-543
   pathophysiology of, 541
   patient-family education for, 546
Radiation therapy, 1-38
Radiographs, 616
Radiologic studies, 438
Radionuclide imaging, 195
Range of motion. See ROM (range of motion).
Rapid HIV tests, 549
RBC (red blood cell) counts, 671
RDS (respiratory distress syndrome), 719-720
Red blood cell counts. See RBC (red blood cell) counts.
Reference resources, 799-812
Reflex urinary incontinence, 339-341
Regional enteritis. See CD (Crohn's disease).
Rehabilitation Act of 1973, 591, 636
Rejection, renal transplants, 230-241. See also Renal
      transplants.
Relaxation techniques, 172
Remodeling, 181-182
Renal function studies, 688, 712
Renal scans, 232
Renal tissue perfusion, ineffective
   CAD and, 175
   circulatory failure and, 157-159
   DIC and, 498
   polycythemia and, 502-503
   thrombocytopenia and, 507
   urinary diversions and, 254-255
Renal transplants, 239-242
   deficient knowledge issues for, 240-241
   diagnoses and interventions for, 239-242
   discharge planning for, 242
   fundamentals of, 239
   health care settings for, 239
   immunosuppression and, 239-240
   infection risks and, 239-240
   pathophysiology of, 239
   patient-family teaching for, 242
   rejection of, 230-241
Renal ultrasound, 218, 232, 243
Renal-urinary care, 207-260, 802-803
   ARF, 231-238
   BPH, 207-216

Renal-urinary care (Continued)
   calculi, ureteral, 243-248
   CKD, 217-222
   dialysis, 223-230
      hemodialysis, 223-226
      peritoneal, 227-230
   diversions, urinary, 249-256
   reference resources for, 802-803
   transplants, renal, 239-242
   urinary tract obstructions, 257-260
Replacement, joints. See Joint replacement surgeries.
Requirement estimations, 566-567
Research Institute on Addictions, 782
Residual limb care, 512-513. See also Amputations.
Respirators, N95 vs. particulate, 783, 792
Respiratory care, 117-148
   ARF, 147-148
   COPD, 117-121
   PE, 137-142
   pneumonia, 123-129
   pneumothorax and hemothorax, 131-136
   reference resources for, 800-801
   TB, 143-146
Respiratory distress syndrome. See RDS (respiratory
      distress syndrome).
Respiratory failure, acute. See ARF (acute respiratory
      failure).
Respiratory syncytial virus bronchiolitis. See RSV (respi-
      ratory syncytial virus) bronchiolitis.
Restorative proctocolectomy, 456. See also Fecal diver-
      sions (colostomy, ileostomy, and IPAA).
Restrictive cardiomyopathy, 182. See also HF (heart
      failure).
Retention, urinary, 339-341
Retrograde urography, 232
Reversible ischemicneurologic deficit. See RIND (revers-
      ible ischemicneurologic deficit).
Rh-immune globulin, 679, 734
Rheumatoid arthritis. See RA (rheumatoid arthritis).
RIND (reversible ischemicneurologic deficit), 349-350.
      See also Stroke.
Role performance, ineffective
   amputations and, 511-512
   bedrest, prolonged and, 70-71
ROM (range of motion), 61-62
Rotazyme tests, 642
RSV (respiratory syncytial virus) bronchiolitis, 593-598
   assessments for, 593
   diagnoses and interventions for, 593-596
      additional considerations for, 596
      airway clearance, ineffective, 593-594
      fluid volume, deficient, 595-596
      gas exchange, impaired, 594-595
   diagnostic tests for, 593
   discharge planning for, 596
   fundamentals of, 593
   health care settings for, 593
   pathophysiology of, 593
   patient-family education for, 596
Rule of nines, modified, 599
Rupture of membranes, preterm premature. See PPROM
      (preterm premature rupture of membranes).

S
SAFE KIDS, 599, 608, 640, 653, 657
SANS (Scale for the Assessment of Negative Symptoms),
      770
SAPS (Scale for the Assessment of Positive Symptoms),
      770
SBS (shaken baby syndrome), 615-616. See also Child
      abuse and neglect.
Scale for the Assessment of Negative Symptoms. See
      SANS (Scale for the Assessment of Negative
      Symptoms).
Scale for the Assessment of Positive Symptoms. See
      SAPS (Scale for the Assessment of Positive
      Symptoms).

Scales and instruments. See Measurement instruments
      and scales.
Schizophrenia, 769-774
   assessments for, 769-770
   deficient knowledge issues for, 771-773
      causes, signs, and symptoms, 771
      medication impacts, 772-773
   diagnoses and interventions for, 771-774
      additional considerations for, 774
      sensory perception, disturbed, 771-772
   diagnostic tests for, 770-771
   discharge planning for, 774
   fundamentals of, 769
   health care settings for, 769
   pathophysiology of, 769
   patient-family education for, 774
Schizophrenia Society of Canada, 774
Scintigraphy, thyroid, 379
SCIs (spinal cord injuries), 333-348
   ASIA impairment scale for, 333-335
   assessments for, 333-335
   diagnoses and interventions for, 335-348
      AD, 335-336
      additional considerations for, 348
      airway clearance, ineffective, 337
      constipation, 342
      disuse syndrome, 343-344
      fecal impaction, 342
      ineffective tissue perfusion, cardiopulmonary,
         338-339
      ineffective tissue perfusion, cerebral, 338
      ineffective tissue perfusion, peripheral, 338-339
      injury risks, 344-345
      reflex urinary incontinence, 339-341
      sexual dysfunction, 346-347
      skin integrity, impaired, 345-346
      urinary retention, 339-341
   diagnostic tests for, 334-335
   discharge planning for, 348
   family-patient education for, 348
   fundamentals of, 333
   health care settings for, 333
   pathophysiology of, 333
SE (status epilepticus), 323. See also Seizures and
      epilepsy.
Second-generation sulfonylureas, 692-693
Secondary hypothyroidism, 407. See also Hypothyroidism.
Secondary OA (osteoarthritis), 529. See also OA
      (osteoarthritis).
Secondary osteoporosis, 535-549. See also Osteoporosis.
Seizures and epilepsy, 323-332
   assessments for, 323-325
   deficient knowledge issues for, 327-330
      AED side effects, 328-330
      life-threatening environmental factors, 327-328
      preventive measures, 327-328
   diagnoses and interventions for, 325-331
      additional considerations for, 331
      therapy noncompliance, 330-331
      trauma risks, 325-327
   diagnostic tests for, 324-325
   discharge planning for, 331
   epileptic syndromes, 324
   fundamentals of, 323
   generalized absence (petit mal) seizures, 324
   generalized myoclonic seizures, 324
   generalized tonic-clonic (grand mal) seizures, 323-324
   health care settings for, 323
   partial complex (psychomotor) seizures, 324
   partial simple (focal) motor seizures, 324
   pathophysiology of, 323
   patient-family education for, 331
   SE, 323-324
   temporal lobe seizures, 324
Selective serotonin reuptake inhibitors. See SSRIs
      (selective serotonin reuptake inhibitors).

Self-care deficits
  bipolar disorder (manic component) and, 747-748
  CP and, 612-613
  fractures and, 519-520
  general neurologic care and, 277-279
  RA and, 543-544
  urinary diversions and, 255-256
Self-esteem, low
  ADHD and, 586
  major depression and, 764-765
Senile osteoporosis, 535-549. See also Osteoporosis.
Sensory perception, disturbed
  cancer care and, 37
  dementia (Alzheimer's type) and, 755-756
  general neurologic care and, 280
  hypothyroidism and, 410-411
  schizophrenia and, 771-772
  stroke and, 355-356
Septic pelvic thrombophlebitis, 703
Septic shock, 157. See also Shock (cardiac vs. noncardiac).
Serum chemistries, 218, 695, 793-795
Serum electrolyte levels, 177-178, 641-642
Serum osmolality, 373-374, 671
Settings, health care. See Health care settings.
Sexual abuse, child, 615-616. See also Child abuse and
  neglect.
Sexual dysfunction
  bedrest, prolonged and, 70
  BPH and, 207-216
  cancer care and, 10-11
  cervical insufficiency and, 685
  OA and, 532-533
  SCIs and, 346-347
Shaken Baby Alliance, 620
Shaken baby syndrome. See SBS (shaken baby syndrome).
SHARE, 680, 686, 718, 726, 736
SHEA (Society for Healthcare Epidemiology of Amer-
  ica), 792
Sheehan Patient Rated Anxiety Inventory, 738, 746
Shock (cardiac vs. noncardiac), 157-160
  anaphylactic shock, 157
  cardiogenic shock, 157
  diagnoses and interventions for, 157-160
    additional considerations for, 160
    ineffective tissue perfusion, cardiopulmonary,
      157-159
    ineffective tissue perfusion, cerebral, 157-159
    ineffective tissue perfusion, peripheral, 157-159
    ineffective tissue perfusion, renal, 157-159
  diagnostic tests for, 157
  discharge planning for, 160
  fundamentals of, 157
  gas exchange, impaired, 160
  health care settings for, 157
  hypovolemic shock, 157
  neurogenic shock, 157
  pathophysiology of, 157
  patient-family education for, 160
  septic shock, 157
SIADH (syndrome of inappropriate antidiuretic
  hormone), 415-418
  assessments for, 415
  diagnoses and interventions for, 415-418
    additional considerations for, 418
    fluid volume, excess, 415-416
    protection, ineffective, 416-417
  diagnostic tests for, 415
  discharge planning for, 418
  fundamentals of, 415
  health care settings for, 415
  pathophysiology of, 415
  patient-family education for, 418
Sickle cell pain crisis, 659-664
  assessments for, 659
  deficient knowledge issues for, 661-663
  diagnoses and interventions for, 660-663

Sickle cell pain crisis (Continued)
  additional considerations for, 663
  ineffective tissue perfusion, cardiopulmonary,
    660-661
  ineffective tissue perfusion, cerebral, 660-661
  pain, acute, 660
  diagnostic tests for, 659
  discharge planning for, 663-664
  fundamentals of, 659
  health care settings for, 659
  pathophysiology of, 659
  patient-family education for, 663-664
Sidelines High Risk Pregnancy Support, 680, 686, 694,
  701, 718, 726, 736
Sigmoid colostomy, 455-456. See also Fecal diversions
  (colostomy, ileostomy, and IPAA).
Sigmoidoscopy, 446
Significant other psychosocial support, 72-92. See also
  Psychosocial support.
Simpson-Angus Rating Scale, 770
Sinus x-rays, 282
Skin integrity, impaired
  abdominal trauma and, 425
  amputations and, 512-513
  BPH and, 211
  burns and, 602-603
  cancer care and, 7-9, 19-22
  CKD and, 220-221
  DM and, 382
  fecal diversions and, 456-457
  fractures and, 518-519, 639
  gastroenteritis and, 643-644
  hepatitis and, 465
  older adult care and, 100-101
  perioperative care and, 59-60
  SCIs and, 345-346
  UC and, 492
  ureteral calculi and, 245-246
  urinary diversions and, 253-254
Skin testing, allergen, 578
Skull fractures, 362. See also TBIs (traumatic brain
  injuries).
Skull x-rays, 282
SLE (systemic lupus erythematosus), 505
Sleep
  patterns, disturbed, 57-58, 73-74, 101-102, 401-402
    hyperthyroidism and, 401-402
    older adult care and, 101-102
    perioperative care and, 57-58
    psychosocial support and, 73-74
  studies, 196
SNRIs, 589, 768
Social isolation
  anxiety disorders and, 740
  HIV/AIDS and, 557
  psychosocial support and, 84
Society for Healthcare Epidemiology of America. See
  SHEA (Society for Healthcare Epidemiology of
  America).
Spasms, chronic, 310
Spastic CP (cerebral palsy), 609. See also CP (cerebral
  palsy).
Special needs care, 547-576, 807-809
  HIV/AIDS, 547-558
  nutritional support, 565-576
  reference resources for, 807-809
  wound management, 559-564
Specific drug names and drug classes. See Drug-related
  impacts.
Spinal cord injuries. See SCIs (spinal cord injuries).
Spine x-rays, 334-335
Spiritual distress
  bipolar disorder (manic component), 745-746
  palliative and end-of-life care and, 114
  psychosocial support and, 78-79
  substance abuse disorders and, 776

Spirometry, 117-118
Spontaneous (closed) pneumothorax, 131-132. See also
  Pneumothorax and hemothorax.
Sputum cultures, 117-118, 578, 622
SSRIs (selective serotonin reuptake inhibitors), 743, 767
ST-segment elevation myocardial infarction. See STEMI
  (ST-segment elevation myocardial infarction).
Standard of Pain Management Nursing Practice, 40-41
Standard Precautions, CDC (Centers for Disease
  Control and Prevention), 783-792, 784t-791t
STARBRIGHT Foundation, 584, 627, 664
State-Trait Anxiety Inventory, 738, 746
Status epilepticus. See SE (status epilepticus).
STEMI (ST-segment elevation myocardial infarction),
  165
Sterile speculum examinations, 720, 730
Stimulants, 588-589
Stomal tissue perfusion, ineffective, 254-255
Stool analyses, 622, 642
Stress
  anxiety disorders and, 737
  cancer care and, 10
  disorder, acute, 737-738. See also Anxiety disorders.
Stress tests, 166, 178, 182-183, 196
Stress urinary incontinence, 213-214
Stroke, 349-360
  assessments for, 350-351
  brain attacks, 349-350
  deficient knowledge issues for, 357-358
    carotid angioplasty/stent procedures, 357-358
    carotid endarterectomy procedures, 357-358
  diagnoses and interventions for, 351-359
    additional considerations for, 358
    physical mobility, impaired, 351-352
    sensory perception, disturbed, 355-356
    unilateral neglect, 354-355
    verbal communication, impaired, 353-354
  diagnostic tests for, 350-351
  discharge planning for, 358
  fundamentals of, 349-350
  health care settings for, 350
  hemorrhagic, 349-350
  ischemic, 349-350
  lacunar, 349-350
  pathophysiology of, 349-350
  patient-family education for, 358
  RIND, 349-350
  TIAs, 349-350
Substance abuse disorders, 775-780
  alcoholism, 775-782
  assessments for, 775-776
  deficient knowledge issues for, 780-781
  diagnoses and interventions for, 776-782
    additional considerations for, 782
    denial, ineffective, 778
    family processes, interrupted, 777-778
    imbalanced nutrition, less than body requirements,
      779-780
    injury risks, 776-777
    sensory perception, disturbed, 779
  diagnostic tests for, 776
  discharge planning for, 782
  fundamentals of, 775
  health care settings for, 775
  medication impacts and, 780-781
  pathophysiology of, 775
  patient-family education for, 782
Suicide risks
  bipolar disorder (manic component) and, 746
  major depression and, 761-764
  schizophrenia and, 770
  substance abuse disorders and, 776
Sulfonylureas, second-generation, 692-693
Superficial burns, 600. See also Burns.

Support, psychosocial, 73-92
　family and significant other, 87-92
　　current health status, patient, 91-92
　　deficient knowledge issues and, 91-92
　　diagnoses and interventions for, 87-92
　　family coping, disabled, 90-91
　　family coping, enhanced, 91
　　family coping, impaired, 89-90
　　family processes, interrupted, 88-89
　　fear, 87-88
　　fundamentals of, 87
　　HIPAA and, 87
　　prescribed therapies, patient, 91-92
　palliative and end-of-life care and, 112-116. See also
　　Palliative and end-of-life care.
　patient, 73-86
　　additional considerations for, 85
　　anxiety, 74-75
　　body image, disturbed, 80-81
　　coping, ineffective, 76-77
　　current health status, 84-85
　　deficient knowledge issues for, 84-85
　　fear, 76
　　fundamentals of, 73
　　grieving, anticipatory vs. dysfunctional, 79-80
　　powerlessness, 77-78
　　prescribed therapies, 84-85
　　sensory perception, disturbed, 82-83
　　sleep patterns, disturbed, 73-74
　　social isolation, 84
　　spiritual distress, 78-79
　　verbal communication, impaired, 81-82
Surgical-medical care plans
　cardiovascular, 149-206
　　aneurysms, 149-150
　　atherosclerotic arterial occlusive disease, 151-156
　　CAD, 165-176
　　cardiac surgeries, 161-164
　　circulatory failure, 157-160
　　dysrhythmias and conduction disturbances, 177-180
　　HF, 181-192
　　hypertension, 193-195
　　hypertension, pulmonary, 195-200
　　venous thrombosis and thrombophlebitis, 201-205
　endocrine, 373-418
　　diabetes, DI, 373-376
　　diabetes, DKA, 387-394
　　diabetes, DM, 377-386
　　HHNK syndrome, 395-398
　　hyperthyroidism, 399-406
　　hypothyroidism, 407-414
　　SIADH, 415-418
　general, 1-116
　　bedrest, prolonged, 61-71
　　cancer, 1-38
　　older adult, 93-104
　　pain management, 39-44
　　palliative and end-of-life, 105-116
　　perioperative, 45-60
　　psychosocial support, family and significant other,
　　　87-92
　　psychosocial support, patient, 73-86
　GI, 419-494
　　abdominal trauma, 419-428
　　appendicitis, 429-432
　　CD, 445-454
　　cholelithiasis, cholecystitis, and cholangitis,
　　　433-436
　　cirrhosis, 437-444
　　fecal diversions, 455-462
　　pancreatitis, 469-476
　　peptic ulcers, 477-480
　　UC, 487-494
　GI care
　　hepatitis, 463-468
　　peritonitis, 481-486

Surgical-medical care plans (Continued)
　hematologic, 495-508
　　anemia of chronic disease, 495-496
　　DIC, 497-500
　　polycythemia, 501-504
　　thrombocytopenia, 505-508
　musculoskeletal, 509-546
　　amputations, 509-514
　　arthritis, OA, 529-534
　　arthritis, RA, 541-546
　　fractures, 515-522
　　joint replacement surgeries, 523-528
　　osteoporosis, 535-540
　neurologic, 261-372
　　GBS, 287-294
　　general, 261-264
　　intervertebral disk disease, 295-304
　　meningitis, bacterial, 281-286
　　MS, 305-312
　　PD, 313-322
　　SCIs, 333-348
　　seizures and epilepsy, 323-332
　　stroke, 349-360
　　TBIs, 361-372
　reference resources for, 799-812
　renal-urinary, 207-260
　　ARF, 231-238
　　BPH, 207-216
　　calculi, ureteral, 243-248
　　CKD, 217-222
　　dialysis, hemodialysis, 223-226
　　dialysis, peritoneal, 227-230
　　diversions, urinary, 249-256
　　transplants, renal, 239-242
　　urinary tract obstructions, 257-260
　respiratory, 117-148
　　ARF, 147-148
　　COPD, 117-121
　　PE, 137-142
　　pneumonia, 123-129
　　pneumothorax and hemothorax, 131-136
　　TB, 143-146
　special needs, 547-576
　　HIV/AIDS, 547-558
　　nutritional support, 565-576
　　wound management, 559-564
Swallowing, impaired
　cancer care and, 28-29
　general neurologic care and, 267-269
　hyperthyroidism and, 405
　intervertebral disk disease and, 303-304
　nutritional support and, 574
Sweat chloride test, 621-622
Sweat gland dysfunction, 621
Symptom exacerbation issues, 306-307
Syndrome of inappropriate antidiuretic hormone. See
　SIADH (syndrome of inappropriate antidiuretic
　hormone).
Systemic lupus erythematosus. See SLE (systemic lupus
　erythematosus).
Systolic dysfunction, 181-182

T
Tactile perception, disturbed. See Disturbed sensory
　perception.
TB (pulmonary tuberculosis), 143-146
　airborne infection isolation procedures and, 144-145
　assessments for, 143-144
　deficient knowledge issues for, 144-145
　diagnoses and interventions for, 144-145
　diagnostic tests for, 144
　discharge planning for, 145
　fundamentals of, 143
　health care settings for, 143
　LTBIs, 143
　MDR, 143

TB (Continued)
　pathophysiology of, 143
　patient-family education for, 145
TBIs (traumatic brain injuries), 361-372
　assessments for, 361-363
　brain death, 363
　brain herniation, 363
　brain lacerations, 362
　cerebral blood vessel rupture, 362-363
　concussions, 361, 364
　contusions, 361-362
　DAIs, 361
　deficient knowledge issues for, 364, 367-371
　　caretaker responsibilities, 364
　　craniotomy procedures, 367-369
　　ventricular shunt procedures, 370-371
　diagnoses and interventions for, 364-372
　　additional considerations for, 371
　　fluid volume, excess, 366-367
　　infection risks, 364-366
　　pain, acute, 367
　diagnostic tests for, 363
　discharge planning for, 372
　fundamentals of, 361
　health care settings for, 361
　IICP, 362-363
　pathophysiology of, 361
　patient-family education for, 372
　skull fractures, 362
TBSA (total body surface area), 599
Teaching, patient-family. See Education, patient-family.
Temporal lobe seizures, 324
Temporary colostomy, 455-456
Temporary ileostomy, 456
TENS (transcutaneous electrical nerve stimulation)
　devices, 274
Tension pneumothorax, 131-132. See also Pneumothorax
　and hemothorax.
Tertiary hypothyroidism, 407. See also Hypothyroidism.
Tests. See Diagnostic tests.
THA (total hip arthroplasty), 523-528. See also Joint
　replacement surgeries.
The Joint Commission. See TJC (The Joint Commission).
Therapy noncompliance issues, 330-331
Thioamide impacts, 403-404
Thoracic aneurysms, 149. See also Aneurysms.
Thought processes, disturbed
　ADHD and, 586
　dementia (Alzheimer's type) and, 754-755
　palliative and end-of-life care and, 109-110
Thrombocytopenia, 505-508
　assessments for, 505
　diagnoses and interventions for, 506-508
　　additional considerations for, 508
　　ineffective tissue perfusion, cerebral, 507
　　ineffective tissue perfusion, peripheral, 507
　　ineffective tissue perfusion, renal, 507
　　pain, acute, 508
　　protection, ineffective, 506-507
　diagnostic tests for, 505-506
　DIC and, 505. See also DIC (disseminated intravascu-
　　lar coagulation).
　discharge planning for, 508
　fundamentals of, 505
　health care settings for, 505
　HIT, 505
　ITP, 505
　pathophysiology of, 505
　patient-family education for, 508
　SLE and, 505
　TTP, 505
　vWF and, 505
Thrombophlebitis and venous thrombosis, 201-205
　assessments for, 201
　deficient knowledge issues for, 204
　diagnoses and interventions for, 201-205

Thrombophlebitis and venous thrombosis (Continued)
   additional considerations for, 205
     ineffective tissue perfusion, cardiopulmonary, 202
     ineffective tissue perfusion, peripheral, 202-203
     pain, acute, 202-203
   diagnostic tests for, 201
   discharge planning for, 205
   fundamentals of, 201
   health care settings for, 201
   pathophysiology of, 201
   patient-family education for, 205
Thrombosis, venous, 201-205. See also Venous thrombosis and thrombophlebitis.
Thrombotic thrombocytopenic purpura. See TTP
   (thrombotic thrombocytopenic purpura).
Thyroid disorders
   hyperthyroidism, 399-406
     assessments for, 399
     deficient knowledge issues for, 403-404
     diagnoses and interventions for, 400-405
     diagnostic tests for, 399
     discharge planning for, 405
     fundamentals of, 399
     health care settings for, 399
     pathophysiology of, 399
     patient-family education for, 405
   hypothyroidism, 407-414
     assessments for, 407
     diagnoses and interventions for, 408-412
     diagnostic tests for, 407
     discharge planning for, 413
     fundamentals of, 407
     health care settings for, 407
     pathophysiology of, 407
     patient-family education for, 413
     primary vs. secondary, 407
Thyroid-stimulating hormone levels, 630
Thyrotropin levels, 379
Thyroxine levels, 630
TIAs (transient ischemic attacks), 349-350. See also
   Stroke.
Tissue integrity, impaired
   atherosclerotic arterial occlusive disease and, 152-154
   burns and, 602-603
   corneal, 270-271, 402-403
   fecal diversions and, 456-457
   general neurologic care and, 270-271
   HIV/AIDS and, 553
   hyperthyroidism and, 402-403
   peptic ulcers and, 479-480
   wound management and, 559-564
Tissue perfusion, ineffective
   aneurysms and, 150
   cardiopulmonary, 7, 157-169, 173, 185-186, 202, 289,
     338-339, 498, 504, 660-661
     CAD and, 173
     cancer care and, 7
     circulatory failure and, 157-159
     DIC, 498
     DIC and, 498
     GBS and, 289
     HF and, 185-186
     polycythemia and, 504
     SCIs and, 338-339
     sickle cell pain crisis, 660-661
     venous thrombosis and thrombophlebitis and, 202
   cerebral, 66-67, 157-159, 173, 185-186, 289, 338, 498,
     502-503, 507, 660-661
     bedrest, prolonged and, 66-67
     CAD and, 173
     circulatory failure and, 157-159
     DIC and, 498
     GBS and, 289
     HF and, 185-186
     polycythemia and, 502-503
     SCIs and, 338

Tissue perfusion, ineffective (Continued)
     sickle cell pain crisis and, 660-661
     thrombocytopenia and, 507
   gastrointestinal, 424-425
   impaired stomal, 254-255
   joint replacement surgeries and, 524-525
   peripheral, 6, 65-66, 154-159, 173-174, 185-186,
     202-203, 224-225, 338-339, 392, 489, 502-503,
     507, 638-639
     atherosclerotic arterial occlusive disease and,
       154-155
     bedrest, prolonged and, 65-66
     CAD and, 173-174
     cancer care and, 6
     circulatory failure and, 157-159
     DIC and, 498
     DKA and, 392
     fractures and, 638-639
     hemodialysis and, 224-225
     HF and, 185-186
     polycythemia and, 502-503
     SCIs and, 338-339
     thrombocytopenia and, 507
     venous thrombosis and thrombophlebitis and,
       202-203
   renal, 157-159, 175, 498, 502-503, 507
     CAD and, 175
     circulatory failure and, 157-159
     DIC and, 498
     polycythemia and, 502-503
     thrombocytopenia and, 507
   urinary diversions and, 254-255
TJC (The Joint Commission), 39-40, 792
TKA (total knee arthroplasty), 523-528. See also Joint
   replacement surgeries.
Tonic-clonic (grand mal) seizures, generalized, 323-324
Torus fractures, 637. See also Fractures.
Total body surface area. See TBSA (total body surface
   area).
Total hip arthroplasty. See THA (total hip arthroplasty).
Total knee arthroplasty. See TKA (total knee arthro-
   plasty).
Total parenteral nutrition. See TPN (total parenteral
   nutrition).
Touch perception, disturbed. See Sensory perception,
   disturbed.
TPN (total parenteral nutrition), 567-568. See also
   Nutritional support.
Transcutaneous electrical nerve stimulation devices. See
   TENS (transcutaneous electrical nerve stimulation)
   devices.
Transient ischemic attacks. See TIAs (transient ischemic
   attacks).
Transitional feedings, 568. See also Nutritional support.
Translabial ultrasound, 681
Transmission-Based Precautions
   Airborne Infection Isolation, 783-792, 784t-791t
   Contact, 783-792, 784t-791t
   Droplet, 283, 783-792, 784t-791t
   Protective Environment, 783-792, 784t-791t
Transmural colitis. See CD (Crohn's disease).
Transplant Recipients International Organization. See
   TRIO (Transplant Recipients International
   Organization).
Transplants, renal, 239-242
   deficient knowledge issues for, 240-241
   diagnoses and interventions for, 239-242
   discharge planning for, 242
   fundamentals of, 239
   health care settings for, 239
   immunosuppression and, 239-240
   infection risks and, 239-240
   pathophysiology of, 239
   patient-family teaching for, 242
   rejection of, 230-241
Transrectal ultrasound, 207

Transvaginal ultrasound, 681
Transverse colostomy, 455-456. See also Fecal diversions
   (colostomy, ileostomy, and IPAA).
Trauma
   abdominal, 419-428
     assessments for, 419-420
     diagnoses and interventions for, 421-427
     diagnostic tests for, 420
     discharge planning for, 427
     fundamentals of, 419
     health care settings for, 419
     pathophysiology of, 419
     patient-family education for, 427
   risks, 59, 325-327
     perioperative care and, 59
     seizures and epilepsy, 325-327
   TBIs, 361-372. See also TBIs (traumatic brain injuries).
     brain death, 363
     brain herniation, 363
     brain lacerations, 362
     cerebral blood vessel rupture, 362-363
     concussions, 361, 364
     contusions, 361-362
     DAIs, 361
     deficient knowledge issues for, 364, 367-371
     diagnoses and interventions for, 364-372
     diagnostic tests for, 363
     discharge planning for, 372
     fundamentals of, 361
     health care settings for, 361
     IICP, 362-363. See also IICP (increased intracranial
       pressure).
     pathophysiology of, 361
     patient-family education for, 372
     skull fractures, 362
   traumatic pneumothorax, 131-132. See also Pneumo-
     thorax and hemothorax.
Tremor studies, 314
Tricyclic antidepressants, 589, 742-743, 766-767
TRIO (Transplant Recipients International
   Organization), 242
TTP (thrombotic thrombocytopenic purpura), 505. See
   also Thrombocytopenia.
Tuberculin skin tests, 144
Tuberculosis. See TB (pulmonary tuberculosis).
Tunneled central venous catheters, 13
TURP syndrome, 210
Tympanocentesis, 647
Tympanometry, 647
Types I and II DM (diabetes mellitus), 629. See also DM
   (diabetes mellitus).

U
UC (ulcerative colitis), 487-494
   assessments for, 487-488
   vs. CD, 445. See also CD (Crohn's disease).
   deficient knowledge issues for, 492-493
   diagnoses and interventions for, 488-489
     additional considerations for, 493
     diarrhea, 491
     fluid volume, deficient, 488-489
     infection risks, 489-490
     injury risks, 489-490
     nausea, 490-491
     pain, acute, 490-491
     skin integrity, impaired, 492
   diagnostic tests for, 488
   discharge planning for, 493
   fundamentals of, 487
   health care settings for, 487
   pathophysiology of, 487
   patient-family education for, 493
Ulcers
   peptic, 477-480
   pressure, 562-564
   ulcerative colitis. See UC (ulcerative colitis).

Ultrasound
    Doppler, 201-202, 379, 407, 509, 720
    intravascular, 166
    obstetric, 674, 682, 688, 695, 712, 730
    pelvic, 704
    renal, 218, 232, 243
    translabial, 681
    transrectal, 207
    transvaginal, 681
Unilateral neglect, 354-355
United Cerebral Palsy Association, 614
United Network for Organ Sharing, 242
United Ostomy Association, 256, 453, 461
United States Fires Association. See USFA (United
    States Fire Association).
Unstable glucose levels, 379-381
Upper GI series, 446
Ureteral calculi, 243-248
    assessments for, 243
    deficient knowledge issues for, 246-247
        calculi formation, 246-247
        dietary impacts, 246-247
    diagnoses and interventions for, 244-247
        additional considerations for, 247
        pain, acute, 244
        skin integrity, impaired, 245-246
        urinary elimination, impaired, 244-245
    diagnostic tests for, 243
    discharge planning for, 247
    fundamentals of, 243
    health care settings for, 243
    pathophysiology of, 243
    patient-family education for, 247
Urge urinary incontinence, 213
Urgency, 244-245
Urinalysis, 138, 207, 231-232, 243, 314, 378, 439,
    671-672, 682, 704, 720
Urinary diversions, 249-256
    continent, 249
    deficient knowledge issues for, 255-256
    diagnoses and interventions for, 249-256
        additional considerations for, 256
        anxiety, 249-250
        ineffective tissue perfusion, impaired stomal,
            254-255
        infection risks, 252
        protection, ineffective, 252-253
        self-care considerations, 255-256
        skin integrity, impaired, 253-254
        urinary elimination, impaired, 250-251
    discharge planning for, 256
    fundamentals of, 249
    health care settings for, 249
    intestinal (ileal conduit), 249
    orthotopic neobladder, 249
    pathophysiology of, 249
    patient-family education for, 256
    pouches, Indiana vs. Kock, 249
Urinary elimination, impaired
    cancer care and, 29-30
    ureteral calculi and, 244-245
    urinary diversions and, 250-251
Urinary incontinence
    BPH and, 213-214
    cancer care and, 10
    reflex, 339-341
    SCIs and, 339-341
    stress, 213-214
    urge, 213
Urinary-renal care, 207-260, 802-803
    ARF, 231-238
    BPH, 207-216

Urinary-renal care (Continued)
    calculi, ureteral, 243-248
    CKD, 217-222
    diversions, urinary, 249-256
    reference resources for, 802-803
    transplants, renal, 239-242
    urinary tract obstructions, 257-260
Urinary retention, 339-341
Urinary tract infections. See UTIs (urinary tract
    infections).
Urinary tract obstructions, 257-260
    assessments for, 257-258
    diagnoses and interventions for, 258-259
        additional considerations for, 259
        fluid volume, deficient, 258-259
        pain, acute, 259
    discharge planning for, 260
    fundamentals of, 257
    health care settings for, 257
    pathophysiology of, 257
    patient-family education for, 260
    UTIs and, 257
Urine
    chemistries, 671-672, 695, 793-795
    cultures and sensitivity, 207, 243
    function studies, 712
Urography, retrograde, 232
USFA (United States Fire Association), 608
Uterine monitoring, external, 720, 730
Uterotonics, 678-679
UTIs (urinary tract infections), 257

V
Vaccines, pneumococcal, 283-284, 286
VADs (venous access devices), 12-14
Vasodilation, 190-191
Vasodilators, 183-185
Vasopressin challenge tests, 373-374
VASs (visual analog scales), 39-40
Venous access devices. See VADs (venous access
    devices).
Venous thrombosis and thrombophlebitis, 201-205
    assessments for, 201
    deficient knowledge issues for, 204
    diagnoses and interventions for, 201-205
        additional considerations for, 205
        ineffective tissue perfusion, cardiopulmonary, 202
        ineffective tissue perfusion, peripheral, 202-203
        pain, acute, 202-203
    diagnostic tests for, 201
    discharge planning for, 205
    fundamentals of, 201
    health care settings for, 201
    pathophysiology of, 201
    patient-family education for, 205
Ventilation
    mechanical, 127
    ventilation-perfusion, 138, 147-148
        mismatches, 147-148
        scans, pulmonary, 138
Ventricular shunt procedures, 370-371
Verbal communication, impaired
    CP and, 613
    general neurologic care and, 275-276
    psychosocial support and, 81-82
    stroke and, 353-354
Violence risks, other-directed, 746-747
Viral resistance testing, 549
Visual analog scales. See VASs (visual analog scales).
Visual perception, disturbed. See Sensory perception,
    disturbed.

Vitamin and mineral supplements, 626
Volume, fluid. See Fluid volume, imbalanced.
vWF (von Willebrand factor), 505

W
Water deprivation tests, 373-374
WBC (white blood cell) counts, 124, 420, 439, 669
Western blot tests, 548-549
White blood cell counts. See WBC (white blood cell)
    counts.
WHO (World Health Organization), 40-41, 143, 378
Whole blood chemistries, 791t-793t, 793-795
WOB (work of breathing), 578-579, 593, 624
Wong-Baker Faces Pain Scale, 39-40
Work of breathing. See WOB (work of breathing).
World Health Organization. See WHO (World Health
    Organization).
Wound management care, 559-564, 703-710
    assessments for, 559, 561-562
    diagnoses and interventions for, 559-564
        additional considerations for, 564
        tissue integrity, impaired, 559-564
    diagnostic tests for, 559, 562
    discharge planning for, 560, 562, 564
    fundamentals of, 559
    health care settings for, 559, 561-562
    patient-family education for, 560, 562
    postpartum wound infection, 70, 703-710
        abdominal, 703
        assessments for, 703
        deficient knowledge issues for, 705-709
        diagnoses and interventions for, 704-710
        diagnostic tests for, 704
        discharge planning for, 710
        episiotomy, 703
        health care settings for, 703
        pathophysiology of, 70
        patient-family education for, 710
        sepsis, 703
        septic pelvic thrombophlebitis, 703
    pressure ulcers, 562-564
    wound closures, 559-564
        by primary intention, 559-560
        by secondary intention (surgical or traumatic),
            561-564

X
X-rays
    abdominal, 149
    chest, 117-118, 123-124, 131-132, 138, 143-144,
        147-148, 166, 182-183, 195, 282, 578, 593,
        621-622, 659
    KUB, 218
    sinus, 282
    skull, 282
    spine, 334-335
Xenon-133 studies, 509
Xerostomia, 111. See also Oral mucous membranes,
    impaired.

Y
Yale-Brown Obsessive Scale, 738, 746
Young Mania Scale, 746

Z
Zung Self-Rating Depression Scale, 762